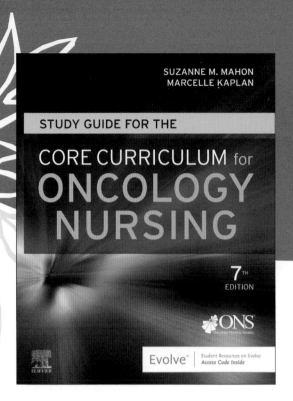

SUZANNE M. MAHON
MARCELLE KAPLAN

STUDY GUIDE FOR THE

CORE CURRICULUM for
ONCOLOGY NURSING

7TH EDITION

ONS
Oncology Nursing Society

Evolve® | Student Resources on Evolve
Access Code Inside

Prepare for the OCN® Exam with the *only* study guide developed in collaboration with the Oncology Nursing Society

T0073884

New Edition!

Oncology Nursing Society
February 2024
ISBN: 978-0-323-93052-9
Also available as an ebook

Based on the latest test blueprint for the OCN® Exam, this study guide is the **only question-and-answer review developed in collaboration with the Oncology Nursing Society.** A new companion Evolve website includes all Study Guide content in a fully interactive quizzing engine that simulates an actual OCN® Exam.

- **NEW! Updated content** reflects the exam blueprint for the very latest OCN® Examination, along with the latest research evidence and important changes in cancer treatment and related nursing care.

- **NEW! Fully interactive quizzing engine on a new Evolve website** includes all Study Guide content, simulating an actual OCN® Exam in either *Study Mode* (with immediate question feedback) or *Exam Mode* (with feedback only at the end of the simulated exam).

- **UNIQUE! In-depth Q&A review** reflects the latest OCN® Test Plan and essential content from the *Core Curriculum for Oncology Nursing*, including the full continuum of cancer care, the scientific basis for practice, palliation of symptoms, oncologic emergencies, and professional performance.

- **900 review questions are written by OCN®-certified experts** to ensure high quality and consistency with the ONS *Core Curriculum* and OCN® Exam, with a strong emphasis on patient safety and quality care.

- **Answer key** includes detailed rationales for correct and incorrect responses.

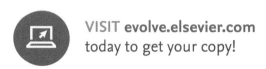

VISIT evolve.elsevier.com
today to get your copy!

23-NHPdp-0411
TM/AF 6/23

ELSEVIER

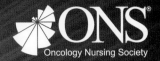

CORE CURRICULUM for ONCOLOGY NURSING

7TH **EDITION**

Editor

JEANNINE M. BRANT, PhD, APRN, AOCN®, FAAN

Executive Director, Clinical Science and Innovation
City of Hope
Duarte, California;
Assistant Affiliate Professor
College of Nursing, Montana State University
Bozeman, Montana

Section Editors

Diane G. Cope, PhD, APRN, BC, AOCNP®

Oncology Nurse Practitioner, Medical Oncology
Florida Cancer Specialists and Research Institute
Fort Myers, Florida

Marlon Garzo Saría, PhD, RN, OCN®, AOCNS®, FAAN

Director of Advanced Nursing Practice
Nurse Scientist
Providence Saint John's Health Center
Santa Monica, California;
Deputy Chief Nurse, United States Air Force
March Air Reserve Base, California

ELSEVIER

ELSEVIER
3251 Riverport Lane
St. Louis, Missouri 63043

CORE CURRICULUM FOR ONCOLOGY NURSING, SEVENTH EDITION

ISBN: 978-0-323-93051-2

Previous editions copyrighted 2020, 2016, 2005, 1998, 1992, 1987. All rights reserved.

Executive Content Strategist: Lee Henderson
Content Development Manager: Danielle Frazier
Senior Content Development Specialist: Maria Broeker
Publishing Services Manager: Deepthi Unni
Project Manager: Thoufiq Mohammed
Senior Book Designer: Renee Duenow

Printed in India

Last digit is the print number: 9 8 7 6 5 4 3 2 1

Working together
to grow libraries in
developing countries

www.elsevier.com • www.bookaid.org

CONTRIBUTORS

Kristine Deano Abueg, RN, MSN, OCN®, CBCN
Leukemia and Lymphoma Nurse Navigator
Hematology and Oncology
Kaiser Permanente
Roseville, California

Aida Akopyan, MS, LCGC
Genetic Counselor
Genetics
Providence St. Joseph Medical Center
Burbank, California

Tahani Al Dweikat, EMHCA, BSN, RN, OCN®, CCRP
Oncology Clinical Research Nurse
Nursing Research
City of Hope
Duarte, California

Nijmeh Al-Atiyyat, PhD, MSC, RN, BC
Advanced Nurse Specialist, Oncology/Nursing Education
Mentor of Oncology Nursing Master Program
Associate Professor
Adult Health Department, Faculty of Nursing
Hashemite University
Zarqa, Jordan;
UNESCO, Vice-Chairperson IBC, UNESCO Chairholder
Amman, Jordan

Nimian Bauder, MSN, APRN, AGCNS-BC, NPD-BC, EBP-C
Clinical Nurse Specialist
Surgical Oncology/Medical Telemetry
City of Hope
Duarte, California

Rosaleen D. Bloom, PhD, APRN, ACNS-BC, AOCNS®
Assistant Professor
School of Nursing
Texas A&M University
Round Rock, Texas

Christine L. Boley, RN, MSN, ACNP-BC
Oncology Nurse Practitioner
Medical Oncology
Saint John's Cancer Institute
Providence Saint John's Health Center
Santa Monica, California

Deborah L. Bolton, MN, RN, AOCNS®, AOCNP®
Clinical Nurse Specialist, Oncology
Kaiser Permanente Foundation Hospital
East Bay Service Area
Oakland, California

Jeannine M. Brant, PhD, APRN, AOCN®, FAAN
Executive Director, Clinical Science and Innovation
City of Hope
Duarte, California;
Assistant Affiliate Professor
College of Nursing, Montana State University
Bozeman, Montana

Adrianzel Mark A. Buan-Lagazo, BSBA, BSN, MSNc, RN, PHN
Clinical Nurse II
BMT/Hematology
Health Care
Stanford, California;
Clinical Nurse II
Oncology/Hematology/BMT
UC Davis Health
Sacramento, California

Nico C. Buan-Lagazo, MSN, RN, OCN®, BMTCN
BMT Quality Assurance Nurse
BMT Program
UC Davis Health
Sacramento, California

Darcy Burbage, DNP, RN, AOCN®, CBCN
Oncology Clinical Nurse Specialist
Oncology Consultant
Newark, Delaware

Dawn Camp-Sorrell, MSN, CRNP, AOCN®
Oncology Nurse Practitioner
Oncology
Children's of Alabama
Birmingham, Alabama

Deena Centofanti, MS, RN, AOCN®
Clinical Nurse Specialist
Nursing Education
Rutgers Cancer Institute of New Jersey
New Brunswick, New Jersey

Kimberly Childers, MS, LCGC
Regional Manager, Genetic Counselor
Genetics and Genomics
Providence Center for Clinical Genetics and Genomics
Los Angeles, California

Diane G. Cope, PhD, APRN, BC, AOCNP®
Oncology Nurse Practitioner, Medical Oncology
Florida Cancer Specialists and Research Institute
Fort Myers, Florida

Stacie Corcoran, RN, MS
Program Director
Adult Cancer Survivorship
Department of Medicine
Memorial Sloan Kettering Cancer Center
New York City, New York

Gail W. Davidson, BSN, MS
Nurse Practitioner
Hepatology
The Ohio State University
Columbus, Ohio

Patti Davis, RN, BSN, OCN®
Manager of Nursing Operations
Cancer Center
Intermountain Healthcare, St. Vincent CCOM
Billings, Montana

Elizabeth Delaney, DNP, CNS, FNP-BC, OCN®, ACHPN
Nurse Practitioner
Hematology/Oncology
Dayton Physicians Network;
Chief Nursing Officer and Vice President
4CancerWellness
Dayton, Ohio

Deena Damsky Dell, MSN, BSN, APRN, AOCN®, LNC
Clinical Nurse Specialist
Sarasota Memorial Hospital Brian D. Jellison Cancer Institute
Sarasota, Florida

Lorraine Drapek, DNP, FNP-BC, AOCNP®
Nurse Practitioner
Radiation Oncology
Massachusetts General Hospital
Boston, Massachusetts

Kristen Elliot, RN, BSN, CHPN
Palliative Care Coordinator
Providence Saint John's Health Center
Santa Monica, California

Jeanne M. Erickson, PhD, RN
Associate Professor Emeritus
University of Wisconsin-Milwaukee College of Nursing
Milwaukee, Wisconsin

Elizabeth Freitas, PhD, MS, BSN
Clinical Nurse Specialist
Pain and Palliative Care
The Queen's Medical Center
Honolulu, Hawaii;
Adjunct Assistant Professor
Nancy Atmospera-Walch School of Nursing
University of Hawaii
Honolulu, Hawaii

Jaya Mini Gill, MD, MHA, BSN, RN
Clinical Research Manager
Pacific Neuroscience Institute/Providence Saint John's
Health Center
Santa Monica, California

Savanna J. Gilson, MSN, RN, OCN®
Clinical Educator
Medical Surgical Oncology
PIH Health Whittier Hospital
Whittier, California

Ora K. Gordon, MD, MS, FACMGG
Medical Director
Clinical Genetics and Genomics
Providence Southern California
Los Angeles, California

Robin I. Green, MSNed, FNP-BC, CMSRN, OCN®
Senior Nurse Educator
Incyte
Mira Loma, California

Jennifer Hadjar, MSN, RN, OCN®
Clinical Program Director, Oncology Quality & Safety
The Mount Sinai Hospital
Mount Sinai Health System
New York, New York

Emily A. Haozous, PhD, RN, FAAN
Research Scientist
Southwest Center
Pacific Institute for Research and Evaluation
Albuquerque, New Mexico

Joshua B. Hardin, PhD, MSN, RN, CCRN, CPAN
Nursing Instructor
Inver Hills Community College
Inver Grove Heights
Minnesota

Jeanne Held-Warmkessel, MSN, RN, AOCN®, ACNS-BC
Clinical Nurse Specialist
Nursing
Fox Chase Cancer Center
Philadelphia, Pennsylvania

Rachel Hirschey, PhD, RN
Assistant Professor
School of Nursing
University of North Carolina at Chapel Hill
Chapel Hill, North Carolina;
Associate Member
Lineberger Comprehensive Cancer Center
Chapel Hill, North Carolina

Anna Howard, PharmD, BCOP
Lead Oncology Pharmacist
Pharmacy
Billings Clinic
Billings, Montana

Martha Inofuentes, MSN, RN, OCN®, CMSRN
Oncology Nurse Navigator
Medical Oncology
Providence Roy and Patricia Disney Family Cancer Center
Burbank, California

Annette Brant Isozaki, MSN
Staff Nurse/Charge Nurse
Bone Marrow Transplant
CAR T Cell Therapy and Investigational Therapy Unit
City of Hope
Duarte, California

Catherine E. Jansen, PhD, RN, AOCNS®
Oncology Clinical Nurse Specialist
Department of Oncology and Hematology
The Permanente Medical Group;
Clinical Professor
Physiological Nursing
University of California, San Francisco
San Francisco, California

Kathryn Johnson, DNP, MSc, FNP-BC
Clinical Program Manager
Tisch Cancer Institute
Icahn School of Medicine at Mount Sinai
New York City, New York

Andrew D. Kass, MSN, APN, AOCNP®
Nurse Practitioner
Infusion Center
Rutgers Cancer Institute of New Jersey
New Brunswick, New Jersey

Pamela Katz, MSN, RN, OCN®
Nurse Clinician
Robert H Lurie Comprehensive Cancer Center
Northwestern Memorial Medical Group
Chicago, Illinois

Brenda Keith, MN, RN, AOCNS®
Breast Therapeutic Area Manager
Genentech
Clinical Nurse Specialist, Oncology
Therapeutic Area Manager
Commercial and Field Sales;
Clinical Nurse Specialist, Oncology
Prescott Valley, Arizona

Shaunna Kersten, MS, APRN, NP, CNS
Adult Nurse Practitioner
Oncology
Independent Practitioner
Bozeman, Montana

Santosh Kesari, MD, PhD
Director, Neuro-oncology
Chair and Professor
Department of Translational Neurosciences
Medical Director
Research Clinical Institute
Providence Southern California
Santa Monica, California

Deborah Kirk, DNP, FNP-BC, NP-C, AOCN®, FAANP
Associate Dean Nursing (Regional)
Associate Professor
Nurse Practitioner
School of Nursing and Midwifery
Edith Cowan University
SW Campus
Bunbury, Western Australia

Timotea Lara, RN, MSN, AOCNP®, NP-C
Oncology Nurse Practitioner
Radiation Oncology
St. John's Health Center
Santa Monica, California

Laura B. LaRose, MSN, RN-BC, AGACNP-BC, AOCNS®
Nurse Practitioner
Hematology/Oncology
Saint John's Health Clinic
Santa Monica, California

Susie Maloney-Newton, APRN, MS, AOCN®, AOCNS®
Oncology Advanced Practice Nurse
Senior Director
The Medical Affairs Company
Dayton, Ohio

Chrystal Martin, BSN, RN, OCN®
Regulatory and Accreditation Specialist
Regulatory and Accreditation
Billings Clinic
Billings, Montana;
President
BigSky ONS, Local Chapter
Oncology Nursing Society
Billings, Montana

Leslie Matthews, RN, MSN, ANP-BC, AOCNP®
Nurse Practitioner
Nursing
Memorial Sloan Kettering Cancer Center
New York City, New York

Melody Mendenhall, RN, MSN
Nurse Practitioner
Hematology/Oncology
Santa Monica UCLA Medical Center
Santa Monica, California

Lourdes Moldre, RN, MSN, ACNP
Patient Care Director
Office of the CNO
UCSF Health
San Francisco, California

Kathleen Murphy-Ende, PhD, PsyD, MSN, FNP-BC, PMHNP-BC
Clinical Psychologist and Nurse Practitioner
Psychiatry
University of Wisconsin-Madison
Madison, WI, United States

Tara J. Ower, RN, MSN, FNP-C
Breast Health Specialist Nurse Practitioner
Margie Petersen Breast Center
Providence Saint John's Health Center
Santa Monica, California

Rachelle Park, BSN, RN, OCN®
Nurse Navigator
Margie Petersen Breast Center
Providence Saint John's Health Center
Santa Monica, California

Karen Hsu Patterson, MSN, FNP-C, ACHPN
Nurse Practitioner
Palliative Care
Providence Saint John's Health Center
Santa Monica, California

Jennifer Peterson, MSN, RN, OCN®, BMTCN
Clinical Practice Education Specialist
Clinical Practice Education and Professional Development
City of Hope
Duarte, California

Tanya Price, MSN, CNS, OCN®
Senior Nurse Liaison
Karyopharm Therapeutics
Newton, Massachusetts

Ana Maricela Rocha, MSN, APRN, AGPCNP, AOCNP®
Nurse Practitioner
Lawrence J. Ellison Institute for Transformative Medicine
Los Angeles, California

Krista M. Rubin, MS, RN, FNP-BC
Nurse Practitioner
Center for Melanoma
Massachusetts General Hospital
Boston, Massachusetts

Margaret Rummel, BSN, MHA
Oncology Nurse Navigator
Head and Neck Cancers
Patient and Family Services
Penn Medicine
Philadelphia, Pennsylvania

Nezar Ahmed Salim, MSN, RN
Oncology
The George Washington University Hospital
Washington, DC

Marlon Garzo Saría, PhD, RN, OCN®, AOCNS®, FAAN
Director of Advanced Nursing Practice
Nurse Scientist
Providence Saint John's Health Center
Santa Monica, California;
Deputy Chief Nurse, United States Air Force
March Air Reserve Base, California

Carla Schaefer, DNP, RN, OCN®, CENP
Associate Chief Nursing Officer
Solid Tumors
Rutgers Cancer Institute of New Jersey
New Brunswick, New Jersey

Rowena N. Schwartz, PharmD
Professor
Pharmacy Practice and Administrative Sciences
University of Cincinnati;
Oncology Clinical Pharmacy Specialist
Pharmacy
University of Cincinnati Medical Center
Cincinnati, Ohio

Marie Christine Seitz, DNP, RN, NP, AOCN®, NE-BC, BMT-CN
Clinical Nurse Consultant
Bristol Myers Squibb
Encino, California;
Clinical Nurse II, Bone Marrow Transplant Unit
Children's Hospital Los Angeles
Los Angeles, California

Kerri Stuart, RN, MSN, OCN®
Director of Cancer Services
Sutter Roseville Hospital
Roseville, California

Geline J. Tamayo, MSN
Clinical Nurse Specialist
Oncology
UC San Diego Health
San Diego, California

Amanda Towell-Barnard, DCur, MCur, BCur (Ed et Adm), CHN, Dip ICU, RN
Senior Lecturer
School of Nursing and Midwifery
Edith Cowan University
Perth, Western Australia;
Adjunct Research Fellow
Centre for Nursing Research
Sir Charles Gairdner Hospital
Perth, Western Australia

Joni L. Watson, DNP, MBA, RN, OCN®
Chief Vision Officer
The Creating Collective
Rockwall, Texas

Tiffany Whetzel, MSN, RN, MEDSURG-BC, OCN®
Nurse Manager
Palliative Medicine
Covenant Medical Center
Lubbock, Texas

Terry Wikle Shapiro, RN, MSN, CRNP
Nurse Practitioner
Pediatric Stem Cell Transplant
Penn State Children's Hospital;
Clinical Instructor
Department of Pediatrics
Penn State College of Medicine
Hershey, Pennsylvania

Sari Williams, MSN, RN, FNP-C
Certified Family Nurse Practitioner
Supportive Care Medicine
City of Hope
Duarte, California

Barbara Wilson, MS, RN, AOCN®, OCN®, ACNS-BC
Director, Oncology Professional Practice
Cancer Network
WellStar Health System
Marietta, Georgia

Katrina Young, MSN, RN, OCN®, MEDSURG-BC
Nurse Manager
Oncology/Stem Cell
Providence Covenant Medical Center
Lubbock, Texas

REVIEWERS

Suzanne Allen, DNP, APRN, AGCNS-BC, AOCNS®, OCN®
Oncology Clinical Nurse Specialist
Winship Cancer Institute
Emory Healthcare
Atlanta, Georgia

Monica L. Beck, PhD, RN, OCN®, CNE
Assistant Professor
College of Nursing
The University of Alabama in Huntsville
Huntsville, Alabama

Christa Braun-Inglis, DNP, APRN-Rx, FNP-BC, AOCNP®
Nurse Practitioner/Assistant Researcher
Clinical Faculty, UH Nancy Atmospera-Walch School of Nursing
University of Hawaii Cancer Center/Hawaii Minority
Underserved NCORP
Honolulu, Hawaii

Ellen Carr, RN, PhD, AOCN®
Editor
Clinical Journal of Oncology Nursing
Oncology Nursing Society
Pittsburgh, Pennsylvania

Patti Davis, RN, BSN, OCN®
Manager of Nursing Operations
Cancer Center
Intermountain Healthcare, St. Vincent CCOM
Billings, Montana

Lorraine Drapek, DNP, FNP-BC, AOCNP®
Nurse Practitioner
Radiation Oncology
Massachusetts General Hospital
Boston, Massachusetts

Beth Faiman, PhD, MSN, APRN-BC, AOCN®, BMTCN, FAAN
Nurse Practitioner
Department of Hematology and Medical Oncology
Cleveland Clinic Taussig Cancer Institute
Cleveland, Ohio

Adrienne Vazquez Guerra, APRN, ACNP-BC, AOCNP®
Nurse Practitioner
Cancer Center
University of Miami, Sylvester Comprehensive Cancer Center
Miami, Florida

Pamela S. Herena, MSN, RN, OCN®
SVP, Clinical Trial Operations
Scientific Medical Affairs
Sacramento, California

Patricia Jakel, RN, MN, AOCN®
Oncology Nurse Specialist Consultant
Medical Oncology
UCLA Health
UCLA School of Nursing
Los Angeles, California

Patricia Kormanik, RN, MSN, NP-C, AOCNP®
Nurse Practitioner, Retired
Encinitas, California

Denise Scott Korn, MSN, RN, OCN®
Nursing Professional Development Specialist
Clinical Education
Atrium Health Wake Forest Baptist High Point Medical Center
High Point, North Carolina

Kathleen Murphy-Ende, PhD, PsyD, MSN, FNP-BC, PMHNP-BC
Clinical Psychologist and Nurse Practitioner
Psychiatry
University of Wisconsin-Madison
Madison, Wisconsin

Debrah Fiona Rigg, RN, BSN, OCN®
Unit Nurse Educator
Hematology/Oncology
Winship Cancer Institute of Emory University
Atlanta, Georgia

Gabriela Rodriguez, MSN, APRN, AGPCNP-BC, OCN®
Nurse Practitioner
Medical Oncology
University of Chicago Medicine
Chicago, Illinois

Brenda K. Shelton, DNP, APRN-CNS, RN, CCRN, AOCN®, NPD-BC
Clinical Nurse Specialist
Kimmel Cancer Center at Johns Hopkins
The Johns Hopkins Hospital
Baltimore, Maryland

Shama Shrestha, BSN, RN, OCN®
Nurse Case Manager
Palliative Care
University of California, San Diego
La Jolla, California

Jennifer A. Tschanz, MSN, RN, FNP-BC, AOCNP®, ACHPN
Nurse Practitioner
Norfolk, Virginia

Ruth E. Van Gerpen, MS, RN, APRN-CNS, AOCNS®, PMGT-BC
Clinical Nurse Specialist, Retired
Bryan Medical Center
Lincoln, Nebraska

Grace Szu-En Wu, MSN-FNPc, BSN-RN, PHN, MPT
Pre Anesthesia
City of Hope
Duarte, California

Vickie Yattaw, RN, BSN, OCN®
Oncology Education and Support Services Manager
C.R. Wood Cancer Center
Glens Falls Hospital
Glens Falls, New York

PREFACE

On behalf of Section Editors Diane G. Cope and Marlon Garzo Saría and myself, we are pleased to bring you the seventh edition of the *Core Curriculum for Oncology Nursing*. Writing this edition was unique in so many ways. As we began, we were just emerging from the COVID-19 pandemic, which presented many challenges for people personally and within the workplace. Staff shortages, low morale, and compassion fatigue were paramount, yet oncology nurses showed up to edit, write, and review this reference. Although the future may be uncertain, I think many of us can acknowledge that we are ready to move forward.

The importance of diversity, equity, and inclusion (DEI) has also emerged since the previous edition. As nurses, we need to embrace diverse ideas and courageously stand against marginalization of all disparate populations. Individually and collectively, we need to address both racism and social determinants of health and their tremendous impact on poor cancer outcomes. Because oncology nurses are everywhere in the healthcare system, we can make a difference. We have woven DEI throughout this seventh edition, as it is a thread in all that we do.

As in the previous editions, the OCN® Test Blueprint is the organizing framework for the book. The parts and chapters reflect specific portions of the Test Blueprint. One of the major uses of this book is to prepare for the OCN® certification examination. The seventh edition features a more streamlined, clinically relevant application of the nursing process, which includes an overview of each problem, assessment, and management. The easy-to-use outline format has been retained in this edition.

As cancer care is rapidly evolving, we have once again updated chapters and book sections to reflect the dynamic trends in cancer care delivery and cancer care. Part 1 includes information from epidemiology to screening and early detection, to palliative and end-of-life care. Shared decision-making and navigation are instrumental in that continuum of care and are included in this section. Part 2 provides information on carcinogenesis, precision health, genetics, and clinical trials. The content has rapidly evolved in this section; therefore, the page counts have been substantially increased to include advances in these areas. In addition, the nomenclature of genetics has evolved, and we have made changes to ensure consistency with the ONS Precision Medicine/Genomics Taxonomy. For example, the word "mutation" is often misunderstood, and the preferred term, depending on the context, is "pathogenic variant." Myelofibrosis was added to Part 3. The cancers in this section are listed alphabetically for easy reference. Part 4 has undergone substantial changes. CAR-T cell therapy was added to Chapter 27, and a section on oral adherence was added to Chapter 29. Part 5 discusses palliation of symptoms. As in the site-specific cancers section, topics are arranged alphabetically for easy use. Part 6 discusses oncologic emergencies, and Part 7 adds Chapter 52 to emphasize the importance of addressing disparities across the cancer experience. The final section of the book, Section 8, is about the Professional Practice of Oncology Nursing and includes the importance of self-care in the chapter on Compassion Fatigue.

Of utmost importance throughout the book was our due diligence to present verifiable evidence that supports the information presented. In wading through the abundance of literature that exists, authors, editors, and reviewers alike focused on obtaining and referencing the most current research, guidelines, and best practices to support equipping nurses in the delivery of high-quality cancer care.

Our thanks to ONS for providing us the opportunity to revise and update this reference. Our special thanks to Bill Tony and Dave Burns from ONS Press, who assisted with this edition of the *Core Curriculum*. Our special thanks to Lee Henderson, Maria Broeker, and Thoufiq Mohammed at Elsevier. As with any endeavor, it takes a village, and many challenges occurred along the way! As previously noted, during the writing of this edition, we were just emerging from the COVID-19 pandemic. In addition, Diane G. Cope lived through a devastating Florida hurricane. Marlon Garzo Saría rotated time between his military service and his oncology leadership position. As for me, I was serving on the ONS Board of Directors and was the ONS President as this book came to a close. For all of us, life is about moving pieces, and yet we maintained our course and accomplished this seventh edition. It has been a pleasure to work with such an efficient and dedicated team.

We also want to thank our families and friends, who caught us editing at odd hours and were patient with us during those essential deadlines! Finally, we thank the contributors who were also dealing with personal and workplace challenges following the COVID-19 pandemic. As busy as their lives were, they said "yes" to writing, and oncology nurses can now glean from their expertise and wisdom within these pages. May this book equip you with the knowledge and skills needed to deliver quality cancer care to patients and families around the world!

Jeannine M. Brant

CONTENTS

1

Epidemiology, Prevention, and Health Promotion

Joni L. Watson

OVERVIEW

I. Cancer epidemiology
  A. Definition
    1. Study of the distribution and determinants of cancer in population groups
    2. Assists in the development of population-based risk profiles
  B. Global cancer statistics (Sung et al., 2021)
    1. Cancer incidence worldwide
      a. The extent of the coronavirus disease 2019 (COVID-19) impact on global cancer data is currently unknown.
        (1) World regions experienced health system closures, screening and detection program suspensions, limited access to care, and individuals' concern for socialization.
        (2) Cancer incidence is expected to decline short-term followed by advanced-stage diagnoses and mortality increases (National Cancer Institute's PROSPR Consortium et al., 2021; Kutikov et al., 2020).
      b. Approximately 19.3 million new cancer cases were diagnosed in 2020.
        (1) Asia makes up 59.5% of the global population, and experiences approximately half of all newly diagnosed global cancer cases.
        (2) The Americas comprise 20.9% of global cancer incidence.
      c. The cancer rate is projected to increase by 47% to 28.4 million new cases in 2040, primarily because of transitioning countries' demographic, globalization, and economic changes linked to modifiable risk behaviors.
      d. The top five most commonly diagnosed cancers are female-sex-assigned-at-birth breast (11.7%), lung (11.4%), colorectal (10.0%), prostate (7.3%), and stomach (5.6%).

(1) Female breast, lung, colorectal, stomach, and prostate cancers make up nearly 50% of all cases diagnosed.
(2) Lung cancer is the most common cancer in males.
  (a) In 2012 approximately 58% of cancer cases occurred in less developed countries.
  (b) Lung cancer rates range widely across the globe as a result of varying stages of the tobacco epidemic as well as varying outdoor ambient air pollution rates.
(3) Breast cancer is the most common cancer in females.
  (a) The 2020 data marks the first time female breast cancer topped the list of most commonly diagnosed cancers across both sexes, surpassing lung cancer.
  (b) Breast cancer incidence is 88% higher in economically transitioned countries than in transitioning countries as a result of reproductive, hormonal, and lifestyle—primarily obesity—risk factors.
    2. Cancer mortality worldwide (Sung et al., 2021)
      a. An estimated 10.0 million people died from the disease in 2020.
        (1) Asia experiences 58.3% of all global cancer mortality.
        (2) The Americas comprise 14.2% of global cancer mortality.
      b. The top five most common causes of death from cancer are lung (18%), colorectal (9.4%), liver (8.3%), stomach (7.7%), and female breast (6.9%).
        (1) Lung cancer is the primary cancer cause of death in men, followed by liver and colorectal cancer.

(2) Breast cancer is the primary cancer cause of death in women, followed by lung and colorectal cancer.

(3) Approximately two-thirds of lung cancer deaths are attributable to smoking.

(4) Some of the most rapidly increasing mortality rates can be linked to poor health infrastructure and limited cancer control programs in low Human Development Index countries.

C. Cancer statistics in the United States (U.S.) (Siegel, Miller, Fuchs, & Jemal, 2022)

1. Cancer incidence in the U.S.

a. The extent of the COVID-19 impact on U.S. cancer data is currently unknown.

(1) States experienced health system closures, screening and detection program suspensions, limited access to care, and individuals' concern for socialization leading to exposure.

(2) Cancer incidence is expected to decline short-term followed by advanced-stage diagnoses and mortality increases (Yabroff et al., 2021).

b. Estimated 1,918,030 new cancer cases in 2022

c. Approximately 5250 new cases every day

d. Estimates exclude basal cell and squamous cell skin cancers

e. For all sexes combined, the top five most commonly diagnosed cancers are breast, prostate, lung and bronchus, colorectal, and uterine corpus (Fig. 1.1).

f. Among females

(1) The five most common cancers are breast (31%), lung and bronchus (13%), colorectal (8%), uterine (7%), and melanoma of the skin (5%)

(2) Breast, lung, and colorectal cancers account for over one-half (51%) of all new cancer diagnoses

g. Among males-sex-assigned-at-birth

(1) The five most common cancers are prostate (27%), lung and bronchus (12%), colorectal (8%), urinary bladder (6%), and melanoma of the skin (6%)

(2) Prostate, lung, and colorectal cancers account for almost one-half (48%) of all new cancer diagnoses

2. Trends in cancer incidence rates (Siegel et al., 2022)

a. For all sexes, cancer incidence rates declined from 1975 to 2018

(1) Males have a higher cancer incidence than females, with incidence decreasing until 2013 and stabilizing through 2018.

(2) Female cancer incidence rates were stable through the mid-2010s but have slowly increased 0.2% per year in recent years.

(3) The male-to-female cancer incidence disparity has decreased from 1.39 in 1995 to 1.14 in 2018.

b. Cancer site with increasing incidence trends

(1) Female breast cancer incidence has increased 0.5% per year for the last 20 years as a result of declining fertility rates and increasing obesity rates.

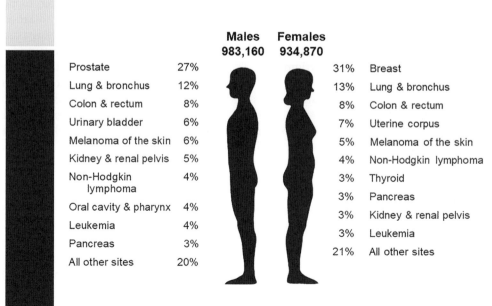

Estimated New Cancer Cases* in the US in 2022

Males 983,160   Females 934,870

Males		Females	
Prostate	27%	31%	Breast
Lung & bronchus	12%	13%	Lung & bronchus
Colon & rectum	8%	8%	Colon & rectum
Urinary bladder	6%	7%	Uterine corpus
Melanoma of the skin	6%	5%	Melanoma of the skin
Kidney & renal pelvis	5%	4%	Non-Hodgkin lymphoma
Non-Hodgkin lymphoma	4%	3%	Thyroid
Oral cavity & pharynx	4%	3%	Pancreas
Leukemia	4%	3%	Kidney & renal pelvis
Pancreas	3%	3%	Leukemia
All other sites	20%	21%	All other sites

*Excludes basal cell and squamous cell skin cancers and in situ carcinoma except urinary bladder.

Fig. 1.1 Estimated new cancer cases in the U.S. in 2022. From *American Cancer Society, 2022. Cancer Statistics 2022 Slide Presentation.* American Cancer Society Inc.

    (2) Colorectal cancer incidence increased by 1.5% in people younger than 50 likely due to modifiable risk factors.

  c. Cancer sites with decreasing incidence trends

    (1) Prostate cancer incidence dropped rapidly from 2004 to 2017 due to early detection and screening. Current incident increases and staging shifts may be a result of overscreening.

    (2) Lung cancer incidence dropped 3% in males and 1% in females from 2009 to 2018, reflecting trends in smoking prevalence.

    (3) Colorectal cancer incidence declined by 2% in people aged 50 and older.

    (4) Thyroid cancer incidence is decreasing 2.5% per year thanks to efforts to mitigate overdetection.

3. Trends in cancer mortality rates (Siegel et al., 2022)

  a. Estimated 609,360 deaths from cancer in 2022.

  b. About 1700 deaths per day.

  c. Cancer is the second leading cause of death in the U.S., second to heart disease.

  d. Cancer is the leading cause of death for women aged 40–79 and men aged 60–79.

  e. One of every four deaths is caused by cancer.

  f. Cancer is the leading cause of death for Hispanic and Asian Americans.

  g. Cervical cancer, one of the most preventable cancers, is the second leading cause of death in women ages 20–39.

  h. Among females-sex-assigned-at-birth, the five leading causes of cancer-related deaths are lung (21%), breast (15%), colorectal (8%), pancreas (8%), and ovary (4%).

  i. Among males-sex-assigned-at-birth, the five leading causes of cancer-related deaths are lung (21%), prostate (11%), colorectal (9%), pancreas (8%), and liver/intrahepatic bile duct (6%).

  j. There is a paucity of cancer data for lesbian, gay, bisexual, transgender, queer, questioning, intersex, asexual, and agender people (Gonzales & Zinone, 2018).

  k. For all cancers combined, cancer mortality rates steadily declined from 215 per 100,000 in 1991 to 146 per 100,000 in 2019, a drop of 32%.

  l. For all races, cancer mortality rates declined from 1992 to 2019.

  m. A reported 3.4 million fewer cancer deaths from 1991 to 2019, resulting from steady progress and advances in prevention, screening, treatment, and survivorship.

  n. Lung cancer mortality declining—as a result of earlier detection and treatment advances from 2010 through 2019—has largely contributed to the overall decreasing mortality rate.

    (1) Lung cancer mortality in males decreased 56% from 1990 to 2019.

    (2) Lung cancer mortality in females decreased 32% from 2002 to 2019.

4. Cancer survival statistics in the U.S. (Siegel et al., 2022; American Cancer Society [ACS], 2019)

  a. The 5-year relative survival rate for all cancers combined is 68%.

  b. Since the 1960s, the 5-year relative survival rate for all cancers has increased from 39% to 68% in White people and from 27% to 63% in Black people

  c. As of January 1, 2019, the NCI estimated 16.9 million cancer survivors in the U.S.

    (1) Sixty-four percent of cancer survivors are 65 years of age or older.

    (2) Only 1 in 10 cancer survivors are younger than age 50.

    (3) For all stages combined, 5-year survival is highest for prostate (98%), melanoma of the skin (93%), and female breast cancer (90%).

    (4) Survival is lowest for lung (22%), liver (20%), and pancreas (11%).

    (5) The chronic myeloid leukemia relative survival rate has gone from 22% in the mid-1970s to 71% in 2017.

    (6) The distant-stage melanoma 5-year survival rate has increased from 15% in 2004 to 30% in 2017.

    (7) After decades of plateau survival rates, lung cancer survival is increasing across all cancer stages. Three-year survival post diagnosis increased from 19% in 2001 to 31% in 2017.

  d. By 2030, there will be an estimated 22.1 million cancer survivors alive in the U.S.

5. Cancer health disparities (National Cancer Institute [NCI], 2020)

  a. Definition of "cancer health disparities"—adverse differences in incidence, prevalence, mortality, survivorship, and burden of cancer or related health conditions that exist among specific population groups in the U.S.

    (1) Population groups may be characterized by age, disability, education, race/ethnicity, gender identity, sexual orientation, income, poverty, lack of health insurance, geographic location, national origin, and other characteristics.

  b. Race/Ethnicity related cancer disparities in the U.S. (NCI, 2020)

    (1) Blacks/African Americans have higher death rates for most cancers.

    (2) Historically for breast cancer, White females have had the highest incidence rate; however, Black/African American female's rates have caught up. Despite now similar incident rates, the highest mortality rate is seen among Black/African American females.

(3) For cervical cancer, Hispanic/Latina females have the highest incidence rate; however, the highest mortality rate is seen among African American females.

(4) For prostate cancer, Black/African American males have the highest incidence and mortality rates than other ethnic groups in the U.S.

(5) For both lung and colorectal cancers, Blacks/African Americans have the highest incidence and mortality compared with other ethnic groups in the U.S.

(6) Asians/Pacific Islanders have the highest incidence and mortality rates of liver and stomach cancers compared with other ethnic groups in the U.S.

(7) American Indians/Alaska Natives have the highest incidence and mortality rates of kidney cancer in the U.S.

(8) Blacks/African Americans have the highest cancer incidence rates, followed by Whites, Hispanic/Latinos, Asian/Pacific Islanders, and American Indian/Alaskan Natives.

(9) African American men are more than twice as likely as white men to die of prostate cancer.

(10) American Indian/Alaska Native and Asian Pacific Islanders have the highest rates of liver and intrahepatic bile duct cancers.

(11) The lowest mortality rate is seen in Asian/Pacific Islander men.

c. Age-related cancer disparities in the U.S. (ACS, 2021; NCI, 2020; Siegel et al., 2022)

(1) The risk of developing cancer increases with age.

(2) Approximately 87% of all cancers are diagnosed in persons 55 years or older.

d. Gender, sexual orientation, and identity-related cancer disparities in the U.S.

(1) Females-sex-assigned-at-birth have a one in three lifetime risk of developing cancer.

(2) Males-sex-assigned-at-birth have a one in two lifetime risk of developing cancer.

(3) As there is a significant data gap for gender-expansive groups, overall lifetime risk of developing cancer is unknown for lesbian, gay, bisexual, transsexual, queer, questioning, intersex, asexual, and agender people (Gonzales & Zinone, 2018).

(4) Smoking and alcohol rates are higher among lesbian, gay, and bisexual youths than heterosexual counterparts.

(5) Gay men and bisexual women are more likely to be diagnosed with cancer than heterosexual counterparts (Gonzales & Zinone, 2018).

e. Geographic cancer disparities in the U.S.

(1) Significant incidence and mortality differences exist in different locations.

(2) White people who live in Appalachia have a significantly higher risk of developing colorectal, lung, and cervical cancers than other White people in the U.S. (NCI, 2020).

(3) Migratory data demonstrate the adoption of the cancer pattern of the area to which migration occurs, suggesting lifestyle, behavioral, and environmental factors as causative or exacerbating.

f. Socioeconomic status (SES) cancer disparities in the U.S.

(1) Low SES is associated with an increased risk of lung cancer, cervical cancer, stomach cancer, and cancer of the head and neck.

(2) Tobacco use has increased among poorer populations.

(3) More advanced disease at diagnosis is found among poor populations and those who live in rural areas.

(4) High SES is associated with an increased risk of breast, prostate, and colon cancers.

g. Education-related cancer disparities in the U.S.

(1) Regardless of race/ethnicity, people with higher education die less prematurely—before age 65—than counterparts with lower education

h. Political, economic, social, and cultural determinants and factors may create barriers to accessing information and cancer care services across the oncology care continuum.

II. Cancer prevention

A. Modifiable cancer risk factors contribute to more than 40% of all cancers (ACS, 2021)

1. Tobacco use (ACS, 2021)

a. Single largest preventable cause of disease and premature death in the U.S.

(1) Accounts for at least 30% of all cancer deaths in the U.S. and close to 40% of all cancer deaths in Appalachia and some Southern U.S. regions

(2) Increases the risk of cancers of the lung, mouth, nasal cavities, larynx, pharynx, oral cavity, esophagus, stomach, colorectum, liver, pancreas, kidney, bladder, uterine cervix, ovary, and acute myeloid leukemia

b. Combustible tobacco products

(1) Cigarettes, cigars, pipes, waterpipes (hookahs or shishas), and self-rolled products.

(2) More than 34 million Americans smoke cigarettes.

(3) Waterpipe smoking delivers the same or higher levels of toxins as cigarettes with growing evidence of similar harm and health effects.

(a) In 2020, 3% of U.S. high school students reported waterpipe smoking within the past month.

(4) Cigar smoking

    (a) Increases the risk of cancers of the lung, oral cavity, larynx, esophagus, and probably pancreas.

    (b) Cigar smokers are 4–10 times more likely to die of laryngeal, oral, or esophageal cancers than nonsmokers.

    (c) Estimated 6% of men and 1% of women currently smoke cigars.

    (d) Cigar use highest among American Indian/Alaska Natives (5%).

    (e) In 2020, 5% of U.S. high school students reported cigar smoking within the past month.

(5) Disparities

    (a) Adults without a high school degree are two to four times more likely to be current smokers than those with a college degree.

    (b) Among current smokers, the highest percentage is found in American Indians/Alaska Natives.

    (c) Those who are uninsured are twice as likely to be current smokers than those who are insured.

c. Second-hand smoke (ACS, 2022)

    (1) Risk factor for lung cancer, cardiovascular disease, and other respiratory diseases.

    (2) There is no safe level of second-hand smoke exposure.

    (3) Exposure causes 5% of lung cancers annually.

    (4) About 21% of nonsmokers in the U.S. have detectable levels of cotinine, a biomarker used to measure exposure to tobacco smoke.

    (5) About 35% of children, aged 3–17 years, are exposed to second-hand smoke.

    (6) Second-hand smoke exposure has declined since 1988 with the rise of tobacco control efforts including comprehensive smoke-free laws.

d. Smokeless tobacco

    (1) Chewing tobacco, snuff, and snus are not safe substitutes for smoking

    (2) Increases the risk of oral, pancreatic, and esophageal cancers

    (3) Electronic nicotine delivery systems (ENDS), also known as *e-cigarettes*

        (a) Battery-operated devices in which the inhaled vapor is produced from cartridges that contain nicotine, flavor, and other chemicals

        (b) Use may lead nonsmokers, especially children, to begin smoking

        (c) As of 2016 the U.S. Food and Drug Administration (FDA) classified ENDS as a tobacco product, bringing them under FDA regulation

        (d) The FDA has not approved any ENDS to date as a cessation aid

        (e) As of 2019, 5% of adults were e-cigarette users

        (f) As of 2020, 3 million U.S. high school students (20%) use ENDS, with appealing flavors as the primary reason for use

2. Excess body weight (ACS, 2021)

a. Definitions

    (1) Overweight/obesity, physical inactivity, and poor nutrition are major risk factors for cancer

    (2) Overweight and obesity classification by body mass index (BMI) (Table 1.1)

        (a) Overweight or preobese: BMI range between 25.0 and 29.9 kg/m^2

        (b) Obese: BMI of 30.0 kg/m^2 or higher

b. Second only to tobacco use as a cancer risk factor

c. Responsible for approximately 18% of cancer cases and 16% of cancer deaths

    (1) Increase the risk of 13 cancers: uterine corpus, esophagus (adenocarcinoma), liver, stomach (gastric cardia), kidney (renal cell), brain (meningioma), multiple myeloma, pancreas, colorectum, gallbladder, ovary, breast (postmenopausal), and thyroid

    (2) May also be linked to risk of non-Hodgkin lymphoma (diffuse large B-cell lymphoma), male breast cancer, and fatal prostate cancer

d. Overweight/obesity and gender

    (1) Overweight prevalence has been stable since the 1960s at about 40% in males and 25%–30% in females.

    (2) Obesity prevalence has increased significantly since the 1960s to about 43% of males and 42% of females.

TABLE 1.1 Classification of Overweight and Obesity by Body Mass Index (BMI) (National Institutes of Health, National Health, Lung, and Blood Institute, n.d.)

	Obesity Class	BMI (kg/m^2)
Underweight		<18.5
Normal		18.5–24.9
Overweight		25.0–29.9
Obesity	I	30.0–34.9
	II	35.0–39.9
Extreme obesity	III	> 40

Data from *National Institutes of Health, National Health, Lung, and Blood Institute. Classification of overweight and obesity by body mass index.* (n.d.). https://www.nhlbi.nih.gov/health/educational/lose_wt/BMI/bmi_dis.htm.

(3) Approximately 5% of cancers in males and 11% of cancers in females are attributed to excess body weight.

e. Obesity and race/ethnicity

(1) Black/African American females (57%) have the highest rates of obesity compared to Hispanic (44%), White (40%), and Asian (17%) females.

(2) Hispanic males (46%) have the highest obesity compared to White (46%), Black/African American (41%), and Asian (18%) males.

f. Obesity and age

(1) Obesity prevalence quadrupled in youths (ages 2–19) from 5% in the 1970s to 19% in 2018.

(2) From 1999 to 2018, adolescent (ages 12–19) obesity prevalence increased in Mexican Americans (22%–31%), Black/African Americans (21%–28%), and Whites (14%–16%).

g. Contributing factors

(1) Foods and beverages high in calories may contribute to altered amounts and distribution of body fat, insulin resistance, and higher concentrations of growth factors that promote cancer growth

(2) Processed and red meats

(a) Associated with increased risk of colorectal, prostate, and pancreatic cancers

(b) Nitrates or other substances used to preserve processed meats involved in carcinogenesis

(3) Decreased fruit and vegetable consumption

(a) Only 13% of adults reported eating three or more servings of vegetables and 27% reported eating two or more servings of fruit daily in 2019.

(b) Increased consumption of fruits and vegetables associated with decreased risk of lung, esophageal, stomach, and colorectal cancers.

(c) High intake of whole-grain foods associated with decreased risk of colorectal cancer.

(4) Decreased physical activity

(a) Extended leisure-time sitting is linked to increased cancer death.

(b) In 2018, 54% of adults reported meeting the recommended 150 minutes of moderate or 75 minutes of vigorous physical activity.

(c) Those with higher education levels were more likely to meet recommended physical activity levels.

3. Alcohol consumption

a. Alcohol is a known carcinogen, classified by the International Agency for Research on Cancer similar to tobacco and ultraviolet (UV) radiation exposure in that there is no safe amount (Rehm & Shield, 2014).

b. Risk factor for cancers of the mouth, pharynx, larynx, esophagus, liver, colorectum, pancreas, stomach, and breast (ACS, 2021).

c. Has synergistic effect with tobacco.

d. The more one drinks over the course of a lifetime, the higher the cancer risk (ACS 2021; NCI, 2021).

e. 67% of adults reported current alcohol consumption in 2018.

f. In 2019, 29% of U.S. high school students report alcohol consumption in the last 30 days, with females (32%) more than males (26%).

4. Type 2 diabetes (ACS, 2021, 2022)

a. A chronic condition in which the body loses insulin response

b. Shares modifiable risk factors of excess body weight, poor nutrition, and physical inactivity

c. Growing evidence suggests it is an independently increased risk for liver, endometrium, pancreas, colorectal, kidney, bladder, breast, and ovary cancers

5. Ultravoilet radiation (UVR) exposure (ACS, 2021, 2022)

a. Primarily from solar UVR exposure

b. Secondarily from artificial UVR exposure (i.e., indoor tanning)

c. Significant risk factor for melanoma, basal, and squamous skin cancers

(1) Basal cell carcinoma—most common skin cancer; is rarely deadly; influenced by both long-term and intermittent sun exposure

(2) Squamous cell carcinoma (also called *keratinocyte carcinoma* or *KC*)—often begins with small scaly lesions called *solar keratoses* or *actinic keratoses;* linked to cumulative time in the sun; both squamous and basal cell cancers typically found on the head, neck, and arms, areas most frequently exposed to sunlight

(3) Melanoma

(a) Accounts for 1% of all skin cancers but 75% of skin cancer deaths (Tripp, Watson, Balk, & Swetter, 2016).

(b) Estimated 99,780 new cancers and 7650 deaths from melanoma in 2022.

(c) Risk factors include consistent UVR exposure (via solar or artificial), multiple moles, fair skin type, family and personal history, older age, and inadequate immune system.

(d) 91% of melanomas are attributable to UVR exposure.

(e) More than 410,000 cases of KC and more than 6000 cases of melanoma can be attributed to indoor tanning.

    (f) Numerous states and the District of Columbia have laws prohibiting tanning for those 18 years old and younger.

    (g) Federal rules and regulations are currently pending to prohibit indoor tanning for those 18 years old and younger.

6. Cancer screening (ACS, 2021)
   a. For people of average risk, recommended cancer screenings are available for breast, cervical, colorectal, lung, and prostate cancers.
   b. See Chapter 2.

7. Virus exposure and vaccines (ACS, 2021, 2022)
   a. Infectious agents account for 13% of all cancers worldwide and 3% of all cancers in the U.S.
   b. Eleven bacteria, viruses, and parasites are classified as cancer-causing agents in humans (Plummer et al., 2016).

   (1) *Helicobacter pylori*
       (a) Associated with 31% of stomach cancers
       (b) About one-third of the U.S. population is infected, often without symptoms
       (c) Transmitted through fecal–oral and oral–oral routes

   (2) Hepatitis B virus (HBV)
       (a) HBV infection is associated with cirrhosis, liver cancer, and non-Hodgkin lymphoma.
         i. Transmitted through blood or mucosal contact with infected body fluids
         ii. It accounts for nearly 6 out of 10 liver cancers in undeveloped countries as opposed to 1 out of 10 liver cancers in the U.S.
         iii. 95% of infected adults clear the virus within 6 months of infection.

   (3) Hepatitis C virus (HCV)
       (a) HCV infection is associated with cirrhosis, liver cancer, and non-Hodgkin lymphoma.
         i. It accounts for nearly 6 out of 10 liver cancers in the U.S.
         ii. Transmitted through sexual or blood contact.

   (4) HIV type 1
       (a) HIV infection results in immunosuppression; increases the risk of Kaposi sarcoma and B-cell lymphomas.
       (b) Transmitted through sexual or blood contact.

   (5) High-risk human papillomavirus (HPV)
       (a) Endemic in human population because more than 90% of adults worldwide are seropositive
       (b) Found in virtually all cases of cervical cancers
         i. More than 150 types of HPV (Markowitz et al., 2014)
         ii. Approximately 70% of cervical cancers caused by HPV types 16 or 18
       (c) Leading cause of oral cancer
         i. HPV-16 detected in a substantial proportion of squamous cell carcinomas of the soft palate, tonsils, and base of the tongue
         ii. HPV-16 detected in 60%–70% of all HPV-associated cancers of the oral cavity and oropharynx (Markowitz et al., 2014)

   (6) Epstein–Barr virus
       (a) Best known for causing infectious mononucleosis, often called "*mono*" or the "*kissing disease*"
       (b) Associated with nasopharyngeal cancer, Burkitt lymphoma, Hodgkin lymphoma, and stomach cancer

   (7) Human herpesvirus type 8
       (a) Also known as Kaposi sarcoma herpesvirus
       (b) Has also been linked to some rare blood cancers

   (8) Human T-cell lymphotropic virus type 1
       (a) Associated with T-cell leukemias

   (9) *Opisthorchis viverrini* (the Southeast Asian river fluke parasite) and *Clonorchis sinensis* (the Chinese river fluke parasite)
       (a) Associated with cholangiocarcinoma

   (10) *Schistosoma haematobium* (found in Africa and the Middle East; causes schistosomiasis)
       (a) Associated with bladder cancer

8. Stress and inflammation (NCI, 2015)
   a. Inflammation is the body's natural process to heal injured tissue
       (1) Acute inflammation—begins when there is an injury and ends once the tissue is healed
       (2) Chronic inflammation—may begin when there is no injury and does not end as expected
   b. Over time, inflammation causes DNA damage that can lead to cancer
   c. Causes of inflammation
       (1) Allergens
       (2) Toxins
       (3) Infectious agents
       (4) Conditions (e.g., Crohn disease and ulcerative colitis)

9. Hormonal agents and antineoplastic drugs
   a. Hormone replacement therapy (HRT)
       (1) Combined estrogen–progesterone HRT given to postmenopausal females increases the risk of breast cancer (Manson et al., 2013).
       (2) Estrogens may have a protective role in preventing colorectal cancer (Barzi, Lenz, Labonte, & Lenz, 2013).

(3) Long-term use of HRT increases the risk of endometrial cancer (Trabert et al., 2013).

b. Gender-affirming hormone therapy (GAHT)

(1) Feminizing and masculinizing hormones given to affirm transgender identity may increase the risk of sex-driven cancers (de Blok et al., 2019)

(2) There is a paucity of data on GAHT cancer risk (McFarlane, Zajac, & Cheung, 2018)

c. Selective estrogen receptor modulators

(1) Include tamoxifen and raloxifene

(2) FDA-approved for use to reduce the risk of breast cancer

(3) Have been shown to reduce breast cancer incidence by up to 50% among high-risk women (Mocellin, Pilati, Briarava, & Nitti, 2015).

d. Use of oral contraceptives is associated with breast cancer but may reduce the risk of cancers of ovary and uterus.

e. Daughters of women who took diethylstilbestrol (DES) during pregnancy had an increased incidence of clear cell adenocarcinoma (CCA) of the vagina, especially in their late teens and early 20s. However, after age 25, the incidence of CCA among DES-exposed daughters has decreased by over 80% (Troisi et al., 2007).

f. Anabolic steroids may be associated with liver cancer.

g. Certain fertility drugs (i.e., menotropins [Pergonal]) may increase the risk for ovarian cancer.

h. Growth hormones given to children may increase the risk for leukemia.

i. Immunosuppressive agents (for organ recipients) increase the risk of non-Hodgkin lymphoma.

j. Prior exposure to antineoplastic agents (especially alkylating agents) and radiation therapy increases the risk of secondary cancers.

B. Nonmodifiable cancer risk factors

1. Radiation exposure

a. Natural radiation sources

(1) Radon gas, x-rays, gamma rays, UV light

b. Artificial radiation sources

(1) Radon gas and x-rays

2. Genetics (see Chapter 10)

3. Occupational and environmental exposures (ACS, 2021)

a. There are currently 121 and 88 agents classified as Group 1 carcinogens (carcinogenic to humans) and Group 2A carcinogens (probably carcinogenic to humans), respectively

b. Occupational cancer risks

(1) Account for about 4% of cancers

(2) Males have four times the occupational-associated cancer deaths than females

(3) Introduction of effective regulation of workplace exposures in the mid-20th century believed to have reduced these risks substantially

(4) Asbestos: single most important known occupational carcinogen

(a) Asbestos-related lung cancer and mesothelioma peaked during the middle to the late 1980s because of extensive occupational exposure in shipyards during World War II.

(b) Occupations exposed to asbestos include mining; shipyards; railroads; constructions; boiler plants; firefighting; oil refineries; and paper, textile, and steel mills (Dodson & Hammar, 2011).

(c) Occupational exposures to asbestos fibers, environmental smoke, or radon have a synergistic role in elevating smoking-related lung cancer risk.

(d) Special population concerns

i. Blue-collar workers—tend to have higher smoking rates that increase risks associated with occupational exposures

ii. African Americans—discriminatory work assignments have historically resulted in placement in more hazardous jobs: steel, rubber, and chemical industries

iii. Steel workers—increased rates of lung cancer

iv. Rubber workers—increased rates of prostate cancer

v. Chemical workers—increased rates of bladder cancer

vi. Miners—increased exposure to uranium and radon with a subsequent increase in gastric cancer and birth defects

c. Environmental cancer risks (ACS, 2021)

(1) Radon

(a) Colorless, odorless gas occurring from the breakdown of radioactive elements in the Earth's crust

(b) Second leading cause of lung cancer

(c) Exposure varies widely across the U.S., with higher naturally occurring rates in the upper middle and eastern U.S.

(2) Outdoor air pollution

(a) Combination of particulate matter, liquid droplets, gases, and other substances

(b) Linked to lung and bladder cancers

(c) Exposure varies by U.S. geography, season, temperature, and proximity to pollution sources

(d) U.S. pollution has declined steadily since 1990
(3) Climate change
(a) Caused by human activities impacting weather patterns
(4) Environmental health disparities and justice

III. Health promotion
A. American Cancer Society guidelines on nutrition and physical activity for cancer prevention (Rock et al., 2020)
1. Nutrition: consume a healthy diet with an emphasis on plant sources.
a. Choose foods and beverages in amounts to achieve and maintain a healthy weight.
(1) Eat smaller portions of high-calorie foods.
(2) Choose vegetables, whole fruit, and other low-calorie foods.
(3) Limit consumption of sugar-sweetened beverages.
(4) Avoid consuming large portion sizes.
b. Limit the consumption of processed and red meats.
(1) Minimize consumption of processed meats.
(2) Choose fish, poultry, or beans as an alternative to red meat.
(3) For red meat, select lean cuts and eat smaller portions.
(4) Prepare meat, fish, or poultry by baking, broiling, or poaching rather than frying or charbroiling.
c. Eat at least $2^{1/2}$ cups of vegetables and fruits per day.
d. Choose whole-grain instead of refined-grain products.
e. Zero alcohol intake is best. Limit alcohol intake to no more than two drinks per day for men and one drink per day for women (ACS, 2021).
2. Physical activity (Rock et al., 2020)
a. Intensity, duration, and frequency of physical activity to reduce cancer risk unknown
b. ACS recommendations.
(1) Adults—150–300 minutes of moderate-intensity activity per week or 75–150 minutes of vigorous-intensity activity per week
(2) Children—at least 60 minutes of moderate- or vigorous-intensity activity each day, with vigorous activity on at least 3 days each week
(3) Limiting sedentary behavior (e.g., sitting, lying down, and watching television)
B. ACS guidelines on nutrition and physical activity for cancer survivors (Rock et al., 2020)
1. Achieve and maintain a healthy weight.
a. Limit consumption of high-calorie foods and beverages.
b. Increase physical activity.
2. Engage in regular physical activity.

a. Return to normal daily activities as soon as possible after diagnosis.
b. Exercise at least 150 minutes per week.
c. Include strength training at least 2 days per week.
d. Consume foods high in vegetables, fruits, and whole grains.
C. Vaccination (ACS, 2021)
1. HPV vaccine for prevention of cervical cancer and five other cancers, in addition to genital warts
a. Three vaccines are currently approved by the FDA for HPV chemoprevention; the most commonly used vaccine in the U.S. protects against nine HPV types.
b. Recommended vaccination age is 9–12 years (and as early as 9 years and as late as 26 years); a higher immune response is seen at this age than later adolescence.
(1) A two-dose series is recommended for children before age 15.
(2) After age 15, a three-dose series is recommended.
c. HPV vaccination uptake is increasing but still lags behind other recommended vaccines potentially attributed to myths and lack of education surrounding the vaccine need.
2. Hepatitis B vaccination is the primary prevention strategy to decrease HBV rates.
a. All unvaccinated children, adolescents, and adults at risk for hepatitis B infection should be vaccinated via a three-dose series.
(1) The standard vaccination schedule is at 0, 3, and 6 months.
b. Nearly 91% of adolescents 17 years and younger have had at least three HBV vaccinations.
D. Measures to prevent skin cancer (ACS, 2021)
1. Avoid direct exposure to the sun between the hours of 10 a.m. and 4 p.m., when UV rays are most intense.
2. Wear hats with a brim wide enough to shade the face, ears, and neck, as well as clothing that covers as much as possible of the arms, legs, and torso.
3. Cover exposed skin with a sunscreen lotion and sun protection factor of ≥ 30.
4. Avoid indoor tanning booths and sun lamps.
E. Screening and early detection of cancer (see Chapter 2)

ASSESSMENT

I. Conduct a thorough medical history and physical examination.
A. Obtain demographic information, including age, race/ethnicity, gender, education, employment status and place of employment, insurance coverage, and area of residence.
B. Assess for comorbidities (e.g., hepatitis infection) and previous and current medications (e.g., HRT).

C. Assess for lifestyle risk factors such as tobacco use, alcohol consumption, exposure to UV radiation, weight, nutrition, and level of physical activity.
D. Assess for occupational exposures (e.g., asbestos, benzene, and other chemicals).
E. Assess for personal and family histories of cancer.
F. Include any previous treatment with radiotherapy, chemotherapy, or both.
G. Assess for motivation for preventive behavior (health belief model)
1. Perceived susceptibility to cancer—evidence indicates individuals at risk often are unaware of their risks. (Ask, "How likely do you feel you are to develop cancer?")
2. Perceived severity of cancer. (Ask, "How serious do you feel cancer is?")
3. Perceived benefits of preventive behavior. (Ask, "Do you think you can decrease your risk for cancer by not smoking [or the habit in question]?")
4. Perceived barriers to preventive action. (Ask, "What problems do you think you may have lowering the fat content in your diet [or the behavior in question]?")

MANAGEMENT

I. Medical management
A. Provide cancer prevention vaccines as indicated.
II. Nursing management
A. Provide education regarding health promotion activities.
B. Refer to specialists (e.g., dietician, tobacco addiction treatment specialist) as needed.
C. Encourage participation in chemoprevention trials.
1. Tobacco cessation
a. U.S. Public Health Service (USPHS) "5 A" model in treating smokers who are willing to quit (Fiore, Jaen, & Baker, 2008)
b. For smokers unwilling to quit, the USPHS recommends brief motivational interventions that can help increase attempts.
(1) Ask patient about smoking status.
(2) Advise to quit.
(3) Assess for willingness or readiness to quit.
(4) Assist in quitting.
(5) Arrange a follow-up visit.
(a) Use motivational interviewing techniques such as asking, "Have you considered quitting?"
(b) Discuss the options for quitting such as use of medications (over-the-counter and prescription) to aid smoking cessation.
(c) Assist patient with developing a quit plan.
(d) Offer relevant and culturally appropriate cessation materials, cessation programs, and public cessation hotlines.
c. Various pharmacologic and nonpharmacologic tools exist

2. Encourage proper nutrition.
3. Promote physical activity.
4. Encourage patients to limit sun exposure.
a. Educate persons of all ages about skin cancer prevention.
5. Prevent viral exposures.
a. Offer age-appropriate vaccinations.
b. Discuss safe sex practices.
c. Counsel against intravenous drug use, or educate about and facilitate access to sterile needle and syringe programs.
6. Encourage the avoidance of occupational carcinogen exposures.
a. Use protective clothing and devices; follow safety procedures when exposure unavoidable.

REFERENCES

American Cancer Society. *Cancer treatment & survivorship facts & figures 2019-2021.* (2019). https://www.cancer.org/content/dam/cancer-org/research/cancer-facts-and-statistics/cancer-treatment-and-survivorship-facts-and-figures/cancer-treatment-and-survivorship-facts-and-figures-2019-2021.pdf.

American Cancer Society. *Cancer prevention & early detection: Facts & figures, 2021-2022.* (2021). https://www.cancer.org/content/dam/cancer-org/research/cancer-facts-and-statistics/cancer-prevention-and-early-detection-facts-and-figures/2021-cancer-prevention-and-early-detection.pdf.

American Cancer Society. *Cancer Facts & Figures 2022 slide presentation.* (2022). https://www.cancer.org/research/cancer-facts-statistics/all-cancer-facts-figures/cancer-facts-figures-2022.html.

Barzi, A., Lenz, A. M., Labonte, M. J., & Lenz, H. J. (2013). Molecular pathways: Estrogen pathway in colorectal cancer. *Clinical Cancer Research, 19*(21), 5842–5848.

de Blok, C. J. M., Wiepjes, C. M., Nota, N. M., van Engelen, K., Adank, M. A., Dreijerink, K. M. A., et al. (2019). Breast cancer risk in transgender people receiving hormone treatment: Nationwide cohort study in the Netherlands. *BMJ, 365,* l1652. https://doi.org/10.1136/bmj.l1652.

Dodson, R. F., & Hammar, S. P. (Eds.). (2011). *Asbestos: Risk assessment, epidemiology, and health effects* (2nd ed.). Boca Raton, FL: CRC Press.

Fiore, M. C., Jaen, C. R., Baker, T. B., et al. (2008). *Treating tobacco use and dependence, 2008 update. Clinical practice guideline.* Rockville, MD: U.S. Department of Health and Human Services. Public Health Service.

Gonzales, G., & Zinone, R. (2018). Cancer diagnoses among lesbian, gay, and bisexual adults: Results from the 2013-2016 National Health Interview Survey. *Cancer Causes Control, 29*(9), 845–854.

Kutikov, A., Weinberg, D. S., Edelman, M. J., Horwitz, E. M., Uzzo, R. G., & Fisher, R. I. (2020). A war on two fronts: Cancer care in the time of COVID-19. *Annals of Internal Medicine, 172*(11), 756–758. https://doi.org/10.7326/M20-1133.

McFarlane, T., Zajac, J. D., & Cheung, A. S. (2018). Gender-affirming hormone therapy and the risk of sex hormone-dependent tumours in transgender individuals—A systematic review. *Clinical Endocrinology, 89*(6), 700–711.

Manson, J. E., Chlebowski, R. T., Stefanick, M. L., Aragaki, A. K., Rossouw, J. E., Prentice, R. L., et al. (2013). Menopausal hormone therapy and health outcomes during the intervention and extended poststopping phases of the Women's Health Initiative randomized trials update and overview of health outcomes for WHI update and overview of health outcomes for WHI. *JAMA: The Journal of the American Medical Association, 310*(13), 1353–1368.

Markowitz, L.E., Dunne, E.F., Saraiya, M., Chesson, H.W., Curtis, C.R., Gee, J., et al. (2014). *Human papillomavirus vaccination: Recommendations of the Advisory Committee on Immunization Practices (ACIP).* Centers for Disease Control and Prevention. Retrieved from https://www.cdc.gov/mmwr/preview/mmwrhtml/rr6305a1.htm.

Mocellin, S., Pilati, P., Briarava, B., & Nitti, D. (2015). Breast cancer chemoprevention: A network meta-analysis of randomized controlled trials. *Journal of the National Cancer Institute, 18*(108), 2.

National Cancer Institute (NCI). Chronic inflammation. (2015). https://www.cancer.gov/about-cancer/causes-prevention/risk/chronic-inflammation.

National Cancer Institute (NCI). Cancer health disparities. (2020). https://www.cancer.gov/about-cancer/understanding/disparities.

National Cancer Institute (NCI). Alcohol and cancer risk. (2021). https://www.cancer.gov/about-cancer/causes-prevention/risk/alcohol/alcohol-fact-sheet.

National Cancer Institute's PROSPR Consortium, Corley, D. A., Sedki, M., Ritzwoller, D. P., Greenlee, R. T., Neslund-Dudas, C., et al. (2021). Cancer screening during the coronavirus disease-2019 pandemic: A perspective from the National Cancer Institute's PROSPR Consortium. *Gastroenterology, 160*(4), 999–1002. https://doi.org/10.1053/j.gastro.2020.10.030.

National Institutes of Health, National Health, Lung, and Blood Institute. Classification of overweight and obesity by body mass index. (n.d.). https://www.nhlbi.nih.gov/health/educational/lose_wt/BMI/bmi_dis.htm.

Plummer, M., de Martel, C., Vignat, J., Ferlay, J., Bray, F., & Francheschi, S. (2016). Global burden of cancers attributable to infections in 2012: A synthetic analysis. *Lancet Global Health, 4*(9), e609–e616.

Rehm, J., & Shield, K. (2014). Alcohol consumption. In B. W. Stewart & C. B. Wild (Eds.), *World cancer report 2014.* Lyon: International Agency for Research on Cancer.

Rock, C. L., Thomson, C., Gansler, T., Gaptsur, S. M., McCullough, M. L., Patel, A. V., et al. (2020). American Cancer Society guidelines for diet and physical activity for cancer prevention. *CA: A Cancer Journal for Clinicians, 70*(4), 245–271. https://doi.org/10.3322/caac.21591.

Siegel, R. L., Miller, K. D., Fuchs, H. E., & Jemal, A. (2022). Cancer statistics, 2022. *CA: A Cancer Journal for Clinicians, 72*(1), 7–33. https://doi.org/10.3322/caac.21708.

Sung, H., Ferlay, J., Siegel, R. L., Laversanne, M., Soerjomataram, I., Jemal, A., et al. (2021). Global Cancer Statistics 2020: GLOBOCAN estimates of incidence and mortality worldwide for 36 cancers in 185 countries. *CA: A Cancer Journal for Clinicians, 71*(3), 209–249.

Trabert, B., Wentzensen, N., Yang, H. P., Sherman, M. E., Hollenbeck, A. R., Park, Y., et al. (2013). Is estrogen plus progestin menopausal hormone therapy safe with respect to endometrial cancer risk? *International Journal of Cancer, 132*(2), 417–426.

Tripp, M. K., Watson, M., Balk, S. J., & Swetter, S. M. (2016). State of the science on prevention and screening to reduce melanoma incidence and mortality. *CA: A Cancer Journal for Clinicians, 66*(6), 460–480.

Troisi, R., Hatch, E. E., Titus-Ernstoff, L., Hyer, M., Palmer, J. R., Robboy, S. J., et al. (2007). Cancer risk in women prenatally exposed to diethylstilbestrol. *International Journal of Cancer, 121*(2), 356–360.

Yabroff, K. R., Wu, X. C., Negotia, S., Stevens, J., Coyle, L., Zhao, J., et al. (2021). Association of the COVID-19 Pandemic with patterns of statewide cancer services. *Journal of the National Cancer Institute, 114*(6), 907–909. http://doi.org/10.1093/jnci/djab122. Advance online publication.

2

Screening and Early Detection

Ana Maricela Rocha

OVERVIEW

I. Levels of prevention
   A. Primary prevention—reduce risk factors or increase an individual's resistance, the most effective management for cancer
      1. The goal of primary prevention is to limit the incidence of cancer (e.g., human papillomavirus [HPV] vaccination)
   B. Secondary prevention—early detection and treatment of cancer through screening activities in asymptomatic individuals (e.g., fecal immunochemical test)
      1. The goal of secondary prevention is to prevent disease progression
   C. Tertiary prevention—diagnosis and application of effective therapy to improve outcomes and decrease morbidity and mortality in affected individuals
II. Definitions
   A. Diagnosis—clinical problem-solving process applied to asymptomatic individuals who either screen positive or present in an already symptomatic state; delays in screening, urgent referrals, and treatment are likely to increase mortality as both indirect and direct effects of the COVID-19 pandemic (Lai et al., 2020).
   B. Epidemiology—the study of the distribution and determinants of health-related states.
   C. Screening—the use of tests (e.g., physical examination and history, imaging procedures, or laboratory tests) to detect early stages of cancer aimed at reducing mortality.
   D. Rates—measure of morbidity, or the rate of illness
      1. Incidence, prevalence, or mortality rates can be used to assess the value of instituting a screening test for a particular disease
         a. Involves identification of risk profiles, use of screening guidelines to enhance screening efficacy and decrease risks and costs of screening test(s)
         b. Multiple organizations publish cancer screening guidelines, including the American Cancer Society, National Comprehensive Cancer Network (NCCN), and United States Preventive Services Task Force
         c. Attempts to balance risks versus benefits of screening tests
            (1) There are clear benefits to screening to diagnose the disease early enough to favorably affect morbidity and mortality.
            (2) Not all screening tests are helpful, and most have the potential for harm; false positive results can lead to anxiety, distress, and worry, particularly for individuals at high risk (Kim, Chung, Keir, & Patrick, 2022). Evaluating risk and reducing potential harms of exposure (e.g., radiation) or unnecessary procedures including overdiagnosis in the asymptomatic individual requires further discussion and shared decision-making (US Preventive Services Task Force [USPSTF] et al., 2021).
      2. Incidence—number of new cases identified in a specified population occurring in a particular time period (such as 1 year)
      3. Prevalence—percentage of all individuals affected with the disease at a given point in time
III. Attributes of effective screening tests
   A. Screening test should be readily available, safe, easy, and inexpensive (Givler & Givler, 2022).
   B. Randomized clinical trials (RCTs) demonstrate the effectiveness of screening tests (i.e., reduction in mortality and/or improvement in quality of life).
   C. Validity—accuracy of a screening test to distinguish individuals who have the disease and those who do not
      1. Sensitivity—the ability of a test to detect disease, a true positive result.
      2. Specificity—the ability of a test to detect no disease, a true negative result.
      3. A test that has high sensitivity and high specificity improves the overall ability of increased accuracy.
   D. Reliability—level of agreement between measurements made at different times
   E. Predictive value—useful to assess the feasibility of screening tests; how likely disease is present or absent
      1. Negative predictive value (NPV)—the percentage of persons who screen negative who do not have the disease (true negatives)
      2. Positive predictive value (PPV)—the percentage of persons who screen positive who actually have the disease (true positives)

3. Predictive values vary according to the prevalence of disease; the higher the prevalence of a disease, the higher the PPV and the lower the NPV

IV. Evidence exists for screening recommendations for breast, cervical, lung, and colorectal cancer (CRC) in defined populations; controversy exists for all cancers.
  A. Types of screening biases
    1. Lead time bias
    2. Length time bias
    3. Selection bias
    4. Overdiagnosis (a person without symptoms with an incidental finding, e.g., lung nodule)
  B. Confounding factors with RCTs include contamination of control group, large number of subjects required for screening diseases with low incidence rate, and ethically unacceptable to randomize subjects to non-screened group.
  C. Effective and recommendations exist for breast, colorectal, cervical, and lung, allowing these cancers the potential to be detected earlier.
    1. The rates of false positive results can be as high as 5%–10%, that is, mammogram, over time the risk of having a false positive substantially increase (Givler & Givler, 2022).
    2. Despite low cost and the availability of testing for cancers, screening rates remain below the national goal of 80% (Dougherty et al., 2018).
    3. Additional studies are needed to evaluate barriers and improve screening. For example, current rates for colonoscopy are 63% for eligible adults, rates are lower in minority, ethnic groups and underinsured/uninsured (Dougherty et al., 2018).

V. Characteristics of the cancers that justify the risks and costs associated with screening
  A. Screening should be directed toward an important health problem.
  B. Effective treatment is available to reduce cause-specific mortality and is more effective if initiated during the presymptomatic stage.
  C. The benefit of screening should outweigh the risks and be cost-effective.
  D. Potential screening participants should receive adequate information regarding the risks and potential benefits of participation.

VI. Screening modalities for early detection of cancer
  A. Imaging
  B. Cytologic specimens
  C. Chemical assays
  D. Biomarkers or tumor markers
  E. Proteomics
    1. Substances that may be produced by the tumor or the body's reaction to the cancer and may be detected in abnormal quantities; most often found in blood, body fluids, or tissues.
    2. Although attractive for screening, most currently available biomarkers or tumor markers are nonspecific and lack sensitivity.

VII. Screening guidelines for specific cancers
  A. Breast cancer
    1. Breast cancer screening recommendations (Table 2.1)
      a. Gail model
        (1) Multivariable statistical model that has been developed to help estimate a woman's personal breast cancer risk
        (2) Model incorporates characteristics (age, age of menarche, age at first live birth, number of first-degree relatives with breast cancer, number of previous benign breast biopsies, atypical hyperplasia in a previous breast biopsy, and race) in an effort to assess 5-year and lifetime risks of developing breast cancer (Gail et al., 1989)
      b. Genetic testing for *BRCA1* and *BRCA2* gene pathogenic variants
        (1) General population risk for breast cancer is 12%; for ovarian cancer, it is 1%–2%, carriers of BRCA 1/2 risk of breast cancer is 70% and ovarian up to 40%. Up to 6% of breast cancer and 15% of ovarian cancer diagnosis are BRCA carriers (Petrova, Cruz, & Sánchez, 2022).
        (2) BRCA testing is recommended for people that meet criteria, including an unaffected individual with a first- or second-degree affected blood relative with specific features, such as under age 45 (National Comprehensive Cancer Network [NCCN], 2022b).
        (3) May be offered at any age to aid with treatment decisions, male breast cancer, triple-negative breast cancer, lobular breast cancer, or Ashkenazi Jewish ancestry (NCCN, 2022b).
    2. Impact of screening
      a. Screening and early diagnoses play a vital role in reducing the mortality of breast cancer; studies have found a 40% reduction in mortality for

---

TABLE 2.1 Breast Cancer Screening Recommendations

Women between 40 and 44 have the option to start screening with a mammogram every year.

Women 45–54 should get mammograms every year.

Women 55 and older can switch to a mammogram every other year, or they can choose to continue yearly mammograms. Screening should continue as long as a woman is in good health and is expected to live at least 10 more years.

All women should understand what to expect when getting a mammogram for breast cancer screening—what the test can and cannot do.

Clinical breast exams are not recommended for breast cancer screening among average-risk women at any age.

From *American Cancer Society. Recommendations for the early detection of cancer.* (2017a). https://www.cancer.org/cancer/breastcancer/screening-tests-and-early-detection/american-cancersociety-recommendations-for-the-early-detection-of-breastcancer.html#written_by.

women ages 40–83 who participate in breast cancer screening compared to no screening (Bashirian, Mohammadi, Barati, Moaddabshoar, & Dogonchi, 2020).

b. Reduction in morbidity, screening detects breast cancer at earlier stages, smaller tumor size, and no lymph node involvement. Five-year prognosis for localized is 99%, regional 86%, and distant 27% (Grimm, Avery, Hendrick, & Baker, 2022).

c. Regional and distant stage often requires more extensive therapy with surgery, radiation, systemic therapy often associated with complications (Grimm et al., 2022).

3. Screening modalities
   a. Screening mammography for women at average risk; women aged 40–44 with an option to start annual mammogram; aged 45–54 annual mammogram; women 55 and older may switch to every other year or annually, as long as they are in good health with a life expectancy of 10 years (Oeffinger et al., 2015; American Cancer Society, 2022).
   b. Breast self-exam (BSE) is recommended for breast cancer average-risk screening at any age, and there is little evidence to support routine BSE. Women should be familiar with their breasts and report any changes to their health care provider (American Cancer Society, 2022).
   c. Annual clinical breast examination (CBE) is recommended by NCCN (Oeffinger et al., 2015).
   d. Breast imaging-reporting and data system (BI-RADS) developed by the American Society of Radiology to provide a standardized description and categorization of breast lesions on mammography, ultrasound, and magnetic resonance imaging (Spick, Bickel, Polanec, & Baltzer, 2018).
      (1) Consists of seven categories of mammographic findings, each with terminology and follow-up recommendations, from category 0 (incomplete) to 6 (suspicious for malignancy/malignancy) (American College of Radiologists [ACR], 2021)

4. Screening controversy
   a. BI-RADs category 3 is associated with a 0%–2% chance of malignancy. This category is associated with negative outcomes including unnecessary follow-up of benign lesions, delayed diagnosis when smaller or earlier stage, and biopsies of lesions that have not changed in size or extent (ACR, 2021).
   b. Clinical breast exam (CBE) associated harm includes false positive results. Use of CBE may be a cost-effective option in low resources' settings (Qaseem et al., 2019).
   c. Digital breast tomosynthesis, while more sensitive and less recall rates than mammography, is associated with benefits and harms, including overdiagnosis (Qaseem et al., 2019).

B. CRC
   1. CRC screening recommendations established moderate net benefit for adults 45–49, thus age was decreased from 50 to 45. For adults at average risk (without a history of CRC, polyps, family history of CRC, IBD, FAP, Lynch, or history of radiation to abdomen/pelvis) screening begins at age 45. Screening for age 50–75 is associated with substantial net benefit. Age 76–85 renders a small net benefit for CRC screening (USPSTF et al., 2021; Table 2.2).
   2. Screening modalities, a conversation with patient to review testing options, benefits and harms, and their preference and availability helps to facilitate screening (NCCN, 2022a).
      a. Stool-based tests—Both high sensitivity guaiac-based fecal occult blood test (chemical detection of blood in stool) and fecal immunochemical test (FIT) (antibody detection of blood in stool). Stool DNA test detects DNA biomarkers of cancer cells; sDNA FIT is the only FDA-approved DNA test (USPSTF et al., 2021).
      b. Direct visualization tests—colonoscopy, CT colonography
      c. Flexible sigmoidoscopy. Any abnormal SBT, CT colonography, or flexible sigmoidoscopy requires additional work up with colonoscopy.
   3. Screening controversy
      a. Most harm of screening is associated with colonoscopy as any abnormality with SBT or direct visualization led to colonoscopy.

TABLE 2.2 Colorectal Cancer Screening Recommendations

Recommendation Summary

Adults aged 50–75 years	The USPSTF recommends screening for colorectal cancer in all adults aged 50–75 years. (Recommendation; Evidence Strength Grade A)
Adults aged 45–49 years	The USPSTF recommends screening for colorectal cancer in adults aged 45–49 years. (Recommendation; Evidence Strength Grade B)
Adults aged 76–85 years	The USPSTF recommends that clinicians selectively offer screening for colorectal cancer in adults aged 76–85 years. Evidence indicates that the net benefit of screening all persons in this age group is small. In determining whether this service is appropriate in individual cases, patients and clinicians should consider the patient's overall health, prior screening history, and preferences. (Recommendation; Evidence Strength Grade C)

CRC, Colorectal cancer; CT, computed tomography; FIT, fecal immunochemical test; gFOBT, guaiac-based fecal occult blood test. From US Preventive Services Task Force. Screening for colorectal cancer. (2016a). https://epss.ahrq.gov/ePSS/TopicDetails.do?topicid=205.

b. Risk of harm with colonoscopy or flexible sigmoidoscopy includes bleeding, infection, and perforation, which occurs <1% (USPSTF et al., 2021).

c. Although colonoscopy is the preferred screening method, no direct evidence suggests that colonoscopy improves mortality (Givler & Givler, 2022).

d. One benefit to direct visualization is the ability to remove precancerous polyps at the time of screening; this preventing that polyp from turning into cancer.

C. Cervical cancer

1. Cervical cancer screening, endorsed by ACOG, ASCCP, and SGO recommendations for average-risk individuals aged 21–29 every 3 years with cytology alone, age 30–65 with cytology alone every 3 years, FDA-approved high-risk HPV (hrHPV) every 5 years, cotesting (cytology+hrHPV) every 5 years, no screening over the age of 65 or in individuals with hysterectomy with cervix removed and no history of high-grade cervical precancerous lesions or cervical cancer (American College of Obstetricians and Gynecologists [ACOG], 2021) (Table 2.3)

2. Screening modalities

a. Cervical cytology/Papanicolaou test (Pap test)

(1) Principal screening tool for cervical cancer

(2) Low sensitivity of single Pap test because of both sampling error, in which cancerous cells do not get collected, and reading error; cumulative sensitivity of several tests is high

(3) Cotesting detects more cervical intraepithelial neoplasia, than cytology alone, although it is associated with increased risks of false positive results and colposcopies (ACOG, 2021).

b. hrHPV test

(1) To be used in people aged 25 and older

(2) Two hrHPV tests are approved by FDA with higher to comparable sensitivity as cervical cytology testing (World Health Organization [WHO], 2021).

c. Colposcopy—primary method for evaluation of abnormal Pap tests

(1) Involves viewing the cervix through a long-focal-length dissecting microscope at magnification

(2) Acetic acid (4%) applied before viewing, which allows a directed biopsy of any grossly visible abnormalities

3. Screening controversy

a. Limited availability of testing, limited access, schedule of testing, lack of knowledge of guidelines, and cost (WHO, 2021)

D. Prostate cancer (PC)

1. PC screening recommendations (Table 2.4)

2. Screening modalities

TABLE 2.3 Cervical Cancer Screening Recommendations (USPSTF, 2018)

Population*	Recommendation	USPSTF Recommendation Grade[†]
Aged less than 21 years	No screening	D
Aged 21–29 years	Cytology alone every 3 years[‡]	A
Aged 30–65 years	Any one of the following: • Cytology alone every 3 years • FDA-approved primary hrHPV testing alone every 5 years • Cotesting (hrHPV testing and cytology) every 5 years	A
Aged greater than 65 years	No screening after adequate negative prior screening results[§]	D
Hysterectomy with removal of the cervix	No screening in individuals who do not have a history of high-grade cervical precancerous lesions or cervical cancer	D

HPV, High-risk human papillomavirus; *USPSTF*, US Preventive Services Task Force.

From *US Preventive Services Task Force. Screening for cervical cancer*. (2018). https://www.uspreventiveservicestaskforce.org/uspstf/recommendation/cervical-cancer-screening.

*These recommendations apply to individuals with a cervix who do not have any signs or symptoms of cervical cancer, regardless of their sexual history or HPV vaccination status.

[†]Grade A denotes that "The USPSTF recommends the service. There is high certainty that the net benefit is substantial." A Grade D definition means that, "USPSTF recommends against the service. There is moderate or high certainty that the service has no net benefit of that the harms outweigh the benefits."

[‡]Primary hrHPV testing is FDA approved for use starting at age 25 years, and ACOG, ASCCP, and SGO advise that primary hrHPV testing every 5 years can be considered as an alternative to cytology-only screening in average-risk patients aged 25–29 years.

[§]Adequate negative prior screening test results are defined as three consecutive negative cytology results, two consecutive negative cotesting results, or two consecutive negative hrHPV test results within 10 years before stopping screening, with the most recent test occurring within the recommended screening interval for the test used.

a. Digital rectal examination (DRE)

(1) Studies have found that a PSA of 3> and a positive DRE was more likely to have PC.

(2) DRE should not be used as a stand-alone test. DRE is a complementary test to be used with PSA in asymptomatic individuals (NCCN, 2022c).

3. Serum PSA

a. PSA is a glycoprotein produced by prostatic epithelial cells.

TABLE 2.4 Prostate Cancer Early Detection Recommendations (American Urological Association, 2018)

Recommendations

The AUA panel recommends against PSA screening in men under age 40 years (Recommendation; Evidence Strength Grade C). In this age group there is a low prevalence of clinically detectable prostate cancer, no evidence demonstrating the benefit of screening and likely the same harms of screening as in other age groups.

The AUA panel does not recommend routine screening in men between ages 40 and 54 years at average risk.

(Recommendation; Evidence Strength Grade C)

For men younger than age 55 years at higher risk, decisions regarding prostate cancer screening should be individualized. Those at higher risk may include men of African American race; and those with a family history of metastatic or lethal adenocarcinomas (e.g., prostate, male and female breast cancer, ovarian, pancreatic) spanning multiple generations, affecting multiple first-degree relatives, and that developed at younger ages.

For men aged 55–69 years the Panel recognizes that the decision to undergo PSA screening involves weighing the benefits of reducing the rate of metastatic prostate cancer and prevention of prostate cancer death against the known potential harms associated with screening and treatment. For this reason, the panel strongly recommends shared decision-making for men aged 55–69 years that are considering PSA screening and proceeding based on a man's values and preferences. (Standard; Evidence Strength Grade B)

The greatest benefit of screening appears to be in men aged 55–69 years.

Multiple approaches subsequent to a PSA test (e.g., urinary and serum biomarkers, imaging, risk calculators) are available for identifying men more likely to harbor a prostate cancer and/or one with an aggressive phenotype. The use of such tools can be considered in men with a suspicious PSA level to inform prostate biopsy decisions.

To reduce the harms of screening, a routine screening interval of 2 years or more may be preferred over annual screening in those men who have participated in shared decision-making and decided on screening. As compared to annual screening, it is expected that screening intervals of 2 years preserve the majority of the benefits and reduce overdiagnosis and false positives. (Option; Evidence Strength Grade C)

Additionally, intervals for rescreening can be individualized by a baseline PSA level.

The panel does not recommend routine PSA screening in men age 70+ years or any man with less than a 10- to 15-year life expectancy. (Recommendation; Evidence Strength Grade C)

Some men aged 70+ years who are in excellent health may benefit from prostate cancer screening.

AUA, American Urological Association; *DRE*, digital rectal examination; *NCCN*, National Comprehensive Cancer Network; *ng/mL*, nanograms per milliliter; *PHI*, Prostate Health Index; *PSA*, prostate-specific antigen; *TRUS*, transrectal ultrasound; *USPSTF*, US Preventive Services Task Force.
Data from *American Urological Association*. (2018). *Early Detection of Prostate Cancer*. https://www.auanet.org//guidelines/guidelines/prostate-cancer-early-detection-guideline.

TABLE 2.5 US Preventive Services Task Force; Lung Cancer Screening Guidelines (USPSTF, 2021)

Population	Recommendation
Adults aged 50–80 years who have a 20 pack-year smoking history and currently smoke or have quit within the past 15 years	The USPSTF recommends annual screening for lung cancer with LDCT in adults aged 50–80 years who have a 20 pack-year smoking history and currently smoke or have quit within the past 15 years. Screening should be discontinued once a person has not smoked for 15 years or develops a health problem that substantially limits life expectancy or the ability or willingness to have curative lung surgery. (Recommendation; Evidence Strength Grade B)

LDCT, Low-dose computed tomography; *USPSTF*, US Preventive Services Task Force.
From *US Preventive Services Task Force. Screening for lung cancer.* (2021). https://www.uspreventiveservicestaskforce.org/uspstf/recommendation/lung-cancer-screening.

4. Transrectal ultrasound-guided or transperineal-guided biopsy is performed after multiparametric MRI and biomarker testing that improves the specificity of screening for high suspicion of PC (Jain & Sapra, 2021).
   a. Multiple areas of the prostate gland are biopsied.
   b. Tumor histologic grade based on Gleason score (Gleason & Mellinger, 1974).
5. Screening controversy
   a. For people at average risk of PC, screening with PSA is not recommended under the age of 54 or over the age of 75.
   b. For people aged 55–69, screening with PSA should be a shared decision-making process with benefits versus risks, and patient's preferences and values (Jain & Sapra, 2021).
   c. False positives can lead to unnecessary tests, invasive procedures, overdiagnosis, and distress.
E. Lung cancer
   1. Lung cancer screening guidelines: in 2020 lung cancer was the second most common cancer and the leading cause of cancer-related death for men and women in the U.S. Smoking accounts for 90% of all lung cancers. Other risk factors include environmental exposure; that is, radon, asbestos, radiation therapy, other noncancer lung diseases, race/ethnicity, and lung cancer history in first degree (Jonas et al., 2021; Table 2.5).
   2. Screening modalities
      a. Low-dose (100–200 kVp and ≤40–60 mAs) computed tomography (LDCT)
         (1) If evaluating mediastinal abnormalities or lymph nodes, conducer standard dose CT with IV as appropriate (NCCN, 2022d).
         (2) Sufficient sensitivity and specificity to detect early-stage lung cancer (USPSTF, 2021).

b. PSA is not cancer specific; most individuals with elevated PSA do not have PC.
c. PSA can be elevated due to infection, ejaculation, or trauma (NCCN, 2022c).
d. Medications such as finasteride or dutasteride may decrease PSA levels by up to 50% (NCCN, 2022c).

(3) LDCT is of moderate benefit for people with high-risk lung cancer based on age, exposure, and years since smoking cessation (USPSTF, 2021).

3. Screening controversy
   a. Screening high-risk people with LDCT can reduce lung cancer mortality, but also causes false positive results, leading to additional tests, costs, invasive procedures, overdiagnosis, incidental findings, distress, and radiation-induced cancers (Jonas et al., 2021).
   b. Changes in screening age eligibility in current or former smokers dropped from 55 to 50, and the smoking criteria was reduced from 30 pack years of smoking history to 20, doubling the population of eligible adults (Horn & Haas, 2022).
   c. Screening guidelines apply to only those who have a 20 pack-year smoking history and currently smoke or have quit within the past 15 years.
   d. For people who quit smoking, screening only applies to those who have stopped smoking within the past 15 years.
   e. Screening does not extend beyond age 80, even though the median age of lung cancer diagnosis is 70 (Marshall, Tiglao, & Thiel, 2021).
   f. Screening disparity and inequities exist among women and people who identify as Black, Indigenous, or Latin (Horn & Haas, 2022).

ASSESSMENT

I. History
   A. Demographics—age, gender, race, date, and place of birth, occupation
   B. Chief complaint—brief description of the reason for seeking care
   C. History of present illness: onset of symptom(s), location, duration, characteristics, any aggravating and relieving factors, and timing
   D. Current medications (prescription, vitamins, herbals)
   E. Allergies (medications and environmental)
   F. Past medical history
   G. Family history—medical and cancer histories in relatives
   H. Social history (e.g., smoking, alcohol, illicit drug use, sexual habits, dietary habits, sleep patterns, and exercise)
   I. Review of systems (Table 2.6)
II. Physical examination
   A. Cancer-related physical assessment should include examination of the skin, mouth, neck, lymph nodes, breasts, cervix, pelvis, testicles, rectum, and prostate.
   B. Specific foci of physical examination are presented in Table 2.7.

MANAGEMENT

I. Health counseling
   A. Teach and reinforce healthy lifestyle behaviors.

TABLE 2.6	Review of Cancer-Related Symptoms
System	**History Components or Symptoms**
Constitutional	Fatigue, malaise, recent weight gain or loss, previous and present level of activity; current performance status
Skin	Changes in warts or moles; bleeding, nonhealing lesions, change in sensation; history of skin cancer
Head and neck	Pain, tenderness; mouth lesions; difficulty swallowing or chewing; hoarseness; discharge from eyes, ears, and nose; epistaxis
Respiratory	Cough, pain, dyspnea, hemoptysis, shortness of breath; date and result of last imaging
Cardiac	Dyspnea, orthopnea, chest pain, edema, palpitations, dizziness
Gastrointestinal	Change in appetite, pain, reflux, nausea, vomiting, change in bowel pattern; dates and results of prior CRC screenings
Genitourinary	Change in urinary pattern, nocturia, dysuria, hematuria, change in force of stream, pain; testicular pain or masses; dates and results of prior PSA
Gynecologic	Vaginal discharge, nonmenstrual or intermenstrual bleeding, bloating, enlarged abdominal girth; dates and results of prior Pap screens
Breasts	Change in appearance, skin, vascular pattern, nipple direction, inversion; mass in breast or axillae; dates and results of prior mammograms
Endocrine	Flushing, sweating, orthostasis, palpitations, polyuria, polydipsia
Hematologic/ immunologic	Bruising, anemia, petechiae, purpura, bleeding disorder, anemia, fatigue, fever, infections, night sweats, chills, frequent infections, vaccines (especially HPV), enlarged lymph nodes, early satiety
Musculoskeletal	Pain and stiffness in bones and joints, limitation of movement
Neurologic	Headache, vertigo, seizures, syncope, visual disturbances; sensory, motor, memory or cognitive deficits; facial weakness, speech problems

CRC, Colorectal cancer; HPV, human papillomavirus; PSA, prostate-specific antigen.

B. Shared decision-making regarding screening for cancers.
II. Interventions to improve patient participation in screening programs
   A. Assess the motivation and willingness of patient to learn.
   B. Identify the cultural influences regarding health and health-seeking behaviors.
   C. Provide patient with a personalized risk of developing cancer by the use of health history and risk profiles.
   D. Provide teaching on the risk and benefits of screening.
III. Interventions for patients with positive screening test results
   A. Identify the resources for cancer education and information.

TABLE 2.7   Physical Examination Foci

System	Components of Examination
Skin	Inspect (cutaneous and mucous membrane surfaces, sun-exposed areas). Note the presence of rash, petechiae, bruising, ulcerations of color and surface.
Head, eyes	Inspect (shape, symmetry, nodules, masses, color of conjunctivae and sclerae, symmetry of pupils, reactivity, eye movements).
Ear, nose, and throat	Inspect (symmetry, presence of discharge, integrity of tissues—note polyps, exudate, friability, bleeding).
Oral cavity	Inspect (for color and integrity of mucous membranes, tongue, under tongue, lesions, or plaques). Palpate (note masses and/or tenderness).
Neck	Inspect and palpate (entire neck for nodes—note, size, shape consistency, mobility, tenderness). Palpate thyroid (enlargement, consistency, nodules).
Chest	Inspect (symmetry, use of accessory muscles). Percuss for dullness. Auscultate (breath sounds—note presence of crackles, rhonchi, wheeze).
Breasts	Perform clinical breast examination. Inspect (symmetry, dimpling, skin changes, irregular venous pattern, nipple direction, and nipple discharge). Palpate (for masses, including axillae for lymph nodes).
Abdomen	Inspect (symmetry, presence of surgical scars, abnormal vascular patterns). Auscultate (bowel sounds). Percuss (liver and spleen size). Palpate (for tenderness, masses, inguinal lymph nodes).
Female genital	Inspect (masses, lesions, discharge, or bleeding). Palpate (tenderness, shape, and consistency of abdominal organs, including uterus, ovaries, and colon).
Pelvic	Inspect (mucosal integrity and color of vaginal wall and cervix; presence of lesions, polyps, or bleeding; discharge; constriction; nodules; masses).
Male genital	Inspect (for masses, cutaneous lesions, nodules.) Palpate (for tenderness, masses, consistency, contour, scrotal contents—testes, epididymis).
Rectal, prostate	Inspect (external lesions, hemorrhoids). Perform DRE (note sphincter tone, masses, tenderness, constriction, bleeding). Assess and order stool test for FOBT or FIT. In males, palpate prostate (note size, symmetry, consistency—firmness, tenderness, nodules).

DRE, Digital rectal examination; *FIT*, fecal immunochemical test; *FOBT*, guaiac-based fecal occult blood test.

B. Discuss the implications of positive screening test results.

C. Ensure the adherence and follow-up for persons with positive screenings for cancer.

IV. Interventions to promote population-based screening programs

A. Target high-risk groups (e.g., older adults, ethnic minority, poor).

B. Use media resources and community organizations to publicize the benefits of screening.

C. Employ skilled health care educators to ensure that the target population understands the disease and the importance of screening and early detection.

REFERENCES

American Cancer Society. *American Cancer Society recommendations for the early detection of breast cancer*. (2022). https://www.cancer.org/cancer/breast-cancer/screening-tests-and-early-detection/american-cancer-society-recommendations-for-the-early-detection-of-breast-cancer.html. Accessed 18.07.22.

American College of Obstetricians and Gynecologists (ACOG). *Updated cervical cancer screening guidelines. Practice advisory*. (2021). https://www.acog.org/clinical/clinical-guidance/practice-advisory/articles/2021/04/updated-cervical-cancer-screening-guidelines.

American College of Radiology (ACR). *Breast imaging reporting and data system (BI-RADS)*. (2021). https://www.acr.org/-/media/ACR/Files/RADS/BI-RADS/Mammography-Reporting.pdf.

American Urological Association. *Early detection of prostate cancer*. (2018). https://www.auanet.org//guidelines/guidelines/prostate-cancer-early-detection-guideline.

Bashirian, S., Mohammadi, Y., Barati, M., Moaddabshoar, L., & Dogonchi, M. (2020). Effectiveness of the theory-based educational interventions on screening of breast cancer in women: A systematic review and meta-analysis. *International Quarterly of Community Health Education*, 40(3), 219–236. https://doi.org/10.1177/0272684X19862148.

Dougherty, M. K., Brenner, A. T., Crockett, S. D., Gupta, S., Wheeler, S. B., Coker-Schwimmer, M., et al. (2018). Evaluation of interventions intended to increase colorectal cancer screening rates in the United States: A systematic review and meta-analysis. *JAMA Internal Medicine*, 178(12), 1645–1658. https://doi.org/10.1001/jamainternmed.2018.4637.

Gail, M. H., Brinton, L. A., Byar, D. P., Corle, D. K., Green, S. B., Schairer, C., et al. (1989). Projecting individualized probabilities of developing breast cancer for white females who are being examined annually. *Journal of the National Cancer Institute*, 81(24), 1879–1886. https://doi.org/10.1093/jnci/81.24.1879.

Givler, D. N., & Givler, A. (2022). Health screening. In: *StatPearls*. Treasure Island, FL: StatPearls Publishing. Retrieved from https://www.ncbi.nlm.nih.gov/books/NBK436014/.

Gleason, D. F., & Mellinger, G. T. (1974). Prediction of prognosis for prostatic adenocarcinoma by combined histological grading and clinical staging. *The Journal of Urology*, 111(1), 58–64. https://doi.org/10.1016/s0022-5347(17)59889-4.

Grimm, L. J., Avery, C. S., Hendrick, E., & Baker, J. A. (2022). Benefits and risks of mammography screening in women ages 40 to 49 years. *Journal of Primary Care & Community Health*, 13, 21501327211058322. https://doi.org/10.1177/21501327211058322.

Horn, D. M., & Haas, J. S. (2022). Expanded lung and colorectal cancer screening – Ensuring equity and safety under new guidelines. *The New England Journal of Medicine*, 386(2), 100–102. https://doi.org/10.1056/NEJMp2113332.

Jain, M. A., Leslie, S. W., & Sapra, A. (2021). Prostate cancer screening. In: *StatPearls*. Treasure Island, FL: StatPearls Publishing. Retrieved from https://www.ncbi.nlm.nih.gov/books/NBK556081/.

Jonas, D. E., Reuland, D. S., Reddy, S. M., Nagle, M., Clark, S. D., Weber, R. P., et al. (2021). Screening for lung cancer with low-dose computed tomography: Updated evidence report and systematic review for the US Preventive Services Task Force. *The Journal of the American Medical Association, 325*(10), 971–987. https://doi.org/10.1001/jama.2021.0377.

Kim, A., Chung, K. C., Keir, C., & Patrick, D. L. (2022). Patient-reported outcomes associated with cancer screening: A systematic review. *BMC Cancer, 22*(1), 223. https://doi.org/10.1186/s12885-022-09261-5.

Lai, A. G., Pasea, L., Banerjee, A., Hall, G., Denaxas, S., Chang, W. H., et al. (2020). Estimated impact of the COVID-19 pandemic on cancer services and excess 1-year mortality in people with cancer and multimorbidity: Near real-time data on cancer care, cancer deaths and a population-based cohort study. *BMJ Open, 10*(11), e043828. https://doi.org/10.1136/bmjopen-2020-043828.

Marshall, R. C., Tiglao, S. M., & Thiel, D. (2021). Updated USPSTF screening guidelines may reduce lung cancer deaths. *The Journal of Family Practice, 70*(7), 347–349. https://doi.org/10.12788/jfp.0257.

National Comprehensive Cancer Network (NCCN), (2022a). Clinical practice guidelines in oncology. In: *Colorectal cancer screening. Version 1, 2022*. NCCN. https://www.nccn.org/professionals/physician_gls/pdf/colorectal_screening.pdf.

National Comprehensive Cancer Network (NCCN), (2022b). Clinical practice guidelines in oncology. In: *Genetic/familial high-risk assessment: Breast, ovarian, and pancreatic. Version, 2, 2022*. NCCN. https://www.nccn.org/professionals/physician_gls/pdf/genetics_bop.pdf.

National Comprehensive Cancer Network (NCCN), (2022c). Clinical practice guidelines in oncology. In: *Lung cancer screening. Version 1, 2022*. NCCN. https://www.nccn.org/professionals/physician_gls/pdf/lung_screening.pdf.

National Comprehensive Cancer Network (NCCN), (2022d). Clinical practice guidelines in oncology. In: *Prostate cancer early detection.*

Version 1, 2022. NCCN. https://www.nccn.org/professionals/physician_gls/pdf/prostate_detection.pdf.

Oeffinger, K. C., Fontham, E. T., Etzioni, R., Herzig, A., Michaelson, J. S., Shih, Y.-C., et al. (2015). Breast cancer screening for women at average risk: 2015 guideline update from the American Cancer Society. *The Journal of the American Medical Association, 314*(15), 1599–1614. https://doi.org/10.1001/jama.2015.12783.

Petrova, D., Cruz, M., & Sánchez, M.-J. (2022). BRCA1/2 testing for genetic susceptibility to cancer after 25 years: A scoping review and a primer on ethical implications. *Breast (Edinburgh, Scotland), 61*, 66–76. https://doi.org/10.1016/j.breast.2021.12.005.

Qaseem, A., Crandall, C. J., Mustafa, R. A., Hicks, L. A., Wilt, T. J., Clinical Guidelines Committee of the American College of Physicians, (2019). Screening for colorectal cancer in asymptomatic average-risk adults: A guidance statement from the American College of Physicians. *Annals of Internal Medicine, 171*(9), 643–654. https://doi.org/10.7326/M19-0642.

Spick, C., Bickel, H., Polanec, S. H., & Baltzer, P. A. (2018). Breast lesions classified as probably benign (BI-RADS 3) on magnetic resonance imaging: A systematic review and meta-analysis. *European Radiology, 28*(5), 1919–1928. https://doi.org/10.1007/s00330-017-5127-y.

US Preventive Services Task Force (USPSTF). *Screening for cervical cancer.* (2018). https://www.uspreventiveservicestaskforce.org/uspstf/recommendation/cervical-cancer-screening.

US Preventive Services Task Force (USPSTF). *Screening for lung cancer.* (2021). https://www.uspreventiveservicestaskforce.org/uspstf/recommendation/lung-cancer-screening.

US Preventive Services Task Force (USPSTF), Davidson, K. W., Barry, M. J., Mangione, C. M., Cabana, M., Caughey, A. B., et al. (2021). Screening for colorectal cancer: US Preventive Services Task Force Recommendation Statement. *The Journal of the American Medical Association, 325*(19), 1965–1977. https://doi.org/10.1001/jama.2021.6238.

World Health Organization (WHO), (2021). *WHO guideline for screening and treatment of cervical pre-cancer lesions for cervical cancer prevention* (2nd ed.). Geneva: World Health Organization.

3

Survivorship

Stacie Corcoran

OVERVIEW

I. Definition of cancer survivor (National Comprehensive Cancer Network [NCCN], 2022; National Coalition for Cancer Survivorship, 2018)
   A. Patients diagnosed with cancer are considered survivors from the time of diagnosis through the rest of their lives.
   B. Significant others, family, and caregivers are also affected by the cancer diagnosis and are included in this definition.
II. Statistics on cancer survivors (Miller et al. 2019; National Cancer Institute [NCI], 2022; Siegel, Miller, & Jemal, 2019)
   A. In 2019 there were over 16.9 million cancer survivors in the United States (U.S.)
      1. Number of cancer survivors in the U.S. predicted to increase to more than 22.1 million by 2030
      2. Sixty-four percent of cancer survivors are 65 years of age or older
      3. Sixty-five percent of cancer survivors have survived 5 years or more
   B. Most common cancer sites among males (Cronin et al., 2018)
      1. Prostate, lung, and colorectal
   C. Most common cancer sites among females
      1. Breast, lung, and colorectal
III. Long-term and late effects of cancer treatment
   A. Definitions (Shapiro, 2018)
      1. Long-term side effects begin as a complication of treatment, persist throughout treatment, and may continue after treatment is completed
      2. Late effects are those that begin after treatment is completed, may be absent or subclinical at the end of treatment, and may manifest years later
   B. Cancer survivors are at risk for long-term and late effects related to their cancer and its treatment (Mayer, 2017; Siegel et al., 2019)
   C. Long-term and late effects associated with cancer—vary according to disease, treatment, comorbid conditions, and age of patient (Nekhlyudov et al., 2019)
   D. Long-term and late effects of cancer treatment
      1. Physical consequences (Miller et al., 2019; Slusser, 2018)
         a. Cardiovascular—cardiomyopathy, congestive heart failure, carotid artery disease, valvular heart disease, arrhythmias, pericardial disease
         b. Pulmonary—pulmonary fibrosis, restrictive lung disease, dyspnea, pneumonitis
         c. Gastrointestinal (GI)—malabsorption, dysphagia, gastroesophageal reflux disease, hepatitis, constipation, diarrhea, weight gain, cachexia, incontinence, GI tract strictures, fistulas
         d. Bone—osteopenia, osteoporosis, avascular necrosis
         e. Endocrine—hypothyroidism, adrenal insufficiency, hypopituitarism
         f. Genitourinary—chronic kidney disease, proteinuria or albuminuria, incontinence, hypertension
         g. Oral—xerostomia, dental caries, osteonecrosis of the jaw
         h. Sensory, neurologic, or other—fatigue, hearing loss, visual changes, taste changes or loss, neuropathy, lymphedema, insomnia, skin changes after radiation
         i. Fertility—early menopause, azoospermia, alterations or injury due to surgery or radiation
         j. Sexuality
            (1) General: problems with orgasm, loss of libido, loss of intimacy, perceived or actual disfigurement, alteration in body image
            (2) Higher rate of miscarriage in women of childbearing age, as well as infertility, even when not in menopause (Shliakhtsitsava, Suresh, Hadnott, & Su, 2017)
            (3) Female: vaginal dryness, stenosis, dyspareunia, vaginismus
            (4) Male: erectile dysfunction, retrograde ejaculation
      2. Psychological concerns (Bevilacqua et al., 2018; NCCN, 2021a)
         a. Anxiety
            (1) Higher rates in women
            (2) Shorter time since diagnosis
            (3) Living alone
            (4) Higher number of comorbidities
         b. Depression
            (1) Underreported symptom
            (2) Impacts younger and older survivors
            (3) Associated with poor health care compliance, increased medical care use, higher mortality rates

c. Distress
  (1) Feelings ranging from vulnerability to sadness, to trauma, to panic
  (2) Interferes with quality of life and ability to cope
  (3) May increase around transitions in care, surveillance appointments/testing, loss, and other significant life events
d. Fear of recurrence (Brown, 2021; Butow et al., 2018)
  (1) Commonly reported problem among survivors
  (2) Strong association with younger age
  (3) Documented in all diagnostic groups
  (4) Can negatively impact the quality of life, adherence to follow-up recommendations
  (5) May be triggered around time of surveillance, appointments, testing, or learning of a friend's/relative's new diagnosis
  (6) Associated with depression and impaired daily functioning

3. Social concerns
  a. Changes in roles and relationships (Keesing, Rosenwax, & McNamara, 2016)
    (1) Survivors, partners, family members, friends may experience changes in relationship, poor communication, and feelings of loss related to:
      (a) Emotional withdrawal
      (b) Isolation
      (c) Guilt
      (d) Depression
      (e) Anxiety
      (f) Intimacy issues
  b. Employment concerns (Blinder & Gany, 2020)
    (1) Higher unemployment rate among survivors
    (2) Impacts income, health insurance, and identity
    (3) Majority of survivors return to work (Heinesen, Imai, & Maruyama, 2018)
    (4) Fear of demotion, decreased wages, changing jobs, losing insurance
    (5) Potential obstacles that may impact job performance and productivity include fatigue, pain, cognitive changes, and anxiety
    (6) Increased physical and psychological work demands associated with a higher rate of unemployment (Wang et al. 2018)
    (7) Americans With Disabilities Act (1990) prohibits discrimination based on disability; individualized adjustments and accommodations may promote the ability to continue or return to work
  c. Financial concerns (Guy et al., 2017)
    (1) Survivors have more chronic conditions than nonsurvivors; negatively impacts productivity and health care expenses

4. Cognitive impairment (Slusser, 2018)
  a. Altered attention
  b. Difficulty concentrating
  c. Mental processing speed
  d. Forgetfulness or problems with memory
  e. Difficulty finding words or expressing thoughts
  f. Visual and auditory disturbances
5. Financial toxicity (Blinder & Gany, 2020; Mongelli et al. 2020; Ver Hoeve, Ali-Akbarian, Price, Lothfi, & Hamann, 2021)
  a. Presents persistent challenges in the posttreatment setting
  b. Bankruptcy, symptom control, premature death
  c. Directly linked to anxiety and depression
  d. Change in employment status—reduced schedule, lack of employment, lost wages, or reduced earning potential
  e. Inability to obtain and retain insurance coverage
  f. Nonadherence related to out-of-pocket expenses: follow-up visits, radiology testing, prescriptions, and device costs
  g. Impact on family and lifestyle
6. Spirituality (Cannon, Dokucu, & Loberiza, 2022)
  a. Positive correlation between greater spiritual/ religious beliefs and physical and mental health and quality of life in cancer survivors
    (1) Meaning of illness—its impact on individual empowerment; ability to cope
    (2) Finding inner strength—connectedness to oneself
      (a) Increased psychological well-being, which impacts relationships with others; reduces stress, depression, and anxiety
    (3) Religious faith—shapes how life events are viewed
      (a) Find hope or meaning in stressful, unpredictable events
      (b) Help maintain the sense of control during illness
      (c) Attending worship services and other activities—finding meaningful support through church community

E. Risk of secondary malignancy
  1. Second malignancies among survivors comprise 15%–20% of all cancer diagnoses (Demoor-Goldschmidt & de Vathaire, 2019).
    a. Patients with Hodgkin lymphoma have an increased risk for recurrence and secondary malignancies related to chemotherapy and radiation
    b. Women who received chest radiation as children or adolescents have a significantly increased risk for developing breast cancer (Bakkach et al., 2021)
      (1) The younger the age at diagnosis and treatment, the higher the risk
      (2) Risk increases with time since treatment

c. Contributing factors include age, genetic predisposition, lifestyle behaviors, immunosuppression, and late effects of chemotherapy and radiotherapy

2. Secondary malignancies associated with radiation therapy within the treatment field (Kamran, Gonzalez, Ng, Haas-Kogan, & Viswanathan, 2016) (see Fig. 3.1).

a. Breast: surveillance recommendations for young women who have received chest radiation as a child, adolescent, or young adult (before age 30)—if received a radiation dose of 20 Gy or higher to the chest, annual breast imaging, including mammography, breast magnetic resonance imaging, or both, should be performed starting at age 25

years or at least 8 years after radiation, whichever occurs last

b. Thyroid: surveillance includes ultrasound screening every 2–5 years versus clinical exam only

c. Cutaneous: NCI recommendations for skin cancer, including melanoma, surveillance include annual skin examination

d. Colon: surveillance recommendations for survivors who have received abdominal, pelvic, or spine radiation as a child, adolescent, or young adult—survivors who received a radiation dose of 30 Gy or higher to their colon or rectum should be screened with colonoscopy every 5 years starting at age 35 years or 10 years after radiation, whichever occurs last

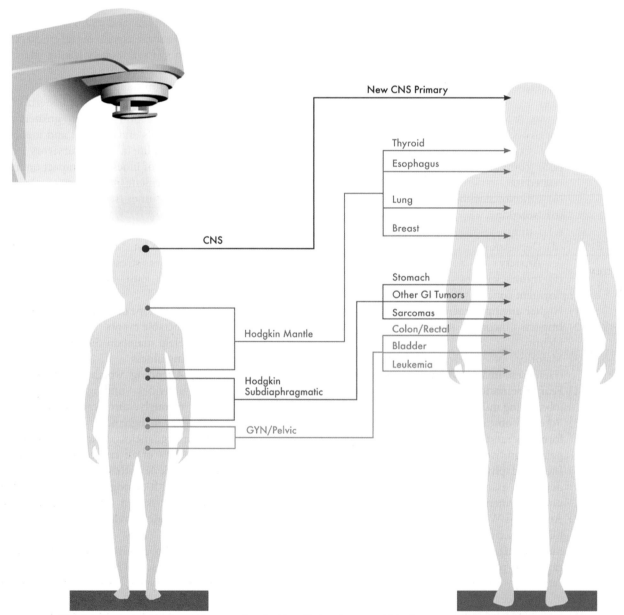

Fig. 3.1 Secondary malignancies associated with radiation therapy within the treatment field. From Kamran, S. C., Gonzalez, A. B. d., Ng, A., Haas-Kogan, D., & Viswanathan, A. N. (2016). Therapeutic radiation and the potential risk of second malignancies. *Cancer, 122*(12), 1809–1821. https://doi.org/10.1002/cncr.29841.

IV. Survivorship care
   A. Survivorship is recognized as a distinct phase of the cancer trajectory, providing multiple opportunities to promote a healthy lifestyle, monitor for recurrence, and identify and manage long-term and late effects (Fig. 3.2) (Vos, Wieldraaijer, van Weert, & van Asselt, 2021)
      1. Many settings institute survivorship care at treatment completion or transition to maintenance therapy (e.g., androgen-blocking treatment for prostate cancer; hormone therapy for breast cancer)
   B. Essential components of survivorship care (Fig. 3.3) (Institute for Medicine [IOM] and National Research Council, 2006)
      1. Assessment to detect recurrence of cancer
      2. Identification and management of long-term and late effects
      3. Screening recommendations for other cancers
      4. Health promotion recommendations (e.g., nutrition, exercise, smoking cessation, sun protection, dental health)
      5. Treatment summary and care plan
      6. Communication with primary care physician and other providers
   C. Barriers to the provision of survivorship care for the future (Jacobs, 2017)
      1. Demand for oncologists will outweigh the supply of providers
         a. Expanding the number of aging Americans
         b. Growing number of cancer survivors
         c. Significant deficits in the oncology workforce

ASSESSMENT

I. History
   A. Clinical data
      1. Demographic information
      2. Providers' names, specialty area (e.g., primary care provider, gynecologist, cardiologist, dentist), and contact information
      3. Past medical history
         a. Comorbidities
         b. Family history, including cancer diagnoses or other major illnesses

   c. Genetic history, if available
   d. Cancer diagnosis, including multiple primaries or relapses
   e. Type and duration of treatment—chemotherapy, immunotherapy, surgery, radiation therapy, hormone therapy
4. Health behaviors
   a. Tobacco/tobacco product use
   b. Alcohol intake
   c. Dietary habits
   d. Physical activity level
   e. Sun exposure
   f. Routine body mass index (BMI) assessment
5. Receipt of preventive and screening health services
   a. Cancer screening (e.g., colonoscopy, mammography)
   b. Immunizations

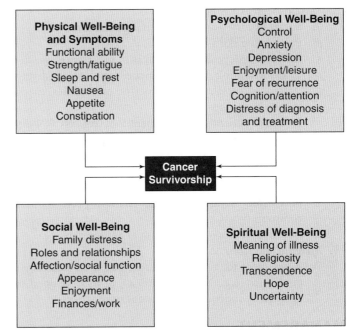

Fig. 3.3 Institute of Medicine (IOM): Components of survivorship care. From Grant, M., Sun, V. (2010). Advances in quality of life at the end of life. *Seminars in Oncology Nursing, 26*(1), 26–35.

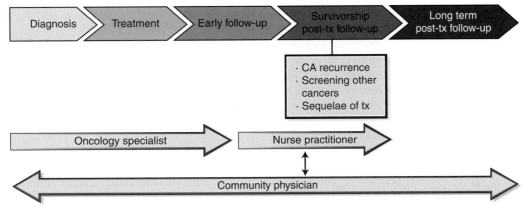

Fig. 3.2 Survivorship as a distinct phase of the cancer trajectory.

6. Genetic testing, as appropriate, for patients with breast, ovarian, or pancreatic cancer (NCCN, 2021b)
B. Focused review of symptoms

II. Physical examination
A. Assessment for long-term and late effects of cancer and its treatment
B. Focused examination to detect recurrence based on disease history and established guidelines (e.g., NCCN, American Society of Clinical Oncology [ASCO], or as developed or adapted by individual institutions or practices)
C. Symptom management assessment
1. Use of patient-reported outcomes tool to assess symptoms/late effects (Morton & Hamilton, 2020)
2. Oncology Nursing Society's Putting Evidence into Practice symptom interventions and guidelines (ONS Guidelines™)
3. National Comprehensive Cancer Network Survivorship Guidelines (NCCN, 2021a)—topics include lymphedema, sleep disorders, and sexual function

III. Psychosocial assessment
A. Social history—occupation, living situation
B. Past coping skills
C. Risk for anxiety, depression, fear of recurrence
1. Contributing factors—fatigue, pain, sleep disturbances, metabolic or endocrine morbidities, medication changes
2. Use of patient self-assessment tool (e.g., NCCN distress thermometer, Patient Health Questionnaire, Hospital Anxiety and Depression Scale) per institutional practices
D. Support systems—identification of available support from family members, friends, peers, church community
E. Neuropsychological evaluation as appropriate

IV. Imaging and laboratory tests
A. Assessment for recurrent disease based on established guidelines (e.g., NCCN or ASCO, or as developed or adapted by individual institutions or practices)

MANAGEMENT

I. Interventions to prevent, mitigate, and relieve adverse effects of cancer and its treatment
A. Assess for any ongoing physiologic, psychological, emotional, social, spiritual, and financial issues
B. Refer to appropriate specialists (e.g., physical or occupational therapist, mental health provider, chaplain, pain and palliative care specialist, speech and swallow therapist), as appropriate (Garmy & Jakobsson, 2018)
1. Rehabilitation: identify impairments associated with cancer history and treatment exposures, develop interventions promoting health and reducing the severity of actual and potential impairments; survivors have many complex needs—physical, cognitive, psychological, sexual, and vocational domains (Stout, Santa Mina, Lyons, Robb, & Silver, 2021)
a. Need for rehabilitation services growing as the number of cancer survivors increases

b. Significant rates of cancer-related physical impairments reported; 53% of adult-onset survivors report functional limitations
c. Rehabilitative services go significantly underutilized
d. Goals are to minimize disability and improve quality of life:
(1) Preventive—lessen effects of expected disabilities
(2) Restorative—return survivors to their previous level of functioning, maximize independence
(3) Supportive—educate survivors regarding accommodations aimed at minimizing debilitating changes
(4) Palliative—minimizing or removing complications, reducing symptom burden, emphasizing comfort
e. Improve ability to work, decrease sick leave, and reduce rates of lost productivity
C. Encourage patients to be physically active; return to daily activities as soon as possible (Box 3.1)
1. Physical activity recommendations for cancer survivors (NCCN, 2021a)
a. At least 150 minutes of moderate-intensity activity or 75 minutes of vigorous-intensity activity or equivalent combination per week
b. Two to three weekly sessions of strength training that involves major muscle groups
c. Stretch major muscle groups and tendons twice weekly
d. Avoid sedentary behaviors
e. Consider limitations for specific populations:
f. Survivors with lymphedema
g. Survivors with ostomy
h. Survivors with bone metastasis or loss
i. Survivors with peripheral neuropathy

BOX 3.1   General Counseling Topics for Survivors

- Be a healthy weight (increasing evidence linking excessive weight to increased cancer risk)
- Be physically active (walk more, sit less)
- Eat well (focus on whole grains, vegetables, fruits, and beans)
- Limit "fast food" consumption (limit or avoid processed food high in fat, starches, or sugars)
- Limit red and processed meat consumption (no more than 12–18 oz/week)
- Limit consumption of sugary drinks (focus on water)
- Limit alcohol consumption
- Don't use supplements for cancer prevention (achieve nutritional needs through diet)
- Do not smoke or use tobacco products
- Avoid excess sun exposure

Adapted from American Institute for Cancer Research (2021). How to Prevent Cancer: 10 Recommendations https://www.aicr.org/cancer-prevention/.

    j. Consider referrals to exercise physiologist or specialist; supervised classes or programs; wearable fitness tracker/pedometer

D. Encourage patients to achieve and maintain healthy eating habits
  1. Plant-based diet
  2. Limit refined sugar and red meat consumption

E. Advise patients on weight management—promote normal BMI
  1. Limit high-calorie foods, especially those with little or no nutritional benefit such as fast foods and fried foods
  2. Substitute with low-calorie, nutrient-rich foods such as fruits, vegetables, and whole grains
  3. Practice portion control
  4. Monitor food labels
  5. Routine weights

F. Counsel patients on tobacco/tobacco product and alcohol use
  1. Avoid tobacco or tobacco products including vaping
  2. Limit alcohol to no more than one drink per day for women and two drinks per day for men

G. Refer to specialists as needed (e.g., nutritionist, smoking cessation counselor, supervised exercise program)

II. Interventions related to knowledge deficit
  A. Assess the motivation and willingness of patient and caregivers to learn
  B. Determine the cultural influences on health teaching
    1. Provide interpreter services as needed
    2. Provide culturally appropriate educational materials to reinforce education
  C. Provide and discuss the survivorship care plan (SCP) (IOM and National Research Council, 2006; Nekhlyudov, Ganz, Arora, & Rowland, 2017)
    1. The SCP should include the following:
      a. Treatment summary—cancer site, type and stage of cancer, date of diagnosis, and any treatment(s) received
      b. Information about long-term and late effects of treatment
      c. Recommend follow-up surveillance and intervals for disease recurrence or progression (e.g.,

NCCN or ASCO, or as developed or adapted by individual institutions or practices)
      d. Recommend health promotion behaviors (e.g., smoking cessation, nutrition, physical activity, sun protection, safe use of complementary and alternative medicine) and health maintenance activities (e.g., cancer screening, bone health screening, and maintaining up-to-date immunizations)
      e. Monitor and manage long-term and late effects
        (1) Per NCCN, ASCO, or other established guidelines, or as developed or adapted by individual institutions or practices for adult survivors
        (2) Children's Oncology Group guidelines may also serve as reference (www.survivorship-guidelines.org)
      f. List of health care team providers with their contact information
      g. Institutional and community resources and referrals based on need

III. Interventions to improve communication and coordination among providers
  A. Clinical updates shared between providers
  B. SCP provided to the patient, primary care provider, and any specialists involved in patient's care

IV. Intervention for adolescent/young adult (AYA) cancer survivors (Lee, Khan, & Salloum, 2018; NCCN, 2022)
  A. Higher-risk population requiring careful follow-up; aged 15–39
    1. Late physical effects (e.g., cardiomyopathy, fatigue, altered cognition, sexual dysfunction, impaired fertility)
    2. Social concerns—relationships, dating, sex, romance, education, career, finances (Janssen, van der Graaf, van der Meer, Manten-Horst, & Husson, 2021)
    3. High rates of being underinsured or uninsured
      a. Unable to afford care
      b. Limited access to treatment and surveillance
      c. Increased reports of medication nonadherence due to cost
  B. Provide age-appropriate assessment, education, and intervention (Table 3.1)

TABLE 3.1 Adolescent/Young Adult Resources

Financial support	• Cancer for College: https://cancerforcollege.org/
	• Expect Miracles Foundation+The Samfund: https://expectmiraclesfoundation.org/samfund-grants
Camps and events	• Camp Make-A-Dream: https://www.campdream.org/about/
	• First Descents: https://firstdescents.org/
Work and career support	• Cancer+Careers: https://www.cancerandcareers.org/en
	• Career Counselors Consortium: http://www.careercc.org/
Emotional support	• Cancare: https://www.cancare.org/
	• Imerman Angels: https://imermanangels.org/
Fertility and family building	• Chick Mission: https://www.thechickmission.org/
	• Livestrong Fertility: https://www.livestrong.org/what-we-do/program/fertility
General	• Cancer.net: https://www.cancer.net/
	• National Coalition for Cancer Survivorship: https://canceradvocacy.org/
	• Stupid Cancer: https://stupidcancer.org/who-we-are/

TABLE 3.2	**Older Adult Survivor Resources**
Emotional support General	• Cancare: https://www.cancare.org/ • Imerman Angels: https://imermanangels.org/ • Administration on Aging: https://acl.gov/about-acl/administration-aging • Cancer.net: https://www.cancer.net/navigating-cancer-care/older-adults/resources-older-adults • The American Geriatrics Society Health in Aging Foundation: https://www.healthinaging.org/ • National Coalition for Cancer Survivorship: https://canceradvocacy.org/

C. Initiate referrals to providers or centers with AYA specialization if possible (e.g., fertility specialist, mental health provider, financial assistance representative)

V. Intervention for older adult survivors
   A. Unique considerations for survivors aged 65 and older
      1. Late effects (e.g., cognitive changes, insomnia, osteoporosis, depression)
      2. Polypharmacy
      3. Caregiver support if needed; independent or supportive living
      4. Increased risk for falls postcancer diagnosis
   B. Provide age-appropriate assessment, education and intervention (Table 3.2)
   C. Collaboration with a trained geriatrician

REFERENCES

Americans With Disabilities Act of 1990, 42 U.S.C. § 12101 et seq. (1990). https://www.ada.gov/pubs/adastatute08.htm.

Bakkach, J., Pellegrino, B., Elghazawy, H., Novosad, O., Agrawal, S., & Bennani Mechita, M. (2021). Current overview and special considerations for second breast cancer in Hodgkin lymphoma survivors. *Critical Reviews in Oncology/Hematology, 157,* 103175. https://doi.org/10.1016/j.critrevonc.2020.103175.

Bevilacqua, L. A., Dulak, D., Schofield, E., Starr, T. D., Nelson, C. J., Roth, A. J., et al. (2018). Prevalence and predictors of depression, pain, and fatigue in older- versus younger-adult cancer survivors. *Psycho-Oncology, 27*(3), 900–907. https://doi.org/10.1002/pon.4605.

Blinder, V. S., & Gany, F. M. (2020). Impact of cancer on employment. *Journal of Clinical Oncology, 38*(4), 302–309. https://doi.org/10.1200/jco.19.01856.

Brown, S. L., Fisher, P., Hope-Stone, L., Damato, B., Heimann, H., Hussain, R., et al. (2021). Fear of cancer recurrence and adverse cancer treatment outcomes: predicting 2- to 5-year fear of recurrence from post-treatment symptoms and functional problems in uveal melanoma survivors. *Journal of Cancer Survivorship.* https://doi.org/10.1007/s11764-021-01129-0.

Butow, P., Sharpe, L., Thewes, B., Turner, J., Gilchrist, J., & Beith, J. (2018). Fear of cancer recurrence: A practical guide for clinicians. *Oncology (Williston Park), 32*(1), 32–38.

Cannon, A. J., Dokucu, M. E., & Loberiza, F. R., Jr. (2022). Interplay between spirituality and religiosity on the physical and mental well-being of cancer survivors. *Support Care Cancer, 30*(2), 1407–1417. https://doi.org/10.1007/s00520-021-06534-w.

Cronin, K. A., Lake, A. J., Scott, S., Sherman, R. L., Noone, A. M., Howlader, N., et al. (2018). Annual report to the nation on the status of cancer, part I: National cancer statistics. *Cancer, 124*(13), 2785–2800. https://doi.org/10.1002/cncr.31551.

Demoor-Goldschmidt, C., & de Vathaire, F. (2019). Review of risk factors of secondary cancers among cancer survivors. *British Journal of Radiology, 92*(1093), 20180390. https://doi.org/10.1259/bjr.20180390.

Garmy, P., & Jakobsson, L. (2018). Experiences of cancer rehabilitation: A cross-sectional study. *Journal of Clinical Nursing, 27*(9–10), 2014–2021. https://doi.org/10.1111/jocn.14321.

Guy, G. P., Yabroff, K. R., Ekwueme, D. U., Rim, S. H., Li, R., & Richardson, L. C. (2017). Economic burden of chronic conditions among survivors of cancer in the United States. *Journal of Clinical Oncology, 35*(18), 2053–2061. https://doi.org/10.1200/jco.2016.71.9716.

Heinesen, E., Imai, S., & Maruyama, S. (2018). Employment, job skills and occupational mobility of cancer survivors. *Journal of Health Economics, 58,* 151–175. https://doi.org/10.1016/j.jhealeco.2018.01.006.

Institute for Medicine (IOM) and National Research Council. (2006). *From cancer patient to cancer survivor: Lost in transition.* Washington, DC: The National Academies Press.

Jacobs, L. (2017). Follow-up care of cancer survivors: Challenges and solutions. *The Lancet Oncology, 18*(1), 19–29.

Janssen, S., van der Graaf, W., van der Meer, D. J., Manten-Horst, E., & Husson, O. (2021). Adolescent and Young Adult (AYA) cancer survivorship practices: An overview. *Cancers, 13*(19), 4847. https://doi.org/10.3390/cancers13194847.

Kamran, S. C., Gonzalez, A. B. d, Ng, A., Haas-Kogan, D., & Viswanathan, A. N. (2016). Therapeutic radiation and the potential risk of second malignancies. *Cancer, 122*(12), 1809–1821. https://doi.org/10.1002/cncr.29841.

Keesing, S., Rosenwax, L., & McNamara, B. (2016). A dyadic approach to understanding the impact of breast cancer on relationships between partners during early survivorship. *BMC Women's Health, 16,* 57. https://doi.org/10.1186/s12905-016-0337-z.57.

Lee, M. J., Khan, M. M., & Salloum, R. G. (2018). Recent trends in cost-related medication nonadherence among cancer survivors in the United States. *Journal of Managed Care & Specialty Pharmacy, 24*(1), 56–64. https://doi.org/10.18553/jmcp.2018.24.1.56.

Mayer, D. (2017). Defining cancer survivors, their needs, and perspectives on survivorship health care in the USA. *The Lancet Oncology, 18*(1), 11–18.

Miller, K. D., Nogueira, L., Mariotto, A. B., Rowland, J. H., Yabroff, K. R., Alfano, C. M., et al. (2019). Cancer treatment and survivorship statistics, 2019. *CA—A Cancer Journal for Clinicians, 69*(5), 363–385. https://doi.org/10.3322/caac.21565.

Mongelli, M. N., Giri, S., Peipert, B. J., Helenowski, I. B., Yount, S. E., & Sturgeon, C. (2020). Financial burden and quality of life among thyroid cancer survivors. *Surgery, 167*(3), 631–637. https://doi.org/10.1016/j.surg.2019.11.014.

Morton, L. M., & Hamilton, B. K. (2020). Using patient-reported outcomes to improve survivorship care. *Blood, 135*(21), 1819–1820. https://doi.org/10.1182/blood.2020005881.

National Cancer Institute (NCI). Statistics and graphs. (2022). https://cancercontrol.cancer.gov/ocs/statistics#:~:text=As%20of%20January%202019%2C%20it,approximately%205.0%25%20of%20the%20population.&text=The%20number%20of%20cancer%20survivors,to%2022.2%20million%2C%20by%202030.

National Coalition for Cancer Survivorship. About us: Our mission. (2018). https://www.canceradvocacy.org/about-us/our-mission/.

National Comprehensive Cancer Network (NCCN). NCCN guidelines. Version 2.2022. Adolescent and young adult (AYA) oncology. (2022). https://www.nccn.org/professionals/physician_gls/pdf/aya.pdf. Accessed 03.05.22.

National Comprehensive Cancer Network (NCCN). NCCN guidelines. Version 2021. Survivorship. (2021a). https://www.nccn.org/professionals/physician_gls/pdf/survivorship.pdf. Accessed 03.05.22.

National Comprehensive Cancer Network (NCCN). NCCN genetic/familial high-risk assessment: Breast, ovarian, and pancreatic. (2021b). https://www.nccn.org/professionals/physician_gls/pdf/genetics_bop.pdf Accessed 03.05.22.

Nekhlyudov, L., Ganz, P. A., Arora, N. K., & Rowland, J. H. (2017). Going beyond being lost in transition: A decade of progress in cancer survivorship. *Journal of Clinical Oncology, 35*(18), 1978–1981. https://doi.org/10.1200/jco.2016.72.1373.

Nekhlyudov, L., Mollica, M. A., Jacobsen, P. B., Mayer, D. K., Shulman, L. N., & Geiger, A. M. (2019). Developing a quality of cancer survivorship care framework: Implications for clinical care, research, and policy. *Journal of the National Cancer Institute, 111*(11), 1120–1130. https://doi.org/10.1093/jnci/djz089.

ONS Guidelines™. https://www.ons.org/ons-guidelines.

Shapiro, C. L. (2018). Cancer Survivorship. *The New England journal of medicine, 379*(25), 2438–2450. https://doi.org/10.1056/NEJMra1712502.

Shliakhtsitsava, K., Suresh, D., Hadnott, T., & Su, H. I. (2017). Best practices in counseling young female cancer survivors on reproductive health. *Seminars in Reproductive Medicine, 35*(4), 378–389. https://doi.org/10.1055/s-0037-1603770.

Siegel, R. L., Miller, K. D., & Jemal, A. (2019). Cancer statistics, 2019. *CA—A Cancer Journal for Clinicians, 69*(1), 7–34. https://doi.org/10.3322/caac.21551.

Slusser, K. M. (2018). *Cancer nursing: Principles and practice* (8th ed.). Burlington, MA: Jones and Bartlett Learning.

Stout, N. L., Santa Mina, D., Lyons, K. D., Robb, K., & Silver, J. K. (2021). A systematic review of rehabilitation and exercise recommendations in oncology guidelines. *CA—A Cancer Journal for Clinicians, 71*(2), 149–175. https://doi.org/10.3322/caac.21639.

Ver Hoeve, E. S., Ali-Akbarian, L., Price, S. N., Lothfi, N. M., & Hamann, H. A. (2021). Patient-reported financial toxicity, quality of life, and health behaviors in insured US cancer survivors. *Support Care Cancer, 29*(1), 349–358. https://doi.org/10.1007/s00520-020-05468-z.

Vos, J. A. M., Wieldraaijer, T., van Weert, H., & van Asselt, K. M. (2021). Survivorship care for cancer patients in primary versus secondary care: A systematic review. *Journal of Cancer Survivorship, 15*(1), 66–76. https://doi.org/10.1007/s11764-020-00911-w.

Wang, L., Hong, B. Y., Kennedy, S. A., Chang, Y., Hong, C. J., Craigie, S., et al. (2018). Predictors of unemployment after breast cancer surgery: A systematic review and meta-analysis of observational studies. *Journal of Clinical Oncology, 36*(18), 1868–1879. https://doi.org/10.1200/jco.2017.77.3663.

4

Palliative and End-of-Life Care

Kristen Elliot and Karen Hsu Patterson

OVERVIEW

I. Palliative care is an essential component of quality care for persons with cancer and their family caregivers
  A. Definition
    1. "Beneficial at any stage of a serious illness, palliative care is an interdisciplinary care delivery system designed to anticipate, prevent, and manage physical, psychological, social, and spiritual suffering to optimize quality of life for patients, their families and caregivers. Palliative care can be delivered in any care setting through the collaboration of many types of care providers. Through early integration into the care plan of seriously ill people, palliative care improves quality of life for both the patient and the family" (National Consensus Project for Quality Palliative Care [NCP], 2018).
  B. Key palliative care components (NCP, 2018; Worldwide Palliative Care Alliance [WPCA], 2020)
    1. Patient and family-centered care across the serious illness trajectory, appropriate at any stage in a serious illness, including along with treatments of curative or life-prolonging intent
    2. Offered in any or all care settings
    3. Goals of care and shared decision-making are essential elements of the palliative care approach
      a. Palliative plan of care is dependent upon patient's preferences, needs, values, expectations, and goals.
      b. Family should be included in conversations, and their concerns identified.
      c. Goals should be reviewed and updated as patient's status or needs change and evolve.
    4. Interdisciplinary team (IDT) (physician, nurse, advanced practice nurse, social worker, chaplain, and other health care professionals) approach to identify and meet the needs of patients and caregivers
    5. Integration of all aspects of patient's care, including physical, psychological, spiritual, emotional, existential, social, cultural, and economic
    6. Assessment and management of, and relief from, pain and other distressing symptoms
    7. Enhancement of quality of life (QOL) for those impacted by serious illness
    8. Support system to help patients live as actively as possible until death
    9. Care of patients and their families when nearing the end of life (EOL), including symptom management, education, expectations
    10. Provide support to help patients and families cope throughout illness, when nearing death, and after the patient has died
    11. Participate in advance care planning (Silveira, 2021)
      a. Discussions held with patients to explore their personal values, goals, and preferences related to future medical care
      b. Provides an opportunity to ensure medical care aligns with these stated values, goals, and preferences
      c. Advance directive: Legal documents about treatment preferences and decisions to be made on the patient's behalf if a patient loses decisional capacity, completed while patient still has decisional capacity
        (1) Living will documents patient preferences around life-sustaining treatments and resuscitation, typically takes effect in the event of irreversible or terminal illness.
        (2) Durable power of attorney for health care documents the choice and authorization of a surrogate medical decision-maker (Hospice and Palliative Nurses Association [HPNA], 2017).
      d. National POLST: Portable Medical Orders (National POLST, 2022)
        (1) Known in many states as Physician Orders for Life-Sustaining Treatment (POLST), may also be called Medical Orders for Scope of Treatment or other names, name varies by state
        (2) Intended for seriously ill or frail persons
        (3) Communicates patient preferences around specific medical interventions in the form of medical orders
        (4) Typically includes orders regarding cardiopulmonary resuscitation (CPR) and medical interventions such as mechanical ventilation and intubation, artificial nutrition, hospitalization
        (5) Valid across a continuum of care settings both inpatient and outpatient, including hospitals,

residential care facilities, clinics, and home; thus, such orders are considered "portable"

C. Standards for palliative care in oncology (National Comprehensive Cancer Network [NCCN], 2022d)
1. Palliative care should be integrated into both usual oncology care and for patients who have specialty palliative care needs.
2. Palliative care needs should be screened for all patients with cancer during their initial visit and reassessed regularly, when clinically indicated.
3. Patients, families, and caregivers should be instructed that comprehensive cancer care includes palliative care.
4. All health care professionals, including trainees, should be provided with educational opportunities to develop palliative care knowledge, skills, and attitudes.
5. Expert care provided by an interprofessional palliative care team should be available for consultation or patient care to patients, families, caregivers, and/or other health care professionals when requested.
6. An interprofessional palliative care team includes, but is not limited to, board-certified physicians, advanced practice providers, social workers, chaplains, and pharmacists.
7. Institutional quality improvement programs should be in place to monitor the quality of palliative care.

D. Domains and competencies for quality palliative care delivery (Dahlin, 2014)
1. Clinical Practice Guidelines for Quality Palliative Care are organized into eight domains (NCP, 2018)
   a. Structure and processes of care
   b. Physical aspects of care
   c. Psychological and psychiatric aspects of care
   d. Social aspects of care
   e. Spiritual, religious, and existential aspects of care
   f. Cultural aspects of care
   g. Care of the patient nearing EOL
   h. Ethical and legal aspects of care

E. Primary, secondary, and tertiary palliative care (Hui & Bruera, 2020; Kaasa et al., 2018; Swami & Case, 2018; von Gunten, 2002)
1. Primary palliative care
   a. Basic palliative care skills provided by general practitioners
   b. Communication regarding advance care planning and prognosis
   c. Basic symptom management
   d. Best provided in community settings; that is, home and clinic
2. Secondary palliative care
   a. Offered in the form of a consultation
   b. Offered by specialist physicians and their medical team; that is, oncologist and interdisciplinary oncology team
   c. Typically provided within a hospital or treatment center/cancer center

3. Tertiary palliative care
   a. Provided by physicians and other team members who have specialty palliative care training
   b. Offered by an interprofessional team composed of physician (board-certified or fellowship-trained specialist), advanced practice registered nurse, nurse, social worker, and spiritual care provider
   c. Address the most complex cases
   d. Formal involvement of interprofessional team in teaching, ongoing quality improvement and safety initiatives, and research to further the palliative care field
   e. Use of evidence-based national guidelines or expert consensus to support patient care processes

F. Specialty palliative care is offered in five major service delivery models (Hui & Bruera, 2020)
1. Acute inpatient consultative teams
2. Acute palliative care units (APCUs)
3. Outpatient palliative care or supportive care clinics integrated within ambulatory care, oncology specialty clinics, radiation oncology, or infusion centers
4. Community-based palliative care programs
5. Hospice care

G. Early integration of palliative care into oncology care
1. Several organizations have discussed the need for and benefit of palliative care in patients with cancer, including the American Society of Clinical Oncology, the Society of Surgical Oncology, the Institute of Medicine, the American College of Surgeons, Commission on Cancer, and the National Comprehensive Cancer Network (Fahy, 2021).
2. Palliative care in congruence with life-prolonging cancer-directed treatment has been shown to allow for better oncology care for both patients and families, specifically in terms of improved symptom management, QOL, satisfaction with care, and less psychological distress (Kaasa et al., 2018).
3. Early integration of palliative care has been shown to not only improve QOL for patients but also improve their survival as well (Temel et al., 2010).
4. Early palliative care referrals improve EOL care and allow for earlier hospice referrals, decrease in readmission rates to acute care centers, and decrease in length of stay, which overall contributes to a reduction of health care costs (Kaasa et al., 2018).
5. Early palliative care increases satisfaction with care in caregivers of patients with advanced cancer (McDonald et al., 2017).
6. Nurses can play a key role in mediating the introduction of early palliative care, building trust, tackling misconceptions of palliative care as equivalent to EOL care or cessation of disease-related treatments, and advocating with oncologists (Mohammed et al., 2020).

II. Palliative care and hospice community resources
  A. Medicare-certified hospice programs
  B. Palliative care programs
    1. Inpatient palliative care consultation in United States (U.S.) hospitals
    2. Outpatient or ambulatory palliative care services are cost-effective or offer cost savings for the health care system by reducing inpatient care and reduced utilization of health care resources (Yadav et al., 2020).
    3. Community-based, nonhospice palliative models of care in the home and nursing home, particularly when integrated with home-based primary care, have the potential to increase the quality of care and reduce health service utilization for persons with cancer and other chronic or serious illnesses, especially for patients who do not meet hospice eligibility criteria but who have significant symptom burden (Daaleman et al., 2019).
      a. Home health aide, homemaker services, or a combination of both may or may not be covered by insurance, depending on identified needs and insurance plan
      b. Social service agencies
      c. Agencies that provide support specifically to persons with a cancer diagnosis (e.g., American Cancer Society)
      d. Agencies that provide services and support to persons with degenerative diseases and their caregivers (e.g., dementia, amyotrophic lateral sclerosis, osteoarthritis)
      e. Layperson-led and professional-led grief support programs—hospices often accept families into their grief support programs, even if the patient was not enrolled in a hospice
III. Palliative care includes and advocates for services and therapeutic modalities to relieve symptom burden, promote and improve functional abilities, and maximize physical comfort and QOL (NCP, 2018).
  A. Rehabilitative therapies such as physical, occupational, and speech therapies
  B. Respiratory therapy
  C. Diet and nutrition counseling
  D. Massage, arts, and music therapies
  E. Complementary, alternative, and integrative medicine therapies
  F. Consideration for palliative chemotherapy and/or radiation aimed at relieving symptom burden, even when curative intent may not be achievable
  G. Home health services
  H. Caregiving support
IV. Hospice care
  A. Definitions
    1. A philosophy of care, a care delivery system, and a regulated insurance benefit. To qualify for hospice care, a patient must be given a prognosis of less than 6 months to live without ongoing disease-directed treatments by two physicians (Tatum & Mills, 2020).

    2. Considered "the model of quality compassionate care for people facing a life-limiting illness, hospice provides expert medical care, pain management, and emotional and spiritual support expressly tailored to the patient's needs and wishes" (National Hospice and Palliative Care Organization [NHPCO], 2021).
    3. Hospice care is part of the palliative care continuum (Fig. 4.1).
  B. Hospice care is based on the understanding that dying is part of the life cycle and that meticulous management of physical, psychosocial, and spiritual symptoms will promote QOL for the patient-family system.
  C. Brief history of hospice as an organized model of care (NHPCO, n.d.a)
    1. The modern hospice movement began through the work of Dame Cicely Saunders, who began her work with the terminally ill in 1948 and founded the first modern hospice, St. Christopher's Hospice, in the United Kingdom, in 1967.
    2. Florence Wald, Dean of the Yale School of Nursing, pioneered the hospice movement in the U.S.
    3. The Connecticut Hospice, founded by Wald, two pediatricians, and a chaplain, opened in 1974 in Branford, Connecticut, and was the first U.S. hospice program.
    4. The Medicare hospice benefit was approved by Congress in 1982 after demonstration projects showed that IDT care focusing on QOL and addressing the symptom burden of terminal illness improved outcomes and cost less than usual care.
    5. Medicare hospice benefit became permanent in 1986, providing a stable source of payment for hospice care; supported a steady growth of hospice programs throughout the U.S.
  D. Similar key features of palliative care apply to hospice care.
  E. The focus of hospice care interventions is relief of distressing symptoms and enhancement of QOL for both patient and family caregivers.
  F. Medicare hospice benefit (NHPCO, n.d.b)

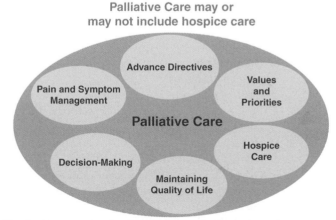

Fig. 4.1 Hospice is part of the palliative care continuum. Palliative care may or may not include hospice care.

1. Patient must have a prognosis of 6 months or less of remaining life to be eligible, as certified by two physicians.
2. There is no limit on the amount of time a patient can spend on hospice care, as long as they continue to meet hospice eligibility with regular reassessments.
3. Top five principal diagnosis categories of patients enrolled in the hospice benefit in the fiscal year 2019 (NHPCO, 2021).
   a. Alzheimer/Dementia/Parkinson disease (20.9%)
   b. Respiratory (7.1%)
   c. Circulatory/heart (6.4%)
   d. Stroke/Cerebrovascular Accident (CVA) (5.4%)
   e. Cancer (4.9%)
4. Late referral to hospice is common (Mulville, Widick, & Makani, 2019).
   a. In 2019 median length of stay in hospice care was 18 days, with 50% of patients dying or discharged within 18 days of admission (NHPCO, 2021).
   b. Hospice referrals may be delayed in pursuit of potentially curative therapies.
   c. Rapid clinical decline at EOL may also make transition to hospice logistically difficult.
   d. Physicians often are reluctant to discuss hospice, as it may be perceived by patients as "giving up".
5. Physicians are often overly optimistic when estimating prognosis and overestimate survival time by a factor of 4 (Soliman et al., 2018).
6. Eligibility criteria (Center for Medicare & Medicaid Services [CMS], 2022a).
   a. The patient must be eligible for Medicare Part A.
   b. The attending physician and hospice physician certify the patient as terminally ill, with a medical prognosis of 6 months or less if the illness runs its natural course.
   c. Patient signs an election statement to choose the hospice benefit and waives all rights to Medicare payments for the terminal illness and related conditions.
   d. Patient receives care from a Medicare-certified hospice
7. Hospice services include (CMS, 2022a)
   a. Services from a hospice-employed physician, nurse practitioner, or other physicians chosen by the patient
   b. Nursing services
   c. Medical equipment and supplies
   d. Medications to manage pain and symptoms
   e. Hospice aide and homemaker services
   f. Physical therapy, occupational therapy, and speech-language pathology services
   g. Medical social services
   h. Dietary counseling
   i. Spiritual counseling
   j. Individual and/or family grief and loss counseling before and after patient's death
   k. Volunteer services
   l. Short-term inpatient care for pain and symptom control
   m. Short-term respite care
8. Levels of hospice care (CMS, 2022a)
   a. Routine home care is provided in the patient's place of residence, including private home, nursing home, and residential care setting, when the patient is not in crisis.
   b. Continuous home care is provided in the patient's place of residence during a brief period of crisis requiring predominantly continuous nursing care and only as needed to maintain patient at home.
   c. Inpatient respite care is provided in an approved inpatient facility on a short-term basis for up to 5 consecutive days to give the caregiver a rest.
   d. General inpatient care is provided in an inpatient facility for pain or symptom control when the symptom(s) cannot be managed at home.

V. Grief and bereavement (refer to Chapter 54 for detailed information) (Corless & Meisenhelder, 2019)
   A. Definitions
      1. Bereavement: The state of having experienced the death of a loved one or family member. Entails loss, grief, and associated processes.
      2. Loss: In the context of palliative care, the permanent absence of a relationship or possession. Value and meaning of loss can vary and are determined by the person sustaining the loss.
      3. Grief: The psychological, social, and somatic responses to loss.
         a. Grief is a normal emotional response to loss.
         b. Anticipatory grief: The psychological, social, and somatic responses to an anticipated loss; an unconscious process.
         c. Complicated or prolonged grief is an intense, intrusive, maladaptive response that persists greater than 1 year beyond the loss.
            (1) Intense grieving beyond 2 weeks can be considered in need of psychiatric intervention in the *Diagnostic and Statistical Manual of Mental Disorders*, fifth edition; however, there is much debate around the overall pathologizing of grief.
         d. Disenfranchised grief occurs when the loss cannot be openly acknowledged, socially validated, or publicly mourned; examples include the death of a person in an unsanctioned relationship such as an extramarital affair or outside of a legally recognized union, loss from miscarriage or abortion, loss of the essence of the individual before actual death (e.g., severe dementia).
      4. Mourning: The outward and active expressions of grief through participation in death and bereavement rituals, social customs, and cultural practices.
   B. Manifestations of grief (Table 4.1)

TABLE 4.1 Manifestations of Grief

Physical	Cognitive	Emotional	Behavioral
Headaches	Sense of depersonalization	Anger	Impaired work performance
Dizziness	Inability to concentrate	Guilt	Crying
Exhaustion	Sense of disbelief and confusion	Anxiety	Withdrawal
Muscular aches	Idealization of the deceased	Sense of helplessness	Avoiding reminders of the deceased
Sexual impotency	Search for meaning of life and death	Sadness	Seeking or carrying reminders of the deceased
Loss of appetite	Dreams of the deceased	Shock	Overreactivity
Insomnia	Preoccupation with image of the deceased	Yearning	Changed relationships
Feelings of tightness or hollowness	Fleeting visual, tactile, olfactory, auditory hallucinatory experiences	Numbness	
Breathlessness		Self-blame	
Tremors		Relief	
Shakes			
Oversensitivity to noise			

Borrowed from Ferrell, B. R., & Paice, J. A. (Eds.). (2019). *Oxford textbook of palliative nursing* (5th ed.). Oxford: Oxford University Press. Adapted from Doka, K. (1989). Grief. In R. Kastenbaum & B. Kastenbaum (Eds.), *Encyclopedia of death* (p. 127). Phoenix, AZ: Oryx Press.

C. Interventions to support persons experiencing grief and bereavement
   1. Formal support
      a. Mourning rituals and practices, which may be associated with religion and/or culture
      b. Support groups
      c. Professional bereavement counseling and/or therapies
      d. Encourage reemergence of hope
   2. Informal support
      a. Occurs among family members, close friends, neighbors, and colleagues
      b. Sharing stories and memories of the deceased
      c. Friendly visits, listening presence, and witnessing of grief process
      d. Assistance with meals, household tasks and maintenance, financial and legal issues
VI. Medical aid in dying (NCCN, 2022d; Ramirez, Fundalinski, Knudson, & Himberger, 2019; Spence, Blanke, Keating, & Taylor, 2017)
   A. May also be known as physician-assisted dying, physician-assisted suicide, or request for hastened death
   B. Upon the voluntary request of a patient deemed to be competent and decisional, a physician provides a prescription for a lethal dose of medication that the patient can self-administer by ingestion, with the explicit intent of ending life
   C. Differs from euthanasia (another individual administers lethal medication to a person with the intent to end life, at that person's voluntary and competent request), which is not legal in any state in the U.S.
   D. Raises complex clinical, legal, and ethical issues
      1. Clinical issues
         a. Explore patient's reason(s) for requesting hastened death and intensify palliative care
         b. Ensure that distressing or overly burdensome symptoms are aggressively well managed

         c. Reassess the psychiatric and psychological issues, existential suffering; referral to a mental health professional when appropriate
         d. Review the patient–family relationships, worries, or concern for family or caregiver burden or abandonment
         e. Offer education about natural disease trajectory and the dying process
         f. Provide information about voluntary withdrawal or refusal of therapies or interventions
         g. Potential benefit of hospice support
      2. Legal issues
         a. As of this writing, the status of medical aid in dying within the U.S. is decided on a state level
         b. Legal in some states and undergoing legislative review in others
         c. Patient request to withdraw or withhold treatment; or request for more aggressive symptom management are not equivalent to medical aid in dying or hastening death
      3. Ethical issues
         a. Autonomy: a patient's right and capacity to make independent decisions for their own well-being
            (1) May be threatened by changes in clinical or physical condition that impair decisional capacity and cognitive abilities
            (2) May be influenced by family, religious, or cultural beliefs or preferences
         b. Beneficence: Benefit to a patient
            (1) Allows patient control and dignity over their dying process
            (2) Duty to protect a patient from, and relieve, intolerable suffering
            (3) Some believe that the availability of medical treatment, including palliative care, invalidates the potential benefit of medical aid in dying

c. Nonmaleficence: An obligation not to inflict harm upon a patient
   (1) Does honoring a request for hastened death prevent harm from undertreated and uncontrolled symptoms and suffering?
   (2) Does honoring a request for hastened death bring harm by explicitly ending one's life?
d. Justice: Providing what is fair and equitable to a patient
   (1) Concern that disabled or socially disadvantaged persons may request hastened death under pressure, duress, or lack of social support
E. Listen to patient concerns and explore options without judgment while offering support, empathy, and kindness

ASSESSMENT

I. Comprehensive assessment of patient and family (Chovan, 2019)
   A. Input gathered from patient, family, and members of the IDT along with information from patient's health records.
   B. Palliative care nursing assessment builds upon standard nursing assessment with additional focus on maximizing patients' comfort and QOL.
   C. Use of active listening, appropriate use of silence, and ensuring self-awareness when speaking with patients about their care are important tools for the palliative care nurse to practice.
   D. Assessments should be performed regularly to recognize evolving needs and changing goals of patients and families who are facing chronic or life-limiting illnesses.
      1. At the time of diagnosis
      2. During treatment and with each consecutive treatment course
      3. After initial treatment, and after additional treatments, or if goals change
      4. At the time of active dying
   E. Palliative care nursing assessments focus on three specific domains with the goal of maximizing patients' QOL.
      1. Physical
      2. Psychosocial
      3. Spiritual
   F. All providers should strive to provide culturally competent care.
      1. Defined as, "[U]sing one's understanding to respect and tailor health care that is equitable and ethical after becoming aware of oneself and others in a diverse cultural encounter. Cultural competence occurs when one is sensitive and embraces openness, has a desire to want to know other cultures, and actively seeks cultural knowledge. Cultural competence is enhanced and sustained through possession of a high level of moral reasoning. Cultural competence results in improved health outcomes, perceived quality healthcare, satisfaction with healthcare and adherence to treatment and advice" (Henderson, Horne, Hills, & Kendall, 2018, p. 599).
   G. Prior to engaging with patient and family, a comprehensive review of patient's electronic health record (EHR) is completed.
      1. Allows for focused assessment and increases the effectiveness of visit
      2. EHR review provides additional insight regarding care
         a. Demographic information
         b. Referring provider and date of referral
         c. Patient's next of kin and their contact information
         d. Primary point of contact or surrogate decision-maker
         e. Religious affiliation
         f. Advance health directive and/or code status
         g. Insurance coverage
         h. Develop an understanding of recent health status and trajectory of care
         i. Medications and allergies
         j. Diagnostic test results
         k. Complementary therapies

II. Nursing assessment throughout the continuum of care
   A. Chronic illness typically follows three trajectories (Fig. 4.2; Lynn & Adamson, 2003)
      1. Cancer progression often follows the pattern of steady functional status and general comfort with a quick and significant drop-off as the EOL nears.
      2. Long-standing illnesses, noncancer related, typically follow an up-down pattern, with an overall downward trajectory. EOL often occurs secondary to an acute exacerbation and/or complication rather suddenly. This is typical for organ failure, such as heart or lung failure.
      3. Frailty, dementia, or debilitating stroke progression can follow many paths but typically exhibits a slow and progressive decline.
   B. Nursing assessment at the time of diagnosis (Chovan, 2019)
      1. Physical assessment
         a. Complete review of systems and patient interview
         b. Complete head-to-toe assessment
         c. Focused assessment to address common symptoms of the disease
         d. Engage patient and family in discussion regarding code status and medical decision-making
      2. Psychosocial assessment
         a. Provide anticipatory grief support to both patient and family
         b. Assess both patient's and family's coping styles
         c. Assess the patient's needs when receiving information, for example, how much or how little information they would like to know
         d. Provide insight and education to patients or families who are not familiar with the health care system

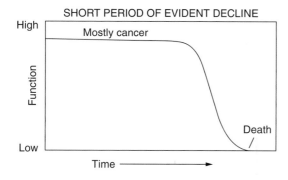

SHORT PERIOD OF EVIDENT DECLINE

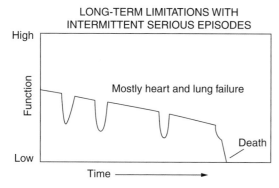

LONG-TERM LIMITATIONS WITH
INTERMITTENT SERIOUS EPISODES

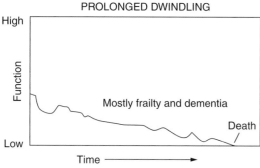

PROLONGED DWINDLING

Fig. 4.2 Dying trajectories. From Lynn, J., & Adamson, D. M. (2003). *Living well at the end of life. Adapting health care to serious chronic illness in old age.* Washington, D.C.: Rand Health. https://www.rand.org/pubs/white_papers/WP137.html.

3. Spiritual assessment
   a. Inquire about any spiritual practices which may allow the health care team to provide better patient-specific care.
   b. Inquire about spiritual practices that promote healthy coping.
   c. Determine if a referral to a spiritual care person is indicated and/or desired by patient and family.
      (1) If patient/family are connected with a spiritual community, they may prefer their established religious leadership, such as minister, priest, rabbi, imam, or other religious figures.
      (2) If not connected with a traditional spiritual community, consider referral to chaplain or spiritual care department.
C. Nursing assessment during treatment (Chovan, 2019)
   1. Physical assessment

a. Focused reassessment of patient, understanding usual disease process, typical side effects of treatment, and body systems affected.
b. Reassess symptoms and advocate for improved management if present.
c. During patient assessment, identify if problems are present and utilize early nursing interventions to confront these problems before they occur or progress.
d. Consider utilizing Palliative Performance Scale (PPS) (see Section II, G1) for ongoing comparison throughout treatment course.
2. Psychosocial assessment
   a. It is imperative that a patient's physical symptoms be managed prior to engaging in discussions about the impact of their illness on their life.
   b. Monitor for signs and symptoms of anxiety and depression; screen for suicidal ideation if depression symptoms are present and make appropriate support referral as needed.
   c. Assess the need for counseling and/or medication that may help promote better coping and symptom management.
   d. Patients with a chronic illness may endure treatment for a prolonged period of time; however, at some point along their disease trajectory, they may wish to reevaluate the benefits versus the burdens of continued aggressive care.
3. Spiritual assessment
   a. Assess the patient's support system and who that may include.
   b. Discuss the QOL and how treatment may be impacting this.
   c. Explore the desire to amend advance directive or code status.
   d. Explore the patient's use of spiritual practices.
   e. Assess the need to refer to chaplain or someone in patient's personal faith community for additional spiritual support.
D. Nursing assessment after treatment (Chovan, 2019)
   1. Physical assessment
      a. Assess for remaining treatment-related or disease process-related symptoms.
      b. Explore the benefits versus the burdens of palliative interventions that may be needed to address these symptoms.
      c. Assess for changes since prior assessments with a focus on systems related to treatment and disease.
      d. May use PPS tool to assess patient's functional status (see Section II, G1).
   2. Psychosocial assessment
      a. When reviewing decisions around the continuation of disease-directed treatments, consider issues of quantity of life versus QOL.
      b. Evaluate the patient's openness to reassess and set new goals of care.

c. Assess the family's coping and overall adaptation to stress

d. Determine if discussion about hospice is appropriate based on patient's goals and priorities

3. Spiritual assessment

a. Determine if there is spiritual suffering present; refer to chaplain if appropriate

b. Reassess the presence of outside or community support and inquire if patient and/or family require additional help

c. Elicit the patient's focus on future hope versus signs of hopelessness

d. Assess the patient or family's desire to discuss worsening condition and even death

E. Nursing assessment during active dying (Chovan, 2019)

1. Physical assessment

a. The primary focus is to assess for and limit patient suffering

b. Identify the signs and symptoms of impending death and intervene when appropriate to ensure patient's comfort (Table 4.2)

2. Psychosocial assessment

a. Determine if there is a need for guidance or assistance with communication among patient and family, friends, and/or caregivers during this transitional period.

b. Determine whether the patient and family need additional education regarding the dying

process, and if so, their readiness to receive this information.

c. Confirm that all important family members and friends have had the opportunity to visit in person, via telephone, or virtually, if this is desired by patient.

d. Determine if there are any complementary or alternative therapies that may be calming or helpful for patient or family.

e. Assess for signs of poor coping among the family and make appropriate support referrals to social worker and/or chaplain as needed.

3. Spiritual assessment

a. Facilitate life review and encourage storytelling with patient and family, if able.

b. Provide family with a calming presence or allow privacy if this is preferred.

c. Allow patient and family the opportunity to express emotions, such as love, forgiveness, appreciation, and grief.

d. Monitor the patient for panic attacks, statements of fear or worsened restlessness, agitation, pain, or shortness of breath, as these may indicate spiritual distress.

e. If warranted, offer resources for hospice services and bereavement support services.

f. Referral to chaplain or spiritual care if necessary.

F. Symptom assessment (refer to Part 5, "Palliation of Symptoms," Chapters 34–47 for detailed information on symptom management and treatment modalities)

1. Fatigue in patients with cancer has been underreported, underdiagnosed, and undertreated. It is common in patients with cancer and is experienced by almost all patients receiving chemotherapy and radiation therapy, bone marrow transplantation, or treatment with biological response modifiers (NCCN, 2022b).

2. Systematic review/metaanalysis found the pain was prevalent in 40% of cancer patients during and up to 3 months after curative cancer treatment (Evenepoel et al., 2022).

3. Common symptoms frequently experienced in advanced cancer include pain, breathlessness, nausea and vomiting, and fatigue (Henson et al., 2020).

4. Other common symptoms experienced while receiving anticancer therapies include peripheral neuropathy, diarrhea, constipation, sleep/wake disturbances such as insomnia or sedation, anorexia and/or cachexia, malignant bowel obstruction, malignant wounds, delirium, depression, and anxiety (NCCN, 2022a, 2022b, 2022c, 2022d).

5. Palliative care patients may experience symptom clusters; therefore it is important not to limit symptom assessment to a report of pain.

6. Complications or symptoms related to the disease process, such as fatigue and anxiety, may exacerbate pain.

TABLE 4.2 Common Physical Symptoms by Persons Who Are Actively Dying

Symptom	Definition
Agitation	Nonpurposeful movements associated with increased anxiety
Anorexia	No interest in eating or drinking
Confusion	Disorientation and lack of orderly thought
Delirium	An acute change in consciousness, cognition, and perceptual disturbances that can fluctuate throughout the day
Dyspnea	Shortness of breath
Fatigue	Overwhelming tiredness
Incontinence	Bladder, bowel
Insomnia	Difficulty sleeping
Mottling	Changes in skin color and temperature due to decreasing circulation that progresses from distal to proximal during the last 2–3 hours of life
Pain	PQRSTU
Restlessness	Uncontrollable increase in motor activity
Skin breakdown	Due to local ischemia secondary to immobility
Terminal secretions	Collection of saliva in the back of the throat that gurgles with each breath

PQRSTU, Precipitates/palliates, quality, region/radiation, severity, timing, understanding.
From Chovan, J. D. (2019). Principles of patient and family assessment. In B. R. Ferrell & J. A. Paice (Eds.), *Oxford textbook of palliative nursing* (5th ed., pp. 32–54). Oxford: Oxford University Press.

7. Interventions to alleviate pain may cause side effects resulting in new or worsening symptoms (Paice, 2019)
   a. Opioids—constipation is the most common side effect; however, opioids may also cause nausea, sedation, pruritis
   b. Radiation therapy—may cause an acute pain flare requiring increased analgesics temporarily
   c. Celiac plexus block—may cause persistent diarrhea
8. Symptom assessment instruments
   a. Edmonton Symptom Assessment System (ESAS) (Hui & Bruera, 2017)
      (1) Has been validated in multiple languages and has been updated to ESAS—Revised (ESAS-r) (Watanabe et al., 2011).
      (2) ESAS-r assesses nine common symptoms in palliative care (pain, tiredness, drowsiness, nausea, lack of appetite, depression, anxiety, shortness of breath, and well-being) (Fig. 4.3)
      (3) Scored on a 0–10 scale, specifying a time frame of "now".
      (4) Accompanying definitions describe various symptoms.
      (5) If patients are unable to complete the form or are unresponsive and incapable of self-reporting (final days of life), observer judgments become necessary and a space is provided for the person completing the assessment.
   b. Distress screening (NCCN, 2022c; Ownby, 2019)
      (1) Distress should be assessed in all palliative care patients and managed in all stages of the disease trajectory.
      (2) NCCN Distress Thermometer is the primary tool to screen for distress and asks user to rate

---

Edmonton Symptom Assessment System:
(revised version) (ESAS-R)

Please circle the number that best describes how you feel NOW:

No Pain	0	1	2	3	4	5	6	7	8	9	10	Worst Possible Pain
No Tiredness *(Tiredness = lack of energy)*	0	1	2	3	4	5	6	7	8	9	10	Worst Possible Tiredness
No Drowsiness *(Drowsiness = feeling sleepy)*	0	1	2	3	4	5	6	7	8	9	10	Worst Possible Drowsiness
No Nausea	0	1	2	3	4	5	6	7	8	9	10	Worst Possible Nausea
No Lack of Appetite	0	1	2	3	4	5	6	7	8	9	10	Worst Possible Lack of Appetite
No Shortness of Breath	0	1	2	3	4	5	6	7	8	9	10	Worst Possible Shortness of Breath
No Depression *(Depression = feeling sad)*	0	1	2	3	4	5	6	7	8	9	10	Worst Possible Depression
No Anxiety *(Anxiety = feeling nervous)*	0	1	2	3	4	5	6	7	8	9	10	Worst Possible Anxiety
Best Well-being *(Well-being = how you feel overall)*	0	1	2	3	4	5	6	7	8	9	10	Worst Possible Well-being
No _____ Other Problem *(for example, constipation)*	0	1	2	3	4	5	6	7	8	9	10	Worst Possible _____

Patient's Name _____

Date _____   Time _____

Completed by - check one:
☐ Patient
☐ Family caregiver
☐ Health care professional caregiver
☐ Caregiver assisted

A

BODY DIAGRAM ON REVERSE SIDE

Fig. 4.3 ESAS-r: (A) Rating scale.

Please mark on these pictures where it is that you hurt:

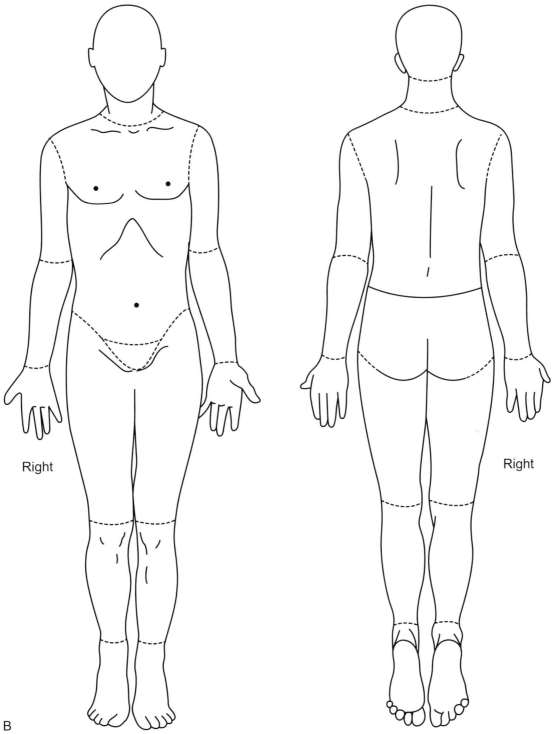

Right   Right

B

Fig. 4.3—Cont'd (B) Anatomic diagram to mark pain. *ESAS-r*, Edmonton Symptom Assessment Scale—Revised.

distress level over the prior week on a scale from 0 (no distress) to 10 (extreme distress).

(3) NCCN Distress Thermometer may be used with the NCCN Problem List that provides a comprehensive supplemental 39-item list of potential sources of distress in the categories

of practical, family, physical, and emotional problems, and spiritual/religious concerns.

(4) A patient should be referred for evaluation and treatment of distress.

(a) Mild distress (<4): referral to primary oncology team with resources available

(b) Moderate to severe distress (≥4): referral to mental health professional, social worker, spiritual care provider, and/or counselor

(5) NCCN Distress Thermometer and Problem List are within the NCCN Guidelines, Distress Management, Version 2.2022 (NCCN, 2022c), available on their website https://www.nccn.org/.

G. Assessment tools used to measure performance and functional status

1. PPS (Fig. 4.4) is a validated tool which measures both performance status and predicts survival of palliative care patients with cancer (Baik et al., 2018)

   a. PPS measures five essential functional domains: ambulation, activity level and burden of disease, self-care, oral intake, and level of consciousness.

   b. Each domain is divided into 11 levels from 0% to 100% and scored in 10%-point increments. A score of 0% indicates death and 100% indicates fully independent and healthy.

2. Eastern Cooperative Oncology Group Performance Status (Table 4.3)

   a. Abnormal: score of 3 or higher

3. Karnofsky Performance Scale (Table 4.3)

   a. Abnormal: score of less than 50%

H. Additional considerations and assessments

1. The Social Work Assessment Tool, administered by social workers, is a validated tool developed by NHPCO to rate psychosocial domains within the context of palliative care and hospice (Reese & Csikai, 2018; Reese et al., 2006). Patients, family members, and/or caregivers are rated on their coping in the following domains: EOL care decisions consistent with patients' religious and cultural norms; patients' thoughts of suicide or wanting hastened death; death anxiety; environmental preferences, social support, financial resources, safety, comfort, complicated anticipatory grief, denial, and spirituality.

2. A number of formal assessment tools are available to examine dimensions of cancer caregiver satisfaction, needs, distress, burden, and QOL (Tanco et al., 2017).

MANAGEMENT

I. Nursing management

A. Physical (Mazanec et al., 2019)

1. Assessment of physical symptoms and provide active symptom management

   a. Pain (NCCN, 2022a)

      (1) Pharmacological interventions: acetaminophen; nonsteroidal antiinflammatory drugs, adjuvant analgesics for neuropathic pain such as antidepressants, anticonvulsants, and topical agents; corticosteroids; opioids; other nonopioid analgesics

      (2) Nonpharmacological interventions: heat, ice, positioning, physical therapy, occupational therapy, massage, acupuncture, acupressure, TENS unit, lymphedema management

      (3) Consider asking about interventional procedures, such as nerve blocks, epidural or intrathecal medications via infusion pump

   b. Dyspnea (NCCN, 2022d)

      (1) Pharmacological interventions: bronchodilators, diuretics, antibiotics, and transfusions to treat potentially reversible causes; oxygen therapy, opioids, and may use benzodiazepines if concurrent anxiety present

      (2) Nonpharmacological interventions: use of fans, maintain cooler temperatures, use of relaxation techniques and stress management

   c. Anorexia/cachexia (NCCN, 2022d)

      (1) Pharmacological interventions: appetite stimulant

      (2) Nonpharmacological interventions: referral to dietician, swallow evaluation, assess for the underlying cause; if patient at EOL, educate family that a decrease in appetite and thirst are a part of the normal dying process

   d. Nausea/vomiting (NCCN, 2022d)

      (1) Potential causes: chemotherapy/radiation-induced; bowel obstruction; gastric outlet obstruction; gastroesophageal reflux disease; electrolyte imbalances; side effects from other medications; psychogenic

      (2) Pharmacologic interventions: corticosteroids, 5-HT3 antagonists, antipsychotic, anticholinergic, antihistamine, antidepressant, oral cannabinoid

   e. Constipation (NCCN, 2022d)

      (1) Preventive measures: fluid intake, dietary fiber, exercise if appropriate/able, prophylactic osmotic, and/or stimulant laxatives

      (2) Potential causes: comorbidities such as diabetes mellitus or hypothyroidism, side effects of medications (such as opioids), fecal impaction, obstruction

      (3) Interventions: titration of laxatives, glycerin or mineral suppository, manual disimpaction, tap water enema, consider peripherally acting mu-opioid receptor antagonist aimed at opioid-induced constipation (avoid in post-op ileus or mechanical bowel obstruction)

   f. Diarrhea (NCCN, 2022d)

      (1) Potential causes: chemotherapy-induced, post-surgical, irritable bowel syndrome/Crohn's disease, recent antibiotic administration, radiation-induced, Graft-versus-host-disease or other immunotherapy-induced colitis, insufficiency of pancreas, infection, and dietary changes

      (2) Treatments vary depending on the cause of diarrhea; however, may include antidiarrheal

Palliative Performance Scale (PPSv2)

PPS Level	Ambulation	Activity Level & Evidence of Disease	Self-care	Intake	Conscious level
PPS 100%	Full	Normal activity & work **No evidence** of disease	Full	Normal	Full
PPS 90%	Full	Normal activity & work **Some evidence** of disease	Full	Normal	Full
PPS 80%	Full	Normal activity & work *with* effort Some evidence of disease	Full	Normal or reduced	Full
PPS 70%	Reduced	Unable normal activity & work **Significant** disease	Full	Normal or reduced	Full
PPS 60%	Reduced	Unable hobby/house work Significant disease	Occasional assistance	Normal or reduced	Full or confusion
PPS 50%	Mainly sit/lie	Unable to do any work **Extensive** disease	Considerable assistance	Normal or reduced	Full or drowsy or confusion
PPS 40%	Mainly in bed	Unable to do most activity Extensive disease	Mainly assistance	Normal or reduced	Full or drowsy +/- confusion
PPS 30%	Totally bed bound	Unable to do any activity Extensive disease	Total care	Reduced	Full or drowsy +/- confusion
PPS 20%	Totally bed bound	Unable to do any activity Extensive disease	Total care	Minimal sips	Full or drowsy +/- confusion
PPS 10%	Totally bed bound	Unable to do any activity Extensive disease	Total care	Mouth care only	Drowsy or coma
PPS 0%	Dead	-	-	-	-

Instructions: PPS level is determined by reading left to right to find a 'best horizontal fit.' Begin at left column reading downwards until current ambulation is determined, then, read across to next and downwards until each column is determined. Thus, 'leftward' columns take precedence over 'rightward' columns. Also, see 'definitions of terms' below.

Definition of Terms for PPS

As noted below, some of the terms have similar meanings with the differences being more readily apparent as one reads horizontally across each row to find an overall 'best fit' using all five columns.

1. **Ambulation** (Use item **Self-Care** to help decide the level)
   - **Full** — no restrictions or assistance.
   - **Reduced ambulation** — degree to which the patient can walk and transfer with occasional assistance.
   - **Mainly sit/lie vs. Mainly in bed** — the amount of time that the patient is *able to* sit up or *needs* to lie down.
   - **Totally bed bound** — unable to get out of bed or do self-care.

2. **Activity & Evidence of Disease** (Use **Ambulation** to help decide the level.)
   - **Activity** — Refers to normal activities linked to daily routines (ADL), house work, and hobbies/leisure.
   - **Job/work** — Refers to normal activities linked to both paid and unpaid work, including homemaking and volunteer activities.
   - Both include cases in which a patient continues the activity but may reduce either the time or effort involved.

   Evidence of Disease
   - **No evidence of disease** — Individual is normal and healthy with no physical or investigative evidence of disease.
   - **'Some,' 'significant,' and 'extensive' disease** — Refers to physical or investigative evidence which shows disease progression, sometimes despite active treatments.

   - Example 1: Breast cancer:
     | some | = a local recurrence |
     | significant | = one or two metastases in the lung or bone |
     | extensive | = multiple metastases (lung, bone, liver, or brain), hypercalcemia or other complication |

   Example 2: CHF:
some	= regular use of diuretic &/or ACE inhibitors to control
significant	= exacerbations of CHF, effusion, or edema, necessitating increases or changes in drug management
extensive	= 1 or more hospital admissions in past 12 months for acute CHF & general decline with effusions, edema, SOB

3. **Self-Care**
   - **Full** — Able to do all normal activities such as transfer out of bed, walk, wash, toilet, and eat without assistance.
   - **Occasional assistance** — Requires *minor* assistance from several times a week to once every day, for the activities noted above.
   - **Considerable assistance** — Requires *moderate* assistance every day, for *some* of the activities noted above (getting to the bathroom, cutting up food, etc.).
   - **Mainly assistance** — Requires *major* assistance every day, for *most* of the activities noted above (getting up, washing face, and shaving, etc.). Can usually eat with minimal or no help. This may fluctuate with level of fatigue.
   - **Total care** — Always requires assistance for all care. May or may not be able to chew and swallow food.

4. **Intake**
   - **Normal** — eats normal amounts of food for the individual as when healthy.
   - **Normal or reduced** — highly variable for the individual; 'reduced' means intake is less than normal amounts when healthy.
   - **Minimal to sips** — very small amounts, usually pureed or liquid, and well below normal intake.
   - **Mouth care only** — no oral intake.

5. **Conscious Level**
   - **Full** — fully alert and orientated, with normal (for the patient) cognitive abilities (thinking, memory, etc.).
   - **Full or confusion** — level of consciousness is full or may be reduced. If reduced, confusion denotes delirium or dementia, which may be mild, moderate, or severe, with multiple possible etiologies.
   - **Full or drowsy +/- confusion** — level of consciousness is full or may be markedly reduced; sometimes included in the term stupor. Implies fatigue, drug side effects, delirium, or closeness to death.
   - **Drowsy or coma +/- confusion** — no response to verbal or physical stimuli; some reflexes may or may not remain. The depth of coma may fluctuate throughout a 24-hour period. Usually indicates imminent death.

Fig. 4.4 Palliative Performance Scale. From Copyright Victoria Hospice Society, BC, Canada. https://www.victoriahospice.org.

TABLE 4.3 Comparison of Eastern Cooperative Oncology Group (ECOG) Performance Status and Karnofsky Performance Status

ECOG Performance Status	Karnofsky Performance Status
0—Fully active, able to carry on all predisease performance without restriction	100—Normal, no complaints; no evidence of disease
1—Restricted in physically strenuous activity but ambulatory and able to carry out work of a light or sedentary nature (e.g., light housework, office work)	90—Able to carry on normal activity; minor signs or symptoms of disease
2—Ambulatory and capable of all self-care but unable to carry out any work activities; up and about more than 50% of waking hours	80—Normal activity with effort, some signs or symptoms of disease
	70—Cares for self but unable to carry on normal activity or to do active work
	60—Requires occasional assistance but is able to care for most of personal needs
	50—Requires considerable assistance and frequent medical care
3—Capable of only limited self-care; confined to bed or chair more than 50% of waking hours	40—Disabled; requires special care and assistance
	30—Severely disabled; hospitalization is indicated, although death not imminent
4—Completely disabled; cannot carry on any self-care; totally confined to bed or chair	20—Very ill; hospitalization and active supportive care necessary
	10—Moribund
5—Dead	0—Dead

From Karnofsky, D., & Burchenal, J. (1949). The clinical evaluation of chemotherapeutic agents in cancer. In C. MacLeod (Ed.), *Evaluation of chemotherapeutic agents* (pp. 191–205). New York, NY: Columbia University Press; Zubrod, C, et al. (1960). Appraisal of methods for the study of chemo-therapy in man: Comparative therapeutic trial of nitrogen mustard and thiophosphoramide. *Journal of Chronic Diseases, 11,* 7–33.

agents, oral or IV hydration, antibiotics, anticholinergic agents, probiotics, or corticosteroids

g. Malignant bowel obstruction (NCCN, 2022d)
   (1) Pharmacological interventions: administration of supplemental fluids, opioids, corticosteroids, antiemetics (if complete bowel obstruction, motility-increasing agents, such as metoclopramide, should not be used)
   (2) Other treatments: surgical, endoscopic, gastrostomy tube, or nasogastric tube for draining

h. Sleep/wake disturbances including insomnia and sedation (NCCN, 2022d)
   (1) Potential causes: stress, anxiety, pain, nausea, depression, delirium, side effects of medication or medication withdrawal, or primary sleep disorders
   (2) Pharmacological interventions for insomnia: antipsychotics, sedatives, benzodiazepines, antidepressants, alpha-adrenergic blockers, melatonin-receptor agonists
   (3) Pharmacological interventions for daytime sedation: central nervous system stimulant

i. Delirium (NCCN, 2022d)
   (1) Potential causes: dehydration, unrelieved pain, metabolic disturbances, hypoxia, bowel obstruction, infection, brain metastases, other neurologic events, medication effects, or medication withdrawal
   (2) Nonpharmacological intervention: decrease disturbances in sleep/wake cycle, ensure patient has their glasses or hearing aid if required
   (3) Pharmacological interventions: utilize haloperidol or other antipsychotics

j. Medical cannabis may be helpful to improve pain, nausea, vomiting, poor appetite, sleep disturbances, and emotional health; may be administered via oral tablets or capsules, oil solutions, oromucosal spray, edible products, inhaled (smoked or vaporized), or topical application (Vinette et al., 2022)

B. Psychosocial (Chovan, 2019)
   1. Complete psychosocial assessment
   2. Complete general assessment of mental status
   3. Ability to differentiate between normal grief response and depression
   4. Encourage patient and family to participate in decision-making, offering some control in care plan
   5. Offer support and primary interventions with a follow-up referral to psychiatry, psychologist, and/or counseling services
   6. Utilize the expertise of palliative care team social worker and/or chaplain

C. Spiritual (Chovan, 2019)
   1. Primary assessment of spiritual coping
   2. Allow the patient and family to tell their story and share their values, beliefs, traditions, and practices
   3. Provide sensitivity to patient's spiritual beliefs and needs
   4. Referral to spiritual care providers as needed

D. Provide education to patients, families, and other health care team members about palliative care

E. Coordinate the plan of care with patient, family, and the treatment team

II. Care for the imminently dying
   A. Patients who are in the last hours of their lives often experience unrelieved physical, emotional, spiritual, and social suffering
   B. Recognizing the signs of imminent death is critical to providing the best care possible during this phase
   C. Identifying this phase is not always easy or straightforward
   D. Patients and families may have preferences for the location of death

1. Among patients receiving home-based palliative care services, home was the most preferred location of death (Cai, Zhang, Guerriere, & Coyte, 2020).
2. More than half of adult cancer patients prefer to die at home (Fereidouni et al., 2021).
3. Acute hospital deaths are associated with lower quality of death, and higher grief and depressive symptoms in caregivers, when compared to home hospice deaths (Hatano et al., 2017).
4. However, preferences for location of death may vary by race and ethnic group; and overly burdensome physical and emotional EOL caregiving needs may be difficult to manage in the home setting; do not assume that home death is always preferred (Wachterman, Luth, Semco, & Weissman, 2022).

E. Clinical signs of impending death may include (Harman, Bailey, & Walling, 2021)
1. Patient becoming bedbound
2. Altered level of consciousness
3. Less interest in foods and fluids
4. Loss of ability to take oral medications
5. Changes in breathing pattern (Cheyne–Stokes respirations)
6. Decreased urine output
7. Nonreactive pupils
8. Decreased response to visual or verbal stimuli
9. Inability to close eyelids
10. Drooping of nasolabial folds
11. PPS of <10% (Fig. 4.4)

F. Honoring preferences for EOL care requires clear communication about the benefits and burdens of medical procedures. Ideally, these goals of care conversations are held early in the disease trajectory and are revisited over time as the disease progresses.
1. Landmark SUPPORT (Study to Understand Prognoses and Preferences for Outcomes and Risks of Treatments) study focused on EOL suffering experienced by those nearing death and identified substantial shortcomings in caring for the seriously ill (The SUPPORT Principal Investigators, 1995). Findings include:
   a. Forty-seven percent of physicians knew when their patients wished to avoid CPR.
   b. Forty-six percent of Do Not Resuscitate orders were written within 2 days of death.
   c. Thirty-eight percent of patients who died spent at least 10 days in an intensive care unit.
   d. Fifty percent of patients experienced moderate to severe pain at least half the time.
2. Mechanical ventilation and CPR are medical procedures of particular importance (Harman et al., 2021).
   a. Preferable for these discussions to take place before the dying phase, if possible.
   b. Although CPR may prolong life in some patients, it will not reverse terminal illness.

c. Patients imminently dying should not be subjected to CPR, as this is a nonbeneficial and potentially harmful procedure.
3. Artificial nutrition and hydration, also called medical administration of nutrition and hydration (MANH), at the EOL is a controversial topic with physical, emotional, spiritual, and ethical considerations (American Academy of Hospice and Palliative Medicine, 2013; HPNA, 2020).
   a. MANH should be considered a medical intervention.
   b. Originally developed to provide short-term support for acutely ill patients, MANH may offer symptomatic benefits in the setting of acute or reversible conditions.
   c. MANH may provide psychological or spiritual benefit to patients and families when they believe that food and fluids are a basic human right and/or a religious necessity.
   d. In EOL situations, MANH is unlikely to prolong life and can lead to complications that increase physical suffering.
   e. Potential burdens or adverse effects of MANH include aspiration and diarrhea (enteral nutrition), sepsis (parenteral nutrition), pressure sores, skin breakdown, complications from fluid overload, and the need for physical restraints in agitated or confused patients.
   f. Recommendations
      (1) Acknowledge and respect the decision made by the patient and/or family caregivers to initiate, withhold, or withdraw MANH.
      (2) Facilitate education about the dying process and its effects on nutrition and fluid status.
      (3) Support the dying person's wishes to drink if that is their wish.
      (4) Offer frequent care of the mouth and lips.
      (5) Foster caregiver involvement in mouth care.
      (6) Discuss the benefits, risks, and burdens of MANH with the dying person and caregivers.
      (7) Consider a therapeutic trial of MANH if goals of care reflect this desire and if distressing symptoms are associated with dehydration, such as thirst or delirium.

G. Symptoms specific to EOL (Harman et al., 2021)
1. Weakness and functional decline.
   a. Burden of illness increasing along with diminished tolerance for physical activity.
   b. Implement scheduled turning or repositioning of the patient to reduce the risk of pressure ulcers and pain.
   c. Offer assistance and education to caregivers for personal hygiene and care.
2. Pain
   a. Opioids are the primary choice for managing pain.

b. Patient's prior opioid use should be considered when dosing for comfort.

3. Dyspnea
   a. Opioids and supplemental oxygen are mainstays in treatment for dyspnea.
   b. Fan therapy (blowing air toward a patient's face) has been shown to be useful for patients when experiencing dyspnea.

4. Nausea
   a. Does not typically occur at EOL spontaneously.
   b. Nausea at EOL is usually related to a known underlying issue such as malignant bowel obstruction, gastroparesis, or radiation/chemotherapy.
   c. Consider rotating opioids if nausea is opioid-induced.

5. Delirium
   a. May present as confusion, restlessness, agitation, and/or sleep-wake disturbances.
   b. May occur with moaning and groaning, which could be misinterpreted as pain.
   c. Options for management of terminal delirium include haloperidol, olanzapine, or risperidone.
   d. For patients with Parkinson disease or parkinsonian side effects from antipsychotics, preferred option is quetiapine.

6. Anxiety or agitation
   a. May be difficult to determine if anxiety/agitation is caused by terminal delirium or by psychological or physical discomfort.
   b. Ativan is benzodiazepine of choice for anxiety/agitation.

7. Seizures
   a. Occasionally, seizures occur at EOL without prior history when brain metastases are present or a neurologic injury increases the risk.
   b. Ativan is used when seizures arise as a new symptom; however, when known seizure disorder exists, the recommendation is to continue the prior effective anticonvulsant regimen.

8. Airway secretions
   a. Often a sign seen as the dying process has progressed, may be referred to as "death rattle".
   b. Halting intravenous fluids and/or enteral feedings may help to decrease secretions.
   c. Positioning of patient on their side may assist in mobilizing secretions from the airway.
   d. If pharmacological approach is used, glycopyrrolate is the preferred medication; however, may also use atropine or scopolamine.

9. Loss of sphincter control
   a. May use urinary catheter if indicated and agreed upon with family.
   b. Can use rectal tube for intractable diarrhea, though rarely necessary.

10. In some cases, symptoms may be so severe that they cannot be adequately managed despite comprehensive conventional treatments (NCCN, 2022d).

   a. Palliative sedation, the intentional lowering of wakefulness toward, and possibly including, unconsciousness, may be considered to treat refractory, uncontrolled severe symptoms.
   b. Utilizes nonopioid medications such as benzodiazepines, barbiturates, or propofol.

H. Care of the patient and family after death (NCCN, 2022d)
   1. Notify the family of death and offer condolences.
   2. Allow the family to have time with the body.
   3. Care of the body after death should be culturally sensitive and respectful.
   4. If autopsy is not desired, remove lines, drains, and tubes.
   5. Offer support to family and refer to bereavement services if desired.
   6. If death occurred while receiving hospice services, Medicare requires hospice to provide comprehensive bereavement care and support services to the caregiver and family for 1 year after the death of the hospice patient (CMS, 2022b).

REFERENCES

American Academy of Hospice and Palliative Medicine. Statement on artificial nutrition and hydration near the end of life. (2013). http://aahpm.org/positions/anh.

Baik, D., Russell, D., Jordan, L., Dooley, F., Bowles, K. H., & Masterson Creber, R. M. (2018). Using the Palliative Performance Scale to estimate survival for patients at the end of life: A systematic review of the literature. Journal of Palliative Medicine, 21(11), 1651–1661. https://doi.org/10.1089/jpm.2018.0141.

Cai, J., Zhang, L., Guerriere, D., & Coyte, P. C. (2020). Congruence between preferred and actual place of death for those in receipt of home-based palliative care. Journal of Palliative Medicine, 23(11), 1460–1467. https://doi.org/10.1089/jpm.2019.0582.

Centers for Medicare & Medicaid Services (CMS). Hospice. (2022a). https://www.cms.gov/Medicare/Medicare-Fee-for-Service-Payment/Hospice.

Centers for Medicare & Medicare Services (CMS). Medicare learning network fact sheet: Creating an effective hospice plan of care. (2022b). https://www.cms.gov/files/document/creating-effective-hospice-plan-care.pdf.

Chovan, J. D. (2019). Principles of patient and family assessment. In B. R. Ferrell & J. A. Paice (Eds.), Oxford textbook of palliative nursing (5th ed., pp. 32–54). Oxford: Oxford University Press.

Corless, I. B., & Meisenhelder, J. B. (2019). Bereavement. In B. R. Ferrell & J. A. Paice (Eds.), Oxford textbook of palliative nursing (5th ed., pp. 390–404). Oxford: Oxford University Press.

Daaleman, T. P., Ernecoff, N. C., Kistler, C. E., Reid, A., Reed, D., & Hanson, L. C. (2019). The impact of a community-based serious illness care program on healthcare utilization and patient care experience. Journal of the American Geriatrics Society, 67(4), 825–830. https://doi.org/10.1111/jgs.15814.

Dahlin, C. (2014). Competencies for the hospice and palliative advanced practice nurse (2nd ed.). Hospice and Palliative Nurses Association.

Evenepoel, M., Haenen, V., De Baerdemaecker, T., Meeus, M., Devoogdt, N., Dams, L., et al. (2022). Pain prevalence during cancer treatment: A systematic review and meta-analysis. Journal of Pain and Symptom Management, 63(3), e317–e335. https://doi. org/10.1016/j.jpainsymman.2021.09.011.

Fahy, B. N. (2021). Current guidelines for integration of palliative care in oncology. Surgical Oncology Clinics of North America, 30(3), 431–447. https://doi.org/10.1016/j.soc.2021.02.002.

Fereidouni, A., Rassouli, M., Salesi, M., Ashrafizadeh, H., Vahedian-Azimi, A., & Barasteh, S. (2021). Preferred place of death in adult cancer patients: A systematic review and meta-analysis. Frontiers in Psychology, 12, 1–12. https://doi.org/10.3389/fpsyg.2021.704590.

Harman, S. M., Bailey, F. A., & Walling, A. M. (2021). Palliative care: The last hours and days of life. Waltham, MA: UpToDate. Retrieved 26.04.22 from https://www.uptodate.com/contents/palliative-care-the-last-hours-and-days-of-life.

Hatano, Y., Aoyama, M., Morita, T., Yamaguchi, T., Maeda, I., Kizawa, Y., et al. (2017). The relationship between cancer patients' place of death and bereaved caregivers' mental health status. Psycho-Oncology, 26(11), 1959–1964. https://doi.org/10.1002/pon.4412.

Henderson, S., Horne, M., Hills, R., & Kendall, E. (2018). Cultural competence in healthcare in the community: A concept analysis. Health & Social Care in the Community, 26(4), 590–603. https://doi.org/10.1111/hsc.12556.

Henson, L. A., Maddocks, M., Evans, C., Davidson, M., Hicks, S., & Higginson, I. J. (2020). Palliative care and the management of common distressing symptoms in advanced cancer: Pain, breathlessness, nausea and vomiting, and fatigue. Journal of Clinical Oncology, 38(9), 905–914. http://ascopubs.org/doi/full/10.1200/JCO.19.00470.

Hospice and Palliative Nurses Association (HPNA). HPNA position statement – Advance care planning. (2017). https://journals.lww.com/jhpn/fulltext/2018/10000/hpna_position_statement_advance_care_planning.15.aspx.

Hospice and Palliative Nurses Association (HPNA). HPNA position statement – Medically administered nutrition and hydration. (2020). https://cpb-us-e1.wpmucdn.com/wordpressua.uark.edu/dist/9/936/files/2022/01/HPNA-Medically-Administered-Nutrition-and-Hydration-Statement.pdf.

Hui, D., & Bruera, E. (2017). The Edmonton Symptom Assessment System 25 years later: Past, present, and future developments. Journal of Pain and Symptom Management, 53(3), 630–643. https://doi.org/10.1016/j.jpainsymman.2016.10.370.

Hui, D., & Bruera, E. (2020). Models of palliative care delivery for patients with cancer. Journal of Clinical Oncology: Official Journal of the American Society of Clinical Oncology, 38(9), 852–865. https://doi.org/10.1200/JCO.18.02123.

Kaasa, S., Loge, J. H., Aapro, M., Albreht, T., Anderson, R., Bruera, E., et al. (2018). Integration of oncology and palliative care: A Lancet Oncology Commission. The Lancet. Oncology, 19(11), e588–e653. https://doi.org/10.1016/S1470-2045(18)30415-7.

Lynn, J., & Adamson, D. M. (2003). Living well at the end of life. Adapting health care to serious chronic illness in old age. Washington, D.C.: Rand Health.

Mazanec P, Reimer R, Bullington J, Coyne PJ, Harris H, Catherine Dubois M, et al. Interdisciplinary palliative care teams: Specialists in delivering palliative care. In: Ferell RB, Paice JA, editors. Oxford Textbook of Palliative Nursing. 5th ed. United States of America: Oxford University Press; 2019. pp. 89–98.

McDonald, J., Swami, N., Hannon, B., Lo, C., Pope, A., Oza, A., et al. (2017). Impact of early palliative care on caregivers of patients with advanced cancer: Cluster randomised trial. Annals of Oncology, 28(1), 163–168. https://doi.org/10.1093/annonc/mdw438.

Mohammed, S., Savage, P., Kevork, N., Swami, N., Rodin, G., & Zimmerman, C. (2020). "I'm going to push this door open. You can close it": A qualitative study of the brokering work of oncology clinic nurses in introducing early palliative care. Palliative Medicine, 34(2), 209–218. https://doi.org/10.1177/0269216319883980.

Mulville, A. K., Widick, N. N., & Makani, N. S. (2019). Timely referral to hospice care for oncology patients: A retrospective review. American Journal of Hospice and Palliative Medicine, 36(6), 466–471. https://doi.org/10.1177/1049909118820494.

National Comprehensive Cancer Network (NCCN). NCCN guidelines adult cancer pain. Version 2.2022. (2022a). https://www.nccn.org/professionals/physician_gls/pdf/pain.pdf.

National Comprehensive Cancer Network (NCCN). NCCN guidelines cancer-related fatigue. Version 2.2022. (2022b). https://www.nccn.org/professionals/physician_gls/pdf/fatigue.pdf.

National Comprehensive Cancer Network (NCCN). NCCN guidelines distress management. Version 2.2022. (2022c). https://www.nccn.org/professionals/physician_gls/pdf/distress.pdf.

National Comprehensive Cancer Network (NCCN). NCCN guidelines palliative care. Version 1.2022. (2022d). https://www.nccn.org/professionals/physician_gls/pdf/palliative.pdf.

National Consensus Project for Quality Palliative Care (NCP). (2018). Clinical practice guidelines for quality palliative care (4th ed.). Richmond, VA: National Coalition for Hospice and Palliative Care. https://www.nationalcoalitionhpc.org/ncp.

National Hospice and Palliative Care Organization (NHPCO). History of hospice. (n.d.a). https://www.nhpco.org/hospice-care-overview/history-of-hospice/.

National Hospice and Palliative Care Organization (NHCPO). Medicare hospice benefit. (n.d.b). https://www.nhpco.org/hospice-care-overview/medicare-hospice-benefit-info/.

National Hospice and Palliative Care Organization (NHPCO). NHPCO facts and figures: 2022 Edition. (2021). https://www.nhpco.org/hospice-care-overview/hospice-facts-figures/.

National POLST. POLST: Portable medical orders for seriously ill or frail individuals. (2022). https://polst.org/.

Ownby, K. K. (2019). Use of the distress thermometer in clinical practice. Journal of the Advanced Practitioner in Oncology, 10(2), 175–179. https://doi.org/10.6004/jadpro.2019.10.2.7.

Paice, J. A. (2019). Pain management. In B. R. Ferrell & J. A. Paice (Eds.), Oxford textbook of palliative nursing (5th ed., pp. 116–131). Oxford: Oxford University Press.

Ramirez, C. T., Fundalinski, K., Knudson, J., & Himberger, J. (2019). Palliative care and requests for assistance in dying. In B. R. Ferrell & J. A. Paice (Eds.), Oxford textbook of palliative nursing (5th ed., pp. 837–841). Oxford: Oxford University Press.

Reese, D. J., & Csikai, E. L. (2018). Social work assessment and outcomes measurement in hospice and palliative care. American Journal of Hospice and Palliative Medicine, 35(12), 1553–1564. https://doi.org/10.1177/1049909118788342.

Reese, D. J., Raymer, M., Orloff, S. F., Gerbino, S., Valade, R., Dawson, S., et al. (2006). The Social Work Assessment Tool (SWAT). Journal of Social Work in End-of-Life & Palliative Care, 2(2), 65–95. https://doi.org/10.1300/J457v02n02_05.

Silveira, M. J. (2021). Advance care planning and advance directives. Waltham, MA: UpToDate. Retrieved 05.07.22 from https://www.uptodate.com/contents/advance-care-planning-and-advance-directives.

Soliman, I. W., Cremer, O. L., de Lange, D. W., Slooter, A. J. C., van Delden, J. (Hans) J. M., van Dijk, D., et al. (2018). The ability of intensive care unit physicians to estimate long-term prognosis in survivors of critical illness. *Journal of Critical Care, 43*, 148–155. https://doi.org/10.1016/j.jcrc.2017.09.007.

Spence, R. A., Blanke, C. D., Keating, T. J., & Taylor, L. P. (2017). Responding to patient requests for hastened death: Physician aid in dying and the clinical oncologist. *Journal of Oncology Practice, 13*(10), 693–699. https://doi.org/10.1200/JOP.2016.019299.

The SUPPORT Principal Investigators. (1995). A controlled trial to improve care for seriously ill hospitalized patients: The study to understand prognoses and preferences for outcomes and risks of treatments (SUPPORT). *Journal of the American Medical Association (JAMA), 274*(20), 1591–1598.

Swami, M., & Case, A. A. (2018). Effective palliative care: What is involved? *Oncology (Williston Park, NY), 32*(4), 180–184.

Tanco, K., Park, J. C., Cerana, A., Sisson, A., Sobti, N., & Bruera, E. (2017). A systematic review of instruments assessing dimensions of distress among caregivers of adult and pediatric cancer patients. *Palliative & Supportive Care, 15*(1), 110–124. https://doi.org/10.1017/S1478951516000079.

Tatum, P. E., & Mills, S. S. (2020). Hospice and palliative care: An overview. *Medical Clinics of North America, 104*(3), 359–373. https://doi.org/10.1016/j.mcna.2020.01.001.

Temel, J. S., Greer, J. A., Muzikansky, A., Gallagher, E. R., Admane, S., Jackson, V. A., et al. (2010). Early palliative care for patients with metastatic non-small-cell lung cancer. *The New England Journal of Medicine, 363*(8), 733–742. https://doi.org/10.1056/NEJMoa1000678.

Vinette, B., Côté, J., El-Akhras, A., Mrad, H., Chicoine, G., & Bilodeau, K. (2022). Routes of administration, reasons for use, and approved indications of medical cannabis in oncology: A scoping review. *BMC Cancer, 22*(1), 319. https://doi.org/10.1186/s12885-022-09378-7.

von Gunten, C. F. (2002). Secondary and tertiary palliative care in US hospitals. *Journal of the American Medical Association (JAMA), 287*(7), 875–881.

Wachterman, M. W., Luth, E. A., Semco, R. S., & Weissman, J. S. (2022). Where Americans die – Is there really "no place like home"? *The New England Journal of Medicine, 386*(11), 1008–1010. https://doi.org/10.1056/NEJMp2112297.

Watanabe, S. M., Nekolaichuk, C., Beaumont, C., Johnson, L., Myers, J., & Strasser, F. (2011). A multicenter study comparing two numerical versions of the Edmonton Symptom Assessment System in palliative care patients. *Journal of Pain and Symptom Management, 41*(2), 456–468. https://doi.org/10.1016/j.jpainsymman.2010.04.020.

Worldwide Hospice Palliative Care Alliance (WPCA). (2020). *Global atlas of palliative care* (2nd ed.). World Health Organization. http://www.thewhpca.org/resources/global-atlas-on-end-of-life-care.

Yadav, S., Heller, I. W., Schaefer, N., Salloum, R. G., Kittelson, S. M., Wilkie, D. J., et al. (2020). The health care cost of palliative care for cancer patients: A systematic review. *Supportive Care in Cancer, 28*(10), 4561–4573. https://doi.org/10.1007/s00520-020-05512-y.

5

Nurse Navigation Across the Cancer Continuum

Darcy Burbage

OVERVIEW

I. Definitions and roles
   A. Definition: the navigator role in the oncology setting includes patient navigator, care navigator, professional nurse navigator, cancer care navigator, nurse navigator, and Oncology Nurse Navigator (ONN) (Table 5.1).
      1. Various standards and guidelines define and recommend navigator role functions, minimum education, and operational practice settings (Oncology Nursing Society [ONS], 2017; Tables 5.1 and 5.2).
      2. Each navigation program differs, based on the needs and resources of the health care facility providing care (Kline et al., 2019).
      3. Oncology Nursing Society (ONS) recognized that ONNs were practicing without a clear definition of the role (ONS, 2017).
      4. According to ONS, an ONN is defined as a professional registered nurse with oncology-specific knowledge who uses the nursing process to provide quality health care to patients with timely education and resources (ONS, 2017).
   B. Role delineation (Lubejko et al., 2017)
      1. Clarification of the role was needed to support its growth and standardization.
      2. In 2012 ONS conducted a role delineation study (RDS) to clearly define the role.
         a. The RDS led to the development of the ONN Core Competencies (Tables 5.3 and 5.4).
      3. A second RDS conducted in 2016 revealed differences between a clinical oncology nurse and an ONN.
         a. ONN assists with patient/family navigation of the plan of care. This includes:
            (1) Education and coaching of colleagues about the navigation role
            (2) Collaboration to identify and establish best practices
   C. Competencies (ONS, 2017)
      1. ONN Core Competencies outline the fundamental and advanced knowledge, skills, and expertise of an ONN. Four competency areas include:
         a. Coordination of the care of patients with a past, current, or potential diagnosis of cancer
         b. Communication—assist patients with cancer, families, and caregivers to overcome health care system barriers
         c. Education and resources—facilitate informed decision-making and timely access to quality health and psychosocial care throughout the cancer care continuum
         d. Establish and maintain the professional role of the ONN—to promote quality improvement of an organization's navigation program
   D. Standards of Professional Practice (Professional Oncology Nurse Navigation Task Force, 2022)
      1. Representatives of select professional organizations involved in navigation identified best practices to guide practice for professional navigators.
      2. Nineteen standards have been identified ranging from qualifications to advocacy, operations, quality improvement, and continuum of care and are applicable to all types of professional navigators.
   E. Certifications
      1. ONN demonstrates strong oncology knowledge
      2. Foundation for ONN certification, based on RDSs
      3. Certifications established by the Oncology Nursing Certification Corporation (ONCC) exist (but not nurse navigator–specific) (Oncology Nursing Certification Corporation, 2018)
      4. From the Academy of Oncology Nurse and Patient Navigators (AONN +) (Academy of Oncology and Patient Navigators [AONN +], 2018)
         a. ONN—Certified Generalist
         b. Oncology Patient Navigator—Certified Generalist
         c. ONN—Certified Generalist Thoracic

II. History
   A. In 1990 first patient navigation program for medically underserved patients with breast cancer developed by Harold Freeman in New York City (Freeman, 2004, 2015).
      1. Goal was to reduce cancer mortality rates by improving access to quality care
      2. High breast cancer mortality rate among poor black women
         a. Fifty percent of the women were uninsured.

TABLE 5.1 Navigator Definitions

	Definition
Oncology Nurse Navigator (ONN)	An ONN is a professional RN with oncology-specific clinical knowledge who offers individualized assistance to patients, families, and caregivers to help overcome health care system barriers. Using the nursing process, an ONN provides education and resources to facilitate informed decision-making and timely access to quality health and psychosocial care throughout all phases of the cancer continuum.
Lay Navigator	A trained nonprofessional or volunteer who provides individualized assistance to patients, families, and caregivers to help overcome health care system barriers and facilitate timely access to quality health and psychosocial care from prediagnosis through all phases of the cancer experience.
Novice ONN	A nurse who has worked 2 years or less in the ONN role and is building upon his or her academic preparation, nursing knowledge, and oncology navigation experience to develop in the ONN role.
Expert ONN	An ONN who has worked at least 3 years, is proficient in the role, and has the education and experience to use critical thinking and decision-making skills pertaining to the evolution of navigation processes and the individual ONN.

From Baileys, K. A., McMullen, L., Lubejko, B., Christensen, D., Haylock, P. J., Rose, T., et al. (2018). Nurse navigator core competencies: An update to reflect the evolution of the role. *Clinical Journal of Oncology Nursing, 22*(3), 272–281. Retrieved from https://doi.org/10.1188/18.CJON.272-281.

TABLE 5.2 Navigator Preparation

Job Title	Recommended Preparation
Lay Patient Navigators	No professional degree, medical licensure, or credentials; education at or below a bachelor's degree
Allied health patient navigators	Professional backgrounds (i.e., medical assistants), educational degrees higher than bachelor's degree but not clinically focused
Nurse navigators	Two-year or BSN or RN, APN, NP, and other nursing backgrounds
Social worker/counselor	Education with at least a BS in social work, MS in counseling; Licensed mental health counselors
Other health navigators	Did not fit the earlier categories

APN, Advanced Practice Nurse; *BS,* Bachelor of Science; *BSN,* Bachelor of Science in Nursing; *MS,* Master of Science; *NP,* Nurse Practitioner; *RN,* Registered Nurse

From Wells, K. J., Valverde, P., Ustjanauskas, A. E., Calhoun, E. A., & Risendal, B. C. (2018). What are patient navigators doing, for whom, and where? A national survey evaluating the types of services provided by patient navigators. *Patient Education and Counseling (PEC), 101*(2), 285–294. Retrieved from https://doi.org/10.1016/j.pec.2017.08.017.

    b. Five-year survival rates improved from 39% to 70%.

B. In 2005 Cancer Patient Navigation Act was established.

    1. In 2010 President Obama signed the Patient Protection and Affordable Care Act, which required navigation programs to become part of health care.

    2. Currently required components of the Oncology Care Model, a novel episode-based payment system developed by the Center for Medicare and Medicaid Services (Professional Oncology Navigation Task Force, 2022).

C. Patient Navigation Research Program (PNRP) data showed no difference in survival outcomes for patients with Medicaid coverage compared with uninsured patients, despite the passage of the Affordable Care Act in 2010 (Freeman, 2015).

    1. Data demonstrated additional nonfinancial barriers to care, including variables associated with poverty:

       a. Unemployment

       b. Lack of adequate social support

       c. Lower education levels

    2. One PNRP study demonstrated delays in cancer diagnosis can be overcome by patient navigation, addressing barriers such as unemployment, housing type, and marital status.

D. Incorporated in 2009, the AONN + provides a network for professionals involved and interested in patient navigation and survivorship care services toward managing complex care over the cancer care treatment continuum (AONN +, 2018).

    1. ONN certification platform to demonstrate their skills, expertise, and knowledge.

    2. The AONN + created a network of nurse navigators and patient navigators interested in enhancing and promoting their roles in navigation.

E. In 2010 the ONS, Association of Oncology Social Work, and National Association of Social Workers published a joint position statement: *Joint Position Statement on the Role of Oncology Nursing and Oncology Social Work in Patient Navigation* (Oncology Nursing Society, Association of Oncology Social Work, and National Association of Social Workers, 2010).

F. American College of Surgeons Commission on Cancer (CoC) added patient navigation as a requirement for CoC accreditation in 2015 (American College of Surgeons, 2016).

    1. Although initially patient navigation included cancer prevention, it now includes the entire health continuum: prevention, detection of disease, diagnosis, treatment, and survivorship care (Freeman, 2015).

G. ONS (ONS, 2017)

    1. In 2015—then revised in 2017—ONS established a position statement: Role of the Oncology Nurse Navigator Throughout the Cancer Trajectory.

TABLE 5.3   Oncology Nurse Navigation (ONN) Competency Categories for Novice Navigator

Competency Category 1: Coordination of Care	The ONN facilitates the appropriate and efficient delivery of health care services, both within and across systems, and serves as the key contact to promote optimal outcomes while delivering patient-centered care.
	Assesses patient needs upon initial encounter and periodically throughout navigation, matching unmet needs with appropriate services, referrals, and support services, such as palliative care, dietitians, medical providers, social work, pre-/rehabilitation, and legal and financial services.
	Identifies potential and realized barriers to care (e.g., transportation, childcare, elder care, housing, language, culture, literacy, role disparity, psychosocial, employment, financial, insurance) and facilitates referrals as appropriate to mitigate barriers.
	Develops knowledge of available local, community, or national resources and the quality of services provided; also establishes relationships with the providers of these services.
	Develops or uses appropriate screening/assessment tools and methods (e.g., Distress Thermometer, pain scale, fatigue scale, performance status, motivational interviewing, financial) to promote a consistent holistic plan of care.
	Facilitates timely scheduling of appointments, diagnostic testing, and procedures to expedite the plan of care and to promote continuity of care.
	Participates in coordination of the plan of care with the multidisciplinary team, promoting timely follow-up on treatment and supportive care recommendations (e.g., cancer conferences/tumor boards).
	Facilitates individualized care within the context of functional status, cultural consideration, health literacy, psychosocial, reproductive/fertility, and spiritual needs for patients, families, and caregivers.
	Applies knowledge of clinical guidelines (e.g., National Comprehensive Cancer Network, American Joint Committee on Cancer) and specialty resources (e.g., ONS Putting Evidence into Practice resources) throughout the cancer continuum.
	Assists in the identification of candidates for molecular testing and/or genetic testing and counseling, and facilitates appropriate referrals.
	Supports a smooth transition of patients from active treatment into survivorship, chronic cancer management, or end-of-life care.
	Assists patients with cancer with issues related to treatment goals, advance directives, palliative care, and end-of-life concerns using an ethical framework that is nonjudgmental and nondiscriminatory.
	Ensures documentation of patient encounters and provided services.
	Applies knowledge of insurance processes (e.g., Medicare, Medicaid, third-party payers) and their impact on staging, referrals, and patient care decisions toward establishing appropriate referrals, as needed.
Competency Category 2: Communication	The ONN demonstrates interpersonal communication skills that enable exchange of ideas and information effectively with patients, families, and colleagues at all levels. This includes writing, speaking, and listening skills.
	Builds therapeutic and trusting relationships with patients, families, and caregivers through effective communication and listening skills.
	Acts as a liaison between the patients, families, caregivers, and the providers to optimize outcomes.
	Advocates for patients to promote patient-centered care that includes shared decision-making and patients' goals of care with optimal outcomes.
	Provides psychosocial support to and facilitates appropriate referrals for patients, families, and caregivers, especially during periods of high emotional stress and anxiety.
	Empowers patients and families to self-advocate and communicate their needs.
	Adheres to established regulations concerning patient information and privacy.
	Promotes a patient- and family-centered care environment for ethical decision-making and advocacy for patients with cancer.
	Ensures that communication is culturally sensitive and appropriate for the identified level of health literacy.
	Facilitates communication among members of the multidisciplinary cancer care team to prevent fragmented or delayed care that could adversely affect patient outcomes.

continued

TABLE 5.3   Oncology Nurse Navigation (ONN) Competency Categories for Novice Navigator—cont'd

Competency Category 3: Education	The ONN provides appropriate and timely education to patients, families, and caregivers to facilitate understanding and support informed decision-making.
	Promotes lifelong learning and evidence-based practice to improve the care of patients with a past, current, or potential diagnosis of cancer.
	Demonstrates effective communication with peers, members of the multidisciplinary health care team, and community organizations and resources.
	Contributes to ONN program and role development, implementation, and evaluation within the health care system and community.
	Participates in the tracking and monitoring of metrics and outcomes, in collaboration with administration, to document and evaluate outcomes of the navigation program and report findings to the cancer committee.
	Collaborates with the cancer committee and administration to perform and evaluate data from the community needs assessment to identify areas of improvement that will affect the patient navigation process and participate in quality improvement based on identified service gaps.
	In collaboration with other members of the health care team, builds partnerships with local agencies and groups that may assist with cancer patient care, support, or educational needs.
	Establishes and maintains professional role boundaries with patients, caregivers, and the multidisciplinary care team in collaboration with manager, as defined by job description.
Competency Category 4: Professional Role	The ONN works to promote and advance the role of the ONN and takes responsibility to pursue personal–professional growth and development. In addition, the ONN facilitates the continual promotion and quality improvement of the organization's navigation program to best meet the needs of their community.
	Promotes lifelong learning and evidence-based practice to improve the care of patients with a past, current, or potential diagnosis of cancer.
	Demonstrates effective communication with peers, members of the multidisciplinary health care team, and community organizations and resources.
	Contributes to ONN program and role development, implementation, and evaluation within the health care system and community.
	Participates in the tracking and monitoring of metrics and outcomes, in collaboration with administration, to document and evaluate outcomes of the navigation program and report findings to the cancer committee.

From Baileys, K. A., McMullen, L., Lubejko, B., Christensen, D., Haylock, P. J., Rose, T., et al. (2018). Nurse Navigator core competencies: An update to reflect the evolution of the role. *Clinical Journal of Oncology Nursing*, *22*(3), 272–281. https://doi.org/10.1188/18.CJON.272-281.

2. ONS established the Nurse Navigator Special Interest Group (SIG) in 2010.
3. ONS Nurse Navigator SIG was renamed the Navigation and Care Coordinator Community to highlight the ONN role in care coordination in 2016 (ONS, 2017).

III. Measuring ONN value
   A. Components of oncology nursing navigation programs (Gordils-Perez, Schneider, Gabel, & Trotter, 2017; Cantril, Christensen, & Moore, 2019; Kline et al., 2019)
     1. Relationship building with providers, patients, and families
       a. Efficient communication
       b. Timely psychosocial support
     2. Provide expertise and education to patients and family members, based on the foundation of oncology patient diagnosis, treatment, and survivorship
   B. Methods and strategies to measure ONN value, patient outcomes of care (Gordils-Perez et al., 2017; National Academies of Sciences, Engineering, and Medicine [NASEM], 2018; Yackzan et al., 2019).
     1. Timeliness of care; access to care
     2. Management and monitoring of plan of care
       a. Symptom management
     3. Provider, patient, and family satisfaction scores
     4. Clinical trial accrual
     5. Health care system utilization
       a. Reduces hospital readmissions
   C. Develop a template to identify essential components of care by ONNs to measure outcomes (Hanes-Lewis et al., 2018; Munoz, Farshidpour, Chaudhary, & Fathi, 2018; Miller & Sheatter, 2020; Temucin & Nahcivan, 2020). Study designs capture:
     1. Cancer patient population focus
     2. Consistent and reliable support for patients and family members
       a. Effective communication
       b. Timely and appropriate psychosocial support
         (1) Initial and ongoing administration of distress tools and evaluation of interventions to address distress, based on distress tool scoring
     3. Outcomes that eliminate barriers to treatment
       a. Expedited referrals

TABLE 5.4 Oncology Nurse Navigation (ONN): Additional Expert Competency Category (#5)	
Competency Category 5: Expert Oncology Nurse Navigator	The expert ONN is proficient in the role and has the education, knowledge, and experience to use critical thinking and decision-making skills pertaining to the evolution of the ONN role and process improvement in the navigation processes.
	Contributes to the development of the cancer program community needs assessment and makes suggestions to the cancer committee on navigation program changes related to community assessment outcomes and cancer program strategic plan.
	Assists in gap analysis, quality improvement, and process improvement measures, data analysis, and makes recommendations to the cancer committee for appropriate navigation program changes related to the data.
	Develops and promotes pathways for ONN patient recruitment by collaborating with internal and external stakeholders.
	Tracks use of internal and external resources of staff and patients and makes recommendations for appropriate or improved use as needed.
	Expands current or develops new processes to survey patient and/or caregiver satisfaction related to navigation services, collects results, and reports to cancer committee.
	Contributes to program growth through collaboration with cancer program administration to develop a marketing strategy to support the navigation program.
	Contributes to the knowledge base of the health care community and in support of the ONN role through activities such as involvement in professional organizations, presentations, publications, and research.
	Disseminates information about the ONN role to other health care team members through peer education, mentoring, and preceptor experiences.
	Collaborates with treating physician(s) and support staff to prevent unnecessary hospitalizations or clinic visits and improve adherence to treatment through the design and implementation of appropriate patient education and follow-up.
	Orients, mentors, and guides novice ONNs.
	Collaborates with cancer program administration and cancer committee to develop strategies to fulfill the requirements and standards of the American College of Surgeons Commission on Cancer.
	Contributes to program sustainability, improvement, and/or development through collaboration with the institutional foundation in grant writing and philanthropy.

From Baileys, K. A., McMullen, L., Lubejko, B., Christensen, D., Haylock, P. J., Rose, T., et al. (2018). Nurse Navigator core competencies: An update to reflect the evolution of the role. *Clinical Journal of Oncology Nursing, 22*(3), 272–281. https://doi.org/10.1188/18.CJON.272-281.

    b. Prompt initiation and continuation of treatment sessions

    4. ONNs provide ongoing conduit to patients and families—orientation, education, and resources.

IV. Research and evidence-based practice/limitations

  A. Limitation of published research; additional published studies need to demonstrate effectiveness, improved patient outcomes due to the contributions of ONN (ONS, 2017)

  B. Replicating existing navigation programs is difficult due to:

    1. Lack of standardized job descriptions

    2. Lack of standardized processes

    3. Lack of standardized ONN qualifications (credentials, competencies, education, preparation, and experience)

  C. When evaluating the benefits of navigation and ONN contributions, consider these strategies and components in study designs (Fessele, 2017; Hanes-Lewis et al., 2018):

    1. Increasing the number of participants/patients

    2. Participants/patients representing ethnic and financial diversity

    3. After initiating navigation, conduct 5-year studies to monitor the recurrence of disease and survivorship care.

    4. Carefully examine processes that link the navigation to improved patient outcomes.

  D. Until recently, ONN outcome studies and metrics to evaluate the role have been limited due to:

    1. Relatively small sample sizes

    2. Poor or incomplete response rates to questionnaires

    3. Questionnaire data: lack of reliable and valid instruments to gather data

    4. Lack of data about patients who have used navigation services

      a. When ONN consulting, what services have been provided? Screening? Assessment? Providing referrals or resources?

  E. Types of practice settings (urban vs. rural) and location in the United States and other countries—additional need for navigation services (Fessele, 2017; Flucke & Sullivan-Moore, 2021; Professional Oncology Navigation Task Force, 2022; Spencer et al., 2018)

    1. Geographic differences and the need for oncology care navigators

    2. Differences in Medicaid expansion that would support navigation services

    3. Oral chemotherapy parity legislation

    4. Financial toxicity

  F. Qualitative research studies are difficult to replicate about nurse navigation and the ONN as an effective role in the delivery of patient care (Melhem & Daneault, 2017).

1. Best to compare qualitative study results to other qualitative studies with same study designs.

G. AONN+ published its navigation metrics toolkit to measure the impact and reach of ONN. Core metrics identified five key areas (AONN+ 2020):
   1. Navigator competencies
   2. Navigator caseload
   3. Barriers to care
   4. Psychosocial distress screening
   5. Intervention

ASSESSMENT

I. Patient history and plan of care (Gordils-Perez et al., 2017; Miller, 2018)
   A. Assess patient's history, clinical status, barriers to care
   B. Caregiver and family support
II. Psychosocial assessment
   A. Distress assessment is the focus of cancer patient clinical care (Hanes-Lewis et al., 2018; National Comprehensive Cancer Network [NCCN], 2022).
      1. Assessment is the foundation for psychosocial support and resources.
      2. Assessment includes family and caregiver support.
      3. National Comprehensive Cancer Network is a frequent source of distress assessment tools.

MANAGEMENT

I. ONN coordinates plan of care, based on health care system, options, and accessible resources.

A. Goals of navigation service (Gordils-Perez et al., 2017; Miller, 2018; Kline et al., 2019):
   1. Provide education about treatment plan that empowers clients to actively engage in decision-making and self-care.
   2. Facilitate timely access to care and treatment, based on treatment guidelines.
      a. Identify and resolve barriers
   3. Provide education on symptom and side effect management to reduce early and late treatment-associated complications.
      a. Access to resources
      b. Expedite referrals
   4. Reduce distress; provide psychosocial support.
   5. Liaison for patient, family members, and patient's health care providers.
      a. Serve as the patient's advocate
B. Navigation models of care
C. Cancer care continuum (Institute of Medicine, 2013; McMullen & Cavone, 2020) (Fig. 5.1).
   1. Prevention and risk reduction
      a. Within survivorship programs—includes some community outreach, education, surveillance programs
   2. Screening—triage newly referred patients
   3. Diagnosis
      a. In conjunction with providers and support staff, the nurse navigator ensures there are orders for stage-appropriate tests: radiology, diagnostic, and molecular tests (e.g., epidermal growth factor receptor testing).
      b. Ensure timely medical and oncology-related clinic appointments.

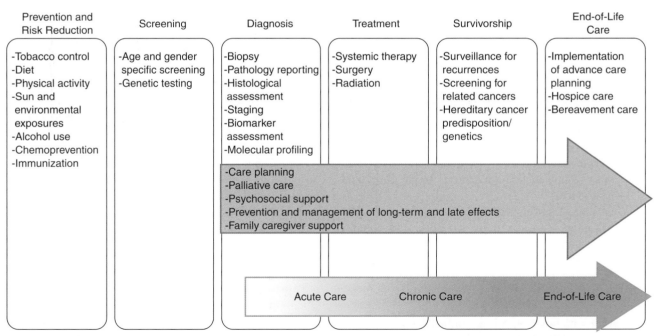

Fig. 5.1 Cancer Care Continuum Model. From Institute of Medicine. 2013. *Delivering High-Quality Cancer Care: Charting a New Course for a System in Crisis.* https://doi.org/10.17226/18359. Reproduced with permission from the National Academy of Sciences, Courtesy of the National Academies Press, Washington, D.C.

c. Follow guidelines for workup; ensure they are complete.

d. Oncology case conferences/tumor board review

e. Molecular profiling

(1) ONN expedited genomic testing to support timely decision-making (Jeyathevan, Lemonde, & Cooper-Brathwaite, 2017).

4. Treatments—consistent and available interpreter of plan of care, once established

5. Survivorship

a. Initiate and maintain surveillance programs.

b. Screen for late and long-term side effects, recurrent disease, secondary malignancies.

6. Palliative care

7. End-of-life care—coordinate and expedite referrals to hospice resources

D. ONN care model (ONS, 2017)

1. Continuity of care and coordination of care, based on providers in the community

2. Includes cultural traditions in the community, survivorship

II. Address barriers to care

A. Access to care—patient navigation is important to reduce or eliminate barriers to access quality cancer care (Munoz et al., 2018; Kline et al., 2019; Flucke & Sullivan-Moore, 2021)

1. Access to timely diagnosis and initiation of treatment are barriers to quality care (Freeman, 2015; Munoz et al., 2018).

B. Barriers to care also include financial, transportation, language differences, cultural and ethnic diversity, and communication among the health care team and patients, as well as barriers to emotional support (NASEM, 2018).

1. Lack of resources, lack of knowledge about resources, ability to complete complex/duplicative paperwork

a. Childcare

b. Lodging

2. Insufficient resources or patient ineligibility for existing resources due to living in rural areas, patients without citizenship, being underinsured, having income levels above specific program thresholds

3. Lack of patient connection with others, reluctance to request assistance, embarrassment about situation

4. Language and literacy as barriers

C. Psychosocial distress (NCCN, 2022)

1. Assess, monitor, document, and intervene at all stages of disease.

2. Assess frequently (i.e., each clinic visit).

3. Follow clinical practice guidelines for assessment and intervention.

D. Managing/alleviating financial toxicity (Fessele, 2017; Spencer et al., 2018)

1. Twenty percent to 48% of patients with cancer report significant financial burden due to their cancer treatment.

2. Patients with cancer are 2.6 times more likely to declare bankruptcy than the general population.

3. Navigators can facilitate financial assistance for patient treatment and costs associated with receiving treatment:

a. Medication or prescription drug assistance programs

b. Charity care

c. Copay assistance

d. Assistance with nonmedical expenses, such as transportation or lodging

III. Management exemplars

A. Example #1: The Oral ONN improves patient care and satisfaction (Anderson, Reff, McMahon, & Walters, 2017).

1. Oral oncolytics account for approximately 25% of current oncology treatments.

2. The role of the oral ONN was developed to meet this shift in cancer care delivery and to provide continuity of care for patients receiving oral chemotherapy by:

a. Assessing the patient's health literacy

b. Securing financial assistance

c. Astute patient and family education to ensure adherence and review supportive medications, such as antiemetics and steroids

d. Ongoing follow-up calls to provide ongoing education, assess side effects, and provide emotional support

3. Integration of the oral ONN role has improved multidisciplinary communication, patient education, and adherence.

B. Example #2: Comparison of satisfaction of services and benefits between patients with and without an ONN (NASEM, 2018; Yackzan et al., 2019)

1. A retrospective chart review was conducted and patient satisfaction indicates higher satisfaction among patients with an ONN as compared to those without ONN contact.

2. Seventy-six percent of the ONN contact group indicated that their emotional needs were addressed as compared to 39% in the non-ONN contact group.

3. Eighty-seven percent of the ONN contact group compared to 56% of the non-ONN contact group indicated the ONN kept their family informed about what to expect.

4. Seventy-eight percent as compared to 59% indicated that their care was coordinated among doctors and caregivers.

5. ED visits between ONN-navigated patients were 31% compared to 58% of non-ONN-navigated patients (NASEM, 2018).

6. Thirty-day readmission rates were 15% in the ONN navigated patients as compared to 31% in non-ONN-navigated patients (NASEM, 2018).

C. Example #3: Expansion of the ONN role through tele-health (Rowett & Christensen, 2020)
1. The ongoing COVID-19 pandemic has created an opportunity to highlight the power of technology to implement creative solutions to address access to health care.
2. Telehealth includes:
   a. Interactive video and audioconferencing
   b. Web-based and mobile applications
3. The ONN's role and telehealth:
   a. Orient patient and family to telehealth process.
   b. Manage the expectations, and keep patient and family members informed.
   c. Assess and address ongoing barriers to care.
   d. Provide emotional support, education regarding treatment, side effects, next steps, survivorship, palliative care, and end of life.
   e. Suggest the use of web-based education and mobile applications.
4. Benefits
   a. Reduced financial stress from not having to take time off from work, gas mileage, parking fees.
   b. Maintain continuity of care while keeping safe from exposure to COVID-19.
5. Limitations
   a. Infrastructure: Lack of internet access in rural areas; lack of technology to access telehealth or web-based platform(s)
   b. Insurance reimbursement
   c. Providing telehealth across state lines
D. Example #4: Palliative care coordination (Melhem & Daneault, 2017)
1. ONN coordinating palliative care was just as important to the patient as the physician in the patient's ongoing care.
2. The ONN can address most relational needs and share/explain disease information.
   a. In addition to their medical needs, patients reported they had psychological, social, and spiritual needs addressed.
3. ONN encounters increased patient satisfaction:
   a. Ensured the patient understands his or her disease
   b. Followed the patient from initial diagnosis, if possible
   c. Provided the patient with emotional support; validated feelings; referred to other professionals, as needed
   d. Listened attentively; was present without judgment; acknowledged the patient's experience and suffering
   e. Ensured the patient's physical comfort; also comfort with the treatment plan and team
   f. Was proactive to cooperate and communicate efficiently and effectively with other care providers

REFERENCES

Academy of Oncology Nurse & Patient Navigators (AONN+). *Certification.* (2018). https://www.aonnonline.org/certification.

Academy of Oncology Nurse & Patient Navigators (AONN+). *Navigation metrics toolkit.* (2020). https://www.aonnonline.org/navigation-metrics.

American College of Surgeons. *Commission on cancer: Standards and resources.* (2016). https://www.facs.org/quality-programs/cancer/coc/standards.

Anderson, M. K., Reff, M. J., McMahon, R. S., & Walters, D. R. (2017). The role of the oral oncology nurse navigator. *Oncology Issues, 32*(5), 26–30. https://www.ncoda.org/wp-content/uploads/bp-attachments/7249/article_nursenavigatorwithcover.pdf.

Cantril, C., Christensen, D., & Moore, E. (2019). Standardizing roles: Evaluating oncology nurse navigator clarity, educational preparation, and scope of work within two healthcare systems. *Clinical Journal of Oncology Nursing, 23*(1), 52–59. https://doi.org/10.1188/19.CJON.52-59.

Fessele, K. L. (2017). Financial toxicity: Management as an adverse effect of cancer treatment. *Clinical Journal of Oncology Nursing, 21*(6), 762–764. https://doi.org/10.1188/17.CJON.762-764.

Flucke, N., & Sullivan-Moore, C. (2021). Patient assessment: Using the oncology nurse navigator patient assessment for rural and other resource-poor settings. *Clinical Journal of Oncology Nursing, 25*(6), 729–734. https://doi.org/10.1188/21.CJON.729-734.

Freeman, H. P. (2004). A model patient navigation program. *Oncology Issues, 19*(5), 44–46.

Freeman, H. P. (2015). Patient navigation as a targeted intervention: For patients at high risk for delays in cancer care. *Cancer, 121*(22), 3930–3932. https://doi.org/10.1002/cncr.29610.

Gordils-Perez, J., Schneider, S. M., Gabel, M., & Trotter, K. J. (2017). Oncology nurse navigation: Development and implementation of a program at a comprehensive cancer center. *Clinical Journal of Oncology Nursing, 21*(5), 581–588. https://doi.org/10.1188/17.CJON.581-588.

Hanes-Lewis, H., Clayton, M. F., Viswanathan, S., Moadel-Robblee, A., Clark, L., & Caserta, M. (2018). Distress and supportive care needs of ethnically diverse older adults with advanced or recurrent cancer. *Oncology Nursing Forum, 45*(4), 496–507. https://doi.org/10.1188/18.ONF.496-507.

Institute of Medicine. (2013). *Delivering high-quality cancer care: Charting a new course for a system in crisis.* Washington, D.C.: National Academies Press.

Jeyathevan, G., Lemonde, M., & Brathwaite, A. C. (2017). The role of oncology nurse navigators in facilitating continuity of care within the diagnostic phase for adult patients with lung cancer. *Canadian Oncology Nursing Journal, 27*(1), 74–80. https://doi.org/10.5737/236880762717480.

Kline, R. M., Rocque, G. B., Rohan, E. A., Blackley, K. A., Cantril, C. A., Pratt-Chapman, M. L., et al. (2019). Patient navigation in cancer: The business case to support clinical needs. *Journal of Oncology Practice, 15*(11), 585–590. https://doi.org/10.1200/JOP.19.00230.

Lubejko, B., Bellfield, S., Kahn, E., Lee, C., Peterson, N., Rose, T., et al. (2017). Oncology nurse navigation: Results of the 2016 role delineation study. *Clinical Journal of Oncology Nursing, 21*(1), 43–50. https://doi.org/10.1188/17.CJON.43-50.

McMullen, L., & Cavone, S. (2020). Navigating each phase of the patient journey. In D. M. Christensen & C. Cantril (Eds.), *Oncology nurse navigation: Delivering patient-centered care across the continuum* (2nd ed., pp. 145–160). Pittsburgh, PA: Oncology Nursing Society.

Melhem, D., & Daneault, S. (2017). Needs of cancer patients in palliative care during medical visits: Qualitative study. *Canadian Family Physician, 63*(12), e536–e542.

Miller, E. (2018). Neuro-oncology nurse navigation: Developing the role for a unique patient population. *Clinical Journal of Oncology Nursing, 22*(3), 347–349. https://doi.org/10.1188/18.CJON.347-349.

Miller, E., & Sheaffer, H. (2020). Academic nurse navigation: Unique aspects and strategies for success. *Clinical Journal of Oncology Nursing, 24*(5), 579–581. https://doi.org/10.1188/20.CJON.579-581.

Muñoz, R., Farshidpour, L., Chaudhary, U. B., & Fathi, A. H. (2018). Multidisciplinary cancer care model: A positive association between oncology nurse navigation and improved outcomes for patients with cancer. *Clinical Journal of Oncology Nursing, 22*(5), e141–e145. https://doi.org/10.1188/18.CJON.E141-E145.

National Academies of Sciences, Engineering, and Medicine (NASEM). (2018). *Establishing effective patient navigation programs in oncology: Proceedings of a workshop.* Washington, D.C.: The National Academies Press. https://pubmed.ncbi.nlm.nih.gov/29847082/.

National Comprehensive Cancer Network (NCCN). *Distress management, [v1.2022].* (2022). www.nccn.org.

Oncology Nursing Certification Corporation. Certifications. (2018). https://www.oncc.org/certifications.

Oncology Nursing Society (ONS). *Oncology nurse navigator core competencies.* (2017). https://www.ons.org/sites/default/files/2017ONNcompetencies.pdf.

Oncology Nursing Society, Association of Oncology Social Work, and National Association of Social Workers. (2010). Joint position statement on the role of oncology nursing and oncology social work in patient navigation. *Oncology Nursing Forum, 37*(3), 251–252.

Professional Oncology Nurse Navigation Task Force. (2022). Oncology navigation standards of professional practice. *Clinical Journal of Oncology Nursing, 26*(3), E14–E25. https://www.ons.org/cjon/26/3/oncology-navigation-standards-professional-practice.

Rowett, K. E., & Christensen, D. (2020). Oncology nurse navigation: Expansion of the navigator role through telehealth. *Clinical Journal of Oncology Nursing (Suppl), 24*(3), 24–31. https://doi.org/10.1188/20.CJON.S1.24-31.

Spencer, J. C., Samuel, C. A., Rosenstein, D. L., Reeder-Hayes, K. E., Manning, M. L., Sellers, J. B., et al. (2018). Oncology navigators' perceptions of cancer-related financial burden and financial assistance resources. *Supportive Care in Cancer, 26*(4), 1315–1321. https://doi.org/10.1007/s00520-017-3958-3.

Temucin, E., & Nahcivan, N. O. (2020). The effects of the nurse navigation program in promoting colorectal cancer screening behaviors: A randomized controlled trial. *Journal of Cancer Education, 35*(1), 112–124. https://doi.org/10.1007/s13187-018-1448-z.

Yackzan, S., Stanifer, S., Barker, S., Blair, B., Glass, A., Weyl, H., et al. (2019). Outcome measurement: Patient satisfaction scores and contact with oncology nurse navigators. *Clincal Journal of Oncology Nursing, 23*(1), 76–81. https://pubmed.ncbi.nlm.nih.gov/30682008/.

6

Communication and Shared Decision-Making

Pamela Katz

I. Shared decision-making (SDM): historical background (Hoving, Visser, Mullen, & van den Borne, 2010)
  A. 1960s–1970s post-World War II: model of care delivery for patient-physician relationship was predominantly patriarchal.
    1. Patients are more passive and unconditionally conform to physician's treatment plans.
    2. Patients who did not comply with their health care provider's recommendations were considered to be deviant and behaving irrationally.
  B. Early 1970s: shared model of care is taking hold, particularly in cancer setting.
    1. Paternalistic model of care is becoming unpopular.
    2. First communication courses for health care professionals being developed.
  C. The 1980s showed an increasing societal emphasis on patients' rights and the growth of patient advocacy organizations.
  D. Major factors for the emergence of SDM as the dominant model of care in today's health care.
    1. Rising cost of health care (Ford, 1977)
    2. Increasing health care consumerism in the United States, Europe, Australia, and Canada (McDevitt, 1986; Price, 1981)
    3. Increased desire for consumer involvement, autonomy, and control over their care (Tariman, Berry, Cochrane, Doorenbos, & Schepp, 2012)
    4. Emphasis of patient-centered care as an indicator of high-quality care (Institute of Medicine, 2001)
    5. Explosion of cancer treatment choices (Tariman et al., 2012)
    6. Disruptive idea, as it demands shifts in power and control of interactions between clinicians and patients (Elwyn et al., 2017)
  E. Model expanded to include improved health care literacy skills.
    1. Cannot assume patients have skills to integrate the evidence and expertise into their decision-making process (Muscat et al., 2021)
II. SDM: definition and components
  A. Process in which health care professionals and patients work together to select tests, treatments, management, or support packages, based on clinical evidence and the patient's values and informed preferences (Muscat,

Shepherd, & Nutbeam, 2021). Decisions are made in a collaborative way, where trustworthy information is provided in accessible formats about a set of options, typically in situations where the concerns, personal circumstances, and contexts of patients and their families play a major role in decisions (Elwyn et al., 2017).
  B. Steps in the SDM process: The SHARE approach (Agency for Healthcare Research and Quality, 2020)
    1. *Step 1: Involve your patient in the treatment decision process:* inform them of choices and invite them to be involved in the decisions.
    2. *Step 2: Assist your patient in comparing and evaluating treatment options:* discuss the risks and benefits of each option.
    3. *Step 3: Assess your patient's goals, values, and priorities:* understand and incorporate what matters most to your patient.
    4. *Step 4: Make a decision with your patient:* decide the best course of treatment as a team.
    5. *Step 5: Evaluate the treatment decision:* plan to follow up and revisit the decision, monitor progress, and revise as needed. Communication is a critical aspect of SDM (Siminoff & Step, 2005).
  C. Critical aspects
    1. Integrates a socially based process into the dynamics of the physician-patient relationship.
    2. Examines antecedent factors that have the potential to influence communication (e.g., prior medical care experiences, language and acculturation, cognitive status, education level).
    3. Emphasizes jointly constructed communication climate.
    4. Outcome focuses on treatment preferences established by the patient and the treatment team (providers, nurses, interdisciplinary team).
    5. Done well, combines different types of expertise—expertise in the world of medicine and expertise in a personal lifeworld where priorities exist (Elwyn et al., 2017).
  D. Key elements (Charles, Gafni, & Whelan, 1999; Slade, 2017)
    1. At least two participants: clinician and patient; often includes other treatment team members and patient's family.

2. Both parties share information. Provider(s) define/explain the health care problem, present options.

3. Both parties take steps to build consensus about preferred treatment, weighing risks and benefits. Parties discuss benefits/risks/costs, clarify patient values/preferences, and discuss patient ability/self-efficacy.

4. Provider(s) present what is known and make recommendations. Provider(s) clarify the patient's understanding.

5. Decision is made via mutual agreement between patient and clinician on treatment approach (verbal and/or written).

E. SDM is the preferred model of care delivery by lawmakers and policymakers because it supports the patient's autonomy and empowers the patient to take responsibility of one's own health (Ubel, Scherr, & Fagerlin, 2018).

1. Relies on good communication between patient and provider, trust, and respect.

F. SDM has demonstrated short- and long-term benefits (Truglio-Londrigan & Slyer, 2018):

1. Short-term benefits
   a. Increased confidence in treatment decisions
   b. Higher satisfaction with treatment decisions
   c. Enhanced trust with providers
   d. Improved self-efficacy
   e. Mental health—less stress and anxiety related to treatment decision-making

2. Long-term benefits
   a. Patient satisfaction and confidence in their health care choices
   b. Patient treatment adherence
   c. Quality of life
   d. Potential disease remission

G. SDM care delivery model is advantageous for older adults (Ramsdale, Csik, Chapman, Naeim, & Canin, 2017):

1. Facilitates collaboration, communication, and patient-centeredness.

2. Minimizes the fragmentation that impairs the current provision of cancer care.

3. This is particularly important with older adults, given their potential for not proactively participating in their care based on a multitude of factors (generational, lessened communication abilities), as well as having multiple providers due to many comorbidities.

III. Barriers to SDM (Pel-Littel, Snaterse, & Teppich, 2021, see Fig. 6.1)

A. Barriers perceived by oncology nurses

1. Practice barrier—nonnursing responsibilities (e.g., charting, administrative tasks) take away time from patients; lack of provider confidence in the ability to participate effectively.

2. Patient barrier—lack of readiness for patient to participate in SDM; lack of knowledge to participate; age-related challenges (cognition and mindset).

3. Institutional policy barrier—lack of institutional policy that allows a specific block of nurse's time for patient education on therapy or lack of support for the process.

4. Scope-of-practice barrier—Federal, state, and board of nursing laws and regulations that prohibit nurse practitioner from autonomous practice.

5. Administration as a barrier—nursing administrators do not provide adequate support for nurses to actively participate in SDM process.

6. Structural barrier—noisy environment (hospital); lack of privacy; lack of systemic alerts/triggers in the electronic medical record (to incorporate decision aids).

B. Barriers perceived by oncologists (Pel-Little et al., 2021)

1. Lack of time.

2. Patient anxiety.

3. Patient lack of information and/or misinformation.

4. Patient unwillingness or inability to participate.

5. Inability to talk in language patients can easily understand, low health literacy.

6. Lack of commonality in approaches to SDM, while maintaining flexibility for modifications.

IV. Patient preferences for decision-making in oncology care

A. Patients with cancer prefer to have a role in cancer care and treatment decision-making (Singh et al., 2010; Tariman, Berry, Cochrane, Doorenbos, & Schepp, 2010).

B. Degner and Beaton's Pattern of Treatment Decision Making questionnaire (Fig. 6.2) (Degner & Beaton, 1987; Degner, Sloan, & Venkatesh, 1997) is the most widely used instrument to elicit patient's preferences for participation in cancer treatment decision-making process (Tariman et al., 2010).

V. Influential factors in treatment decision-making in older adults; aged 60+ (Puts et al., 2015):

A. Convenience and success rate of treatment

B. Seeing the necessity of treatment

C. Trust in the physician

D. Following the physician's recommendation

VI. Patient information needs

A. Information priorities in patients diagnosed with cancer (Tariman, Doorenbos, Schepp, Singhal, & Berry, 2014):

1. Diagnosis

2. Prognosis

3. Treatment options

B. Assertion of independence and how to maintain self-care are priority information needs in older adults diagnosed with cancer (Sattar et al., 2018; Tariman, Doorenbos, Schepp, Singhal, & Berry, 2015)

VII. Quality of communication and clinician factors

A. Clinician characteristics that have a positive impact on the quality of communication and/or patient outcomes (De Vries et al., 2014)

1. Communication skills training

2. An external locus of control (focus on outward aspects from their own being, such as institutional and administrative factors)

3. Empathy

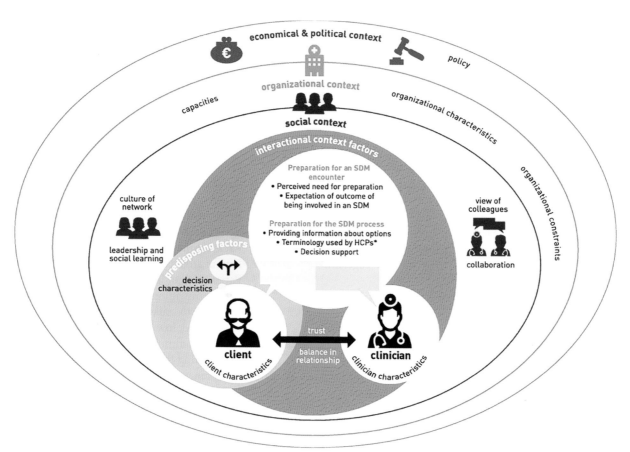

Fig. 6.1 Adapted taxonomy for barriers of and facilitators to shared decision-making. From Pel-Littel, R. E., Snaterse, M., Teppich, N. M., et al. (2021). Barriers and facilitators for shared decision making in older patients with multiple chronic conditions: A systematic review. *BMC Geriatrics, 21*(1), 112. https://pubmed.ncbi.nlm.nih.gov/33549059/.

DEGNER and BEATON's Pattern of Decision-Making

Active: Patient Controlled
Card A

I prefer to make the final treatment decision.

Card B

I prefer to make the final treatment decision after seriously considering my doctor's opinion.

Collaborative: Jointly Controlled
Card C

I prefer that my doctor and I share responsibility for deciding which treatment is best.

Passive: Provider Controlled
Card D

I prefer my doctor to make the final treatment decision, but only after my doctor has seriously considered my opinion.
Card E

I prefer to leave all treatment decisions to my doctor.

Fig. 6.2 The most widely used instrument to elicit patient's preferences for participation in health care decision-making. From Degner, L. F., & Beaton, J. I. (1987). *Life death decisions in health care*. New York: Hemisphere Publishing.

4. Socioemotional approach
5. SDM style
B. Clinician characteristics that have a negative impact on patient outcomes
1. Increased level of fatigue
2. Burnout
3. Expression of worry

VIII. Decision aids and SDM (Kojovic & Tariman, 2017)
A. Decision aids for health treatment and screening decisions (Stacey et al., 2014)
1. Explicit values clarification exercises improve informed values-based choices
2. Positive effect on patient-practitioner communication

   3. Variable effect on length of consultation
   4. Increase patient's involvement and improve knowledge and realistic perception of outcomes
   5. Less is known about the degree of detail that decision aids need in order to have positive effects on attributes of the decision or decision-making process, but they are proven to have positive effects.
IX. Nursing roles during SDM (Tariman & Szubski, 2015; Tariman et al., 2016)
   A. Patient needs assessment
   B. Information sharing with oncology team
   C. Patient education
   D. Advocacy
   E. Psychological support
   F. Outcome evaluation
   G. Management of side effects
   H. Complex role contingent on several variables within the context of uncertainty
X. Opportunities to improve outcomes related to SDM
   A. Develop institutional policy supporting SDM model in current practice
   B. Delineate the roles of nurses during SDM, particularly advocacy and patient education on treatment options
   C. Annual education and training of nurses on SDM (as well as all treatment team members)
   D. Develop and test a conceptual model of the roles of oncology nurses during SDM
   E. Develop/utilize a measurement tool to assess the role competence of oncology nurses in SDM; nurses need more support and training to feel competent as part of the process (Katz, Tariman, Hartle, & Szubski, 2017)
   F. Three-talk model of SDM including conversational steps, initiated by providing support when introducing options, followed by strategies to compare and discuss trade-offs, before deliberation based on informed preferences (Elwyn et al., 2017)
   G. Increased efforts to reduce "risk" by removing literacy-related barriers in decision aids (Muscta et al., 2021)

REFERENCES

Agency for Healthcare Research and Quality. (2020). *The SHARE Approach—Essential steps of shared decisionmaking: Quick reference guide.* Rockville, MD: Agency for Healthcare Research and Quality. https://www.ahrq.gov/health-literacy/professional-training/shared-decision/tools/resource-1.html. Last reviewed September 2020.

Charles, C., Gafni, A., & Whelan, T. (1999). Decision-making in the physician-patient encounter: Revisiting the shared treatment decision-making model. *Social Science & Medicine, 49*(5), 651–661.

De Vries, A. M., de Roten, Y., Meystre, C., Passchier, J., Despland, J.-N., & Stiefel, F. (2014). Clinician characteristics, communication, and patient outcome in oncology: A systematic review. *Psycho-Oncology, 23*(4), 375–381. https://doi.org/10.1002/pon.3445.

Degner, L. F., & Beaton, J. I. (1987). *Life-death decisions in health care.* New York: Hemisphere Publishing.

Degner, L. F., Sloan, J. A., & Venkatesh, P. (1997). The Control Preferences Scale. *Canadian Journal of Nursing Research, 29*(3), 21–43.

Elwyn, G., Durand, M. A., Song, J., Aarts, J., Barr, P. J., Berger, Z., et al. (2017). A three-talk model for shared decision making: Multistage consultation process. *BMJ, 359,* j4891. https://doi.org/10.1136/bmj.j4891.

Ford, H. (1977). The rising cost of health care: The health services "crisis"—Reality or fantasy? *Journal of the Tennessee Medical Association, 70*(11), 822–827.

Hoving, C., Visser, A., Mullen, P. D., & van den Borne, B. (2010). A history of patient education by health professionals in Europe and North America: From authority to shared decision making education. *Patient Education and Counseling, 78*(3), 275–281. https://doi.org/10.1016/j.pec.2010.01.015.

Institute of Medicine. (2001). *Crossing the quality chasm: A new health system for the 21st century.* Washington, D.C.: The National Academies Press.

Katz, P., Tariman, J. D., Hartle, L., & Szubski, K. (2017). Development and testing of cancer treatment shared decision-making scale for nurses (SDMS-N). In: *STTI 28th international nursing research congress.* https://www.ons.org/sites/default/files/2022-01/Chapter6_CoreCurriculum.pdf.

Kojovic, B., & Tariman, J. D. (2017). Decision aids: Assisting patients with multiple myeloma and caregivers with treatment decision making. *Clinical Journal of Oncology Nursing, 21*(6), 660–664. https://doi.org/10.1188/17.CJON.660-664.

McDevitt, P. K. (1986). Health care consumerism: The new force. *Journal of Hospital Marketing, 1*(1–2), 43–57.

Pel-Littel, R. E., Snaterse, M., Teppich, N. M., Buurman, B. M., van Etten-Jamaludin, F. S., van Weert, J. C. M., et al. (2021). Barriers and facilitators for shared decision making in older patients with multiple chronic conditions: A systematic review. *BMC Geriatrics, 21,* 112. https://doi.org/10.1186/s12877-021-02050-y.

Price, R. (1981). Consumerism in health—Are we accountable and if so, how? *Australian Nurses' Journal, 10*(9), 50–52.

Muscat, D. M., Shepherd, H. L., Nutbeam, D., Trevena, L., & McCaffery, K. J. (2021). Health literacy and shared decision-making: Exploring the relationship to enable meaningful patient engagement in healthcare. *Journal of General Internal Medicine, 36*(2), 521–524. https://doi.org/10.1007/s11606-020-05912-0.

Puts, M. T., Tapscott, B., Fitch, M., Howell, D., Monette, J., Wan-Chow-Wah, D., et al. (2015). A systematic review of factors influencing older adults' decision to accept or decline cancer treatment. *Cancer Treatment Reviews, 41*(2), 197–215. https://doi.org/10.1016/j.ctrv.2014.12.010.

Ramsdale, E. E., Csik, V., Chapman, A. E., Naeim, A., & Canin, B. (2017). Improving quality and value of cancer care for older adults, *American Society of Clinical Oncology Education Book, 37,* 383–393. https://doi.org/10.14694/EDBK_175442.

Sattar, S., Alibhai, S. M. H., Fitch, M., Krzyzanowska, M., Leighl, N., & Puts, M. T. E. (2018). Chemotherapy and radiation treatment decision-making experiences of older adults with cancer: A qualitative study. *Journal of Geriatric Oncology, 9*(1), 47–52. https://doi.org/10.1016/j.jgo.2017.07.013.

Siminoff, L. A., & Step, M. M. (2005). A communication model of shared decision making: Accounting for cancer treatment decisions. *Health Psychology, 24*(4 Suppl), S99–S105. https://doi.org/10.1037/0278-6133.24.4.S99.

Singh, J. A., Sloan, J. A., Atherton, P. J., Smith, T., Hack, T. F., Huschka, M. M., et al. (2010). Preferred roles in treatment decision making among patients with cancer: A pooled analysis of studies using the Control Preferences Scale. *American Journal of Managed Care, 16*(9), 688–696.

Slade, M. (2017). Implementing shared decision making in routine mental health care. *World Psychiatry, 16*(2), 146–153. https://doi.org/10.1002/wps.20412.

Stacey, D., Legare, F., Col, N. F., Bennett, C. L., Barry, M. J., Eden, K. B., et al. (2014). Decision aids for people facing health treatment or screening decisions. *Cochrane Database of Systematic Reviews,* (1), CD001431. https://doi.org/10.1002/14651858.

Tariman, J. D., Berry, D. L., Cochrane, B., Doorenbos, A., & Schepp, K. (2010). Preferred and actual participation roles during health care decision making in persons with cancer: A systematic review. *Annals of Oncology, 21*(6), 1145–1151. https://doi.org/10.1093/annonc/mdp534.

Tariman, J. D., Berry, D. L., Cochrane, B., Doorenbos, A., & Schepp, K. G. (2012). Physician, patient, and contextual factors affecting treatment decisions in older adults with cancer and models of decision making: A literature review. *Oncology Nursing Forum, 39*(1), E70–E83. https://doi.org/10.1188/12.ONF.E70-E83.

Tariman, J. D., Doorenbos, A., Schepp, K. G., Singhal, S., & Berry, D. L. (2014). Information needs priorities in patients diagnosed with cancer: A systematic review. *Journal of the Advanced Practitioner in Oncology, 2014*(5), 115–122.

Tariman, J. D., Doorenbos, A., Schepp, K. G., Singhal, S., & Berry, D. L. (2015). Top information need priorities of older adults newly diagnosed with active myeloma. *Journal of the Advanced Practitioner in Oncology, 6*(1), 14–21.

Tariman, J. D., Mehmeti, E., Spawn, N., McCarter, S. P., Bishop-Royse, J., Garcia, I., et al. (2016). Oncology nursing and shared decision making for cancer treatment. *Clinical Journal of Oncology Nursing, 20*(5), 560–563. https://doi.org/10.1188/16.CJON.560-563.

Tariman, J. D., & Szubski, K. L. (2015). The evolving role of the nurse during the cancer treatment decision-making process: A literature review. *Clinical Journal of Oncology Nursing, 19*(5), 548–556. https://doi.org/10.1188/15.CJON.548-556.

Truglio-Londrigan, M., & Slyer, J. T. (2018). Shared decision-making for nursing practice: An integrative review. *The Open Nursing Journal, 12,* 1–14. https://doi.org/10.2174/1874434601812010001.

Ubel, P. A., Scherr, K. A., & Fagerlin, A. (2018). Autonomy: What's shared decision making have to do with it? *The American Journal of Bioethics, 18*(2), W11–W12. https://doi.org/10.1080/15265161.2017.1409844.

Carcinogenesis

Marie Christine Seitz

I. *Carcinogenesis:* normal cells are transformed into cancer cells through a complex and dynamic process that starts with pathogenic changes in regulatory cells and is promoted by genomic instability, inflammation, and interactions within the tumor microenvironment (Fig. 7.1; McCance, 2019). These pathogenic alterations were formerly referred to as mutations but variant with a qualifier about pathogenicity is preferred (Oncology Nursing Society, 2023). Recent theories identify factors as enabling agents of cancer and hallmarks of cancerous cells (Fouad & Aanei, 2017; Hanahan, 2022; Hanahan & Weinberg, 2011).

A. Causes of pathogenic cellular alterations

1. Deoxyribonucleic acid (DNA) pathogenic cellular alterations can be caused by environmental factors known as *carcinogens*. Most DNA somatic pathogenic variants are not inherited (acquired); also known as *somatic pathogenic variants*. Somatic pathogenic variants can accumulate over a lifetime, contributing to the increased cancer incidence as we age (Rote, 2019).

2. Pathogenic variants can also be inherited or germline pathogenic variants.

a. Currently, 5%–10% of cancer of all cancers are thought to be linked to germline pathogenic variants, with over 50 hereditary cancer syndromes identified (National Institute, 2022).

B. Pathogenic alterations of regulatory genes/chromosomes in cells (Table 7.1; Rote, 2019):

1. *Proto-oncogenes:* genes that code for proteins involved in normal cell growth. When altered, they may enable a cancer cell to be self-sufficient in growth. A commonly used analogy is that the genes, when altered, are like a car's gas pedal that is stuck.

a. *Ras* is a commonly pathogenically altered proto-oncogene, especially in pancreatic and colorectal cancers. A point variant (which happens at a single location of DNA or a single base pair) can change *Ras* from a proto-oncogene to an oncogene.

2. *Tumor-suppressor genes:* genes that control proliferation by preventing uncontrolled growth. When altered, these genes no longer suppress proliferation. In the car analogy, these genes, when altered, are like the brake pedal that does not work.

a. The *RB* gene normally inhibits cell division, with pathogenic alterations of this gene leading to persistent cell growth. Pathogenic variants in this gene are associated with childhood retinoblastoma and many lung, breast, and bone cancers (Rote, 2019).

b. The tp53 tumor-suppressor gene (*TP53*), when functioning normally, activates caretaker genes. When pathogenically altered, the *TP53* gene loses its ability to activate the caretaker genes leading to increased pathogenic alterations and development of cancer.

3. *Caretaker genes:* DNA repair genes that correct mistakes in normal cells that might be caused by carcinogens during replication. In some individuals, these genes may not be functional, which makes it easier for a pathogenic variant to result in cancer.

4. Chromosome translocations result when pieces of one chromosome move to another chromosome as the cell divides. This type of genetic alteration may activate an oncogene.

a. The *MYC* proto-oncogene is normally located on chromosome 8. In the Burkitt lymphoma cells, this portion of DNA is relocated to chromosome 14. This translocation allows the *MYC* gene to be overexpressed, driving proliferation and blocking differentiation of the B-lymphocyte (Rote, 2019).

b. In chronic myeloid leukemia the *BCR* gene on chromosome 22 is fused to the *Abl* gene on chromosome 9. This translocation is also known as the *Philadelphia chromosome*. This fusion makes a protein called a *tyrosine kinase*, which promotes the proliferation of myeloid cells. Imatinib, the originally targeted tyrosine kinase inhibitor, was designed to specifically inhibit this pathway.

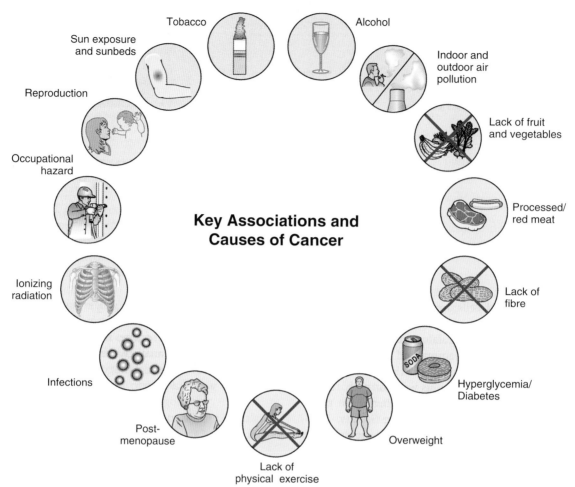

Fig. 7.1 Key associations and causes of cancer. From McCance, K. L. (2019). Cancer epidemiology. In K. L. McCance, S. E. Huether, V. Brashers, & N. Rote (Eds.), *Pathophysiology: The biologic basis for disease in adults and children* (8th ed., pp. 379–425). Amsterdam: Elsevier.

TABLE 7.1 Comparison of Cancer Gene Types

Gene Type	Normal Function	Effect of Pathogenic Alterations
Caretaker	DNA and chromosome stability	Chromosome instability and increased rates of Pathogenic alterations
Dominant oncogenes[a]	Encode proteins that promote growth (e.g., growth factors)	Overexpression or amplification causes gain of function
Tumor suppressors (recessive oncogenes)	Encode proteins that inhibit proliferation and prevent or repair pathogenic alterations	Requires loss of function of both alleles to increase cancer risk

DNA, Deoxyribonucleic acid.
[a]Pathogenic changes or alterations a proto-oncogene may cause it to become an oncogene, which can cause the growth of cancer cells. From Rote, N. S. (2019). Cancer biology. In K. L. McCance, S. E. Huether, V. Brashers, & N. S. Rote (Eds.), *Pathophysiology: The biologic basis for disease in adults and children* (8th ed., pp. 346–378). Amsterdam: Elsevier.

II. Process of carcinogenesis (Fig. 7.2)
  A. Enabling factors: facilitate the development of cancer cells and tumor progression (Hanahan & Weinberg, 2019)
    1. Genomic instability and pathogenic variants: cancer cells have defects in mechanisms that regulate genome replication and chromosomal segregation, like the Pathogenic variants previously mentioned. This defective regulation results in an increased rate of harmful genetic alterations compared with normal cells. The genetic makeup of cancer cells is less stable than that of normal cells.
      a. Hereditary nonpolyposis colon cancer syndrome is characterized by microsatellite instability. Microsatellites are a series of tandem repeated nucleotides. The variation in the number of these tandem repeated nucleotides can be identified in pathology. Normal cells have a consistent length of nucleotides (Kumar, Abbas, & Aster, 2021).
    2. Epigenetic variant: A change in the chemical structure of DNA that does not change the DNA coding sequence.

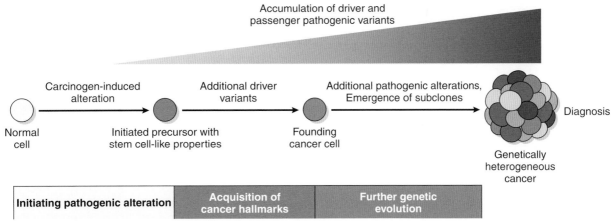

Fig. 7.2 Development of a cancer through the stepwise acquisition of multiple pathogenic alterations. A tumor is formed from a single precursor cell with genetic alterations that undergoes clonal expansion. Clonal evolution describes the process of cells within a tumor accumulating genetic changes over time that are different from one cell to the next. Thus, a tumor may be heterogeneous and consist of cells that arose from the same mother cell that are genotypically different from one another. Tumors arise from the survival of the fittest collection of cancer cells. From Kumar, V., Abbas, A. K., & Aster, J. C. (2021). Neoplasia. In V. Kumar, A. K. Abbas, & J. C. Aster (Eds.), *Robbins and Cotran pathologic basis of disease* (10th ed., pp. 268–338). Philadelphia, PA: Elsevier Saunders.

(1) An example of an epigenetic mechanism is DNA methylation. Adding or removing methyl groups from DNA affects the transcription of genes. The addition or subtraction of methyl groups may be affected by diet, the environment, and certain medications. One example of a medication that hypomethylates is decitabine, which is used in the treatment of myelodysplastic syndrome (Townsley & Battiwalla, 2019). If DNA is not transcribed, it is essentially silenced. Some cancers are associated with hypermethylation of the regulatory regions of genes.

(2) Other cancers (e.g., some colon cancers) are associated with a lack of methylation, which makes it easier for genes to be overexpressed (Hanahan, 2022). Hypomethylation may contribute to cancer when it is a tumor-suppressor gene not being transcribed (Kumar et al., 2021).

3. Tumor-promoting inflammation: various inflammatory cells from both the innate and adaptive immune systems are often identified within and around tumor tissue (Hanahan & Weinberg, 2019).

a. Inflammatory cells supply signaling molecules to the tumor microenvironment, including growth factors, survival factors, proangiogenic factors, extracellular matrix (ECM)-modifying enzymes, and inductive signals that lead to activation of epithelial–mesenchymal transition (EMT) and other hallmark-promoting programs (Hanahan & Weinberg, 2019).

b. During inflammation reactive oxygen and nitrogen species are created to combat pathogens and to stimulate tissue repair and regeneration, but these chemicals can also damage DNA, which lead to pathogenic alterations that initiate and promote cancer (Hanahan & Weinberg, 2019).

c. One example is tumor necrosis factor, a chemical released by white blood cells in response to inflammation. This cytokine may have an antitumor effect (in immune surveillance); however, it plays a role in carcinogenesis as well.

d. Some chronic inflammatory conditions are associated with tumor formation (Table 7.2).

e. Interactions between tumor cells and the surrounding normal tissue's stroma or the environment (Fig. 7.3).

f. The stroma consists of connective tissue, blood vessels, immune inflammatory cells such as macrophages and lymphocytes, and associated fibroblasts.

g. Communication and signaling between tumor cells and normal stroma cells lead to tumor growth and metastasis through a multitude of reciprocal pathways that transform both normal tissue and the tumor. For example, tumors may elicit immune and stromal responses to stimulate the formation of new blood vessels (angiogenesis).

h. Example: transforming growth factor alpha (TGF-α) or the epidermal growth factor receptor (EGFR) signaling pathway plays a role in some colon cancer metastases (Langley & Fidler, 2011).

(1) Some metastatic colon cancer cells produce five times more EGFR compared with non-metastatic cells.

(2) TGF-α initiates angiogenic processes in normal endothelial cells.

(3) Signal mediated by EGFR in colon cancer and resident endothelial populations.

TABLE 7.2   Chronic Inflammatory Conditions and Infectious Agents Associated With Neoplasms

Inflammatory Condition	Associated Neoplasm(s)
Asbestosis, silicosis	Mesothelioma, lung carcinoma
Bronchitis	Lung carcinoma
Cystitis, bladder inflammation	Bladder carcinoma
Gingivitis, lichen planus	Oral squamous cell carcinoma
Inflammatory bowel disease, Crohn disease, chronic ulcerative colitis	Colorectal carcinoma
Lichen sclerosus	Vulvar squamous cell carcinoma
Chronic pancreatitis, hereditary pancreatitis	Pancreatic carcinoma
Reflux esophagitis, Barrett esophagus	Esophageal carcinoma
Sialadenitis	Salivary gland carcinoma
Sjögren syndrome, Hashimoto thyroiditis	MALT lymphoma
Skin inflammation	Melanoma
Infection Agent (Nonviral)	
Helicobacter pylori	Gastric adenocarcinoma, MALT lymphoma
Chronic bacterial cholecystitis	Gallbladder cancer
Schistosomiasis	Bladder, liver, rectal carcinoma; follicular lymphoma of spleen
Liver flukes	Cholangiocarcinoma
Infectious Agent (Viral)	
HIV-1	Non-Hodgkin lymphoma, squamous cell carcinomas, Kaposi sarcoma
Hepatitis B and hepatitis C	Hepatocellular carcinoma
Epstein–Barr virus	B-cell non-Hodgkin lymphoma, Burkitt lymphoma, nasopharyngeal carcinoma
Kaposi Sarcoma–associated Herpesvirus (KSHV/HHV8)	Kaposi sarcoma
HPV-16, -18, -31, others	Cervical, anogenital warts
HTLV-1	Adult T-cell leukemia/lymphoma

HIV-1, Human immunodeficiency virus type 1; *HPV*, human papilloma virus; *HTLV-1*, human T-cell lymphotropic virus-1; *MALT*, mucosa-associated lymphoid tissue.
From Rote, N. S. (2019). Cancer biology. In K. L. McCance, S. E. Huether, V. Brashers, & N. S. Rote (Eds.), *Pathophysiology: The biologic basis for disease in adults and children* (8th ed., pp. 346–378). Amsterdam: Elsevier.

(4) When combined with vascular endothelial growth factor (VEGF) production, lymphangiogenesis is stimulated; tumor cells may spread to regional lymph nodes.

(5) Cetuximab, a monoclonal antibody, blocks ligand binding to EGFR; used in EGFR-positive patients to reduce primary tumor size and lymphatic spread.

4. Polymorphic microbiomes: Polymorphic variability in the microbiomes of individual patients can impact the cancer phenotype, including cancer development, malignant progression, and response to therapy (Hanahan, 2022).

   a. *Direct mutagenesis: Escherichia coli* carrying the *PKS* locus can induce cancerous changes in colonic epithelium via impairment of normal DNA replication and repair mechanisms.

   b. *Ligand mimetics*: Different bacteria can bind to the surface of colonic epithelial cells and induce increased epithelial proliferation.

   c. Metabolite production: Bacterial families produce various byproducts that can induce changes to both differentiated and undifferentiated cells (Hanahan, 2022).

B. Hallmarks of cancer: Refer to the biologic capabilities that a cancer cell acquires in a progressive multistep process that transforms a normal cell to a malignant cell (Fouad & Aanei, 2017; Hanahan & Weinberg, 2011, 2019). Tumors consist of cancer cells with various pathogenic variants supportive tissues (the tumor microenvironment) that interact and evolve together. The process is enabled by genomic instability and inflammation as described earlier. When the tumor gains a variety of clonally evolved and pathogenically altered cells that collectively have all these hallmarks of cancer, it is considered malignant (Hanahan & Weinberg, 2019).

1. Cancer cells sustain proliferative signaling.

   a. Normal cells regulate proliferation with growth-promoting signals that start and stop mitosis.

   b. Some cancer cells deregulate the signals through various means, including the following:

      (1) Production of growth factors themselves.

      (2) Transmission of signals to stimulate normal cells to supply cancer cells with growth factors.

      (3) Presence of pathogenic variants may create proto-oncogenes, inactivate tumor-suppressor genes, or disrupt negative feedback signaling.

         (a) The *Ras* oncoprotein normally signals cells to stop proliferating. Pathogenically altered *Ras* inactivates the negative

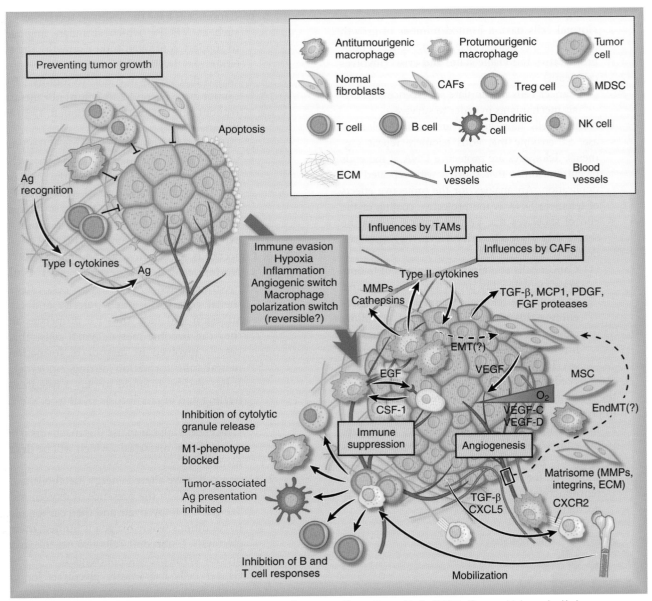

Fig. 7.3 Cancers live in a complex microenvironment. From Rote, N. S. (2019). Cancer biology. In K. L. McCance, S. E. Huether, V. Brashers, & N. S. Rote (Eds.), *Pathophysiology: The biologic basis for disease in adults and children* (8th ed., pp. 346–378). Amsterdam: Elsevier.

feedback mechanism, and cancer cells consequently keep proliferating or producing. This is a prevalent pathogenic variant in many human cancers, such as pancreatic and colorectal cancers.

(4) May counterbalance excessive proliferative signaling by forcing some cells into senescence. This may allow high growth and avoidance of cell death pressures that ultimately allow the cancer cells to persist (Hanahan & Weinberg, 2019).

2. Cancer cells evade growth suppressors.

a. Normal cells regulate growth with tumor-suppressor genes that lead to senescence (cellular aging) and apoptosis (programmed cell death). Cell growth is also limited by contact inhibition (cell growth and division stop on physical contact with other cells).

b. Some cancer cells have pathogenic variants that disable gatekeeper proteins controlling mitoses, inactivating cancer inhibition.

3. Cancer cells resist cell death.

a. Normal cells experience apoptosis or programmed cell death. A process called *autophagy* allows normal cells to be broken down during cellular stress so that organelles and cell contents can be reused in other cells.

b. Necrotic cells release proinflammatory signals. Cancer cells use these proinflammatory signals to recruit inflammatory cells and enhance tumor growth through the microenvironment (Hanahan & Weinberg, 2019).

4. Enabling replicative immortality.
   a. Normal cells have a limited number of growth and division cycles because of senescence (a non-proliferative but viable state) and crisis (involves cell death).
      (1) Cancer cells manipulate senescence and crisis mechanisms in order to survive.
   b. Normal cells have limited amounts of telomerase, an enzyme that adds telomere repeat segments. Telomeres are protective DNA at the ends of chromosomes that shorten with repeated cell duplication. An analogy for the protective effects of telomere DNA is the protective coating at the end of shoelaces that prevent fraying. When the shortened ends reach a critical level, they signal cell death.
      (1) Cancer cells contain high amounts of telomerase, which adds protective telomeres and prevents the telomere segment from shortening. This process is believed to allow continued cell replication; contributes to immortalization—cells avoid or survive crises (Fig. 7.4).
5. Cancer cells induce angiogenesis. Angiogenesis is the creation of new blood vessels from existing ones to provide nutrients and remove waste products.
   a. In normal tissues, angiogenesis takes place during embryogenesis with tissue and organ development. The process happens transiently in adulthood for wound healing and during female reproductive cycling. Otherwise, the process is dormant (Fig. 7.5).

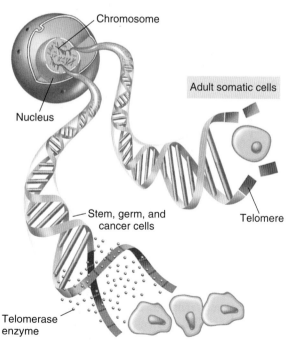

Fig. 7.4 Control of immortality: telomeres and telomerase. From Rote, N. S. (2019). Cancer biology. In K. L. McCance, S. E. Huether, V. Brashers, & N. S. Rote (Eds.), *Pathophysiology: The biologic basis for disease in adults and children* (8th ed., pp. 346–378). Amsterdam: Elsevier.

   b. Cancer cells have the ability to secrete substances such as VEGFs, which stimulate angiogenesis to support continued tumor growth. The stimulation may lead to the creation of new growing vessels that supply nutrients to tumors. "Tumors cannot grow beyond 2 to 3 mm^3 nor metastasize without new vasculature" (Folkman, 1971; Fouad & Aanei, 2017).
   c. Tumor vasculature is less organized than normal vasculature. Consequently, blood flow is chaotic, leading to hypoxia—considered the most important trigger of angiogenesis—and acidosis that stimulates angiogenesis, decreases therapeutic effectiveness, and contributes to resistant clonal expansion (Fouad & Aanei, 2017).
6. Cancer cells activate invasion and metastasis.
   a. Normal cells have a developmental regulatory program called *EMT*. This process causes epithelial cells to lose cell polarity and cell–cell adhesion and have invasive properties so that they can become mesenchymal cells. This process is involved in mesoderm formation and neural tube formation during embryogenesis. It has also been found to play a role in wound healing and organ fibrosis (Kalluri & Weinberg, 2009).
   b. Cancer cells appear to use this mechanism during invasion and metastasis, which will be described further.
7. Cancer cells have altered energy metabolism.
   a. Normal cells in the presence of oxygen metabolize glucose to pyruvate and then carbon dioxide. In conditions where oxygen is limited, they favor glycolysis. Embryonic cells also use the glycolysis process in the presence of oxygen.
   b. Cancer cells use mostly glycolysis for energy production, even in the presence of oxygen, also called the *Warburg effect*.
8. Cancer cells evade immune destruction.
   a. Evidence indicates that deficiencies in T lymphocytes, T-helper cells, and natural killer cells increase the risk of cancer development (Mandal & Viswanathan, 2015).
      (1) Example: cancer cells can evade the T-cell response by expressing PDL1 to block T-cell recognition of the cancer cell that would usually initiate a cytotoxic response. There is a class of anticancer therapy called *checkpoint inhibitors* that targets PDL1 (Fig. 7.6).
9. Unlocking phenotypic plasticity.
   a. Normal cells go through a process of differentiation to a terminal cell type.
   b. In cancer, cells are able to escape from a normal differentiation process in three ways (Fig. 7.7).
      (1) *Dedifferentiation:* Cells that are terminally differentiated are able to revert to a progenitor cell form.

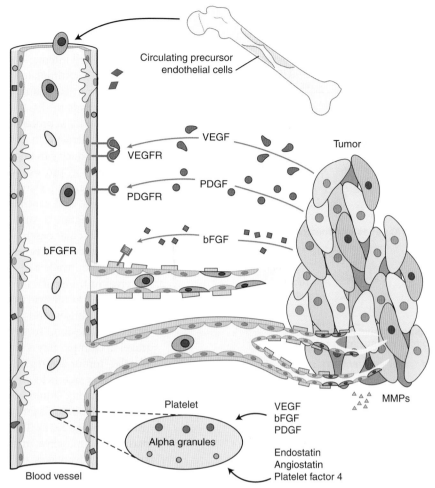

Fig. 7.5 Tumor-induced angiogenesis. From Rote, N. S. (2019). Cancer biology. In K. L. McCance, S. E. Huether, V. Brashers, & N. S. Rote (Eds.), *Pathophysiology: The biologic basis for disease in adults and children* (8th ed., pp. 346–378). Amsterdam: Elsevier.

(a) In melanoma, suppression of the *MITF* master regulator of melanocyte differentiation leads to the reactivation of neural crest progenitor genes and a dedifferentiation of a terminal melanocyte (Hanahan, 2022).

(2) *Blocked differentiation:* Cells that are incompletely differentiated progenitor cells can be blocked from further differentiation into their mature state.

(a) In acute promyelocytic leukemia, a translocation of the *PML* gene locus with the retinoic acid α nuclear receptor blocks the terminal differentiation of the myeloid progenitor stem cells (Hanahan, 2022).

(3) *Transdifferentiation:* Cells that are terminally differentiated change from one cell type to a different cell type. Pathologists termed this process metaplasia.

(a) Genetic changes in various pancreatic cell genes can lead to pancreatic acinar cells transdifferentiating to a ductal cell phenotype (Jiang et al., 2016).

10. Senescent cells.

a. Irreversible form of cellular proliferative arrest that allows for the inactivation of diseased or damaged cells, and causes the production of different chemokines, cytokines, and proteases.

b. When dysregulated, these senescent cells can support neoplastic changes and tumor progression.

(1) Cancer-associated fibroblasts are demonstrated to undergo senescence, releasing a senescence-associated secretory phenotype that provides a paracrine effect to surrounding tissue stimulating tissue invasion and metastasis (Faget, Ren, & Stewart, 2019).

III. Metastasis is the spread of cancer cells from the site of the original tumor or organ to distant tissues and organs in the body.

A. The presence of metastatic disease at diagnosis is an important prognostic factor because it indicates advanced disease. It is estimated that 30% of newly diagnosed solid tumors (excluding skin cancers other than melanomas) present with metastatic disease (Kumar et al., 2021). The majority of cancer-related deaths are related to metastatic disease.

ANTITUMOR IMMUNITY

IMMUNE EVASION BY TUMORS

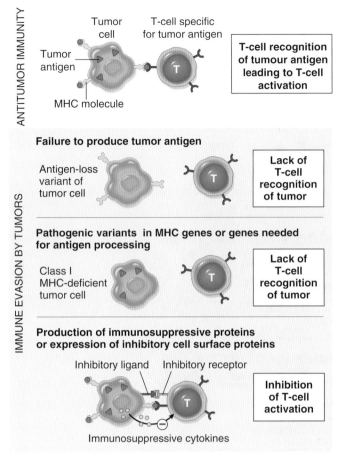

Fig. 7.6 Mechanisms by which tumor cells evade the immune system. From Rote, N. S. (2019). Cancer biology. In K. L. McCance, S. E. Huether, V. Brashers, & N. S. Rote (Eds.), *Pathophysiology: The biologic basis for disease in adults and children* (8th ed., pp. 346–378). Amsterdam: Elsevier.

B. Major factors of the metastatic cascade
1. Invasion of the ECM by tumor cells (Fig. 7.8).
   a. Downregulate cadherin glycoproteins that mediate cell–cell interactions.
   b. Produce or stimulate stromal cells such as fibroblasts or inflammatory cells to secrete proteases that degrade the ECM.
   c. Attach to ECM proteins that can assist with mobility and interact with the ECM to create an environment conducive to migration of the tumor cells.
   d. Through a process called *locomotion*, which includes complex signaling involving proteases, cytokines, and motility factors, tumor cells are able to migrate through the ECM and gain access to the vascular basement membrane.
   e. Process occurs in reverse when tumor cell emboli reach and invade a distant site (Fig. 7.9).
2. Survival in transport: tumor cells in circulation are susceptible to destruction by mechanical stress, immune defenses, and apoptosis because of lack of cell–cell adhesion. To survive, tumor cells tend to travel in clumps, may combine with platelets to form platelet–tumor aggregates, and may interact with coagulation factors to create emboli.
3. Research using "liquid biopsy" is ongoing, examining patient's biofluids for cancer-derived components (Martins et al., 2021). These biofluids include blood, plasma, serum, saliva, urine, and gastric juices. There are many advantages to liquid biopsies, including easy collection and the opportunity for serial collection over time. Liquid biopsy samples are thought to represent a population of heterogeneous tumor

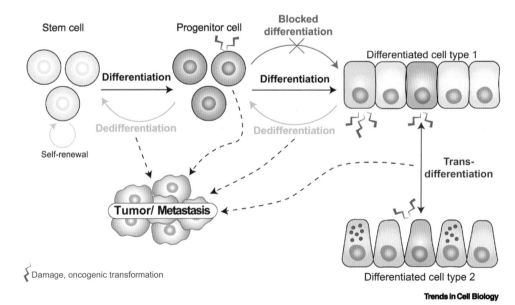

Fig. 7.7 Unlocking phenotypic plasticity. Phenotypic plasticity is arguably an acquired hallmark capability that enables various disruptions of cellular differentiation, including (1) dedifferentiation from mature to progenitor states, (2) blocked (terminal) differentiation from progenitor cell states, and (3) transdifferentiation into different cell lineages. From Jehanno, C., Vulin, M., Richina, V., Richina, F., & Bentires-Alj, M. (2022). Phenotypic plasticity during metastatic colonization. *Trends in Cell Biology, 32*(10), P854–867. https://doi.org/10.1016/j.tcb.2022.03.007.

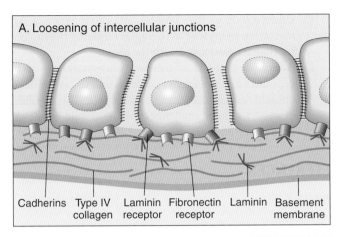

A. Loosening of intercellular junctions

Cadherins | Type IV collagen | Laminin receptor | Fibronectin receptor | Laminin | Basement membrane

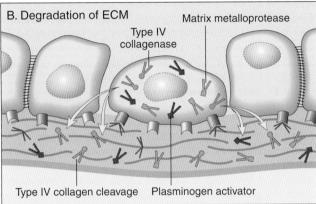

B. Degradation of ECM

Matrix metalloprotease

Type IV collagenase

Type IV collagen cleavage | Plasminogen activator

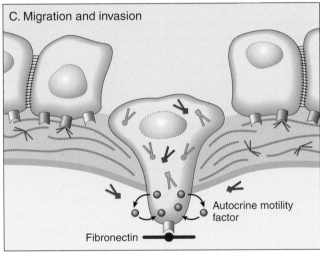

C. Migration and invasion

Autocrine motility factor

Fibronectin

Fig. 7.8 Sequence of events in the invasion of epithelial basement membranes by tumor cells. From Kumar, V., Abbas, A. K., & Aster, J. C. (2021). Neoplasia. In V. Kumar, A. K. Abbas, & J. C. Aster (Eds.), *Robbins and Cotran pathologic basis of disease* (10th ed., pp. 268–338). Philadelphia, PA: Elsevier Saunders.

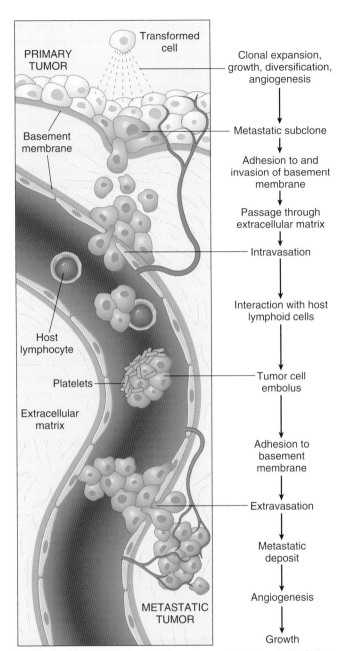

Transformed cell

PRIMARY TUMOR

Basement membrane

Host lymphocyte

Platelets

Extracellular matrix

METASTATIC TUMOR

Clonal expansion, growth, diversification, angiogenesis

Metastatic subclone

Adhesion to and invasion of basement membrane

Passage through extracellular matrix

Intravasation

Interaction with host lymphoid cells

Tumor cell embolus

Adhesion to basement membrane

Extravasation

Metastatic deposit

Angiogenesis

Growth

Fig. 7.9 The metastatic cascade. From Kumar, V., Abbas, A. K., & Aster, J. C. (2021). Neoplasia. In V. Kumar, A. K. Abbas, & J. C. Aster (Eds.), *Robbins and Cotran pathologic basis of disease* (10th ed., pp. 268–338). Philadelphia, PA: Elsevier Saunders.

cells more accurately than tissue biopsy (Hirahata et al., 2022). Liquid biopsy testing is currently FDA approved in different cancer types to determine actionable pathogenic variants for treatment decision-making (Weintraub, 2020). Pathways of cancer dissemination:

a. Direct invasion to an adjoining organ

b. Seeding throughout a body cavity such as the peritoneal cavity (e.g., ovarian cancer)

c. Dissemination through the lymphatic system
   (1) Entrapment at the first lymph node, or the "sentinel lymph node"
   (2) "Skip metastasis," where cells bypass the first node and reach more distant sites

d. Dissemination through the blood vessels
   (1) Arterial spread
      (a) Tumor cells may be spread through the pulmonary capillary beds or pulmonary arteriovenous shunts, or when pulmonary tumors metastasize and create tumor emboli.

(b) Because arteries have thicker walls, they are less readily penetrated than veins (Kumar et al., 2021).

(2) Venous spread

(a) Tumor cells often go to the first capillary bed encountered. Liver and lungs are the most frequent sites of metastasis (Rote, 2019).

4. Common sites for metastasis include bones, the lungs, the liver, and the central nervous system. Predilection for certain tumors to metastasize to specific sites may be influenced by the following:

a. Patterns of blood flow.

b. Cell receptors and genes that direct the cell to travel to specific sites.

c. Tumor cell production of adhesion molecules that prefer certain distant organs.

d. Chemical signals and growth factors, which are found only in selected organs.

e. Inhibitor substances produced by organs not typically sites for metastatic growth.

f. Collectively, items b to e may be a result of "crosstalk" between cancer cells and normal host cells. That is, cancer cells may release cytokines that induce the host cells to produce substances that recognize receptors on the cancer cells. Hence, the cancer cells may have a "homing device" that attracts them to select host organs and may promote their growth in these distant tissues (Kumar et al., 2021 Rote, 2019; Table 7.3).

IV. Key points

A. Cancer is a heterogeneous group of diseases that are caused by environment exposures, lifestyle, and genetic factors (McCance, 2019).

B. Metastasis contributes to the pain and suffering caused by cancer and is the major cause of death from cancer (Rote, 2019).

C. Understanding the process of carcinogenesis and metastasis helps lead to therapies targeting the molecular changes associated with the disease.

D. Although there is a growing understanding of the genomics and the factors contributing to cancer development, cancer cells remain adaptable. This flexibility of cancer creates challenges for the development of a single cure-all therapy.

REFERENCES

Faget, D. V., Ren, Q., & Stewart, S. A. (2019). Unmasking senescence: Context-dependent effects of SASP in cancer. *Nature Reviews Cancer, 19*(8), 439–453. https://doi.org/10.1038/s41568-019-0156-2.

Folkman, J. (1971). Tumor angiogenesis: Therapeutic implications. *The New England Journal of Medicine, 285*(21), 1182–1186. https://doi.org/10.1056/nejm197111182852108.

Fouad, Y. A., & Aanei, C. (2017). Revisiting the hallmarks of cancer. *American Journal of Cancer Research, 7*(5), 1016–1036.

Hanahan, D. (2022). Hallmarks of cancer: New dimensions. *Cancer Discovery, 12*(1), 31–46. https://doi.org/10.1158/2159-8290.Cd-21-1059.

Hanahan, D., & Weinberg, R. A. (2011). Hallmarks of cancer: The next generation. *Cell, 144*(5), 646–674. https://doi.org/10.1016/j.cell.2011.02.013.

Hanahan, D., & Weinberg, R. A. (Eds.). (2019). *Hallmarks of cancer: An organizing principle for cancer medicine* (11th ed.). Wolters Kluwer.

Hirahata, T., ul Quraish, R., ul Quraish, A., ul Quraish, S., Naz, M., & Razzaq, M. A. (2022). Liquid biopsy: A distinctive approach to the diagnosis and prognosis of cancer. *Cancer Informatics, 21*, 1–7. https://doi.org/10.1177/11769351221076062.

Jiang, M., Azevedo-Pouly, A. C., Deering, T. G., Hoang, C. Q., DiRenzo, D., Hess, D. A., et al. (2016). MIST1 and PTF1 collaborate in feed-forward regulatory loops that maintain the pancreatic acinar phenotype in adult mice. *Molecular and Cellular Biology, 36*(23), 2945–2955. https://doi.org/10.1128/mcb.00370-16.

Kalluri, R., & Weinberg, R. A. (2009). The basics of epithelial-mesenchymal transition. *The Journal of Clinical Investigation, 119*(6), 1420–1428. https://doi.org/10.1172/JCI39104.

Kumar, V., Abbas, A. K., & Aster, J. C. (2021). Neoplasia. In V. Kumar, A. K. Abbas, & J. C. Aster (Eds.), *Robbins and Cotran pathologic basis of disease* (10th ed., pp. 268–338). Amsterdam: Elsevier.

Langley, R. R., & Fidler, I. J. (2011). The seed and soil hypothesis revisited – The role of tumor-stroma interactions in metastasis to different organs. *International Journal of Cancer, 128*(11), 2527–2535. https://doi.org/10.1002/ijc.26031.

Mandal, A., & Viswanathan, C. (2015). Natural killer cells: In health and disease. *Hematology/Oncology and Stem Cell Therapy, 8*(2), 47–55. https://doi.org/10.1016/j.hemonc.2014.11.006.

Martins, I., Ribeiro, I. P., Jorge, J., Gonçalves, A. C., Sarmento-Ribeiro, A. B., Melo, J. B., et al. (2021). Liquid biopsies: Applications for cancer diagnosis and monitoring. *Genes, 12*(3), 349. https://doi.org/10.3390/genes12030349.

McCance, K. L. (2019). Cancer epidemiology. In K. L. McCance, S. E. Huether, V. Brashers, & N. Rote (Eds.), *Pathophysiology: The biologic basis for disease in adults and children* (8th ed., pp. 379–425). Amsterdam: Elsevier.

TABLE 7.3 Common Sites of Metastasis

Cancer Type	Main Sites of Metastasis
Bladder	Bone, liver, lung
Breast	Bone, brain, liver, lung
Colon	Liver, lung, peritoneum
Kidney	Adrenal gland, bone, brain, liver, lung
Lung	Adrenal gland, bone, brain, liver, other lung
Melanoma	Bone, brain, liver, lung, skin, muscle
Ovary	Liver, lung, peritoneum
Pancreas	Liver, lung, peritoneum
Prostate	Adrenal gland, bone, liver, lung
Rectal	Liver, lung, peritoneum
Stomach	Liver, lung, peritoneum
Thyroid	Bone, liver, lung
Uterus	Bone, liver, lung, peritoneum, vagina

From *National Cancer Institute at the National Institute for Health. Metastatic cancer.* (2020). https://www.cancer.gov/types/metastatic-cancer. Accessed 11.03.22.

National Cancer Institute. (2022). *The genetics of cancer*. National Institutes of Health. Retrieved from https://www.cancer.gov/about-cancer/causes-prevention/genetics.

National Cancer Institute. (2020). *Metastatic cancer: When cancer spreads*. Retrieved from https://www.cancer.gov/types/metastatic-cancer.

Oncology Nursing Society (2023). Genomics and Precision Oncology Learning Library. Retrieved from: https://www.cancer.gov/types/metastatic-cancer.

Rote, N. S. (2019). Cancer biology. In K. L. McCance, S. E. Huether, V. Brashers, & N. S. Rote (Eds.), *Pathophysiology: The biologic basis for disease in adults and children* (8th ed., pp. 346–378). Amsterdam: Elsevier.

Townsley, D. M., & Battiwalla, M. (2019). Myleodysplastic syndromes. In G. P. Rodgers & N. S. Young (Eds.), *The Bethesda handbook of clinical hematology* (4th ed., pp. 90–103). Wolters Kluwer.

Weintraub, K. (2020, September 3). 'Coming into their own': FDA approval of liquid biopsy tests puts early, less invasive cancer detection in broader reach. *USA Today*. https://www.usatoday.com/story/news/health/2020/09/03/cancer-fda-approves-liquid-biopsy-tests-can-improve-treatment/5644829002/.

8

Immunology

Christine L. Boley

I. Definition of immunology (Actor, 2019)
   A. Study of health maintenance and homeostasis based on identification and eradication of foreign microbes, repair of tissue damage, and defense of the host through the capacity to distinguish self from nonself, while preventing malignant proliferation
      1. Impairment or lack of these components disrupts homeostasis by lack of immune response to allergens, antigens, infectious microbes, or tumor cells, leading to the development of various disease processes.
II. Basic concepts
   A. Organ and tissue components of the immune system (Doan, Lievano, Swanson-Mungerson, & Viselli, 2022)
      1. Primary lymphoid organs—allow for the maturation of lymphocytes and includes the following organs:
         a. Bone marrow (BM)—location of B-cell differentiation and maturation
         b. Thymus—location of T-cell differentiation and maturation
      2. Secondary lymphoid organs and tissues—sites where antigens are captured, processed, and removed (Actor, 2019)
         a. Lymph nodes—filters cellular waste and initiates immune responses to antigens circulating in the lymph, skin, or mucosal surfaces
            (1) Part of unidirectional lymphatic circulation, which is dependent on body's movement to circulate lymph and carry it to vascular system via thoracic duct and subclavian artery.
            (2) Normal lymph nodes increase and decrease in size throughout life.
            (3) Damaged or destroyed lymph nodes/tissues do not regenerate; swelling can result from the accumulation of lymph fluid, called lymphedema.
         b. Spleen—responds to bloodborne antigens and contains plasma cells
         c. BM—functions as both primary and secondary lymphoid organ
         d. Lymphoid tissue—gastrointestinal mucosa (Peyer patches), tonsils/adenoids (Waldeyer ring), and other body systems' mucosa-associated lymphoid tissue
         e. The brain is part of the lymphatic and immune systems
   B. Hematopoiesis—regulation, production, and development of blood cells (Johnston, 2022). Fig. 8.1 provides an overview of the hematopoietic hierarchy (Zhang, Gao, Xia, & Liu, 2018).
      1. Hematopoiesis begins with a single cell, a self-renewing pluripotent stem cell.
         a. Protein markers on surfaces called the cluster of differentiation (CD)
            (1) CD identifies cell type and function and provides molecular signaling
      2. Cells divide into undifferentiated hematopoietic stem cells that are committed to one of two cell lineages or pathways: lymphoid or myeloid progenitor cells.
         a. Lymphoid—B cell, helper T cell, cytotoxic T cell, natural killer (NK) cells
         b. Myeloid—dendritic cell, macrophage, neutrophil, eosinophil, mast cell, megakaryocyte, erythrocyte (red blood cell [RBC]), basophils, and monocytes
III. Cellular components of the immune system (Doan et al., 2022; Johnston, 2022)
   A. Myeloid stem cell lineage—further divided into two lineages:
      1. Granulocyte-monocyte lineage
         a. Granulocytes—have granules in cytoplasm with enzymes that aid in the digestion of foreign particles (phagocytosis) and cause inflammation.
            (1) Neutrophils or polymorphonuclear neutrophil: rapidly produced and are first responders to bacterial and fungal microbes.
               (a) Short lived—about 7 hours, but most abundant granulocyte
               (b) Cause inflammatory response due to engulfing/destroying foreign particles/debris
            (2) Basophils: have IgE receptors that are involved in allergic responses and cause the release of histamine/prostaglandins.
            (3) Eosinophils: attack parasites, secrete leukotrienes/cytokines that cause inflammation during allergic responses.

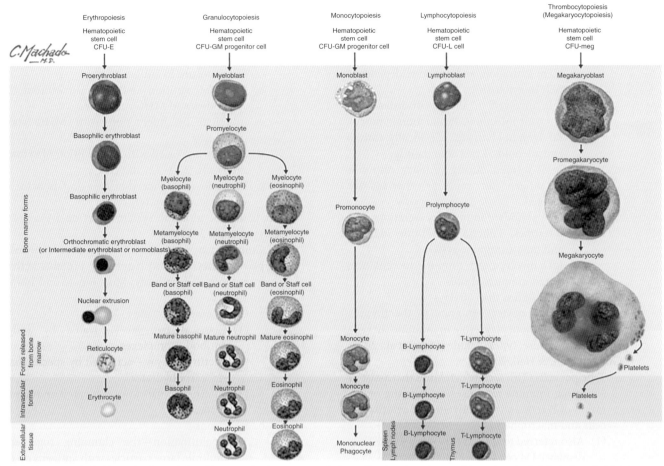

Fig. 8.1 Hematopoietic hierarchy. From https://www.netterimages.com/schematic-showing-stages-of-hematopoiesis-labeled-ovalle-histology-carlos-a-g-machado-13651.html.

b. Monocytes—migrate from BM to inflammatory site, where they divide and become macrophages (Johnston, 2022).
  (1) Macrophages—rapidly recognize, ingest, and kill microbes
    (a) Present these processed antigens to T cells, called antigen-presenting cell (APC).
    (b) Release proinflammatory cytokines called M1 to initiate an immune response.
    (c) Release antiinflammatory cytokines called M2 to initiate wound healing and maintain homeostasis.
  (2) Mononuclear phagocytes—fixed and mobile phagocytic cells associated with blood monocytes and tissue macrophages
c. Dendritic cells (DCs)—capture foreign cells and process antigens (Johnston, 2022).
  (1) Immature DCs found in peripheral tissue possess phagocytic functions for innate immunity
  (2) Function as major APC and travel from tissue to secondary lymphoid tissue to present antigen to naïve T and B cells; this process activates T cells

  (3) Functions as a direct link between innate and adaptive immunity
2. Megakaryocyte-erythrocyte lineage
  a. Megakaryocyte—forms into platelets before circulation
    (1) Has immunologic function that releases inflammatory mediators, recruits leukocytes to tissue damage, prevents excessive bleeding
  b. Erythrocytes (RBCs)—involved in tissue nourishment, oxygenation, and blood viscosity
  c. Mast cells—produce inflammatory response within tissues, not bloodborne, and release tumor necrosis factor/interleukin-8 (TNF/IL-8)
B. Lymphoid stem cell lineage has three types of lymphocytes that are key for immune responses:
1. B cells (B lymphocytes)—develop in the BM. Two types of B cells (Doan et al., 2022)
  a. Memory B cells: activated B cells specific to an antigen
    (1) Quickly respond after a second exposure of the host
    (2) Long-term immune cells
  b. Plasma cells: produce and secrete antibodies against antigens after exposure (Gutzeit, Chen, & Cerutti, 2018)

(1) Secretes one of the five different specific immunoglobulins (Igs):
   (a) IgG: 75% of a person's antibodies. Involved with neutralization, opsonization, complement activation, and antibody-dependent cellular cytotoxicity.
   (b) IgE: involved in allergic disorders and parasitic infections. Production in mucosal lymphoid tissue, specifically tonsils and adenoids. Least abundant Ig.
   (c) IgM: formed during primary response to antigen and wanes as other Igs are formed.
   (d) IgA: abundant in mucous secretions and intestines. Functions in both adaptive and innate immune systems.
   (e) IgD: involved with immune surveillance; found in mucosal sites.
(2) Usually live less than 30 days

2. T cells (T lymphocytes)—migrate to the thymus gland for maturation; play a role in immune surveillance and response; types include (Doan et al., 2022; Guyton, Hall, & Hall, 2021):
   a. T-helper cells (Th): secrete cytokines that assist in activating immune responses, such as the maturation of B cells and the activation of cytotoxic T cells and macrophages.
      (1) Also referred to as CD4+ T cells because they display CD4 cell surface molecules
      (2) Account for two-thirds of mature T cells
      (3) Recognize antigens in conjunction with class II major histocompatibility complex (MHC) molecules
      (4) Th cell type I (Th1)—secretes cytokines (interferon [IFN], IL, TNF) and develops cell-mediated immunity Tc cells (Petersone & Walker, 2022)
      (5) Th cell type II (Th2)—secretes antiinflammatory cytokines and B-cell maturation
   b. Cytotoxic T cells (Tc): destroy viral infections, cancer; play a role in autoimmunity and allogenic organ rejection.
      (1) Called CD8+ T cells because they display CD8 protein on their surface
      (2) Recognize antigens in conjunction with class I MHC molecules
      (3) Induce apoptosis of foreign cells through the release of enzymes
   c. T regulatory cells (Tregs): previously called suppressor T cells.
      (1) Suppress T-cell-mediated immunity, as well as suppress autoreactive T cells against self, called immune tolerance.
      (2) Treg and Th cells help maintain immunologic homeostasis within host.
   d. Memory T cells: induce secondary cell-mediated immune response.

3. NK cells—develop in BM (Johnston, 2022)
   a. Large granular cells that release cytokines, rapidly migrate to the site of inflammation, and directly kill tumor- or viral-infected cells without previous exposure to antigens.
   b. Faster recognition and response without using antibodies and MHC molecules.
   c. Inhibited by interaction with MHC class I molecules.
   d. Activity increased with the addition of cytokines such as IL-2, IL-12, and IFN-γ.
   e. Immunosenescence due to aging is associated with a decrease in NK cells.

C. Mediators of immune system function (Actor, 2019; Guyton et al., 2021)
   1. Complement system—an interactive network of plasma enzymes and regulatory proteins activated in a controlled pathway; links innate and humoral immunity
      a. Complement cascade
         (1) Classical pathway—activated by antigen-antibody complexes
         (2) Lectin pathway—activated by specific bacterial carbohydrates
         (3) Alternative pathway—activated on microbial surfaces
      b. Functions
         (1) Agglutination—the clumping together of multiple large particles with antigens on their surface
         (2) Precipitation—a large antigen and antibody complex that are insoluble and precipitate
         (3) Opsonization—phagocytosis of antigen-antibody complexes when products of the complement cascade interact with neutrophils and macrophages
         (4) Cell lysis—destruction of targeted pathogen
   2. Cytokines
      a. A large variety of proteins secreted by immune cells to assist with cell-cell signaling during different immune responses, such as cellular proliferation and migration, apoptosis, and inflammation (Actor, 2019)
         (1) Lymphokines—produced by lymphocytes to attract macrophages and other lymphocytes to site of infection for immune response, including:
            (a) IFNs—released in response to pathogens, such as viral infections, and are produced early in response to infection
            (b) ILs—help T and B lymphocytes and hematopoietic cells divide, differentiate, and activate
            (c) Colony-stimulating growth factors—assist with differentiation of all BM progenitor stem cells
         (2) Chemokines—induce chemotaxis, which is the activation and movement of leukocytes

throughout the body in response to a chemical release

   (3) TNFs—play key roles in mediating inflammation; cause fevers, apoptosis, and acute-phase cytotoxic reactions

     (a) Produced by eosinophils, mast cells, neutrophils, NK cells, macrophages, CD4+ cells, and lymphocytes

   (4) Transforming growth factors—control cell division and repair

  3. MHC—group of genes that controls the production of glycoproteins found on the surface of all species' nucleated cells (except RBCs); help distinguish as "self-antigens" (Actor, 2019; Guyton et al., 2021)

   a. Two classes:

    (1) MHC class I molecules: displayed on almost all nucleated cells

    (2) MHC class II molecules: more specialized, or "professional" APCs, such as DCs, monocytes, macrophages, and B cells

   b. In humans, this is called human leukocyte antigen (HLA) and consists of more than 200 genes located on chromosome 6 inherited from both parents.

    (1) HLA typing of donor and recipient lymphocytes is performed prior to BM transplant to obtain the best HLA match, improving engraftment and decreasing immune reaction.

   c. Immune response can be mounted against foreign MHC molecules.

IV. Immune system responses—body's defense against foreign substances

  A. Involves both innate and adaptive immunity

   1. Innate immunity—or natural immunity, is the immediate, first line of defense against invasion; does not rely on previous exposure, or "memory," to be initiated. (Johnston, 2022)

    a. Natural barriers—inborne to prevent damage by environmental substances and prevent infection by pathogens

     (1) Physical—epithelial cells of intact skin and mucous membranes

     (2) Chemical—bile, mucus, perspiration, tears (lysozyme), normal flora

     (3) Cellular—leukocytes, cytokines

    b. Inflammatory response—nonspecific process that results in rapid activation of several plasma protein systems; mast cell degranulation; vascular changes; and the influx of macrophages, neutrophils, NK cells, and DCs in direct response to tissue damage once natural barrier is broken

     (1) Prevents infection and further damage by binding to microbes

     (2) Cascade of cells released for phagocytosis, promote inflammatory mediators, release of cytokines, and remove cellular debris

     (3) Host innate immune cells have surface receptors, called pattern recognition receptors, that distinguish between self and pathogens which have pathogen-associated molecular patterns and cell damage/death molecules, called damage-associated molecular patterns

     (4) Feedback inhibition mechanisms to control damage to tissues

     (5) Unable to differentiate or memorize different types of pathogens

     (6) Macrophages and DCs produce cytokines that facilitate the development of the adaptive immune response

   2. Adaptive immunity—occurs in later stages of immune response with specific immune cells and has memory, which allows for longer lived immune response. Two types of adaptive immunity: humoral and cell mediated (Actor, 2019)

    a. Humoral immunity—antibodies produced by B lymphocytes.

     (1) Antigens in lymphatic fluid pass through secondary lymphatic organs, which activates B cells; antigen is processed and presented on surface with MHC-II molecule.

     (2) Each B-cell lymphocyte recognizes only one type of antigen; this is called specificity.

     (3) Specific B-cell lymphocytes quickly multiply and differentiate to become either memory or plasma cells with help from helper T cells.

     (4) Each specialized plasma cell produces one specific antibody; these committed, highly differentiated cells are not phagocytic.

      (a) These antibodies circulate, encounter antigens, and bind to them, producing cytokine reaction, which attracts macrophages/NK cells

     (5) Memory B cells are capable of recognizing a particular antigen at either future exposures or at other body sites; they produce plasma cells to generate an antibody specific to the antigen

    b. Cell-mediated immunity: T lymphocytes (Petersone & Walker, 2022).

     (1) T precursor cells migrate to thymus (primary lymphoid tissue) to mature into CD4+ helper T cells or CD8+ cytotoxic T cells, which then migrate to the secondary lymphoid organs as inactivated or naïve cells.

     (2) Antigens are presented to naïve T cells by APCs (macrophages or DCs).

     (3) T lymphocytes specific to the presented antigen are produced: MHC class II molecules on APCs activate CD4+ T cells, and MHC class I molecules on APCs activate CD8+ T cells in the presence of costimulatory signals. This process activates T cells.

c. Activated T cells multiply, producing cytokines, and are released into lymphatic fluid from the bloodstream to navigate back and forth and perform their functions as previously mentioned.

d. T-lymphocyte memory cells are produced and respond by activating T lymphocytes when exposed to the same antigen in the future.

e. Cytotoxic T cells and NK cells are capable of directly attacking other cells and destroying them.

B. Autoimmunity—loss of immune tolerance to the body's own tissues

1. Occurs after destruction of body's own tissues when self-antigens are circulated, and cause acquired immunity with activated T cell or antibodies.

V. Tumor immunology (Desai, Coxon, & Dunn, 2022)

A. Tumor recognition and rejection:

1. Cytotoxic immune response requires a complex interaction of the innate and adaptive immune systems to identify malignant cells and kill them.

a. Cancer progression occurs due to the evolution of mutated tumor cells, which evades the immune system over time, leading to immune-resistant clones, called cancer immunoediting

b. Extrinsic tumor suppressor mechanism (NK cells, T cells, B cells, and DCs) engages in three sequential phases:

(1) Elimination—innate and adaptive immunity destroy growing tumors before they are clinically measurable.

(a) Called immune surveillance

(b) The host remains cancer free due to the host immune system

(2) Equilibrium—a rare cancer clone acquires resistance to elimination by the immune system, where its growth is stabilized by the adaptive immune system; the innate system can no longer keep tumor in check.

(a) Rare tumor clones persist and can enter into the escape phase if immune balance is tipped towards suppression in tumor microenvironment.

(b) Usually the longest phase.

(3) Escape—persistent tumor clones have acquired the ability to evade the adaptive immune system, and clinical disease is apparent. Tumor cells that emerge are:

(a) No longer recognized by the adaptive immune system due to antigen loss/alteration of variants, and/or defects in tumor antigen processing or presentation.

(b) Insensitive to immune effector mechanisms, such as upregulating immune checkpoint molecules, like PD1 and PDL-1, which promote T-cell exhaustion and dysfunction.

(c) Able to induce an immunosuppressive state within the tumor microenvironment by manipulation of cytokines.

(d) Goal of treatment in this phase is to return to elimination or equilibrium phase.

B. Tumor immunogenicity (Aburg, 2018; Liu & Sun, 2021)

1. Defined as the ability of a tumor to induce an antitumor adaptive immune response.

a. Influenced by the infiltration of T cells into the tumor. Increasing T cells into a tumor allows for tumor antigen release, tumor antigen processing and presentation, T-cell priming and activation, the movement of T cells in circulation to tumors.

2. Vaccination—passive immunity through artificial injection of selected molecules to elicit a T-cell and B-cell-mediated responses.

a. Laboratory processed solution containing tumor-associated antigen, harvested from a tumor's surface, loaded with a substance that signals the immune system to stimulate an immune response. Solution is injected into host and taken up by APC and presented to MHC complex; this presents to naïve CD4+ and CD8+ T cells and B cells in the lymph nodes to sign their maturation and differentiation. Circulating antigen-specific cytotoxic T cells lyse the "foreign" antigen through immune-mediated pathways and produce lasting antitumor memory B and T cells.

b. Two types:

(1) Prophylactic vaccine to protect against carcinogenic viruses

(2) Therapeutic vaccine injected directly into tumors

REFERENCES

Aburg, K. D. (2018). Active immunity: vaccine therapy. In S. Walker & E. P. Dunphy (Eds.), *Guide to cancer immunotherapy*. Pittsburgh, PA: Oncology Nursing Society.

Actor, J. K. (2019). *Introductory immunology* (2nd ed.). San Diego, CA: Elsevier Inc.

Desai, R., Coxon, A. T., & Dunn, G. P. (2022). Therapeutic applications of the cancer immunoediting hypothesis. *Seminars in Cancer Biology, 78*, 63–77. https://doi.org/10.1016/j.semcancer.2021.03.002.

Doan, T., Lievano, F., Swanson-Mungerson, M., & Viselli, S. (2022). *Immunology* (3rd ed.). Philadelphia, PA: Wolters Kluwer.

Gutzeit, C., Chen, K., & Cerutti, A. (2018). The enigmatic function of IgD: Some answers at last. *European Journal of Immunology, 48*(7), 1101–1113. https://doi.org/10.1002/eji.201646547.

Guyton, A. C., Hall, J. E., & Hall, M. E. (2021). Resistance of the body to infection: *Guyton and Hall textbook of medical physiology* (14th ed.). Philadelphia, PA: Elsevier Inc.

Johnston, R. B. (2022). *An overview of the innate immune system*. Waltham, MA: UpToDate. https://www.uptodate.com/contents/an-overview-of-the-innate-immune-system?search=innate%20immune%20system&source=search_result&selectedTitle=1~150&usage_type=default&display_rank=1.

Liu, Y.-T., & Sun, Z.-J. (2021). Turning cold tumors into hot tumors by improving T-cell infiltration. *Theranostics, 11*(11), 5365–5386. https://www.thno.org/v11p5365.htm.

Petersone, L., & Walker, L. S. K. (2022). Activation of CD4+ T lymphocyte. In L. H. Butterfield, H. K. Kaufman, & F. M. Marincola (Eds.), *Cancer immunotherapy principles and practice* (2nd ed.). New York, NY: Springer Publishing Company.

Zhang, Y., Gao, S., Xia, J., & Liu, F. (2018). Hematopoietic hierarchy – An updated roadmap. *Trends in Cell Biology, 28*(12), 976–986. https://doi.org/10.1016/j.tcb.2018.06.001.

9

Precision Medicine

Marlon Garzo Saría and Santosh Kesari

I. Definition
   A. Use of specific information about an individual's biology, environment, and lifestyle choices to prevent, diagnose, and treat disease (Lee, Hamideh, & Nebeker, 2019).
   B. Customized treatment according to the biological characteristics of individuals or population subgroups increases efficiency and reduces health care costs (Lopes-Júnior, 2021).
   C. Not to be confused with *personalized medicine*, where the patient is viewed as an individual from diagnosis to therapy; does not intrinsically depend on large data sets or population-based approaches to redefine disease (Ho et al., 2020).
   D. Precision Medicine Initiative (PMI) was first introduced in 2015 to support research that explores the genetics of cancer, improve access to personalized health information, and collect data from a diverse national cohort (Lee et al., 2019).
      1. All of Us Research Program, a major component of the PMI, seeks to create a research repository consisting of biospecimens, electronic health records, physical measurements, and lifestyle data from 1 million US participants (For further reading, visit https://allofus.nih.gov/)
   E. Table 9.1 provides a glossary of terms to help understand precision medicine.
II. Applications of precision medicine
   A. Hereditary cancer risk assessment: identifying patients and families who may be at increased risk of developing certain types of cancer (ACOG, 2019).
      1. Hereditary Breast and Ovarian Cancer Syndrome: *BRCA1* and *BRCA2* (most common); *ATM, BRIP1, CDH1, CHEK2, NBN, NF1, PALB2, RAD51C, RAD51D*
      2. Lynch Syndrome (hereditary nonpolyposis colorectal cancer): *MLH1, MSH2, MSH6, PMS2,* and *EPCAM*
      3. Li–Fraumeni syndrome: *TP53*
      4. Cowden syndrome: *PTEN*
      5. Peutz–Jeghers syndrome: *STK11*
      6. Hereditary diffuse gastric cancer: *CDH1*
   B. Cancer prediction models and tools: key element of precision medicine and population health management; predicts disease risk and clinical outcomes to tailor preventive strategies and therapeutic treatments for individuals most likely to benefit (Waters et al., 2020)
      1. Breast Cancer Risk Assessment Tool: estimates a woman's risk of developing invasive breast cancer over the next 5 years and up to age 90 (National Cancer Institute, 2017)
         a. Age
         b. Age at the start of menstruation
         c. Age at first live birth of a child
         d. Number of first-degree relative (mother, sisters, daughters) with breast cancer
         e. Number of previous breast biopsies (whether positive or negative)
         f. Presence of atypical hyperplasia in a biopsy
      2. Melanoma Risk Assessment Tool: estimates a person's risk of developing invasive melanoma (National Cancer Institute, 2008)
         a. Demographics (age, gender, race)
         b. Prior sunburns
         c. Complexion
         d. Current number and size of skin moles
         e. Extent of freckling
      3. Partin tables: show the probability that prostate cancer is confined to the prostate, presence of lymphatic invasion, seminal vesicle involvement, or lymph node metastases (Johns Hopkins University, 2022)
         a. Serum prostate-specific antigen level
         b. Clinical stage
         c. Gleason score
      4. Colorectal cancer risk assessment tool: uses the information about risk and preventive factors to calculate a patient's absolute risk of colorectal cancer for a specific time period (National Cancer Institute, 2019)
         a. Demographics
         b. Diet and physical activity
         c. Medical history
         d. Family history
      5. Cancer of the Lung Evaluation and Assessment of Risk: determines a smoker's risk for developing lung cancer in the next 5, 10, or 15 years (Doyle-Lindrud, 2015). Many other lung cancer risk assessment tools are available, including Spitz, Liverpool Lung Project,

TABLE 9.1 Precision Medicine Glossary

Mechanisms of Decision

Precision medicine	Use of therapeutics that are expected to confer benefit to a subset of patients whose cancer displays specific molecular or cellular features
Pharmacogenomics	The study of how genomic variation within the individual or their disease (including gene expression, epigenetics, germline, and somatic pathogenic variants) influences his/her response to drugs
Stratified medicine	The use of a molecular assay to define subpopulations, rather than individuals, who are likely to benefit from a treatment intervention
Molecular tumor board	A multidisciplinary tumor board encompassing molecular biologists, geneticists, and bioinformaticians discussing not only the classical radiological, clinical, and standard biological data of the patient but also the modern molecular diagnostic tests

Characteristics of Molecular Alterations

Mutation/genomic Variant	An alteration in the most common DNA/RNA nucleotide sequence. Variants are defined based on the type of DNA/RNA error. The term variant can be used to describe an alteration that may be benign, pathogenic, or of unknown significance. Variants may be germline (inherited) or somatic (acquired). The term variant is used in place of the term mutation.
Cancer gene	Altered forms of normal cell genes that through pathogenic changes can promote cancer development and progression
Driver variant	A somatic genomic alteration that provides a critical role in the development and/or maintenance of the tumor malignant phenotype, including cancer initiation, progression, maintenance, or growth
	Provides a growth advantage of the cell and is involved in oncoogenesis
Passenger variant	A somatic genomic alteration within either a coding or non-coding region of the genome that does not confer a selective growth advantage under a given set of selective pressures
Oncogene addiction	Describes tumor that becomes dependent on the expression and function of driver genes and its ablation negatively impacts tumor maintenance and progression
Pathogenic variant	An alteration that may be inherited (germline) or acquired (somatic) and predisposes an individual to a specific disease
	Directly contributes to the development of disease. Additional evidence is not expected to alter the classification of this variant.
Deleterious variant	Older term that has been replace with pathogenic or likely pathogenic variant. See pathogenic variant
Targetable genomic alteration/druggable genomic alteration	A genomic alteration that encodes an altered protein against which a drug exists or can be synthesized
Actionable genomic alteration	Includes both targetable alterations and genomic alterations that cannot be directly targeted but that lead to dysregulation of a pathway in which there are possible targets
Point variant	Focal alteration in genomic DNA including single or double nucleotide substitutions
Insertion/deletion Variants	Insertions and deletions of (referred to as "indels") that are typically small (1–5 bp) and less frequently medium, from 100 bp up to 30 kb or long (more than 30 kb)
	Insertion is a type of variant involving the addition of genetic material. An insertion variant can be small, involving a single extra DNA base pair, or large, involving a piece of a chromosome. Deletion is a type of variant involving the loss of genetic material. It can be small, involving a single missing DNA base pair, or large, involving a piece of a chromosome
Structural variant (preferred)/genomic rearrangement	Changes in the orientation, location, or number of copies of segments of genomic DNA
Copy number variation (germline)	Germline copy number variants that contribute toward interindividual genomic variability and may predispose to various inherited medical disorders
Copy number alteration (somatic)	A change in copy number that has arisen in somatic cells including cancer cells
	A copy number variation (CNV) is when the number of copies of a particular gene varies from one individual to the next. Following the completion of the Human Genome Project, it became apparent that the genome experiences gains and losses of genetic material. The extent to which copy number variation contributes to human disease is not yet known. It has long been recognized that some cancers are associated with elevated copy numbers of particular genes
Gene amplification	A copy number increase of a restricted chromosomal region
Copy number gain	Gain of a chromosomal segment or even whole chromosome/chromosome arm resulting in a regional copy number that exceeds the background genome ploidy
Homozygous deletion	Bi-allelic loss of a segment of DNA arising through independent overlapping deletions involving both chromosomes

Tumor Characteristics

Intratumor heterogeneity	Multiple subclonal populations of cancer cells that differ in their genomic, epigenomic, transcriptional, morphological, or behavioral features within an individual tumor

continued

TABLE 9.1   Precision Medicine Glossary—cont'd

Intertumor heterogeneity	Genomic, epigenomic, transcriptional, pathological, or clinical differences between individuals' cancers
Clonal evolution	The mechanism by which a cancer develops from a once normal cell, through a reiterative process of pathogenic variant accumulation, clonal selection, and clonal expansion
Cancer clone	Cancer cells derived from the same ancestral cell
Cancer subclone	The progeny of a pathogenically altered cell arising within a cancer clone
Circulating tumor cells	Cells that have been shed from a tumor into body fluids (i.e., blood, cerebrospinal fluid) and can provide information about the molecular characteristics of the tumor of the patient
Cell-free circulating tumor DNA	DNA derived from tumor cells that is found extracellular, circulating in bodily fluids (i.e., blood, cerebrospinal fluid) that can provide information about the molecular characteristics of the tumor of the patient
Extracellular vesicles	Cell-derived nano-sized vesicles generated by cell membrane shedding or vesicle exocytosis that carry tumor-derived nucleic acids and proteins and can provide information about the molecular characteristics of the tumor of the patient
Clinical Trials and Statistics	
Basket trial	Biomarker-based, randomized, or nonrandomized clinical trial that includes multiple histologies investigating a therapeutic intervention, such as a drug or a drug combination targeting a specific molecular aberration across different cancer types
Umbrella trial	Biomarker-based, randomized, or nonrandomized clinical trial that is histology-specific investigating different therapeutic interventions, such as different drugs or drug combinations, matched to different molecular aberrations in a single cancer type
Adaptive trial	Clinical trial that includes a prospectively planned opportunity for modification of one or more specified aspects of the study design and hypotheses based on analysis of data (usually interim data) from subjects in the study
N-of-one trial	Clinical trial of a single subject investigating a specific therapeutic intervention, such as a drug or a drug combination

Adapted from Yates, L. R., Seoane, J., Le Tourneau, C., Siu, L. L., Marais, R., Michiels, S., et al. (2018). The European Society for Medical Oncology (ESMO) precision medicine glossary. *Annals of Oncology, 29*(1), 30–35, ISSN 0923-7534. https://doi.org/10.1093/annonc/mdx707.

Hoggart, and Prostate, Lung, Colorectal, and Ovarian (American Association for Thoracic Surgery, 2016).
  a. Smoking history
  b. Age and gender
  c. Medical history
  d. Family history of cancer
  e. Prior exposures to asbestos
C. Individualization of diagnosis, prognosis, and therapy for each patient by using sophisticated molecular diagnostics and imaging made possible by recent technologic advances (McAlister, Laupacis, & Armstrong, 2017)
D. Pharmacogenomics (Dodson, 2017)
  1. Integration of pharmacology and genomics in developing safe and effective medications
  2. Dose determination based on genomics
  3. Types of tests include
    a. Drug disposition testing: drug disposition genes can alter the pharmacokinetics of a drug
      (1) *CYP2D6*, a drug disposition gene, generates the metabolite endoxifen from tamoxifen
      (2) Endoxifen is 100 times more potent than the parent drug tamoxifen
      (3) High CYP2D6 activity (rapid metabolizers) has significantly higher serum concentrations of endoxifen
      (4) High CYP2D6 activity has been associated with higher relapse-free survival rates
    b. Drug target testing: drug target genes can change the pharmacodynamics of a drug
      (1) UGT1A1 is an active metabolite of irinotecan
      (2) Low activity of UGT1A1 enzyme associated with increased serum concentration of the active metabolite, which increases the risk of adverse events, particularly neutropenia
      (3) Patients with two identical UGT1A1*28 alleles, which have a lower enzyme expression and activity, have a significantly higher risk of neutropenia compared with patients carrying UGT1A1*1 (normal allele)
      (4) Food and Drug Administration (FDA) recommended reduced irinotecan dose for patients with UGT1A1*28/*28
    c. Targeted cancer therapies: most common type of test within oncology practice; involves the use of genetic and genomic information of the cancer tissue to guide the selection of an appropriate targeted drug therapy
E. Identification of therapeutic targets (Akhoon, 2021)
  1. Design therapies to more precisely target cancer cells through two primary methods:
    a. selectively disrupting pathways necessary for cancer cell survival or growth (pathway-based targeted therapy)
    b. artificially modulating patients' immune systems to generate a response against cancer cells (immunotherapy)
  2. Table 9.2 provides a list of common cancers, actionable pathogenic variants, and targeted therapies.

TABLE 9.2 Selected Common Cancers, Actionable Pathogenic Variants, and Targeted Therapy (Brant, & Mayer, 2017)

Actionable Pathogenic Variant	Cancer Type	Targeted Therapy
ALK	Lung (nonsmall cell), lymphoma (large cell), neuroblastoma	Alectinib, brigatinib, crizotinib, ceritinib
BCL-2	Chronic lymphocytic leukemia	Venetoclax
BCR-ABL	Chronic myelogenous leukemia	Bafetinib, bosutinib, dasatinib, imatinib, nilotinib, ponatinib
BRAF	Colorectal, melanoma, ovarian, thyroid	Cobimetinib, dabrafenib, trametinib, vemurafenib
EGFR	Lung, colon	Afatinib, gefitinib, imatinib, osimertinib
FLT3	Acute myeloid leukemia, mastocytosis	Lestaurtinib, midostaurin, sorafenib, sunitinib
Histone deacetylase	Lymphoma (T-cell cutaneous), multiple myeloma	Panobinostat, romidepsin, vorinostat
Her2	Brain, breast, lung, ovarian, stomach	Pertuzumab, trastuzumab
KRAS	Colorectal, lung, pancreatic	Cetuximab and panitumumab
mTOR	Astrocytoma (subependymal giant cell), breast, pancreatic (neuroendocrine), renal	Everolimus, ridaforolimus, temsirolimus
MET (c-MET)	Lung (nonsmall cell), medullary thyroid	Cabozantinib, crizotinib
PARP	*BRCA* pathogenic variants (germline or somatic), fallopian tube, ovarian (epithelial), peritoneal	Niraparib, olaparib, rucaparib
PDL-1	Head and neck squamous cell, Hodgkin lymphoma, Merkel cell carcinoma, urothelial carcinoma	Atezolizumab, avelumab, durvalumab, nivolumab, pembrolizumab

Author's note: The development of new anticancer agents is one of the most rapidly changing aspects of cancer research. Information provided in this table may not be the most current after publication. Refer to the National Cancer Institute for the most up-to-date information: https://www.cancer.gov/about-cancer/treatment/types/targeted-therapies/targeted-therapies-fact-sheet.
Modified from Brant, J. M., & Mayer, D. K. (2017). Precision medicine: Accelerating the science to revolutionize cancer care. *Clinical Journal of Oncology Nursing, 21*(6), 722–729. https://doi.org/10.1188/17.CJON.722-729.

3. For the most current list of FDA-approved targeted therapies and indications, refer to the Targeted Therapies Fact Sheet from the National Cancer Institute at https://www.cancer.gov/about-cancer/treatment/types/targeted-therapies/targeted-therapies-fact-sheet.

F. Ethical considerations (Jonsson & Stefansdottir, 2019)
   1. Consent: data collected and research aims often change over time; dynamic consent may solve some issues; presumed consent can be considered
   2. Additional findings: incidental results, also referred to as secondary findings, are findings that have potential health or reproductive importance and discovered during testing for an unrelated problem; issues related to communicating medically actionable additional findings
   3. Privacy in databanks used in precision medicine
   4. Justice: delivering the gains and progress of precision medicine consistent with equal rights to health care

G. Patient care considerations (Fu et al., 2019)
   1. Collection and inclusion of family health history and other social factors with *omic* data into patient care and electronic health record documentation
   2. Develop accurate and understandable information content and patient education tools about precision health
   3. Integrated precision health interventions into patient care workflows
   4. Establish reimbursement from third-party payors for precision health assessments
   5. Develop reliable and valid patient outcome measures that can be used to evaluate effective precision health implementation

REFERENCES

Akhoon, N. (2021). Precision medicine: A new paradigm in therapeutics. *International Journal of Preventive Medicine, 12*(1), 2. https://www.ncbi.nlm.nih.gov/pmc/articles/PMC8106271/.

American Association for Thoracic Surgery. Lung cancer risk assessment tool. (2016). https://www.sts.org/resources/lung-nodule-resources/lung-cancer-screening-guidelines.

American College of Obstetricians and Gynecologists. (2019). Hereditary cancer syndromes and risk assessment: ACOG committee opinion, number 793. *Obstetrics and Gynecology, 134*(6), e143–e149. https://doi.org/10.1097/AOG.0000000000003562.

Brant, J. M., & Mayer, D. K. (2017). Precision medicine: Accelerating the science to revolutionize cancer care. *Clinical Journal of Oncology Nursing, 21*(6), 722 -729. https://doi.org/10.1188/17.CJON.722-729.

Dodson, C. H. (2017). Pharmacogenomics: Principles and relevance to oncology nursing. *Clinical Journal of Oncology Nursing, 21*(6), 739–745. https://doi.org/10.1188/17.CJON.739-745.

Doyle-Lindrud, S. (2015). Risk prediction tools in oncology. *Clinical Journal of Oncology Nursing, 19*(6), 665–666. https://doi.org/10.1188/15.CJON.665-666.

Fu, M. R., Kurnat-Thoma, E., Starkweather, A., Henderson, W. A., Cashion, A. K., Williams, J. K., et al. (2020). Precision health: A nursing perspective. *International Journal of Nursing Sciences, 7*(1), 5–12. https://doi.org/10.1016/j.ijnss.2019.12.008.

Ho, D., Quake, S. R., McCabe, E., Chng, W. J., Chow, E. K., Ding, X., et al. (2020). Enabling technologies for personalized and precision medicine. *Trends in Biotechnology, 38*(5), 497–518. https://doi.org/10.1016/j.tibtech.2019.12.021.

Johns Hopkins University. New Partin nomogram. (2022). https://www.hopkinsmedicine.org/brady-urology-institute/conditions_and_treatments/prostate_cancer/risk_assessment_tools/partin-tables.html.

Jonsson, J. J., & Stefansdottir, V. (2019). Ethical issues in precision medicine. *Annals of Clinical Biochemistry, 56*(6), 628–629. https://doi.org/10.1177/0004563219870824.

Lee, J., Hamideh, D., & Nebeker, C. (2019). Qualifying and quantifying the precision medicine rhetoric. *BMC Genomics, 20*(1), 868. https://doi.org/10.1186/s12864-019-6242-8.

Lopes-Júnior, L. C. (2021). Personalized nursing care in precision-medicine era. *SAGE Open Nursing, 7*, 23779608211064713. https://doi.org/10.1177/23779608211064713.

McAlister, F. A., Laupacis, A., & Armstrong, P. W. (2017). Finding the right balance between precision medicine and personalized care. *Canadian Medical Association Journal, 189*(33), E1065–E1068. https://doi.org/10.1503/cmaj.170107.

National Cancer Institute. Melanoma risk assessment tool. (2008). https://www.cancer.gov/melanomarisktool/.

National Cancer Institute. Breast cancer risk assessment tool. (2017). https://www.cancer.gov/bcrisktool/.

National Cancer Institute. Colorectal cancer risk assessment tool. (2019). https://ccrisktool.cancer.gov/index.html.

Oncology Nursing Society. *Genomics Taxonomy Terms Table of Contents.* (2023). https://www.ons.org/genomics-taxonomy/genomics-taxonomy-terms-table-contents.

Waters, E. A., Taber, J. M., McQueen, A., Housten, A. J., Studts, J. L., & Scherer, L. D. (2020). Translating cancer risk prediction models into personalized cancer risk assessment tools: Stumbling blocks and strategies for success. *Cancer Epidemiology, Biomarkers & Prevention, 29*(12), 2389–2394. https://doi.org/10.1158/1055-9965.EPI-20-0861.

10

Genetics and Cancer

Aida Akopyan, Kimberly Childers, Ora K. Gordon, and Martha Inofuentes

OVERVIEW

I. The "central dogma" of molecular biology, that is, "DNA makes RNA, and RNA makes protein," guides the production of protein for all bodily functions (Nussbaum, McInnes, & Willard, 2016).

  A. Cancer has a multifactorial etiology with genetic, environmental, lifestyle, aging, hormonal, and other factors all interacting to produce a malignant transformation.

  B. All cancer is "genetic"—meaning that it is due to changes in the deoxyribonucleic acid (DNA). Genetic pathogenic variants and genetic instability are at the core of cancer development (Mahon, 2020).

  C. The genetic changes that cause cancer can be either inherited or acquired over a person's lifetime. In most cases, they are acquired.

    1. Inherited genetic changes are called "germline"—meaning they are present from the time of birth. These are passed down through generations and cause an increased risk for various kinds of cancer. Inherited cancer encompasses both "hereditary" and "familial" cancer types.

    2. Acquired genetic changes are called "somatic." They arise due to factors like environmental exposures, lifestyle (alcohol, smoking, obesity/diet), hormonal factors, or simply the aging process. They are present in the cell that eventually becomes a cancer and are NOT passed down through the generations. This is also called "sporadic" cancer (Mahon, 2020).

  D. It typically takes many genetic changes to cause cancer to develop. Inherited genetic changes present at birth increase an individual's risk, but additional acquired genetic changes must still occur in a cell for cancer to develop (Mahon, 2020).

II. Genetics primer (Nussbaum et al., 2016)

  A. Chromosomes are threadlike structures of DNA containing genetic information.

  B. There are 46 chromosomes per cell which include 23 chromosome pairs—one copy from each parent.

    1. The small arm of the chromosome is identified as the "petite," or "p," arm.

    2. The long arm is labeled the "q" arm because "q" follows "p" in the alphabet.

  C. Two types of nucleic acid exist.

    1. DNA comprises two nucleotide chains, which are held together by oxygen bonds, and coiled around one another to form a double helix. Two bases:

      a. Purines: adenine (A) and guanine (G).

      b. Pyrimidines: thymine (T) and cytosine (C).

      c. DNA base pairs are complementary: A attaches to T, and G attaches to C.

    2. Ribonucleic acid (RNA) consists of a single nucleotide chain and represents a complimentary copy of a strand of DNA.

      a. DNA sequence order determines the RNA sequence, which codes for amino acids and the protein.

      b. In RNA, the base uracil (U) replaces thymine (T).

      c. Transcription refers to the process of making RNA from DNA (Fig. 10.1).

        (1) Loosening DNA wound around the histone allows transcription.

        (2) Tightening the DNA around the histone prevents transcription.

      d. Primary types of RNA

        (1) Messenger RNA (mRNA) directs the order of the amino acids in a protein.

        (2) A codon is a sequence of three mRNA nucleotides which yields one of the 20 amino acids (e.g., the codon ACG is translated into the amino acid threonine).

        (3) There is redundancy in the code. Multiple codons can code for the same amino acid (e.g., ACC and ACG both code for threonine).

        (4) A change in the first position of the codon will usually cause a different amino acid to be produced, causing an error in building the protein.

        (5) An mRNA nucleotide change in the third position of the codon rarely causes an amino acid change.

        (6) Changes in the DNA sequence result in changes to the mRNA sequence. Harmful changes are frequently referred to as pathogenic variants, or more formally known as pathogenic variants. Conversely, polymorphisms are common and oftentimes do not have a negative impact on protein function (clinically benign).

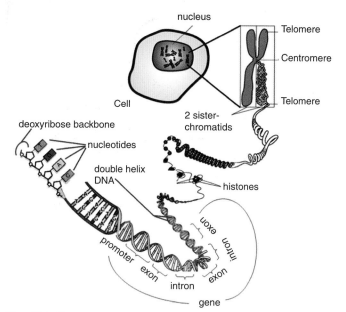

Fig. 10.1 Chromosome and gene structure. Courtesy the National Human Genome Research Institute, Bethesda, MD.

D. Single nucleotide variant (SNV; also referred to as a single nucleotide polymorphism [SNP]): a single nucleotide change causing variation in the DNA sequence (these affect at least 1% of the population) (National Cancer Institute [NCI], n.d.c; Nussbaum et al., 2016).

1. Genome-wide association studies (GWAS) help scientists identify genes associated with a particular disease (or another trait). This method studies the entire set of DNA (the genome) of a large group of people, searching for small variations (SNVs). Each study can look at hundreds or thousands of SNVs at the same time. Scientists can then identify SNVs that occur more frequently in people with a certain disease than in people without it.

2. An SNV may or may not have an influence on traits or health conditions. Alone, an SNV may cause a small increase in risk for disease (including cancer). Cumulatively, however, many SNVs together can cause a more significant risk for cancer. To date, this is best described in "familial" breast, prostate, and colorectal cancer cohorts (Black et al., 2020; Jenkins et al., 2019; Mavaddat et al., 2019).

3. Pathogenic Variant: a permanent alteration of nucleotide sequence of a gene causing a rare and abnormal variant; more likely responsible for a disease. Pathogenic Variants are now called pathogenic variants on clinical molecular tests.

    a. Translation refers to the process of creating protein using chains of amino acids coded for by mRNA.

    (1) A variety of RNA types are involved in the protein development process, including transfer RNA (tRNA), ribosomal RNA (rRNA), small silencing RNAs (smRNA), piwi interacting RNAs (piRNA), and small interfering RNA (siRNA) (Gorski, Vogel, & Doudna, 2017; Siomi et al., 2016).

    (2) The amino acid sequence determines the structure of the protein.

    (3) Genetic changes leading to changes in the amino acid sequence and subsequent protein structure can be a contributing factor to the development of cancer.

E. Genes are individual units of hereditary information located at a specific position on a chromosome.

1. Genes consist primarily of exons and introns.

    a. Exons: protein-coding segments of a gene

    b. Introns: non–protein-coding segments; the sequence-interrupting piece of a gene

F. Epigenetics: the process of switching genes on and off with a variety of "chemical tails" attached to the DNA structure without changing the DNA sequence (Centers for Disease Control [CDC], 2022).

1. DNA transcription is controlled by opening or closing tightly wound histone structures.

2. This occurs by opening (allowing transcription) and closing the histone structure to alter the "DNA to RNA to protein" outcome.

3. Diet, exercise, aging, drugs, and environmental exposures can affect epigenetics positively or negatively.

4. Genomic imprinting is a form of epigenetic inheritance in which the regulation of a gene or chromosomal region is dependent on the sex of the transmitting parent. During gametogenesis, imprinted regions of DNA are differentially marked in accordance to the sex of the parent, resulting in parent-specific expression. This "parent-of-origin" effect is observed in certain hereditary cancer syndromes, such as with the SDHD gene in hereditary paraganglioma-pheochromocytoma (PGL-PCC) syndrome. SDHD pathogenic variants cause an increased risk for PGL/PCC when paternally inherited, but NOT when maternally inherited (Baysal, 2004).

III. Types of genetic changes and mechanism of cancer development

A. Pathogenic Variants (Mahon, 2020)

1. Pathogenic Variants significantly impact protein function. A variety of pathogenic variants types result in an altered form or different protein than required for the correct function of a gene; pathogenic variant include frameshift, missense, nonsense, splicing changes (Griffiths, Miller, & Suzuki, 2000).

2. Germline pathogenic variants occur in the reproductive cells (egg or sperm) of a person with an inherited predisposition to cancer. These cause hereditary cancer.

3. Somatic pathogenic variants occur in body cells (except gametes) after conception and are acquired over a lifetime. These cause sporadic cancer.

B. Chromosomal abnormalities—all of which can cause cancer development but are typically somatic (Nussbaum et al., 2016)

1. Translocations refer to segments of one chromosome that break off and attach themselves to other chromosomes, resulting in altered protein production. Occur often in some types of cancer—like hematologic malignancies.
2. Aneuploidy is an abnormal number of chromosomes.
3. Loss of heterozygosity refers to the loss of the second segment of both copies (alleles) of a chromosome.
4. Microsatellite instability (MSI) is a change in the DNA in some cells, like tumor cells, where short, repeated sequences of nucleotide repeats (microsatellites) are different from the inherited DNA. MSI is a signature feature to indicate the possibility of Lynch syndrome (LS)—a germline abnormality in mismatch-repair (MMR) genes related to risk for colorectal, endometrial, and other cancers (NCCN, 2021). Importantly, MSI can also occur sporadically. The presence of MSI is an indication of a better response to certain kinds of immunotherapies in cancer treatment. MSI is a surrogate for MMR deficiency (MMRd), and MMRd is now routinely reported on anatomic pathology reports and somatic tumor molecular tests.

C. Types of genes involved in cancer risk and development
1. A malignant tumor is derived from genetic instability and pathogenic variants in genes that control cell growth and proliferation.
2. Regulatory genes (NCI, n.d.b; Nussbaum et al., 2016)
   a. Proto-oncogenes: normal genes essential for usual cell growth and regulation. pathogenic variants occurring in proto-oncogenes convert to oncogene activation to cause uncontrolled cell division. These are almost always somatic pathogenic variants and NOT inherited (e.g., *HER2*). There are rare germline inherited cancer risks caused by proto-oncogenes (e.g., *RET*).
   b. Tumor suppressor genes: function as regulators of cell growth (e.g., *TP53*). Some tumor suppressor genes appear to play a role in cell cycle regulation or DNA repair. Pathogenic Variant of a tumor suppressor gene may cause uncontrolled cell growth. Pathogenic Variants in these kinds of genes occur in both germline and somatic settings.
   c. DNA repair genes
      (1) MMR genes: a type of DNA repair gene responsible for keeping the DNA free of erroneous insertions or deletions during DNA synthesis; associated with MSI and LS. This can be tested for in the tumor through immunohistochemical (IHC) testing or MSI testing. LS is the result of a germline pathogenic variant in any gene in the MMR family—MLH1, MSH2, MSH6, and PMS2. Pathogenic Variants in these genes make patients eligible for certain kinds of immunotherapy (Keytruda) regardless of whether inherited or somatic.
      (2) Homologous recombination repair genes: a type of DNA repair gene responsible for repairing double-strand breaks during DNA synthesis; associated with *many* inherited cancer genes including *BRCA1/2*, *PALB2*, and *RAD51C*. pathogenic variants in these genes make patients eligible for certain kinds of immunotherapy (PARPi therapy) whether inherited or somatic.
      (3) Mutator gene-phenotype/high mutational burden
         (a) Allows increased pathogenic variant of genes due to poor proofreading or insertion of incorrect nucleotides left unrepaired.
         (b) Efficient at acquiring pathogenic variants with both clonal and random pathogenic variants allowing thousands of pathogenic variants versus lower rates seen with normal cells (Loeb, 2016).
         (c) On somatic testing for cancer, this is known as "high pathogenic variant burden" and can indicate certain chemotherapeutic choices.
      (4) Driver and passenger pathogenic variants.
         (a) Driver pathogenic variants unrepaired DNA damage with an increased chance of oncogene pathogenic variants. These pathogenic variants offer a selective growth advantage and are the targets for specific therapies such as ALK, EGFR, tyrosine kinase inhibitors, and PIK3.
         (b) Passenger pathogenic variants nucleotide changes that *do not* provide a growth advantage. These are not expected to predict response to individual therapies.

IV. Types of inherited cancer risk—hereditary versus familial
A. At least 10% of all cancers are considered to be hereditary. This percentage varies based on cancer type. Certain cancers, such as ovarian and medullary thyroid, are more likely to be hereditary than other types of cancer (upwards of 20% of these cases may be hereditary) (NCI, 2017; Walsh et al., 2011).
B. More than 100 genes have been found to cause hereditary cancer syndromes (NCCN, 2020).
C. Familial cancer may represent cases where a single hereditary cause is not identified but a significant family history remains, such as multiple individuals on the same side of the family with breast cancer. This is often due to a combination of environmental and inherited factors (like SNVs). Familial cancers make up ~15%–20% of all cancers diagnosed. This percentage again varies based on cancer type. Familial risk is typically lower than the risk associated with a hereditary syndrome.

V. Genetic testing
A. Germline testing for hereditary cancer risk
1. Historically, single genes or related genes were tested by sequencing one at a time (e.g., BRCA1/2

or LS-MLH1/MSH2/MSH6/PMS2). Though this still occurs, most hereditary testing is now done as part next-generation sequencing (NGS) panels that included either all genes related to an organ site (breast or colon) or are "pan cancer" up to very comprehensive 100 gene panels (Laduca et al., 2020).

2. Patients who had hereditary cancer testing in the past (prior to 2014) should thus be offered updated testing to a more current comprehensive gene panel.

B. Tumor profiling

1. Offered by many commercial laboratories to identify a range of things from risk of recurrence to tumor type to medication targets.

2. Utilizes varying technologies—RNA expression assays, sequencing, methylation, pathogenic variant burden.

3. Can identify both somatic and germline pathogenic variants depending on the gene and/or pathogenic variants identified, this may trigger separate germline testing (e.g., *BRCA1/2* pathogenic variant on tumor profiling regardless of the cancer type) (DeLeonardis, Hogan, Cannistra, Rangachari, & Tung, 2019).

4. Somatic tumor profiles can evolve over time—both as the cancer develops and in response to various therapies.

   a. Therefore, tumor profiling may be done multiple times over a given cancer course—often to identify novel chemotherapeutic agents.

   b. "Liquid biopsy" is one way in which tumor profiling can be done on a blood sample to monitor the course of disease over time (Siravegna et al., 2019).

C. Paired tumor/germline testing (Salvador et al., 2019)

1. For individuals with absence of IHC (e.g., loss of MSH6) or MSI on tumor testing, this can be either acquired (somatic) or hereditary (LS) (see the section on "MMR genes" above).

2. Some labs offer parallel (paired) testing of both the tumor and germline to clarify whether the patient has LS—associated with risks for other malignancies in the patient and hereditary risk for relatives—or somatic loss—not associated with additional cancer risks/family risks.

3. Outside of this, some somatic testing labs also offer germline testing (either paired or as reflex) for a variety of other somatic findings. Use caution, as germline testing may be limited in these cases. The patient may still benefit from further germline panel testing.

D. Direct-to-consumer (DTC) testing

1. Food and Drug Administration (FDA) approved *BRCA1/2* testing from 23andMe (U.S. Food & Drug Administration [FDA], 2019).

2. Includes only the three *BRCA1/2* (selected variants) pathogenic variants most common in persons of Ashkenazi descent (U.S. Food & Drug Administration [FDA], 2018).

3. DTC testing does often look at SNPs, related to possible "familial" diseases like breast cancer. Important to note that this may include SNPs in genes like BRCA1/2 that are NOT pathogenic variants and do NOT cause high inherited breast/ovarian cancer risk. Read reports carefully.

4. DTC testing is not meant to be used for the diagnosis of disease and/or clinical decision-making (FDA, 2018).

5. Many pathogenic variants identified on DTC testing are actually false positives; there can also be false negatives (Tandy-Connor et al., 2018).

6. "Raw data" from DTC testing can run through outside algorithms (like promethease) to obtain more data on SNPs, etc. This is even less reliable (Moscarello, Murray, Reuter, & Demo, 2019).

E. Predisposition genetic testing and tumor profiling techniques

1. Next-generation DNA sequencing (second-generation sequencing)

   a. Most commonly used now for hereditary cancer panels and tumor profiling.

   b. Can sequence many genes at once with appropriate coverage to identify pathogenic variants.

   c. Lower-cost, higher-efficiency technique to Sanger sequencing (described below).

   d. Detects single nucleotide changes as well as small insertions, deletions, variations in copy number (like a misspelled word, or a single word switched around or missing in a novel).

   e. More "variants of unknown significance" are identified given the large number of genes tested.

2. Direct sequencing (Sanger sequencing)

   a. Determines the sequence of a gene being tested and detects sequence changes in regions being analyzed.

   b. May miss pathogenic variants outside the coding region or pathogenic variants that are large genomic rearrangements (LGRs) or large deletions.

   c. The base of initial hereditary cancer testing offered; primarily used now to confirm pathogenic variants identified on NGS or other techniques.

3. LGRs via multiplex ligation-dependent probe amplification: detect large rearrangements, deletions, and duplications (like pages or paragraphs missing or rearranged in a novel) (Park et al., 2017).

   a. These alterations were not often identified on hereditary cancer testing prior to ~2010 as this testing only used Sanger sequencing. Now, it is common to have included on hereditary cancer panels. NOT commonly included on tumor profiling.

4. RNA analysis:

   a. Recently (~2020) launched with NGS for hereditary cancer testing to 1-classify VUSs by determining whether the RNA transcript is intact and 2-identify novel pathogenic variants in the introns of DNA which impact the RNA transcript.

   b. Relative increase in yield of ~9% over DNA testing alone (Landrith et al., 2020).

5. Whole-exome or whole-genome sequencing.
   a. Low-cost alternative technique to Sanger sequencing if necessary to sequence all exons (gene to protein-coding regions) of the genome or the entire genome
   b. Often used in "population screening" for hereditary cancer and other diseases; may thus incidentally identify individuals with inherited cancer risk
6. GWAS (NCI, n.d.a; Nussbaum et al., 2016).
   a. Used in research/discovery to survey the entire genome for small nucleotide alterations
   b. Purpose is to:
      (1) Detect SNVs (SNPs) or small pathogenic variants to determine association with disease.
      (2) Review for changes with specific disease (cancer type) versus people without the disease.
      (3) Aim is to obtain genetic data, with potential impact on personalized profiling for identifying risk, aiding in diagnosis, pharmacogenomics, and disease monitoring (Soon, Hariharan, & Snyder, 2013).
7. Cytogenetic reports include number of chromosomes, sex chromosome designation (XX or XY or aberrations of these chromosomes); abnormality abbreviation—first chromosome separated with a semicolon from the second chromosome t(14;16), then the arm and band number (q32; q23) (Palumbo & Russo, 2016).
   a. Not typically used in hereditary cancer testing—used in diagnosing hematologic malignancies and following bone marrow transplantation
8. Other genetic testing is available, including microarrays, transcriptome, protein truncation assays, histone modifications, and chromosome conformation.

VI. Ethical, legal, and social issues associated with genetic information (Nussbaum et al., 2016; Zaami et al., 2021)
A. Implications of predisposition genetic testing
   1. Predisposition genetic testing can empower patients by allowing them to take early steps in both cancer detection and prevention. A positive genetic test result may have important implications for the patient's cancer screening methodology and regimen. A positive result may be difficult to accept for some patients; for others, it may ease some of the patient's anxiety since the ambiguity of not knowing their pathogenic variant status is resolved.
   2. A negative test result can also have a powerful impact on an individual. When a patient undergoes genetic testing for a known familial variant, a "true negative" result provides necessary reassurance regarding the patient's own cancer risks (one would be at population risk in this case). Additionally, a negative genetic result may eliminate the need for enhanced surveillance and allow a patient to proceed with general population screening instead.
   3. Some individuals may feel guilt, anxiety, or depression associated with a positive genetic testing result in themselves or a relative. Appropriate pre-test genetic counseling aids in assessing the patient's readiness in pursuit of genetic testing and to allow the patient to express any concerns or questions.
   4. Intrafamilial issues may arise because predisposition genetic testing affects all family members.
   5. Various support groups and resources exist for individuals and families who are impacted by a genetic syndrome. It is of utmost importance to provide these types of resources to patients whenever appropriate.
B. Financial considerations:
   1. Genetic testing is now covered by most insurers when genetic testing criteria (NCCN, 2020) are met based on the patient's personal and/or family history.
   2. Many genetic testing laboratories offer reduced-cost testing or patient assistance for individuals whose insurance does not cover the cost of testing or for individuals who do not meet genetic testing criteria.
   3. Some genetic testing laboratories offer no-cost testing to family members of an individual who has tested positive for a pathogenic variant within a certain time frame from the report release date.
   4. Providers and patients work together with the patient's insurer to advocate for coverage of necessary screening and surgical intervention for individuals who test positive for a pathogenic variant. Coverage of necessary medical management is oftentimes based on medical guidelines (NCCN, 2021, 2022b).
C. Quality assurance of genetic testing laboratories:
   1. Most major clinical laboratories today are both certified by the Clinical Laboratory Improvement Amendments and accredited by the College of American Pathologists, ensuring quality and safety in the laboratory and laboratory results.
   2. Clinical genetic testing laboratories may vary in their testing methodology and interpretation of genetic variants. Certain differences may include, but are not limited to, the inclusion of additional genes, RNA analysis, polygenic risk score, and extent of sequencing and deletions/duplication analysis of various genes. Different labs may have slightly differing point systems with regard to the classification of variants, thus resulting in conflicting classifications of the same variant at times. Most labs follow ACMG guidelines for the classification of variants (https://www.ncbi.nlm.nih.gov/pmc/articles/PMC4544753/).
   3. It is important to note that DTC laboratories may or may not meet the standards/certifications that are followed by clinical laboratories.
      a. DTC testing laboratories often perform genotyping rather than full gene sequencing and deletion/duplication analysis. Caution should be exercised in the interpretation of these results,

which generally are not appropriate for clinical management decision-making.

D. Legal issues may involve the following:
1. State and federal legislative approaches have been proposed or enacted, depending on the issue and state (NCCN, 2020).
   a. The Genetic Information Nondiscrimination Act (GINA), federal legislation enacted in 2008, applies to health insurance and employment discrimination based on genetic information (NCCN, 2020).
      (1) Health insurance protections include protection against accessing an individual's genomic information, requirements for an individual to undergo a genetic or genomic test, and using genomic information against a person during medical underwriting.
      (2) Employment protections include prohibiting employers from accessing an individual's genetic information, use of genomic information to deny employment, or collecting genomic information without consent.
      (3) GINA does not supersede state legislation that provides for more extensive protection.
      (4) GINA does not apply to active-duty military personnel, Veterans Administration, or Indian Health Service because the laws amended for GINA do not apply to these groups.
      (5) Of note, GINA does not protect the patient from potential discrimination from life, long-term care, and disability insurers. Oftentimes, it is recommended for a patient to obtain these policies, if desired, prior to pursuing predisposition genetic testing.
   b. The US Equal Employment Opportunity Commission released guidelines in March 1995 on the definition of "disability" under the Americans with Disabilities Act (ADA), which is now extended to include discrimination based on genetic information. This set of guidelines is not law but is an interpretation of the language of the ADA and may be overturned in a court of law (FDA, 2018).
2. Self-insured employers may also be exempt from state laws and regulations on health insurance because of the Employee Retirement Income Security Act of 1974, which governs employer pension plans as well as other benefits (U.S. Department of Labor, n.d.).

ASSESSMENT

I. Computer Prediction Models:
A. There are two types of computer prediction models used in genetics:

1. Those that identify the risk of having an inherited cancer risk pathogenic variant
2. Those that estimate the risk of developing a specific cancer
3. Some models do both

B. The following are commonly used models for risk assessment/pathogenic variant probability. This is not a comprehensive list as there are many additional models currently available.

C. Cancer Risk Assessment Models:
1. Breast: Gail (Breast Cancer Risk Assessment Tool)—assesses the risk to develop invasive breast cancer based on the number of first-degree relatives with breast cancer diagnosis, current age, race/ethnicity, age at menarche, age at menopause, age at first live birth, number of breast biopsies plus history of atypical hyperplasia, race/ethnicity (NCI, n.d.c).
   a. A Gail 5-year risk of >1.67% for breast cancer was used as threshold for chemoprevention trials with tamoxifen and raloxifene (Vogel, 2009).
   b. USPSTF no longer recommends a specific level of risk but generally benefits to risk favors greater than 3% 5-year risk.
2. Breast: Tyrer–Cuzick/IBIS—Now the most widely accepted model to determine screening guidelines for breast cancer. Assesses risk to develop invasive breast cancer with more comprehensive inputs than Gail. In addition to Gail inputs, TC/IBIS also accounts for the woman's family history (maternal and paternal) for first, second, and select third-degree relatives, breast density, height and body mass index, hormone replacement therapy use, and BRCA1/2 pathogenic variant status in patient/relatives. A lifetime risk of >20% is used by NCCN/ACS to determine women eligible for breast MRI screening (ACS, 2022; NCCN, 2021; 2022b).
3. Colorectal: NCI Colorectal Cancer Risk Assessment Tool—estimates the risk of colorectal cancer for men and women between ages of 50 and 85, or from African American, Asian American/Pacific Islander, Hispanic/Latino, or white ethnic groups. Accounts for age, sex, height/weight, diet and physical activity, screening and polyp history, medication use, and first-degree relatives with colorectal cancer. Unable to accurately estimate the risk of colorectal cancer in those with a diagnosis of ulcerative colitis, Crohn disease, LS, HNPCC, or familial adenomatous polyposis (FAP) (NCI, n.d.c).
4. Melanoma Risk Assessment Tool—estimates a person's risk of developing invasive melanoma. The variables of demographics (age, gender, race), tanning ability, complexion, and current number and size of skin moles, plus the extent of freckling are used to calculate risk (NCI, n.d.d).

D. Pathogenic Variant Probability Models:
1. *BRCA1/2*: BRCAPRO—a computer program that calculates the possibility of an individual having

an inherited pathogenic variant in the *BRCA1* or *BRCA2* gene (Harvard University, 2022).

2. LS: PREMM5: A model used to identify the likelihood of pathogenic variants in the MMR genes (LS). Accounts for patient sex, current age, and personal/family history of Lynch-associated cancers (first- and second-degree relatives) (https://premm.dfci.harvard.edu/).

II. Assess indications for cancer predisposition testing
   A. There are various guidelines for testing eligibility.
      1. The most commonly referenced are NCCN: Genetic/Familial High Risk Assessment: Breast, Ovarian and Pancreatic (also includes Prostate and other cancers, NCCN, 2022b) and Genetic/Familial High-Risk Assessment Colorectal (also includes polyposis and other cancers, NCCN, 2021). NCCN also has recommendations for genetic testing in various disease-specific guidelines—for example, Kidney cancer (NCCN, 2022c). These are updated regularly, and so it is important to ensure you are looking at the most updated version of these guidelines.
      2. Other professional society guidelines also exist—for example, ASBrS recommending consideration of genetic testing for all women with breast cancer (Manahan et al., 2019).
   B. Single indicators for hereditary cancer risk assessment (NCCN, 2021, 2022b).
      1. The following adult-onset cancers are single indicators for a genetic evaluation:
         a. Ovarian cancer
         b. Pancreatic adenocarcinoma
         c. Triple-negative breast cancer
         d. Breast cancer diagnosed at ≤45 years old or ≤50 years old with additional personal/family history or unknown family history
            (1) Consider if breast cancer diagnosed <60 or bilateral disease
         e. Breast or prostate cancer in the setting of Ashkenazi Jewish ancestry
         f. Male breast cancer
         g. Metastatic, intraductal/cribriform, or high/very-high-risk group (Gleason 8+) for prostate cancer
         h. Colonic polyposis (recommend if >20 colon adenomas, consider if >10 colon adenomas)
         i. Colon cancer diagnosed <50 years old
         j. Uterine cancer diagnosed <50 years old
         k. Diffuse gastric cancer diagnosed <40 years old
         l. Medullary thyroid cancer
         m. PGL/PCC
         n. LFS tumor spectrum (i.e., soft tissue sarcoma, osteosarcoma, CNS tumor, adrenocortical carcinoma, breast cancer), particularly diagnosed ≤45 years old
      2. Genetic testing may be reasonable to consider in various other circumstances beyond those listed above. For example, there are a number of pediatric-onset cancers that warrant genetic testing (e.g.,

Retinoblastoma, Wilms tumor) (Schiffman et al., 2013).
   C. Molecular tumor profiling results as an indicator for hereditary germline testing (DeLeonardis et al., 2019).
      1. Pathogenic Variants identified on tumor profiling can be either somatic (acquired) or germline (inherited).
      2. There are some pathogenic variants, like those in *TP53*, that are almost always somatic and rarely indicate the need for germline testing.
      3. There are other pathogenic variants, like those in *BRCA1.2*, that are more often germline, and so any identified *BRCA1/2* pathogenic variant on tumor profiling should be followed by germline testing *regardless of the cancer type and/or family history*.
      4. There has been literature developed to guide clinicians in determining what tumor profiling results should prompt germline testing.
   D. Family history-based indications for germline testing (NCCN, 2021).
      1. Family history of any of the single indicators (see "B" above) in close relatives (first, second, and third degrees)
      2. Multiple close relatives (first, second, and third degrees) with the same or related types of cancer (i.e., breast and ovarian cancer, or cancers that can be seen occurring due to a single genetic syndrome such as endometrial and colon)
      3. Degrees of relationship:
         a. First-degree relatives are full siblings, children, and parents.
         b. Second-degree relatives include aunts/uncles and grandparents.
         c. Cousins and great-aunts/great-uncles are third-degree relatives.
      4. Autosomal-dominant inheritance: multiple generations with the same or related type of cancers.
         a. A trait can be maternally or paternally inherited. Most cancer syndromes are inherited in an autosomal-dominant fashion, meaning that there is a 50% chance that the pathogenic variant may be passed down to each child of an individual who has a genetic pathogenic variant (the risk is independent for each child).
         b. De novo pathogenic variant a change in a gene, present for the first time in one family member due to a new pathogenic variant in a germ cell (egg or sperm) of one of the parents or in the fertilized egg. The genetic change will henceforth be inherited in an autosomal-dominant fashion in the family.
   E. A large selection of hereditary cancer genes and their associated cancers are highlighted in Table 10.1.
   F. Classically described autosomal-dominant hereditary cancer syndromes and unique clinical manifestations are highlighted in Table 10.2.

TABLE 10.1 Hereditary Cancer Genes and Their Associated Cancers

Genes	Breast	Ovarian	Colorectal	Endometrial	Skin	Pancreatic	Gastric	Prostate	Kidney	Paraganglioma and Pheochromocytoma	Heme	Lung	Brain or Nervous System	Other
APC			●				●						●	Polyposis; thyroid
ATM	●					●	●	●						
AXIN2			●			●		●						Oligodontia; polyposis
BAP1					●				●			●		
BARD1	●													
BMPR1A			●											Polyposis
BRCA1	●	●				●		●						
BRCA2	●	●			●	●		●						
BRIP1	○	●												
CDH1	●						●							
CDK4					●									
CDKN2A					●	●								
CHEK2	●		●					●						
CTNNA1							●							
DICER1		●										●	●	
EPCAM			●	●			●						●	
FH					●				●	○				
FLCN					●				●					
GREM1			●											
HOXB13								●						
LZTR1													●	
MEN1						●				●				Endocrine tumors
MET									●					
MITF					●				●					
MLH1		●	●	●	●	●	●	●	●				●	
MSH2		●	●	●	●	●	●	●	●				●	
MSH3**			●											Polyposis
MSH6			●	●	●	●	●	●	●				●	
MUTYH**			●											Polyposis
NF1	●									●			●	GIST
NF2										●			●	
PALB2	●	●				●		●						
PMS2		○	●	●	○	○	○	○	○					
POLD1			●	●										
POLE			●											
POT1					●								●	
PTCH1					●								●	
PTEN	●		●	●	●				●				●	Polyposis; thyroid

Column headings (conditions/tumors):

- Retinoblastoma
- Thyroid
- GIST
- GIST
- GIST
- GIST
- GIST
- Polyposis; hemorrhagic telangiectasia
- Polyposis
- (Osteo)sarcoma; adrenocortical carcinoma
- Parathyroid
- Endocrine tumors
- Erythrocytosis
- Polyposis
- GIST
- Carney complex
- Sessile serrated polyposis

Genes:

- RAD51D
- RB1
- RET
- RUNX1
- SDHA
- SDHAF2
- SDHB
- SDHC
- SDHD
- SMAD4
- SMARCA4
- SMARCB1
- STK11
- TP53
- TSC1
- TSC2
- VHL

Limited Evidence Genes

- BLM*
- CEBPA
- CDC73
- CDKN1B
- EGLN1
- FANCC
- GALNT12
- GATA2
- KIF1B
- MAX
- MUTYH*
- NBN*
- NTHL1**
- PDGFRA
- PHOX2B
- PRKAR1A
- RECQL
- RNF43
- TMEM127
- XRCC2

* indicates monoallelic/heterozygous state (autosomal-dominant condition).
** indicates biallelic/homozygous state (autosomal recessive condition).
● indicates established association with specified cancer.
○ indicates limited evidence for association with specified cancer.

TABLE 10.2   Classic Hereditary Cancer Syndromes and Unique Clinical Manifestations

Syndrome	Clinical Manifestations	Common Gene(s)
Birt–Hogg–Dube syndrome [OMIM, 2018]	Classic noncancerous skin lesions, that is, fibrofolliculoma (30–40 years), bilateral and multifocal renal tumors, and multiple bilateral lung cysts associated with spontaneous pneumothorax.	FLCN
Cowden syndrome, also known as PTEN hamartoma tumor syndrome [OMIM, 2018]	Characterized by benign skin findings, increased lifetime risks for breast, follicular thyroid, renal cell, endometrial, and colorectal cancers, and possibly melanoma. Macrocephaly >97th percentile; 58 cm for women and 60 cm for men. Mucocutaneous lesions, trichilemmomas, lipomas. Multiple colon hamartomas.	PTEN
Familial adenomatous polyposis and attenuated familial adenomatous polyposis (Gardner syndrome) [OMIM, 2018]	Colon polyposis (adenomas), desmoid tumors, osteomas, thyroid cancer, and hepatoblastoma Increased the lifetime risk of colorectal cancer (nearly 100% for classic FAP [>100 adenomatous polyps in colon] and 70% for attenuated FAP [30–100 adenomatous polyps]). Elevated lifetime risk for duodenal, pancreatic, papillary thyroid cancer, and medulloblastoma. Childhood hepatoblastoma risk.	APC
Li–Fraumeni syndrome [OMIM, 2018]	Cancers of brain, breast, adrenal cortex, and non-Ewing sarcoma with onset before age 50.	TP53
Multiple endocrine neoplasia type I [OMIM, 2018]	Endocrine and nonendocrine tumors, including parathyroid glands, pituitary gland, and the pancreas.	MEN1
Multiple endocrine neoplasia type II [OMIM, 2018]	Medullary thyroid cancer and pheochromocytoma. Subtypes 2A = hyperparathyroidism 2B = FMTC 4 = similar to MEN type 1, especially hyperparathyroidism, pituitary gland, and other endocrine glands and organs.	RET
Neurofibromatosis type 1 [OMIM, 2018]	Malignant peripheral neural sheath tumors, neurofibromas, pheochromocytomas, meningiomas, gastrointestinal stromal tumors, optic gliomas, café-au-lait macules, axillary or inguinal freckles, iris hamartomas, and sphenoid wing dysplasia or congenital bowing or thinning of long bones	NF1
Neurofibromatosis type 2 [OMIM, 2018]	Gliomas, vestibular schwannoma, schwannomas of other cranial and peripheral nerves, meningioma, ependymomas, and astrocytoma	NF2
Nevoid basal-cell carcinoma syndrome (Gorlin syndrome) [OMIM, 2018]	Multiple basal-cell carcinomas beginning in the 20s, jaw keratocysts beginning in the teens. Dysmorphic features include macrocephaly, bossing of the forehead (unusually pronounced), coarse facial features, facial milia, and skeletal anomalies	PTCH
Peutz–Jeghers syndrome [OMIM, 2018]	GI polyposis—PJS-type hamartomatous polyps are most common in the small intestine but can also occur in the stomach, large bowel, and extraintestinal sites. Risk for recurrent obstruction and intussusception childhood or young adulthood. Colorectal, gastric, pancreatic, breast cancer Mucocutaneous pigmentation—dark blue to brown macules around the mouth, on buccal mucosa, eyes, nostrils, perianal area, and fingers. The macules may fade in puberty and adulthood. Females: risk for ovarian SCTAT, and adenoma malignum of the cervix. Males: risk for Sertoli cell tumors of the testes.	STK11
Tuberous sclerosis complex ([OMIM, 2018])	Characteristic skin findings—hypomelanotic macules, confetti skin lesions, facial angiofibromas, shagreen patches, fibrous cephalic plaques, ungual fibromas CNS features—subependymal nodules, cortical tubers, and SEGA, seizures, intellectual disability/developmental delay, psychiatric illness Renal—angiomyolipomas, cysts, renal cell carcinoma Pulmonary—LAM Cardiac—rhabdomyomas, arrhythmias	TSC1 and TSC2
Von Hippel–Lindau ([OMIM, 2018])	Renal cell cancer; hemangioblastoma of brain, spinal cord, and retina; renal cysts; pheochromocytomas; endolymphatic sac tumors; and pancreatic islet cell tumors	VHL

FAP, Familial adenomatous polyposis; FMTC, familial medullary thyroid carcinoma; GI, gastrointestinal; LAM, lymphangioleiomyomatosis; SCTAT, sex cord tumors with annular tubules; SEGA, subependymal giant cell astrocytomas.

G. CDC Tier 1 Genomics Applications (CDC, 2014):
1. The CDC's Office of Public Health Genomics defines Tier 1 genomic applications as "those having significant potential for positive impact on public health based on available evidence-based guidelines and recommendations." Approximately 2 million people in the United States are at increased risk for adverse health outcomes because they have genetic pathogenic variants associated with one of the following conditions:
   a. Hereditary Breast and Ovarian Cancer Syndrome (HBOC)—increased risk for breast, ovarian, prostate, and pancreatic cancers due to pathogenic variants in *BRCA1* or *BRCA2* genes
   b. LS—increased risk for colorectal, endometrial, ovarian, and other cancers associated with pathogenic variants in MMR genes
   c. Familial hypercholesterolemia—increased risk for heart disease or stroke due to pathogenic variants leading to very-high cholesterol levels from an early age
2. See Table 10.3 for additional information regarding risks and management recommendations for Hereditary Breast and Ovarian Cancer syndrome and LS.
H. Pedigree documentation (NCCN, 2021, 2022b).
1. A recorded disease history for at least three generations of the family.
2. Utilize common pedigree nomenclature (Fig. 10.2).
3. Paternal lineage on the left side and maternal lineage on the right side of the pedigree.
4. Include three generations, minimum, for both lineages with at least first- and second-degree relatives.
5. Add distant relatives (greater than third-degree relatives) in one lineage when information is available. "Singleton" children can affect gender-related disease probabilities (e.g., male children when there is ovarian cancer history in females of the earliest generation or prostate cancer with primarily female generations).
6. Include ancestry of all grandparents.
7. Relatives with cancer diagnosis should also be designated with:
   a. Primary site of cancer(s) with treatment type
   b. Age at diagnosis for primary cancers
   c. History of surgery or treatments that may have reduced the risk of cancer
   d. Bilateral salpingo-oophorectomy in premenopausal women to decrease the risk of ovarian and breast cancers, or colectomy to decrease the risk of colorectal cancer
   e. Chemoprevention (e.g., tamoxifen, raloxifene for breast, or aspirin for colon cancer)
   f. Current age, or age at and cause of death (if deceased)

g. Carcinogenic exposures (e.g., tobacco or alcohol use, asbestos exposure, radiation, and viral mutagens such as HPV and prolonged hormone replacement therapy)
h. Physical characteristics indicative of hereditary cancer (e.g., macrocephaly, café-au-lait spots or other cutaneous findings, and history of spontaneous pneumothorax)
i. Other significant health problems (e.g., history of blood clots in the patient/family could be related to factor V Leiden; need for genetic testing before colectomy)
8. Relatives without cancer (pertinent negatives)
   a. Current age or age at death with cause (if deceased).
   b. History of surgeries or treatment that may have reduced the risk of cancer.
   c. Cancer screening practices.
   d. Nonmalignant features associated with the syndrome in question (e.g., benign tumors of the parathyroid gland are associated with multiple endocrine neoplasia type II syndrome).
   e. Carcinogenic exposures.

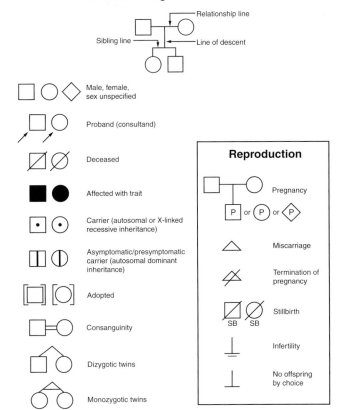

Fig. 10.2 Pedigree nomenclature symbols. Symbols used in drawing pedigrees of persons with family history of cancer. *National Cancer Institute. Pedigree nomenclature: Image details.* (2015). https://visualsonline.cancer.gov/details.cfm?imageid=10346. Retrieved 26.07.22.

TABLE 10.3   Cancer Risks and Management Recommendations for Hereditary Breast and Ovarian Cancer Syndrome and Lynch Syndrome

	Cancer Risks	Management Guidelines
HBOC *BRCA1* *BRCA2*	**Females (AFAB)** Breast cancer: *BRCA1* up to 72% by age 80 *BRCA2* up to 69% by age 80 Ovarian cancer: *BRCA1* up to 44% by age 80 *BRCA2* up to 17% by age 80 **Males (AMAB)** Breast cancer: *BRCA1* ~1%–2% lifetime risk *BRCA2* ~6%–7% lifetime risk Prostate cancer: *BRCA1* ~20% lifetime risk *BRCA2* ~20%–25% lifetime risk **Both** Pancreatic cancer: *BRCA1* ≤5% lifetime risk *BRCA2* ~5%–10% lifetime risk Melanoma: *BRCA1* risk not well-established *BRCA2* <5% lifetime risk	Enhanced breast cancer screening with annual mammogram and breast MRI alternating every 6 months is recommended beginning at age 25–30. Consider referral to breast surgery for further discussion of surgical options, such as bilateral prophylactic mastectomy. Ovarian cancer screening has low sensitivity and specificity, thus prophylactic BSO is recommended between ages 35–40 (BRCA2 carriers can consider postponing until 40–45 due to later average age of onset). Enhanced prostate cancer screening is recommended in *BRCA2* carriers beginning at age 40 and can be considered in *BRCA1* carriers. Pancreatic cancer screening may be recommended, dependent on family history. Please refer to NCCN (2022b) for complete and detailed management guidelines.
Lynch syndrome or HNPCC *MLH1* *MSH2* and *EPCAM* *MSH6* *PMS2*	Colorectal cancer: *MLH1:* 46%–61% *MSH2* and *EPCAM:* 33%–52% *MSH6:* 10%–44% *PMS2:* 8.7%–20% Endometrial cancer (AFAB): *MLH1:* 34%–54% *MSH2* and *EPCAM:* 21%–57% *MSH6:* 16%–49% *PMS2:* 13%–26% Ovarian cancer (AFAB): *MLH1:* 4%–20% *MSH2* and *EPCAM:* 8%–38% *MSH6:* ≤1%–13% *PMS2:* 1.3%–3% Renal pelvis/ureter cancer: *MLH1:* 0.2%–5% *MSH2* and *EPCAM:* 2.2%–28% *MSH6:* 0.7%–5.5% *PMS2:* ≤1%–3.7% Bladder cancer: *MLH1:* 2%–7% *MSH2* and *EPCAM:* 4.4%–12.8% *MSH6:* 1.0%–8.2% *PMS2:* ≤1%–2.4% Gastric cancer: *MLH1:* 5%–7% *MSH2* and *EPCAM:* 0.2%–9% *MSH6:* ≤1%–7.9% *PMS2:* Inadequate data Small bowel cancer: *MLH1:* 0.4%–11% *MSH2* and *EPCAM:* 1.1%–10% *MSH6:* ≤1%–4% *PMS2:* 0.1%–0.3%	Enhanced screening recommendations vary based on the specific MMR gene pathogenic variant present. High-quality colonoscopy screening is recommended at increased interval for all carriers, as frequently as every 1–2 years. EGD can be considered, particularly in the presence of family history or certain risk factors, every 3–5 years. Risk-reducing total hysterectomy and bilateral salpingo-oophorectomy can be considered after the completion of childbearing; encourage shared decision-making between the patient and the provider with regard to surgical timing. Enhanced screening, such as endometrial biopsy, can be considered every 1–2 years beginning at age 30–35 in individuals who have not undergone prophylactic surgery. Please refer to NCCN (2021) for complete and detailed management guidelines.

TABLE 10.3 Cancer Risks and Management Recommendations for Hereditary Breast and Ovarian Cancer Syndrome and Lynch Syndrome

Cancer Risks	Management Guidelines
Pancreatic cancer:	
MLH1: 6.2%	
MSH2 and *EPCAM:* 0.5%–1.6%	
MSH6: 1.4%–1.6%	
PMS2: ≤1%–1.6%	
Biliary tract cancer:	
MLH1: 1.9%–3.7%	
MSH2 and *EPCAM:* 0.02%–1.7%	
MSH6: 0.2%–≤1%	
PMS2: 0.2%–≤1%	
Prostate cancer:	
MLH1: 4.4%–13.8%	
MSH2 and *EPCAM:* 3.9%–23.8%	
MSH6: 2.5%–11.6%	
PMS2: 4.6%–11.6%	
Brain cancer (Turcot syndrome):	
MLH1: 0.7%–1.7%	
MSH2 and *EPCAM:* 2.5%–7.7%	
MSH6: 0.8%–1.8%	
PMS2: 0.6%–≤1%	
Skin cancer/sebaceous neoplasms (Muir-Torre syndrome):	
MLH1: increased risk	
MSH2 and *EPCAM:* increased risk (higher in *MSH2* c.942+3A>T variant carriers)	
MSH6: potential increased risk	
PMS2: potential increased risk	

HBOC, Hereditary breast and ovarian cancer syndrome; *HNPCC,* hereditary nonpolyposis colorectal cancer syndrome.

f. Other significant health problems (e.g., history of multiple adenomatous colon polyps).

9. Tests that are ordered should have results information that:
   a. Can be interpreted with sufficient sensitivity and specificity
   b. Is "actionable" to assist in medical decision-making
   c. Will assist in diagnosis and management of cancer/risk
   d. Can assist with clarification of cancer risk in family member

10. Offer genetic testing and services as indicated
    a. Provide genetic counseling—physicians, nurses, or genetic counselors with specialized training in genetics (NCCN, 2020).
    b. Inform patients regarding their potential for increased cancer risk from an inherited susceptibility and the availability of predisposition genetic testing (NCCN, 2020).
    c. Assistance to help patients make informed decisions (without coercion or personal opinions) about genetic testing with consideration for their health care needs, preferences, and values.

11. Provide informed consent—precedes genetic testing for the patient to be tested and should include the following:
    a. Purpose of the genetic test
    b. Motivation for testing
    c. Risks and benefits of genetic testing
    d. Limitations of genetic testing
    e. Inheritance pattern of the gene(s) being tested
    f. Risk of misidentified paternity, if applicable
    g. Accuracy and sensitivity of genetic testing method
    h. Outcomes of genetic testing
    i. Confidentiality of genetic testing results
    j. Possibility of discrimination
    k. Alternatives to genetic testing
    l. How testing will impact health care decision-making
    m. Cost of testing
    n. Right to refuse
    o. Testing in children (<18 years of age)—performed only when clinical utility has been established (Bavdekar et al., 2013; Kesserwan, Friedman Ross, Bradbury, & Nichols, 2016)

MANAGEMENT

I. Interpreting results of inherited cancer predisposition testing (Nussbaum et al., 2016)
   A. Negative Results: The predictive value of a negative test result varies, depending on whether a known genetic pathogenic variant exists in the family.
      1. A negative test result with a known familial genetic pathogenic variant is referred to as a "true negative." This can indicate:
         a. The patient is within the "general population risk of cancer" associated with that branch of the family. No additional high-risk screening required.
         b. Family history from the other parent can still influence the risk of developing cancer.
         c. Potential for other genomic/environmental modifiers, for example, tobacco and polygenic (SNP) related risk.
      2. A negative result with "no known family genetic pathogenic variant" may occur because:
         a. Genetic testing performed was unable to identify the pathogenic variant present in the family due to technological limitations (i.e., coverage of a particular region of the gene is not adequate, RNA analysis vs. DNA analysis).
         b. The cancer in the family may be associated with a cancer susceptibility gene other than the one tested or in a gene(s) yet to be discovered in science.
         c. The cancer in the family is not the result of a germline genetic pathogenic variant, but rather is "familial" or "sporadic" disease—due to a combination of less penetrant inherited risk factors (like SNPs) as well as shared environment, lifestyle, or other risk factors.
         d. Important to recommend testing for relevant relatives on both sides of the family in this case in an attempt to identify which of these is true.
   B. "Variant of uncertain clinical significance" (VUS) (Maxwell et al., 2016; NCI, n.d.a, Strom, 2016)
      1. A change in a gene in which the association with cancer risk cannot be established.
      2. VUS is NOT a pathogenic variant; testing did not identify an inherited risk for disease.
      3. Over time (sometimes months, sometimes many years) VUSs are "reclassified" either UP to pathogenic/likely pathogenic (harmful) or DOWN to benign/likely benign (harmless).
      4. A VUS finding is COMMON (up to ~40% on larger panels).
      5. MOST (>90%) or VUSs are reclassified down to benign/likely benign (harmless) as science obtains more data. In this case, they are just part of normal variation.
      6. Use of Clinvar (Park et al., 2021) to see how other labs may classify that same variant.
      7. Labs report VUS and reclassifications differently; some always, some never, and some only when specific conditions are met or by provider request.
         a. Because a VUS may be reclassified as benign or pathogenic in the future, it is important for patients to keep in contact with their ordering provider. Explain how the patient/family will be notified (e.g., phone call from the clinic or office if the office is notified by the lab of a VUS reclassification). Patients can also reach out to the lab directly about VUS updates.
      8. Offer genetic testing to certain members of the family (especially relatives with cancer), if appropriate, to determine whether the VUS is associated with a disease in other members of the family. However, do NOT offer testing to relatives without cancer as a way to identify cancer risk. Depending on laboratory policy, it may be free to certain members of the family to help with variant classification.
   C. Positive results:
      1. "Penetrance" refers to the proportion of all individuals with a specific genotype that expresses the phenotype (e.g., cancer). For almost all cancer susceptibility genes, penetrance is not 100%.
      2. "Expressivity" refers to the degree to which a single individual with a specific genotype will exhibit a specific trait (e.g., hundreds versus thousands of polyps in someone with inherited polyp predisposition), presenting with breast versus ovarian versus pancreatic cancer in a family with a *BRCA1/2* pathogenic variant.
      3. Penetrance and expressivity may be different for different genetic pathogenic variants in the same cancer susceptibility gene (e.g., an *APC* I1307K pathogenic variant, common in Ashkenazi Jewish individuals, raises the risk of colorectal cancer by ~2×; other APC pathogenic variants which cause FAP result in 100s–1000s of polyps and ~100% risk of colorectal cancer).
         a. Penetrance and expressivity may also be affected by other genetic variations, as well as by the environment and other personal factors (e.g., difference in breast cancer risk in a family with BRCA1/2 pathogenic variants due to additional breast cancer risk SNPs, difference in polyp count due to diet/lifestyle amongst relatives).
         b. A positive test result may or may not be a significant "cause" of cancer in the patient/family, depending on the type of genetic pathogenic variant identified. This is now more common with larger panel testing, so-called "off target" or "incidental" findings.

II. Medical Management of Identified Risk
  A. Chemoprevention (American Society of Clinical Oncology Cancer.Net, 2022)
    1. Tamoxifen, raloxifene (for *BRCA1/2*, other hereditary breast cancer–associated pathogenic variants and empirically elevated breast cancer risk)
    2. Hormonal contraceptive pills for ovarian cancer risk reduction (for *BRCA1/2*, other hereditary ovarian cancer–associated pathogenic variants and empirically elevated ovarian cancer risk)
    3. Aspirin and nonsteroidal antiinflammatory drugs for colorectal cancer prevention
    4. Finasteride for prostate cancer prevention
  B. Diet and exercise
    1. Advise against exposures which may increase the risk of certain cancers. For example, smoking increases the risk of lung and bladder cancer, while alcohol consumption increases the risk of breast, pancreatic, liver, and other cancers. The World Health Organization has classified processed meats including ham, bacon, and salami as a Group 1 carcinogen, which means that there is strong evidence that processed meats cause cancer (International Agency for Research on Cancer, 2015).
    2. Plant-based and antiinflammatory diet and 150 minutes of exercise per week have been shown to reduce cancer incidence and recurrence.
    3. Studies on vitamins and supplements are difficult to assess. Turmeric, lycopene, and vitamin D have significant data on cancer prevention and risk; other vitamins and supplements data more limited.
  C. Provide ongoing surveillance that detects cancer as early as possible, when chances for cure are greatest (i.e., enhanced breast cancer screening with annual mammogram and breast MRI alternating every 6 months in *BRCA1, BRCA2, PALB2, CHEK2, ATM* carriers) (NCCN, 2022a).
  D. Risk-reducing surgery (also called *prophylactic surgery*) as indicated, which is the removal of as much of the tissue at risk as possible to reduce the risk of developing a cancer. Follow evidence-based guidelines and literature (e.g., a 23-year-old female with a *BRCA2* pathogenic variant can have children and breastfeed prior to consideration of risk-reducing bilateral mastectomy and completion of salpingo-oophorectomy by age 40) (NCCN, 2022b).

REFERENCES

American Cancer Society (ACS). *American Cancer Society recommendations for the early detection of breast cancer.* (2022). https://www.cancer.org/cancer/breast-cancer/screening-tests-and-early-detection/american-cancer-society-recommendations-for-the-early-detection-of-breast-cancer.html.

American Society of Clinical Oncology. (2022). *Chemoprevention. Cancer.Net.* https://www.cancer.net/navigating-cancer-care/prevention-and-healthy-living/chemoprevention.

Bavdekar, S. B. (2013). Pediatric clinical trials. *Perspectives in Clinical Research, 4*(1), 89–99. https://doi.org/10.4103/2229-3485.106403.

Baysal, B. E. (2004). Genomic imprinting and environment in hereditary paraganglioma. *American Journal of Medical Genetics. Part C: Seminars in Medical Genetics, 129C*(1), 85–90. https://doi.org/10.1002/ajmg.c.30018.

Black, M. H., Li, S., LaDuca, H., Lo, M.-T., Chen, J., Hoiness, R., et al. (2020). Validation of a prostate cancer polygenic risk score. *The Prostate, 80*(15), 1314–1321. https://doi.org/10.1002/pros.24058. Epub 2020 Aug 17. PMID: 33258481; PMCID: PMC7590110.

Centers for Disease Control (CDC). *Tier 1 genomics applications and their importance to public health.* (2014). https://www.cdc.gov/genomics/implementation/toolkit/tier1.htm.

Centers for Disease Control (CDC). *What is epigenetics?* (2022). https://www.cdc.gov/genomics/disease/epigenetics.htm#:~:text=Epigenetics%20is%20the%20study%20of,body%20reads%20a%20DNA%20sequence.

DeLeonardis, K., Hogan, L., Cannistra, S. A., Rangachari, D., & Tung, N. (2019). When should tumor genomic profiling prompt consideration of germline testing? *Journal of Oncology Practice, 15*(9), 465–473. https://pubmed.ncbi.nlm.nih.gov/31509718/.

Gorski, S. A., Vogel, J., & Doudna, J. A. (2017). RNA-based recognition and targeting: sowing the seeds of specificity. *Nature Reviews: Molecular Cell Biology, 18*, 215–228. https://doi.org/10.1038/nrm.2016.174.

Griffiths, A. J. F., Miller, J. H., Suzuki, D. T., et al. (2000). An introduction to genetic analysis. In: *How DNA changes affect phenotype* (7th ed.). New York, NY: W. H. Freeman.

Harvard University. *BayesMendel Lab BRCAPRO.* (2022). https://projects.iq.harvard.edu/bayesmendel/brcapro.

Hirakata, S., & Siomi, M. C. (2016). piRNA biogenesis in the germline: From transcription of piRNA genomic sources to piRNA maturation. *Biochimica et Biophysica Acta, 1859*(1), 82–92. https://doi.org/10.1016/j.bbagrm.2015.09.002.

International Agency for Research on Cancer. *IARC monographs evaluate consumption of red meat and processed meat.* (2015). https://www.iarc.who.int/wp-content/uploads/2018/07/pr240_E.pdf.

Jenkins, M. A., Win, A. K., Dowty, J. G., MacInnis, R. J., Makalic, E., Schmidt, D. F., et al. (2019). Ability of known susceptibility SNPs to predict colorectal cancer risk for persons with and without a family history. *Familial Cancer, 18*(4), 389–397. PMID: 31209717; PMCID: PMC6785388. https://doi.org/10.1007/s10689-019-00136-6

Kesserwan, C., Ross, L. F., Bradbury, A. R., & Nichols, K. E. (2016). The advantages and challenges of testing children for heritable predisposition to cancer. *American Society of Clinical Oncology educational book* (36, pp. 251–269). American Society of Clinical Oncology. Annual Meeting. https://doi.org/10.1200/EDBK_160621.

LaDuca, H., Polley, E. C., Yussuf, A., Hoang, L., Gutierrez, S., Hart, S. N., et al. (2020). A clinical guide to hereditary cancer panel testing: Evaluation of gene-specific cancer associations and sensitivity of genetic testing criteria in a cohort of 165,000 high-risk patients. *Genetics in Medicine: Official Journal of the American College of Medical Genetics and Genomics, 22*(2), 407–415. https://doi.org/10.1038/s41436-019-0633-8.

Landrith, T., Li, B., Cass, A. A., Conner, B. R., LaDuca, H., et al. (2020). Splicing profile by capture RNA-seq identifies pathogenic germline variants in tumor suppressor genes. *NPJ Precision Oncology, 4*(1), 1–9. https://doi.org/10.1038/s41698-020-0109-y.

Loeb, L. A. (2016). Human cancers express a mutator phenotype: Hypothesis, origin, and consequences. *Cancer Research, 76*(8), 2057–2059. https://doi.org/10.1158/0008-5472.CAN-16-0794.

Mahon, S. (2020). *Germline and somatic variants: What is the difference?* ONS Voice. Retrieved from https://voice.ons.org/news-and-views/germline-and-somatic-variants-what-is-the-difference.

Manahan, E. R., Kuerer, H. M., Sebastian, M., Hughes, K. S., Boughey, J. C., Euhus, D. M., et al. (2019). Consensus guidelines on genetic testing for hereditary breast cancer from the American Society of Breast Surgeons. *Annals of Surgical Oncology, 26*(10), 3025–3031. https://doi.org/10.1245/s10434-019-07549-8.

Mavaddat, N., Michailidou, K., Dennis, J., Lush, M., Fachal, L., Lee, A., et al. (2019). Polygenic risk scores for prediction of breast cancer and breast cancer subtypes. *American Journal of Human Genetics, 104*(1), 21–34. https://doi.org/10.1016/j.ajhg.2018.11.002.

Maxwell, K. N., Hart, S. N., Vijai, J., Schrader, K. A., Slavin, T. P., Thomas, T., Wubbenhorst, B., et al. (2016). Evaluation of ACMG-guideline-based variant classification of cancer susceptibility and non-cancer-associated genes in families affected by breast cancer. *The American Journal of Human Genetics, 98*(5), 801–817. https://doi.org/10.1016/j.ajhg.2016.02.024.

Moscarello, T., Murray, B., Reuter, C. M., & Demo, E. (2019). Direct-to-consumer raw genetic data and third-party interpretation services: More burden than bargain? *Genetics in Medicine: Official Journal of the American College of Medical Genetics and Genomics, 21*(3), 539–541. https://doi.org/10.1038/s41436-018-0097-2.

National Cancer Institute (NCI). *The genetics of cancer.* (2017). https://www.cancer.gov/about-cancer/causes-prevention/genetics.

National Cancer Institute (NCI). *Dictionary of genetics terms.* (n.d.a). https://www.cancer.gov/publications/dictionaries/genetics-dictionary.

National Cancer Institute (NCI). *Dictionary of cancer terms.* (n.d.b). https://www.cancer.gov/publications/dictionaries/cancer-terms/.

National Cancer Institute (NCI). *Breast cancer risk assessment tool.* (n.d.c). https://bcrisktool.cancer.gov/calculator.html.

National Cancer Institute (NCI). *The Melanoma Risk Assessment Tool.* (n.d.d). https://mrisktool.cancer.gov/#:~:text=The%20Melanoma%20Risk%20Assessment%20Tool%20was%20developed%20for%20use%20by,in%20this%20case%205%20years.

NCCN. (2020). NCCN updates guidelines for hereditary cancer risks. *American Journal of Medical Genetics: Part A, 182*(12), 2813–2814. https://doi.org/10.1002/ajmg.a.61253.

NCCN. *NCCN guidelines genetic/familial high-risk assessment: Colorectal V.1.* (2021). https://www.NCCN.genetics_colon.pdf.

NCCN. *NCCN guidelines for breast cancer V.1. Screening and diagnosis.* (2022a). https://www.NCCN.breast-screening.pdf.

NCCN. *NCCN guidelines genetic/familial high-risk assessment: Breast, ovarian and pancreatic V.2.* (2022b). https://www.NCCN.genetics_bop.pdf.

NCCN. *NCCN guidelines kidney cancer V.4.* (2022c). https://www.NCCN.kidney.pdf.

Nussbaum, R. L., McInnes, R. R., & Willard, H. F. (2016). *Thompson & Thompson genetics in medicine* (8th ed.). Philadelphia, PA: Elsevier.

Online Mendelian Inheritance in Man (OMIM). *An Online Catalog of Human Genes and Genetic Disorders.* (2018). https://www.omim.org/.

Palumbo, E., & Russo, A. (2016). Chromosome imbalances in cancer: Molecular cytogenetics meets genomics. *Cytogenetic and Genome Research, 150*(3–4), 176–184. https://doi.org/10.1159/000455804. Retrieved from.

Park, B., Sohn, J. Y., Yoon, K. A., Lee, K. S., Cho, E. H., Lim, M. C., et al. (2017). Characteristics of BRCA1/2 mutations carriers including large genomic rearrangements in high risk breast cancer patients. *Breast Cancer Research and Treatment, 163*(1), 139–150. https://doi.org/10.1007/s10549-017-4142-7.

Park, K.-J., Lee, W., Chun, S., & Min, W.-K. (2021). The frequency of discordant variant classification in the human gene mutation database: A comparison of the American College of Medical Genetics and Genomics Guidelines and ClinVar. *Laboratory Medicine, 52*(3), 250–259. https://doi.org/10.1093/labmed/lmaa072.

Salvador, M. U., Truelson, M., Mason, C., Souders, B., LaDuca, H., Dougall, B., et al. (2019). Comprehensive paired tumor/germline testing for Lynch syndrome: Bringing resolution to the diagnostic process. *Journal of Clinical Oncology, 37*(8), 647–657. https://doi.org/10.1200/JCO.18.00696.

Schiffman, J. D., Geller, J. I., Mundt, E., Means, A., Means, L., & Means, V. (2013). Update on pediatric cancer predisposition syndromes. *Pediatric Blood & Cancer, 60*(8), 1247–1252. https://doi.org/10.1002/pbc.24555.

Siravegna, G., Mussolin, B., Venesio, T., Marsoni, S., Seoane, J., Dive, C., et al. (2019). How liquid biopsies can change clinical practice in oncology. *Annals of Oncology: The Journal of the European Society for Medical Oncology, 30*(10), 1580–1590. https://doi.org/10.1093/annonc/mdz227.

Soon, W. W., Hariharan, M., & Snyder, M. P. (2013). High-throughput sequencing for biology and medicine. *Molecular Systems Biology, 9*(1), 640. https://doi.org/10.1038/msb.2012.61.

Strom, S. P. (2016). Current practices and guidelines for clinical next-generation sequencing oncology testing. *Cancer Biology & Medicine, 13*(1), 3–11.

Tandy-Connor, S., Guiltinan, J., Krempely, K., LaDuca, H., Reineke, P., Gutierrez, S., et al. (2018). False-positive results released by direct-to-consumer genetic tests highlight the importance of clinical confirmation testing for appropriate patient care. *Genetics in Medicine, 20*(12), 1515–1521. https://doi.org/10.1038/gim.2018.38. Epub 2018 Mar 22. PMID: 29565420; PMCID: PMC6301953.

U.S. Department of Labor. Emplwoyee Retirement Income Security Act of 1974 (ERISA). (n.d.). https://www.dol.gov/general/topic/health-plans/erisa#:~:text=The%20Employee%20Retirement%20Income%20Security,for%20individuals%20in%20these%20plans.

U.S. Food & Drug Administration (FDA). *FDA authorizes, with special controls, direct-to-consumer test that reports three mutations in the BRCA breast cancer genes.* (2018). https://www.fda.gov/NewsEvents/Newsroom/PressAnnouncements/ucm599560.htm.

U.S. Food & Drug Administration (FDA). *Direct-to-consumer tests.* (2019). https://www.fda.gov/medical-devices/in-vitro-diagnostics/direct-consumer-tests.

Vogel, V. G. (2009). The NSABP Study of Tamoxifen and Raloxifene (STAR) trial. *Expert Review of Anticancer Therapy, 9*(1), 51–60. https://doi.org/10.1586/14737140.9.1.51.

Walsh, T., Casadei, S., Lee, M. K., Pennil, C. C., Nord, A. S., Thornton, A. M., et al. (2011). Mutations in 12 genes for inherited ovarian, fallopian tube, and peritoneal carcinoma identified by massively parallel sequencing. *Proceedings of the National Academy of Sciences of the United States of America, 108*(44), 18032–18037. https://doi.org/10.1073/pnas.1115052108.

Zaami, S., Orrico, A., Signore, F., Cavaliere, A. F., Mazzi, M., & Marinelli, E. (2021). Ethical, Legal and Social Issues (ELSI) associated with non-invasive prenatal testing: Reflections on the evolution of prenatal diagnosis and procreative choices. *Genes, 12*(2), 204. https://doi.org/10.3390/genes12020204.

11

Research Protocols and Clinical Trials

Marlon Garzo Saría and Santosh Kesari

I. Definitions
  A. Research protocol: written description of a clinical study (ClinicalTrials.gov, 2021)
  B. Clinical research: also referred to as clinical study; studies that involve human volunteers intended to contribute to medical knowledge (ClinicalTrials.gov, 2021)
  C. Clinical trials: studies that test new treatments or new ways of using existing treatments, also referred to as *experimental* or *interventional studies* (ClinicalTrials.gov, 2021)
  D. Types of clinical research
    1. Observational studies: goal is to understand a situation to develop a hypothesis that can be evaluated using a clinical trial (National Cancer Institute [NCI], 2020b; National Institutes of Health [NIH], 2022)
    2. Case report/case study/case series: explore a single individual (case report) or small group (case series) to determine the likelihood of an association between an observed effect and a specific event
    3. Ecological study: often used to measure the prevalence and incidence of disease or condition
    4. Cross-sectional studies: describe the association between a condition and other characteristics that may exist in a specific group
    5. Case-control studies: compare cases (subjects with outcome of interest) to controls (similar subjects who do not have the disease or condition) with respect to exposure
    6. Cohort studies: subjects who do not have the outcome or condition are followed and compared based on the exposure
    7. Natural history studies: subjects with cancer or those who are at high risk for developing cancer (e.g., because of their family history) are followed over a long period of time
    8. Cancer Care Delivery Research: multidisciplinary studies that explore the impact of patient, clinician, and organizational factors on clinical outcomes, access to care, cost of care, and patient well-being; studies are conducted and funded through the National Cancer Institute Community Oncology Research Program (Geiger et al., 2020)
  E. Clinical Trials (experimental or interventional studies): participants receive specific interventions; each type is designed to answer different research questions (NCI, 2020b; NIH, 2022)
    1. Prevention trials: evaluate the safety and efficacy of various risk reduction strategies
      a. Action studies (e.g., being more active, quitting smoking, eating more fruits and vegetables)
      b. Agent or chemoprevention studies (e.g., taking certain medications, vitamins, and supplements)
    2. Screening trials: evaluate the effectiveness of new techniques for early detection of cancer in the general population
    3. Diagnostic trials: evaluate tests or procedures that may better identify cancer in symptomatic individuals
    4. Treatment or therapeutic trials: evaluate the safety and efficacy of new drugs, vaccines, biological agents, approaches to surgery or radiation therapy, treatment combinations, educational approaches, or other interventions
    5. Quality-of-life or supportive care trials: explore pharmacologic or nonpharmacologic therapies to minimize cancer- and cancer treatment-related toxicities on persons with cancer and their families
    6. Behavioral trials: evaluate interventions to promote behavioral changes to improve health
  F. Expanded access or compassionate use (Food and Drug Administration [FDA], 2019a)
    1. Expanded access: also referred to as "compassionate use"; a potential pathway for a patient with an immediately life-threatening condition or serious disease or condition to gain access to an investigational medical product (drug, biologic, or medical device) for treatment outside of clinical trials when no comparable or satisfactory alternative therapy options are available
II. Clinical trials
  A. Randomized clinical trial designs (Nair, 2019)
    1. Parallel group trial design: participant is randomized to one of several treatment groups and each group will be allocated a different intervention; most commonly used study design (Fig. 11.1)

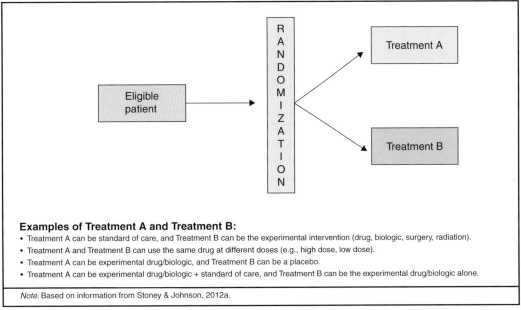

Examples of Treatment A and Treatment B:
- Treatment A can be standard of care, and Treatment B can be the experimental intervention (drug, biologic, surgery, radiation).
- Treatment A and Treatment B can use the same drug at different doses (e.g., high dose, low dose).
- Treatment A can be experimental drug/biologic, and Treatment B can be a placebo.
- Treatment A can be experimental drug/biologic + standard of care, and Treatment B can be the experimental drug/biologic alone.

Note. Based on information from Stoney & Johnson, 2012a.

Fig. 11.1 Parallel design: two study groups (Stoney & Johnson, 2012). Based on data from Stoney, C. M., & Johnson, L. L. (2012). Design of clinical studies and trials. In J. I. Gallin & F. P. Ognibene (Eds.), *Principles and practice of clinical research* (3rd ed., pp. 225–242). New York: Elsevier. https://doi.org/10.1016/B978-0-12-382167-6.00019-9.

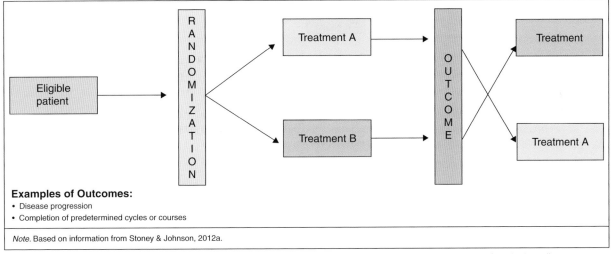

Examples of Outcomes:
- Disease progression
- Completion of predetermined cycles or courses

Note. Based on information from Stoney & Johnson, 2012a.

Fig. 11.2 Crossover design. Based on data from Stoney, C. M., & Johnson, L. L. (2012). Design of clinical studies and trials. In J. I. Gallin & F. P. Ognibene (Eds.), *Principles and practice of clinical research* (3rd ed., pp. 225–242). New York: Elsevier. https://doi.org/10.1016/B978-0-12-382167-6.00019-9.

2. Crossover design: allows participants to receive more than one treatment, the order of the interventions is randomized; addresses ethical limitations of a placebo control (Fig. 11.2)
3. Factorial design: allows for multiple factors (i.e., multiple treatments) to be studied simultaneously; can answer two or more questions with one trial (Fig. 11.3)
4. Randomized withdrawal design: all participants receive experimental treatment during an open-label period, nonresponders are dropped from the trial, and the responders are randomized to receive intervention or placebo in the second phase of the trial (Fig. 11.4)

B. Newer study designs (Nair, 2019)
1. Adaptive randomization methods: best described as play the winner, drop the loser designs; favors the group with the best chance of success by increasing the probability of patients being randomized to that group
2. Seamless design: a type of continuous trial process by "connecting" different trial phases, especially from Phase II to Phase III
3. Internal pilot design: the first phase of the study is designated a "pilot phase," and the study is continued until the sample size is achieved (definitive phase); analysis incorporates the pilot subjects
4. Stepped-wedge cluster randomized trial: used to evaluate health service delivery interventions or

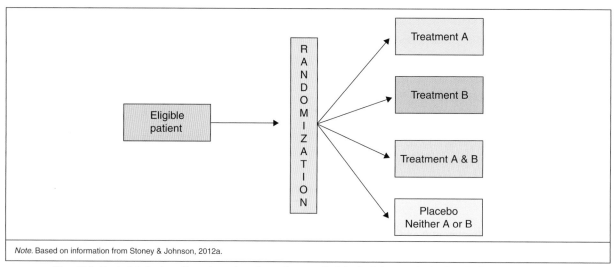

Note. Based on information from Stoney & Johnson, 2012a.

Fig. 11.3 Factorial design. Based on data from Stoney, C. M., & Johnson, L. L. (2012). Design of clinical studies and trials. In J. I. Gallin & F. P. Ognibene (Eds.), *Principles and practice of clinical research* (3rd ed., pp. 225–242). New York: Elsevier. https://doi.org/10.1016/B978-0-12-382167-6.00019-9.

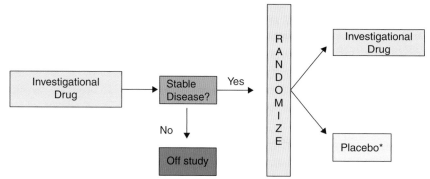

Fig. 11.4 Randomized withdrawal design. Redrawn from Nair, B. (2019). Clinical trial designs. *Indian Dermatology Online Journal, 10*(2), 193–201. https://doi.org/10.4103/idoj.IDOJ_475_18
*Placebo should only be used if no other treatment is available.

other cluster-level interventions; clusters are randomized to one of several different sequences which dictate the time at which the cluster will switch from the control condition to the intervention condition, with all clusters eventually receiving the intervention condition (Hemming, Taljaard, & Grimshaw, 2019)

C. Master protocol trials—innovative clinical trial framework that allows for the evaluation of one or more investigational treatments in multiple subgroups of a study population within the same overall clinical trial structure; expedites clinical drug development, enhances trial efficiency, and brings medicines to patients faster (Lu et al., 2021; Meyer et al., 2020)

 1. Basket trial: one targeted therapy or treatment combination is evaluated in the context of multiple diseases or disease subtypes (Fig. 11.5)
 2. Umbrella trial: multiple targeted therapies or treatment combinations are evaluated in the context of a single disease or several diseases (Fig. 11.6)
 3. Platform trial: multiple investigational treatments or treatment combinations are evaluated in the context

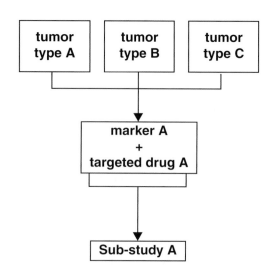

Fig. 11.5 Basket trial (Hirakawa, Asano, Sato, & Teramukai, 2018). Adapted from Hirakawa, A., Asano, J., Sato, H., & Teramukai, S. (2018). Master protocol trials in oncology: Review and new trial designs. *Contemporary Clinical Trials Communications, 12*, 1–8. https://doi.org/10.1016/j.conctc.2018.08.009.

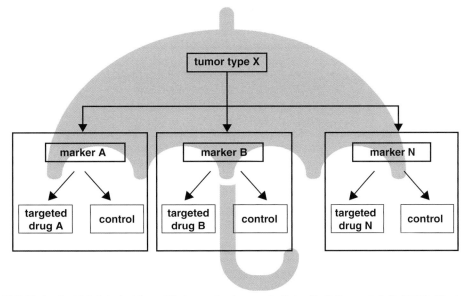

Fig. 11.6 Umbrella trial. Adapted from Hirakawa, A., Asano, J., Sato, H., & Teramukai, S. (2018). Master protocol trials in oncology: Review and new trial designs. *Contemporary Clinical Trials Communications, 12,* 1–8. https://doi.org/10.1016/j.conctc.2018.08.009.

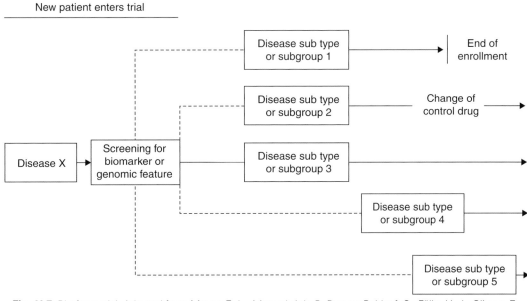

Fig. 11.7 Platform trial. Adapted from Meyer, E. L., Mesenbrink, P., Dunger-Baldauf, C., Fülle, H.-J., Glimm, E., Li, Y., Posch, M., & König, F. (2020). The evolution of master protocol clinical trial designs: A systematic literature review. *Clinical Therapeutics, 42*(7), 1330–1360. https://doi.org/10.1016/j.clinthera.2020.05.010.

of a single disease, possibly within several substudies for different disease subtypes (Fig. 11.7)

D. Phases of clinical trials (Table 11.1)

E. Considerations in clinical trials

1. Research team: led by a principal investigator (PI) and consists of professionals who study the safety and efficacy of drugs, devices, and interventions before approval for use with confidence on the public (NCI, 2020a)

   a. PI supervises all aspects of a clinical trial

   b. Other members of the research team include research nurse, data manager, and staff physician or nurse

   c. Additional members may include project manager, medical adviser, clinical research associate, regulatory affairs manager, trial supplies pharmacist, and statistician (Certified Clinical Research Professionals Society, 2021)

2. Ethics of clinical research: clinical research has the potential to exploit patient volunteers; ethical guidelines protect patient volunteers and preserve the integrity of the science (National Institutes of Health [NIH] Clinical Center, 2021)

   a. Research studies must demonstrate social and scientific value, address relevant problems or significant health-related questions

TABLE 11.1   Phases of Clinical Trials (Ness & Cusack, 2015)

Phase	Description	Goals	Approximate Subjects
0	• Exploratory study using small doses of investigational agent • Very limited drug exposure with limited duration of dosing (approx. ≤ 7 days) • No therapeutic (or diagnostic) intent • Conducted before traditional phase I study • Conducted under an exploratory IND application	• Provide human PK or PD data • Determine whether the mechanism of action defined in preclinical models could be observed in humans • Refine biomarker assay using human tumor tissue, surrogate tissue, or both • Enhance efficiency and increase the chance of success of subsequent development of the agent	• 10–12
I	• Traditional FIH dose-finding study for single agent • Dose-finding study when using multiple agents or multiple interventions (e.g., drug+radiation)	• Evaluate the safety and tolerability • Determine MTD: • Single agent • Combination of agents • Combination interventions • Determine DLT • Define optimal BAD • Evaluate PK or PD data • Observe preliminary response (e.g., antitumor activity)	• 20–100 • Healthy volunteer • Patient volunteer • Usually many cancer types (e.g., solid tumors) • Refractory to standard therapy or no remaining standard therapy • Adequate organ function, specifically bone marrow, liver, kidney • Pediatric studies conducted after safety and toxicity evaluation in adults
II	Phase IIA • Proof-of-concept study to provide initial information on the activity of intervention to justify conducting a larger study Phase IIB • Optimal dosing study to target population	Phase IIA • Demonstrate the activity of the intervention in the intended patient condition or targeted population • Establish proof of concept Phase IIB • Establish optimal dosing for the intended patient condition or targeted population to be used in phase III study • Evaluate for safety	• 80–300 • More homogenous population deemed likely to respond based on phase I data, preclinical models, and/or mechanisms of action • Subject needs to have a disease that can be accurately and reproducibility measured • May limit number of prior treatments
III	RCT	• Compare the efficacy of intervention being studied to a control group • Evaluate for safety	• Hundreds to thousands • Homogenous population
IV	Postmarketing study	• Evaluate safety during postmarketing period • May or may not be required by the US FDA • Compare the drug to another similar product that is already being marketed • Monitor for long-term and additional safety, efficacy, and quality of life • Assess drug-food interactions • Assess the effect in specific populations (e.g., pregnant women, children) or determine cost-effectiveness	• Hundreds to thousands • With the labeled indication of the newly marketed drug or biologic

BAD, Biologically active dose; *DLT*, dose-limiting toxicity; *FDA*, Food and Drug Administration; *FIH*, first-in-human; *IND*, investigational new drug; *MTD*, maximum tolerated dose; *PD*, pharmacodynamic; *PK*, pharmacokinetic; *RCT*, randomized controlled trial.
Adapted from Ness, E., & Cusack, G. (2015). Types of clinical research: Experimental. In A. D. Klimaszewski, M. Bacon, J. A. Eggert, E. Ness, J. G. Westendorp, & K. Willenberg (Eds.), *Manual for clinical trials nursing* (3rd ed.). Pittsburgh, PA: Oncology Nursing Society.

b. Investigators should be trained in the conduct of research—most commonly used is the Collaborative Institutional Training Initiative (CITI Program)

c. Research studies must be methodologically rigorous

d. Codes of ethics and codes of conduct
   (1) Nuremberg Code: voluntary consent of the human subject is absolutely essential
   (2) Declaration of Helsinki: respect for the individual, right to self-determination, and the right to make informed decisions
   (3) Belmont Report: respect for persons, beneficence, and justice
   (4) US Common Rule (Protection of Human Research Subjects [2009] 45 C.F.R. pt. 46, subpt. A, §§ 46.101–46.124): institutional review boards (IRBs); protections for

pregnant women, fetuses, neonates, children, and prisoners

(5) Council for International Organizations of Medical Sciences: conduct of research for developing countries

e. Issues with the ethical conduct of research

(1) Therapeutic misconception: research participants fail to distinguish the goals of clinical research from standard personal care (Abernethy et al., 2021)

(2) Scientific integrity: authenticity, transparency, and honesty in all aspects of the research process, from study design to dissemination of results; fairness in peer review, collegiality, and adherence to standards of practice

(3) Research misconduct: fabrication, falsification, or plagiarism in proposing, performing, or reviewing research, or in reporting research results

(4) Conflict of interest: personal, financial, professional, or political interests that are likely to undermine the ability to meet or fulfill primary professional, ethical, or legal obligations

f. Protection of human subjects in clinical trials (FDA, 2019b)

(1) IRBs, sometimes referred to as research ethics committees or research ethics boards, review and monitor biomedical research involving human subjects.

(2) An IRB has the authority to approve, require modifications in (to secure approval), or disapprove research.

(3) Institutional Animal Care and Use Committee is responsible for oversight of humane care and use of laboratory animals (National Institutes of Health [NIH] Office of Laboratory Animal Welfare, 2021).

(4) The International Council for Harmonization—Good Clinical Practice protects the rights, safety, and welfare of human subjects; used by most companies to write clinical trial policies and procedures.

III. Research protocol

A. Clear, detailed, and transparent action plan that guides the conduct of a clinical trial (Saría, 2017)

1. For investigators: written plan to carry out the clinical trial

2. For trial participants: precise description of the methodology

3. For ethics committees and IRBs: information on a safety plan and assurances to protect participants' welfare and rights

4. For funding agencies: mechanism to evaluate proposed methodologies

5. For reviewers: description of a priori methods to address potential biases

---

BOX 11.1   Elements of a Protocol

- Title page
- Schema
- Objectives
- Background and rationale
- Patient eligibility criteria
- Pharmaceutical information
- Treatment plan
- Procedures for patient entry on study
- Adverse events list and reporting requirements
- Dose modifications for adverse events
- Criteria for response assessment
- Monitoring of patients
- Off-study criteria
- Statistical considerations
- Records to be kept
- Participation
- Multicenter trials

From *National Cancer Institute Cancer Therapy Evaluation Program. A handbook for clinical investigators conducting therapeutic clinical trials supported by CTEP, DCTD, NCI [v.1.2].* (2014). http://ctep.cancer.gov/investigatorResources/docs/InvestigatorHandbook.pdf.

B. Essential elements of a protocol (Box 11.1; Mitchell & Smith, 2015)

1. Schema: brief description of the treatment plan provided in a diagram format (see Figs. 11.1–11.7)

2. Eligibility criteria: characteristics that potential participants must meet to be enrolled in the trial; includes demographic, disease-specific, and treatment-related variables (Saría, 2017)

a. Common inclusion criteria: must be satisfied before a patient can enter a trial

(1) Cancer status or stage of disease, for example, remission, progressive disease, failed previous treatment

(2) Health and performance status, for example, laboratory values, Eastern Cooperative Oncology Group, or Karnofsky Performance status

(3) Measurable disease, for example, tumor size measured using computed tomography (CT) or positron emission tomography/CT scans

(4) Presence or absence of tumor biomarkers

b. Common exclusion criterion: history of certain prior treatment, confusion/dementia, and other comorbidities

3. Pharmaceutical information: details on experimental agents (i.e., investigational or commercial agent)

4. Treatment plan: includes aspects of experimental treatment, including dose, route, and schedule

5. Adverse events list and reporting requirements: identify previously reported side effects associated with the experimental treatment; include procedures for reporting (i.e., method, time frame, regulatory and administrative agencies)

TABLE 11.2 Clinical Trial Endpoints (Madsen & Ness, 2016)

Endpoint	Definition
Overall survival	Time from randomization until death
	Intent-to-treat population
Disease-free survival	Randomization until recurrence of tumor or death from any cause
	Adjuvant setting after definitive surgery or radiotherapy
	Large percentage of patients achieve complete response after chemotherapy
Objective response rate	Proportion of patients with reduction of tumor size of a predefined amount and for a minimum period
	Measure from time of initial response until progression
	Sum of partial-response patients and complete-response patients
	Uses standardized criteria when possible
Progression-free survival	Randomization until objective tumor progression or death
	Preferred regulatory endpoint
	Assumes deaths are related to progression
Time to progression	Randomization until objective tumor progression, excluding deaths
Time to treatment failure	Randomization to discontinuation of treatment for any reason (e.g., progressive disease, toxicity, death)
	Not recommended for regulatory drug approval

From Madsen, L. & Ness, E. (2016). Protocol development and response assessment. In A. D. Klimaszewski, M. Bacon, J. Eggert, E. Ness, J. Westendorp, & K. Willenberg (Eds.), *Manual for clinical trials nursing*. Pittsburgh: Oncology Nursing Society.

a. Common Terminology Criteria for Adverse Events (CTCAE v5.0): provides standardization and consistency in the definition of treatment-related toxicity

6. Criteria for response assessment: objective study endpoints, including definitions of complete and partial response, stable disease, and progressive disease
   a. Clinical trial endpoints (Table 11.2)
   b. Response evaluation criteria in solid tumors: solid tumor response assessment
      (1) Complete response: disappearance of all target lesions, and any pathologic lymph nodes (whether target or nontarget) must have reduction in short axis to less than 10 mm
      (2) Partial response: at least a 30% decrease in the sum of the diameters of target lesions
      (3) Progressive disease: at least a 20% increase in the sum of the diameters of target lesions
      (4) Stable disease: neither partial response nor progressive disease
   c. Internationally agreed-upon response standards exist for hematologic malignancies (refer to Chapters 18, 20, and 21)
7. Off-study criteria: circumstances that prevent the participant from continuing the trial (e.g., progressive disease, adverse events, or delay in study treatment)

IV. Nursing implications
   A. Provide information related to clinical trials participation
      1. Reinforce information received from PI, clinical trial nurse (CTN), or members of the research team regarding the research study in which they are considering participation.
      2. Discuss the risks and benefits of the research study.

3. Explain that participating is voluntary and that refusal to participate or withdrawal later will not result in penalty or loss of benefits to which the research participant is otherwise entitled.
4. Review alternatives for treatment.

   B. Assist patient and family in decision-making
      1. Encourage patient to discuss the research study with family, friends, and a trusted non-family member advisor (i.e., pastor, attorney).
      2. Instruct patient and family to write down pros and cons of, and alternatives to, participation in the research study.
      3. Read and discuss with significant others the informed consent form and educational information provided by the PI or CTN.
      4. Instruct patient and family to write down questions for PI or research nurse. Provide patient with sample questions.
      5. Encourage patient and family to approach PI or CTN to ask questions.
      6. Allow patient and family time to make a decision.
      7. Provide resources, including websites that have patient information about clinical trials.

REFERENCES

Abernethy, E. R., Campbell, G. P., Hianik, R. S., Thomson, M. C., Blee, S. M., Sibold, H. C., Dixon, M. D., Switchenko, J. M., & Pentz, R. D. (2021). Reassessing the measurement and presence of therapeutic misconception in a phase 1 setting. *Cancer, 127*(20), 3794–3800. https://doi.org/10.1002/cncr.33746.

Certified Clinical Research Professionals Society. The clinical trials team – Roles & responsibilities. (2021). https://ccrps.org/clinical-research-blog/the-clinical-trials-team-roles-amp-responsibilities.

ClinicalTrials.gov. Glossary of common site terms. (2021). https://clinicaltrials.gov/ct2/about-studies/glossary.

Food and Drug Administration (FDA). Expanded access. Keywords, definitions, and resources. (2019a). https://www.fda.gov/news-events/expanded-access/expanded-access-keywords-definitions-and-resources.

Food and Drug Administration (FDA). Institutional review boards (IRBs) and protection of human subjects in clinical trials. (2019b). https://www.fda.gov/about-fda/center-drug-evaluation-and-research-cder/institutional-review-boards-irbs-and-protection-human-subjects-clinical-trials.

Geiger, A. M., O'Mara, A. M., McCaskill-Stevens, W. J., Adjei, B., Tuovenin, P., & Castro, K. M. (2020). Evolution of cancer care delivery research in the NCI Community Oncology Research Program. *Journal of the National Cancer Institute, 112*(6), 557–561. https://doi.org/10.1093/jnci/djz234.

Hemming, K., Taljaard, M., & Grimshaw, J. (2019). Introducing the new CONSORT extension for stepped-wedge cluster randomised trials. *Trials, 20*(1), 68. https://doi.org/10.1186/s13063-018-3116-3.

Hirakawa, A., Asano, J., Sato, H., & Teramukai, S. (2018). Master protocol trials in oncology: Review and new trial designs. *Contemporary Clinical Trials Communications, 12*, 1–8. https://doi.org/10.1016/j.conctc.2018.08.009.

Madsen, L., & Ness, E. (2016). Protocol development and response assessment. In A. D. Klimaszewski, M. Bacon, J. Eggert, E. Ness, J. Westendorp, & K. Willenberg (Eds.), *Manual for clinical trials nursing.* Pittsburgh, PA: Oncology Nursing Society.

Lu, C. C., Li, X. N., Broglio, K., Bycott, P., Jiang, Q., Li, X., McGlothlin, A., Tian, H., & Ye, J. (2021). Practical considerations and recommendations for master protocol framework: Basket, umbrella and platform trials. *Therapeutic Innovation & Regulatory Science, 55*(6), 1145–1154. https://doi.org/10.1007/s43441-021-00315-7.

Meyer, E. L., Mesenbrink, P., Dunger-Baldauf, C., Fülle, H.-J., Glimm, E., Li, Y., Posch, M., & König, F. (2020). The evolution of master protocol clinical trial designs: A systematic literature review. *Clinical Therapeutics, 42*(7), 1330–1360. https://doi.org/10.1016/j.clinthera.2020.05.010.

Mitchell, W., & Smith, Z. (2015). Elements of a protocol. In A. D. Klimaszewski, M. Bacon, J. A. Eggert, E. Ness, J. G. Westendorp, & K. Willenberg (Eds.), *Manual for clinical trials nursing* (3rd ed.). Pittsburgh, PA: Oncology Nursing Society.

Nair, B. (2019). Clinical trial designs. *Indian Dermatology Online Journal, 10*(2), 193–201. https://doi.org/10.4103/idoj.IDOJ_475_18.

National Cancer Institute (NCI). Research team members. (2020a). https://www.cancer.gov/about-cancer/treatment/clinical-trials/what-are-trials/team.

National Cancer Institute (NCI). Types of clinical trials. (2020b). https://www.cancer.gov/about-cancer/treatment/clinical-trials/what-are-trials/types.

National Institutes of Health (NIH). NIH clinical research trials and you. (2022). https://www.nih.gov/health-information/nih-clinical-research-trials-you/basics.

National Institutes of Health (NIH) Clinical Center. Patient recruitment: Ethics in clinical research. (2021). https://clinicalcenter.nih.gov/recruit/ethics.html.

National Institutes of Health (NIH) Office of Laboratory Animal Welfare. The Institutional Animal Care and Use Committee. (2021). https://olaw.nih.gov/resources/tutorial/iacuc.htm.

Ness, E., & Cusack, G. (2015). Types of clinical research: Experimental. In A. D. Klimaszewski, M. Bacon, J. A. Eggert, E. Ness, J. G. Westendorp, & K. Willenberg (Eds.), *Manual for clinical trials nursing* (3rd ed.). Pittsburgh, PA: Oncology Nursing Society.

Saría, M. G. (2017). Clinical trials. In S. Newton, M. Hickey, & J. M. Brant (Eds.), *Mosby's oncology nursing advisor* (2nd ed.). St. Louis, MO: Elsevier.

Stoney, C. M., & Johnson, L. L. (2012). Design of clinical studies and trials. In J. I. Gallin & F. P. Ognibene (Eds.), *Principles and practice of clinical research* (3rd ed., pp. 225–242). New York: Elsevier. https://doi.org/10.1016/B978-0-12-382167-6.00019-9.

Bone and Soft Tissue Cancers

Katrina Young and Tiffany Whetzel

OVERVIEW

I. Definition
  A. Bone cancer
    1. Most common types—Osteosarcoma and Ewing tumors
      a. Osteosarcoma—most common type of cancer which begins in the bones. The most common sites include the bones around the knee (distal femur and proximal tibia) and upper arm bone (proximal humerus) (American Cancer Society [ACS], 2020).
      b. Ewing tumor—group of cancer that begins in the bone or nearby soft tissues. The most common sites include the pelvis, chest wall, and legs (ACS, 2021a).
    2. Some rare types include chondrosarcoma, high-grade undifferentiated pleomorphic sarcoma of bone, fibrosarcoma of bone, giant cell tumor of bone and chordoma (ACS, 2018).
  B. Soft tissue sarcoma (ACS, 2021b)
    1. Develop in soft tissues such as fat, muscle, nerves, fibrous tissue, blood vessels, or deep skin tissues. Most begin in the arms or legs.
II. Epidemiology
  A. Bone cancer—2022 estimates (bone and joints)—3910 new cases; 2100 deaths (ACS, 2022a)
    1. Approximately 68%–73% survival at 5 years (ACS, 2022a)
    2. Bone cancers in pediatrics/adolescents:
      a. Osteosarcoma (2% of all childhood cancers) (ACS, 2020)
      b. Ewing sarcoma (1% of all childhood cancers) (ACS, 2021a)
  B. Soft tissue sarcoma—2022 estimates—13,190 new cases; 5130 deaths; incidence slightly higher for men (ACS, 2021b)
III. Pathophysiology
  A. Primary bone cancer and soft tissue sarcomas
    1. Primary bone cancer (Prater & McKeon, 2021)
      a. Usually occur in the metaphysis of long bones

b. There are various subtypes based on the location of the tumor—central (intramedullary), surface (periosteal/cortical), and extra skeletal
    2. Patterns of growth (Samuel, 2018)
      a. Compression of normal tissue
      b. Resorption of bone by reactive osteoclasts
      c. Destruction of normal tissue (when malignant)
    3. Soft tissue sarcomas (ACS, 2021b)
      a. Can be found in soft tissues such as fat, muscle, nerves, fibrous tissues, blood vessels, or deep skin tissues
      b. More than 50 different types of soft tissue sarcoma
  B. Metastatic spread to bone from primary solid tumors. Common primary cancers that metastasize to the bone are bladder, breast, kidney, lung, melanoma, prostate, thyroid, and uterus (National Cancer Institute [NCI], 2020).
IV. Prevention and risk factors
  A. Soft tissue sarcoma (ACS, 2021b)
    1. Risk factors include radiation, certain family cancer syndromes, a damaged lymph system, and exposure to certain chemicals.
  B. Osteosarcoma (osteogenic sarcoma, osseous tissue) (ACS, 2020)
    1. Risk factors include age (highest for those between ages of 10 and 30), height (usually taller for their age), gender (more common in males), race/ethnicity (slightly more common in African Americans and Hispanics/Latinos), radiation, certain bone diseases (Paget, hereditary multiple osteochondromas, fibrous dysplasia), and certain family cancer syndromes (retinoblastoma, Li–Fraumeni syndrome, Rothmund–Thomson syndrome, Bloom syndrome, Werner syndrome, Diamond–Blackfan anemia) (ACS, 2020).
    2. There are no known lifestyle or environmental changes which impact Osteosarcoma.
  C. Ewing family tumors (EFT, reticuloendothelial tissue) (ACS, 2021a)

1. Risk factors include race/ethnicity (more common in Whites, either non-Hispanic or Hispanic), gender (more common in males), and age (more common in older children and teens).
2. There are no known lifestyle or environmental changes which impact the EFT.

D. Kaposi sarcoma (ACS, 2018)
   1. Caused by infectious virus: Kaposi sarcoma–associated herpesvirus (KSHV). Virus also known as *human herpesvirus 8*.
      a. KSHV is in the same family as Epstein–Barr virus
   2. Most cases occur in people who have HIV and AIDS. Prevention includes protected sex, daily antiviral drugs for those at high risk for HIV, using clean needles to inject recreational drugs, and treating HIV-positive pregnant mothers and babies with anti-HIV drugs and avoiding breastfeeding.

V. Diagnosis
   A. Clinical symptoms
      1. Bone (NCI, 2022a)
         a. Can present as painful or painless swollen mass
         b. Variety of presenting symptoms include a lump that may feel soft or warm, unexplained fever, a pathological fracture
      2. Soft tissue sarcoma (ACS, 2021b)
         a. New lump anywhere in body
            (1) Half start on an arm or leg
         b. Worsening abdominal pain (location retroperitoneum)
            (1) Blood in stool or vomit
   B. Physical examination
      1. Characteristics (ACS, 2022a)
         a. Mass may or may not be visible, palpable; may be firm, nontender, warm
         b. Size noted, bilateral comparison
         c. Limited range of motion
   C. Diagnostic imaging (NCI, 2022a)
      1. Radiography (cannot see changes until tumor is advanced)
         a. Bone scan—shows additional skeletal lesions
         b. Other imaging: computed tomography (CT) of chest and abnormal area, magnetic resonance imaging, positron emission tomography, angiogram, CHEST X-RAY (if CT chest not done), X-ray of bone (usually done first)
   D. Biopsy (NCI, 2022a)
      1. May perform a needle biopsy, excisional biopsy, or an incisional biopsy
   E. Laboratory values (NCI, 2022a)
      1. Elevated serum alkaline phosphatase and elevated lactate dehydrogenase level because of increased osteoblastic activity

VI. Histopathology
   A. Classified or staged by cell type, origin-connective tissue (fat, muscle, tendons, fibrous tissue) (American Joint Committee on Cancer [AJCC], 2022)

B. Sarcomas classified by histology, not location (ACS, 2022b)
C. Pathology evaluation can include (NCI, 2022b, 2022c)
   1. Cell type or tissue of origin
   2. Genetic factors: alterations and variants
   3. Immunohistochemistry testing results

VII. Staging
   D. Staging based on biologic behavior and tumor aggressiveness
      1. Musculoskeletal Tumor Society staging system is commonly used to stage bone cancer. Based on three key components (ACS, 2021b).
         a. Grade (G)—either low grade (G1) or high grade (G2)
            (1) Low grade (G1) looks more like a normal cell and is likely to grow and spread slowly
            (2) High grade (G2) looks more abnormal and is likely to grow and spread more rapidly
         b. Extent of the primary tumor (T)—either intracompartmental (T1) or extracompartmental (T2)
            (1) Intracompartmental (T1) remained within the bone
            (2) Extracompartmental (T2) has spread beyond the bone
         c. Metastasized (M)—spread to any lymph nodes or other organs.
      2. The other staging system which can be used is the American Joint Committee on Cancer TNM system (AJCC, 2022).
         a. Tumor (T)—Extent of tumor
         b. Nodes (N)—Has it spread to nearby lymph nodes?
         c. Metastasis (M)—The spread to distant sites?
         d. Grade (G)—How abnormal the cells look?
      3. The system used for staging is based on the physician preference.

VIII. Prognosis and survival
   A. Sarcomas
      1. Prognosis depends on tumor size, grade, resection margin (NCI, 2022b, 2022c).
         a. Prognosis poor with metastasis
         b. Spread from primary lesions to lung, breast, colon, pancreas, kidney, thyroid, prostate, stomach, and testes (NCI, 2022b, 2022c)
         c. Other early metastatic sites—spine, ribs, pelvis (90% in axial skeleton) (ACS, 2022b)
         d. Tumor infiltrates may be distant from the site of origin
   B. EFT (reticuloendothelial tissue) (NCI, 2022b, 2022c)
      1. For Ewing sarcoma, the 5-year survival rate has increased from 59% to a range of 75%–80% for children younger than 15 and for adolescents (15–19); 5-year survival rate increased from 20% to approximately 65%.
   C. Kaposi sarcoma (NCI, 2022b, 2022c)
      1. Five-year overall survival rate on chemotherapy 85%
   D. Osteosarcoma (NCI, 2022b, 2022c)

1. Between 1975 and 2010 childhood osteosarcoma mortality decreased by more than 50%
2. In adolescents (15–19), 5-year survival rate increased 56% to approximately 66%

E. Soft tissue sarcoma (NCI, 2022b, 2022c)
1. Highly malignant (approximately 25% with metastases at time of diagnosis to lungs, lymph nodes, and other bones) (NCI, 2022b, 2022c)
2. 5-year relative survival rates for all stages combined is 65% because of multimodality therapies, precision in surgery (wide resections) (ACS, 2022b)
3. In 2022 in the United States, about 13,190 new cases diagnosed; 5130 will die

MANAGEMENT

A. Treatment (ACS, 2022b; Samuel, 2018)
1. Goals: survival, removal of tumor, preserve functioning

B. Treatment: surgery
1. Treatment of choice with osteosarcoma, fibrosarcoma, chondrosarcoma
2. Types of surgery:
   a. Amputation
   b. Limb salvage
   c. Rotationplasty
3. Amputation versus limb salvage issues—increased effort to salvage rather than amputate; issues that affect the decision include:
   a. Acceptable surgical margins
   b. Blood vessels and nerves involved with the tumor
   c. Age (in children younger than 10 years, surgery affects limb growth)
   d. Typical treatment strategy: if limb salvage, radiation therapy follows
4. Amputation issues
   a. When tumor extends to incisional surface
   b. When location necessitates (e.g., tumor extends to vertebral body and pelvis)
   c. Infection, skeletal immaturity
   d. Major neurovascular involvement
5. Reconstruction (Samuel, 2018)
   a. Bone autografts, allografts
   b. After soft tissue resection, three common methods:
      (1) Arthrodesis or fusion (with implants or grafts)
      (2) Arthroplasty for joints
      (3) Allografts (since the 1960s)—bone, tendon, ligament, connective tissue
6. Issues—nonunion, infections, healing, functional concerns (especially with limb salvage)

C. Treatment: adjuvant radiotherapy (RT) (Samuel, 2018)
1. Soft tissue tumors can be radiosensitive and radio responsive
2. Usually, external-beam RT, before or after surgery

a. Used when tumor is localized or after surgical debulking or tumor removal
3. For palliative care, pain relief (NCI, 2022b, 2022c)

D. Treatment: chemotherapy or immunotherapy (National Comprehensive Cancer Network [NCCN], 2022a, 2022b)
1. Adjuvant or neoadjuvant with surgery/RT (Samuel, 2018)
   a. Outcomes show better local control, increased time to treatment failure, especially in EFT, rhabdomyosarcoma, and osteosarcomas (NCI, 2022b, 2022c)
   b. Treats occult micro-metastases (Samuel, 2018)
   c. In advanced tumors, treatments can include sequential and/or multiagent protocols (Samuel, 2018)
      (1) Exception—highly active antiretroviral therapy for Kaposi sarcoma (NCI, 2022b, 2022c)
   d. Targeted molecular therapies are promising (oncogene activation triggered by viruses or antibodies) (Samuel, 2018)
2. Food and Drug Administration–approved chemotherapeutic agents—doxorubicin (Adriamycin), cisplatin (Platinol), cyclophosphamide (Cytoxan), dacarbazine (DTIC-Dome), ifosfamide (Ifex), methotrexate (Mexate), vincristine (Oncovin), cosmegen (Dactinomycin), and denosumab (Xgeva) (NCI, 2022b, 2022c)
   a. Combination regimens: soft tissue sarcoma subtypes, nonspecific histologies. Selected therapies (NCCN, 2022b):
      (1) AD: doxorubicin, dacarbazine
      (2) AIM: doxorubicin, ifosfamide, Mesna
      (3) MAID: Mesna, doxorubicin, ifosfamide, dacarbazine
      (4) gemcitabine; docetaxel, vinorelbine or dacarbazine (unresectable or metastatic)
3. Systemic treatment using molecular and cell biology (antiangiogenesis, monoclonal antibodies, vaccines, T cells) (NCCN 2022b):
   a. As an example, for gastrointestinal stromal tumor with disease progression after standard therapies, some selected molecular/cell biology therapies (NCCN, 2022b; Vallilas et al., 2021):
      (1) Sorafenib
      (2) Nilotinib
      (3) Pazopanib
      (4) Avapritinib
      (5) Cabozantinib
      (6) Dasatinib
      (7) Everolimus
      (8) Larotrectinib

X. Nursing implications
A. Care related to phantom limb pain or sensation (Samuel, 2018)
1. One to 4 weeks postoperatively; usually resolves in a few months; can be chronic

2. Client aware of itching, pressure, tingling, severe cramping, throbbing, burning pain
3. Usually triggered by fatigue, stress, excitement, and other stimuli

B. Care related to preoperative care when client will lose limb (Samuel, 2018)

1. For anticipated amputation, many psychological needs exist (especially with adolescents); issues to address include anxiety, depression; grief about lost limb; physical as well as emotional and social losses; altered body image; fear of disability; coping with deformity; short-term loss of independence and self-sufficiency

2. Rehabilitation plan after surgery—awareness of possible symptoms after surgery, including phantom limb sensation, pain (throbbing, burning), itching pressure, tingling, and severe cramping

3. Postoperative care when client has lost limb (Xu et al., 2020)
   a. Observation of drainage from the site for redness, hemorrhage, increased pain, tenderness and swelling, blisters, abrasion
   b. If need for stump care
      (1) Elevation of stump (usually at least 24–48 hours) to prevent edema and promote venous return
      (2) Unwrap stump dressing every 4–6 hours for the first 2 days post op, then daily: assess for color, temperature, and most proximal pulse on the stump before rewrapping it. Compare findings to the contralateral extremity
      (3) Dangling and transfer to chair after the day of surgery
         (a) Assisting client into prone position three or four times per day for 15 minutes minimum to prevent hip contractures, turning every 2 hours
         (b) Coordination of collaborative services (e.g., physical therapy, social services, occupational therapy)

4. Postoperative management of limb salvage (Xu et al., 2020)
   a. Neurovascular checks distal to surgical site
   b. Monitor for blood loss and anemia from extensive tumor resection and reconstruction
   c. Monitor wound site for signs of infection
   d. Pain management

5. Many other areas for nurses to address in their plan of care (Samuel, 2018)
   a. Pathologic fractures/weight-bearing
   b. Radiation effects
   c. Chemotherapy effects

d. Body image
e. Impaired sexuality and fertility
f. Psychosocial support and coping
g. Survivorship and follow-up

REFERENCES

American Cancer Society (ACS). *Kaposi sarcoma*. (2018). https://www.cancer.org/cancer/kaposi-sarcoma.html.

American Cancer Society (ACS). *Osteosarcoma*. (2020). https://www.cancer.org/cancer/osteosarcoma.html.

American Cancer Society (ACS). *Ewing family of tumors*. (2021a). https://www.cancer.org/cancer/ewing-tumor.html.

American Cancer Society (ACS). *Bone cancer stages*. (2021b). https://www.cancer.org/cancer/bone-cancer/detection-diagnosis-staging/staging.html.

American Cancer Society (ACS). *Cancer facts and statistics*. (2022a). https://www.cancer.org/research/cancer-facts-statistics.html.

American Cancer Society (ACS). *Soft tissue sarcoma*. (2022b). https://www.cancer.org/cancer/soft-tissue-sarcoma.html.

American Joint Committee on Cancer (AJCC). (2022). *Cancer staging systems*. American College of Surgeons. Retrieved from https://www.facs.org/quality-programs/cancer/ajcc/cancer-staging.

National Cancer Institute (NCI). Metastatic cancer: When cancer spreads. (2020). https://www.cancer.gov/types/metastatic-cancer#:~:text=Where%20Cancer%20Spreads%20%20%20%20Cancer%20Type,brain%2C%20liver%2C%20lung%20%209%20more%20rows%20.

National Cancer Institute (NCI). *Primary bone cancer*. (2022a). https://www.cancer.gov/types/bone/bone-fact-sheet.

National Cancer Institute (NCI). *Soft tissue sarcoma treatment (PDQ) – Health professional version*. (2022b). https://www.cancer.gov/types/soft-tissue-sarcoma/hp/adult-soft-tissue-treatment-pdq.

National Cancer Institute (NCI). *Bone cancer – Health professional version*. (2022c). https://www.cancer.gov/types/bone/hp.

National Comprehensive Cancer Network (NCCN). (2022a). Bone cancer *[v1.2022]*. Retrieved from. https://www.nccn.org/professionals/physician_gls/pdf/bone.pdf

National Comprehensive Cancer Network (NCCN). (2022b). Soft Tissue Sarcoma *[v2.2022]*. Retrieved from https://www.nccn.org/professionals/physician_gls/pdf/sarcoma.pdf.

Prater, S., & McKeon, B. (2021). Osteosarcoma. In: *StatPerals*. Treasure Island, FL: StatPearls Publishing. Retrieved from https://www.ncbi.nlm.nih.gov/books/NBK549868/.

Samuel, L. C. (2018). Bone and soft tissue sarcomas. In C. H. Yarbro, D. Wujcik, & B. H. Gobel (Eds.), *Cancer nursing: principles and practice* (8th ed., pp. 1243–1277). Sudbury, MA: Jones & Bartlett.

Vallilas, C., Sarantis, P., Kyriazoglou, A., Koustas, E., Theocharis, S., Papavassiliou, A. G., et al. (2021). Gastrointestinal stromal tumors (GISTs): Novel therapeutic strategies with immunotherapy and small molecules. *International journal of molecular sciences*, 22(2), 493. https://doi.org/10.3390/ijms22020493.

Xu, M., Wang, Z., Yu, X. C., Lin, J. H., & Hu, Y. C. (2020). Guideline for limb-salvage treatment of osteosarcoma. *Orthopaedic Surgery*, 12(4), 1021–1029. https://doi.org/10.1111/os.12702.

13

Breast Cancer

Tara J. Ower and Rachelle Park

OVERVIEW

I. Anatomy and physiology (National Cancer Institute [NCI], 2022a)
  A. Both men and women develop breasts from the same embryologic tissues. At puberty, female sex hormones, mainly estrogen, promote the development of tissue; this does not occur in men because of higher amounts of testosterone. Women's breasts become more prominent than those of men.
     1. Size and shape of breasts vary from woman to woman and will change over the course of her life.
     2. Breast tissue consists mostly of adipose tissue. Within this tissue are lobes, lobules, ducts, blood vessels, lymph vessels, lymph nodes, nerves, connective tissue, and ligaments; externally are the nipple and areola (Fig. 13.1).
        a. Adipose tissue—determines breast size and shape; becomes more prominent after menopause; 2:1 ratio of milk glands to fat in lactating breast; 1:1 ratio of milk glands to fat in nonlactating breast.
        b. Glandular tissue—consist of 15–20 lobes with lobules and milk ducts that head toward the nipple and produce breast milk.
        c. Lymphatic tissues—consist of lymph nodes and lymph vessels; 75% of lymph fluid flows toward the axilla (pectoral, subscapular, humeral); 25% flows toward the parasternal lymph nodes, other breast, or abdomen.
        d. Breast tissue overlies the chest (pectoral) muscles; it lies between the sternum and the midaxillary line (axilla) from the second to the sixth ribs and below the clavicle.
     3. Males may develop a condition called *gynecomastia*, which is an increase in breast tissue. It is most often the result of hormonal imbalance (Vandeven & Pensler, 2022).
II. Epidemiology
  A. Worldwide—Most prevalent cancer; 2.3 million new cases in 2020 (WHO, 2022).
  B. United States—Estimated new cases in 2022, approximately 290,560 (287,850 women and 2710 men); estimated deaths in 2022 about 43,780 (43,250 women and 530 men) (Siegel, Miller, Fuchs, & Jemal, 2022).
     1. Accounts for 31% of new cancer cases in US women (Siegel et al., 2022).
     2. Second leading cause of cancer-related death in US women (American Cancer Society [ACS], 2022).
  C. Mortality trends
     1. Death rate peaked in 1989. Declining 1.3% per year from 2010 to 2019, attributed to improvements in screening and treatment (ACS, 2022; NCI, 2022b).
     2. Mortality rate 41% higher for Black women than White women, despite lower incidence (ACS, 2022; NCI, 2022b).
  D. Trends in incidence rates
     1. Between 2002 and 2003, breast cancer incidence rate dropped by 7%, largely because of a reduction in the use of hormone replacement therapy.
     2. Since the mid-2000s, the rate of new cases has increased by approximately 0.5% per year (ACS, 2022).
     3. An estimated 51,400 US women newly diagnosed with in situ breast cancer in 2022 (ACS, 2022).
III. Risk factors (ACS, 2022; National Comprehensive Cancer Network [NCCN], 2022)
  A. Female gender—Men can get breast cancer too, but it's much more common in women.
  B. Age—Risk increases with age; median age is 62.
  C. Race and ethnicity
     1. One in 8 White women will develop breast cancer from birth until death.
     2. One in 10 African American women will develop breast cancer.
        a. More African American women are diagnosed with breast cancer at a younger age (<40 years old).
     3. Lower rates in Hispanic, Asian/Pacific Islander, and Native American women.
  D. Genetic factors—Family history of inherited breast cancer. Less common, 5% to 10% of all breast cancers. One out of five men who develop breast cancer has a family history of the disease. All eligible patients should undergo genetic testing after the diagnosis of breast cancer. Multigene testing should be done (NCCN, 2022).
     1. BRCA1: Greater than 60% lifetime risk of developing breast cancer, with a predisposition to triple-negative breast cancer.

Anatomy of the Female Breast

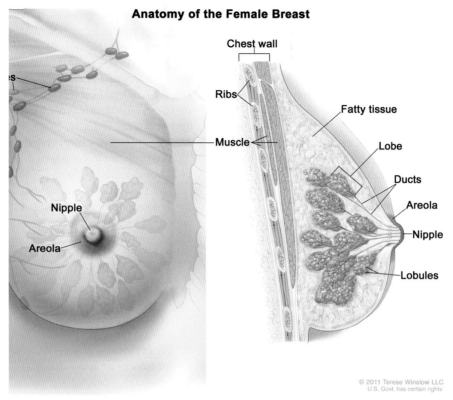

Chest wall

Ribs

Muscle

Nipple

Areola

Fatty tissue

Lobe

Ducts

Areola

Nipple

Lobules

© 2011 Terese Winslow LLC
U.S. Govt. has certain rights

Fig. 13.1 Anatomy of the female breast. From https://nci-media.cancer.gov/pdq/media/images/415520.jpg.

2. BRCA2: Greater than 60% lifetime risk of developing breast cancer, with a predisposition to ER-positive breast cancers.
3. TP53: Li–Fraumeni syndrome risk; risk is greater than 60%, with a predisposition to triple-positive breast cancer.
4. ATM (ataxia-telangiectasia mutated): Causes ataxia-telangiectasia disease, which is associated with a 15%–40% increased rate of developing breast cancer.
5. BARD1: Increased 15%–40% risk of developing breast cancer in lifetime. Strong evidence for triple-negative breast cancer.
6. PTEN: Causes Cowden disease; lifetime risk of developing breast cancer is 40%–60%.
7. STK11: Can cause Peutz–Jeghers syndrome; lifetime risk is 40%–60%.
8. CHEK2: Increased lifetime risk of 15%–40% of developing breast cancer, with a predisposition of developing ER-positive carcinoma.
9. Lynch syndrome: Hereditary nonpolyposis colorectal cancer.
10. PALB2: Making a protein called partner and localizer of BRCA2. Increased lifetime risk of 41%–60% of developing breast cancer, with overrepresentation of triple-negative breast cancer.
11. BRIP1: Insufficient data to define lifetime risk, potential increase for breast cancer.
12. RAD51C and RAD51D: Increased lifetime risk of 15%–40%, strong for ER/progesterone-receptor (PR) negative cancer.
13. NF1: Increased lifetime risk of 15%–40% of developing breast cancer. Recommended to start annual mammograms at age 30, with consideration of Breast MRI until age 50.
14. CDH1: Increased lifetime risk of 41%–60% of developing breast cancer, with a predisposition for lobular carcinoma.
15. Klinefelter syndrome: Extra X chromosome has increased risk of breast cancer due to higher levels of estrogen and lower levels of male hormones, androgens.

E. Personal history
1. Reproductive/hormonal factors
   a. Age—Late age of first full-term pregnancy (after 30); less risk if first pregnancy before 20.
   b. Nulliparity—Never pregnant increases risk.
   c. Number of births—Lower risk seen with a higher number of births.
   d. Lactation or breastfeeding—Decreased risk in women who breastfed their babies, especially for long duration.
   e. Age at menarche/menopause—Increased risk with early menstruation (before age 12), and late menopause (after age 55).
2. Postthoracic radiation therapy to chest (e.g., radiation therapy to the chest for Hodgkin lymphoma and non-Hodgkin lymphoma, especially as a teen or young adult).
3. Family history—Increased risk in women who have first-degree relative(s) (mother, father, sister,

daughter, brother) with breast cancer. Having one first-degree relative almost doubles the risk. Having two first-degree relatives increases the risk threefold.

    4. Breast implants—Increase the risk of developing breast implant-associated anaplastic large cell lymphoma (BIA-ALCL). This rare type of non-Hodgkin lymphoma appears to happen more often with textured implants.

  F. Lifestyle factors (ACS, 2022; NCCN, 2022)

    1. Use of hormone replacement therapy (including bioidenticals) and oral contraceptives.

    2. Lack of exercise—Exercise lowers body weight, affects hormone levels, alters metabolism.

    3. Diets high in fat, especially polyunsaturated fats (Maisonneuve, 2017).

    4. Monounsaturated fats such as olive oil may be protective (Maisonneuve, 2017).

    5. Obesity/weight gain—Being overweight or obese after menopause increases your risk of developing breast cancer. Before menopause, estrogen is primarily made in your ovaries. After menopause, most estrogen comes from fat tissue. Having more fat tissue after menopause can raise estrogen levels and increase the chances of developing breast cancer.

    6. Alcohol consumption—Women who have one drink per day have a 7%–10% increase in risk compared with those who do not drink. Two to three drinks per day increases the risk to about 20%.

IV. Primary prevention of breast cancer in *high-risk* individuals (NCCN, 2022)

  A. Risk-reducing medications:

    1. Tamoxifen—First-generation selective ER modulator (SERM) used in pre- and postmenopausal women, as well as men. While on Tamoxifen, women have an increased risk (less than 1% per year) of developing endometrial cancer.

    2. Raloxifene—SERM used to reduce risk in postmenopausal women.

    3. Aromatase inhibitors (AI)—used in women but not commonly used in men.

      a. Exemestane—Showed benefit in reducing invasive breast cancers in postmenopausal women who were at moderate risk for breast cancer

      b. Anastrozole

    4. Contraindications for tamoxifen and raloxifene—History of deep vein thrombosis, pulmonary embolus, thrombotic stroke, transient ischemic attack, or known inherited clotting trait.

  B. Risk-reduction surgery—Bilateral mastectomy; typically only recommended if patient has a pathogenic variant.

  C. Increased screening measures—For those patients who have a risk model lifetime score of >20% or a genetic pathogenic variant, consider an annual mammogram to begin 10 years prior to when the youngest family member was diagnosed with breast cancer and consider an annual MRI with contrast to begin 10 years prior to

when the youngest family member was diagnosed with breast cancer, not prior to age 25 or age 40 (whichever comes first) (NCCN, 2022).

V. Early detection—Increased chance of survival if breast cancer diagnosed at an early stage. Use of risk models (i.e., Tyrer–Cuzick or Gail model) important to develop personalized screening protocols based on patient's overall lifetime risk score (NCCN, 2022).

  A. Signs of breast cancer (NCI, 2022a)

    1. Lump or thickening in or near the breast or near the underarm (axilla)

    2. Change in the size or shape of the breast

    3. Dimpling or puckering of the skin

    4. New onset nipple inversion (nipple turned inwards toward the breast)

    5. Nipple discharge

    6. Scaly, red, or swollen skin on the breast, areola, or nipple

    7. Dimples in the skin that look like the skin of an orange (peau d'orange)

VI. Diagnostic measures (NCI, 2022a; ACS, 2022)

  A. Clinical breast exam—Palpate breast and axillary tissue for masses or acute changes.

  B. Imaging

    1. Mammogram—Machine compresses the breast and uses x-rays to look at breast tissue; can detect masses, calcifications, asymmetries, and distortions. Recommended annually at age 40. Undergoing a mammogram has the same radiation exposure as an individual would expect to receive from natural (background) radiation over 7 weeks.

      (1) Screening mammogram: Performed on women who have no symptoms or active breast problems. Includes views from two angles.

      (2) Diagnostic mammogram: Performed when a woman has symptoms or there is a finding on a screening mammogram. Includes extra views.

      (3) Tomosynthesis (3D) mammogram: Lowers the chance of the patient being "called back"; considered more comfortable for the patient; better at viewing abnormalities in dense breast tissue.

    2. Ultrasound—Uses sound waves to produce images of internal structures of the breast to help identify masses or other abnormalities. Can determine if a mass is solid or fluid-filled.

    3. MRI—Mammogram and ultrasound typically done first. MRI can help determine the extent of a known breast cancer and look for other areas of concern (contralateral breast, axillary lymph nodes). Uses contrast dye.

  C. Biopsy—Removal of tissue for microscopic evaluation by pathologist.

    1. MRI, mammogram, or ultrasound may be used to localize biopsy site.

    2. Types of biopsies:

      a. Core needle biopsy (ultrasound or MRI guided)

b. Vacuum-assisted stereotactic biopsy (mammography guided)

c. Excisional biopsy (surgical excision)

3. If biopsy positive for cancer, biomarker tests done to determine estrogen-receptor (ER) status, PR status, HER2 status, and Ki67 (marker of proliferation), which will guide treatment.

VII. Classic histopathologic classifications of breast cancer (ACS, 2022; NCCN, 2022)

A. Invasive ductal carcinoma (IDC)

1. Most common type. Approximately 80% of all breast cancer cases.

2. Starts in the cells that line the ducts.

3. Clinical prognosis highly variable; depends on cellular morphologic characteristics: ER, PR, Ki67, and HER2.

B. Invasive lobular carcinoma (ILC)

1. Approximately 10% of breast cancer cases.

2. Starts in the cells that line the lobules.

3. Difficult to diagnose because of radial pattern of spread, not easily detected on mammography, usually nonpalpable, and more likely to affect bilateral breasts compared with IDC.

C. Subtypes of invasive carcinoma (less than 5% of cases)

1. More favorable prognosis—papillary, tubular, mucinous, medullary carcinoma.

2. Less favorable prognosis—metaplastic carcinoma, micropapillary carcinoma, mixed carcinoma.

D. Inflammatory breast cancer (NCCN, 2022)

1. Aggressive and rare subtype of IDC, 1%–5% of all breast cancers

2. Clinical signs include edema, erythema, skin thickening, peau d'orange (dimpled appearance); resulting from fluid build-up caused by blocked lymph channels.

E. Paget disease of the breast—characterized by unilateral eczematous changes in the nipple; seen with ductal carcinoma in situ (DCIS) and invasive breast cancer.

F. Cystosarcoma phyllodes—Less than 1% of breast neoplasms.

1. 90% benign and 10% malignant; surgical excision recommended.

2. Rarely metastasizes but may recur locally.

G. Rare tumors—Include squamous cell carcinoma, lymphoma, and angiosarcoma.

H. Nonmalignant/noninvasive tumors

1. DCIS, also called intraductal carcinoma (NCCN, 2022).

a. Proliferation of cells inside the ducts

b. Stage 0

c. Surgical excision recommended to prevent progression to invasive cancer.

d. Usually not palpable, often detected by mammography and pleomorphic (broken glass dispersal pattern) calcifications; highly suspicious of malignancy and need further evaluation; biopsy recommended.

e. Architectural patterns—micropapillary, solid, comedo, papillary, cribriform. Comedonecrosis often more aggressive and at higher risk of recurrence or becoming invasive.

2. Lobular carcinoma in situ, also called lobular neoplasia.

a. Proliferation of cells lining the lobules

b. Increases risk of developing breast cancer

c. Often multicentric (more than one tumor) and multifocal (involves more than one quadrant of the breast).

d. Usually not detected on mammography or in physical examination but may be an incidental finding on pathology report or may be seen on breast MRI

e. Surgical excision recommended

3. Atypical ductal hyperplasia and atypical lobular hyperplasia.

a. Surgical excision recommended

4. Other high-risk breast lesions:

a. Flat epithelial atypia

b. Fibroepithelial lesions: fibroadenomas and phyllodes tumor

c. Pseudoangiomatous stromal hyperplasia

d. Sclerosing lesion

e. Radial scar

f. Papillary lesions

VIII. Molecular classification of breast cancer (Fragomeni, Sciallis, & Jeruss, 2018)

A. The molecular subtypes are based on the genes the cancer cells express, which controls how the cells behave. Molecular classification of breast tumors may be based on:

1. Single-gene arrays: ER, PR, HER2, Ki67

2. Multigene expression

a. Multigene transcript profiles use gene chip expression microarray (e.g., Oncotype DX Assay) or real-time polymerase chain reaction (e.g., Mammaprint, Prosigna, EndoPredict, Breast Cancer Index, and other tests).

3. Recent reports indicate distinct gene expression profiles for inflammatory breast cancer, HER2-positive breast cancer, lobular breast cancer, and BRCA-mutant breast cancer.

B. Breast cancer has been divided into at least five subgroups with distinct clinical outcomes and biologic features.

1. Luminal A tumors

a. ER positive and PR positive (high expression), HER2 negative

b. Tend to be low grade, low Ki67 (<20%)

c. Most likely to respond to endocrine therapy and have a favorable prognosis

d. 30%–40% of all invasive breast cancers

2. Luminal B tumors

a. ER positive, PR positive (lower expression), HER2 negative, high Ki67 (>14%–20%)

b. Grade 2 or 3; less well differentiated

c. 20%–30% of all invasive breast cancers

3. Luminal B–like tumors

a. ER positive, PR positive/negative, any Ki67, HER2 positive

4. HER2-amplified

a. Tumors have amplification of *HER2* gene on chromosome 17q and may have overexpression of other genes adjacent to HER2.

b. Clinical prognosis of these tumors was poor, but with the advent of trastuzumab (Herceptin) therapy, clinical outcome has improved.

c. 12%–20% of all invasive breast cancers.

d. HER2 subtypes:
HER2 enriched—ER/PR negative, HER2 positive
HER2 luminal—ER/PR positive, HER2 positive

5. Basal tumors

a. Tumors negative for ER, PR, and HER2 overexpression, or "triple-negative."

b. *BRCA1* breast cancers, younger women, and African Americans commonly fall into this group.

c. Often have a poor prognosis; therefore will likely benefit from chemotherapy.

d. 15%–20% of all invasive breast cancers.

IX. Histologic grade (ACS, 2022; NCCN, 2022).

A. Bloom–Richardson or Nottingham grading system most often used.

1. Grade 1: low grade or well differentiated.

2. Grade 2: intermediate grade or moderately differentiated.

3. Grade 3: high grade or poorly differentiated.

X. Staging (NCCN, 2022)

A. Stages of breast cancer give anatomic, pathologic, or prognostic staging; will determine the risk of recurrence.

B. The American Joint Committee on Cancer devised a way to explain how much cancer is in the body, where it is located, and what is the subtype (American College of Surgeons, 2018; NCCN, 2022).

1. Staging is done twice. *Clinical stage* is based on the biopsy, physical exam, and imaging. *Pathologic stage* is determined by the tissue removed during surgery.

2. Tumor, node, and metastasis (TNM) is used to describe an individual's staging.

a. T (tumor): size of the main tumor.

b. N (node): if the cancer has spread to the regional lymph nodes.

c. M (metastasis): if the cancer has spread to distant parts of the body.

3. Stage 0: noninvasive, such as DCIS.

4. Stage 1: Invasive, tumors are <2 cm with no lymph node involvement.

5. Stage 2: Invasive, tumors are 2–5 cm with some evidence of lymph node involvement.

6. Stage 3: Invasive; heavy burden of breast and axilla lymph node involvement; inflammatory breast cancer is considered stage 3.

7. Stage 4: Metastatic; evidence that the cancer has spread to distant organs.

C. Staging workup includes the following:

1. Computed tomography (CT) of chest (if pulmonary symptoms are present). Abdominal pelvic ± CT or MRI (if there is elevated alkaline phosphatase, abnormal liver function test, abdominal symptoms, or clinical stage IIA or higher).

2. Bone scan (if indicated for bone pain or elevated alkaline phosphatase).

3. Positron emission tomography or CT (optional)—not recommended for all women.

4. Bilateral breast MRI (stages I–III optional)—not recommended for all women.

5. Blood work, including complete blood cell count, platelets (plts), liver, and alkaline phosphatase.

D. Metastatic pattern

1. The most common organs involved in metastases in the local area are regional lymph nodes (axillary, internal mammary, inferior, supraclavicular lymph nodes) or in the skin.

a. Internal mammary nodes—involved in about 25% of patients with tumors in the upper inner quadrant and 15% with outer quadrant lesions.

2. Contralateral breast—most common in ILCs.

3. Distant metastatic sites—most commonly bone, lungs, liver, and brain.

a. Hematogenous spread—to liver, lung, bone, brain, and abdomen.

b. Lymphatic spread—to intramammary lymph nodes, axillary nodes, mediastinal nodes, other lymphatics.

4. Unusual sites of distant metastasis (frequency of <1% at each site): eye, bladder, genital organs, placenta, soft tissue, head and neck, GI tract, other thoracic organs such as heart, abdominal organs, nervous system (Di Micco et al., 2019).

XI. Prognosis and survival rates

A. 5-year relative survival rate (at time of diagnosis): All stages combined 90%. Localized (confined to primary site) 99%; regional (lymph node involvement) 86%; distant (metastasis) 29% (NCI, 2022b).

B. Factors affecting prognosis and treatment (NCCN, 2022):

1. Lymph node status—Poorer prognosis with more lymph node involvement.

2. Tumor size—Better prognosis with smaller tumors.

3. Histologic grade—More aggressive disease with higher grade tumors.

4. Hormone-receptor status—Better prognosis with ER-positive and/or PR-positive tumors.

5. Histologic tumor type—Invasive tumors have ability to metastasize.

6. Ki67—A marker of proliferation. Most useful for early-stage, ER-positive, HER2-negative patients. Ki67 of 5% or less, or 30% or more, used to estimate the prognosis and usefulness of chemotherapy (Nielsen et al., 2021).

7. Oncogene HER2 and EGFR overexpression.

8. Breast cancer gene expression testing—The following tests are performed on a patient's tumor tissue to assess the risk of distant recurrence and to guide systemic treatment (NCCN, 2022).

   a. OncoType DX—A 21-gene assay used to predict chemotherapy benefit (in addition to endocrine therapy) and estimate 10-year risk of distant recurrence in women with early-stage, ER positive, HER2 negative, lymph node–negative or between 1 and 3 positive lymph nodes, invasive breast cancer (NCCN, 2022; Precision Oncology, 2022; Sun, Wu, Bean, Hagemann, & Lin, 2021).

      (1) Postmenopausal patients: Recurrence score <26 no benefit from addition of chemotherapy. Recurrence score ≥26 chemotherapy recommended.

      (2) Premenopausal patients with negative lymph nodes: Recurrence score ≤15 no benefit from adding chemotherapy. Recurrence score 16–25 benefit of adding chemotherapy may be considered. Recurrence score ≥26 chemotherapy recommended.

      (3) Premenopausal patients with 1–3 positive lymph nodes: Recurrence score <26 consider chemotherapy. Recurrence score ≥26 chemotherapy recommended.

   b. MammaPrint—70-gene microarray-based assay that identifies women with early-stage breast cancer at risk of distant recurrence in 10 years (ACS, 2022; NCCN, 2022; Soliman, Shah, & Srkalovic, 2020).

      (1) Can be performed on any hormone receptor or HER2 status.

      (2) Result provided as *low* or *high* risk of metastasis.

   c. BluePrint—Used in combination with Mamma-Print. 80-gene microarray-based subtyping assay that categorizes tumors as Luminal or Basal type. Categorizes Luminal-type tumors as Luminal A (low risk) or Luminal B (high risk) (Soliman et al., 2020).

   d. Prosigna—50-gene assay to assess the risk of recurrence and potential response to chemotherapy. Early-stage, ER-positive, lymph node–negative, or lymph node–positive cancers (ACS, 2022; Sonic Genetics, 2022).

   e. EndoPredict—12-gene assay to assess the 10-year risk of recurrence, chemotherapy benefit, and benefit of extended endocrine therapy. Early-stage, ER-positive, HER2-negative, node-negative, and node-positive (1–3 nodes) breast cancers (Myriad, 2021; NCCN, 2022).

   f. Breast Cancer Index—Predicts benefit of additional endocrine therapy (past 5 years) to reduce distant recurrence. For early-stage, hormone receptor–positive breast cancers (Biotheranostics, 2022; NCCN, 2022).

MANAGEMENT

I. Locoregional treatment of clinical stages I–III, N0, or N+M0 disease (NCCN, 2022; NCI, 2022a).

   A. Breast-conserving surgery (also known as lumpectomy, partial mastectomy)—with surgical axillary staging, followed by radiation therapy, and possible chemotherapy, targeted therapy, or endocrine therapy.

      1. Removal of the cancer and a rim of normal tissue, while preserving as much breast tissue as possible.

      2. Negative margins important to prevent local recurrence.

      3. Breast-conserving surgery may result in deformity of the breast (asymmetry, indentation).

      4. Oncoplastic breast reconstruction can be performed at the time of surgery by reshaping the remaining breast tissue after the cancer is removed. Oncoplastic reconstruction uses a wide variety of plastic surgery incisions/techniques (e.g., breast lift, breast reduction). If desired by the patient, a similar procedure on the contralateral breast may be performed to provide symmetry (Chu, Hanson, Hwang, & Wu, 2021).

   B. Mastectomy—with surgical axillary staging, with or without reconstruction.

      1. Consider chemotherapy.

      2. Consider radiation if surgical margin positive or < 1 mm, tumor > 5 cm, positive lymph nodes.

      3. Breast reconstruction for mastectomy can be performed at the same time as mastectomy or after completion of cancer treatment.

         (a) Options for breast reconstruction include the following:

            (1) 1 stage: Breast implants inserted at the time of surgery (direct to implant)

            (2) 2 stage: Tissue expanders, with implants inserted during a second surgery

            (3) Latissimus dorsi alone

            (4) Transverse rectus abdominus myocutaneous or deep inferior epigastric perforator tissue flap

            (5) Pedicle or gluteal flap

   C. Sentinel lymph node biopsy—preferred method of axillary lymph node staging.

      1. Sentinel lymph node—most likely the first lymph nodes to which cancer may spread from a primary tumor.

   D. Axillary lymph node dissection—done if sentinel lymph nodes positive or if palpable or biopsy-proven positive lymph nodes in axilla.

II. Adjuvant endocrine therapy—ER-positive and/or PR-positive cancers (NCCN, 2022).
   A. Premenopausal at diagnosis:
      1. Tamoxifen for 5–10 years, with or without ovarian suppression or ablation. If ovarian suppression or ablation, may use aromatase inhibitor for additional 3–5 years (anastrozole, letrozole, exemestane).
   B. Postmenopausal at diagnosis:
      1. Aromatase inhibitor for 5 years: anastrozole, letrozole, exemestane. Consider extending treatment 3–5 years. Can also use tamoxifen first and then AI, or AI and then tamoxifen to complete 5–10 years of treatment. Uncertainty regarding the sequence and total duration of treatment at this time; though patients with lymph node involvement may benefit from taking an aromatase inhibitor greater than 5 years. AI and tamoxifen are not meant to be taken at the same time.
      2. For postmenopausal patients with contraindication to AI, or who cannot tolerate AI due to side effects, may consider tamoxifen for 5–10 years. Potential side effects of endocrine therapy include hot flashes, joint aches, loss of bone density, dry skin, vaginal dryness, and decreased libido. Bone density test recommended prior to initiation of aromatase inhibitor if age >65, personal or family history of osteoporosis.
III. Common chemotherapy agents used to treat invasive breast cancer (NCCN, 2022).
   a. May use a single agent or combination regimen
   b. Number of cycles and days between cycles vary with drug(s) used
      1. Alkylating agents—for example, cyclophosphamide
      2. Platinum-based alkylating agents—for example, carboplatin, cisplatin
      3. Anthracyclines—for example, doxorubicin, epirubicin
      4. Antimetabolites—for example, capecitabine, fluorouracil, gemcitabine, methotrexate
      5. Microtubule inhibitors—for example, docetaxel, eribulin, ixabepilone, paclitaxel, vinorelbine
IV. Targeted therapies for HER2-positive breast cancers (NCCN, 2022)
   a. HER2 antibodies
      1. Pertuzumab
      2. Trastuzumab
      3. Trastuzumab substitutes
   b. HER2 inhibitors
      1. Lapatinib
      2. Neratinib
   c. HER2 conjugates
      1. Ado-trastuzumab emtansine
      2. Fam-trastuzumab deruxtecan-nxki
V. Targeted therapies for advanced breast cancer (NCCN, 2022)

a. Cyclin-dependent kinase 4 and 6 inhibitors (CDK4/6)—for example, palbociclib, ribociclib, abemaciclib.
      1. For hormone receptor–positive/HER2-negative cancer
      2. Used in combination with an aromatase inhibitor or fulvestrant
   b. mTOR inhibitors—for example, everolimus
      1. For hormone receptor–positive cancer
      2. Used in combination with an aromatase inhibitor; may be used with tamoxifen or fulvestrant
   c. PARP inhibitors—for example, olaparib, talazoparib
      1. For patients with a *BRCA1* or *BRCA2* gene pathogenic variant, and HER2 negative
   d. PIK3CA inhibitor—alpelisib
      1. Must test for PIK3CA pathogenic variant
      2. For hormone receptor–positive/HER2-negative cancer; postmenopausal women; men
      3. Used in combination with fulvestrant
VI. Nursing implications (ACS, 2022)
   A. Oncology Nurse Navigator role: provides education and resources to facilitate informed decision-making and timely access to quality health and psychosocial care throughout all phases of the cancer continuum (Oncology Nursing Society, 2017).
      1. Patient navigation programs in the United States have led to improvement in diagnostic or treatment timelines, particularly for women in lower socioeconomic classes or minority groups (Yeoh et al., 2018).
   B. Nurses play a vital role in educating patients regarding disease process, treatment options, side effects, self-care, body image, fertility, and pregnancy during and after treatment.
      1. Interventions to increase patient knowledge regarding disease process, treatment, and side effects.
         a. Explaining disease process and treatment options in a nonjudgmental way and at the patient's level of understanding.
         b. Encouraging discussion regarding potential physical and emotional changes resulting from treatment and exploration of personal values and beliefs as they relate to treatment options.
         c. Facilitating patient's involvement in treatment decision-making to the extent desired.
         d. Providing education regarding the risk for lymphedema; teaching the patient how to measure the circumference of the affected arm and to notify the provider if it increases.
         e. Informing the patient about altered arm and breast sensations (numbness and tingling of arm, lack of sensation on chest wall, phantom breast sensation after mastectomy) that may persist indefinitely after surgery.
         f. Assessing for menopausal symptoms (hot flashes, vaginal dryness) that may be associated with adjuvant endocrine therapy or chemotherapy-induced ovarian failure.

g. Monitoring for and managing side effects of surgery, radiation, chemotherapy, and endocrine therapy.

2. Interventions to promote self-care and enhance adaptation and rehabilitation.

a. Facilitating communication between patient and health care providers; alerting the health care team to the patient's concerns about breast cancer and its treatment.

b. Assessing coping skills, support system, feelings about body image, sexual identity, role relationships.

c. Providing the patient with information regarding community resources available for support, rehabilitation, breast prostheses, or wigs.

d. Survivorship visit (see Chapter 3) with provider for transition visit and discussing long-term follow-up, surveillance, exercise, diet, and symptoms to be aware of, as well as future office visits.

e. Teaching the patient about the importance of practicing breast self-examination, maintaining annual imaging recommendations, and examining the axilla for lymphadenopathy.

REFERENCES

American Cancer Society (ACS). Breast cancer. (2022). https://www.cancer.org/cancer/breast-cancer.html.

American College of Surgeons (ACoS). (2018). *AJCC cancer staging manual* (8th ed.) ACoS: Chicago, IL.

Biotheranostics, Inc. (2022). *Breast Cancer Index.* https://www.breastcancerindex.com/.

Chu, C. K., Hanson, S. E., Hwang, R. F., & Wu, L. C. (2021). Oncoplastic partial breast reconstruction: Concepts and techniques. *Gland Surgery, 10*(1), 398–410. https://doi.org/10.21037/gs-20-380.

Di Micco, R., Santurro, L., Gasparri, M. L., Zuber, V., Fiacco, E., Gazzetta, G., et al. (2019). Rare sites of breast cancer metastasis: A review. *Translational Cancer Research, 8*(Suppl 5), S518–S552. https://doi.org/10.21037/tcr.2019.07.24.

Fragomeni, S. M., Sciallis, A., & Jeruss, J. S. (2018). Molecular subtypes and local-regional control of breast cancer. *Surgical Oncology Clinics of North America, 27*(1), 95–120. https://www.ncbi.nlm.nih.gov/pmc/articles/PMC5715810/.

Maisonneuve, P. (2017). Epidemiology, lifestyle, and environmental factors. In U. Veronesi & P. Veronesi (Eds.), *Breast cancer: Innovations in research and management.* Milan: Springer International Publishing.

Myriad. *Hereditary Breast Cancer.* (2021). https://myriad.com/patients-families/disease-info/breast-cancer/.

National Cancer Institute (NCI). *Breast cancer treatment (adult).* (2022a). www.cancer.gov/types/breast/patient/breast-treatment-pdq.

National Cancer Institute (NCI). *Cancer stat facts: Female breast cancer.* (2022b). https://seer.cancer.gov/statfacts/html/breast.html.

National Comprehensive Cancer Network (NCCN). *NCCN clinical practice guidelines in oncology: Breast cancer [v2.2022].* (2022). https://www.nccn.org/professionals/physician_gls/pdf/breast.pdf.

Nielsen, T. O., Leung, S. C. Y., Rimm, D. L., et al. (2021). Assessment of Ki67 in breast cancer: Updated recommendations from the international Ki67 in breast cancer working group. *Journal of the National Cancer Institute, 113*(7), 808–819. https://doi.org/10.1093/jnci/djaa201.

Oncology Nursing Society. *2017 Oncology nurse navigator core competencies.* (2017). https://www.ons.org/sites/default/files/2017ONNcompetencies.pdf.

Precision Oncology. *Oncotype DX Breast Recurrence Score test.* (2022). https://precisiononcology.exactsciences.com/patients-and-caregivers/understanding-your-diagnosis/breast-cancer/breast-recurrence-score?gclid=CjwKCAiAu5agBhBzEiwAdiR5tFI3aZ-oG5RybBICLhzhuZBM-Vv7hHOaSaRfPtaN2Nb-mS8O7CSSeRoC53kQAvD_BwE.

Siegel, R. L., Miller, K. D., Fuchs, H. E., & Jemal, A. (2022). Cancer statistics, 2022. *CA: A Cancer Journal for Clinicians, 72*(1), 7–33. https://doi.org/10.3322/caac.21708.

Soliman, H., Shah, V., Srkalovic, G., et al. (2020). MammaPrint guides treatment decisions in breast cancer: Results of the IMPACt trial. *BMC Cancer, 20*(1), 1–13. https://doi.org/10.1186/s12885-020-6534-z.

Sonic Genetics. *Breast cancer gene expression; also known as Prosigna, PAM50.* (2022). https://www.sonicgenetics.com.au/our-tests/all-tests/breast-cancer-gene-expression/.

Sun, L., Wu, A., Bean, G. R., Hagemann, I. S., & Lin, C.-Y. (2021). Molecular testing in breast cancer: Current status and future directions. *The Journal of Molecular Diagnostics, 23*(11), 1422–1432.

Vandeven, H. A., & Pensler, J. M. (2022). Gynecomastia. [Updated 2021 Aug 13]. In: *StatPearls [Internet].* Treasure Island, FL: StatPearls Publishing. https://www.ncbi.nlm.nih.gov/books/NBK430812/.

WHO. (2022). *Breast Cancer.* https://www.who.int/news-room/fact-sheets/detail/breast-cancer.

Yeoh, Z.-Y., Jaganathan, M., Rajaram, N., Rawat, S., Tajudeen, N. A., Rahim, N., et al. (2018). Feasibility of patient navigation to improve breast cancer care in Malaysia. *Journal of Global Oncology, 4*, 1–13. https://doi.org/10.1200/jgo.17.00229.

14

Gastrointestinal Cancers

Timotea Lara

ESOPHAGEAL CANCER

Overview

I. Arise from either the glandular or the squamous epithelium and have different risk factors for each.

II. Epidemiology
  A. Estimated 20,640 new esophageal cancer cases diagnosed; 16,410 deaths from esophageal cancer in 2022 (American Cancer Society [ACS], 2022a, 2022b, 2022c, 2022d, 2022e, 2022f, 2022g).
  B. Esophageal cancer—1% of all cancers diagnosed in the United States; much more common in some other parts of the world (ACS, 2022d).
  C. Older adults at higher risk, peak incidence in the sixth to the seventh decade of life (Jain & Dhingra, 2017).

III. Pathophysiology
  A. Esophageal squamous cell cancer arises through esophageal lining through the progression of premalignant precursor lesions due to irritation and inflammation caused by risk factors (Jain & Dhingra, 2017).
  B. Modifiable risk factors
    1. Barrett esophagus (BE) (adenocarcinoma) (ACS, 2022d)
    2. Obesity (adenocarcinoma)
    3. Diet—low consumption of fruits and vegetables
    4. Gastroesophageal reflux disease (GERD) (adenocarcinoma)
    5. Smoking (squamous cell); alcohol (squamous cell)
    6. Occupational exposure (dry cleaners, asbestos)
  C. Nonmodifiable risk factors
    1. Gender—more prevalent in males (adenocarcinoma)
    2. Genetic syndromes (e.g., tylosis, Howel–Evans syndrome, Bloom syndrome, Fanconi anemia, familial BE) (ACS, 2022a, 2022b, 2022c, 2022d, 2022e, 2022f, 2022g)
    3. Achalasia—cancers are found about 15–20 years after the achalasia began
    4. Plummer–Vinson Syndrome (esophageal webs)
    5. History of other cancers
    6. Hiatal hernia (National Comprehensive Cancer Network [NCCN], 2022c)
    7. Lack of physical activity

IV. Prevention
  A. Healthy lifestyle
  B. Maintain physical activity.
  C. Avoid alcohol and tobacco.
  D. Incorporate fruits and vegetables in diet.
  E. Maintain healthy body weight.
  F. Treat Barrett's esophagitis and/or GERD.
  G. Twice daily proton pump inhibitor and aspirin or other nonsteroidal antiinflammatory drugs (NSAIDs) are a promising approach for high-risk patients with BE (Moayyedi & El-Serag, 2021).

V. Diagnosis
  A. Endoscopy, laparoscopy, thoracoscopy
  B. Computed tomography (CT) scan of chest and abdomen with oral and intravenous (IV) contrast, magnetic resonance imaging (MRI), positron emission tomography (PET) scan
  C. Endoscopic ultrasound (EUS)
  D. Bronchoscopy (NCCN, 2022c)
  E. Biopsy must be performed to confirm the diagnosis

VI. Histopathology
  A. Squamous cell carcinoma
    1. Arises from squamous cell epithelium
    2. More common in developing countries
    3. Most common in mid esophagus
  B. Adenocarcinoma
    1. Arises from glandular epithelium
    2. Affects mostly distal esophagus; esophagogastric junction (EGJ)
    3. Appears to be related to GERD and BE (ACS, 2022d; NCCN, 2022c)
  C. Molecular classification
    1. MSI-H/dMMR testing if metastatic disease is suspected
    2. HER2 and PD-L1 testing if metastatic adenocarcinoma suspected (NCCN, 2022c)

VII. Staging
  A. American Joint Committee on Cancer (AJCC) (American Joint Committee on Cancer [AJCC], 2018)
  B. Separate staging for adenocarcinoma versus squamous cell carcinoma (NCCN, 2022c)

VIII. Prognosis and survival
  A. The 5-year survival rate is 19.9% (National Cancer Institute [NCI], 2022).
  B. Favorable prognostic factors: early-stage disease and complete resection (NCI, 2022).

C. 5-year survival rates for stages I and II are 46.4% (NCI, 2022).

D. HER2-positive tumors associated with poor overall survival (OS) and a higher 5-year mortality rate (Nagaraja & Eslick, 2015).

E. Prognostic significance of epidermal growth factor receptor overexpression remains controversial (Guo, Yu, Zhu, & Guo, 2015).

F. Mortality rates higher for black males.

Management

I. Surgery
   A. Endoscopic resection/ablation for carcinoma in situ or tumor in situ (TIS) in selected stage I patients
   B. Esophagectomy for patients with stages I–III
II. Radiation
   A. Concurrent with chemotherapy—usually in neoadjuvant setting
   B. May be used with concurrent chemotherapy as definitive therapy if patient declines surgery or is not a surgical candidate
   C. In palliative setting for pain control, alleviate obstruction/restore swallowing
III. Systemic therapy
   A. Chemotherapy is used with radiation therapy as neoadjuvant or definitive therapy
   B. Chemotherapy is the primary treatment for stage IV disease
   C. Trastuzumab added to chemotherapy for HER2+ metastatic adenocarcinoma
   D. Ramucirumab alone or in combination with paclitaxel
   E. Pembrolizumab for patients with MSI-H/dMMR for the second-line therapy and the third-line therapy for patients PD-L1 positive (NCCN, 2022c)
   F. Common chemotherapy regimens for esophageal cancer (Table 14.1) (NCCN, 2022c)

STOMACH CANCER

Overview

I. In Western countries, the proximal lesser curvature, cardia, and EGJ are the most common sites. Gastric cancer is not common in North America; however, it is rampant in other parts of the world.
II. Epidemiology
   A. Estimated 26,560 cases of stomach cancer diagnosed, and about 11,180 people will die of this type of cancer in 2021 (NCI, 2022)
   B. Higher incidence in Hispanic Americans, African Americans, Native American, and Asian/Pacific Islanders than non-Hispanic whites (ACS, 2022g)
III. Pathophysiology
   A. Chronic gastric inflammation caused by risk factors and virulence of bacteria or viruses can contribute to the development of gastric cancer. For example, *Helicobacter pylori* can inhibit tumor suppression

TABLE 14.1 Common Chemotherapy Regimens Used in Esophageal and Gastric Cancers

Type of Chemotherapy	Preferred Regimen per NCCN
Preoperative chemoradiation	Paclitaxel and carboplatin; cisplatin and 5-FU; oxaliplatin and 5-FU
Perioperative chemotherapy (three cycles preoperative and three cycles postoperative)	Cisplatin and 5-FU; epirubicin, cisplatin, 5-FU (ECF), oxaliplatin, and 5-FU
Definitive chemoradiation	Cisplatin and 5-FU; oxaliplatin and 5-FU,[a] cisplatin and paclitaxel and carboplatin
Postoperative chemoradiation	Infusional 5-FU or capecitabine
Metastatic	Docetaxel, cisplatin, 5-FU (DCF); ECF, cisplatin, and 5-FU or capecitabine; oxaliplatin and 5-FU or capecitabine; irinotecan and 5-FU

5-FU, 5-Fluorouracil; *NCCN*, National Comprehensive Cancer Network.
[a]May use capecitabine instead of 5-FU.
Data from *National Comprehensive Cancer Network. NCCN practice guidelines in oncology: Esophageal and esophagogastric junction cancer [v.2.2018].* (2018). https://www.nccn.org/professionals/physician_gls/pdf/esophageal.pdf; *National Comprehensive Cancer Network. NCCN practice guidelines in oncology: Gastric cancer [v.2.2018].* (2018). https://www.nccn.org/professionals/physician_gls/pdf/gastric.pdf
These are always tricky because you need to sign in to get there.

pathways that can increase the risk of developing gastric cancer (Seeneevassen et al., 2021).
   B. Modifiable risk factors
      1. Diet high in salted and smoked foods, low in fruits and vegetables
      2. Alcohol use greater than four drinks per day
      3. Smoking
      4. Obesity—high body mass index (BMI) associated with gastric cardia cancer
      5. *H. pylori*; gastric ulcers (ACS, 2022g)
   C. Nonmodifiable risk factors
      1. Age, 60–80 years of age
      2. Male sex, family history
      3. Epstein–Barr virus
      4. Previous gastric surgery
      5. Gastric polyps
      6. Inherited cancer syndromes
         a. Hereditary diffuse gastric cancer (rare)
         b. Familial adenomatous polyposis (FAP)
         c. Peutz–Jeghers syndrome (PJS)
         d. Juvenile polyposis syndrome
         e. Lynch syndrome (NCCN, 2022d)
IV. Prevention
   A. Avoid diet high in smoked/pickled foods and salted meats/fish
   B. Consume diet high in fresh fruits and vegetables
   C. Regular exercise
   D. Healthy body weight
   E. Treat *H. pylori*, gastric ulcers (ACS, 2022g)

V. Diagnosis
   A. Endoscopy; histologic examination is required to establish diagnosis
   B. CT chest, abdomen, and pelvis; PET scan
   C. EUS
VI. Histopathology
   A. 95% are adenocarcinomas
   B. Molecular classification
      1. MSI-H/dMMR testing if metastatic disease is suspected
      2. HER2 and PD-L1 testing if metastatic adenocarcinoma suspected (NCCN, 2022d)
VII. Staging
   A. Staging (AJCC, 2018)
      1. Prognostic staging for gastric cancer is complex; based on multiple principles—clinical, pathologic, and response to neoadjuvant therapy
VIII. Prognosis and survival
   A. Poor prognosis, as it is typically diagnosed in later stages
   B. 5-year relative survival rate in the United States is about 32% (ACS, 2022g)

Management

I. Surgery
   A. TIS or T1 may be eligible for ER
   B. Stage T1B to T3: gastric resection
   C. Stage T4: en-bloc resection
II. Radiation
   A. Used in adjuvant setting with concurrent chemotherapy
   B. May be used in neoadjuvant setting with concurrent chemotherapy
   C. Given concurrently with chemotherapy in nonsurgical candidates (definitive)
   D. Palliative
III. Systemic therapy—same principles as discussed for esophageal cancer
   A. See Table 14.1 for common chemotherapy regimens used for gastric cancer
   B. Trastuzumab added for HER2-overexpressing metastatic adenocarcinoma
   C. Ramucirumab alone or in combination with paclitaxel
   D. Pembrolizumab for patients with MSI-H/dMMR for the second-line therapy and the third-line therapy for patients PD-L1 positive (NCCN, 2022d)

COLORECTAL CANCER

Overview

I. Colorectal cancer (CRC) usually begins as a noncancerous growth called a *polyp*; develops on the inner lining of the colon or rectum and grows slowly over a period of 10–20 years. Typical slow growth pattern is why screening is so important
II. Epidemiology
   A. Estimated 106,180 new cases of colon cancer, 44,850 of rectal cancer in the United States in 2022 (ACS, 2022c)
   B. Third most common cancer diagnosed in both men and women in the United States
   C. Third leading cause of cancer-related deaths in men and women in the United States and world
   D. Expected to cause about 52,580 deaths in 2022 (ACS, 2022c)
   E. CRC highest in Black communities, higher than any other racial/ethnic group in the United States (ACS, 2022c)
   F. African Americans 20% more likely to be diagnosed and about 40% high risk of mortality (ACS, 2022c)
III. Pathophysiology
   A. Inflammatory process and genetic and environmental risk factors contribute to CRC development
   B. Modifiable risk factors
      1. Smoking
      2. Alcohol intake
      3. High-fat diet
      4. High intake of red and processed meats
      5. Obesity
      6. Inadequate intake of fruits and vegetables
      7. Physical inactivity
   C. Nonmodifiable risk factors
      1. Age >50
      2. Race, blacks at higher risk
      3. Familial clustering—20% of cases associated
         a. Personal or family history of colon cancer or inflammatory bowel disease
         b. Hereditary cancer syndromes—5% of cases have germline pathogenic variants
            (1) FAP—attenuated familial polyposis, MUTYH-associated polyposis (MAP-1)
            (2) Lynch syndrome (hereditary nonpolyposis CRC)
      4. Other syndromes can also increase CRC risk, including PJS-1, serrated polyposis syndrome (SPS-1), colonic adenomatous polyposis of unknown etiology (CPUE-1)
      5. Presence of edematous polyps (Jochem & Leitzman, 2016; NCCN, 2022b)
IV. Prevention
   A. Maintain a healthy weight.
   B. Limit red and processed meats.
   C. Eat more vegetables and fruits.
   D. Limit alcohol intake—fewer than two drinks/day for males, one drink/day for females.
   E. Avoid tobacco.
   F. Exercise regularly.
   G. Chemoprevention: acetylsalicylic acid, NSAIDs may be considered for high patients; however, risks outweigh the benefits (Mohammed, Nagendra Sastry Yarla, Madka, & Rao, 2018).
   H. Dairy and milk consumption.
V. Screening and diagnosis
   A. Colonoscopy (every 10 years); most accurate and versatile diagnostic test
   B. Flexible sigmoidoscopy (every 5 years)
   C. Air contrast barium enema (every 5 years)

D. Fecal occult blood (annually)

E. Fecal immunochemical test (annually)

F. Stool DNA test (every 3 years)

G. Biopsy; histologic examination

H. CT chest, abdomen, and pelvis

VI. Histopathology

A. Adenocarcinoma accounts for 95% of all cases, originates from the glandular epithelium.

B. Molecular classification

1. KRAS/NRAS (in patients with metastatic disease)

2. BRAF (in patients with metastatic disease)

3. MMR or MSI in appropriate patients (NCCN, 2022b, 2022e)

VII. Staging

A. AJCC staging; TNM (AJCC, 2018)

1. Tumor invasion of colon and rectal muscle layers

2. Node involvement

3. Metastatic disease presence

B. Colectomy with a minimum of 12 lymph nodes (LNs) for correct staging (NCCN, 2022b)

VIII. Prognosis and survival

A. Prognosis depends on the stage at which the CRC is diagnosed.

B. The 5-year survival rate for CRC is 65%; localized disease is as high as 90%, but only 39% of patients are diagnosed at an early stage.

C. Stage IV 14% (ACS, 2022c)

Management

I. Surgery for resectable disease

A. Colon cancer

1. Colectomy with en-bloc removal of regional LNs (Fig. 14.1)

B. Rectal

1. Transanal resection

2. Transabdominal resection

II. Radiation

A. Colon cancer

1. Neoadjuvant setting, concurrent with chemotherapy for bulky disease

2. May allow for resection

B. Rectal cancer

1. Used in adjuvant setting due to high risk for local recurrence

2. Neoadjuvant for unresectable disease, concurrent with chemotherapy

C. Palliative setting for both colon and rectal for pain control, obstruction

III. Systemic

A. Colon Cancer

1. Neoadjuvant setting concurrent with radiation therapy for unresectable disease

B. Rectal Cancer

1. Adjuvant setting FOLFOX, CAPEOX, capecitabine/5-FU/leucovorin

2. Neoadjuvant setting for unresectable disease—capecitabine preferred

C. Metastatic setting

1. FOLFOX, FOLFIRI±bevacizumab or cetuximab/panitumumab (targeted therapy) depending on the KRA/NRAS status

2. Regorafenib as the targeted therapy

3. Trifluridine/tipiracil

4. PD-1 inhibitors pembrolizumab or nivolumab—dMMR/MSI-H (NCCN, 2022b, 2022e)

5. PD-L1-inhibitors atezolizumab (TECENTRIQ®)

6. CTLA-4 inhibitors ipilimumab (YERVOY®)

ANAL CANCER

Overview

I. Rare cancer arising from the squamocolumnar epithelium; directly linked to human papillomavirus infection (HPV) (particularly serotypes 16 and 18) (ACS, 2022a)

II. Epidemiology

A. Estimated 9440 new cases and 1670 deaths related to anal cancer in 2022 (ACS, 2022a)

B. More common in women than men

C. Higher risk in white women and black men (ACS, 2022a)

D. Incidence is rising (ACS, 2022a)

III. Pathophysiology

A. Anogenital infections with HIV

B. Chronic immunosuppression

C. Risk factors

1. HPV-16—nearly universal in men who have sex with other men (MSM)

2. Other cancers associated with HPV

3. HIV infection

4. Smoking

5. Anal sex

6. Lowered immunity (ACS, 2022a)

7. Gender and race/ethnicity

IV. Prevention

A. HPV vaccination—recommended in boys and girls 11–12 years, females 13–26, males 13–21, and for MSM up to age 26

B. Condom use

C. Treat HIV

D. Cease smoking (NCCN, 2022a)

V. Diagnosis

A. Biopsy—needs to confirm squamous cell origin

B. CT chest, abdomen, and CT pelvis or MRI pelvis

C. Anoscopy

D. Rigid proctosigmoidoscopy (ACS, 2022a, 2022b, 2022c, 2022d, 2022e, 2022f, 2022g)

E. Endoscopy

F. HIV test

G. Transrectal or endorectal ultrasound

H. PET

1. Gynecologic examination for women

VI. Histopathology

A. Squamous cell cancer, HIV associated or non-HIV associated

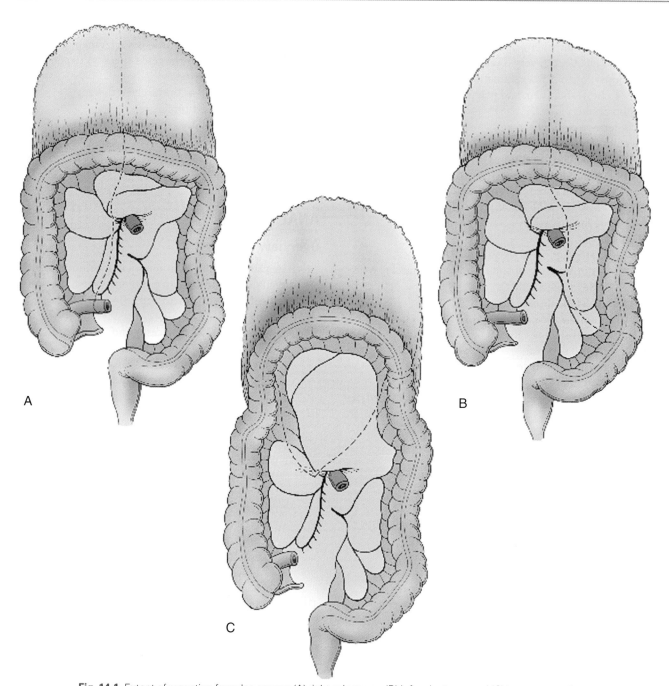

Fig. 14.1 Extent of resection for colon cancer: (A) right colectomy, (B) left colectomy, and (C) transverse colectomy. From Rothrock, J. (2011). *Alexander's care of the patient in surgery* (14th ed.). Philadelphia, PA: Mosby.

VII. Staging (AJCC, 2018)
  A. Most are clinical staging due to limit of surgery as primary treatment (NCCN, 2022a)
VIII. Prognosis and survival—5-year survival for stage I about 80%; stage IV is estimated at 35% (ACS, 2022a)

Management

  I. Surgery—local excision for stage I well-differentiated tumors
  II. Radiation
      A. Definitive therapy with stages I–III with concurrent chemotherapy
      B. Palliative for stage IV disease if indicated
  III. Systemic therapy
      A. Definitive chemotherapy with stages I–III 5-FU/mitomycin concurrent with radiation therapy
      B. Palliative chemotherapy stage IV disease—cisplatin/5-FU, FOLFOX, carboplatin/paclitaxel
      C. Palliative immunotherapy—nivolumab, pembrolizumab (NCCN, 2022a)

HEPATOCELLULAR CANCER

Overview

I. Occurs predominantly in patients with underlying chronic liver disease and cirrhosis. Hepatocellular cancer (HCC) begins as a single tumor that grows larger, spreads late in the disease to other parts of the liver. Second type seems to start as small cancer nodules throughout the liver, not just a single tumor—seen most often in people with cirrhosis (chronic liver damage), most common in the United States (ACS, 2022e).

II. Epidemiology
   A. HCC is the second leading cause of cancer death worldwide.
   B. Estimated 41,260 new cases diagnosed, 30,520 deaths in the United States in 2022.
   C. Liver cancer incidence has more than tripled since 1980; peak of the epidemic may have passed due to improved treatments for hepatitis C and hepatitis B immunization.
   D. Trends: increased obesity, type 2 diabetes, and nonalcoholic fatty liver disease (NAFLD) replacing viral and alcohol-related liver disease.

III. Pathophysiology
   A. The process of dysplastic hepatocytes to hepatic neoplasm is a complex process that develops from inflammation and injury to the liver (Alqahtani et al., 2019).
   B. Modifiable risk factors
      1. High-fat diet, obesity, including childhood obesity
      2. NAFLD
      3. Diabetes
      4. Alcohol, smoking
      5. Exposure to chemical carcinogens
      6. Anabolic steroids
   C. Nonmodifiable risk factors
      1. Primary biliary cirrhosis
      2. Nonalcoholic steatohepatitis
      3. Hepatitis B or C
      4. Genetic disorders such as hemochromatosis and Wilson's disease can cause chronic inflammation leading to liver damage and increased HCC risk
      5. Parasitic infection (ACS, 2022e; NCCN, 2021a)
      6. Gender: more common in males
      7. Asian Americans and Pacific Islanders higher rates (ACS, 2022e)

IV. Prevention
   A. Avoiding/treating hepatitis infection
   B. Limiting alcohol and tobacco use
   C. Maintaining healthy weight
   D. Limiting exposure to cancer-causing chemicals
   E. Treating diseases that increase HCC risk (ACS, 2022e; NCCN, 2021a)

V. Diagnosis
   A. Ultrasound
   B. Angiography
   C. Bone scan
   D. Abdominal multiphasic CT
   E. MRI
   F. Alpha fetoprotein is a predictor of advanced disease and poor prognosis
   G. Biopsy
      1. Diagnostic approach to a solid liver lesion in a high-risk patient is determined initially by the size of the lesion
      2. Biopsy for histologic confirmation is not required if lesion fulfills typical imaging criteria for HCC

VI. Histopathology
   A. Gross morphology
      1. Nodular—associated with cirrhosis
      2. Massive—noncirrhosis type
      3. Diffuse—small distinct areas throughout the liver (NCCN, 2021a)

VII. Staging—AJCC, TNM
   Additional staging systems consideration (ACS, 2022e):
   A. Child–Pugh score (cirrhosis staging system)
   B. Model for end-stage liver disease
   C. Okuda, Cancer of the Liver Italian Program and Barcelona Clinic Liver Cancer (ACS, 2022e)

VIII. Prognosis and survival
   A. Prognosis based on tumor burden, liver function, and general health status
   B. Generally poor—majority of patients are diagnosed with advanced disease
   C. Localized tumors have approximately 30% survival at 5 years
   D. Advanced tumors have an estimated 3% 5-year survival (ACS, 2022e)

Management

I. May be limited because of underlying liver function

II. Surgery
   A. Partial hepatectomy—potentially curative in patients with early-stage HCC, only in setting of preserved liver function, Child–Pugh score A (assess the prognosis of chronic liver disease)

III. Transplantation
   A. Additional potentially curative option for early-stage HCC
   B. Removes both detectable and undetectable tumor lesions and treats underlying cirrhosis
   C. Treatment before transplantation may include bridge therapy or downstaging therapy with transarterial chemoembolization (TACE) or thermal/radiofrequency ablation (RFA)

IV. Local-regional therapies
   A. Ablation—RFA, microwave ablation, cryoablation
   B. Arterially directed therapies—transarterial bland embolization, TACE, yttrium-90 transarterial radioembolization (TARE), TACE with drug-eluting beads (DEB)

V. Radiation—external beam radiation allows high-dose radiation to focal liver tumors while sparing surrounding tissue
   A. Intensity-modulated radiation therapy
   B. Stereotactic body radiation therapy (SBRT)

VI. Systemic
  A. First line—sorafenib
  B. Second line—regorafenib, nivolumab
    1. Child–Pugh score A to B7 only
  C. Systemic chemotherapy recommended in the context of clinical trial only (NCCN, 2021a)

PANCREATIC CANCER

Overview

I. Pancreatic adenocarcinoma is the most common form of pancreatic cancer. It is one of the most aggressive and lethal cancers. It accounts for almost 95% of cases and arises from the exocrine pancreas.
II. Epidemiology
  A. In 2022 an estimated 62,210 people will be diagnosed with pancreatic cancer and 49,830 people will die of the disease in the United States (ACS, 2022f).
  B. Fourth most common cause of cancer death in the United States (ACS, 2022f)
III. Pathophysiology
  A. Pancreatic adenocarcinoma is most commonly found in the head of the pancreas but may also be found in the body and the tail. It is often found at advanced stages, when it is found in the tail as it does not typically produce symptoms until it has spread. It typically first metastasizes to regional LNs, then to the liver and, less commonly, to the lungs. It may also directly invade surrounding visceral organs such as the duodenum, stomach, and colon. It may also spread via the peritoneal cavity causing peritoneal carcinomatosis (NCCN, 2021b). Pancreatic neuroendocrine is less common.
  B. Modifiable risk factors
    1. Tobacco use; smoking increases the risk of pancreatic cancer by approximately 25% (ACS, 2022f)
    2. Obesity (BMI >30)
    3. Lack of exercise
    4. Chemical exposure (heavy metals, benzidine, pesticides, asbestos, benzene)—seen in dry cleaning and metal working industries (ACS, 2022f)
    5. Alcohol consumption
    6. Poor diet
    7. Increase in abdominal girth
    8. Periodontal disease
  C. Nonmodifiable risk factors
    1. Age (approximately 70 years of age)
    2. Higher incidence in African Americans (50%–90%)
    3. Higher risk in males
    4. Family history of pancreatic cancer
    5. Inherited genetic syndromes such as hereditary breast and ovarian cancer syndrome (BRCA 1 & 2 and PALB2), Lynch syndrome, FAP, PJS, familial atypical multiple mole melanoma, hereditary pancreatitis, cystic fibrosis, and ataxia-telangiectasia
    6. Diabetes, both types 1 and 2
    7. Chronic pancreatitis, which is usually related to alcohol abuse
    8. Liver cirrhosis (NCCN, 2021b)
IV. Prevention
  A. Avoid tobacco.
  B. Keep healthy weight.
  C. Exercise regularly.
  D. Avoid heavy alcohol use.
  E. Limit exposure to certain chemicals in the workplace (ACS, 2022f).
V. Diagnosis
  A. Clinical presentation
  B. Pancreatic protocol CT—helps to see tumor in relation to blood vessels, which is critical for surgical planning
  C. Multidisciplinary review
  D. Biopsy (CT guided or EUS), if indicated
    1. Histologic confirmation is required to establish a diagnosis
    2. Staging evaluation to establish disease extent and resectability rather than biopsy in cases where the diagnosis is yet to be histologically confirmed
  E. Chest CT
  F. Biomarkers—CA 19-9 (NCCN, 2021b)
  G. Molecular profiling—KRAS>90%
  H. Genetic (germline) testing
VI. Histopathology
  A. Adenocarcinoma—accounts for 95% of all cases
  B. Neuroendocrine tumors—rare (carry better prognosis) (NCCN, 2021b)
VII. Staging
  A. AJCC; TNM
  B. Usually found in later stages
VIII. Prognosis and survival
  A. Typically carries poor prognosis, as less than 20% of patients are surgical candidates at the time of diagnosis and the median OS for nonresected patients is 3.5 months.
  B. 5-year survival rate for stage 1 disease is approximately 13%, and for stage 4 disease is 1% (ACS, 2022f).

Management

I. Disease is typically classified as resectable, borderline resectable, locally advanced unresectable, or disseminated.
II. Surgery—due to late presentation, 15%–20% of patients are unable to have surgery (Zhang, Sanagapalli, & Stoita, 2018).
  A. Pancreatoduodenectomy (Whipple procedure) is the most common procedure done. It removes the head of the pancreas, duodenum, a portion of the common bile duct, gallbladder, and sometimes part of the stomach.
  B. Distal pancreatectomy. A procedure in which the tail of the pancreas and/or portion of the body of the pancreas is removed but not the head.
  C. Total pancreatectomy. A procedure in which the entire pancreas and spleen are surgically removed. Rarely performed.

D. Goals of surgery are for negative margins, as a positive margin is associated with poor OS.

III. Radiation
   A. Neoadjuvant setting with concurrent chemotherapy or SBRT (clinical trial or experienced center with high volume of liver cancer)
   B. Adjuvant setting with chemotherapy
   C. Palliative therapy

IV. Systemic therapy
   A. Adjuvant chemotherapy
      1. Gemcitabine, 5-FU, gemcitabine/capecitabine
   B. Unresectable and/or metastatic setting
      1. FOLFIRINOX (5-FU, leucovorin, irinotecan, oxaliplatin), gemcitabine/nab-paclitaxel, gemcitabine/cisplatin (BRCA 1 and BRCA 2 or PALB2 pathogenic variants)
      2. Second-line FOLFOX, 5-fluorouracil/Nal-Irinotecan
      3. Immunotherapy (Pembrolizumab)—second line for MSI-H, dMMR type tumors, *NTRK* gene fusion (NCCN, 2021b)

CHOLANGIOCARCINOMA

Overview

I. Cholangiocarcinomas encompass all tumors originating from the epithelium of the bile duct. Cholangiocarcinomas are diagnosed throughout the biliary tree and are typically classified as intrahepatic or extrahepatic. Intrahepatic cholangiocarcinomas are located within the hepatic parenchyma. Extrahepatic occurs anywhere within the extrahepatic bile duct, from the junction of the right and left hepatic ducts to the common bile duct (NCCN, 2021a).

II. Epidemiology
   A. Rare—only about 8000 cases diagnosed in the United States annually.
   B. The incidence is increasing but may be due to the ability to accurately diagnose intrahepatic cholangiocarcinoma.
   C. More common in Southeast Asia due to parasitic infections (ACS, 2022b).

III. Pathophysiology
   Risk factors
   A. No predisposing risk factors can be identified in most patients. However, associations have been found to include hepatitis C virus (HCV), HBV, cirrhosis, diabetes, obesity, alcohol, NAFLD, and tobacco.

IV. Prevention: Preventive measures
   A. Avoid tobacco.
   B. Keep healthy weight.
   C. Exercise regularly.
   D. Avoid heavy alcohol use.

V. Diagnosis
   1. Clinical presentation, incidental finding during a gallbladder surgery
   2. Multiphasic abdominal/pelvic CT/MRI
   3. CT chest
   4. Liver function tests, carcinoembryonic antigen, and CA19-9

   5. Necessity of establishing a tissue diagnosis prior to surgery depends upon the clinical situation

VI. Histopathology—more than 90% are adenocarcinomas
   A. Extrahepatic more common than intrahepatic
   B. Broadly divided into three histologic types based on growth patterns: mass forming, periductal infiltrating, and intraductal growing (NCCN, 2022b)

VII. Staging:
   A. AJCC; TNM:
   B. Staging dependent on the origin of cancer: Intrahepatic, perihilar, and distal bile duct cancers (ACS, 2022a, 2022b, 2022c, 2022d, 2022e, 2022f, 2022g)

VIII. Prognosis and survival
   A. Prognosis typically better for extrahepatic compared with intrahepatic
   B. Local disease 5-year survival rate is approximately 52% but the distant spread 5-year survival rate is 2% (ACS, 2022a, 2022b, 2022c, 2022d, 2022e, 2022f, 2022g)

Management

I. Surgery
   A. Complete resection only potentially curative treatment for intrahepatic and extrahepatic cholangiocarcinoma; if possible, carries a much better prognosis.
   B. Liver transplantation sometimes a curative option with LN negative, nondisseminated, locally advanced hilar cholangiocarcinomas.

II. Local–regional therapies for intrahepatic cholangiocarcinoma similar to HCC; include RFA, TACE, DEB-TACE, and TARE; hepatic arterial infusion also used in certain settings

III. Radiation
   A. Employed as local-regional therapy in intrahepatic
   B. Sometimes used in adjuvant setting combined with chemotherapy

IV. Systemic therapies—used in adjuvant and advanced settings: capecitabine (preferred adjuvant), or 5-fluorouracil, oxaliplatin, gemcitabine, and cisplatin (preferred advanced) (NCCN, 2021a)

REFERENCES

Alqahtani, A., Khan, Z., Alloghbi, A., Said Ahmed, T. S., Ashraf, M., & Hammouda, D. M. (2019). Hepatocellular carcinoma: Molecular mechanisms and targeted therapies. *Medicina (Kaunas, Lithuania)*, 55(9), 526. https://doi.org/10.3390/medicina55090526.

American Cancer Society (ACS). *Anal cancer detailed guide*. (2022a). http://www.cancer.org/cancer/anal-cancer.html.

American Cancer Society (ACS). *Bile duct cancer detailed guide*. (2022b). https://www.cancer.org/cancer/bile-duct-cancer.html.

American Cancer Society (ACS). *Colorectal cancer detailed guide*. (2022c). http://www.cancer.org/cancer/colon-rectal-cancer.html.

American Cancer Society (ACS). *Esophagus cancer detailed guide*. (2022d). http://www.cancer.org/cancer/esophagus-cancer.html.

American Cancer Society (ACS). *Liver cancer detailed guide*. (2022e). http://www.cancer.org/cancer/liver-cancer.html.

American Cancer Society (ACS). *Pancreatic cancer detailed guide.* (2022f). http://www.cancer.org/cancer/pancreatic-cancer.html.

American Cancer Society (ACS). *Stomach cancer detailed guide.* (2022g). http://www.cancer.org/cancer/stomach-cancer.html.

American Joint Committee on Cancer (AJCC). *Implementation of AJCC 8th edition cancer staging system.* (2018). https://www.facs.org/media/2zvlrdmi/ajcc_staging_rules_8th_ed.pdf.

Guo, Y.-M., Yu, W.-W., Zhu, M., & Guo, C.-Y. (2015). Clinicopathological and prognostic significance of epidermal growth factor receptor overexpression in patients with esophageal adenocarcinoma: A meta-analysis. *Diseases of the Esophagus, 28*(8), 750–756. https://doi.org/10.1111/dote.12248.

Jain, S., & Dhingra, S. (2017). Pathology of esophageal cancer and Barrett's esophagus. *Annals of Cardiothoracic Surgery, 6*(2), 99–109. https://doi.org/10.21037/acs.2017.03.06.

Jochem, C., & Leitzmann, M. (2016). Obesity and colorectal cancer. In T. Pshon & K. Nimptsch (Eds.), *Obesity and cancer.* Cham: SUI: Springer.

Mohammed, A., Yarla, N. S., Madka, V., & Rao, C. V. (2018). Clinically relevant anti-inflammatory agents for chemoprevention of colorectal cancer: New perspectives. *International Journal of Molecular Sciences, 19*(8), 2332. https://doi.org/10.3390/ijms19082332.

Moayyedi, P., & El-Serag, H. B. (2021). Current status of chemoprevention in Barrett's esophagus. *Gastrointestinal Endoscopy Clinics of North America, 31*(1), 117–130. https://doi.org/10.1016/j.giec.2020.08.008.

National Cancer Institute (NCI). *Surveillance, epidemiology, and end results program.* (2022). https://seer.cancer.gov/.

Nagaraja, V., & Eslick, G. D. (2015). HER2 expression in gastric and oesophageal cancer: A meta-analytic review. *Journal of Gastrointestinal Oncology, 6*(2), 143–154. https://doi.org/10.3978/j.issn.2078-6891.2014.107.

National Comprehensive Cancer Network (NCCN). *NCCN practice guidelines in oncology: Hepatobiliary cancer [v.2.2018].* (2021a). https://www.nccn.org/professionals/physician_gls/pdf/hepatobiliary.pdf.

National Comprehensive Cancer Network (NCCN). *NCCN practice guidelines in oncology: Pancreatic adenocarcinoma cancer [v.5.2021].* (2021b). https://www.nccn.org/professionals/physician_gls/pdf/pancreatic.pdf.

National Comprehensive Cancer Network (NCCN). *NCCN practice guidelines in oncology: Anal cancer [v.2.2022].* (2022a). https://www.nccn.org/professionals/physician_gls/pdf/anal.pdf.

National Comprehensive Cancer Network (NCCN). *NCCN practice guidelines in oncology: Colon cancer [v.1.2022].* (2022b). https://www.nccn.org/professionals/physician_gls/pdf/colon.pdf.

National Comprehensive Cancer Network (NCCN). *NCCN practice guidelines in oncology: Esophageal and esophagastric junction cancer [v.2.2022].* (2022c). https://www.nccn.org/professionals/physician_gls/pdf/esophageal.pdf.

National Comprehensive Cancer Network (NCCN). *NCCN practice guidelines in oncology: Gastric cancer [v.2.2022].* (2022d). https://www.nccn.org/professionals/physician_gls/pdf/gastric.pdf.

National Comprehensive Cancer Network (NCCN). *NCCN practice guidelines in oncology: Rectal cancer [v.1.2022].* (2022e). https://www.nccn.org/professionals/physician_gls/pdf/rectal.pdf.

Seeneevassen, L., Bessède, E., Mégraud, F., Lehours, P., Dubus, P., & Varon, C. (2021). Gastric cancer: Advances in carcinogenesis research and new therapeutic strategies. *International Journal of Molecular Sciences, 22*(7), 3418. https://doi.org/10.3390/ijms22073418.

Zhang, L., Sanagapalli, S., & Stoita, A. (2018). Challenges in diagnosis of pancreatic cancer. *World Journal of Gastroenterology, 24*(19), 2047–2060. https://doi.org/10.3748/wjg.v24.i19.2047.

15

Genitourinary Cancers

Robin I. Green

KIDNEY CANCER

Overview

I. Physiology and pathophysiology (OpenStax, 2018)
   A. Anatomy
      1. The kidneys are on either side of the spine in the retroperitoneal space between the parietal peritoneum and the posterior abdominal wall.
      2. Protected by muscle, fat, and ribs
      3. The adrenal gland is located on the superior aspect of each kidney, with the adrenal cortex influencing renal function through aldosterone production.
      4. The inner structure consists of the renal cortex, medulla, renal columns separating the renal pyramids, and renal papillae.
      5. Receive about 25% of cardiac output at rest
   B. Physiology
      1. The nephron is the basic structural and functional unit of the kidney.
         a. Cleanses blood and balances constituents in circulation through filtration, reabsorption, and secretion
         b. Regulates blood pressure
         c. Controls red blood cell production and calcium absorption
         d. Comprises glomerulus, a tuft of high-pressure capillaries formed from the afferent arterioles, surrounded by the proximal end of a continuous, sophisticated tubule creating Bowman capsule
   C. Kidney cancer classifications (Atkins 2022)
      1. Clear cell carcinoma, also known as *conventional* or *nonpapillary*
         a. Comprises 75%–85% of cases
         b. Thought to arise from proximal renal tubule
         c. Hereditary and sporadic form
         d. Prognosis based on stage
      2. Papillary renal cell carcinoma (RCC)
         a. Comprises 10%–15% of cases
         b. Thought to arise from proximal renal tubular epithelium
         c. Hereditary and sporadic forms
         d. Prognosis based on stage and type of papillary cell
      3. Chromophobe RCC
         a. Comprises 5%–10% of cases
         b. Arises from renal tubular epithelium; proposed to originate in collecting ducts
         c. Excellent prognosis—better than papillary or clear cell carcinoma
      4. Oncocytic RCC
         a. Comprises 3%–7% of cases
         b. Arises from intercalculated cells of the collecting duct
         c. Behave in a benign fashion, rarely metastatic
   D. Collecting duct carcinoma or Bellini duct carcinoma of the kidney
      1. Comprises fewer than 1% of all cases
      2. Arises in medullary collecting ducts
      3. Younger age, more frequently in African American individuals
      4. Aggressive with rapid metastasis
      5. Subtype of collecting duct carcinoma
         a. Renal medullary carcinoma
         b. Occurs almost exclusively in African American men with sickle cell disease (Jonasch, Gao, & Rathmell, 2014; NORD, 2021)
   E. Unclassified RCC
      1. Remains as diagnostic category for tumors that do not fit into other categories
      2. Sarcomatoid is no longer considered a distinct category but is viewed as a manifestation of high-grade carcinoma.
      3. Includes rare tumors—may be misclassified subtypes of RCC (Jonasch et al., 2014; Mirsadraei & Chen, 2017)
   F. Tumors of the renal pelvis (National Cancer Institute [NCI], 2020)
      1. Very rare
      2. 5% or less of all cases (Liu, Lin, & Chang, 2013; Khoo & Tang, 2019)
   G. Urothelial or transitional cell carcinomas
      1. May occur at any site within the upper urinary collecting system
      2. Generally multifocal
      3. Decreased incidence over past decades (NCI, 2020)
   H. Renal cell cancers—tend to grow toward the medullary portion of the kidney and spread via direct extrusion to the renal vein or the vena cava

1. Metastasis at diagnosis in 30% of patients; recurrence in 40%, even among those with early-stage disease (Motzer et al., 2022)

II. Epidemiology
   A. Kidney cancers rare in the United States, accounting for only 4.2% of all cancers (Padala et al., 2020)
      1. Incidence and death rates have been rising since 1998.
      2. Average age of diagnosis in the United States is 64 years old.
      3. Rising incidence may be related to common use of high-resolution imaging and incidental finding of tumors among asymptomatic persons.
      4. Two-thirds of renal carcinomas are now discovered incidentally during pelvic and abdominal scanning (Padala et al., 2020).
      5. Renal cell cancer incidence rates vary by race/ethnicity (Padala et al., 2020).
   B. Male predominance, two-thirds of diagnosis of RCC (Padala et al., 2020)

III. Risk factors (Padala et al., 2020)
   A. Tobacco use, obesity, hypertension, unopposed estrogen use, diuretic treatment, prior radiation therapy (RT), occupational exposure to petroleum products or heavy metals, asbestos exposure, and dialysis-acquired cystic kidney disease
   B. Dietary factors: high-fat diets, high-protein diets, diets low in antioxidants
   C. Genetic predisposition, von Hippel–Lindau (VHL) disease (usually diagnosed 20 years earlier than average), non-Hodgkin lymphoma, and sickle cell disease linked to an increased risk of kidney cancer
   D. Clear cell carcinomas associated with loss/inactivation of short arm of chromosome 3p (Hsieh et al., 2018; Liu et al., 2013)
      1. Alterations found in 91%–94% of patients (Atkins, 2022; Hsieh et al., 2018; Liu et al., 2013)
      2. Association also found with VHL disease
         a. Papillary RCC
            (1) Normal 3p but often trisomies 3q, 8, 12, 17, and 20 noted
            (2) Trisomies 7 and 17 and the loss of the Y chromosome also reported (Jonasch et al., 2014)
         b. Chromophobe RCC associated with loss of chromosomes 1, 2, 6, 10, 13, and 21 and alterations of chromosome 17
         c. Common metastatic sites: lungs, abdominal and mediastinal lymph nodes, liver, and bone (Fig. 15.1; Motzer et al., 2022)

IV. Prevention
   1. Smoking cessation
   2. Maintain healthy weight and diet rich in fruits and vegetables (Padala et al., 2020)
   3. Control of hypertension

V. Histopathology

   A. Grading (Jonasch et al., 2014; Swami, Nussenzveig, Haaland, & Agarwal, 2019)
      1. Fuhrman grading system on a scale of 1 (least aggressive) to 4 (most aggressive)
      2. Higher nuclear grade associated with worse 5-year overall survival

VI. Diagnosis and staging (Motzer et al., 2022)
   A. Screening—no screening tests available for kidney cancer; patients with multiple affected relatives should be referred for genetic counseling, possible surveillance
   B. Classic triad symptoms: Only 10% of patients present with hematuria, flank pain, and palpable mass
   C. Diagnostic measures (Table 15.1)
      1. Kidney, ureter, and bladder (KUB) radiography
      2. Intravenous pyelography (also referred to as excretory urography): commonly used to evaluate patients presenting with hematuria
      3. Renal ultrasonography
      4. Pelvic or abdominal computed tomography—diagnostic test of choice
      5. Renal angiography—less commonly performed; may be necessary because of large vascular mass if renal artery embolization is planned
      6. Magnetic resonance imaging (MRI)—especially important if vena cava involvement
      7. Retrograde urography
   D. Staging
      1. Staging—based on tumor size, lymph node involvement, and distant metastasis
      2. American Joint Committee on Cancer (AJCC) staging system used for grading (Amin et al., 2017; Motzer et al., 2022)
      3. No known tumor or molecular marker to confirm diagnosis, remission, progression, or relapse
      4. Research for potential urinary and serum biomarkers promising (Pastore et al., 2015)

VII. Prognosis and survival
   A. Prognostic factors: patient age, histologic grade and type, disease stage, performance status, low hemoglobin level, elevated serum calcium and lactate dehydrogenase (LDH or LD) levels, number and location of metastatic sites, time to appearance of metastasis, and prior nephrectomy (Motzer et al., 2022)
   B. Immunohistochemically stains: determine systemic therapy (Padala et al., 2020)
      1. Programmed death ligand-1
      2. Vascular endothelial growth factor (VEGF)
   C. Antithyroid antibodies stimulated by interleukin-2 (IL-2) immunotherapy may be associated with improved survival (Motzer et al., 2022).
   D. The 5-year survival rate based on the SEER database which does not group cancers by AJCC TNM stages (stage 1, stage 2, stage 3, etc.) but rather into localized, regional, and distant stages: localized 93%, regional

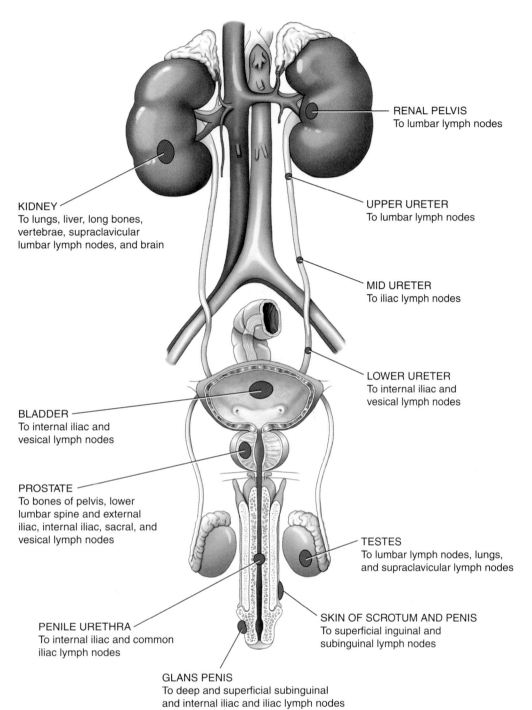

RENAL PELVIS
To lumbar lymph nodes

KIDNEY
To lungs, liver, long bones,
vertebrae, supraclavicular
lumbar lymph nodes, and brain

UPPER URETER
To lumbar lymph nodes

MID URETER
To iliac lymph nodes

LOWER URETER
To internal iliac and
vesical lymph nodes

BLADDER
To internal iliac and
vesical lymph nodes

PROSTATE
To bones of pelvis, lower
lumbar spine and external
iliac, internal iliac, sacral, and
vesical lymph nodes

TESTES
To lumbar lymph nodes, lungs,
and supraclavicular lymph nodes

SKIN OF SCROTUM AND PENIS
To superficial inguinal and
subinguinal lymph nodes

PENILE URETHRA
To internal iliac and common
iliac lymph nodes

GLANS PENIS
To deep and superficial subinguinal
and internal iliac and iliac lymph nodes

Fig. 15.1 Sites of tumor origin and metastases in the male.

71%, distant 14%, all stages combined 76% (ACS, 2022c; Siegel et al., 2022).

Management

I. NCCN guidelines Version 4.2022 give the most updated guidelines for the complex management and multiple drug options (NCCN, 2022b).

II. Active surveillance (stage 1A RCC)—option should be considered for patients with decreased life expectancy or extensive comorbidities that would place them at risk for more invasive treatment (Motzer et al., 2022).

III. Surgery

A. Radical nephrectomy—primary treatment since 1960 (Motzer et al., 2022)

B. Partial nephrectomy—preferred whenever feasible, especially in patients with limited renal function, bilateral tumors, or a solitary kidney (Motzer et al., 2022).

C. Open, laparoscopic, robotic surgical techniques are used to perform radical and partial nephrectomies.

D. Cryosurgery and radiofrequency ablation—option for patients with clinical stage T1 lesions who are not surgical candidates (Motzer et al., 2022).

TABLE 15.1   Urologic Diagnostic Tests and Nursing Interventions

Test	Preparation	Nursing Interventions
Radiographic examination of KUB	None—plain film of abdomen	Explain to the patient the need to lie flat on examination table. Do not schedule after barium studies (will obscure kidneys).
Excretory urography	Dye excreted unchanged by kidneys; notify radiologist if kidney function is impaired; limit fluid intake to assist the kidneys in concentrating the substance in the urine. Dye injected intravenously; anaphylactic or allergic reaction to dye may occur; may need to premedicate with antihistamines.	Assess history of allergy to iodine dyes or contrast media before test; pretesting may be indicated. Use of iodine dyes may be contraindicated in patients with severe renal or hepatic disease or clinical hypersensitivity (severe allergies, asthma). Have emergency equipment and personnel available before injection (anaphylaxis and cardiovascular reactions may occur) and 30–60 minutes after test (delayed reactions). Observe for adverse reactions to dye—angina, chest pain, arrhythmias, hypotension, dizziness, blurred vision, headache, fever, convulsions, dyspnea, rhinitis, laryngitis, and nausea.
Retrograde urography	General anesthesia or opioid analgesia may be used; cystoscope is inserted; iodinated dye is injected via the urethral catheter. Laxatives at bedtime before test may be used to cleanse bowel.	Observe for reaction to anesthetic or analgesic. Monitor for bleeding, symptoms of urinary tract infections, dysuria, or difficulty voiding after test.

KUB, Kidneys, ureter, bladder.

E. Cytoreductive nephrectomy before systemic therapy for patients with surgically resectable primary tumor and multiple metastatic sites (Motzer et al., 2022)
  1. Patients most likely to benefit are those with lung-only metastases, good prognostic features, and good performance status.
IV. RT (ACS, 2022c; Motzer et al., 2022)
  A. Renal cell cancers unresponsive to radiotherapy
  B. May be used for palliation (e.g., skeletal metastasis, brain metastasis)
V. Chemotherapy—has not been shown to improve survival (ACS, 2022c)
VI. Immunotherapy
  A. IL-2
    1. Overall response rate of 14%, with 5% complete responses
      a. Majority who had complete response had durable complete remissions (ACS, 2022c; Motzer et al., 2022).
      b. Patients should have good performance status, normal organ function.
  B. Interferon-alpha (ACS, 2022c)
    1. Produced response rates of 10%–15% given as a single agent
    2. Can be given in combination with IL-2 or bevacizumab
  C. Immune checkpoint inhibitors (ACS, 2022c; Motzer et al., 2022)
    1. Checkpoints turn on or off to start an immune process
    2. Prevents immune system from attacking normal cells

  3. Cancer cell may use checkpoints to avoid being attacked
  4. Drugs being developed to target checkpoints
VII. Targeted therapies
  A. Everolimus (RAD001), axitinib (Inlyta), sorafenib (Nexavar), sunitinib (Sutent), temsirolimus (Torisel), bevacizumab (Avastin), and pazopanib (Votrient), to name a few
  B. Common side effects—fatigue, skin rash, diarrhea, hand–foot syndrome, increased glucose and cholesterol levels, cardiovascular and delayed wound healing
VIII. Nursing implications
  A. Maximize safety postoperatively.
    1. Pulmonary hygiene—teach patients to perform cough and deep-breathing exercises.
    2. Observe for signs of hemorrhage.
    3. Monitor vital signs, hemoglobin, hematocrit, kidney function tests, and urine output.
    4. Provide pharmacologic and nonpharmacologic pain relief measures.
    5. Nursing to assist with patient navigation of surgical procedures, oncology, and treatment. May be treated in hospital or oncology clinic.
  B. Provide patient education regarding follow-up care and surveillance.
    1. Teach patient to identify and manage symptoms, including when to report symptoms.
    2. Refer to mental health specialist, community resources, support groups as needed.
    3. Provide education and cancer survivorship care plan, which includes treatment summary, pycho-social support, and follow-up plan.

BLADDER CANCER

Overview

I. Physiology and pathophysiology
   A. Primary function
      1. The bladder is a hollow muscular organ that serves as a temporary reservoir for urine, which is then discharged through the urethra.
      2. In men, critical adjacent structures include the prostate, seminal vesicles, urethra, ureter, nerves at the base of the penis, and local lymph nodes (see Fig. 15.1).
      3. In women, critical adjacent structures include the uterus, ureter, ovaries, fallopian tubes, urethra, and local lymph nodes (Fig. 15.2).
   B. Changes associated with cancer
      1. Proliferation of abnormal tissue in one or more places within the bladder
      2. Clinical manifestations—grossly visible or microscopic hematuria (especially with bladder wall invasion), dysuria, burning, frequency, suprapubic and/or pelvic pain (ACS, 2022a)
   C. Major classifications of bladder cancer (ACS, 2022a)
      1. Urothelial carcinoma (formerly known as *transitional cell carcinoma*)
         a. Arises from epithelial layer of the bladder, which rests on basement membrane
         b. Comprises about 95% of bladder tumors (ACS, 2022a)
         c. Can be further subdivided—carcinoma in situ, noninvasive papillary carcinoma, invasive papillary carcinoma, and solid tumors
            (1) 70%–80% considered "superficial" disease—World Health Organization has recommended the term be abandoned; referred to as *non–muscle-invasive bladder cancer* (NMIBC) (NCI, 2018a)
            (2) Papillary tumors confined to the first two layers of the bladder but project toward the lumen (ACS, 2022a)
               (a) These tumors demonstrate changes to chromosome 9 and an overexpression of VEGF, leading to angiogenesis (NCI, 2018a).

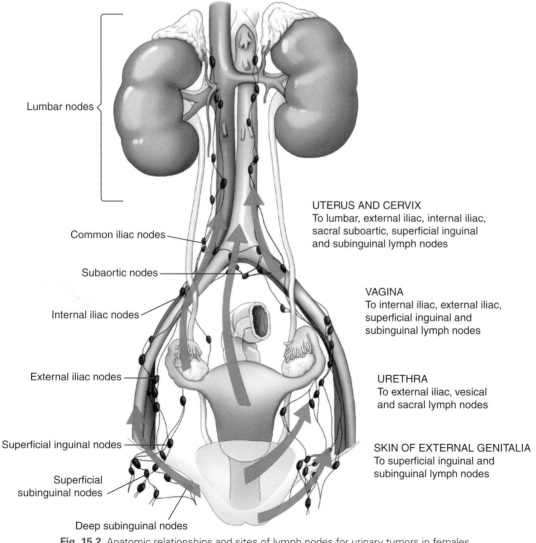

Lumbar nodes

Common iliac nodes

Subaortic nodes

Internal iliac nodes

External iliac nodes

Superficial inguinal nodes

Superficial subinguinal nodes

Deep subinguinal nodes

UTERUS AND CERVIX
To lumbar, external iliac, internal iliac, sacral suboartic, superficial inguinal and subinguinal lymph nodes

VAGINA
To internal iliac, external iliac, superficial inguinal and subinguinal lymph nodes

URETHRA
To external iliac, vesical and sacral lymph nodes

SKIN OF EXTERNAL GENITALIA
To superficial inguinal and subinguinal lymph nodes

Fig. 15.2 Anatomic relationships and sites of lymph nodes for urinary tumors in females.

2. Squamous cell carcinomas—make up approximately 1%–2% of cases; this is related to schistosomiasis infection that is endemic in Egypt
3. Adenocarcinomas—make up approximately 1% of cases
4. Small cell tumors—make up less than 1% of cases (ACS, 2022a)

II. Epidemiology
   A. Incidence rates high in the United States and Africa (ACS, 2022a)
   B. Most common malignancy of the urinary system
   C. Estimated new cases in the United States in 2022—81,180 (ACS, 2022b)
   D. Male-to-female ratio nearly 4:1 (Saginala et al., 2020)
   E. Median age at diagnosis 73 years; rarely diagnosed before age 40 years (Saginala et al., 2020)
   F. African Americans lag behind Whites in 5-year survival rates (ACS, 2022b)

III. Risk factors
   A. Tobacco use
      1. Most significant risk factor, accounting for 50%–65% of all bladder tumors in men, 25% in women (Saginala et al., 2020)
   B. High body mass index may increase risk and risk of recurrence, but results are inconsistent (Westhoff et al., 2017, 2018)
   C. Dietary supplements containing aristocholic acid (ACS, 2022a)
   D. Arsenic in drinking water (ACS, 2022a)
   E. Not drinking enough fluids (ACS, 2022a)
   F. Chronic bladder irritations and infections have unclear link (NCI, 2018a)
   G. History of bladder or other urothelial cancer (NCI, 2018a)
   H. Genetics and family history (Saginala et al., 2020)
   I. No strong evidence suggesting that supplementation with any micronutrient reduces bladder cancer risk (Piyathilake, 2016)
   J. Diets rich in fruits and vegetables, low in processed meats, in addition to smoking cessation may be somewhat protective for bladder cancer (Piyathilake, 2016)
   K. Common metastatic sites—lymph nodes, bones, lung, liver, and peritoneum (NCI, 2018a)

IV. Prevention
   A. 81.8% of cases could be attributed to known preventable causes (Saginala et al., 2020).
   B. 7% cases are predicted to arise from heritable genetic influence (Saginala et al., 2020).

V. Histopathology
   A. Grading
      1. Tumor grade (grades X, 1, 2, 3, 4)—refers to the degree of tumor cell differentiation and aggressive nature of the tumor cells
         a. This grading system has changed to a low- and high-grade designation to match the current World Health Organization/International Society of Urologic Pathology (WHO/ISUP)–recommended grading system
         b. High-grade tumors tend to grow more quickly and are more likely to metastasize

VI. Diagnosis and staging
   A. Screening—not currently recommended by any major preventive group in the United States
      1. No specific serologic tumor markers
      2. Urinary assays for bladder cancer
         a. Food and Drug Administration (FDA)–approved nuclear matrix protein 22 assay: a noninvasive test used for the surveillance and monitoring of patients with bladder cancer (Xylinas et al., 2014).
         b. Other FDA-approved urinary assays for bladder cancer detection and monitoring—bladder tumor–associated antigen (BTA) assays, ImmunoCyt test, and UroVysion fluorescence in situ hybridization assay. The sensitivity and specificity of the BTA stat test are 57%–83% and 60%–92%, respectively.
         c. Elevated urine levels of COL4A1 and COL13A1 show promise for diagnosis and prognosis (Miyake et al., 2017).
         d. Urinary biomarkers are insufficiently effective when used in isolation, and cytology remains the gold standard in many practices (Ng, Stenzl, Sharma, & Vasev, 2021).
   B. Staging
      1. AJCC staging system (Amin et al., 2017)

VII. Prognosis and survival
   A. Prognostic indicators—tumor grade, size, location, biomarkers such as the *p21* gene and ki67 antigen, cellular adhesion models, and response to therapy
   B. 5-year survival rate by stage of bladder cancer—stage 0 (98%), stage I (88%), stage II (63%), stage III (46%), and stage IV (15%) (ACS, 2022a)

Management

I. NCCN guidelines Version 1.2022 give the most updated guidelines for the complex management and multiple drug options (National Comprehensive Cancer Network [NCCN], 2022a)
II. Neoadjuvant chemotherapy
   A. Preferred: DDMVAC (dose-dense methotrexate, vinblastine, doxorubicin, and cisplatin) with growth factors for support 3–6 cycles
   B. Other: Gemcitabine and cisplatin for 4 cycles
III. NMIBC
   A. Goal—prevent disease progression/invasion, avoid bladder loss, increase survival and possible cure
   B. Primary mode of treatment—cystoscopy to confirm tumor presence, then transurethral resection (TUR) of bladder tumor; tumor removal achieved by fulguration (burning with electrical current) or laser therapy
      1. Most common side effects—bleeding and infection

2. Perforation of surrounding tissues also risk of treatment
IV. Intravesical therapy—includes intravesical chemotherapy and immunotherapy
   A. Indications based on the probability of recurrence and progression to muscle-invasive disease such as size, number, and grade (NCCN, 2022a)
   B. Intravesicular chemotherapy has been found to be more effective than TUR alone in preventing tumor recurrence.
   C. Most common agents: mitomycin C (MMC), Bacillus Calmette–Guerin (BCG), thiotepa (Thioplex), valrubicin, doxorubicin (Adriamycin)
      1. Combination of these drugs has also been used.
      2. Thiotepa is infrequently used in clinical practice due to higher systemic side effects, such as myelosuppression.
V. Treatment of muscle-invasive disease
   A. Radical cystectomy with urinary diversion
      1. Removal of the bladder and prostate in men
      2. Hysterectomy in women
      3. Bilateral pelvic lymphadenectomy, including at a minimum common internal iliac, external iliac, and obturator nodes in both men and women
      4. Potential complications—infection, bleeding, and sexual dysfunction
      5. Presurgical chemotherapy using DDMVAC (methotrexate [Mexate], vinblastine [Velban], doxorubicin [Adriamycin], cisplatin [Platinol]) demonstrated to double survival rates in patients with advanced bladder cancer compared with surgery alone (NCI, 2018a)
      6. Cisplatin-based combination chemotherapy strongly recommended by NCCN guidelines (NCCN, 2022a)
      7. Types of urinary diversions (see Chapter 38)
         a. Ileal conduit (Fig. 15.3)—urinary diversion performed with cystectomy
            (1) A portion of the terminal end of the ileum is isolated, the proximal end is closed, and the distal end is brought out through an opening in the abdominal wall and sutured to the skin, creating a stoma.
            (2) Ureters are implanted into the ileal segment, urine flows into the conduit, and peristalsis propels urine out through the stoma.
         b. Continent ileal reservoir (Fig. 15.4)—technique that provides an intraabdominal pouch for storage of urine
            (1) Typically, the stoma has a nipple valve to prevent ureteral reflux. The stoma is generally placed below the undergarment line.
            (2) No external collecting device needed; urine remains in reservoir until patient self-catheterizes through stoma, approximately every 6 hours.

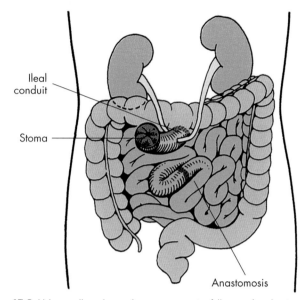

Fig. 15.3 Urinary diversion using a segment of ileum. As short a segment as possible is used and positioned in the right lower quadrant of the abdomen in an isoperistaltic direction. From Christensen, B. L., & Kockrow, E. O. (2010). *Adult health nursing care* (6th ed.). St. Louis, MO: Mosby.

         c. Orthotopic neobladder—a technique that provides a creation of a new bladder that is made from the intestine; better quality of life reported compared with ileal conduit.
   B. Bladder preservation therapy
      1. Although radical cystectomy is the current primary treatment modality, some patients cannot tolerate cystectomy or are unwilling to undergo the procedure
      2. Bladder preservation strategies include the following:
         a. External beam RT
         b. Trimodality therapy—TUR, RT, and systemic chemotherapy
   C. Chemotherapy
      1. Advanced bladder cancer is often treated with systemic chemotherapy.
         a. NCCN guidelines indicate the first-line combination chemotherapy for metastatic disease includes the following (NCCN, 2022a):
            (1) Dose-dense DDMVAC with growth factor support
            (2) Gemcitabine and cisplatin (carboplatin if unable to take cisplatin)
         b. For the second-line therapy, single-agent taxane or gemcitabine preferred
         c. For concurrent treatment with RT, radiosensitizing chemotherapy regimens include the following:
      2. Cisplatin alone or in combination with 5-fluorouracil (5-FU).
      3. Mitomycin C in combination with 5-FU.

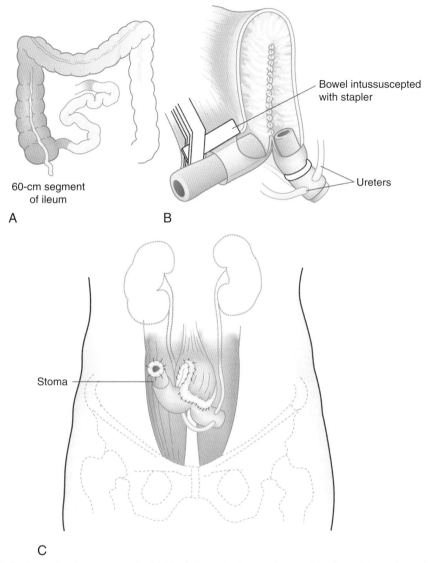

60-cm segment
of ileum

A   B

Bowel intussuscepted
with stapler

Ureters

Stoma

C

Fig. 15.4 Kock pouch urinary reservoir. (A) Shaded area indicates the section of small intestine selected for reservoir construction. (B) Afferent (nonrefluxing) limb for ureteral implantation and efferent limb (with nippled valve) for stoma are created by using stapling devices. (C) Completed reservoir with the efferent limb drawn through the abdominal wall and stoma created. From Tanagho, E. A., & McAninch, J. W. (Eds.) (1992). *Smith's general urology* (13th ed.). San Mateo, CA: Appleton & Lange.

4. Immunotherapy may be added after chemotherapy or given alone depending on the disease and patient factors (including those that cannot take cisplatin).
   a. Immune checkpoint inhibitor
      (1) PD-1
      (2) PD-L1
   b. Targeted therapy
      (1) FGFR3
      (2) FGFR2
5. Clinical trial
D. RT
   1. Useful in the management of invasive disease
   2. Linear accelerator with multiple fields, daily or twice daily

3. An empty bladder required for both simulation and treatment
4. Radiation usually preceded by TUR
5. Often used as combined-modality therapy with chemotherapy
6. Dose range to whole bladder—40–50.4 gray (Gy), with an additional boost to 66–70 Gy for gross disease and gross nodal disease to 54–66 Gy. All doses depend on patient's tolerance (NCCN, 2022a).
IX. Nursing implications
   A. Maximize safety postoperatively
      1. Pulmonary hygiene—teach patient to perform cough and deep-breathing exercises; use of incentive spirometry.

2. Increase in activity as tolerated to help with prevention of clots.
3. Observe for signs of hemorrhage.
4. Monitor vital signs, hemoglobin, hematocrit, kidney function tests, and urine output.
5. Provide pharmacologic and nonpharmacologic pain relief measures.
6. Information on support group and psychosocial needs.
7. Nurse to assist with navigation of surgery, oncologist, urologist, and oncology clinic. Patient may be treated in urology office, infusion center, or hospital setting.
B. Interventions related to the management of RT (see Chapter 27); targeted therapies and biotherapies (see Chapter 29)
C. Interventions for patients receiving intravesical chemotherapy
   1. BCG—contraindicated in patients with immune system compromise because of HIV or steroid use, urinary tract infection, or past reactions to tuberculosis strains; systemic tuberculosis may develop.
   2. Thiotepa—low molecular weight leads to high rates of systemic absorption and severe myelosuppression.
   3. Mitomycin C—may cause dysuria, frequency, and, less commonly, allergic reactions and myelosuppression.
D. Management of common ileal conduit problems (Table 15.2).

PROSTATE CANCER

Overview

I. Physiology and pathophysiology
   A. Primary function
      1. Located posterior to the symphysis pubis, inferior to the bladder, in front of the rectum (see Fig. 15.1)
      2. Prostate gland—encircles the urethra as it leaves the bladder
      3. Comprises three zones—transitional zone, central zone, and peripheral zone
      4. Functions as a secondary sex organ that secretes a component of seminal fluid
   B. Changes associated with cancer
      1. Most cancers develop in the peripheral zone.
      2. Malignant cell growth spreads locally to the seminal vesicles, bladder, and peritoneum (see Fig. 15.1).
         a. Lymphatic, hematogenous spread is also common; pelvic lymph node invasion
   C. Major classifications
      1. Adenocarcinomas—95%
      2. Remaining 5% are sarcomas, mucinous or signet ring tumors, adenoid cystic carcinomas, and small cell undifferentiated cancers (ACS, 2022b).
II. Epidemiology
   A. National trend in prostate cancer incidence—increased rates from 1988 to 1992 coinciding with the advent of widespread prostate-specific antigen (PSA) testing;

sharp declines from 1992 to 1995, followed by a leveling off from 1995 to 2013; decrease of 8% from 2009 to 2013 likely due to the United States Preventive Services Task Force (USPSTF) recommendation against routine testing (ACS, 2022b).
   B. Approximately 268,490 men newly diagnosed and 34,500 are estimated to die of the disease yearly; the third leading cause of cancer death among men (ACS, 2022b).
   C. Accounts for one-third of all male cancers; most commonly diagnosed noncutaneous cancer among men.
   D. 5-year survival rates—steady improvement since 1974 for both Whites and African Americans; however, continuing lower 5-year survival rates for all stages of prostate cancer among African Americans (ACS, 2022b).
   E. African American men have the highest incidence rates and more aggressive type of prostate cancer compared to White men (Rawla, 2019).
III. Risk factors
   A. Increasing age—only well-established risk factor (ACS, 2022b)
      1. More than 60% of prostate cancers are diagnosed in men 65 years or older.
      2. Autopsy studies reveal 30% of men aged 50 have evidence of adenocarcinoma of the prostate; by age 90 that percentage rises to 57%.
   B. Ethnicity
      1. Higher mortality rates in Western/developed countries compared with developing countries (e.g., developing countries such as in Asia and the Middle East) (Kumst, Singh, Malik, Manne, & Mishra, 2017)
      2. Highest incidence and mortality rates in the world among African Americans (ACS, 2022b; Kumst et al., 2017)
   C. Dietary factors

TABLE 15.2 Management of Common Ileal Conduit Problems

Problem	Interventions
Urinary odor	Avoid the use of rubber pouch
	Soak appliance in vinegar and water, 1:4
Rash around stoma or under pouch	Dry and powder skin except under adhesive
	Use a skin barrier (e.g., Stomahesive)
Macerated skin around stoma	Dry skin, and apply a hydroponic skin barrier
	Decrease the size of pouch opening
Crystals on or around stoma	Apply vinegar compresses on stoma and inside pouch
Ulcerated stoma	Enlarge pouch opening
	Consult enterostomal therapist if not partially healed in 1 week
Monilial infection after antibiotic therapy	Dry skin, and apply nystatin (Mycostatin) powder
	Encourage oral fluids
Hyperplasia of skin around stoma	Decrease pouch-opening size
Fistula	Revise stoma at new site

1. Possible role of high-fat or high-dairy diets in promotion of prostate cancer.
2. Diets high in vitamins E, D, and selenium possibly inhibit or prevent prostate cancer (Chhabra et al., 2018).
3. Studies are inconsistent on the role of obesity (ACS, 2022b).
4. Diets high in lycopene linked to a low incidence of prostate cancer (ACS, 2022b).

D. Occupational exposures
   1. Farming and cadmium exposure through welding and battery manufacturing associated with increased risk, as is Agent Orange exposure in Vietnam veterans and firefighters increases risk (ACS, 2022b; Chamie, DeVere White, Lee, Ok, & Ellison, 2008)

E. Genetic factors
   1. Prostate cancer susceptibility locus, called HPC1, located on chromosome 1—thought to be responsible for 33% of all hereditary prostate cancer and 3% of cases overall
   2. Pathogenic variants of *BRCA1* and *BRCA2* genes—implicated in breast cancer, as well as in prostate cancer
   3. Having a single first-degree relative with prostate cancer—increases risk twofold to threefold; having a first- and second-degree relative affected increases risk sixfold

F. Common metastatic sites—lung, liver, adrenal glands, kidneys, and bones

IV. Prevention
   A. No evidence yet on how to prevent prostate cancer (Rawla, 2019)
   B. Lower risk by limiting high-fat foods, exercise, and increase vegetables and fruits (Rawla, 2019)

V. Histopathology
   A. Grading—based on the Gleason score (Amin et al., 2017; Mohler et al., 2016)
      1. Primary grade—based on evaluation of architecture of malignant glands in the largest portion of the specimen; most common cell grade seen
      2. Secondary grade—assigned to the next largest area of malignant growth; second most common cell grade seen
      3. Score computed by adding the primary and secondary grades together; order reveals most common cell grade (i.e., 3 + 4 = 7 vs. 4+3 = 7); scores 2–10 possible
      4. Higher scores (8–10) indicate aggressive disease, with a poor prognosis

VI. Diagnosis and staging
   A. Screening
      1. High level of controversy continues at the national level with regard to routine screening for prostate cancer with PSA testing.
         a. Central issue—PSA testing may reveal clinically insignificant tumors; ensuing treatment causes significant side effects, resulting in diminished quality of life.
      2. Following USPSTF recommendations, the American Urologic Association published new guidelines for prostate cancer screening in 2019 (Cheuck, 2019).
         a. PSA screening in men younger than 40 years not recommended
         b. Routine screening in men 40–54 years at average risk not recommended; at-risk men may benefit from shared decision-making at this earlier age
         c. Shared decision-making about PSA screening for men aged 55–69 years; greatest screening benefit in this age group
         d. Screening interval of 2 or more years for those deciding on screening
         e. PSA screening not recommended for men 70 years or older or for those with less than a 10- to 15-year life expectancy
      3. Normal range for PSA varies by age, race, and prostate size—0 to 4 ng/mL considered standard norm. Other markers: PSA density, PSA velocity.

   B. Diagnostic tests
      1. Digital rectal examination (DRE)—assess for size, lesions, symmetry, texture
         a. Simple and inexpensive, but only the posterior and lateral areas can be palpated
      2. Transrectal ultrasound (TRUS)—evaluation of the prostate volume
      3. Biopsy
         a. Performed with TRUS for guidance
         b. Transrectal route preferred; six specimens obtained from both sides of the prostate
      4. Pelvic MRI to evaluate capsular penetration, seminal vesicle involvement, lymph node metastasis
      5. Bone scans—to evaluate possible bone metastasis; generally not performed unless PSA level is above 10 ng/mL or patient complaints of skeletal symptoms (Mohler et al., 2016)
      6. Laboratory studies
         a. PSA—increased levels may be significant as an adjunct in differential diagnosis or as a marker for disease progression
            (1) Men should avoid ejaculation for 48 hours before test
            (2) Finasteride (Propecia), androgen receptor blockers, PC-SPES may also affect PSA levels (Mohler et al., 2016)

   C. Staging
      1. AJCC staging system (Amin et al., 2017)

VII. Prognosis
   A. 5-year survival rate by stage of prostate cancer—local (near 100%), regional (near 100%), and distant disease (31%) (ACS, 2022b)
   B. 5-year survival for all stages combined—89.9% for Whites, 65.5% for African Americans (Kumst et al., 2017)

Management

I. NCCN guidelines Version 4.2022 give the most updated guidelines for the complex management and multiple drug options (NCCN, 2022b).

II. Management will depend on disease, risk group, age, and life expectancy.
III. Early-stage disease
   A. Treatment options—active surveillance, observation or expectant management, radical prostatectomy with lymph node dissection, three-dimensional conformal radiotherapy (3D-CRT), or brachytherapy
      1. Radical prostatectomy—complete removal of prostate; lymph node sampling
         a. Alternative approaches—laparoscopic prostatectomy and robotic laparoscopic prostatectomy (Mohler et al., 2016)
      2. 3D-CRT—radiation doses to prostate greater than 81 Gy (Mohler et al., 2016) intensity-modulated RT replacing 3D
      3. Androgen deprivation therapy increasingly being used adjuvantly with radiation (Mohler et al., 2016)
      4. Brachytherapy—guided by TRUS, radioactive seed placement into the prostate gland via the perineum through a grid template (Mohler et al., 2016)
         a. Isotopes used—iodine-125 or palladium-103
      5. Active surveillance, expectant management for lower Gleason score (<6)—follow-up with PSA testing, needle biopsy, DRE, followed by active treatment if disease progression noted (Mohler et al., 2016)
      6. Cryosurgery—direct application of freezing temperatures to the prostate via percutaneously inserted cryogenic probes (Mohler et al., 2016)
      7. Clinical trial
   B. Complications of treatment
      1. Incontinence—conflicting data because of imprecise measurement; estimated range from 3% to 87% after radical prostatectomy, 3% to 7% for external beam radiotherapy, 6% for brachytherapy; other complications: urethral stricture, urethral sloughing, and bladder outlet obstruction.
      2. Erectile dysfunction—nerve-sparing prostatectomy techniques lessen incidence; comparisons difficult because of imprecise definitions and measurement; high rates reported after surgery, and some form of impotence seen in 6%–61% of cases after brachytherapy.
      3. Gastrointestinal dysfunction—diarrhea, proctitis, and rectal bleeding associated with both RT and brachytherapy.
   C. Treatment for advanced prostate cancer
      1. Hormonal manipulation—accepted standard for metastatic prostate cancer and in patients at high risk for relapse; also used in neoadjuvant setting
         a. Orchiectomy—surgical removal of testicles; produces rapid response; for patients unreliable in taking medication or when estrogen is contraindicated
            (1) Not acceptable as an option for many men
            (2) Psychological trauma as a result of surgical castration
         b. Luteinizing hormone–releasing hormones (LHRH) (LHRH analogs; such as leuprolide [Lupron], goserelin [Zoladex], Triptorelin [Trelstar])—decrease the production of testosterone; may produce fewer side effects compared with estrogens; used with flutamide (Eulexin) to reduce "flare," which is the sudden exacerbation of symptoms (NCCN, 2022b)
            (1) Flare can be life threatening, with spinal cord compression and ureteral obstruction (NCCN, 2022b)
            (2) Other side effects: hot flashes, loss of libido, erectile dysfunction, gynecomastia
         c. Antiandrogens (flutamide [Eulexin], enzalutamide [Xtandi], megestrol acetate [Megace], Flutamide [Eulexin], Bicalutamide [Casodex], Nilutamide [Nilandron])—interfere with intracellular androgen activity; effects may be delayed 1–2 months
         d. Estrogen therapy—generally, diethylstilbestrol
            (1) Used in castration-resistant prostate cancer
            (2) Results in decreased pain, decreased tumor size, decreased urinary symptoms (Mohler et al., 2016)
            (3) Complications—gynecomastia, sodium retention, weight gain, and severe cardiovascular and thrombotic complications
            (4) Associated with relapse within 2–3 years; at the time of relapse, disease often becomes resistant to further hormone treatment
         e. Ketoconazole (Nizoral)—suppresses adrenal testosterone production
            (1) Used in castration-resistant prostate cancer
            (2) Administered with hydrocortisone to reduce the risk of adrenal insufficiency (NCCN, 2022b)
            (3) Abiraterone (Zytiga)—used in combination with prednisone for castration-resistant prostate cancer (NCCN, 2022b)
      2. Clinical trial
   D. RT—for local extension and distant metastases
      1. External or internal (radioactive beeds) radiation
      2. Primary treatment option for stage D lesions if hormone manipulation ineffective or contraindicated; may be used as a component of combined-modality therapy
      3. Used for palliation of pain from bone metastasis or spinal cord compression
      4. Radium-223 for symptomatic bone metastases
   E. Chemotherapy
      1. Optimal timing of initiation of chemotherapy in men with castration-resistant prostate cancer undetermined (Mohler et al., 2016; NCCN 2022b)
      2. Docetaxel (Taxotere) preferred (Mohler et al., 2016; NCCN, 2022b)
      3. Other options—sipuleucel-T, mitoxantrone, cyclophosphamide, estramustine, vinblastine, and vinorelbine; cabazitaxel preferred after docetaxel
      4. Clinical trial

IX. Nursing implications
   A. Manage physical, psychological, social, and spiritual distress during and after treatment
      1. Nurse to assist with navigation of surgery, oncologist, urologist, radiation oncology, and oncology clinic. Patient may be treated in urology office, infusion center, radiation oncology, or hospital setting.
      2. Encourage patient to verbalize feelings about disease and treatment.
      3. Refer to mental health specialist, community resources, support groups (e.g., ACS, UsToo), as needed.
      4. Teach patient to identify and manage symptoms and when to report.
      5. Manage pain and other side effects.
   B. Promote optimal sexual functioning
      1. Facilitate discussion among the physician, nurse, patient, and caregiver about the potential impact of treatment on sexual functioning, interventions to minimize effects.
         a. Obtain permission, before and after treatment, to discuss functional and anatomic changes with treatment and resultant sexual concerns.
         b. Respect the patient's reticence in discussing sexual concerns.
      2. Use terminology appropriate to social and cultural level.
      3. Provide written information and anatomic drawings, as indicated, for clarifications and to reinforce teaching.
      4. Provide specific suggestions related to the treatment used and alternatives.
         a. Teach patient and caregiver about options for the treatment of impotence—pharmacologic, mechanical, surgical. See Chapter 38 for the management of genitourinary symptoms.
         b. Refer to physical therapy, sexual counseling, if indicated.

REFERENCES

American Cancer Society. *Bladder cancer*. (2022a). https://www.cancer.org/cancer/bladder-cancer.html.

American Cancer Society. *Cancer facts and figures 2022*. (2022b). https://www.cancer.org/content/dam/cancer-org/research/cancer-facts-and-statistics/annual-cancer-facts-and-figures/2022/2022-cancer-facts-and-figures.pdf.

American Cancer Society. *Kidney cancer*. (2022c). https://www.cancer.org/cancer/kidney-cancer.html.

Amin, M. B., Edge, S., Greene, F., Byrd, D. R., Brookland, R. K., & Washington, M. K. (Eds.). (2017). *American Joint Committee on Cancer (AJCC) cancer staging manual* (8th ed.). Berlin: Springer International Publishing.

Atkins, M. B., Richie, J. R., Shah, S. (2022). *Epidemiology, pathology, and pathogenesis of renal cell carcinoma*. Waltham, MA: UpToDate. https://www.uptodate.com/contents/epidemiology-pathology-and-pathogenesis-of-renal-cell-carcinoma.

Chamie, K., DeVere White, R. W., Lee, D., Ok, J.-H., & Ellison, L. M. (2008). Agent Orange exposure, Vietnam War veterans, and the risk of prostate cancer. *Cancer, 113*(9), 2464–2470. https://doi.org/10.1002/cncr.23695.

Cheuck, L. (January 14, 2019). What are the USPSTF guidelines on prostate cancer screening? *Medscape*. https://emedicine.medscape.com/article/458011-overview.

Chhabra, G., Singh, C. K., Ndiaye, M. A., Fedorowicz, S., Molot, A., & Ahmad, N. (2018). Prostate cancer chemoprevention by natural agents: Clinical evidence and potential implications. *Cancer Letters, 422*, 9–18. https://doi.org/10.1016/j.canlet.2018.02.025.

Hsieh, J. J., Le, V. H., Oyama, T., Ricketts, C. J., Ho, T. H., & Cheng, E. H. (2018). Chromosome 3p loss-orchestrated VHL, HIF, and epigenetic deregulation in clear cell renal cell carcinoma. *Journal of Clinical Oncology, 36*(36), 3533–3539. https://doi.org/10.1200/JCO.2018.79.2549. Advance online publication.

Jonasch, E., Gao, J., & Rathmell, W. K. (2014). Renal cell carcinoma. *BMJ, 349*, g4797. https://doi.org/10.1136/bmj.g4797.

Khoo, A. C. H., & Tang, W. H. (2019). Renal pelvis urothelial carcinoma with bowel metastases. *Clinical Nuclear Medicine, 44*(12), 983–984. https://doi.org/10.1097/RLU.0000000000002797.

Kumar, S., Singh, R., Malik, S., Manne, U., & Mishra, M. (2017). Prostate cancer health disparities: An immuno-biological perspective. *Cancer Letters, 414*, 153–165.

Liu, K.-W., Lin, V. C.-H., & Chang, I.-W. (2013). Clear cell adenocarcinoma of the renal pelvis: an extremely rare neoplasm of the upper urinary tract. *Polish Journal of Pathology, 64*(4), 308–311.

Mirsadraei, L., & Chen, Y.-B. (2017). Unclassified renal cell carcinoma: Diagnostic and molecular updates. *AJSP: Reviews & Reports, 22*(6), 301–304. https://doi.org/10.1097/PCR.0000000000000215.

Miyake, M., Morizawa, Y., Hori, S., Tatsumi, Y., Onishi, S., Owari, T., et al. (2017). Diagnostic and prognostic role of urinary collagens in primary human bladder cancer. *Cancer Science, 108*(11), 2221–2228. https://doi.org/10.1111/cas.13384.

Mohler, J. L., Armstrong, A. J., Bahnson, R. R., D'Amico, A. V., Davis, B. J., Eastham, J. A., et al. (2016). Prostate cancer, version 1.2016: Featured updates to the NCCN guidelines. *Journal of the National Comprehensive Cancer Network, 14*(1), 19–30.

Motzer, R. J., Jonasch, E., Agarwal, N., Alva, A., Baine, M., Beckermann, K., et al. (2022). Kidney cancer, Version 3.2022, NCCN clinical practice guidelines in oncology. *Journal of the National Comprehensive Cancer Network, 20*(1), 71–90. https://doi.org/10.6004/jnccn.2022.0001.

National Cancer Institute (NCI). Bladder cancer. (2018). https://cancer.gov/types/bladder.

National Cancer Institute (NCI). Transitional cell cancer of the renal pelvis and ureter treatment (PDQ®)–Health professional version. (2020). https://www.cancer.gov/types/kidney/hp/transitional-cell-treatment-pdq.

National Comprehensive Cancer Network (NCCN). Bladder cancer [v.2.2022]. (2022a). https://www.nccn.org/professionals/physician_gls/pdf/bladder.pdf.

National Comprehensive Cancer Network (NCCN). Prostate cancer [v.4.2022]. (2022b). https://www.nccn.org/professionals/physician_gls/pdf/prostate.pdf.

National Organization for Rare Disorders (NORD). Renal medullary carcinoma. (2021). https://rarediseases.org/rare-diseases/renal-medullary-carcinoma/#:~:text=Renal%20medullary%20carcinoma%2C%20also%20known,of%20the%20red%20blood%20cells.

Ng, K., Stenzl, A., Sharma, A., & Vasdev, N. (2021). Urinary biomarkers in bladder cancer: A review of the current landscape and future directions. *Urologic Oncology: Seminars and Original Investigations, 39*(1), 41–51. https://doi.org/10.1016/j.urolonc.2020.08.016.

OpenStax. Anatomy & physiology. OpenStax CNX. (2018). https://cnx.org/contents/FPtK1zmh@8.119:7l9EIHui@4/Gross-Anatomy-of-the-Kidney.

Padala, S. A., Barsouk, A., Thandra, K. C., Saginala, K., Mohammed, A., Vakiti, A., et al. (2020). Epidemiology of renal cell carcinoma. *World Journal of Clinical Oncology, 11*(3), 79–87. Published online May 14, 2020. https://doi.org/10.14740/wjon1279.

Pastore, A. L., Palleschi, G., Silvestri, L., Moschese, D., Ricci, S., Petrozza, V., et al. (2015). Serum and urine biomarkers for human renal cell carcinoma. *Disease Markers, 2015,* 251403. 9 pages. https://doi.org/10.1155/2015/251403.

Piyathilake, C. (2016). Dietary factors associated with bladder cancer. *Investigative and Clinical Urology, 57*(Suppl 1), S14–S25. https://doi.org/10.4111/icu.2016.57.S1.S14.

Rawla, P. (2019). Epidemiology of prostate cancer. *World Journal of Oncology, 10*(2), 63–89. Published online April 20, 2019. https://doi.org/10.14740/wjon1191.

Saginala, K., Barsouk, A., Aluru, J. S., Rawla, P., Padala, S. A., & Barsouk, A. (2020). Epidemiology of bladder cancer. *Medical Sciences (Basel), 8*(1), 15. Published online March 13, 2020. https://doi.org/10.3390/medsci8010015.

Siegel, R. L., Miller, K. D., Fuchs, H. E., & Jemal, A. (2022). Cancer statistics, 2022. *CA: A Cancer Journal for Clinicians, 72*(1), 7–33. https://doi.org/10.3322/caac.21708.

Swami, U., Nussenzveig, R. H., Haaland, B., & Agarwal, N. (2019). Revisiting AJCC TNM staging for renal cell carcinoma: Quest for improvement. *Annals of Translational Medicine, 7*(Suppl 1), S18. https://doi.org/10.21037/atm.2019.01.50.

Westhoff, E., Witjes, J. A., Fleshner, N. E., Lerner, S. P., Shariat, S. F., Steineck, G., et al. (2018). Body mass index, diet-related factors, and bladder cancer prognosis: a systematic review and meta-analysis. *Bladder Cancer, 4*(1), 91–112. https://doi.org/10.3233/BLC-170147.

Westhoff, E., Wu, X., Kiemeney, L. A., Lerner, S. P., Ye, Y., Huang, M., Dinney, C. P., et al. (2017). Dietary patterns and risk of recurrence and progression in non-muscle-invasive bladder cancer. *International Journal of Cancer, 142*(9), 1797–1804. https://doi.org/10.1002/ijc.31214.

Xylinas, E., Kluth, L. A., Rieken, M., Karakiewicz, P. I., Lotan, Y., & Shariat, S. F. (2014). Urine markers for detection and surveillance of bladder cancer. *Urologic Oncology: Seminars and Original Investigations, 32*(3), 222–229. Epub September 17, 2013. Review. https://doi.org/10.1016/j.urolonc.2013.06.001.

Head and Neck Cancers

Margaret Rummel

16

OVERVIEW

I. Definition
   A. Cancers of the oral cavity, oropharynx, nasal cavity, paranasal sinuses, nasopharynx, larynx, hypopharynx, salivary glands, and lymph nodes in the upper part of the neck
   B. Includes cancers of the thyroid and parathyroid glands
II. Epidemiology (American Cancer Society [ACS], 2022a, 2022e; American Society of Clinical Oncology [ASCO], 2022a; UpToDate, 2022a)
   A. Sixth most common cancer in the United States
      1. Accounts for 3% of malignancies, with approximately 66,000 cases annually and 15,000 deaths
   B. Estimated incidence and death rates, 2021:
      1. Larynx cancer: 12,470 (incidence); 3280 (death rate)
      2. Oral cavity and pharynx cancers: 51,540 (incidence); 10,030 (death rate)
      3. Thyroid cancer: 43,800 (incidence); 2230 (death rate)
   C. Most tumors occur in the oral cavity, oropharynx, larynx, nasal cavity, paranasal, nasopharynx, laryngeal, and hypopharyngeal
   D. Higher incidence rates (National Cancer Institute [NCI], 2022a)
      1. Over 40 years of age
      2. Men 2× higher incidence than women
III. Pathophysiology
   A. Anatomy of the head and neck (H–N) (Fig. 16.1)
      1. Oral cavity—extends from the lips to the hard palate above and the circumvallate papillae below; structures include lips, buccal mucosa, the floor of the mouth, upper and lower alveoli, retromolar trigone, hard palate, and anterior two-thirds of the tongue
      2. Oropharynx—extends from the circumvallate papillae below and hard palate above to the level of the hyoid bone; structures include the base of the tongue (posterior one-third), soft palate, tonsils, and posterior pharyngeal wall
      3. Nasal cavity and paranasal sinuses—include nasal vestibule; paired maxillary, ethmoid, and frontal sinuses; and a single sphenoid sinus
      4. Nasopharynx—located below the base of the skull and behind the nasal cavity; continuous with the posterior pharyngeal wall
      5. Larynx—extends from the epiglottis to the cricoid cartilage; protected by the thyroid cartilage, which encases it; subdivided into three areas
         a. Supraglottis—below the base of the tongue, extending to but not including the true vocal cord; includes epiglottis, aryepiglottic folds, arytenoid cartilages, and false vocal cords
         b. Glottis—area of the true vocal cord
         c. Subglottis—below the true vocal cord, extending to the cricoid cartilage
      6. Hypopharynx—extends from the hyoid bone to the lower border of the cricoid cartilage; structures include pyriform sinuses, postcricoid region, and the lower posterior pharyngeal wall
   B. Critical adjacent structures
      1. Regional lymph nodes of the neck drain the anatomic structures of the H-N; the area includes the submental submaxillary, upper and lower jugular, posterior triangle (spinal accessory), and preauricular nodes (Fig. 16.2)
      2. H-N structures are contiguous with the lower aerodigestive tract—trachea, lungs, and esophagus.
      3. The nasopharynx and paranasal sinuses are close to the brain.
   C. Risk factors (ASCO, 2022b; NCI, 2022b)
      1. Tobacco use—all types including smokeless tobacco types; chewing, oral, or spit tobacco; snuff or dipping tobacco; dissolvable tobacco.
      2. Excessive alcohol intake increases the risk of developing oral or pharyngeal cancer.
      3. Use of tobacco and alcohol together poses a greater risk of developing these cancers than people who use either tobacco or alcohol alone.
      4. Use of e-cigarettes remains controversial as a risk factor.
      5. Use of Paan (betel quid) which is common in Southeast Asia.
      6. Epstein–Barr virus is a risk factor for nasopharyngeal cancer and cancer of the salivary glands.
      7. 60%–70% of cancers of the oropharynx may be linked to human papillomavirus (HPV). The rate of HPV oral cancer is increasing.
      8. Higher incidence of HPV cancers in men than women.

9. Additional risk factors (ASCO, 2022b)
   a. Gastroesophageal reflux
   b. Diet
   c. History of neck radiation
   d. Familial history of cancer
   e. Environmental exposure (wood, dust, asbestos)
   f. Poor dental hygiene
   g. Use of marijuana
   h. Previous H–N cancer (HNC)
   i. Sun exposure—lip and skin cancers

IV. Primary prevention
   A. Smoking cessation; limiting alcohol intake; preventing exposure to tobacco, nicotine, and environmental carcinogenic agents; early detection of infection by HPV (ACS, 2022b).
   B. Smoking cessation programs are encouraged to successfully help at-risk HNC patients to quit smoking (ACS, 2022c; National Comprehensive Cancer Network [NCCN], 2022a; Smokefree.gov, 2022).
   C. Tobacco addiction is both mental and physical. Treatment involves a combination of medicine, a method to change personal habits, and emotional support.
   D. Treatment and counseling for excessive alcohol use (National Institute on Alcohol Abuse and Alcoholism, 2022).
   E. HPV vaccinations (CDC, 2022a)
      1. HPV vaccine is recommended for routine vaccination at age 11 or 12 years. (Vaccination can be started at age 9.) The vaccine works best prior to any HPV exposure.
      2. Recommended vaccination for everyone through age 26 years if not adequately vaccinated when younger.
      3. HPV vaccination is given as a series of either two or three doses, depending on age at initial vaccination.

V. Diagnosis
   A. Screening
      1. Detection: many laryngeal and some hypopharyngeal cancers can be found early
         a. Hoarseness, voice changes, or dysphagia
         b. Painless white patch or red patch in the mouth
         c. Painless lump in the mouth or neck
         d. Difficulty chewing, swallowing, or breathing

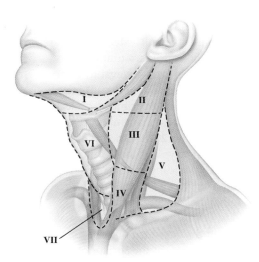

Fig. 16.1 Regional lymphatic pattern in the head and neck. From Friedman, M., Kelley, K., & Maley, A. (2011). Central neck dissection. *Operative Techniques in Otolaryngology—Head and Neck Surgery, 22*(2), 169–172. https://doi.org/10.1016/j.otot.2011.04.001.

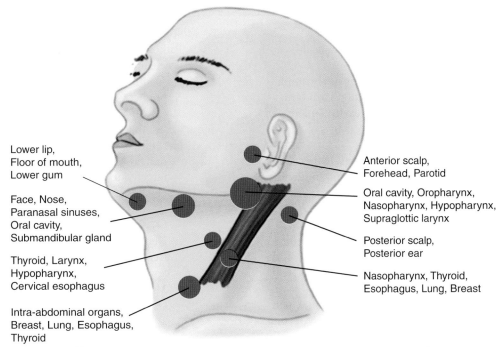

Fig. 16.2 Likely sites of metastasis from various areas of the head and neck.

2. Screening strategies: inspection of the oral cavity is often part of the physical examination by a primary care physician (PCP) and/or dentist.
3. There are no standard screening guidelines for HNCs (United States Preventive Task Force, 2022).

B. Diagnosis of H–N tumors (NCCN, 2022a)
   1. History (risk factors)
      a. Signs and symptoms of disease
      b. A lump or sore that does not heal in the mouth, lip, or throat
      c. A sore throat that does not go away
      d. A change or hoarseness in the voice
      e. A white or red patch in the mouth
      f. A feeling that something is caught in the throat
      g. Difficulty chewing or swallowing
      h. Difficulty moving the jaw or tongue
      i. Swelling in the jaw
      j. Numbness in the tongue or other areas of the mouth
      k. Pain in one ear without hearing loss
   2. Other possible symptoms
      a. White or red patch on the gums, tongue, or lining of the mouth
      b. Bleeding, pain, or numbness in the lip, mouth, or nose
      c. Loose teeth or dentures that no longer fit well
      d. Blocked sinuses that do not clear, or sinus pressure or pain
      e. Double vision or the eyes pointing in different directions
      f. Pain in the upper teeth
      g. Pain, pressure, or drainage in the ear
      h. A lump (usually painless) in the area of the ear, cheek, jaw, lip, or inside the mouth
      i. Fluid draining from the ear
      j. Weight loss for no known reason
      k. Ear pain or hearing loss
   3. Any symptoms should be evaluated by a health care professional.

C. Physical examination: visualization, mirror examination of the pharynx and larynx, palpation via a bimanual examination to assess the oral cavity and upper neck

D. Radiologic studies
   1. Computed tomography (CT)—to assist in determining the extent of the primary tumor and to identify metastasis to the cervical lymph nodes
   2. Magnetic resonance imaging—superior to CT in staging nasopharyngeal primaries
   3. Positron emission tomography with CT—useful in determining specific areas for biopsy, lymph node involvement, and extent of disease to aid in treatment planning

E. Laboratory studies—complete blood cell count, chemistry studies, liver function tests, liquid biopsy testing for circulating tumor HPV (Gu et al., 2020)

F. For histologic diagnosis, procedures to obtain specimen:

1. Fine-needle aspiration—preferred over open biopsy for treatment planning and management
2. Excisional biopsy of the lesion
   a. On small oral cavity, lip, or skin lesions
   b. Open or excisional biopsy of suspicious neck nodes can be contraindicated because it may alter or interfere with subsequent treatment
   c. Exception—when all other examinations fail to identify a primary site or when lymphoma is suspected
3. Incisional biopsy—tumor sample along with adjoining normal tissue
4. Panendoscopy (passing an endoscope along the entire mucosa of the upper aerodigestive tract)—to examine and perform a biopsy on suspicious areas, determine the full extent of disease, and identify synchronous primary tumors
5. Lymph node biopsies/eval to determine the spread of tumor regionally or distant metastasis

G. From biopsies and specimens, molecular and genetics studies (Eskander, Ghanem, & Agrawal, 2018; Fulcher, Haigentz, & Ow, 2018; Gill, Vasan, Givi, & Joshi, 2018; Multidisciplinary Larynx Cancer Working Group [MLCWG], Mulcahy, & Mohamed, 2018; NCCN, 2022a)

VI. Histopathology
A. Histology classification of HNCs
   1. Most HNCs are squamous cell carcinomas (SCC) that start in the flat squamous cells that make up the thin layer of tissue on the surface of the structures in the H–N.
   2. Other histology includes verrucous SCC, adenocarcinoma, minor salivary gland tumors, spindle cell carcinoma, fibrosarcomas, chondrosarcomas, neuroendocrine tumors, melanomas, lymphomas, and metastatic disease (Tamaki, Miles, Lango, Kowalski, & Zender, 2018; UpToDate, 2022b).

B. Molecular classification
   1. Pathology/histologic diagnosis from molecular pathway expression, targeted markers (NCCN, 2022b)
      a. Identification of p16 and p53 protein expression predictive of HNC outcomes.
         (1) HPV-positive disease has a better outcome than HPV-negative disease.
      b. Multiple molecular pathways better predict the outcomes and potentially the type of treatment targeted to those markers.
         (1) Based on pathology results and clinical staging, treatment based on algorithms.
         (2) Example: HPV+SCC base of the tongue.
      c. Depending on the clinical stage (i.e., T1–T2 N0), treatment can be surgery, radiation chemotherapy, or a combination (NCCN, 2022a).
      d. Molecular testing should be done on all tissues.
         (1) PD-L1 weak positive is defined PD-L1 expression in 1%–49% of tumor cells, and PD-L1 strong positive is defined as expression in ≥50% of tumor cells (Paintal & Brockstein, 2020).

VII. Staging
  A. TNM (tumor–node–metastasis) classification system for specific diagnoses developed by the American Joint Committee on Cancer (Lydiatt et al., 2017)
  B. Metastatic patterns
    1. HNC is a locally aggressive disease that can spread regionally to the lymphatics of the neck.
    2. Most patients present with stage III or IV disease (tumor is very large, has invaded adjacent tissue, or is a primary tumor that has spread to the lymphatics).
    3. At the time of initial diagnosis, distant metastases are uncommon at presentation (NCCN, 2022a).
      a. HNCs tend to recur locally; can also develop second primary HNCs; usually of the upper aerodigestive tract or lung; depends on the original cancer site and if patients continue to use tobacco and drink alcohol
    4. The most common sites of distant metastasis for laryngeal cancer are the lungs followed by the liver and bones (Tamaki et al., 2018).
VIII. Prognosis and survival
  A. Survival rates
    1. The 5-year relative survival rate for all stages of oral cavity and pharynx cancers combined is 68% but is much lower in Blacks (36%) than in Whites (56%). Studies indicate survival is better for patients with cancer who test positive for HPV (ACS, 2022d; ASCO, 2022c; NCI 2022c; National Institute of Dental and Craniofacial Research, 2022).
    2. For laryngeal cancer (all stages), 5-year survival rate is 61% (NCI 2022c).
    3. For thyroid cancer, 5-year relative survival rate is 98% (ACS, 2022d).
  B. The rate of new cases of laryngeal cancer is decreasing by about 2%–3% a year, most likely because fewer people are smoking (ASCO, 2022c).

MANAGEMENT

  I. Developments
  II. General Principles
    A. Developments in care and treatment—reduced deformities and improved cosmetic effect because of prosthetic devices and surgical flaps (myocutaneous and free flaps) (McEwen, Dunphy, & Rios, 2018; Tamaki et al., 2018)
      1. Since the early 1970s, more conservative surgical technique and reconstruction has improved quality of life (QOL)—decreasing dysfunctional airway, communication, swallowing (NCCN, 2022d).
      2. Transoral robotic surgery is an innovative, minimally invasive treatment option to remove HNCs through the mouth, especially those related to the HPV (NCCN, 2022d).
    B. General principles
      1. Based on TNM classification tumor volume and grade, as well as patient age, performance status, and goals of care (Eskander et al., 2018; Fulcher et al., 2018; Gill et al., 2018; MLCWG et al., 2018; NCCN, 2022a)
      2. Surgery and radiation—the primary treatment modalities for managing malignant H–N tumors; adjuvant chemotherapy for recurrent and metastatic disease (NCCN, 2022d)
        a. Best to implement an interdisciplinary (interprofessional) approach to managing the patient and family with HNCs on admission (e.g., nurses, various physicians, dental, social workers, palliative care, physical therapist [PT], occupational therapist [OT], nurse navigator, counselors, audiologists, registered dietitian) (Brunner et al., 2015; Guy et al., 2019; NCCN, 2022c; Sørensen, 2021; Takes et al 2020).
        b. In general, for early-stage HNCs (i.e., T1 and T2 lesions of the oral cavity, larynx, nose, and paranasal sinuses), treatment is surgery or radiation (Fulcher et al., 2018; Gill et al., 2018; NCCN, 2022c).
        c. T2 can involve metastasis (NCCN, 2022d).
      3. For later-stage HNCs (i.e., T3 and T4 tumors), treatment is combination therapy either surgery followed by chemoradiation or chemoradiation alone (NCCN, 2022a).
      4. For clinically negative neck nodes and a large primary lesion (T2, N0) of the oral cavity, oropharynx, hypopharynx, or larynx, treatment is either lymphadenectomy or radiation with or without concurrent chemotherapy (because tumor cells can spread) (NCCN, 2022d).
    C. Surgery
      1. Common surgical procedures (Table 16.1)
    D. Radiation therapy (RT) (see Chapter 27)
      1. Primary treatment to control the primary tumor and adjacent lymph nodes while maintaining structure and function—external beam (over 5–7 weeks) in dose fractions; dose range 62–72 gray (Gy) for gross disease, 44–63 Gy for subclinical disease (NCCN, 2022e).
      2. Adjuvant treatment for stage III and IV disease and tumors that can spread toward the midline (e.g., oropharyngeal lesions)
        a. On average 50–66 Gy (in 2.0-Gy dose fractions) over 5–6 weeks is adjuvant treatment for locally advanced HNCs (NCCN, 2022e)
      3. External beam RT performed approximately 4–6 weeks after surgery
      4. RT methods include photons and protons
        a. Protons deliver a more directed radiation beam with less scatter to surrounding tissues.
      5. Preoperative radiation or permanently placed iodine-125 seeds are used to debulk large or unresectable lesions.
      6. Treatment for nasopharyngeal cancer is multifaceted.
        a. Surgical resection is preferred for early-stage disease if feasible.

TABLE 16.1   Surgical Procedures for Head and Neck Cancers

Procedure	Physical Alteration	Nursing Implications
Laser	Little to none	Minimal bleeding
Composite resection	Resection of oral cavity, oropharyngeal lesion in continuity with neck dissection Portion of mandible is resected Reconstruction with myocutaneous flaps is usually required, with resections of large amounts of tissue	May experience problems with speech (decreased articulation with tongue involvement), swallowing (impaired mastication, salivary drooling, aspiration), altered facial contour
Cordectomy	Removal of all or part of the vocal cords	All: normal speech no longer possible Part: may cause hoarse voice
Supraglottic laryngectomy	Resection of structures above the false vocal cords, including the epiglottis (preserves the true vocal cords)	Aspiration until swallowing techniques are learned Maintains a relatively normal voice
Hemilaryngectomy	Vertical excision of one true and one false cord and underlying cartilage	Hoarse voice Minimal or no swallowing problems
Total laryngectomy	Excision of the entire larynx from the hyoid bone to the second tracheal ring	Permanent tracheostomy Aphonia Decreased sense of smell Unable to perform Valsalva maneuver
Maxillectomy	Partial or total en-bloc resection of the cavity May include the ethmoid sinus, lateral nasal wall, palate, and floor of orbit	Preoperatively, maxillofacial prosthodontist makes dental obturator to fill the large surgical defect and to facilitate swallowing Requires daily care to cavity and placement of obturator
Orbital exoneration	Resection of orbit secondary to extension of maxillary sinus tumor or recurrent disease	Facial defect Unilateral vision loss Requires daily care and cleansing of cavity
Craniofacial, skull base resection	Surgical approach to inaccessible midfacial and extensive paranasal sinus and nasopharyngeal lesions	May have facial defect and cranial nerve (III, IV, V) deficits
Radical neck dissection	Resection of sternocleidomastoid muscle, jugular vein, spinal accessory nerve, and cervical lymph nodes	Shoulder droop Concave contour of neck
Modified neck dissection	Radical neck dissection with preservation of the sternocleidomastoid muscle, jugular vein, or spinal accessory nerve	Shoulder droop if spinal accessory nerve resected Concave contour of neck
Lymphadenectomy	Resection of lymph nodes in neck	Surgical scars
Thyroidectomy	Removal of all or part of the thyroid gland	Surgical scars Possibly radioactive iodine (radioiodine therapy) daily thyroid hormone (levothyroxine) pill

Data from American Cancer Society (ACS). (2022). *Laryngeal and hypopharyngeal cancer.* https://www.cancer.org/cancer/laryngeal-and-hypopharyngeal-cancer.html; National Cancer Institute (NCI). (2022). *Head and neck cancers.* https://www.cancer.gov/types/head-and-neck/head-neck-fact-sheet; National Comprehensive Cancer Network (NCCN). (2022). *Head and neck cancers 2.2018.* https://www.nccn.org/professionals/physician_gls/pdf/head-and-neck.pdf; National Comprehensive Cancer Network (NCCN). (2022). *Thyroid cancers, 1.2018.* https://www.nccn.org/professionals/physician_gls/pdf/thyroid.pdf.

b. Carefully selected clients who experience treatment failure with RT can be treated with base-of-skull resection of the tumor.

c. Radiation or concurrent systemic therapy may be used for unresectable tumors or poor surgical candidates.

7. Brachytherapy—treatment for lesions of the anterior and posterior tongue, floor of mouth, and nasal vestibule (implanted iridium-192 or cesium-137)

8. A low dose of radioactive iodine given after surgery for thyroid cancer destroyed (ablated) residual thyroid tissue as effectively as a higher dose, but with fewer side effects and less exposure to radiation (NCCN, 2022e).

E. Chemotherapy

1. Chemotherapy alone is not curative.

a. Reduces tumor volume or rids clinically detectable SCCs.

b. Treatment for recurrent or metastatic disease

2. As adjuvant and neoadjuvant therapy, single-agent or combination chemotherapy regimens—cisplatin (Platinol), bleomycin (Blenoxane), fluorouracil (5-fluorouracil, 5-FU), paclitaxel (Taxol), and methotrexate (Mexate); also used for palliative therapy for recurrent or unresectable lesions (NCCN, 2022a)

a. First-line single agents: cisplatin (Platinol), carboplatin (Paraplatin), 5-FU, docetaxel (Taxotere), paclitaxel (Taxol), epirubicin (Ellence) (NCCN, 2022a)

b. Combination protocols of chemotherapy with RT used because of the sensitizing effect of chemotherapy

(1) Example—RADPLAT (protocol for mouth cancers; strategy is concurrent RT, cisplatin-based infusion to the tumor and systemic neutralization)

F. Targeted therapies
   1. Treatment for those diagnosed with HPV-positive oropharyngeal cancer may be different from that for those with oropharyngeal cancers that are HPV-negative. Patients with HPV-positive oropharyngeal tumors may have a better prognosis and may do just as well on less intense treatment (Boggs, 2015; Haddad & Glass, 2017).
   2. Food and Drug Administration has approved targeted therapies for HNC: cetuximab (Erbitux), pembrolizumab (Keytruda), and nivolumab (Opdivo) (NCCN, 2022a).
   3. Targeted therapies may be combined with RT (NCCN, 2022a).
   4. Patients should be assessed for clinical trials; eligibility for all treatment modalities.

G. Combined chemotherapy and RT (NCCN, 2022a)
   1. Concomitant treatment provides synergy to treatment strategy.

H. Palliative therapy (Hendriks-Ferguson & Ott, 2016)
   1. Surgery, radiation, chemotherapy, or combination therapy for unresectable lesions or recurrent tumors or when surgery is considered high risk
   2. To relieve pain, bleeding, or obstruction, short courses of radiation may be given in various protocols (NCCN, 2022e).

I. Nursing implications
   1. Assessment: H–N function (McEwen et al., 2018; NCCN, 2022a)
      a. Respiration
         (1) HNCs affect the structures of the upper airway, which transports warmed, filtered, and humidified air into the lungs.
         (2) When disease and treatment affect this area, the natural air-conditioning function of the upper air passageways is bypassed. The effect—cooling and dryness of the trachea and lungs—may lead to infection.
         (3) When the upper airway is altered, the sense of smell changes (e.g., inability to sniff).
      b. Speech
         (1) When all or part of the larynx is removed, it results in loss of the vibrating component for speech; thus, sound waves cannot be produced (total laryngectomy) or are diminished (partial).
         (2) Surgery to the mouth, tongue, or palate causes alterations in the person's ability to articulate clear, understandable speech.
         (3) Cancer or treatment of the nose or paranasal sinuses impacts the tone and quality of speech.
         (4) Altered speech: phonation (from larynx), articulation (from the lips, tongue, and soft palate), resonation (tone and quality of speech from resonators—pharynx, mouth, nose, paranasal sinuses).
      c. Swallowing (Balusik, 2014; NCCN, 2022a)
         (1) Swallowing is a highly regulated and coordinated physiological act.
         (2) Components—coordination of 22 muscle groups and six cranial nerves facilitate the transport of food from the mouth to the stomach in four phases of swallowing.
            (a) Oral preparatory—in the oral cavity, the bolus of food is chewed and combined with saliva; the tongue, using front and back movement, propels the bolus into the pharynx
            (b) Taste receptors are on the tongue, soft palate, glossopalatine arch, and posterior wall of the pharynx
            (c) Pharyngeal—the bolus moves through the pharynx and is propelled toward the esophagus; the vocal cords close, and the larynx moves upward and forward, preventing aspiration
            (d) Esophageal—the bolus moves through the esophagus and enters the stomach
         (3) Supraglottic laryngectomy affects the pharyngeal phase of swallowing, undermining the protection of the glottis. Until swallowing techniques are mastered, aspiration is a risk.
         (4) When the structures in the oral cavity and oropharynx undergo extensive resections (requiring flap reconstruction), swallowing phases (oral preparatory and oral) change and may result in drooling of saliva, decreased/difficulty with mastication, aspiration, and pooling of food and fluids.
         (5) RT to this area causes decreased saliva production (xerostomia), with loss of lubrication of food bolus and taste changes.
            (a) Dental hygiene is necessary before RT treatment begins and continuously through life.
            (b) With RT, the risk for dental caries or osteoradionecrosis is increased.
            (c) With RT, it is important to adhere to the prescribed fluoride treatment protocol (trays, dental gel, fluoride toothpaste).
      d. Trismus (restriction in opening the mouth)—may be caused by surgery or RT
         (1) Affects the ability to eat a regular diet. It also may affect speech, swallowing, mastication, and adequate oral hygiene.
         (2) Jaw exercises to increase the opening of the mouth may help reduce the stiffness of trismus.
         (3) PT/OT may help in decreasing trismus.

(4) Ongoing evaluation with a speech therapist may also help.

  e. Hormone regulation

   (1) Thyroid—the thyroid makes hormones that help control heart rate, blood pressure, body temperature, and weight

   (2) Parathyroid—the parathyroid glands make parathyroid hormone, which helps the body use calcium and keeps the amount of calcium in the blood at normal levels

   (3) May need an endocrinology referral to help manage thyroid hormones

2. Preoperative care (Bressler, 1999; Dort et al., 2017)

  a. Preoperative teaching; discuss disease, treatment, side effects, pain management, and anticipated postoperative changes including body image changes and communication challenges

  b. Preoperative nutrition assessment with a registered dietitian to optimize nutritional status

  c. Preoperative speech evaluation if having a partial/total laryngectomy

  d. Fertility counseling and preservation if the patient is of childbearing age

  e. Provide instruction about equipment (tracheostomy tube, drains, nasogastric (NG) tube, percutaneous endoscopic gastrostomy (PEG) tube, intravenous (IV) pumps, suction catheter)

  f. Provide counseling, support, and other resources.

  g. Counseling regarding smoking cessation and alcohol use

  h. Consult social work for supportive counseling and psychosocial distress screening.

  i. Determine the reading ability and the language barriers in planning for postoperative communication preoperatively.

   (1) Options: paper and pencil, magic slate, picture board, nonverbal cues, smartphones, iPads, computers, or other electronic communication devices

  j. Discuss possible discharge planning options post hospitalization.

3. Postoperative care: maximize safety (Baehring & McCorkle, 2012; Bressler, 1999; NCCN, 2022a)

  a. Patient in proximity to nurses' station to monitor client with altered airway

  b. For tracheotomy patients, tracheotomy is securely held in place.

   (1) Keep an extra tracheostomy tube of the same size (inner and outer cannulas and obturator), scissors, cotton-free gauze, and a tracheal dilator at the bedside.

  c. Call bell within reach at all times

  d. If a patient has a tracheostomy, identify a method of communication.

  e. Observe for signs and symptoms of delirium tremens in patients with a recent history of alcohol abuse.

  f. Observe for aspiration in patients who have had a supraglottic laryngectomy (includes resection of structures in the oropharynx, or cranial nerve [IX, X, XII] deficits).

  g. For patients at risk for carotid rupture (i.e., after neck dissection), implement carotid precautions.

  h. Manage the airway (Bressler, 1999; Hyzy & McSparron, 2021; Loerzel, Woodfin, Reising, & Sole, 2014).

   (1) Tracheostomy (i.e., total laryngectomy):

     (a) Airway

       i. Use of a cuffed tracheostomy tube when the client needs mechanical ventilation; may be removed by postoperative day 2 or 3

       ii. Laryngectomy tube used if stoma begins to narrow

     (b) Humidity

       i. Humidified air or oxygen via a tracheostomy collar to prevent mucosa drying and crusting of secretions.

       ii. Apply moistened 4×4 gauze pads over the stoma.

       iii. A stoma bib worn over the stoma helps lessen the drying of mucosa.

       iv. Teach about symptoms of inadequate humidity—thick, tenacious secretions that are difficult to expectorate.

     (c) Stoma care

       i. Cleanse stoma with 50% peroxide/50% normal saline solution.

       ii. Remove all mucus crusting twice each day and as needed.

       iii. Remove visible mucus plugs with a Kelly clamp.

       iv. Apply a thin layer of prescribed ointment around the stoma twice each day, if recommended.

     (d) Suction to clear airway

       i. To prevent hypoxemia and arrhythmia, the lungs are hyperoxygenated, hyperinflated, or both before and after suctioning.

       ii. To precipitate coughing and mobilize secretions if needed, 2–5 mL of normal saline solution is instilled into the tracheostomy for lavage. Then the trachea and bronchi are stimulated.

       iii. To mobilize secretions and prevent atelectasis, an incentive spirometer is attached via a female adapter to a plastic tracheostomy tube, chest physical therapy is provided (as indicated), or both.

       iv. Record the color, amount, and odor of sputum produced, and frequency of suctioning.

(e) Tracheostomy care
  i. Initially remove and cleanse the inner cannula of all mucus and crusts with a solution of 50% peroxide/50% normal saline every 4–8 hours, then twice daily and as needed.
  ii. Replace soiled tracheostomy ties, as needed. To determine tightness, one fingerbreadth should be allowed underneath the ties.
(f) Respiratory hygiene
  i. Coughing, turning, and deep breathing
  ii. Use of incentive spirometry
i. Wound care (Armstrong & Meyr, 2022; Baehring & McCorkle, 2012; Bressler, 1999)
  (1) Every 3–4 hours, assess the surgical wounds, noting color (pink versus cyanotic), temperature, and capillary refill (immediately after blanching) of skin and muscle flaps.
  (2) Avoid excessive pressure that interferes with flap perfusion and viability (e.g., tight tracheostomy ties, oxygen collars, hyperextension of the neck, and the client lying on the flap).
  (3) Assess the integrity of suture lines, both external and intraoral (if applicable); breakdown may be the first sign of wound infection or fistula formation.
  (4) Clean the external suture lines with a solution of 50% peroxide/50% normal saline; then the prescribed ointment is applied every 4–8 hours.
  (5) If the patient has had nasal surgery, a maxillectomy, an orbital exoneration, or a combination of all these, as ordered by the physician, clean the cavities to remove accumulated crusts.
    (a) Use a solution of 50% normal saline/50% sodium bicarbonate or normal saline solution.
  (6) Assess wound drains for color, amount, and odor of drainage, and drain patency.
    (a) If not prevented or treated early, clotting and air leaks may lead to wound infections.
4. Posttreatment nursing care
  a. Oral care (NCCN, 2022a; NCI, 2022d; Oncolink, 2022)
    (1) Prevention—thorough and frequent mouth care and ongoing follow-up with a dental provider
    (2) Rinse mouth (swish and spit) before and after meals and at bedtime with either: Normal saline (1 tsp of table salt to 1 quart [32 oz.] of water) or salt and soda (1 tsp of salt and 1 tsp of baking soda in 1 quart of water).
    (3) Use nonabrasive (waxed) dental floss.

    (4) Use a fluoridated toothpaste or a fluoride treatment recommended by the dentist.
    (5) Use of nonalcoholic mouthwashes
    (6) To gently cleanse the cavity, use a gravity gavage or jet-spray dental cleansing system.
  b. Nutrition (Chasen et al., 2009; NCCN, 2022f; van den Berg et al., 2014; Ye, Chang, Findlay, Brown, & Bauer, 2021)
    (1) Assess patients for nutritional risks. 75%–80% of patients have significant weight loss, and 35%–60% are malnourished at diagnosis (Nugent, Lewis, & O'Sullivan, 2013).
      (a) Nutrition should be protein-rich, easy to swallow (e.g., protein shakes, soups, pudding), given in small and frequent meals (if needed) to meet daily caloric requirements and promote adequate, continuous hydration.
    (2) All patients should receive nutritional counseling from a registered dietitian (NCCN, 2022f).
    (3) Identify patients who have nutritional deficiencies and require oral, enteral, or parenteral nutritional supplements.
      (a) Greater than 5% weight loss in a month or 10% or more over the past 6 months
      (b) More than 20% below ideal body weight
      (c) Treatment with various nutritional interventions such as feeding tubes, for example, NG tubes, PEG, or IV nutrition support (but only if enteral feeding is not feasible)
    (4) With the physician, coordinate methods of nutritional support—enteral tube feedings, other methods.
    (5) Assess after surgery for swallowing dysfunction and evaluation by a speech therapist (NCCN, 2022f).
  c. Mobility (Gane, McPhail, Hatton, Panizza, & O'Leary, 2018)
    (1) Neck dissection—the spinal accessory nerve (SAN) and the sternocleidomastoid muscles may be resected; physical therapy referral needed to evaluate and treat
      (a) Could result in shoulder droop, atrophy of the trapezius muscle, forward curvature of the spine, and limited range of motion (approximately 90 degrees) of the shoulder
      (b) Treatment—after wound drains are removed and the patient has progressed to resistive exercises, initiate active and passive range of motion shoulder exercises; the optimal goal is a functional range of 150 degrees
      (c) Physical dysfunction affects QOL
  d. Symptom management

(1) Review strategies to manage side effects: chemoradiation, immunotherapy, or radiation alone (NCI, 2022d).

(2) On discharge, nursing should provide patient education and support to the patient and caregiver to avoid emergency room visits and readmissions due to posttreatment complications (Baskin et al., 2018; Wu & Hall, 2018).

(3) Focus on issues of survivorship (Berkowitz et al., 2018).

    (a) Disease and treatment side effect management

    (b) Ways to address hearing loss, sleep, fatigue, and anxiety

    (c) Strategies to reduce alcohol and tobacco intake (ACS, 2022c; Penfold, Thomas, Waylen, & Ness, 2018)

e. Body image changes (Baehring & McCorkle, 2012; McEwen et al., 2018; Ringash et al., 2018)

(1) Promote control of secretion and odor; teach wound, oral, and tracheostomy care.

(2) Encourage self-care activities (e.g., tracheostomy care, tube feeding, suctioning) and activities of daily living (e.g., grooming, hair combing, shaving, applying makeup).

(3) Promote physical activity.

(4) Encourage resocialization: social interactions, support group participation either in person or virtual (e.g., Voice Masters, Lost Chord Club, Support for People with Oral and Head and Neck Cancer [SPONC], Cancer Support Community).

(5) Inform the patient of resources to purchase tracheostomy covers, scarves, makeup, or other cosmetic assistance; consulting with the ACS Look Good, Feel Better programs (e.g., hair care, scarves).

(6) Support patients and their families to grieve; allowing them to voice concerns, fears, and anxieties. Provide caregiver resources.

f. Communication (Balusik, 2014; van den Berg et al., 2014)

(1) Cancers in the oral cavity affect the function of articulation; therapy includes:

    (a) Exercises to increase strength, range of motion, coordination, and accuracy of tongue movement

    (b) Use of oral prostheses to compensate for tissue loss and allow for greater contact of the tongue with the palate, creating more intelligible speech

(2) Cancers in the larynx affect phonation.

    (a) After a partial laryngectomy, exercises to improve voice quality, pitch, and loudness

        i. After a total laryngectomy (Loerzel et al., 2014)

        ii. Use of a battery-operated electronic device that provides an artificial vibration to replace vibration of the vocal cords. The device is placed against the skin or in the mouth, which vibrates the tissue and creates an artificial voice while the patient mouths the words to create speech (Electrolarynx).

    (b) Use of esophageal speech—air is swallowed and trapped in the esophagus, then released, allowing air to vibrate against the walls of the esophagus.

    (c) Use of tracheoesophageal prosthesis—placement of a prosthesis in a surgically created tracheoesophageal fistula; the sound is formed by air from the lungs, creating a better quality of esophageal speech.

g. Swallowing (Baijens et al., 2020; Balusik, 2014)

(1) Surgeries, chemotherapy, and RT as a treatment for HNC can affect swallowing.

(2) Baseline speech evaluation should be done.

(3) To assess the oral and pharyngeal stages of the swallow, a barium swallow or videofluoroscopy may be performed in radiology. It provides a moving image of your swallowing in real-time using different food/liquid consistencies. A speech therapist may be present during the study.

(4) Swallowing plan for the patient (Baijens et al., 2020; Balusik, 2014)

    (a) Compensatory strategies—postural changes that facilitate passage of food into the oral cavity and pharynx (head elevated, upper body upright positioning); changes in food consistency (i.e., thin versus thick fluids, semisolid versus pureed foods).

    (b) Indirect swallowing therapy—jaw and tongue range of motion exercises; adduction of tongue exercises to improve laryngeal closure.

    (c) Direct swallowing therapy using supraglottic swallow.

        i. Patient instructions:

            (a) Prepare the bolus of food in the oral preparatory phase.

            (b) Before initiating the swallow, hold breath to close the vocal cords.

            (c) Swallow while still holding breath.

            (d) Cough while exhaling after the swallow to expectorate remaining food or fluids on top of vocal cords.

            (e) Repeat steps (c) and (d) (swallow and cough).

        ii. To avoid aspiration, inflate the cuff on the tracheostomy tube partially or totally during meals and 30 minutes afterward.

    iii. With some patients, remove the tracheostomy tube to improve swallowing, allowing the larynx to elevate.

    iv. Until the patient can take adequate amounts by mouth, enteral tube feedings maintain nutritional requirements.

    v. Speech and swallowing: assessment and management (NCCN, 2022a)

      (a) Evaluation at baseline with follow-up recommendations for speech and/or swallowing dysfunction

      (b) Regular evaluation/assessment by speech pathologists

      (c) Periodic videofluoroscopic and/or swallowing studies as indicated

h. Pain Management (NCCN, 2022f)

  (1) Assess pain every 4 hours or more as needed and reassess after giving pain medication to evaluate effectiveness.

  (2) Provide optimal pain management utilizing both nonpharmaceutical and pharmacological treatments.

  (3) Utilization of Gabapentin (Neurontin) or Pregabalin (Lyrica) for management of nerve-related pain

  (4) Referral to palliative care may be indicated to assist with pain and symptom management.

i. Psychosocial issues (Berkowitz et al., 2018; McEwen et al., 2018; PDQ Supportive and Palliative Care Editorial Board, 2022)

  (1) HNC are at higher risk of having emotional distress than any other form of cancer (Kar, Asheem, Bhaumik, & Rao, 2020).

  (2) Psychological impact is significant, affects physical functioning, mental health status, and QOL (Hammermüller et al., 2021).

  (3) Mental health issues in cancer patients are often underreported.

    (a) Depression (Fan, Chao, & Lin, 2018; Rhoten, Murphy, Dietrich, & Ridner, 2018)

      i. H–N patients are more likely to suffer depressive disorders than non-HNC patients.

      ii. Estimated to range from 6% to 48% of patients suffer from depression

      iii. Other factors besides cancer diagnosis may contribute to depression.

    (b) Quality of life (Lechelt, Rieger, & Cowan, 2018)

      i. Constant adjustment to balance treatment side effects, body image changes, long-term toxicities of treatment, and QOL

j. Resources (ACS, 2022f)

  (1) American Cancer Society (ACS)

  (2) SPONC

  (3) Head and Neck Cancer Alliance

  (4) Oley Foundation

  (5) Oral Cancer Foundation

  (6) Local community resources

k. Survivorship: 5-year survival rate for HNC is 68% (CDC, 2022b; McEwen et al., 2018; NCCN, 2022g, 2022h; Oncolink, 2022)

  (1) Assessment and management of physical and psychosocial long-term and late effects of HNC and its treatment

  (2) Ongoing surveillance and monitoring by PCP for long-term toxicities of treatment per NCCN guidelines

    (a) Screening and early detection of second primary cancers

    (b) Dental evaluations every 6 months due to the risk of dental issues and osteonecrosis of the jaw post-RT

  (3) Rehabilitation needs for posttreatment issues

    (a) Trismus/dysphagia—continued speech therapy and physical therapy (PT) to improve outcomes

    (b) Nutritional counseling to maximize nutritional status and assure adequate intake

    (c) Referral to a prosthodontist for prosthetic devices such as obturators, and other prosthetic devices

  (4) SAN palsy/cervical dystonia/muscle spasms/neuropathies/shoulder dysfunction

    (a) PT/OT evaluations and treatment to improve range of motion and decrease pain and stiffness from radiation fibrosis and surgery

    (b) Pain management referral if indicated

  (5) Lymphedema

    (a) Referral to PT/OT to a certified lymphedema therapist who is familiar with treating HNC patients for therapy or compression garment

  (6) Fatigue

    (a) Daily physical activity to combat fatigue such as walking

    (b) Referral to PT/OT for a cancer rehabilitation program

  (7) Psychosocial distress

    (a) Referral to counseling or support groups such as SPONC or laryngectomy groups for both the patient and caregiver

  (8) Laboratory monitoring

    (a) Monitoring for thyroid levels post radiation as patients may need replacement therapy

(9) Smoking cessation
 (a) Referral to smoking cessation program if needed
(10) Integrative therapies
 (a) May play a role in the management of posttreatment toxicities
  i. Botox has been used for the management of neck fibrosis and vocal cord paralysis.
  ii. Acupuncture has been utilized for xerostomia and trismus.
(11) Total laryngectomy patients should have an emergency safety plan in place due to impaired communication.

REFERENCES

American Cancer Society (ACS). (2022a). *Cancer facts & figures 2022.* https://www.cancer.org/content/dam/cancer-org/research/cancer-facts-and-statistics/annual-cancer-facts-and-figures/2022/2022-cancer-facts-and-figures.pdf . Accessed March 2022.

American Cancer Society (ACS). (2022b). *How to quit smoking.* https://www.cancer.org/latest-news/how-to-quit-smoking.html. Accessed March 2022.

American Cancer Society (ACS). (2022c). *Health risks of smokeless tobacco.* https://www.cancer.org/cancer/cancer-causes/tobacco-and-cancer/smokeless-tobacco.html. Accessed March 2022.

American Cancer Society (ACS). (2022d). *Head and neck cancer statistics.* https://cancerstatisticscenter.cancer.org/#!/cancer-site/Larynx. Accessed March 2022.

American Cancer Society (ACS). (2022e). *Key statistics for thyroid cancer.* https://www.cancer.org/cancer/thyroid-cancer/about/key-statistics.html. Accessed May 2022.

American Cancer Society (ACS). (2022f). *Resources.* https://www.cancer.org/. Accessed May 2022.

American Society of Clinical Oncology (ASCO). (2022a). Head and neck cancer: Statistics. *Cancer.Net.* https://www.cancer.net/cancer-types/head-and-neck-cancer/statistics. Accessed March 2022.

American Society of Clinical Oncology (ASCO). (2022b). Head and neck cancer: Risk factors and prevention. *Cancer.Net.* https://www.cancer.net/cancer-types/head-and-neck-cancer/risk-factors-and-prevention. Accessed March 2022.

American Society of Clinical Oncology (ASCO). (2022c). Laryngeal and hypopharyngeal cancer: Statistics. *Cancer.Net.* https://www.cancer.net/cancer-types/laryngeal-and-hypopharyngeal-cancer/statistics. Accessed April 2022.

Armstrong, D. G., & Meyr, A. J. (2022). *Basic principles of wound management.* Waltham, MA: UpToDate. Retrieved from https://www.uptodate.com/contents/basic-principles-of-wound-management?search=wound%20care&source=search_result&selectedTitle=1~150&usage_type=default&display_rank=1.

Baehring, E., & McCorkle, R. (2012). Postoperative complications in head and neck cancer. *Clinical Journal of Oncology Nursing, 16*(6), E203–E209. https://doi.org/10.1188/12.CJON.E203-E209.

Baijens, L. W. J., Walshe, M., Aaltonen, L.-M., Arens, C., Cordier, R., Cras, P., et al. (2021). European white paper: Oropharyngeal dysphagia in head and neck cancer. *European Archives of Oto-rhino-laryngology, 278*(2), 577–616. https://doi.org/10.1007/s00405-020-06507-5.

Balusik, B. (2014). Management of dysphagia in patients with head and neck cancer. *Clinical Journal of Oncology Nursing, 18*(2), 149–150. https://doi.org/10.1188/14.CJON.149-150.

Baskin, R. M., Zhang, J., Dirain, C., Lipori, P., Fonseca, G., Sawhney, R., et al. (2018). Predictors of returns to the emergency department after head and neck surgery. *Head & Neck, 40*(3), 498–511. https://doi.org/10.1002/hed.25019.

Berkowitz, C. M., Allen, D., Tenhover, J., Zullig, L. L., Fischer, J., Pollak, K. I., et al. (2018). Head and neck cancer survivors: Specific needs and their implications for survivorship care planning. *Clinical Journal of Oncology Nursing, 22*(5), 523–528. https://doi.org/10.1188/18.CJON.523-528.

Boggs, K. L. (2015). Significance of human papillomavirus in head and neck cancers. *Journal of the Advanced Practitioner in Oncology, 6*(3), 256–262. https://doi.org/10.6004/jadpro.2015.6.3.7.

Bressler, C. (1999). Post operative care of the laryngectomy patient. *Perspectives, 2*(1), 1–8. Retrieved from https://www.yumpu.com/en/document/view/4356719/post-operative-care-of-the-laryngectomy-patient-perspective-in-.

Brunner, M., Gore, S. M., Read, R. L., Alexander, A., Mehta, A., Elliot, M., et al. (2015). Head and neck multidisciplinary team meetings: Effect on patient management. *Head & Neck, 37*(7), 1046–1050. https://doi.org/10.1002/hed.23709. Epub 2014 Jul 11.

Centers for Disease Control and Prevention (CDC). (2022a). *Vaccine and preventable diseases.* https://www.cdc.gov/vaccines/vpd/hpv/hcp/recommendations.html. Accessed April 2022.

Centers for Disease Control and Prevention (CDC). (2022b). *Cancer survivors.* https://www.cdc.gov/cancer/survivors/index.htm. Accessed May 2022.

Chasen, M. R., & Bhargava, R. (2009). A descriptive review of the factors contributing to nutritional compromise in patients with head and neck cancer. *Supportive Care in Cancer, 17*(11), 1345–1351.

Dort, J. C., Farwell, D. G., Findlay, M., Huber, G. F., Kerr, P., Shea-Budgell, M. A., et al. (2017). Optimal perioperative care in major head and neck cancer surgery with free flap reconstruction: A consensus review and recommendations from the Enhanced Recovery After Surgery Society. *JAMA Otolaryngology–Head & Neck Surgery, 143*(3), 292–303.

Eskander, A., Ghanem, T., & Agrawal, A. (2018). AHNS Series: Do you know your guidelines? Guideline recommendations for head and neck cancer of unknown primary site. *Head & Neck, 40*(3), 614–621. https://doi.org/10.1002/hed.25026. Epub 2017 Nov 21.

Fan, C.-Y., Chao, H.-L., Lin, C.-S., et al. (2018). Risk of depressive disorder among patients with head and neck cancer: A nationwide population-based study. *Head & Neck, 40*(2), 312–323. https://doi.org/10.1002/hed.24961.

Fulcher, C. D., Haigentz, M., Jr., & Ow, T. J. (2018). AHNS Series: Do you know your guidelines? Principles of treatment for locally advanced or unresectable head and neck squamous cell carcinoma. *Head & Neck, 40*(4), 676–686. https://doi.org/10.1002/hed.25025. Epub 2017 Nov 24.

Gane, E. M., McPhail, S. M., Hatton, A. L., Panizza, B. J., & O'Leary, S. P. (2018). The relationship between physical impairments, quality of life and disability of the neck and upper limb in patients following neck dissection. *Journal of Cancer Survivorship: Research and Practice, 12*(5), 619–631. https://doi.org/10.1007/s11764-018-0697-5.

Gill, A., Vasan, N., Givi, B., & Joshi, A. (2018). AHNS Series: Do you know your guidelines? Evidence-based management of oral cavity cancers. *Head & Neck, 40*(2), 406–416. https://doi.org/10.1002/hed.25024. Epub 2017 Dec 5.

Gu, Y., Wan, C., Qiu, J., Cui, Y., Jiang, T., & Zhuang, Z. (2020 Feb 6). Circulating HPV cDNA in the blood as a reliable biomarker for cervical cancer: A meta-analysis. *PLoS ONE, 15*(2), e0224001. https://doi.org/10.1371/journal.pone.0224001. PMID: 32027658; PMCID: PMC7004305.

Guy, J.-B., Benna, M., Xia, Y., Daguenet, E., Mrad, M. B., Jmour, O., et al. (2019). Quality Assurance in head and neck cancer multidisciplinary team meetings: A watchful eye on real-life experience. *Oral Oncology, 91*, 35–38. https://doi.org/10.1016/j.oraloncology.2019.02.020.

Haddad, R., & Glass, J. (2017). Advances in collaborative practice for patients with head and neck cancers. *Journal of the Advanced Practitioner in Oncology, 8*(3), 261–265.

Hammermüller, C., Hinz, A., Dietz, A., Wichmann, G., Pirlich, M., Berger, T., et al. (2021). Depression, anxiety, fatigue, and quality of life in a large sample of patients suffering from head and neck cancer in comparison with the general population. *BMC Cancer, 21*(1), 94.

Hendricks-Ferguson, V. L., & Ott, R. (2016). Palliative care considerations for patients with head and neck cancer with children at home. *Clinical Journal of Oncology Nursing, 20*(6), 585–587. https://doi.org/10.1188/16.CJON.585-587.

Hyzy, R. C., & McSparron, J. I. (2021). Tracheostomy: Postoperative care, maintenance, and complications in adults. *UpToDate.* Waltham, MA. Retrieved from https://www.uptodate.com/contents/tracheostomy-postoperative-care-maintenance-and-complications-in-adults?search=tracheostomy%20care&source=search_result&selectedTitle=1~150&usage_type=default&display_rank=1.

Kar, A., Asheem, M. R., Bhaumik, U., & Rao, V. U. S. (2020). Psychological issues in head and neck cancer survivors: Need for addressal in rehabilitation. *Oral Oncology, 110*, 104859. https://doi.org/10.1016/j.oraloncology.2020.104859.

Lechelt, L. A., Rieger, J. M., Cowan, K., et al. (2018). Top 10 research priorities in head and neck cancer: Results of an Alberta priority setting partnership of patients, caregivers, family members, and clinicians. *Head & Neck, 40*(3), 544–554. https://doi.org/10.1002/hed.24998.

Loerzel, V. W., Crosby, W. W., Reising, E., & Sole, M. L. (2014). Developing the Tracheostomy Care Anxiety Relief Through Education and Support (T-CARES) program. *Clinical Journal of Oncology Nursing, 18*(5), 522–527. https://doi.org/10.1188/14.CJON.522-527.

Lydiatt, W. M., Patel, S. G., O'Sullivan, B., Brandwein, M. S., Ridge, J. A., Migliacci, J. C., et al. (2017). Head and Neck cancers-major changes in the American Joint Committee on cancer eighth edition cancer staging manual. *CA: a cancer journal for clinicians, 67*(2), 122–137. https://doi.org/10.3322/caac.21389.

McEwen, S. E., Dunphy, C., Rios, J. N., et al. (2018). Evaluation of a rehabilitation planning consult for survivors of head and neck cancer. *Head & Neck, 40*(7), 1415–1424. https://doi.org/10.1002/hed.25113. Epub 2018 Mar 22.

Multidisciplinary Larynx Cancer Working Group (MLCWG), Mulcahy, C. F., Mohamed, A. S. R., et al. (2018). Age-adjusted comorbidity and survival in locally advanced laryngeal cancer. *Head & Neck, 40*(9), 2060–2069.

National Cancer Institute (NCI). (2022a). *How common are head and neck cancers?* https://www.cancer.gov/types/head-and-neck/head-neck-fact-sheet. Accessed March 2022.

National Cancer Institute (NCI). (2022b). *Cancer risk factors.* https://www.cancer.gov/types/head-and-neck/head-neck-fact-sheet. Accessed March 2022.

National Cancer Institute (NCI). (2022c). *Cancer survival rates.* https://www.cancer.gov/types/head-and-neck/head-neck-fact-sheet. Accessed April 2022.

National Cancer Institute (NCI). (2022d). *Oral complications of chemotherapy and head/neck radiation (PDQ®)–Health professional version.* https://www.cancer.gov/about-cancer/treatment/side-effects/mouth-throat/oral-complications-hp-pdq. Accessed March 2022.

National Comprehensive Cancer Network (NCCN). (2022a). *Head and neck cancers, 2.2022.* https://www.nccn.org/professionals/physician_gls/pdf/head-and-neck.pdf.

National Comprehensive Cancer Network (NCCN). (2022b). *Smoking cessation.* https://www.nccn.org/professionals/physician_gls/pdf/smoking.pdf.

National Comprehensive Cancer Network (NCCN). (2022c). *NCCN Guidelines® Insights: Head and Neck Cancers.* https://jnccn.org/view/journals/jnccn/20/3/article-p224.xml. Accessed March 2022.

National Comprehensive Cancer Network (NCCN). (2022d). *Principles of surgery.* https://www.nccn.org/professionals/physician_gls/pdf/head-and-neck.pdf. Accessed May 2022.

National Comprehensive Cancer Network (NCCN). (2022e). *Principles of radiation techniques.* https://www.nccn.org/professionals/physician_gls/pdf/head-and-neck.pdf. Accessed May 2022.

National Comprehensive Cancer Network (NCCN). (2022f). *Principles of nutrition: Management and supportive care.* https://www.nccn.org/professionals/physician_gls/pdf/head-and-neck.pdf. Accessed May 2022.

National Comprehensive Cancer Network (NCCN). (2022g). *Principles of adult pain management.* https://www.nccn.org/professionals/physician_gls/pdf/pain.pdf. Accessed May 2022.

National Comprehensive Cancer Network (NCCN). (2022h). *Survivorship guidelines.* https://www.nccn.org/professionals/physician_gls/pdf/survivorship.pdf. Accessed May 2022.

National Institute on Alcohol Abuse and Alcoholism. (2022). *Treatment for Alcohol Problems: Finding and Getting Help.* https://www.niaaa.nih.gov/publications/brochures-and-fact-sheets/treatment-alcohol-problems-finding-and-getting-help.

National Institute of Dental and Craniofacial Research. (2022). *Oral cancer.* https://www.nidcr.nih.gov/health-info/oral-cancer/more-info. Accessed April 2022.

Nugent, B., Lewis, S., & O'Sullivan, J. M. (2011). Enteral feeding methods for nutritional management in patients with head and neck cancers being treated with radiotherapy and/or chemotherapy. *The Cochrane Database of Systematic, 2013*(1), CD007904. https://doi.org/10.1002/14651858.CD007904.pub3

Paintal, A. S., & Brockstein, B. E. (2020). PD-L1 CPS scoring accuracy in small biopsies and aspirate cell blocks from patients with head and neck squamous cell carcinoma. *Head and Neck Pathology, 14*(3), 657–665. https://doi.org/10.1007/s12105-019-01097-z. Epub 2019 Nov 13. PMID: 31721075; PMCID: PMC7413953.

PDQ Supportive and Palliative Care Editorial Board. (2022). Nutrition in cancer care (PDQ®): Health professional version. In: *PDQ cancer information summaries.* Bethesda, MD: National Cancer Institute (US). Available from: https://www.ncbi.nlm.nih.gov/books/NBK65854/.

Penfold, C. M., Thomas, S. J., Waylen, A., & Ness, A. R. (2018). Change in alcohol and tobacco consumption after a diagnosis of head and neck cancer: Findings from Head and Neck 5000. *Head & Neck*, 40(7), 1389–1399. https://doi.org/10.1002/hed.25116. Epub 2018 Feb 27.

Rhoten, B. A., Murphy, B. A., Dietrich, M. S., & Ridner, S. H. (2018). Depressive symptoms, social anxiety, and perceived neck function in patients with head and neck cancer. *Head & Neck*, 40(7), 1443–1452. https://doi.org/10.1002/hed.25129. Epub 2018 Mar 23.

Ringash, J., Bernstein, L. J., Devins, G., Dunphy, C., Giuliani, M., Martino, R., et al. (2018). Head and neck cancer survivorship: Learning the needs, meeting the needs. *Seminars in Radiation Oncology*, 28(1), 64–74. https://doi.org/10.1016/j.semradonc.2017.08.008.

Smokefree.gov. (2022). *Clearing the Air: Quit Smoking Today*. https://smokefree.gov/sites/default/files/pdf/clearing-the-air-accessible.pdf.

Sørensen, K. (2021). The head and neck multidisciplinary team. *Oxford textbook of plastic and reconstructive surgery* (pp. 853–854). Oxford: Oxford University Press. https://doi.org/10.1093/med/9780199682874.003.0200.

Takes, R. P., Halmos, G. B., Ridge, J. A., Bossi, P., Merkx, M. A. W., Rinaldo, A., et al. (2020). Value and quality of care in head and neck oncology. *Current Oncology Reports*, 22(9). https://doi.org/10.1007/s11912-020-00952-5.

Tamaki, A., Miles, B. A., Lango, M., Kowalski, L., & Zender, C. A. (2018). AHNS Series: Do you know your guidelines? Review of current knowledge on laryngeal cancer. *Head & Neck*, 40(1), 170–181. https://doi.org/10.1002/hed.24862. Epub 2017 Oct 27.

United States Preventive Task Force. (2022). *Oral Cancer: Screening.* https://www.uspreventiveservicestaskforce.org/uspstf/document/RecommendationStatementFinal/oral-cancer-screening.

UpToDate. (2022a). *Epidemiology and risk factors for head and neck cancer.* https://www.uptodate.com/contents/epidemiology-and-risk-factors-for-head-and-neck-cancer. Accessed March 2022.

UpToDate. (2022b). *Pathology of head and neck neoplasms.* https://www.uptodate.com/contents/pathology-of-head-and-neck-neoplasms. Accessed April 2022.

van den Berg, M. G. A., Rütten, H., Rasmussen-Conrad, E. L., Knuijt, S., Takes, R. P., van Herpen, C. M. L., et al. (2014). Nutritional status, food intake, and dysphagia in long-term survivors with head and neck cancer treated with chemoradiotherapy: A cross-sectional study. *Head & Neck*, 36(1), 60–65. https://doi.org/10.1002/hed.23265.

Wu, V., & Hall, S. F. (2018). Rates and causes of 30-day readmission and emergency room utilization following head and neck surgery. *Journal of Otolaryngology—Head & Neck Surgery*, 47(1). https://doi.org/10.1186/s40463-018-0283-x.

Ye, X., Chang, Y.-C., Findlay, M., Brown, T., & Bauer, J. (2021). The effect of timing of enteral nutrition support on feeding outcomes and dysphagia in patients with head and neck cancer undergoing radiotherapy or chemoradiotherapy: A systematic review. *Clinical Nutrition ESPEN*, 44, 96–104. https://doi.org/10.1016/j.clnesp.2021.05.017.

17

Infection-Related Cancers

Rosaleen D. Bloom

OVERVIEW

I. Definition
   A. Cancers caused either directly (e.g., infection disrupting regulation of cell growth and proliferation) or indirectly (e.g., infection weakening the immune system; causing chronic inflammation) by infectious agents (National Cancer Institute [NCI], 2019)
      1. Bacterial
         a. *Helicobacter pylori* (NCI, 2019)
            (1) Gastric
            (2) Gastric mucosa-associated lymphoid tissue lymphoma
         b. Research is exploring links between gut microbiota and colorectal cancer (de Souza et al., 2022).
      2. Parasitic
         a. Blood flukes—schistosomiasis (Centers for Disease Control and Prevention [CDC], 2020b; Costain, MacDonald, & Smits, 2018; NCI, 2019):
            (1) *Schistosoma haematobium*
               (a) Bladder
            (2) Other potential schistosomiasis infections: *Schistosoma mansoni* and *Schistosoma japonicum*
               (a) Possibly infectious causes of intestinal and liver cancer (Costain et al., 2018)
         b. Liver flukes—*Opisthorchis viverrini* and *Clonorchis sinensis* (*Clonorchis*) (CDC, 2020a; NCI, 2019)
            (1) Bile duct—Cholangiocarcinoma (*O. viverrini* and *Clonorchis*)
            (2) Liver (*Clonorchis*)
      3. Viral
         a. Human papillomavirus (HPV) (NCI, 2019)
            (1) Anal
            (2) Bladder (Cantalupo et al., 2018)
            (3) Cervical cancer (cervical carcinoma)
            (4) Head and neck
            (5) Penile
            (6) Vaginal
            (7) Vulvar
         b. Hepatitis B virus (HBV)/Hepatitis C virus (HCV) (NCI, 2019)
            (1) Liver
            (2) HCV-associated B-cell non-Hodgkin lymphoma (NHL)
         c. Epstein–Barr virus (EBV) (NCI, 2019)
            (1) Head and neck (nose and throat)
            (2) Lymphoma
         d. Human herpesvirus type 8 (HHV8), also known as Kaposi sarcoma (KS)–associated herpesvirus (KSHV) (NCI, 2019)
            (1) B-cell NHL (primary effusion lymphoma)
            (2) KS
         e. Human T-cell lymphotropic virus, type 1 (HTLV1) (NCI, 2019)
            (1) NHL (adult T-cell leukemia/lymphoma)
         f. Human immunodeficiency virus (HIV) (NCI, 2019)
            (1) Anal
            (2) Cervical
            (3) KS
            (4) Liver
            (5) Lung
            (6) Lymphomas (non-Hodgkin and Hodgkin disease)
            (7) Throat

II. Epidemiology
   A. Incidence—infections are estimated to cause 15% of all cancer cases annually (Plummer et al., 2016)
      1. Bacterial—*H. pylori* 35.4% (Plummer et al., 2016)
      2. Parasitic—*S. haematobium* 0.3%; *O. viverrini* or *Clonorchis* 0.1% (Plummer et al., 2016)
      3. Viral—HPV 29.5%; HBV 19.2%; HCV 7.8%; EBV 5.5%; HHV8 2%; HTLV1 0.1% (Plummer et al., 2016)
   B. Risk—cancer burden from infectious causes varies greatly depending on developmental status of a country (Plummer et al., 2016)
      1. Less developed countries—66% of cancers are infection related (Plummer et al., 2016)
         a. Sub-Saharan African countries—50% of cancers versus North American and European countries—less than 5% (Plummer et al., 2016)

BACTERIAL

I. Pathophysiology
   A. *H. pylori* irritates gastric and duodenal endothelial cells and increases gastric acid production reducing the mucosal barrier and increasing inflammation. Chronic

inflammation results in carcinogenesis (de Souza et al., 2022; Stern, Miller, Li, & Saxena, 2019).

II. Primary prevention

A. About 60 % of the worldwide population is currently infected with *H. pylori* (Hooi et al., 2017). Prevention strategies include access to clean water, adequate housing (prevent crowded conditions), and access to sanitation.

B. Screening

1. There are no clear screening guidelines for *H. pylori*.

C. Treatment

1. Antibiotic treatment for *H. pylori* may reduce gastric cancer risk; however, there is risk for drug resistance (Chiang et al., 2021; Liou, Lee, El-Omar, & Wu, 2019).

PARASITIC

I. Pathophysiology

A. Blood flukes penetrate the hosts' skin when in freshwater (CDC, 2020b). *S. haematobium* enter the veins of the bladder (Costain et al., 2018). Once in the bladder the parasite causes damage to the bladder endothelium and inflammation, which both may allow for entry and uninhibited growth of cancer-causing viruses and bacteria. *S. haematobium* also leads to gene transcription changes to bladder cells, potentially causing cancer.

B. Flatworms (liver flukes) such as *O. viverrini* and *Clonorchis* enter the bile duct following ingestion of raw or undercooked fish (Prueksapanich et al., 2018). The liver flukes damage the duct, leading to chronic irritation and inflammation, resulting in cancerous cell formation (Prueksapanich et al., 2018).

C. Geography

1. Africa and Middle East—*S. haematobium* (CDC, 2020b)

2. Asia

a. Thailand, Laos, Cambodia, and Vietnam—*O. viverrini* (CDC, 2020a)

b. Korea, China, Taiwan, Vietnam, Japan, and Russia—*Clonorchis* (CDC, 2020a)

3. Changing climate may increase the risk of spread of parasites (CDC, 2020b).

II. Primary Prevention

A. Prevent transmission

1. For *S. haematobium* avoid entering freshwater in affected areas (CDC, 2020b).

2. For *O. viverrini* and *Clonorchis* follow adequately freeze or cook fish from affected areas (CDC, 2020a).

VIRAL

I. Pathophysiology

A. Direct effects

1. DNA and RNA from viruses can alter human cell DNA by impacting proliferation, stopping apoptosis, and identifying ways to escape the immune system by affecting host genes (Chang, Moore, & Weiss, 2017; Schiller & Lowy, 2021).

2. Viruses can create oncoproteins, which lead to host cells becoming cancer cells (e.g., HPV, EBV, HTLV1, and possibly HCV and HBV) (Schiller & Lowy, 2021).

3. MicroRNA can lead to cancer formation (e.g., HHV8 and EBV) (Schiller & Lowy, 2021).

4. Insertion or pathogenic variant of viral genetic material into host DNA can stop replication (e.g. HPV) (Schiller & Lowy, 2021).

B. Indirect effects

1. Immunosuppression caused by HIV prevents immune surveillance and allows other oncogenic viruses to grow unchecked leading to cancer (Schiller & Lowy, 2021).

2. HCV and HBV infections causing inflammation and damaging tissue (Schiller & Lowy, 2021)

II. Primary prevention

A. Vaccination

1. EBV

a. No approved vaccines; however, a phase I clinical trial testing an mRNA vaccine is expected to be completed in 2023 (National Library of Medicine, 2022a)

2. HBV

a. Three-dose schedule, first dose recommended at birth, second dose between 1 and 2 months, and third dose between 6 and 18 months of age (CDC, 2022)

3. HCV

a. There is no vaccine for HCV (Workowski et al., 2021).

4. HHV8

a. There is no approved vaccine for HHV8; however, research is ongoing (Chauhan, Rungta, Goyal, & Singh, 2019).

5. HIV

a. No approved vaccines (therapeutic or preventative); however, a phase I clinical trial testing three mRNA vaccines is expected to be completed in 2023 (National Library of Medicine, 2022bb; NIH Office of AIDS Research, 2021a, 2021b)

6. HPV

a. Vaccination is recommended to start between 11 and 12 years old (can start at 9 years old; recommended to start at 9 if victim of sexual abuse) (CDC, 2022).

b. Two-dose schedule, if between 9 and 14 years old, at the start of vaccination first dose should be followed with second dose within 6–12 months (CDC, 2022)

c. Three-dose schedule, if 15 years old or older or immunocompromised and between ages 9 and 14 years old, at the start of vaccination first dose should be followed with second dose at 1–2 months, and third dose at 6 months (CDC, 2022)

7. HTLV1
   a. There is no approved vaccine for HHV8; however, research is ongoing (Raza, Mizan, Yasmin, Akash, & Shahik, 2021).
B. Prevent transmission
   1. EBV and HHV8 are primarily spread through saliva;
      a. If in presence of known EBV infection, avoid sharing food or beverages, kissing, or sharing personal items (e.g., toothbrush) (CDC, 2020c).
      b. No current recommendation for transmission prevention for HHV8 as individuals are often asymptomatic (NIH Office of AIDS Research, 2022a)
   2. HBV, HCV, HIV, HPV, and HTLV1 - avoid sharing needles, injecting drugs, and unprotected sex (Workowski et al., 2021)
C. Screening
   1. There are no routine screening recommendations for EBV, HHV8, or HTLV1 currently.
   2. HBV screening is recommended at the first prenatal visit for pregnant females and for individuals at high risk with no known vaccination history. No treatment is available for acute hepatitis B; however, there are treatments available for chronic hepatitis B to reduce viral replication and slow liver disease (Workowski et al., 2021).
   3. Universal HCV screening, at least once in an individual's lifetime and with each pregnancy for pregnant females, is recommended if community prevalence is greater than 0.1%; HCV is highly treatable and can be cured with treatment within 8–12 weeks (Workowski et al., 2021).
   4. Universal HIV screening, at least once in an individual's lifetime for ages 15–65, is recommended; annual HIV screening is recommended for individuals at higher risk for infection, specifically males who have sex with males (Workowski et al., 2021).
   5. Routine HPV screening is recommended with Papanicolaou (Pap) smear (Workowski et al., 2021) See Chapter 2.
III. Oncogenic potential of COVID-19
A. Previous infection with severe acute respiratory syndrome–coronavirus-2 (i.e., COVID-19) has not been linked to cancer (Rahimmanesh, Kouhpayeh, Azizi, & Khanahmad, 2022).
B. COVID-19 infection impacts the immune system, but the association with cancer is unknown (Rahimmanesh et al., 2022)
   1. With COVID-19 infection, T cells have impaired response.
   2. Cytokines are elevated.
   3. Growth factors are elevated.
   4. Chemokines during acute phase
   5. Tissue damage and chronic inflammation from "long-COVID-19"
   6. Integration of COVID-19 genetic material in host cells

HUMAN IMMUNODEFICIENCY VIRUS

Overview

I. Pathophysiology
A. HIV—viral illness that produces widespread immune dysfunction due to viral DNA replacement of the normal immune cells
B. Normal immunologic structures (see Chapter 8)
C. Physiologic basis of HIV infection (NIH Office of AIDS Research, 2021b)
   1. Infects vital cells of the immune system (wwww T cells, macrophages, dendritic cells)
   2. Direct viral destruction of affected cells and CD8 cytotoxic lymphocyte recognition and destruction of infected cells
   3. Results in reduced immune cells and immune surveillance competence
D. Pathophysiology of malignancy with HIV
   1. Cytopathic retrovirus member of retroviridae, genus *Lentivirus* (Relf, Shelton, & Jones, 2017)
   2. Transmission (Relf et al., 2017)
      a. Two species of HIV—HIV-1 (more virulent and infective) and HIV-2 (U.S. Department of Health and Human Services, 2019)
         (1) Most HIV-2 found only in West Africa
         (2) Viral combinations—assume HIV-1 unless confirmatory diagnostic criteria met through use of Food and Drug Administration–approved HIV-1/2 differentiating antibody test interpreted as HIV-2 by expert pathologist (U.S. Department of Health and Human Services, 2019)
            (a) HIV-1 positive, HIV-2 negative
            (b) HIV-1 negative, HIV-2 positive
            (c) HIV-1 positive and HIV-2 positive
            (d) Undifferentiated
         (3) Major subtypes of HIV-1: M (major), N (non-M and non-O), O (outlier), and other subtypes labeled by letters A, B, C, D, E, F, G, H, I, J, and K that are associated primarily by geographic region of prevalence (Bbosa, Kaleebu, & Ssemwanga, 2019)
            (a) M subtype replicates in macrophages and CD4+ T lymphocytes and is active in almost 90% HIV-1 viral strains; early infection manifests as high amounts of disease in tonsils and adenoids.
            (b) Other subtypes correlate only to viral infecting mechanisms and origin of transmission; however, increasing genetic variations are of concern for future drug resistance (Bbosa et al., 2019).
         (4) Major groups (formerly subtypes) of HIV-2: A, B, C, D, E, F, G, H, I (Bbosa et al., 2019)
      b. Long incubation and gradual progression typical (NIH Office of AIDS Research, 2021c, 2021d; Shiels et al., 2018; Thrift & Chiao, 2018)

(1) Average time from HIV infection to symptomatic disease depends on inoculation method, exposure, preexisting health, and prompt initiation of treatment for antiretroviral disease.

(2) Average time from infection to active AIDS is approximately 10 years, but shorter with children and older adults.

(3) Average life expectancy is near normal if viral illness is well controlled and associated cancers or adverse effects of antiretroviral therapy do not occur.

c. Transmission through body fluids (blood, semen, vaginal secretions, breast milk)

d. Virus entry via the bloodstream; infection occurs with transmission across mucosal barriers, attaching to dendritic or Langerhans cells

e. Surface antigen gp120—attracted to host CD4 surface marker

f. Human cells with the most abundant CD4—T lymphocytes; CD4 cell surface marker also found on macrophages, monocytes, microglial cells, Langerhans, and dendritic cells

g. Initial occurrence in partially activated CD4 cells, followed by spread via the CD4 cells in gut-associated lymphoid tissue

h. For replication—HIV uses reverse transcriptase, an enzyme that mediates transcription of viral RNA to DNA in infected CD4 cell

i. Viral protein integrated into the cells by integrase

j. After incorporation into cells' DNA, cellular components broken down into functional infectious virions by the enzyme protease

k. Components for more virions made by host cells

l. Process called coating undergone by the new virions, which are then expelled from the host cell by budding

m. Daughter cells disseminate in the bloodstream, infecting new cells

n. Approximately 30% of the viral burden in HIV-positive patients regenerated daily, weakening cellular stability of normal CD4 and progenitor cells, causing apoptosis and reduced circulating CD4 cells (Relf et al., 2017)

3. HIV effect on CD4 lymphocytes—apoptosis and reduced quantity

4. May remain dormant for variable period, or immediate viral production by infected cell may occur

5. Clinical staging and classification of HIV infection

a. Three stages

(1) Acute infection

(2) Chronic/progressive infection—leads to qualitative and quantitative T4-lymphocyte dysfunction, with resultant defect in both cellular and humoral immunity as immunoregulatory function of T4 cells is gradually impaired (Relf et al., 2017)

(3) AIDS—disorder of severe immune deficiency

b. Cofactors in disease progression (Relf et al., 2017)

(1) Lifestyle factors—for example, inadequate nutrition, general poor health, smoking, activities that may result in infection with other strains of HIV, may also influence course of infection

(2) Definitive role of specific cofactors in disease progression controversial; may be difficult to distinguish between comorbid infection and true causal relationship

(3) Infectious cofactors including presence of cytomegalovirus, EBV, HCV, HPV, herpes simplex 6 (HSV-6), HSV-8, and other viruses (D'Aleo et al., 2017)

(4) Approximately 67% of cases in gay, bisexual, and other men who have sex with men; comprises 69% of newly infected HIV infections and half of people living with the disease (CDC, 2021; Peruski et al., 2020)

(5) Increased risk of infection in uncircumcised males related to dendritic cells on foreskin (Workowski et al., 2021)

c. Clinical status—may change rapidly and improve or decline

(1) Centers for Disease Control (CDC) classification system for disease staging—guides therapeutic intervention and support.

(2) Impaired immune surveillance function and chronically stimulated B cells may result in growth of malignantly transformed cells.

(3) Patients may experience abnormal sites of presentation and poor duration of response to therapy (Reid et al., 2018).

II. Incidence and risk

A. HIV (Shiels et al., 2018; Thrift & Chiao, 2018)

1. Estimated 1.2 million people in the United States living with HIV, and one in seven did not know they were infected (NIH Office of AIDS Research, 2021e).

2. In 2019, 36,801 Americans newly infected with HIV, decreasing yearly from 2015 to 2019 (NIH Office of AIDS Research, 2021e).

3. Incidence among multiracial individuals decreased while other races/ethnicities remained stable, but overall new diagnoses decreased in 2019 compared to 2015 (CDC, 2021).

4. Prevalence of HIV in the United States also remained stable from 2010 compared to 2015 (CDC, 2021).

5. Heterosexual contact with HIV-infected individual accounts for about 83% of new HIV diagnoses in females in 2019; male-to-male sexual contact accounts for 61% of new HIV diagnoses in males in 2019 (CDC, 2021).

6. Those older than 50 years are the fastest-growing HIV-positive population and are at increased risk for diseases and cancers not included among the defining AIDS malignancies. Increases attributable to prolonged survival with disease, age-related physiologic changes enhancing the risk of transmission, and propensity to engage in unprotected sex (NIH Office of AIDS Research, 2021f).

7. Approximately one-third of individuals with HIV infection will die of cancer during their disease trajectory (Jensen, Oette, Haes, & Haussinger, 2017).

8. Cancer, liver disease, and concomitant cardiovascular disease are the most common causes of death among HIV-infected individuals whose viral load is effectively managed (Goehringer et al., 2017; Jensen et al., 2017).

B. Malignancy risks—presence of typical malignancy risks enhances likelihood of developing cancer with HIV infection (Reid et al., 2018; Shiels et al., 2018; Suneja et al., 2018; Thrift & Chiao, 2018; Yarchoan & Uldrick, 2018).

1. AIDS-defining malignancies—malignancies related specifically to HIV infection and the subsequently altered immune system
   a. AIDS-defining cancers include NHL, Burkitt lymphoma, KS, and cervical cancer.
   b. B-cell lymphoma is the most frequently diagnosed AIDS-defining malignancy.
   c. HIV-infected women are at increased risk for cervical dysplasia that rapidly progresses to cervical cancer; histology is often characterized by more aggressive disease progression (NIH Office of AIDS Research, 2022b).
   d. Proportional decreases in HIV-related cervical cancers may have not matched other AIDS-related cancers because of the link to HPV (NIH Office of AIDS Research, 2022b).
   e. AIDS-defining malignancies are more common shortly after initiation of active retroviral therapy, particularly among patients with low CD4 counts.

2. Non–AIDS-defining malignancies (D'Aleo et al., 2017; Jensen et al., 2017; Palefsky, 2017; Reid et al., 2018; Shiels et al., 2018; Sigel, Makinson, & Thaler, 2017; Thrift & Chiao, 2018)
   a. Cancers classified as non–AIDS defining—cancers of the anus, head and neck, kidney, liver, and lung and Hodgkin lymphoma
   b. Others with possible association—acute myelogenous leukemia colon, esophageal, and gastric cancers; melanoma; oral cancer, prostate cancer, and squamous cell skin cancer
   c. Increased incidence of non–AIDS-defining malignancies with extended time living with the disease
   d. Malignancies associated with viral infection (e.g., hepatitis B and C and hepatocellular cancer, EBV, Hodgkin disease)—more accelerated conversion to malignancy in HIV-infected individuals (Reid et al., 2018)
      (1) Longer life expectancy with antiretroviral therapy; chronic immune suppression leads to late lymphoproliferative cancers
      (2) May be related to lifestyle commonalities—higher incidence with sexually transmitted diseases, hepatitis; smoking has led to the emergence of other cancers
      (3) Increased incidence of non–AIDS-defining malignancies—disproportionate compared with incidence in the normal population (Yarchoan & Uldrick, 2018)
      (4) Comprise 58% of all cancers in HIV (in 1990 was 31%)
      (5) Less likely related to viral load or CD4 count compared with AIDS-defining malignancies
      (6) More likely to present with aggressive disease and higher risk of metastasis compared with other non–HIV-infected patients
      (7) More common in Whites, males
      (8) Occur at a younger age compared with the same cancers in non-HIV malignancies

C. General principles of HIV-related malignancies (Goncalves, Uldrick, & Yarchoan, 2017; Jensen et al., 2017; Reid, 2018; Shiels et al., 2018)

1. HIV-infected patients are also at risk for other age- and behavior-associated malignancies related to smoking and alcohol intake.

2. Decreased overall incidence of HIV-related malignancies attributed to antiretroviral therapy (Yarchoan & Uldrick, 2018).

3. Since the advent of highly active cART and recognized connection to HSV-8, the incidence of KS has declined dramatically (Goncalves et al., 2017).
   a. Found equally in all subpopulations of HIV-infected persons; reflects same epidemiology as non–HIV-related lymphoma
   b. Still prevalent disease in Africa

4. The coexistence of cancer and HIV may be related to the presence of HIV or other cofactors or lifestyle factors.

5. Staging and diagnosis of HIV-associated cancers are the same as with non–HIV-related cancers of the same pathology (Reid et al., 2018).
   a. Imaging is more complex to interpret due to concomitant HIV-related lymphadenopathy.
   b. Brain and bone lesions often nonmalignant in this population.
   c. Concurrent diagnosis of HIV infection may affect treatment planning.

Management

I. General Principles
   A. The treatment of cancer usually follows nearly the same therapy plan as would be used even in the absence of HIV (Reid et al., 2018).

TABLE 17.1 Overlapping Toxicities Between Antiretroviral and Antineoplastic Agents that May Require Changing the Antiretroviral

Toxicity Concern	Antiretrovirals	Antineoplastic Interactions
Diarrhea	Darunavir, fosamprenavir, lopinavir, saquinavir, tipranavir	When given with antineoplastic agents such as fluoropyrimidines, irinotecan, may produce intolerable diarrhea
Hepatotoxicity	Didanosine, maraviroc, raltegravir, stavudine, tipranavir, zidovudine	Do not administer concomitantly with antineoplastic agents that have hepatic metabolism at standard doses
Hyperbilirubinemia	Didanosine, stavudine, zidovudine	Overlapping toxicities with chemotherapy may produce confusion about source of elevated bilirubin and premature discontinuation of antineoplastic therapies
Hyperglycemia	Atazanavir, darunavir, fosamprenavir, indinavir, ritonavir, saquinavir, tipranavir	Exacerbated hyperglycemia with mTOR inhibitors
Myelosuppression, neutropenia	Zidovudine	Approximately 8% of patients will develop severe neutropenia. Antiretroviral may be discontinued if antineoplastic therapy is also myelosuppressive. Antineoplastics have been associated with exacerbated neutropenia when given with zidovudine include bevacizumab, etoposide, gemcitabine, irinotecan, pemetrexed, platinum agents, taxanes, topotecan
Pancreatitis	Didanosine, stavudine	Avoid concomitant administration with antineoplastics such as L-asparaginase
Peripheral neuropathy	Didanosine, stavudine	May want to discontinue if preferred antineoplastic therapy includes platinum, taxanes, vinca agents
Prolonged QT segment	Atazanavir, ritonavir, lopinavir, saquinavir	May be altered if given concomitantly with antineoplastics causing prolonged QT segment—anthracyclines, arsenic trioxide, dasatinib, lapatinib, nilotinib, sunitinib, tamoxifen
Renal toxicity	Tenofovir, zidovudine	Platinols
Vasculitis	Atazanavir, darunavir, fosamprenavir, indinavir, ritonavir, saquinavir, tipranavir	May enhance radiosensitivity, but may also enhance hypertension and idiosyncratic bleeding tendency of VEGF inhibitors such as bevacizumab, lenalidomide, and thalidomide

VEGF, Vascular endothelial growth factor.

(1) Steroids often avoided in usual cancer treatment regimens due to the high risk of immune reconstitution syndrome (IRIS)
(2) Vaccines during or after cancer treatment may be modified due to continued immune defect
(3) Ideally should be comanaged with an HIV specialist
B. Every attempt should be made to continue cART through antineoplastic therapy because a temporary reduction in CD4 + lymphocyte counts is likely to occur during antineoplastic therapy and CD4 + levels correlate to long-term outcomes (Reid et al., 2018).
   a. Interactions between antiretroviral and antineoplastic agents may be caused by disruption of the CYP pathways.
   b. Even when the metabolism is not disrupted by concomitant antiretroviral and antineoplastic medications, overlapping toxicities may be problematic with combination therapy (Table 17.1).
   c. Nononcologic medications may also be affected by cART (Patel, Borg, Haubrich, & McNicholl, 2018).
     (1) Frequent and thorough assessment of concomitant medications that result in inadequate absorption or altered effectiveness is recommended.

     (2) Nononcologic medications have adverse interactions with antiretroviral agents such as alcohol, amiodarone, anticonvulsants, antihyperlipidemics, antimicrobials (metronidazole, rifabutin, rifampin), azole antifungals (posaconazole, voriconazole), benzodiazepines, cocaine, contraceptives, dexamethasone, digitalis derivatives, histamine-2 receptor agonists, methamphetamine opioids, proton pump inhibitors, and warfarin.

HIV-RELATED LYMPHOMA

Overview

I. Pathophysiology (Carbone, Volpi, Gualeni, & Gloghini, 2017; Reid et al., 2018; Yarchoan & Uldrick, 2018)
  A. Traditionally considered a late manifestation of HIV infection, occurring in the setting of significant immune suppression with CD4 counts less than 200/mm³.
  B. Characteristics specific to HIV include lower CD4 counts (below 200/mm³), older age, lack of CD20+ marker, and lack of cART-related lymphoma (Reid et al., 2018).
  C. Systemic lymphomas seem to have a more complex pathophysiology (Reid et al., 2018).
  D. EBV is present in 33%–67% of HIV lymphomas (Carbone et al., 2017).

E. Genetic analyses of patient cohorts have begun to reveal host-related factors relevant to the risk of lymphoma.

F. Tat protein is an HIV gene product implicated in the pathogenesis of Burkitt and Burkitt-like lymphomas.

II. Common presentation and metastatic sites

A. In systemic disease, extranodal involvement is common; the most commonly affected sites are the gastrointestinal (GI) tract, central nervous system (CNS), and bone marrow.

B. The presentation of primary effusion lymphoma (body cavity lymphoma) is associated with human herpesvirus type 8 (HHV8) (Goncalves et al., 2017; Goncalves, Ziegelbauer, Uldrick, & Yarchoan, 2017).

C. Metastasis—CNS, GI tract, and bone marrow involvement more frequent in HIV-infected persons; every organ system may be involved.

D. Primary CNS involvement—only the CNS involved; no other organs or tissues involved (Gupta et al., 2017).
   1. Multifocal lesions are common; ocular involvement occurs in 20%.
   2. BCL6 pathogenic variant is common.
   3. Primary CNS lymphoma (PCNSL) highly associated with HIV and EBV; linked to lower CD4+ counts

III. Diagnostic measures—usual diagnostic testing with inclusion of serum and tumor HIV testing

IV. Prognosis based on control of HIV disease, specific disease-related variables (Carbone et al., 2017; Goncalves et al., 2017; Reid et al., 2018; Yarchoan & Uldrick, 2018)

V. Classification of HIV-related lymphomas is not altered from the usual malignancy classification (Reid et al., 2018) (see Chapter 20).

VI. Staging and grading are not altered from usual malignancy staging and grading.

Management

VII. Principles of management

A. Treatment based on approaches used for uninfected persons; underlying immune deficiency, presence of opportunistic infections, polypharmacy, and generalized poor health status may require dose reduction, scheduling modifications, and selection of alternative approaches (Reid et al., 2018).
   1. Need to confirm HIV positivity—diagnosis of HIV infection usually made on the basis of a positive antibody test, although tumor biopsy is helpful when other lymphoma risk factors are present, or the causal link is unclear
   2. Diagnosis of HIV-related lymphoma—similar to testing for non–HIV-related infection; because of the wide variance in presenting symptoms, workup in HIV-infected person may have a more aggressive disease
      a. Because HIV-related malignancies may occur at abnormal sites, diagnostic imaging, endoscopic examinations, or both may be more extensive than in HIV-negative persons.
      b. Histology same as immunocompetent hosts—Burkitt, Burkitt-like, diffuse large cell, peripheral T-cell, extranodal marginal zone

   c. Staging for HIV-related lymphoma typically follows the same schema as that for non–HIV-related lymphoma (see Chapter 20)
   d. Majority intermediate or high-grade B-cell tumors
   3. Presentation factors to consider with diagnosis
      a. Brain biopsy may be performed to establish a diagnosis of PCNSL versus opportunistic infection; night sweats may be related to infection with *Mycobacterium avium-intracellulare*, and CNS symptoms are related to cerebral toxoplasmosis (Gupta et al., 2017).
      b. In the absence of brain biopsy, diagnosis of PCNSL is by exclusion. Response to treatment for toxoplasmosis may indicate infection. Lack of response presumes PCNSL (Gupta et al., 2017).
      c. CNS lesions may cause changes in cognitive function, memory loss, decreased attention span, headaches, personality change, focal neurologic deficits, or generalized seizure activity.
      d. GI tract lesions may cause malabsorption, diarrhea, constipation, or focal or diffuse abdominal discomfort; may present as an asymptomatic abdominal mass.
      e. Patients with primary effusion lymphomas present with effusions (pericardial, pleural, or ascites) and no discrete mass.
      f. Involvement of the oral cavity is linked to HIV disease, low CD4+ counts (<100 μL), associated with EBV.
      g. Blood counts are usually normal despite bone marrow involvement.
   4. Survival depends on multiple factors, including cART, degree of immunosuppression, presence of opportunistic infection(s), nutritional status, presenting lesion location, lifestyle, and accessibility of adequate care.
      a. Factors associated with shorter survival include CD4 cell count below 100 cells/mm³, stage III or IV disease, age older than 35 years, history of intravenous drug use, and elevated lactate dehydrogenase. The International Prognostic Index for aggressive lymphoma has also been validated in patients with AIDS-related lymphoma.
      b. Median survival time ranges from 4 to 10 months. Shortest survival time is with CNS primary tumor (median, 1–2 months); longest survival time is with low-grade lymphomas (1–4 years). Lymphomas specific to HIV—primary effusion lymphoma, plasmablastic lymphoma of the oral cavity or other variants.
   5. Lymphomas occurring in other patients with immune suppression; for example, polymorphic B-cell lymphoma (posttransplant lymphoproliferative disorder)
   6. Hodgkin disease, multiple myeloma, and B-cell acute lymphocytic leukemia are examples of other

lymphoid malignancies diagnosed in HIV-infected persons.

7. Large-cell lymphomas mostly found in the GI tract; small-cell lymphomas more likely to involve the bone marrow and meninges

8. Aggressive disease, poor prognosis; better outcomes with early clinical stage and complete response to therapy
   a. Lesions painful and rapidly proliferative; occasionally mistaken for KS
   b. May be preceded by Castleman disease or plasmacytoma (Goncalves et al., 2017)

9. PCNSL (Gupta et al., 2017)

10. Systemic NHL
    a. Typically, a CD4 count less than 100 cells/mm³, often less than 50 cells/mm³; less common since the advent of cART
    b. Uniformly associated with EBV
    c. Less dramatically reduced by cART; overall estimated twofold to sevenfold decline in incidence
    d. Declines in specific subsets of NHL, specifically immunoblastic lymphoma and PCNSL; incidence of Burkitt lymphoma and Hodgkin disease unchanged, suggests possible variable involvement of immune function in tumor development

11. Antiretroviral therapy should be continued during antineoplastic therapy

12. Surgery—rarely used; exceptions include excisional or incisional biopsy in patients with HIV-related NHL

13. Chemotherapy—regimens are unchanged from usual therapies used to treat NHL, although choices may vary based upon the prescribed antiretroviral agents and their potential interactions with antineoplastic agents, and steroids are avoided

14. Radiotherapy
    a. For palliation or consolidation (e.g., involved-field radiotherapy after chemotherapy)
    b. May be used to attempt to control otherwise unresponsive disease

15. Biologic response modifiers—the addition of rituximab a standard therapy for HIV-related NHL; no dose adjustments appear to be necessary, but increased incidence of hemophagocytic syndrome has been noted (Reid et al., 2018)

16. Combined-modality treatment not well documented; synergistic therapeutic effects and side effects must be weighed carefully
    a. Continuation of cART therapy during anticancer treatment desirable, if tolerated by patient; ability to treat cancer while continuing cART therapy associated with reduced incidence of opportunistic infections and higher complete response rates
    b. Increased risk if resistance with inconsistent administration or absorption of cART; sometimes

influences response to entire categories of cART medications

c. Immune recovery inflammatory response syndrome/IRIS (Goncalves et al., 2017; Reid et al., 2018)
   (1) A brisk inflammatory response when the white blood cell count rapidly increases
   (2) Manifestations—fever, edema and effusions, weight loss, myalgias, fatigue, hepatomegaly, lymphadenopathy, splenomegaly, respiratory symptoms, mental status changes, diarrhea and GI distress, anemia, hypoalbuminemia, thrombocytopenia, and hyponatremia
   (3) More often occurs with initial cART therapy or with severe inflammatory or infectious reactions; has occurred with toxoplasmosis, pneumocystis, other opportunistic infections in HIV disease, and EBV reactivation
   (4) More often reported with lymphoma compared with other cancer; has been linked to the administration of rituximab, although also commonly reported with KS
   (5) cART delayed in patients with simultaneously diagnosed HIV and malignancy because of the risk of severe IRIS (Reid et al., 2018)

d. Dose adjustment indicated on the basis of CD4 count, treatment-related side effects, response, and concomitant infections

e. HIV-related lymphoma treated with combination chemotherapy using agents such as cyclophosphamide (Cytoxan), vincristine (Oncovin), methotrexate (Mexate), etoposide (VP-16, VePesid), cytosine arabinoside (Ara-C, Cytosar), bleomycin (Blenoxane), and steroids; methotrexate, bleomycin, doxorubicin (Adriamycin), cyclophosphamide, vincristine (Oncovin), and dexamethasone (M-BACOD) regimen common (Reid et al., 2018)

f. Burkitt lymphoma common in HIV disease; outcomes equivalent to other patients

g. PCNSL usually resistant to systemic chemotherapy because few agents cross the blood–brain barrier; exceptions are high-dose methotrexate (>3 g/m²) and high-dose cytarabine (Ara-C) (>2 g/m²); rituximab recommended and usually well tolerated (Reid et al., 2018)

h. Intrathecal administration of chemotherapy considered to treat lymphomatous meningitis; not useful in bulky disease

i. Concomitant cART plus chemotherapy to be used cautiously when giving chemotherapy with zidovudine (AZT) because of significant bone marrow compromise; increased febrile neutropenia risk with older age, lower CD4 counts

j. Hematopoietic stem cell transplantation may be a treatment option for lymphoma with well-controlled viral load (Reid et al., 2018)

k. Response short lived in high-grade tumors; in low-grade tumors, good control of symptoms, often with longer duration of response

HIV-RELATED KAPOSI SARCOMA

Overview

I. Pathophysiology—soft tissue malignancy characterized by malignant growth of reticuloendothelial cell origin in HIV-infected persons
   A. Before HIV, KS endemic in geographic regions such as the Mediterranean basin and sub-Saharan Africa
   B. Persons receiving immunosuppressive agents after organ transplantation
   C. Malignantly transformed cells reproducing as a result of underlying immune defect in patients with HIV-related KS (epidemic KS)
      1. Disproportionate risk for KS among select immunodeficient populations raised suspicion of secondary infectious factor
      2. KSHV genome—encodes several gene products; host response to the virus critical in determining the outcome of infection and tumor development
      3. HIV-associated tat gene product—may enhance KSHV replication, increase expression of various chemokines, potentiate KSHV effects, and indirectly contribute to oncogenesis
         a. Confirmed by the identification of HHV8, also known as KSHV
         b. Causative association of KSHV with KS
         c. KSHV infection necessary but not sufficient for KS; malignant potential appears to be quite low outside the setting of immune compromise
II. Clinical manifestations and metastatic sites (Suneja et al., 2018)
   A. Types of KS
      1. Endemic KS—locoregional and related to viral cause
      2. Classic KS—rare angiogenic malignancy
      3. Pediatric (lymphadenopathic) KS—occurs in children in developing countries
      4. Epidemic KS (AIDS-related)
   B. Presentation—includes skin lesions ranging from pink to purple to brownish, flat or raised, usually painless (unless in a sensitive area), and do not blanch with pressure; body organ lesions usually nodular and hemorrhagic (Goncalves et al., 2017)
   C. Common locations—lower extremities or face, oral cavity and palate, GI tract, respiratory tract (especially endobronchial)
III. Diagnostic measures (Goncalves et al., 2017)
   A. Similar to testing done when not related to HIV infection
   B. Once tissue diagnosis of KS lesions confirmed, biopsy of new skin lesions not always performed; biopsy of visceral lesions may be performed

IV. Prognosis (Goncalves et al., 2017)
   A. Dramatic increase in survival in the era of cART
   B. Survival for several years possible; shorter in patients with GI tract lesions or B symptoms (fever, night sweats, unintentional weight loss); worse with prior or comorbid major opportunistic infection, with a median survival time of less than 1 year
   C. Survival—depends on cART, degree of immunosuppression, presence of opportunistic infection(s), nutritional status, presenting lesion location, lifestyle, care accessibility
V. Classification, staging, and histology (Goncalves et al., 2017)
   A. All schemas include parameters of cutaneous, lymph node, and visceral involvement and the occurrence of B symptoms.
   B. Classic KS is typically indolent; HIV-related KS may be aggressive and progress rapidly.
   C. Spectrum of tumors varies by risk group; dramatically influenced by HAART.
   D. The incidence of KS was already on the decline in the United States even before the introduction of cART; since then, KS has become a relative rarity in the United States.
   E. Estimates of reduction of KS in HIV-infected persons are as much as 80-fold; in areas where cART is not available (sub-Saharan Africa), KS remains a major problem, and in some areas, it is the major cancer diagnosis.

Management

VI. Principles of management
   A. Risk stratification into good risk and poor risk is helpful (Suneja et al., 2018).
      1. Good risk—confined to skin or lymph nodes or minimal oral disease, CD4 greater than 200/μL, no oral thrush or B symptoms; Karnofsky performance greater than 70
      2. Poor risk—edema or ulceration of tumor; extensive oral, GI, non-node visceral tumors; CD4 less than 200/μL, history of oral thrush or B symptoms, poor performance status, other HIV-related illness
      3. Treatment based on approaches used for uninfected persons; treatment adjustment required for underlying immune deficiency, presence of other opportunistic infections, polypharmacy, and poor health status
   B. Surgery—rarely used in the treatment of KS; exceptions include removal of lesions that interfere with function or cause significant pain
   C. Chemotherapy (Suneja et al., 2018)
      1. Most contain an anthracycline; often liposomal formulation or doses adjusted for overlapping myelosuppression
      2. Taxanes, etoposide, biological response modifiers (e.g., pomalidomide, thalidomide) also commonly used in conjunction with anthracyclines
      3. mTOR inhibitors show promise but interact with antiretroviral therapy

D. Radiotherapy—may be given as photon radiotherapy or superficial electron beam (Suneja et al., 2018)
 1. Doses from 10 to 30 Gy by 45–70 kV x-ray or 4-MV photon
 2. Better response rates with multiple fractions
 3. Effective short to moderate local control may be achieved, especially for cosmetic effects or relief of lymphedema caused by lymphatic lesions; response rates 92% for cutaneous lesions; 100% for oral lesions; 89% for eyelids, conjunctiva, and genitals
 4. Permanent alteration in the radiated skin and lymphatics, with subsequent persistent edema and tissue breakdown
 5. Interferon-alpha, with or without concomitant zidovudine, approved as treatment for HIV-related KS
E. Biologic response modifiers
 1. Dose adjustment possibly indicated on the basis of CD4 count, treatment-related side effects, response, concomitant infections
 2. HIV-related KS treated with cART (up to 86% response rate, durable responses); if recurrent or persistent, may be treated with single-agent therapy (liposomal doxorubicin, paclitaxel) or combination chemotherapy (vincristine, doxorubicin, and bleomycin)
 3. mTOR inhibition (e.g., sorafenib, sunitinib)—reduces tumor angiogenesis and leads to tumor regression (Suneja et al., 2018)
 4. Because of the vascular nature of KS lesions, antiangiogenic compounds are a natural strategy for treatment; ongoing trials include thalidomide (Thalomid), fumagillin, and metastat (a matrix metalloproteinase inhibitor) (Suneja et al., 2018)

OTHER MALIGNANCIES

I. Cervical cancer (Palefsky, 2017; Reid et al., 2018; see also Chapter 23)
 A. Squamous cell carcinoma (SCC) of the cervix added to HIV-related malignancies in 1993 because of the incidence of HPV and cervical dysplasia found in women infected with HIV
 B. Cervical cancer screening in HIV-infected individuals low—influenced by age, ethnicity/race, tobacco use, weight, education, economic issues, risky behaviors (Nega, Woldetsadik, & Gelagay, 2018)
 C. HPV increases the risk of development of, or rapid progression to, cervical cancer
 D. HIV infection increases the risk for cervical cancer recurrence after treatment
 E. Management
 1. Lesions may regress or be controlled with antiretroviral therapy alone
 2. Colposcopy—primary therapy if lesions persist on cART
 3. Cryotherapy—for persistent lesions
 4. Radiation therapy—in the form of brachytherapy; may be administered for locally advanced disease;

radiation toxicity increased in the population receiving antiretroviral agents
II. Anal cancer (Jensen et al., 2017; Michaud, Zhang, Shireman, Lee, & Wilson, 2020; Palefsky, 2017; Reid et al., 2018; see also Chapter 14)
 A. Incidence normally 1.5% of GI malignancies, increased in HIV-infected persons
 B. More common among men practicing anal-receptive intercourse
 C. Like cervical cancer, has been highly associated with HIV infection with HPV
 D. Minimal regression with cART
 E. Prophylactic screening of high-risk individuals recommended but not validated as helpful to reduce incidence or associated mortality. Poor compliance with screening recommendations (<40% among highest risk) (D'Souza et al., 2016).
 F. Management—combined chemotherapy and radiation
III. Hepatocellular carcinoma (HCC) (D'Aleo et al., 2017; Jensen et al., 2017; Reid et al., 2018; see also Chapter 14)
 A. Three to six times increased incidence of HCC in HIV-infected patients; if HCC is related to HIV disease, longevity of survival is better
 B. More common in hepatitis C and HIV dual infection than hepatitis B and HIV infection
 C. More likely in HIV-1 disease
 D. Increased risk with advanced age and hepatic cirrhosis, suggesting the contribution of progressive liver dysfunction
 E. HCC with HIV more aggressive and refractory to treatment, with shorter life expectancy compared with HCC from other causes
 F. Highly responsive to sorafenib
IV. Lung cancer (Reid et al., 2018; Sigel et al., 2017; see also Chapter 19)
 A. Third most common malignancy in patients with HIV
 B. Presentation usually at a younger age compared with lung cancer; mean age 46 years
 C. Highest incidence of mortality among HIV-related cancers
 D. Average life expectancy 6–7 months after diagnosis; usually diagnosed at a late stage with significant symptoms (cough, chest pain, dyspnea, hemoptysis)
 E. Lung infection, which often precedes diagnosis, delays diagnosis because of overlapping symptoms; up to 30% of one cohort had radiographic changes more typical of lung infection
 F. Possible link to chronic pulmonary inflammation and infection unclear
 G. Increased survival with concomitant cART
 H. Significant hematologic toxicity in most patients receiving concomitant cART
V. Hodgkin disease (Reid et al., 2018; Yarchoan & Uldrick, 2018; see also Chapter 20)
 A. Most common non–AIDS-defining malignancy; relative risk 11–31.7 times that for normal population

B. Often occurs within 1 year of diagnosis and cART initiation

C. Common pathology—mixed cellularity and lymphocyte-depleted subtypes; most express herpesvirus

D. More aggressive and less responsive than non-HIV Hodgkin disease

E. Late-stage presentation

F. Common for multiple node groups

G. Less sensitive to chemotherapy or radiotherapy compared with de novo Hodgkin disease

NURSING IMPLICATIONS

I. Maximize patient safety.

  A. Ensure environmental safety for patients experiencing sensorimotor changes (e.g., adequate lighting, especially at night).

  B. Instruct patient about avoidance of potential environmental sources of opportunistic infection—for example, animal waste from pets; or uncooked, undercooked, or improperly stored food (Relf et al., 2017).

II. Decrease incidence and severity of symptoms.

  A. Assess for peripheral neuropathies that may occur from HIV, antiretroviral, or antineoplastic therapy.

  B. Baseline and ongoing assessment for neurocognitive disorders may be related to HIV disease, neurologic malignancies, opportunistic infections, and adverse effects of therapy.

  C. Assess for balance and strength; cachexia and muscle wasting common in combined HIV and cancer cluster; referral to physical and occupational therapy with functional deficits.

  D. Teach (or referral for teaching) about ways to enhance appearance—for example, use of covering cosmetics to hide KS lesions in cosmetically sensitive areas; use of scarves or other clothing to cover swollen lymph nodes; use of clothing appropriate to changing body mass with weight loss.

  E. Instruct the patient to avoid aspirin because it may interfere with platelet function, and recommend the use of acetaminophen instead to control fevers and pains.

  F. Monitor for jaw pain in patients receiving vinca alkaloids; this neuropathy seems to occur more frequently in the HIV population.

  G. Overlapping toxicities between antiretroviral therapy and chemotherapy must be considered in determining the best treatment plan and supportive measures (see Table 17.1).

    1. Diarrhea—lopinavir, tenofovir

    2. Hepatotoxicity—nonnucleoside reverse transcriptase inhibitors, nucleoside reverse transcriptase inhibitors, protease inhibitors

    3. Myelosuppression—zidovudine

    4. Neuropathy—didanosine, stavudine

    5. Nephrotoxicity—indinavir, tenofovir

    6. Nausea and vomiting—didanosine, protease inhibitors, zidovudine

  H. Many antiretroviral medications affect the CYP pathway enzymes and may interfere with chemotherapy-related therapeutic or toxic effects.

    1. CYP inhibitors may require dose reductions.

    2. CYP inducers may require lead to reduced benefit of specific chemotherapy agents, but insufficient research is available with most malignancies to make recommendations. Changes in antiretroviral therapy may be preferable in these situations.

  I. Palliative care referral—particularly helpful for patients experiencing significant physical symptoms or distress (Relf et al., 2017)

    1. Helps patients with multiple or overlapping symptoms

    2. Assists with the management of complexities of polypharmacy

    3. Pain complex in this population because of multiple causes

    4. May help patients explore and rally support systems and informal care resources

    5. Sensitive assessment and interventions for spiritual distress

    6. Supportive and consistent caregivers helpful in recognizing psychosocial distress or mental incapacity related to disease

III. Prevent infection due to immune suppression from disease and treatment.

  A. Assess for opportunistic infections that occur from HIV but are compounded in patients undergoing cancer treatment.

  B. Oral lesions may be due to HIV-related malignancies, opportunistic infections, nutrition deficits (American Dental Association, 2021).

  C. Immunosuppressive effects of chemotherapy are associated with up to 50% temporary reduction in CD4 counts, even if lymphopenia is not a normal adverse effect of that chemotherapy agent. CD4 counts should be monitored during chemotherapy and more frequently in high-risk groups (e.g., older age).

  D. Appropriate antimicrobial prophylaxis based on CD4 counts, if indicated.

  E. Concomitant administration of hematopoietic growth factors is based on increased risk of HIV-related cancer.

IV. Interventions to enhance nutritional status

  A. Teaching techniques to enhance nutritional intake (e.g., use of supplements, keeping ready-to-eat foods available, smaller and more frequent meals)

  B. Providing or encouraging frequent oral hygiene

V. Interventions to monitor for sequelae of disease and treatment that may be different from those for non–HIV-related malignancies

  A. Assess and document the location, appearance, size of KS lesions, lymphadenopathy, organomegaly, or other tumor effects (e.g., abdominal masses, oral lesions, ascites).

  B. Monitor for changes in size or appearance of the abnormalities.

C. Monitor for tumor lysis syndrome in patients with HIV-related NHL as presentation, with bulky disease common and highly responsive to treatment.

D. Assess neurologic status frequently, as neurologic symptoms may signal advanced HIV disease, chemotherapy toxicity, or opportunistic infections.

VI. Monitor response to medical management.

A. Assess usual tolerance to antineoplastic therapies.

B. Consider overlapping toxicities between antiretroviral agents and antineoplastic agents (see Table 17.1).

C. Assess absorption and metabolic drug interactions between antiretroviral and antineoplastic agents (many antiretroviral agents are metabolized through CYP pathways).

D. Careful consideration of initiation of antiretroviral therapy with concomitant newly diagnosed cancer and HIV disease given risk for IRIS or with significant opportunistic infections

VII. Provide cancer screening and disease prevention (Reid et al., 2018).

A. Organizational recommendations for cancer screening—not delineated for HIV-infected patients despite clear risks for specific cancers. Evidence-based literature suggests the following enhanced screening activities in HIV-infected individuals:

1. Pap testing—every 6–12 months for early detection of cervical cancer (Workowski et al., 2021)

2. Anal screening with cytology or high-resolution anoscopy for early detection of SCC—has not been adopted by professional organizations, but a growing body of literature suggests that at-risk individuals can benefit from screening: digital anal examination also a proven cost-effective method to screen for this cancer in high-risk individuals (Workowski et al., 2021)

3. Computed tomography of the chest—as indicated to assess high-risk individuals for lung cancer

4. Sigmoidoscopy—controversy about value in patients with HIV disease because most cancers are right-sided; full colonoscopy required to assess for colon cancer

5. Periodic oral or dental examination—to detect early oropharyngeal masses that can signal HPV-related squamous cell head and neck cancers

VIII. Address the psychosocial issues of HIV and its malignancies.

A. Thorough psychosocial assessment of all patients

B. Assess self-image in patients with KS who have visible lesions that may contribute to distress and social isolation.

C. Determine past experience with HIV disease; in areas of high incidence, multiple losses may occur without adequate time for effective grieving.

D. Recognize that a significant other not infected with HIV may experience feelings of guilt, uncertainty about own health, concern for the future.

E. Monitor for maladaptive coping strategies, especially if the history of substance use disorder is present;

assisting with learning alternative behaviors to manage stress and cope.

IX. Incorporate patient and significant other in care (Relf et al., 2017).

A. Recognize that the patient's family of choice may not be the biologic family of origin.

B. Include persons identified by the patient as significant others in teaching and care decisions when appropriate.

X. Teach to reduce the possibility of HIV transmission (Relf et al., 2017).

A. Provide education about the use of latex condom with a water-based lubricant to reduce risk (petroleum-based lubricants or cosmetic creams weaken the condom, increasing the chance of breakage during use) during every episode of vaginal, rectal, or oral intercourse.

B. Provide information about avoidance of sharing toothbrushes, razors, personal care items.

C. Wearing gloves and using a solution of 1 part household bleach to 10 parts water during cleanup of emesis or other body fluid spills

D. Use universal precautions as recommended by the CDC to reduce the risk of occupational exposure to HIV.

E. Assess the health literacy and ability to comply with complex therapies, multiple appointments with medical specialists.

1. Low literacy associated with only 17%–40% maintaining regular medical care

2. Low literacy associated with lack of understanding of CD4 counts, viral load, medications

3. Studies of antiretroviral adherence reflect low rates of medication adherence among individuals with low health literacy

4. Low health literacy associated with English not being the first language, mental health disorder, lack of understanding of how to access care and support

REFERENCES

American Dental Association. (2021). *Human immunodeficiency virus (HIV)*. https://www.ada.org/resources/research/science-and-research-institute/oral-health-topics/hiv.

Bbosa, N., Kaleebu, P., & Ssemwanga, D. (2019). HIV subtype diversity worldwide. *Current Opinion in HIV and AIDS, 14*(3), 153–160. https://doi.org/10.1097/COH.0000000000000534.

Cantalupo, P. G., Katz, J. P., & Pipas, J. M. (2018). Viral sequences in human cancer. *Virology, 513,* 208–216. https://doi.org/10.1016/j.virol.2017.10.017.

Carbone, A., Volpi, C. C., Gualeni, A. V., & Gloghini, A. (2017). Epstein-Barr virus associated lymphomas in people with HIV. *Current Opinion in HIV and AIDS, 12*(1), 39–46.

Centers for Disease Control and Prevention (CDC). (2020a). *Clonorchis – Resources for health professionals*. https://www.cdc.gov/parasites/clonorchis/health_professionals/index.html.

Centers for Disease Control and Prevention (CDC). (2020b). *Schistosomiasis – Resources for health professionals*. https://www.cdc.gov/parasites/schistosomiasis/health_professionals/index.html.

Centers for Disease Control and Prevention (CDC). (2020c). *Epstein-Barr virus and infectious mononucleosis: About Epstein-Barr virus (EBV)*. https://www.cdc.gov/epstein-barr/about-ebv.html.

Centers for Disease Control and Prevention (CDC). (2021). Estimated HIV incidence and prevalence in the United States, 2015–2019. *HIV Surveillance Supplemental Report 2021, 26*(1). https://www.cdc.gov/hiv/library/reports/hiv-surveillance/vol-33/index.html.

Centers for Disease Control and Prevention (CDC). (2022). *Child and adolescent immunization schedule: Recommendations for ages 18 years or younger, United States, 2022*. https://www.cdc.gov/vaccines/schedules/hcp/imz/child-adolescent.html.

Chang, Y., Moore, P. S., & Weiss, R. A. (2017). Human oncogenic viruses: Nature and discovery. *Philosophical Transactions of the Royal Society B, 372*(1732), 20160264. https://doi.org/10.1098/rstb.2016.0264.

Chauhan, V., Rungta, T., Goyal, K., & Singh, M. P. (2019). Designing a multi-epitope based vaccine to combat Kaposi Sarcoma utilizing immunoinformatics approach. *Scientific Reports, 9*(1), 2517. https://doi.org/10.1038/s41598-019-39299-8.

Chiang, T.-H., Chang, W.-J., Chen, S. L.-S., Yen, A. M.-F., Fann, J. C.-Y., Chiu, S. Y-H., et al. (2021). Mass eradication of *Helicobacter pylori* to reduce gastric cancer incidence and mortality: A long-term cohort study on Matsu Islands. *Gut, 70*(2), 243–250. https://doi.org/10.1136/gutjnl-2020-322200.

Costain, A. H., MacDonald, A. S., & Smits, H. H. (2018). Schistosome egg migration: Mechanisms, pathogenesis and host immune responses. *Frontiers in Immunology, 9*, 3042. https://doi.org/10.3389/fimmu.2018.03042.

D'Aleo, F., Ceccarelli, M., Venanzi Rullo, E., Facciolà, A., Di Rosa, M., Pinzone, M. R., et al. (2017). Hepatitis C-related hepatocellular carcinoma: Diagnostic and therapeutic management in HIV-patients. *European Review for Medical and Pharmacological Sciences, 21*(24), 5859–5867. https://doi.org/10.26355/eurrev_201712_14035.

de Souza, J. B., Brelaz-de-Castro, M. C. A., & Cavalcanti, I. M. F. (2022). Strategies for the treatment of colorectal cancer caused by gut microbiota. *Life sciences, 290*, 120202. https://doi.org/10.1016/j.lfs.2021.120202.

D'Souza, G., Wentz, A. M., Wiley, D., Shah, N. M., Barrington, F., Darragh, T. M., et al. (2016). Anal cancer screening in men who have sex with men in the Multicenter AIDS Cohort Study. *Journal of Acquired Immune Deficiency Syndrome, 71*(5), 570–576. https://doi.org/10.1097/QAI.0000000000000910.

Goehringer, F., Bonnet, F., Salmon, D., Cacoub, P., Paye, A., Chêne, G., et al. (2017). Causes of death in HIV-infected individuals with immunovirologic success in a national prospective survey. *AIDS Research and Human Retroviruses, 33*(2), 187–193. Accessed at https://www.liebertpub.com/doi/full/10.1089/aid.2016.0222.

Goncalves, P. H., Uldrick, T. S., & Yarchoan, R. (2017). HIV-associated Kaposi sarcoma and related diseases. *AIDS, 31*(14), 1903–1916. https://doi.org/10.1097/QAD.0000000000001567.

Gonçalves, P. H., Ziegelbauer, J., Uldrick, T. S., & Yarchoan, R. (2017). Kaposi sarcoma herpesvirus-associated cancers and related diseases. *Current Opinion in HIV and AIDS, 12*(1), 47–56.

Gupta, N. K., Nolan, A., Omuro, A., Reid, E. G., Wang, C.-C., Mannis, G., et al. (2017). Long-term survival in AIDS-related primary central nervous system lymphoma. *Neuro-Oncology, 19*(1), 99–108. https://doi.org/10.1093/neuonc/now155.

Hooi, J. K. Y., Lai, W. Y., Ng, W. K., Suen, M. M. Y., Underwood, F. E., Tanyingoh, D., et al. (2017). Global prevalence of *Helicobacter pylori* infection: Systematic review and meta-analysis. *Gastroenterology, 153*(2), 420–429. https://doi.org/10.1053/j.gastro.2017.04.022.

Jensen, B. E.-O., Oette, M., Haes, J., & Häussinger, D. (2017). HIV-associated gastrointestinal cancer. *Oncology Research and Treatment, 40*(3), 115–118. https://doi.org/10.1159/000456714.

Liou, J.-M., Lee, Y.-C., El-Omar, E. M., & Wu, M.-S. (2019). Efficacy and long-term safety of *H. pylori* eradication for gastric cancer prevention. *Cancers, 11*(5), 593. https://doi.org/10.3390/cancers11050593.

Michaud, J. M., Zhang, T., Shireman, T. I., Lee, Y., & Wilson, I. B. (2020). Hazard of cervical, oropharyngeal, and anal cancers in HIV-infected and HIV-uninfected Medicaid beneficiaries. *Cancer Epidemiology, Biomarkers & Prevention, 29*(7), 1447–1457. https://doi.org/10.1158/1055-9965.EPI-20-0281.

National Cancer Institute (NCI). (2019). *Infectious agents*. https://www.cancer.gov/about-cancer/causes-prevention/risk/infectious-agents.

National Library of Medicine (U.S.). (2022a). A study of an Epstein-Barr Virus (EBV) candidate vaccine, mRNA-1189, in 18- to 30-year-old healthy adults. Identifier: NCT05164094. *ClinicalTrials.gov*. https://clinicaltrials.gov/ct2/show/NCT05164094.

National Library of Medicine (U.S.). (2022b). *A clinical trial to evaluate the safety and immunogenicity of BG505 MD39.3, BG505 MD39.3 gp151, and BG505 MD39.3 gp151 CD4KO HIV trimer mRNA vaccines in healthy, HIV-uninfected adult participants*. Identifier: NCT05217641. *ClinicalTrials.gov*. https://clinicaltrials.gov/ct2/show/NCT05217641.

Nega, A. D., Woldetsadik, M. A., & Gelagay, A. A. (2018). Low uptake of cervical cancer screening among HIV positive women in Gondar University referral hospital, Northwest Ethiopia: Cross-sectional study design. *BMC Women's Health, 18*(1), 87. https://doi.org/10.1186/s12905-018-0579-z.

NIH Office of AIDS Research. (2021a). *What is a therapeutic HIV vaccine?* https://hivinfo.nih.gov/understanding-hiv/fact-sheets/what-therapeutic-hiv-vaccine.

NIH Office of AIDS Research. (2021b). *Understanding HIV: Fact sheets: What is a preventative HIV vaccine?* https://hivinfo.nih.gov/understanding-hiv/fact-sheets/what-preventive-hiv-vaccine.

NIH Office of AIDS Research. (2021c). *Understanding HIV: Fact sheets: HIV and AIDS: The basics*. https://hivinfo.nih.gov/understanding-hiv/fact-sheets/hiv-and-aids-basics.

NIH Office of AIDS Research. (2021d). *Understanding HIV: Fact sheets: The stages of HIV infection*. https://hivinfo.nih.gov/understanding-hiv/fact-sheets/stages-hiv-infection.

NIH Office of AIDS Research. (2021e). *U.S. statistics*. https://www.hiv.gov/hiv-basics/overview/data-and-trends/statistics.

NIH Office of AIDS Research. (2021f). *Understanding HIV: Fact sheets: HIV and older people*. https://hivinfo.nih.gov/understanding-hiv/fact-sheets/hiv-and-older-people.

NIH Office of AIDS Research. (2022a). *Guidelines for the prevention and treatment of opportunistic infections in adults and adolescents with HIV: Human herpesvirus-8 disease*. https://clinicalinfo.hiv.gov/en/guidelines/adult-and-adolescent-opportunistic-infection/human-herpesvirus-8-disease.

NIH Office of AIDS Research. (2022b). *Guidelines for the prevention and treatment of opportunistic infections in adults and adolescents with HIV: Human papillomavirus disease*. https://clinicalinfo.hiv.gov/en/guidelines/adult-and-adolescent-opportunistic-infection/human-papillomavirus-disease.

Palefsky, J. M. (2017). Human papillomavirus-associated anal and cervical cancers in HIV-infected individuals: Incidence and prevention in the antiretroviral era. *Current Opinion in HIV and AIDS, 12*(1), 26–30.

Patel, N., Borg, P., Haubrich, R., & McNicholl, I. (2018). Analysis of drug-drug interactions among patients receiving antiretroviral regimens using data from a large open-source prescription database. *American Journal of Health-System Pharmacy, 75*(15), 1132–1139. https://doi.org/10.2146/ajhp170613.

Peruski, A. H., Wesolowski, L. G., Delaney, K. P., Chavez, P. R., Owen, S. M., Granade, T. C., et al. (2020). Trends in HIV-2 diagnoses and use of the HIV-1/HIV-2 differentiation test – United States, 2010–2017. *Morbidity and Mortality Weekly Report, 69*(3), 63–66. https://doi.org/10.15585/mmwr.mm6903a2.

Plummer, M., de Martel, C., Vignat, J., Ferlay, J., Bray, F., & Franceschi, S. (2016). Global burden of cancers attributable to infections in 2012: a synthetic analysis. *The Lancet Global Health, 4*(9), e609–e616. https://doi.org/10.1016/S2214-109X(16)30143-7.

Prueksapanich, P., Piyachaturawat, P., Aumpansub, P., Ridtitid, W., Chaiteerakij, R., & Rerknimitr, R. (2018). Liver fluke-associated biliary tract cancer. *Gut and Liver, 12*(3), 236–245. https://doi.org/10.5009/gnl17102.

Rahimmanesh, I., Kouhpayeh, S., Azizi, Y., & Khanahmad, H. (2022). Conceptual framework for SARS-CoV-2-related lymphopenia. *Advanced Biomedical Research, 11*, 16. https://doi.org/10.4103/abr.abr_303_20.

Raza, Md. T., Mizan, S., Yasmin, F., Akash, A.-S., & Shahik, S. Md. (2021). Epitope-based universal vaccine for human T-lymphotropic virus-1 (HTLV-1). *PLoS One, 16*(4), e0248001. https://doi.org/10.1371/journal.pone.0248001.

Reid, E., Suneja, G., Ambinder, R., Ard, K., Baiocchi, R., Barta, S., et al. (2018). *NCCN guidelines: Cancer in people living with cancer. Version 1.2018.* www.nccn.org. Accessed 01.07.18.

Relf, M. V., Shelton, B. K., & Jones, K. M. (2017). Common immunological disorders (oncologic emergencies). In P. G. Morton & D. K. Fontaine (Eds.), *Critical Care Nursing* (11th ed., pp. 949–981). Philadelphia, PA: Elsevier Publishing.

Schiller, J. T., & Lowy, D. R. (2021). An introduction to virus infections and human cancer. Recent results in cancer research. *Fortschritte der Krebsforschung. Progres dans les recherches sur le cancer, 217*, 1–11. https://doi.org/10.1007/978-3-030-57362-1_1.

Shiels, M. S., Islam, J. Y., Rosenberg, P. S., Hall, H. I., Jacobson, E., & Engels, E. A. (2018). Projected cancer incidence rates and burden of incident cancer cases in HIV-infected adults in the United States through 2030. *Annals of Internal Medicine, 168*(12), 866–873. https://doi.org/10.7326/M17-2499.

Sigel, K., Makinson, A., & Thaler, J. (2017). Lung cancer in persons with HIV. *Current Opinion in HIV and AIDs, 12*(1), 31–38.

Stern, J., Miller, G., Li, X., & Saxena, D. (2019). Virome and bacteriome: Two sides of the same coin. *Current Opinion in Virology, 37*, 37–43. https://doi.org/10.1016/j.coviro.2019.05.007.

Suneja, G., Reid, E., Ambinder, R.F., Ard, K., Baiocchi, R., Barta, S.K., et al. (2018). *NCCN guidelines: AIDS-related Kaposi sarcoma, Version 1.2018.* www.nccn.org. Accessed 01.07.18.

Thrift, A. P., & Chiao, E. Y. (2018). Are non-HIV malignancies increased in the HIV-infected population? *Current Infectious Disease Reports, 20*(8), 22. https://doi.org/10.1007/s11908-018-0626-9.

U.S. Department of Health and Human Services. (2019). *Guidelines for the use of antiretroviral agents in adults and adolescents living with HIV: Considerations for antiretroviral use in special patient populations: HIV-2 infection.* https://clinicalinfo.hiv.gov/sites/default/files/guidelines/documents/adult-adolescent-arv/guidelines-adult-adolescent-arv.pdf.

Workowski, K. A., Bachmann, L. H., Chan, P. A., Johnston, C. M., Muzny, C. A., Park, I., et al. (2021). Sexually transmitted infections treatment guidelines, 2021. *Morbidity and Mortality Weekly Report, 70*(4), 1–187. https://doi.org/10.15585/mmwr.rr7004a1.

Yarchoan, R., & Uldrick, T. S. (2018). HIV-associated cancers and related diseases. *The New England Journal of Medicine, 378*(11), 1029–1041. https://doi.org/10.1056/NEJMra1615896.

18

Leukemia

Lourdes Moldre, Nico C. Buan-Lagazo, and Adrianzel Mark A. Buan-Lagazo

OVERVIEW

I. Leukemia (Leukemia & Lymphoma Society, 2017a)
   A. Blood cancer that is caused by an accumulation of neoplasms in the bone marrow, blood cells, and lymph nodes.
   B. Pathogenic variants in the DNA stimulate abnormal cells to replicate without recognition by the adaptive immune system.
   C. This cascade results in the multiplication of abnormal cells and interferes with the production and function of the white blood cells (WBC), red blood cells, and platelets.
   D. Acute leukemia grows rapidly with sudden onset. It is composed of immature cells. Chronic leukemia progresses slowly with slower onset and composed of mature cells.

ACUTE LYMPHOBLASTIC LEUKEMIA

Overview

I. Definition
   A. A rapidly growing cancer of blood, bone marrow, and other organs. It does not have a clear cause and can be fatal if not treated.
II. Epidemiology (Leukemia & Lymphoma Society, 2017a; National Comprehensive Cancer Network [NCCN], 2022)
   A. Approximately 5690 new cases and 1580 deaths estimated in 2021 in the United States.
   B. It is the most common form of leukemia among children and adolescents representing 20% of all cancers among persons <20 years, or >3000 new cases annually (Siegel et al., 2017). The risk declines after 5 years of age until the middle twenties and then rises again after the age of 50. Adults have a prevalence of 4 out of 10 cases of acute lymphoblastic leukemia (ALL) (American Cancer Society, 2018b).
   C. Improvements in survival for children and adolescents and young adults (AYAs: individuals between 15 and 39) with 5-year overall survival rates of 89% and 61%, respectively.
   D. Survival rates for adults are approximately 20%–40%, with a 20% rate for older adults.
III. Pathophysiology
   A. Originates from the immature lymphocytes and inhibits the body's ability to fight bacterial and viral infections.

B. Lymphocytes do not develop into mature cells and therefore impair human immunity.
   B. Three subtypes include the B cells, T cells, and natural killer cells.
IV. Prevention
   A. Risk factors (Leukemia & Lymphoma Society, 2017a; NCCN, 2022)
      1. Germline and Chromosomal Abnomalities
         a. Down syndrome, Li–Fraumeni syndrome, neurofibromatosis, Klinefelter syndrome, Fanconi anemia, Shwachman–Diamond syndrome, Bloom syndrome, and ataxia telangiectasia.
      2. Age
         a. 53.5% of patients are diagnosed <20 years old.
            (1) Most common form of childhood leukemia
         b. 29.6% ages 45–65
         c. 13.7% >65 years
      3. Race
         a. Caucasians have a twofold increased risk compared with African Americans.
         b. Hispanic children have the highest incidence of developing ALL.
      4. High-dose radiation
         a. Exposure to atomic bombs.
      5. Viruses
         a. Epstein–Barr virus
         b. Human T-cell leukemia virus-1
V. Diagnosis
   A. Assessment (Leukemia & Lymphoma Society, 2017a; NCCN, 2022)
      1. Fatigue or lethargy
      2. Constitutional symptoms
         a. Fever
         b. Night sweats
         c. Weight loss
      3. Dyspnea
      4. Dizziness
      5. Infections
      6. Easy bruising or bleeding
      7. In children, the only presenting symptom may be pain in the extremities or joints.
      8. 20% of patients may present with lymphadenopathy, splenomegaly, and/or hepatomegaly on physical examination.

9. Chin numbness due to cranial nerve involvement is suggestive of mature B-cell ALL (B-ALL)
B. Workup (NCCN, 2022)
1. Thorough medical history and physical examination
2. Laboratory
a. Complete blood count (CBC) with differential
b. Blood chemistry profile
c. Liver function tests
d. Disseminated intravascular coagulation (DIC) panel
(1) D-Dimer
(2) Fibrinogen
(3) Prothrombin time
(4) Partial thromboplastin time
e. Tumor lysis syndrome panel
(1) Lactate Dehydrogenase (LDH)
(2) Uric acid
(3) Potassium
(4) Phosphate
(5) Calcium
f. Hepatitis B and C
g. Hydrophobic interaction chromatography
h. Cytomegalovirus
i. Pregnancy testing
j. Testicular involvement
(1) Scrotal ultrasound (most common cases of T-ALL)
3. Imaging studies
a. Computed tomography (CT) scans of the neck, chest, abdomen, and pelvis with IV contrast (recommended)
b. Positron emission tomography/CT for diagnosis and follow-up
c. CT/magnetic resonance imaging of the head with contrast

VI. Histopathology
A. The bone marrow is usually hypercellular with auer rods in 70% of blasts
B. Erythroid and megakaryocyte precursors may have dysplastic abnormalities
C. Eosinophil precursors and basophils are increased with rare mast cell hyperplasia
D. Molecular classification
1. ALL is classified histologically as follows:
a. B-cell lymphoblastic leukemia/lymphoma not otherwise specified
b. B-cell lymphoblastic leukemia/lymphoma, with recurrent genetic abnormalities
c. B-cell lymphoblastic leukemia/lymphoma with hypodiploidy
d. B-cell lymphoblastic leukemia/lymphoma with hyperdiploidy
e. B-cell lymphoblastic leukemia/lymphoma with t(9;22) (q34;q11.2) (BCR-ABL1)
f. B-cell lymphoblastic leukemia/lymphoma with t (v;11q23) (MLL rearranged)
g. B-cell lymphoblastic leukemia/lymphoma with (12;21) (p13;q22) (ETV6-RUNX1)
h. B-cell lymphoblastic leukemia/lymphoma with t(1;19) (q23;p13.3) (TCF3-PBX1)
i. B-cell lymphoblastic leukemia/lymphoma with intrachromosomal amplification of chromosome (iAMP21)
j. B-cell lymphoblastic leukemia/lymphoma with translocations involving tyrosine kinases or cytokine receptors (BCR-ABL1-like ALL)
k. T-cell lymphoblastic leukemia/lymphomas
l. Early T-cell precursor lymphoblastic leukemia

VII. Staging
A. Histologic-grade French–American–British classification (Seiter, 2021) (Table 18.1)
1. L1—small cells with a homogeneous chromatin and a regular nuclear shape and a scanty cytoplasm. Occurs in 25%–30% of adults with leukemia.
2. L2—large and heterogeneous cells with an irregularly shaped nucleus; seen in 25%–30% of patients and is the most common.
3. L3—large, homogenous cells with multiple nucleoli; accounts for 1%–2% of adults with leukemia.

VIII. Prognosis and survival
A. The survival rate in children is 94%, while in adults is 40%.
B. Unfavorable prognosis is seen in patients with an elevated white blood cell count greater than 50,000 at diagnosis, central nervous system (CNS) involvement, early relapse, and lack of response to chemotherapy measured by the minimal residual disease (MRD) on bone marrow biopsy.
C. Predictors for survival include age and genetic abnormalities (Hrones & Tsang, 2018). Patients younger than 50 years of age have a more favorable prognosis due to fewer chromosomal abnormalities.

Management

IX. Management
A. Induction, consolidation, and maintenance (NCCN, 2022)
1. Induction
a. Vincristine, anthracyclines (daunorubicin, doxorubicin), and corticosteroids (prednisone,

TABLE 18.1 French–American–British Classification

French–American–British Morphology	Bone Marrow Involvement	Cerebrospinal Fluid
L1 homogeneous blasts, minimal cytoplasm	M1 <5% blasts	CNS 1 no blasts
L2 heterogeneity, prominent nucleoli	M2 5%–25% blasts	CNS 2 WBC <5 UL with blasts
L3 basophilic cytoplasm with prominent vacuolization	M3 >25% blasts	CNS 3 WBC ≥5 UL with blasts

Data from Seiter, K. (2021). What is the French-American-British (FAB) classification of acute lymphoblastic leukemia (ALL)? *Medscape.* https://www.medscape.com/answers/207631-105131/what-is-the-french-american-british-fab-classification-of-acute-lymphoblastic-leukemia-all.

dexamethasone) with or without L-asparaginase (4-drug regimen) and/or cyclophosphamide (5-drug regimen).
  b. Dexamethasone as part of the 4- or 5-drug induction regimen showed a decreased risk of isolated CNS relapse and improved EFS outcomes compared with prednisone in children with ALL.
    (1) Significantly reduced event rate (death, refractory, or replaced leukemia, or secondary malignancy)
    (2) However, no advantage was seen regarding the risk of bone marrow relapse or overall mortality.
    (3) Higher risk of mortality during induction therapy
  2. Consolidation/intensification therapy
    a. Methotrexate, cytarabine, 6-mercaptopurine (6-MP), cyclophosphamide, vincristine, corticosteroids, and L-asparaginase
  3. Maintenance
    a. 6-MP and weekly MTX (with periodic vincristine and corticosteroids) for 2–3 years. Omitted for mature B-ALL.
    b. Targeted therapy
      (1) Tyrosine kinase inhibitors (TKIs) (imatinib, dasatinib, nilotinib, ponatinib, and bosutinib)
      (2) Anti-CD20 monoclonal antibody (rituximab) for CD20-expressing B-cell lineage ALL
      (3) Purine nucleoside analog nelarabine
B. Systemic therapy (NCCN, 2022)
  1. Induction Philadelphia-positive: to induce complete remission (CR)
    a. AYAs and patients <65 years of age
      (1) TKI—targeted therapy that blocks the action of BCR-ABL fusion gene (imatinib, dasatinib, ponatinib, or nilotinib); given with corticosteroids.
      (2) Multiagent chemotherapy may be given with a TKI—vincristine, pegaspargase, steroid (prednisone or dexamethasone), and an anthracycline (doxorubicin or daunorubicin). This regimen may also include cyclophosphamide.
      (3) CNS prophylaxis or treatment—methotrexate or cytarabine is given during a lumbar puncture (IT chemotherapy).
      (4) Clinical trials are also an option for patients who meet the inclusion criteria.
    b. Patients >65 years of age or those with significant comorbidities
      (1) These patients are not eligible for intensive therapy.
      (2) General health, organ function, and comorbidities must be considered by the provider to determine the best regimen for this population.

  2. Induction Philadelphia-negative:
    a. AYA and patients <65 years of age—clinical trial, pediatric chemotherapy regimen, or multiagent chemotherapy
    b. >65 years of age
      (1) Clinical trial or multiagent chemotherapy
      (2) Multiagent chemotherapy or palliative corticosteroids with significant comorbidities
  3. Postremission consolidation and maintenance therapy—treatment given to maintain remission
    a. AYA and patients <65 years of age
      (1) Philadelphia-positive: consolidation should be considered with an allogeneic hematopoietic cell transplantation (HCT) if a donor is available; if a donor is unavailable, multiagent chemotherapy and a TKI will be given.
      (2) Philadelphia-negative: blinatumomab for B-ALL, HCT, or multiagent chemotherapy depending on MRD.
    b. Patients >65 years of age
      (1) Philadelphia-positive: allogeneic HCT or continue the TKI with or without corticosteroids, or TKI plus or minus chemotherapy for consolidation chemotherapy.
      (2) Maintenance chemotherapy includes a TKI for 1 year for Philadelphia-positive.
C. Radiation therapy (NCCN, 2022)
  1. Treatment may be needed to destroy cancer cells that have invaded the brain and spine. CNS involvement is seen in 90% of children (Cousins, Olivares, Michie, Gottlieb, & Halsey, 2017) and 5% of adults (Del Principe et al., 2014).
D. Allogeneic HCT (NCCN, 2022)
  1. Stem cell transplant is a curative treatment for patients with complex cytogenetics with likelihood of relapsing disease that provides patients with human leukocyte–matched hematopoietic stem cells from a relative or unrelated donor after administration of high-dose chemotherapy and/or radiation.
E. Chimeric antigen receptor therapy (CAR T cells) (NCCN, 2022)
  1. Tisagenlecleucel (Kymriah) is a CD 19–directed, genetically modified, T-cell immunotherapy used to treat patients with pre–B-ALL up to age 25 but <26. This therapy was approved in July 2017 for patients who have refractory disease, failed two prior lines of chemotherapy, or relapsed. Associated side effects include cytokine release syndrome, neurologic toxicity (CRES), hypersensitivity reactions, prolonged cytopenias, and hypogammaglobulinemia (Novartis Pharmaceuticals Corporation, 2018).
  2. Brexucabtagene autoleucel (Tecartus) was approved in October 2021 by the Food and Drug Administration (FDA) as the second CAR T-cell therapy for adult patients with relapsed or refractory B-ALL. First-line treatment for patients 26 or older.

F. Nursing implications
   1. Conduct ongoing assessments to monitor for pancytopenia.
   2. Safely administer systemic therapy based on the Oncology Nursing Society (ONS) chemotherapy/biotherapy guidelines for administration.
   3. Monitor for adverse events related to stem cell transplantation.
   4. Discuss the impact of decreased drug adherence in taking oral medications.
   5. Medication education that includes medication schedule, side effect recognition, and timely reporting.

ACUTE MYELOID LEUKEMIA

Overview

I. Definition (National Cancer Institute, n.d.-a)
   A. A fast-growing cancer in which too many myeloblasts (a type of immature white blood cell) are found in the bone marrow and blood
II. Epidemiology (American Cancer Society, 2022)
   A. The American Cancer Society estimated 20,050 new cases of Acute Myeloid Leukemia (AML) in 2022.
   B. Most common among male adults over 45 years of age, with average age being 68.
   C. Average lifetime risk in both sexes is about 0.5%.
III. Pathophysiology
   A. Heterogenous disease with a rapid onset characterized by abnormal hematopoietic stem cells of the myeloid layer of the bone marrow.
IV. Prevention
   A. Assess risk factors (American Cancer Society, 2018c; Leukemia & Lymphoma Society, 2017b).
      1. Germline and chromosomal abnormalities—Fanconi anemia, Bloom syndrome, ataxia-telangiectasia, Down syndrome, Li–Fraumeni syndrome, Diamond–Blackfan anemia, neurofibromatosis type 1, Kostmann syndrome, Trisomy 8
      2. Age
      3. Male
      4. Familial history of AML
      5. History of myelodysplastic syndrome (MDS)
      6. Long-term exposure to benzene. Benzene is a chemical used in oil refineries, chemical plants, gasoline industries, cigarette smoke, vehicle exhaust, glue, detergent, art supplies, and paint.
      7. Smoking
      8. Chemotherapy
         (1) Alkylating agents—cyclophosphamide, mechlorethamine, procarbazine, chlorambucil, melphalan, busulfan, carmustine
         (2) Platinum agents—cisplatin and carboplatin
   B. Possible risk factors
      1. Electromagnetic fields, such as living near power lines
      2. Workplace exposure to diesel, gasoline, and other chemicals
      3. Herbicides or pesticides

V. Diagnosis (American Cancer Society, 2018d; Leukemia & Lymphoma Society, 2017b)
   A. History and physical
      1. Onset of symptoms
      2. Assessment of eyes, mouth, skin, lymph nodes, spleen, and nervous system
      3. Areas of bleeding (nosebleed or skin cuts that will not stop oozing)
   B. Types of samples
      1. CBC with peripheral smear
      2. Bone marrow aspiration and biopsy
      3. Skin biopsy when there is suspected myeloid sarcoma
      4. Lumbar puncture (CNS involvement)
      5. Cytogenetic analysis
      6. Laboratory studies (Hourigan & Malkovska, 2013)
         a. CBC with differential
         b. Hyperuricemia
         c. Elevated blood urea nitrogen
         d. High lactic dehydrogenase
         e. Hypokalemia or hyperkalemia
         f. Lactic acidosis
         g. Hypercalcemia
         h. Hypoglycemia
         i. Hypoxemia
VI. Histopathology (Arbor et al., 2016)
   A. AML with recurrent genetic abnormalities
      1. AML with t(8;21) (q22;q22); RUNX-1-RUNX1T1
      2. AML with inv(16) (p13q22) or t(16;16) (p13;q22) (CBFB-MYH11)
      3. Acute promyelocytic leukemia (APL) with promyelocytic leukemia–retinoic acid receptor (RAR) alpha (PML-RARA)
      4. AML with t(9;11)(p21.3q26.2) or t(3;3) (q21.3;q26.2); GATA2, MECOM
      5. AML (megakaryoblastic) with t(1;22)(p13.3;q13.3); RBM15-MKL1
      6. AML with BCR-ABL1
      7. AML with a pathogenic variant in NPM1
      8. AML with biallelic pathogenic variants in CEBPA
      9. AML with a pathogenic variant in RUNX1
      10. AML with MDS-related changes
   B. AML with myelodysplasia-related changes
   C. Therapy-related myeloid neoplasms
   D. AML, NOS (not otherwise specified)
      1. AML with minimal differentiation
      2. AML without maturation
      3. AML with maturation
      4. Acute myelomonocytic leukemia
      5. Acute monoblastic/monocytic leukemia
      6. Pure erythroid leukemia
      7. Acute megakaryoblastic leukemia
      8. Acute basophilic leukemia
      9. Acute panmyelosis with myelofibrosis
   E. Myeloid sarcoma
   F. Myeloid proliferations related to Down syndrome
      1. Transient abnormal myelopoiesis

2. Myeloid leukemia associated with Down syndrome

VII. Staging (American Cancer Society, 2018a)

A. AML is divided into subtypes, depending on the type of cell the leukemia develops and how mature the cells are.

1. M0: Undifferentiated acute myeloblastic leukemia
2. M1: Acute myeloblastic leukemia with minimal maturation
3. M2: Acute myeloblastic leukemia with maturation
4. M3: APL
5. M4: Acute myelomonocytic leukemia
6. M4 eos: Acute myelomonocytic leukemia with eosinophilia
7. M5: Acute monocytic leukemia
8. M6: Acute erythroid leukemia
9. M7: Acute megakaryoblastic leukemia

VIII. Prognosis and survival

A. To achieve a CR, the treatment for AML should be aggressive.

B. Approximately 60%–70% of adults can achieve a CR after induction therapy.

C. 25% of adults survive 3 or more years and can be cured.

D. Shorter duration of remission and advanced age may indicate decreased survival.

E. Prognostic factors associated with survival include systemic infections, white blood cell count greater than 100,000/mm³, history of MDS, neurologic involvement with leukemia, and treatment-related leukemia development.

F. Patients who have an FLT3 gene pathogenic variant have higher rates of relapse.

G. Survival (American Cancer Society, 2018a)

1. The 5-year survival of adults with AML is approximately 24%. Statistics vary based on biologic features of the disease, advanced age, and comorbidities of the patient.

Management

IX. Management (NCCN, 2021; Hourigan & Malkovska, 2013)

A. Systemic therapy

1. Induction chemotherapy is based on age and favorable/unfavorable risk status

a. Cytarabine and an anthracycline antibiotic (most often daunorubicin; can use doxorubicin or idarubicin)—traditional 7+3 regimen

b. Additional agents: clofarabine, azacytidine, decitabine, fludarabine, and lenalidomide

c. Gemtuzumab ozogamicin

(1) FDA approved for newly diagnosed AML with tumors that express CD33-positive antigens

d. Midostaurin

(1) FDA approved for FLT3 pathogenic variants in combination with standard cytarabine and daunorubicin induction and consolidation chemotherapy

e. Daunorubicin and cytarabine (Vyxeos)

(1) FDA approved for the treatment of therapy-related AML or MDS. Patients who are newly diagnosed with this form of leukemia will receive the standard 7+3 regimen.

B. Day 14 evaluation

1. A bone marrow biopsy is performed on day 14 of postinduction chemotherapy to assess for response to induction chemotherapy. Reinduction chemotherapy is recommended for patients with a residual leukemia of >5% blasts.

2. Postremission chemotherapy—dependent on risk and age

a. Consolidation chemotherapy

(1) High-dose cytarabine (HDAC)

C. Hematopoietic stem cell transplantation

1. Patients with a poor prognosis and complex cytogenetics receive allogeneic stem cells from a human leukocyte antigen–matched donor, which includes siblings, parents, unrelated donors, and cord blood.

2. This form of transplantation has two types. The first type is using own body's stem cell, and the second type is donor-provided stem cells.

D. Nursing implications

1. Assess for modifiable and nonmodifiable risk factors of AML.

2. Assess for pancytopenia and additional new-onset symptoms of leukemia.

3. Assess for oral chemotherapy adherence to minimize risk for medication resistance.

4. Educate patient on the proper schedule with oral chemotherapy.

5. Appropriate pharmacologic and nonpharmacologic management through chemotherapy administration and safe infusion of stem cell transfusion.

ACUTE PROMYELOCYTIC LEUKEMIA

Overview

I. Definition (National Cancer Institute, n.d.-b)

A. An aggressive type of AML in which there are too many immature blood-forming cells in the blood and bone marrow.

B. It is usually marked by an exchange of parts of chromosomes 15 and 17.

II. Epidemiology (Kotiah & Besa, 2021)

A. In the United States, APL accounts for 5%–15% of all adult leukemias.

III. Pathophysiology

A. APL is a biologically and clinically distinct variant of AML that is characterized by a translocation involving the RARA gene on chromosome 17 (Stock & Thirman, 2022).

IV. Prevention (Yetman, 2021)

A. Consult a medical professional if you see warning signs of leukemia.

1. Unexplained fever
2. Chronic fatigue
3. Pale complexion

4. Unusual bleeding
5. Frequent infections
6. Bruising more easily than usual
7. Bone or joint pain

V. Diagnosis (Kotiah & Besa, 2021)
  A. Requires one of the following in addition to diagnostic tests for AML
    1. t(15:17) by cytogenetics
    2. PML/RARA by molecular testing

VI. Histopathology (Kotiah & Besa, 2021)
  A. Hypergranular (Classic M3)
  B. Microgranular (M3v)
  C. Hyperbasophilic
  D. PLZF-RAR alpha (M3r)

VII. Staging (Larson, 2022)
  A. Low-risk: WBC count <10,000/µL and platelet count >40,000/µL
  B. Intermediate risk: WBC count <10,000/µL and platelet count <40,000/µL
  C. High risk: WBC count >10,000/µL

VIII. Prognosis and survival (Kotiah & Besa, 2021)
  A. Good prognosis with long-term survival rates following treatment (90%).
  B. Incidence of early death remains high without treatment (29%).
  C. When intrathecal chemotherapy is given during consolidation for patients with high-risk APL to treat APL, the curative rate is >90%.

Management

IX. Management (Larson, 2022)
  A. Without treatment, APL is the most malignant form of AML, with a median survival of less than 1 month
  B. Induction
    1. Low- or intermediate-risk APL
      a. All-transretinoic acid (ATRA) plus arsenic trioxide (ATO)
    2. High-risk APL
      a. ATRA plus chemotherapy (ongoing trials)
        (1) Gemtuzumab ozogamicin
        (2) Cytotoxic chemotherapy with either hydroxyurea or an anthracycline
        (3) Daunorubicin/cytarabine with or without ATRA
  C. Consolidation
    1. After ATRA plus ATO
      a. ATO-based consolidation
    2. After chemotherapy-based induction
      a. Two cycles of an anthracycline (daunorubicin or idarubicin) plus ATRA
  D. ATRA plus ATO is the initial treatment for APL. It may be given with an anthracycline in low-risk disease and is recommended in high-risk disease in the absence of cardiac disease. This therapy restores the normal growth of cells and promotes the differentiation of hematopoietic cells.

  E. Other options: cytarabine for high risk; cytarabine/anthracycline combination for relapsed APL; gemtuzumab ozogamicin for high risk, relapse, or inability to tolerate ATO due to QT prolongation or other reason.
  F. Intrathecal chemotherapy is given during consolidation for patients with high-risk APL.
  G. Nursing considerations
    1. Coagulopathy
      a. APL can result in DIC and/or primary fibrinolysis.
      b. Monitor coagulation studies and transfuse as necessary.
        (1) Fibrinogen
        (2) D-Dimer
        (3) PT
        (4) aPTT
        (5) Platelet
    2. Differentiation syndrome (aka retinoid acid syndrome or cytokine storm)
      a. Can occur with the absence of ATRA
        (1) Fever
        (2) Peripheral edema
        (3) Pulmonary infiltrates
        (4) Hypoxemia
        (5) Respiratory distress
        (6) Hypotension
        (7) Renal/hepatic dysfunction
        (8) Serositis resulting in pleural/pericardial effusions
      b. Early recognition and aggressive management with dexamethasone therapy
    3. Hyperleukocytosis
      a. Occurs in up to 50% of patients treated with ATRA alone
      b. Prompt treatment of cytarabine and daunorubicin
    4. High intracranial pressure
      a. More common in children and adolescents treated with ATRA
      b. Symptoms may include
        (1) Headache
        (2) Papilledema
        (3) Vision loss

CHRONIC LYMPHOCYTIC LEUKEMIA

Overview

I. Definition (Leukemia & Lymphoma Society, 2021a, 2021b)
  A. Type of blood cancer that begins in the bone marrow.
  B. Can progress either slowly or quickly depending on the form it takes.

II. Epidemiology (American Cancer Society, 2021a)
  A. 21,250 new cases of chronic lymphocytic leukemia (CLL) estimated to occur in 2021 with 4320 deaths in 2021.
  B. The lifetime risk of CLL is 1 in 175 (0.57%) and is most commonly diagnosed at 70 years of age. It is rarely seen in people under 40, and extremely rare in children.
  C. CLL risk is slightly higher in men than women.

III. Pathophysiology
  A. CLL is the most frequent form of leukemia and originates from mature B lymphocytes. The median age at diagnosis is 60, and less than 15% are diagnosed under the age of 50.
IV. Prevention (American Cancer Society, 2021a; Farooqui, Wiestner, & Aue, 2013; Leukemia & Lymphoma Society, 2021a, 2021b)
  A. Family history (first-degree relatives are four times more likely to develop CLL than people who do not have first-degree relatives with the disease)
  B. Exposure to Agent Orange
  C. Age
  D. Gender
  E. Race/ethnicity
V. Diagnosis (Hallek & Al-Sawaf, 2021; Kajtar, 2021)
  A. Peripheral blood—presence of at least 5000 peripheral clonal B cells/μL (5×10^9/L) of at least 3 months; confirmed by flow cytometry
  B. Lymph node and bone marrow biopsy
  C. Immunohistochemistry
  D. Flow cytometry
  E. Cytogenetics
VI. Diagnosis
  A. Assessment (American Cancer Society, 2021a; Farooqui et al., 2013; Leukemia & Lymphoma Society, 2021a, 2021b)
  B. Symptoms—fever, night sweats, weight loss, short of breath during normal activity, anemia, and fatigue
  C. Lymphadenopathy—abdominal discomfort, fullness, and malaise
  D. Splenomegaly
  E. Hepatomegaly
  F. Gastrointestinal bleeding
  G. Extranodal involvement—pulmonary nodules or skin lesions
  H. Recurrent infections
  I. Autoimmune disorders—hemolytic anemia, immune thrombocytopenia purpura
VII. Histopathology (Inamdar & Bueso-Ramos, 2007)
  A. Clusters of round lymphoid cells protrude beneath endothelial veins and enlargement of mantle zone.
  B. The nuclear contours of lymphocytes are irregular, and there is a presence of extensive granulomas. Lymphoma may be masked by the presence of abnormal granulomas (Kajtar, 2021).
  C. Molecular classification (Lamanna, Weiss, & Dunleavy, 2015)
    1. There is a rearrangement of immunoglobulin (Ig) genes, somatic hypermutation, or unmutated subtype.
    2. Unmutated Ig heavy-chain variable subtype accounts for 80% of patients with a ZAP70 expression (Kajtar, 2021).
    3. Histologic grade (none).
VIII. Staging
  A. Rai staging system for CLL is more often used in the United States (Table 18.2) (Rai et al., 1975).

B. Binet staging system is widely used in Europe (Binet et al., 1981).
IX. Prognosis and survival (Kajtar, 2021)
  A. The 5-year survival is 83%; 10-year survival, 59.5% (American Cancer Society, 2021a; Pulte et al., 2016)
  B. Favorable factors: nondiffuse pattern of bone marrow involvement of a pathogenic variant in the IGHV gene, wild type TP53, isolated del 13q; low clinical staging based per Rai and Binet (American Cancer Society, 2021a; Amin & Malek, 2016)
  C. Unfavorable factors: diffuse pattern of bone marrow involvement, advanced age, trisomy 12, TP53 pathogenic variants, (del 11q and del 17p); increased CD38, ZAP70, and CD49d expression; elevated B-2 microglobulin; high clinical stage based on Rai and Binet (American Cancer Society, 2021a; Amin & Malek, 2016)

Management

X. Management (American Cancer Society, 2021a; Farooqui et al., 2013; Leukemia & Lymphoma Society, 2021a; 2021b; NCCN, 2018a)
  A. Factors: Age, overall health, prognostic factors (deletions in chromosomes 17 or 11, or high levels of ZAP70 and CD38) (American Cancer Society, 2021a)
  B. Systemic therapy—dependent on 17p deletion and TP53 pathogenic variant
    1. Standard chemotherapy
      a. Antimetabolites: Cladribine, fludarabine, and pentostatin
      b. Alkylating agents: Bendamustine hydrochloride and chlorambucil
      c. DNA-damaging agent: Cyclophosphamide
      d. Corticosteroids: Prednisone and dexamethasone
    2. Targeted therapies
      a. Ibrutinib: used for patients with 17p deletion (NCCN, 2018a)
      b. Idelalisib: for younger patients and those with significant comorbidities
      c. Venetoclax, acalabrutinib
    3. Monoclonal antibodies
      a. Rituximab: humanized antibody that targets CD20 (ofatumumab and obinutuzumab): Antigen target

TABLE 18.2	Rai Staging System	
Rai Staging System	Risk Group	Clinical Presentation
0	Low	Lymphocytosis
I	Intermediate	Adenopathy and lymphocytosis
II	Intermediate	Splenomegaly, lymphocytosis, or hepatomegaly
III	High	Anemia Hgb <11 g/dL and lymphocytosis
IV	High	Thrombocytopenia <100,000 μL and lymphocytosis

From Rai, K. R., Sawitsky, A., Cronkite, E. P., Chanana, A. D., Levy, R. N., & Pasternack, B. S. (1975). Clinical staging of chronic lymphocytic leukemia. *Blood*, *46*(2), 219–234.

site is CD 20—used in patients with relapsed or refractory disease (NCCN, 2018a).
  b. Alemtuzumab—targets CD 52.
  c. Obinutuzumab, ofatumumab, rituximab, and hyaluronidase human.
C. Allogeneic HCT
  1. This is a potentially curable treatment that provides patients with a graft-versus-tumor effect. The risk versus benefit must be evaluated, given that the patient population is older.
D. Others: Leukapheresis, localized low-dose radiation therapy or surgery (American Cancer Society, 2021a)
E. Clinical trials: new targeted treatments, immunomodulatory drug, early CLL treatment with high-risk patients with less toxic novel agents CAR T-cell therapy, PD-1 checkpoint inhibitors (Leukemia & Lymphoma Society, 2021a, 2021b)
F. Nursing implications
  1. Assess for signs and symptoms of CLL.
  2. Safe administration of systemic therapy according to the ONS chemotherapy/biotherapy administration guidelines
  3. Prompt management of any adverse events related to chemotherapy, targeted therapies, and monoclonal antibodies
  4. Medication education that includes administration, side effect recognition, and safe handling in the home setting to maximize adherence

CHRONIC MYELOGENOUS LEUKEMIA

Overview

I. Definition (Leukemia & Lymphoma Society, 2021a, 2021b)
  A. Cancer of the bone marrow and blood
  B. Usually diagnosed in its chronic phase when treatment is very effective for most patients. Has three phases.
II. Epidemiology (American Cancer Society, 2021b)
  A. 8860 new cases of chronic myelogenous leukemia (CML) estimated to be diagnosed in 2022 (5120 in men and 3740 in women).
  B. About 15% of new leukemia cases are CML. About 1 in 526 will get CML in their lifetime in the United States.
  C. Average age at diagnosis is 64 years old, with half of the total cases being over the age of 65 and older.
  D. Imatinib mesylate (Gleevec) became widely known for causing arrest of the tyrosine kinase activity and producing favorable outcomes.
III. Pathophysiology
  A. CML is a clonal disorder that originates from the Philadelphia chromosome translocation BCR-ABL oncogene. The translocation between chromosome 9 and 22 fuses together, causing tyrosine kinase activity, which results in initiation of leukemia (Philadelphia chromosome). There are three phases of this disorder, which include chronic, accelerated, and blast crisis phase (Leukemia & Lymphoma Society, 2017c).

IV. Prevention (Leukemia & Lymphoma Society, 2017c; Yong & Barrett, 2013)
  A. Gender—CML is slightly more common in men than women
  B. Age—risk of CML increase with age
  C. Radiation exposure
    1. Patients who have been treated with radiation in the past for other cancers have a risk of developing chronic leukemia.
V. Diagnosis (Leukemia & Lymphoma Society, 2017c)
  A. CBC with differential
  B. Bone marrow aspiration and biopsy
  C. Cytogenetic analysis (including BCR-ABL)
  D. Fluorescence in situ hybridization
  E. Quantitative polymerase chain reaction for *BCR-ABL* gene
  F. Assessment (Leukemia & Lymphoma Society, 2017c; Yong & Barrett, 2013)
    1. Weakness, fatigue
    2. Bone pain
    3. Unexplained weight loss
    4. Fevers
    5. Fullness below the ribs
    6. Night sweats
    7. Petechiae, bruising
    8. Chloroma
  G. Laboratory studies (Leukemia & Lymphoma Society, 2017c; Yong & Barrett, 2013)
    1. CBC with differential
      a. Patients may have a slightly elevated white blood cell count over 200×10^9/L.
      b. Anemia
      c. Normal platelets or thrombocytopenia
    2. Peripheral blood smear
      a. Abnormal size of the WBC
      b. Larger amount of blast counts
      c. Normal or giant platelets
VI. Histopathology
  A. Greater than 100,000 WBC with neutrophilia, significant involvement of the metamyelocytes, basophilia, eosinophilia, and monocytosis. Thrombocytosis will be present in 50% of patients.
  B. Up to 100% increased precursors of granulocytes, basophils, and eosinophils in the bone marrow; no visible nodules present; infarcts present in the spleen (Choudhury, 2020).
  C. Molecular classification
    1. (q34;q11) t(9;22) Philadelphia chromosome or *ABL* gene (#9q34) and *BCR* gene (#22q11) fusion is necessary for a diagnosis to be made (Choudhury, 2020)
VII. Staging (Leukemia & Lymphoma Society, 2017c)
  A. Stages of CML (Table 18.3)
VIII. Prognosis and survival
  A. The 5-year survival for CML depends on the phase of disease, response to treatment, and biological features.

TABLE 18.3 Stages of Chronic Myelogenous Leukemia

Chronic Phase	Accelerated Phase	Blast Phase
Increased leukocyte count	≥15% to <30% myeloblasts in the blood 30% myeloblasts and promyelocytes combined ≥20% basophils ≤100,000 platelets	≥30% blasts in the blood, bone marrow, or both
Symptoms may or may not be present	B symptoms: fever, night sweats, weight loss Fatigue Splenomegaly	B symptoms Fatigue Shortness of breath Bone and abdominal pain Splenomegaly Bleeding Infection

From Leukemia & Lymphoma Society. (2017c). *Chronic myeloid leukemia.* https://www.lls.org/leukemia/chronic-myeloid-leukemia/diagnosis/cml-phases-and-prognostic-factors; National Comprehensive Cancer Network. (2018d). *Chronic myeloid leukemia, v. 1.2019.* https://www.nccn.org/professionals/physician_gls/pdf/cml.pdf. Retrieved 04.10.18.

B. Given the evolution of imatinib, survival has doubled from 31% in the 1990s to 90% in those who take their medications consistently (American Cancer Society, 2021b).

Management

IX. Management
  A. Systemic therapy (NCCN, 2018b; Yong & Barrett, 2013)
    1. TKI
      a. First generation: Imatinib
      b. Second generation: Bosutinib, dasatinib, and nilotinib
    2. Low-risk disease—TKI or clinical trial
    3. High-risk disease—second-generation TKI or clinical trial
    4. Second-line therapy depending on detection of an actionable somatic variant
      a. Dasatinib, nilotinib, bosutinib, ponatinib, omacetaxine, and asciminib
    5. Remission induction
      a. Daunorubicin, cytosine arabinoside
  B. Allogeneic transplantation—survival 70%
  C. Nursing implications
    1. Assess patient adherence to oral chemotherapy and knowledge of medication regimen.
    2. Discuss the importance of follow-up and the significance of the treatment plan.
    3. Discuss the importance of continuing therapy and the risk of nonadherence to therapy.
    4. Educate the patient and family on environmental risk factors and exposure to hazardous drugs in the home setting.

REFERENCES

American Cancer Society. (2018a). *Acute myeloid leukemia (AML) subtypes and prognostic factors.* https://www.cancer.org/cancer/acute-myeloid-leukemia/detection-diagnosis-staging/how-classified.html.

American Cancer Society. (2018b). *Facts and figures 2018.* https://www.cancer.org/content/dam/cancer-org/research/cancer-facts-and-statistics/annual-cancer-facts-and-figures/2018/cancer-facts-and-figures-2018.pdf.

American Cancer Society. (2018c). *Risk factors for acute myeloid leukemia (AML).* https://www.cancer.org/cancer/acute-myeloid-leukemia/causes-risks-prevention/risk-factors.html.

American Cancer Society. (2018d). *Tests for acute myeloid leukemia (AML).* https://www.cancer.org/cancer/acute-myeloid-leukemia/detection-diagnosis-staging/how-diagnosed.html.

American Cancer Society. (2021a). *Chronic lymphocytic leukemia (CLL).* https://www.cancer.org/cancer/chronic-lymphocytic-leukemia.html.

American Cancer Society. (2021b). *Chronic myeloid leukemia (CML).* https://www.cancer.org/cancer/chronic-myeloid-leukemia.html.

American Cancer Society. (2022). *Key statistics for acute myeloid leukemia (AML).* https://www.cancer.org/cancer/acute-myeloid-leukemia/about/key-statistics.

Amin, N. A., & Malek, S. N. (2016). Gene mutations in chronic lymphocytic leukemia. *Seminars in Oncology, 43*(2), 215–221. https://doi.org/10.1053/j.seminoncol.2016.02.002.

Arber, D. A., Orazi, A., Hasserjian, R., Thiele, J., Borowitz, M. J., Le Beau, M. M., et al. (2016). The 2016 revision to the World Health Organization classification of myeloid neoplasms and acute leukemia. *Blood, 127*(20), 2391–2405. https://doi.org/10.1182/blood-2016-03-643544.

Binet, J. L., Auquier, A., Dighiero, G., Chastang, C., Piguet, H., Goasguen, J., et al. (1981). A new prognostic classification of chronic lymphocytic leukemia derived from a multivariate survival analysis. *Cancer, 48*(1), 198–206.

Choudhuri, J., & Shi, Y. (2020). Chronic myeloid leukemia (CML), BCR-ABL1 positive. PathologyOutlines.com website. https://www.pathologyoutlines.com/topic/myeloproliferativecml.html. Accessed February 13th, 2023.

Cousins, A. F., Olivares, O., Michie, A. M., Gottlieb, E., & Halsey, C. (2017). Association of CNS involvement in childhood acute lymphoblastic leukaemia with cholesterol biosynthesis upregulation. *The Lancet, 389*, S35. https://doi.org/10.1016/S0140-6736(17)30431-2.

Del Principe, M. I., Maurillo, L., Buccisano, F., Sconocchia, G., Cefalo, M., De Santis, G., et al. (2014). Central nervous system involvement in adult acute lymphoblastic leukemia: Diagnostic tools, prophylaxis, and therapy. *Mediterranean Journal of Hematology and Infectious Diseases, 6*(1), e2014075. https://doi.org/10.4084/MJHID.2014.075.

Farooqui, M., Wiestner, A., & Aue, G. (2013). Chronic lymphocytic leukemia. In G. Rodgers & N. Young (Eds.), *The Bethesda handbook of clinical hematology* (pp. 186–196). Philadelphia, PA: Lippincott Williams & Wilkins.

Hallek, M. & Al-Sawaf, O. (2021). Chronic lymphocytic leukemia: 2022 update on diagnostic and therapeutic procedures *American Journal of Hematology, 96*(12), 1679–1705. https://doi.org/10.1002/ajh.26367.

Hourigan, F., & Malkovska, V. (2013). Acute myeloid leukemia. In G. Rodgers & N. Young (Eds.), *The Bethesda handbook of clinical oncology* (pp. 137–157). Philadelphia, PA: Lippincott Williams & Wilkins.

Hrones, M., & Tsang, P. (2021). Acute lymphoblastic leukemia / lymphoma. PathologyOutlines.com website. https://www.pathologyoutlines.com/topic/lymphnodesALL.html. Accessed February 13th, 2023.

Inamdar, K. V., & Bueso-Ramos, C. E. (2007). Pathology of chronic lymphocytic leukemia: An update. *Annals of Diagnostic Pathology, 11*(5), 363–389. https://doi.org/10.1016/j.anndiagpath.2007.08.002.

Kajtar, B. (2021). Lymphoma & related disorders Mature B cell neoplasms Small B cell lymphomas with a circulating component CLL / SLL. https://www.pathologyoutlines.com/topic/lymphomaCLL.html.

Kotiah, S. D., & Besa, E. C. (2021). Acute promyelocytic leukemia. *Medscape.* Retrieved from https://emedicine.medscape.com/article/1495306-overview.

Lamanna, N., Weiss, M. A., & Dunleavy, K. (2015). *Chronic lymphocytic leukemia and hairy-cell leukemia.* Cancer Network. Retrieved from https://www.cancernetwork.com/cancer-management/chronic-lymphocytic-leukemia-and-hairy-cell-leukemia.

Larson, R. A. (2022). Initial treatment of acute promyelocytic leukemia in adults. UpToDate. https://www.uptodate.com/contents/4498. Retrieved 10.05.22.

Leukemia & Lymphoma Society. (2017a). *Acute lymphoblastic leukemia.* https://www.lls.org/leukemia/acute-lymphoblastic-leukemia.

Leukemia & Lymphoma Society. (2017b). *Acute myeloid leukemia.* https://www.lls.org/leukemia/acute-myeloid-leukemia.

Leukemia & Lymphoma Society. (2017c). *Chronic myeloid leukemia.* https://www.lls.org/leukemia/chronic-myeloid-leukemia.

Leukemia & Lymphoma Society. (2021a). *Chronic lymphocytic leukemia.* https://www.lls.org/leukemia/chronic-lymphocytic-leukemia.

Leukemia & Lymphoma Society. (2021b). *Chronic myeloid leukemia.* https://www.lls.org/leukemia/chronic-myeloid-leukemia.

National Cancer Institute. (n.d.-a). *Acute myeloid leukemia.* https://www.cancer.gov/publications/dictionaries/cancer-terms/def/acute-myeloid-leukemia.

National Cancer Institute. (n.d.-b). *APL.* https://www.cancer.gov/publications/dictionaries/cancer-terms/def/apl.

National Comprehensive Cancer Network (NCCN). (2018a). *Chronic lymphocytic leukemia, v. 1.2019.* https://www.nccn.org/professionals/physician_gls/pdf/cll.pdf. Retrieved 04.10.18.

National Comprehensive Cancer Network (NCCN). (2018b). *Chronic myeloid leukemia, v. 1.2019.* https://www.nccn.org/professionals/physician_gls/pdf/cml.pdf. Retrieved 04.10.18.

National Comprehensive Cancer Network (NCCN). (2021). *Acute myeloid leukemia, v. 2.2018.* https://www.nccn.org/professionals/physician_gls/pdf/aml.pdf.

National Comprehensive Cancer Network (NCCN). (2022). *Acute lymphoblastic leukemia, v. 4.2021.* https://www.nccn.org/professionals/physician_gls/pdf/all.pdf.

Novartis Pharmaceuticals Corporation (2018). *KYMRIAH® (tisagenlecleucel) [package insert].* East Hanover, NJ.

Pulte, D., Castro, F. A., Jansen, L., Luttmann, S., Holleczek, B., Nennecke, A., et al. (2016). Trends in survival of chronic lymphocytic leukemia patients in Germany and the USA in the first decade of the twenty-first century. *Journal of Hematology & Oncology, 9,* 28. https://doi.org/10.1186/s13045-016-0257-2.

Rai, K. R., Sawitsky, A., Cronkite, E. P., Chanana, A. D., Levy, R. N., & Pasternack, B. S. (1975). Clinical staging of chronic lymphocytic leukemia. *Blood, 46*(2), 219–234.

Seiter, K. (2021). What is the French-American-British (FAB) classification of acute lymphoblastic leukemia (ALL)? *Medscape.* https://www.medscape.com/answers/207631-105131/what-is-the-french-american-british-fab-classification-of-acute-lymphoblastic-leukemia-all Retrieved 11.03.19.

Siegel, D. A., Henley, S. J., Li, J., Pollack, L. A., Van Dyne, E. A., & White, A. (2017). Rates and trends of pediatric acute lymphoblastic leukemia – United States, 2001–2014. *Morbidity and Mortality Weekly Report, 66*(36), 950–954. https://doi.org/10.15585/mmwr.mm6636a3.

Stock, W., & Thirman, M. J. (2022). In R. A. Larson & A. G. Rosmarin (Eds.), *Molecular biology of acute promyelocytic leukemia.* Waltham, MA: UpToDate. Retrieved February 18, 2022 from https://www.uptodate.com/contents/molecular-biology-of-acute-promyelocytic-leukemia.

Yetman, D. (2021). Everything you want to know about acute promyelocytic leukemia. *Healthline.* Retrieved from https://www.healthline.com/health/leukemia/acute-promyelocytic-leukemia.

Yong, A., & Barrett, A. (2013). Chronic myelogenous leukemia. In G. Rodgers & N. Young (Eds.), *The Bethesda handbook of clinical oncology* (pp. 170–185). Philadelphia, PA: Lippincott Williams & Wilkins.

19

Lung Cancer

Melody Mendenhall

OVERVIEW

I. Definition
   A. Lung cancer, or bronchogenic carcinoma, refers to malignancies that originate in the airways or pulmonary parenchyma (Knoop, 2018; Siddiqui, Vaqar, & Siddiqui, 2022).
      1. Cancer may be incidentally diagnosed with a chest radiography or other radiographic views that may capture an image of the lungs.
      2. Early signs and symptoms may be absent in part because of the large lung surface area. The most common metastatic sites are the liver, adrenal glands, bones, and brain.

II. Epidemiology (Nemesure, Albano, & Nemesure, 2021; Rudin, Brambilla, Faivre-Finn, & Sage, 2021; Siegel, Miller, Fuchs, & Jemal, 2022)
   A. The two major types of lung cancer are non–small-cell lung cancer (NSCLC) and small-cell lung cancer (SCLC).
      1. Approximately 80% of all lung cancer cases are NSCLC.
         a. Two major subtypes: squamous and nonsquamous (including adenocarcinoma, large-cell carcinoma, and misc subtypes)
         b. Adenocarcinoma is the most common subtype and is also the most common in nonsmokers.
      2. SCLC is most often diagnosed in later stages and is associated with a poor prognosis.
   B. As of 2021 lung cancer was the second most common invasive cancer for both men and women and the most common cause of cancer death in the United States.
      1. In 2022 new cases are estimated at 236,740 (49.8% in men, 50.2% in women).
      2. Estimated mortalities in 2022 are 130,180 (53% men, 47% women).
      3. Both incidence and mortality rates are slowly declining in the United States for both genders, with a sharper decline in men; correlated to a decrease in smoking.
   C. The median age of diagnosis is 71 years old.
   D. Non-Hispanic black men have the highest incidence, as well as poor outcomes, and are diagnosed at a more advanced stage of disease.
   E. Nonsmokers account for 10%–30% of lung cancer cases and are predominantly women.

III. Pathophysiology (Knoop, 2018; Siddiqui et al., 2022)
   A. Anatomy
      1. Lung
         a. The right and the left lung are contained within the thorax and separated by the mediastinum.
         b. The right lung has three lobes (upper, middle, and lower) and 10 segments.
         c. The left lung has two lobes (upper and lower) and eight segments.
         d. The airway consists of the trachea, which breaks off into the bronchus (right and left), the bronchiole, and terminates at the alveoli.
         e. The main function of the lung is to get oxygen from the air to the blood via the alveoli.
      2. Pleura
         a. The pleura is a thin membrane lining the surface of the lungs and the inside of the chest wall.
         b. The pleural space is bounded by the parietal (lining of the lung surface) and visceral (lining the chest wall) membranes.
         c. The volume of fluid in the pleural space results from a balance of fluid production thought to be made by the visceral pleura and absorption by the lymphatics of the parietal pleura.
         d. Pleural effusion occurs when the production of fluid in the pleural space exceeds the absorption.
   B. Risk factors (de Groot, Wu, Carter, & Munden, 2018; National Comprehensive Cancer Network [NCCN] 2022a, 2022b; Shukuya & Takahashi, 2019; Zappa & Mousa, 2016)
      1. Smoking
         a. Cigarette smoking remains the predominant risk factor for developing lung cancer; 70%–90% of cases.
         b. Evidence shows a 20%–30% increase in the risk for lung cancer from exposure to secondhand smoke associated with living with a smoker.
         c. Risk increases with number of years smoked and number of cigarettes per day. To quantify tobacco exposure, the number of packs of cigarettes per day is multiplied by the number of years smoked to obtain pack history.
            (1) For example, one pack per day for 30 years = 30 pack/year smoking history.

d. Tobacco smoke also promotes the carcinogenic effect of other carcinogens, such as radon, asbestos, and air pollution.

e. Electronic cigarettes have been sold in the United States since 2007, and the risk factor for developing lung cancer from this is not well established.

2. Environmental and occupational factors that increase the risk of developing lung cancer
   a. Asbestos exposure (especially for mesothelioma)
   b. Radon gas
   c. Air pollution

3. Genetic risk factors have also been identified.
   a. Patients who smoke and have TP53 germline sequence variations are three times more likely to develop lung cancer than nonsmokers; three genes within chromosome 15 risk for lung cancer—30% increased risk with one marker, 70%–80% increased risk with all three markers.
   b. Whole exome sequencing has become essential in lung cancer and has helped to identify patients with germline pathogenic variants, and is an area of ongoing research.
   c. Lung cancer risk increased two to four times in first-degree relatives of lung cancer patients, controlled for personal smoking history.

4. Preexisting pulmonary disease (chronic obstructive pulmonary disease, pulmonary fibrosis, tuberculosis) is associated with an increased incidence.

IV. Primary prevention (Fintelmann et al., 2015; Knoop, 2018; NCCN, 2022a; Wiener et al., 2015)
A. Lung cancer screening guidelines based on the National Lung Screening Trial (NLST)
   1. The NLST completed in 2011 found fewer lung cancer deaths with spiral low-dose computed tomography (LDCT).
   2. Lung cancer screening is recommended by National Comprehensive Cancer Network (NCCN), Centers for Medicare and Medicaid Services, American Cancer Society, US Preventive Services Task Force (USPSTF), American College of Chest Physicians, and European Society for Medical Oncology.
   3. Current screening guidelines are for current or former smokers (≥30 pack-years or quit <15 years), asymptomatic, age 55–74, to have annual screening with LDCT.
   4. LDCT must be performed in settings that have expertise in lung cancer screening, diagnosis, and treatment.
   5. Screening guidelines do not recommend routine use of chest radiography or sputum cytology because these have not been shown to reduce the risk of mortality.
   6. Early-stage lung cancer may be curable; effective population-based screening could decrease mortality rates.

B. Smoking cessation (Knoop, 2018)

1. Smoking cessation can decrease the risk of developing comorbidities such as cardiovascular disease and other malignancies such as head and neck cancers, colorectal cancer, and liver cancer.

2. Five or more years must lapse before an appreciable decrease in risk occurs.

3. Supportive therapy
   a. Assessing a patient's desire to stop smoking
   b. Teaching stress management and relaxation techniques
   c. Referring patients to tobacco cessation resources such as the national quitline network (1-800-QUIT-NOW)

4. Pharmacologic treatments: nicotine replacement therapy, for example, varenicline and bupropion.

5. Behavioral counseling and cognitive behavioral therapy.

V. Diagnosis and staging (American College of Chest Physicians, 2013; NCCN, 2022a, 2022b)
A. Clinical manifestations (Anwar, Jafri, Ashraf, Jafri, & Fanucchi, 2019; Knoop, 2018)
   1. Patients may not exhibit symptoms until they have locally advanced or metastatic disease.
   2. Symptoms can result from local effects of the tumor, from regional or distant spread, or from distant effects not related to metastasis (paraneoplastic syndromes).
   3. There are intrathoracic and extrathoracic effects of lung cancer.
      a. Intrathoracic effects: it is common for individuals to have both respiratory and constitutional symptoms, including cough, hemoptysis, chest pain, and dyspnea.
         (1) Pleural effusions can cause dyspnea and cough.
         (2) Superior vena cava (SVC) syndrome is more common in SCLC. Symptoms include facial swelling, upper extremity edema, headache, and venous distension.
         (3) Pancoast syndrome is characteristic of lung cancer arising in the superior sulcus and is manifested by shoulder pain.
      b. Extrathoracic metastases can cause the following:
         (1) Liver: enzyme abnormalities
         (2) Bone: pain to the back, chest, or extremities, as well as elevated serum alkaline phosphatase and elevated serum calcium.
         (3) Adrenal: rarely symptomatic. Sometimes detected on staging computed tomography (CT) scans.
         (4) Brain: headache, vomiting, visual field loss, hemiparesis, and seizures.
         (5) Paraneoplastic syndromes are somewhat common in lung cancer, affecting approximately 10% of patients, most often in the late stages. The most common paraneoplastic syndromes are syndrome of inappropriate

antidiuretic hormone (SIADH) and humoral hypercalcemia of malignancy.

    (6) This group of patients can also experience oncologic emergencies such as hypercalcemia, hyponatremia from SIADH, spinal cord compression, superior vena cava (SVC) syndrome, and cardiac tamponade.

B. Complete history and physical examination to include:
1. Identification of findings related to local or systemic spread
2. Evaluation of pulmonary status
3. Identification of any comorbidities, all of which influence treatment options

C. To date, no specific tumor markers for disease status have been identified.

D. Imaging begins with a chest x-ray and CT of the chest, liver, and adrenal glands.
1. If spread is suspected, additional imaging may include positron emission tomography (particularly helpful for nodal evaluation and to identify metastatic sites) and additional imaging of suspicious sites (bone scan, abdominal imaging).
2. Magnetic resonance imaging is recommended for stage II to IIIA lung cancer to evaluate for brain metastasis.

E. Tissue sample to be obtained for diagnosis
1. The least invasive and safest method that is likely to provide the highest yield of tissue for histopathology is recommended.
2. Bronchoscopy is recommended for a centrally located lung lesion to confirm the diagnosis. If negative, further tests are recommended.
   a. Transbronchial needle aspiration
   b. Navigation bronchoscopy
   c. Endobronchial ultrasound–guided needle aspiration
3. Endoscopic ultrasound–guided needle aspiration
4. Transthoracic needle aspiration
5. Mediastinoscopy: a minor procedure used to obtain samples of all accessible lymph nodes

F. In the presence of pleural effusion, a thoracentesis is performed to determine malignancy. Malignant cells present in the pleural fluid alter the stage of lung cancer.

VI. Histopathology
A. Molecular classification (NCCN, 2022a, 2022b)
1. Since the early 2000s, there has been an increased understanding of molecular pathways that have contributed to the development of targeted therapy.
2. Adequate tissue availability is necessary to complete multiple molecular testing; liquid biopsy has been used to identify blood-based tumor markers or circulating biomarkers.
3. Various methods of molecular testing are available to evaluate for gene alterations, including next-generation sequencing (NGS), polymerase chain reaction, and fluorescence in situ hybridization.

4. Gene alterations with available targeted therapies include EGFR, ALK, ROS1, KRAS G12C, MET ex14, BRAF V600E, and NTRK.
5. Other targets are under development; NGS evaluates many other biomarkers, which may help direct patients to an appropriate clinical trial.

B. Histologic grade
1. Unlike other cancers, lung cancer does not have a widely accepted grading system.
2. The most common grading system for NSCLC is based on how different the cancer cell appears, when compared to the cell of origin.
3. SCLC is considered a high-grade neuroendocrine lung cancer.
   a. KI-67 staining is useful in differentiating SCLC and carcinoid (low- and intermediate-grade neuroendocrine carcinomas).

C. Histopathology/morphology (NCCN, 2022a, 2022b)
1. Cancer classification systems commonly in use include the identification of the primary site or anatomic location in the body (lung) and the tissue of origin (histologic type).
   a. Establishment of lung cancer as the primary diagnosis may be challenging, as the lung is a common metastatic site and lung cancer may first appear elsewhere in the body (e.g., brain).
   b. Cell morphology (appearance) is the most common distinguishing factor when differentiating SCLC and NSCLC.
   c. IHC is essential in determining the primary site of cancer and cell lineage. TTF-1, Napsin-A, P40, and p63 are often used to distinguish squamous and nonsquamous lung cancers.

VII. Staging
A. Lung cancer is staged clinically on the basis of clinical examination and imaging findings, and pathologically on surgical and pathologic findings.
1. A biopsy is not required before surgery if a strong clinical suspicion of stage I or II lung cancer exists.
2. Mediastinoscopy (invasive mediastinal staging) is recommended before surgical resection for most patients with clinical stage I or II lung cancer. Performed as the initial step before planned resection (during the same anesthetic procedure).
3. For strong clinical suspicion of N2 or N3 nodal disease, a preoperative invasive mediastinal staging is appropriate.
4. Bronchoscopy is recommended to be performed during the planned surgical resection to limit procedural risks, limit costs, and avoid multiple procedures (NCCN, 2022a).

B. Staging system (refer to American Joint Committee on Cancer [AJCC] Lung Cancer Staging, eighth edition, www.cancerstaging.org)
1. Stage of disease at the time of diagnosis is a critical element in determining appropriate treatment, as well as a key factor in defining prognosis.

2. SCLC uses a simplified staging system of clinically limited or clinically extensive disease.
3. TNM (T=tumor size, N=nodal status, M=metastasis) staging was revised for lung cancer in the AJCC Cancer Staging, eighth edition.
   a. Changes were based on the analysis of a large multinational data set of lung cancer cases.
   b. More accurately differentiate staging and prognosis
   c. Primary changes made in cutoff for tumor size and subdivisions in T staging
   d. Changes in M category made to include contralateral lung nodules and pleural effusions, with subdivisions added

VIII. Prognosis and survival (American Cancer Society, 2022)
   A. Leading cause of cancer-related deaths worldwide, in part because the disease is diagnosed at advanced stages and survival is poor, although improving.
      1. Worldwide, lung cancer remains an epidemic, and deaths from lung cancer are four times more common than from any other cancer.
      2. The overall survival rate for lung cancer at 5 years is only 22.9% in all patients.
      3. Five-year relative survival rates for NSCLC
         a. 26% overall (all stages)
         b. 64% for localized disease
         c. 37% for regional disease
         d. 8% for distant disease
      4. SCLC is difficult to cure because at the time of diagnosis, it is already widely disseminated.
         a. 7% overall (all stages)
         b. 29% localized disease
         c. 18% regional disease
         d. 3% distant metastases
      5. Positive prognostic factors include early stage of disease, good performance status (PS), less than 5% weight loss, and female gender.

MANAGEMENT

(Detterbeck, Lewis, Diekemper, Addrizzo-Harris, & Alberts, 2013; NCCN, 2022a, 2022b)
   I. Principles for medical management
      A. Delivery of care should be timely and efficient.
      B. A multidisciplinary team approach is recommended for lung cancer patients who require multimodality therapy.
      C. Treatment decisions are influenced by the stage of disease, histologic subtype, PS, pulmonary status, comorbidities, age, and patient-informed decisions.
      D. Evidence-based treatment algorithms are readily available electronically from multiple national organizations:
         1. American Society of Clinical Oncology (American Society of Clinical Oncology, 2022)
         2. NCCN
         3. National Cancer Institute

      4. Clinical trials: NCCN recommends the participation of anyone with cancer in a clinical trial; clinical trials can be found at http://clinicaltrials.gov.
   II. Surgery (NCCN, 2022a; Knoop, 2018)
      A. Surgery is the primary treatment for the management of early-stage NSCLC (stages I and II).
         1. Surgery is the best option for curative therapy.
         2. The role of surgery in stage III disease is controversial; reserved for select cases.
            a. Stage IIIA: lymph nodes involved, no distant metastatic disease
            b. Stage IIIB: tumor size is larger, more lymph nodes involved, no distant metastatic disease
         3. Only 25%–35% of cases are candidates for surgical resection.
         4. Surgery also plays a major role in the establishment of the diagnosis by obtaining tissue and has a role in the palliation of symptoms.
         5. Individuals considered for lung surgery should undergo pulmonary function tests to measure forced expiratory volume in the first second and diffusing capacity of the lungs for carbon monoxide.
         6. As primary treatment, the surgical procedure selected depends on both the extent of the disease and the patient's cardiopulmonary status.
            a. In general, lung-sparing resection is preferred; lobectomy remains the standard approach.
            b. Minimally invasive techniques such as video-assisted thoracic surgery are recommended; this surgery may be done in conjunction with wedge resection and has been associated with decreased morbidity.
            c. Systematic lymphadenectomy is recommended (rather than complete lymph node dissection).
            d. Not all patients with lung cancer are candidates for surgery, and in those who are undergoing surgery, resection may be halted if evidence of metastasis is found.
            e. Surgery may also be indicated for metastatic sites of disease that are symptomatic (i.e., resection of a solitary brain metastasis).
         7. Patients who are considered for surgery after neoadjuvant therapy should undergo pulmonary function tests to measure diffusion capacity.
   III. Radiation therapy (RT) (NCCN, 2022a)
      A. In all stages of NSCLC, RT has a potential role for either definitive or palliative therapy.
      B. For early-stage NSCLC (stage I or node-negative stage IIa disease), stereotactic body RT or stereotactic ablative radiotherapy is recommended for the individual who is not a surgical candidate or refuses surgery.
      C. Postoperative radiation administered to those with positive surgical margins.
      D. May be administered for stage III and stage IV disease.
      E. May be effective for the palliation of symptoms and the management of brain metastasis.

F. Advanced techniques—conformal simulation and intensity-modulated radiotherapy, which reduce toxicity and increase survival.
1. Commonly prescribed dosing is 60–70 gray (Gy) in 2-Gy fractions.
2. Treatment planning standard is a minimum of three-dimensional conformal RT.
3. Radiofrequency ablation involves whole-brain RT and stereotactic radiosurgery for the management of brain metastasis and improves the quality of life.

IV. Chemotherapy—NSCLC (NCCN, 2022a)
A. Chemotherapy may be administered as neoadjuvant therapy, concurrently with RT, with immunotherapy, or as a single modality (see NCCN guidelines for treatment recommendations).
B. Rapid advancements in targeted therapy specific to the tumor histology have been developed to treat lung cancer; multiple changes have been made to therapy options and first-line recommendations. It is important to seek out the latest information and nationally recommended guidelines.
C. Chemotherapy can be indicated for individuals with a performed status measured by the Eastern Cooperation Oncology Group of 0 to 2 and may be contraindicated in individual scenarios.
D. Chemotherapy is considered in as many as 80% of NSCLC cases.
E. The backbone for chemotherapy in both NSCLC and SCLC is a platinum doublet (carboplatin or cisplatin) in combination with a secondary agent including pemetrexed (nonsquamous NCLC), navelbine, gemcitabine, etoposide, paclitaxel, nab-paclitaxel, and docetaxel.
F. Nonplatinum agents are often used in subsequent lines, in combination or as single agents.

V. Molecular targeted is appropriate in certain NSCLC cases (NCCN, 2022a).
A. There are effective therapies in the metastatic setting for the following mutations: EGFR, ALK, ROS1, KRAS G12C, MET ex14, BRAF V600E, and NTRK.
B. Adjuvant osimertinib is now standard in certain patients with resected EGFR-mutated NSCLC.
C. Future genetic alteration targets are being investigated, including ERRB1 (HER2) and high-level met amplification.
D. Bevacizumab (nonsquamous only)/ramucirumab—inhibits VEGF (a protein, rather a mutation), are more broadly used in metastatic NSCLC.

VI. Immune-checkpoint inhibitors (NCCN, 2022a, 2022b)
A. Immune-checkpoint inhibitors are now widely used in the treatment of NSCLC and SCLC. Many drugs are approved with a variety of indications.
B. Immune-checkpoint inhibitors are drugs that block specific proteins involved in the downregulation of immune response in cancer cells. Examples are PD1/PDL1 inhibitors and CTLA4 inhibitors.

C. In the metastatic setting, checkpoint inhibitors are used in combination with chemotherapy, as dual agents (2 checkpoint inhibitors combined), and as single agents (PD1 or PDL1 inhibitors).
D. Recently, multiple PD1 inhibitor drugs have been approved before and after surgery and or chemo/radiation (see NCCN guidelines for specific recommendations).
E. Immune-checkpoint inhibitors have side effects related to the inhibition of immune response and can include: thyroid dysfunction, rash, type I diabetes, and inflammation of solid organs, commonly seen in colon, liver, skin, lung, and thyroid.

VII. Palliative care (NCCN, 2022a)
A. Early palliative care combined with standard therapy is recommended because it improves the quality of life, mood, and, in one study, survival.

VIII. Recurrent disease (NCCN, 2022a, 2022b)
A. If solitary site of recurrence local therapy can be considered (surgery, radiation, ablation).
B. For more widespread recurrence, see NCCN guidelines for metastatic lung cancer.

IX. SCLC (NCCN, 2022b)
A. There are several caveats to the treatment of SCLC.
B. Standard of care for individuals with limited disease—concurrent combined modality with chemotherapy or RT.
C. Prophylactic cranial RT indicated for individuals with complete response to chemotherapy or RT to reduce the risk of developing brain metastases, thus improving overall survival.
D. PD1 inhibitors have now been approved following chemo-RT in limited-stage disease and combined with chemotherapy, as well as maintenance in the metastatic setting.
E. In the metastatic setting, targetable mutations are typically not found, and VEGF inhibitors are not used.
F. Standard chemotherapy includes platinum doublet for first line with RT; the most common subsequent treatments include lurbinectedin and topotecan.

X. Nursing implications
A. Patient or family understanding of diagnosis and treatment options
1. Establish goals of care.
2. Assess coping with diagnosis and prognosis.
3. Allow the patient to maintain roles and activities most important to him or her.
4. Emphasize short-term goals in daily care and priority setting.
5. Refer to community resources as appropriate and available.
6. Teach supportive care skills.
7. Maintain realistic hope and yet prepare for changes in lifestyle if prognosis is poor.
8. Recognize needs related to anticipatory grieving.
9. Assist to resume previous roles and responsibilities if prognostic factors are favorable.

B. Treatment
1. Communication is essential in the coordination of care within the multidisciplinary team.
2. Includes teaching, side effect prevention, and monitoring.
3. Pain management with metastatic disease, pleural catheter management, and reinforcement of deep-breathing exercises helpful to increase physical activity.
4. Individuals who receive RT may experience localized skin reactions, esophagitis, fatigue, and symptoms specific to the treatment field.
5. Individuals who receive chemotherapy or targeted agents will have side effect profiles specific to the regimen.
    a. In addition to the risk for neutropenia, cisplatin-based regimens may cause nausea and vomiting and peripheral neuropathies, which require monitoring of kidney functioning.
    b. Some of the targeted therapies may cause rash, diarrhea, or both.
C. Decrease the severity of symptoms associated with the disease, treatment, or both.
1. Individuals diagnosed with lung cancer are known to be at high risk for pain and multiple other symptoms such as shortness of breath, fatigue, and weakness.
2. Maximal palliative care interventions for all symptoms are essential.
3. Refer to Oncology Nursing Society PEP resources (https://www.ons.org/the-pep-topics) for evidence-based guidelines for symptom management.

REFERENCES

American Cancer Society. (2022). *Cancer facts & figures 2022*. Atlanta, GA: American Cancer Society. https://www.cancer.org/content/dam/cancer-org/research/cancer-facts-and-statistics/annual-cancer-facts-and-figures/2022/2022-cancer-facts-and-figures.pdf.

American College of Chest Physicians. (2013). *Lung cancer*. https://www.chestnet.org/Publications/CHEST-Publications/Guidelines-Consensus-Statements.

American Society of Clinical Oncology. (2022). *Thoracic cancer*. https://www.asco.org/practice-patients/guidelines/thoracic-cancer.

Anwar, A., Jafri, F., Ashraf, S., Jafri, M. A. S., & Fanucchi, M. (2019). Paraneoplastic syndromes in lung cancer and their management. *Annals of Translational Medicine, 7*(15), 359. https://doi.org/10.21037/atm.2019.04.86.

de Groot, P. M., Wu, C. C., Carter, B. W., & Munden, R. F. (2018). The epidemiology of lung cancer. *Translational Lung Cancer Research, 7*(3), 220–233. https://doi.org/10.21037/tlcr.2018.05.06.

Detterbeck, F. C., Lewis, S. Z., Diekemper, R., Addrizzo-Harris, D., & Alberts, W. M. (2013). Executive summary: Diagnosis and management of lung cancer, 3rd ed: American College of Chest Physicians evidence-based clinical practice guidelines. *Chest, 143*(5 Suppl), 7S–37S. https://doi.org/10.1378/chest.12-2377.

Fintelmann, F. J., Bernheim, A., Digumarthy, S. R., Lennes, I. T., Kalra, M. K., Gilman, M. D., et al. (2015). The 10 pillars of lung cancer screening: Rationale and logistics of a lung cancer screening program. *RadioGraphics, 35*(7), 1893–1908. https://doi.org/10.1148/rg.2015150079.

Knoop, T. (2018). Lung cancer. In C. H. Yarbro, D. Wujcik, & B. H. Gobel (Eds.), *Cancer nursing: Principles and practice* (8th ed., pp. 1679–1720). Boston: Jones and Bartlett.

National Comprehensive Cancer Network (NCCN). (2022a). *Non-small cell lung cancer [v. 3.2022]*. https://www.nccn.org/professionals/physician_gls/pdf/nscl.pdf.

National Comprehensive Cancer Network (NCCN). (2022b). *Small cell lung cancer [v. 2.2022]*. https://www.nccn.org/professionals/physician_gls/pdf/sclc.pdf.

Nemesure, B., Albano, D., & Nemesure, A. (2021). Short- and long-term survival outcomes among never smokers who developed lung cancer. *Cancer Epidemiology, 75*, 102042. https://doi.org/10.1016/j.canep.2021.102042.

Rudin, C. M., Brambilla, E., Faivre-Finn, C., & Sage, J. (2021). Small-cell lung cancer. *Nature Reviews. Disease Primers, 7*(1), 3. https://doi.org/10.1038/s41572-020-00235-0.

Shukuya, T., & Takahashi, K. (2019). Germline mutations in lung cancer. *Respiratory Investigation, 57*(3), 201–206. https://doi.org/10.1016/j.resinv.2018.12.005.

Siddiqui, F., Vaqar, S., & Siddiqui, A. H. (2022). Lung cancer. In: *StatPearls*. Treasure Island, FL: StatPearls Publishing.

Siegel, R. L., Miller, K. D., Fuchs, H. E., & Jemal, A. (2022). Cancer statistics, 2022. *CA: A Cancer Journal for Clinicians, 72*(1), 7–33. https://doi.org/10.3322/caac.21708.

Wiener, R. S., Gould, M. K., Arenberg, D. A., Au, D. H., Fennig, K., Lamb, C. R., et al. (2015). An official American Thoracic Society/American College of Chest Physicians policy statement: Implementation of low-dose computed tomography lung cancer screening programs in clinical practice. *American Journal of Respiratory and Critical Care Medicine, 192*(7), 881–891. https://doi.org/10.1164/rccm.201508-1671ST.

Zappa, C., & Mousa, S. A. (2016). Non-small cell lung cancer: Current treatment and future advances. *Translational Lung Cancer Research, 5*(3), 288–300. https://doi.org/10.21037/tlcr.2016.06.07.

20

Lymphoma

Tanya Price

HODGKIN LYMPHOMA

Overview

I. Definition
   A. Malignancies of the lymphoid system—a heterogeneous group of malignancies arising from lymphocytes, B cells, T cells, and, rarely, natural killer (NK) cells; usually originates in the lymph nodes or tissue in other sites.
   B. Hodgkin lymphoma (HL) is a rare B-cell malignancy.
II. Epidemiology (American Cancer Society [ACS], 2022; Ansell, 2018; Centers for Disease Control and Prevention [CDC], 2022; National Cancer Institute [NCI], 2022a)
   A. Estimated 8540 new cases diagnosed and 920 deaths from HL in 2022. Overall, incidence rates dropped 1.4% from 2009 to 2018. HL represents approximately 10% of all lymphomas in the United States.
   B. Age-related bimodal incidence—most common among teens and adults aged 15–35 years and adults aged 55 years and older.
   C. Mortality—death rates declining since 1975; falling on average 4.5% each year between 2010 and 2019.
III. Pathophysiology (Ansell, 2018; DeVita, Lawrence, & Rosenberg, 2018; Kaseb, 2022; O'Malley et al., 2019)
   A. The two distinct types are classic HL (cHL) and nodular lymphocyte–predominant HL (NLPHL).
   B. cHL—large multinucleated Reed–Sternberg cell within a reactive cellular background.
      1. Immunohistochemistry stains for CD 30+ CD15+, CD20−.
   C. NLPHL lacks typical Reed–Sternberg cells but has lymphocytic and histiocytic cells.
      1. Characterized by larger cells with folded multilobulated nuclei
      2. Immunohistochemistry stains CD20+, CD45+, CD79a+, CD75+, BCL6+, BOB1+, OCT2+, and J chain −/−
IV. Prevention (ACS, 2022; Ansell, 2018; NCI, 2022a)
   A. The exact cause of HL is unknown.
   B. Factors that increase the risk of HL
      1. Age—most often between ages 15 and 35 years and in those 55 years or older
      2. Infection with the Epstein–Barr virus (EBV), human immunodeficiency virus (HIV), infections with the bacteria such as *Helicobacter pylori*, *Chlamydophila psittaci*, and hepatitis C

      3. More common in males
      4. Family history of lymphoma; same-sex siblings of an HL patient have 10 times the risk of developing HL
      5. Primary immunodeficiencies, prior solid organ and allogeneic bone marrow transplantation
      6. Prior treatment with cytotoxic chemotherapy drugs for other diseases
   C. No known preventive measures
V. Diagnosis (Ansell, 2018; National Comprehensive Cancer Network [NCCN], 2022b)
   A. Clinical presentation—enlarged lymph nodes, spleen, and other immune tissue, with/without systemic symptoms; each histologic subtype has its own clinical features.
      1. cHL—the most common presentation (half of patients) is localized disease (stage I or II) in painless cervical and supraclavicular nodes and mediastinal regions.
      2. NLPHL—more than 80% present with localized disease in cervical, axillary, or inguinal nodes; extranodal disease rare; earlier-stage disease has a more indolent course than those with cHL.
      3. Tends to spread first to adjacent lymph nodes.
      4. Systemic symptoms (B symptoms)—fever, weight loss, fatigue, and night sweats; present in approximately 40% of patients, less common with NLPHL. Another characteristic symptom can be generalized pruritus, and some patients report pain at the nodal site after drinking alcohol, but the significance of these symptoms is unknown.
   B. Diagnostic measures
      1. Excisional lymph node biopsy required
      2. Presence of Reed–Sternberg cells on pathologic examination with cHL
      3. Fluorodeoxyglucose positive emission tomography (FDG-PET)±radiographic studies (contrast computed tomography [CT] of the chest, abdomen, and pelvis); FDG-PET shown to be an important tool in staging to support treatment selection and monitoring treatment response
      4. Bone marrow biopsy may be required for accurate staging
      5. Immunohistochemistry and cytogenetic evaluation

6. HIV testing and additional testing based on recommended treatment plan (e.g., evaluation of ejection fraction and pulmonary function tests)

VI. Histopathology (Kaseb, 2022; Martig, 2022; O'Malley et al., 2019; Swerdlow et al., 2016)
   A. 95% HL are cHL, which includes four subtypes: nodular sclerosis HL, mixed-cellularity HL, lymphocyte depletion HL, and lymphocyte-rich cHL.
   B. Typical immunophenotype for cHL is CD15 +, CD30 +, CD25+, PAX-5+, HLA-DR+, ICAM-1+, Fascin+, CD95+, TRAF1+, CD40+, and CD86+.
   C. NLPHL clinicopathologic entity of B-cell origin is distinct from cHL.
   D. Common immunophenotype for NLPHL is CO20+, CD45+, CD79a+, CD75+, BCL+, BOB.1+, OCT2+, and J chain+.
   E. World Health Organization (WHO) classification of lymphoid neoplasms (Box 20.1).

VII. Staging (Ansell, 2018; NCCN, 2022b)
   A. The Lugano classification modification of the Ann Arbor Staging System. Staging based on the extent of disease and the presence of systemic symptoms (B symptoms).
   B. Patients divided into three major prognostic groups that support treatment decisions (Leukemia and Lymphoma Society [LLS], 2022; NCCN, 2022b; NCI, 2022a; NCI, 2022a)
   C. Hodgkin lymphoma prognostic categories by stage and clinical features (Box 20.2)

VIII. Prognosis and survival (Ansell, 2018; NCI, 2022a)
   A. Combination chemotherapy and/or radiation therapy (RT) cures >80% of newly diagnosed HL patients.
   B. Adverse prognostic factors for advanced HL. An International Prognostic Score (IPS) has been defined by the number of adverse prognostic factors identified at diagnosis. The IPS helps support treatment

---

BOX 20.1 2016 WHO Classification of Mature B-Cell, T-Cell, and NK-Cell Neoplasm

Mature B-Cell Neoplasms
Chronic lymphocytic leukemia/small lymphocytic lymphoma
Monoclonal B-cell lymphocytosis
B-cell prolymphocytic leukemia
Splenic marginal zone lymphoma (MZL)
Hairy cell leukemia
Extranodal MZL of mucosa-associated lymphoid tissue lymphoma
Nodal MZL
Follicular lymphoma
   In situ follicular neoplasia
   Duodenal-type follicular lymphoma
Pediatric-type follicular lymphoma
Primary cutaneous follicle center lymphoma
Mantle cell lymphoma
   In situ mantle cell neoplasia
Diffuse large B-cell lymphoma (DLBCL), not otherwise specified (NOS)
   Germinal center B-cell type
   Activated B-cell type
T-cell/histiocyte-rich large B-cell lymphoma
Primary DLBCL of the central nervous system
Primary cutaneous DLBCL, leg type
Epstein–Barr virus (EBV)–positive DLBCL, NOS
DLBCL associated with chronic inflammation
Lymphomatoid granulomatosis
Primary mediastinal (thymic) large B-cell lymphoma
Intravascular large B-cell lymphoma
ALK-positive large B-cell lymphoma
Plasmablastic lymphoma
Primary effusion lymphoma
HHV8-positive DLBCL, NOS
Burkitt lymphoma
High-grade B-cell lymphoma with MYC and BCL2 and/or BCL6 rearrangements
High-grade B-cell lymphoma, NOS

B-cell lymphoma, unclassifiable, with features intermediate between DLBCL and classical Hodgkin lymphoma

Mature T-Cell and NK-Cell Neoplasms
T-cell prolymphocytic leukemia
T-cell large granular lymphocytic leukemia
Aggressive NK-cell leukemia
Systemic EBV-positive T-cell lymphoma of childhood
Hydroa vacciniforme–like lymphoproliferative disorder
Adult T-cell leukemia/lymphoma
Extranodal NK-/T-cell lymphoma, nasal type
Enteropathy-associated T-cell lymphoma
Monomorphic epitheliotropic intestinal T-cell lymphoma
Hepatosplenic T-cell lymphoma
Subcutaneous panniculitis–like T-cell lymphoma
Mycosis fungoides
Sézary syndrome
Primary cutaneous CD30-positive T-cell lymphoproliferative disorders
   Lymphomatoid papulosis
   Primary cutaneous anaplastic large cell lymphoma
Primary cutaneous gamma-delta T-cell lymphoma
Peripheral T-cell lymphoma, NOS
Angioimmunoblastic T-cell lymphoma
Anaplastic large cell lymphoma, ALK-positive
Anaplastic large cell lymphoma, ALK-negative

Hodgkin Lymphoma
Nodular lymphocyte–predominant Hodgkin lymphoma (NLPHL)
Classical HL
   Nodular sclerosis classical HL
   Lymphocyte-rich classical HL
   Mixed-cellularity classical Hodgkin lymphoma
   Lymphocyte-depleted classical Hodgkin lymphoma

Note: Several histologic types were identified as provisional in the 2016 WHO classification system. They have been left out of this box. Plasma cell neoplasms are not included here; see Chapter 21. Two additional categories *not* included are the rare posttransplant lymphoproliferative disorders and histiocytic and dendritic cell neoplasms.
From Swerdlow, S. H., Campo, E., Pileri, S. A., Harris, N. L., Stein, H., Siebert, R., et al. (2016). The 2016 revision of the World Health Organization classification of lymphoid neoplasms. *Blood*, *127*(20), 2375–2390. https://doi.org/10.1182/blood-2016-01-643569.

BOX 20.2 Hodgkin Lymphoma Prognostic Categories by Stage and Clinical Features

- *Early favorable*: Clinical stage I or II without any risk factors
- *Early unfavorable*: Clinical stage I or II with one or more of the following risk factors:
  - Large mediastinal mass (>33% of the thoracic width on the chest radiography; ≥10 cm on CT scan)
  - Extranodal involvement
  - Involvement of three or more lymph node areas
  - Elevated erythrocyte sedimentation rate (≥50 mm/h)
  - B symptoms
- *Advanced*: Clinical stage III or IV with zero to seven adverse risk factors[1]:
  - Male gender
  - Age ≥45 years
  - Albumin level <4.0 g/dL
  - Hemoglobin level <10.5 g/dL
  - Stage IV disease
  - White blood cell (WBC) count ≥15,000/mm³
  - Absolute lymphocytic count <600/mm³ or lymphocyte count that was <8% of the total WBC count

Data from National Cancer Institute (NCI). (2022). *Adult Hodgkin lymphoma treatment (PDQ®)–Health professional version.* https://www.cancer.gov/types/lymphoma/hp/adult-hodgkin-treatment-pdq; National Comprehensive Cancer Network (NCCN). (2022). *Hodgkin lymphoma, version 2.2022.* https://www.nccn.org/professionals/physician_gls/pdf/hodgkins.pdf.

[1] An IPS has been defined by the number of these adverse prognostic factors identified at diagnosis. The IPS helps support treatment decisions and predict prognosis for patients with stage III to IV disease.

decisions and predict prognosis for patients with stage III to IV disease.

Management

A. Standard treatment approaches defined by prognostic groups (Ansell, 2018; Gallamini, 2021; NCCN, 2022b)
  1. Initial therapy based on the histology, anatomic stage, presence of poor prognostic features, "B" symptoms, and bulky disease.
  2. Because this disease often affects young people, the goal of treatment is to avoid preventable long-term side effects while achieving maximum tumor control.
  3. During treatment, FDG-PET scanning supports treatment decisions to complete therapy as planned or add or omit treatment, response-adapted therapy.
  4. Early favorable stages—limited amount of chemotherapy (typically two cycles) plus involved-field radiation.
  5. Unfavorable stages—moderate amount of chemotherapy (typically four cycles) plus involved-field radiation.
  6. Advanced stages—extensive chemotherapy (typically eight cycles), with or without consolidation RT (usually to residual tumors).
  7. Management of relapsed/refractory disease.

  a. High-dose chemotherapy (HDCT) followed by an autologous stem cell (ASCT) transplant
  b. Other options include the drugs everolimus, brentuximab vedotin, bendamustine, tislelizumab, or lenalidomide.
  8. For patients who fail HDCT with ASCT, options include nivolumab, pembrolizumab, or clinical trials.
  9. Survivorship issues and monitoring for long-term effects (see Chapter 3).
  10. Fertility counseling

NON-HODGKIN LYMPHOMA

Overview

I. Definition
  A. Heterogeneous group of lymphoproliferative cancers with a wide range of histologic appearances, clinical features, behavior, and response to treatment.
  B. Diffuse large B-cell lymphoma (DLBCL) is the most common.
II. Epidemiology
  A. Estimated 80,470 new cases diagnosed and 20,250 deaths from non-HL (NHL) in 2022 (ACS, 2022; CDC, 2022).
    1. Incidence rates falling on average 1% each year between 2010 and 2019.
    2. NHL encompasses a wide variety of disease subtypes for which incidence patterns may vary (ACS, 2022).
    3. Twenty-two percent of NHL cases in the United States are follicular lymphoma (FL) (LLS, 2022).
  B. Mortality rates—Ninth most common cause of cancer death (ACS, 2022). 73.8% survive 5 years (NCI, 2022b).
  C. Most frequently diagnosed among people aged 65–74; median age at diagnosis is 67 years (NCI, 2022b).
III. Pathophysiology (DeVita et al., 2018; Sapkota, 2022)
  A. Arises from B cell, T cell, NK cell due to chromosomal translocation, pathogenic variant, deletion.
    1. Translocation (14:18) is the most common in NHL mostly seen in FL.
    2. t(11:14) is associated with mantle cell lymphoma.
    3. t(8:14) is associated with Burkitt lymphoma.
    4. Alterations in BCL2, BCL6, are associated with diffuse large B-cell.
    5. Primary central nervous system (CNS) lymphoma is most commonly associated with HIV/acquired immune deficiency syndrome.
  B. 85%–90% arise from B lymphocytes, the rest from T lymphocytes or NK lymphocytes.
IV. Prevention
  A. Cause of most cases of NHL unknown
  B. Risk factors for NHL (ACS, 2022; American Society for Clinical Oncology [ASCO], 2021)
    1. Age—may occur in children and young adults although the median age of diagnosis is 67

2. Gender—higher in men than in women
3. Obesity
4. Immunodeficiency disorders—inherited, acquired, and solid organ transplantation
5. Infectious agents
   a. Infection with EBV—associated with Burkitt lymphoma
   b. Infection with the human T-cell leukemia virus, type 1 (HTLV-1)—increases the risk for T-cell lymphoma
   c. Hepatitis viruses B and C—seropositivity higher in DLBCL and FL
   d. HIV
   e. *H. pylori* bacterial infection linked to mucosa-associated lymphoid tissue lymphoma in the stomach
6. Environmental and occupational exposure to radiation, chemicals, pesticides, and solvents
7. Breast implants

V. Diagnosis
   A. Clinical presentation
      1. Dependent on the site of involvement and the natural history of the subtype
      2. Painless lymphadenopathy more generalized, less predictable than HL; more commonly spreads to extranodal sites
      3. Other possible symptoms—pruritus, fatigue, abdominal pain (enlarged spleen or liver; bulky adenopathy), bone pain
      4. Involvement of bone marrow, liver, or other extranodal site common; most often presents as disseminated disease
   B. Diagnostic measures (NCI, 2022b; NCCN, 2022a)
      1. Excisional lymph node core biopsy required.
      2. Radiographic studies: CT scan of the neck, chest, abdomen, and pelvis and/or PET scan. MRI of brain and spinal cord; ultrasound (contrast CT of the chest, abdomen, and pelvis) to assess disease burden. PET used for initial staging and for follow-up after therapy as a supplement to CT scanning.
      3. Bone marrow biopsy may be required for accurate staging.
      4. Lumbar puncture.
      5. Immunohistochemistry, cytogenetics, fluorescent in situ hybridization, flow cytometry, polymerase chain reaction, and molecular profiling/gene sequencing evaluation.
      6. HIV and hepatitis B virus testing and additional testing based on a recommended treatment plan (i.e., evaluation of ejection fraction, pulmonary function tests).
      7. Laboratory monitoring (complete blood count, comprehensive metabolic panel, beta-2-microglobulin, lactate dehydrogenase [LDH], uric acid) to monitor for tumor lysis syndrome as therapy initiated.

VI. Histopathology (ASCO, 2021; LLS, 2022; Swerdlow et al., 2016)
   A. New diseases and subtypes added in the updated 2016 WHO classification system

B. Cell of origin B-cell lymphoma about 90%, T cell about 10%, and NK cell less than 1%
C. Divided into indolent and aggressive NHL
D. Further divided into greater than 60 subtypes by precursor lymphocyte versus mature lymphocyte; further refinement based on immunophenotype and genetic and clinical features

VII. Staging
   A. Lugano Classification modification of Ann Arbor Staging System—based on the extent of disease and on which side of the diaphragm (Sapkota, 2022).
      1. Recent analyses show that the presence of systemic symptoms (B symptoms) does not have prognostic significance for NHL.
   B. Most patients with advanced (stage III or stage IV) disease at presentation.

VIII. Prognosis and survival (LLS, 2022; NCI, 2022b; Sapkota, 2022)
   A. Prognosis: NHL prognosis is dependent on histopathology, the extent of disease and patient factors.
      1. The International Prognostic Index (IPI) is the main tool used with NHL.
      2. IPI uses age, LDH, Eastern Cooperative Oncology Group performance status, stage, and extranodal involvement.
      3. Low risk=0–1, intermediate risk=2, poor risk=3 or more.
   B. Survival: NHL can be divided into two prognostic groups: the indolent lymphomas and the aggressive lymphomas.
      1. Low-grade lymphomas have an indolent course with median survival as long as 20 years without aggressive therapy; not considered curable and characterized by recurrences, especially in advanced stages; occasionally can transform into high-grade NHL.
      2. Aggressive or high-grade lymphomas—prognosis depends on tumor bulk, responsiveness to therapy, and patient's ability to tolerate treatment; majority of patients with localized disease curable with radiation plus chemotherapy or combination chemotherapy alone; overall survival at 5 years is over 60%.
         a. Of patients with aggressive NHL, more than 50% can be cured.
         b. Most relapses occur in the first 2 years after therapy.
   C. Relapse—may occur; requires biopsy and restaging.

Management

(Kumar, Pickard, & Okosun, 2021; NCCN, 2022a; NCI, 2022b; Sapkota, 2022)
   A. Therapeutic choices are increasingly tailored to the immunologically classified lymphoma.
   B. The most common NHL types are indolent (FL 20%) and aggressive (DLBCL 30%) NHL; treatment plans are representative for NHL.
   C. Standard treatment options for indolent FL include the following:
      1. For stage I or II disease:
         a. RT to involved site

b. Monoclonal antibodies (rituximab [Rituxan]) alone or in combination with chemotherapy (single-agent or combination therapy)

c. Observation

2. For stage III or IV disease—optimal treatment is controversial, not curative

a. Observation recommended for asymptomatic patients

b. Numerous drug therapy options available, including rituximab, lenalidomide and rituximab, maintenance rituximab, Obinutuzumab alone or in combination with cytotoxic agents, phosphatidylinositol 3-kinase inhibitors, EZH2 inhibitor, radiolabeled anti-CD-20 monoclonal antibodies, alkylating agents, bendamustine, combination therapy

c. RT for palliation of symptomatic disease

D. Intermediate- and high-grade DLBCL are considered systemic disease. Standard treatment options include the following:

1. For stage I or contiguous II disease

a. Chemotherapy with or without involved-field RT (IF-XRT)

b. R-CHOP (rituximab [Rituxan], cyclophosphamide, doxorubicin [Adriamycin], vincristine, and prednisone)

2. Treatment for aggressive, noncontiguous stage II, III, or IV disease:

a. R-CHOP or other combination chemotherapy

b. Antibody–drug conjugates, radiolabeled antibodies, and CD-19 monoclonal antibodies

c. Chimeric antigen receptor T-cell therapy

E. Recurrent NHL

1. Other chemotherapy regimens (single agent or combination)

2. Autologous peripheral blood stem cell (PBSC) or allogeneic PBSC for aggressive NHL

3. Palliative RT

F. CNS prophylaxis for patients at high risk of CNS disease

G. Supportive care

X. Nursing implications

A. An individualized and holistic plan of care is needed when caring for the patient with a lymphoid malignancy.

B. The plan of care is developed and implemented from the shared decision-making in cooperation with the patient, family, and multidisciplinary team.

C. Interventions related to physical, emotional, psychological, social, and spiritual distress during extensive diagnostic testing and treatment regimen.

1. Encourage patient to verbalize feelings about disease and treatment.

2. Explore coping options with the patient and family, and validate effective mechanisms.

3. Refer to mental health specialist, community support groups (Leukemia and Lymphoma Society, American Cancer Society, and adolescent and young adult cancer programs) as needed.

4. Teach patient to identify and manage symptoms and to report symptoms to health care providers.

5. Provide pharmacologic and nonpharmacologic interventions to managing side effects.

D. Interventions related to the prevention of complications

1. Ongoing assessment for potential disease and treatment-related complications is important: tumor lysis syndrome, superior vena cava syndrome, anemia, and infection. The type of complications depends on the subtype of lymphoma, treatment, and patient variables.

2. Long-term survival, especially for young HL patients, results in increased risk for long-term complications; that is, second malignancies, various organ toxicities (pulmonary, cardiac, renal), fatigue, and sexuality/fertility issues. Teach patients about the importance of monitoring for late effects and yearly evaluations (NCCN, 2022b).

REFERENCES

American Cancer Society (ACS). (2022). *Cancer facts & statistics.* https://cancerstatisticscenter.cancer.org/?_ga=2.62051756.1659083569.1654448065-430032959.1653225936&_gac=1.216752612.1654448067.CjwKCAjw4ayUBhA4EiwATWyBrgaitJlamWcLtotquivKtD_2jnFDfzwJVCs6hkgSIIDX9ijXAbAQLhoCVYMQAvD_BwE#!/. Retrieved 05.06.22.

American Society for Clinical Oncology (ASCO). (2021). *Lymphoma – Non-Hodgkin.* https://www.cancer.net/cancer-types/lymphoma-non-hodgkin.

Ansell, S. M. (2018). Hodgkin lymphoma: 2018 update on diagnosis, risk-stratification, and management. *American Journal of Hematology, 93*(5), 704–715. https://doi.org/10.1002/ajh.25071.

Centers for Disease Control and Prevention (CDC). (2022). *Cancer statistics at a glance.* https://gis.cdc.gov/Cancer/USCS/?CDC_AA_refVal=https%3A%2F%2Fwww.cdc.gov%2Fcancer%2Fdataviz%2Findex.htm#/AtAGlance/. Retrieved 02.04.22.

DeVita, V. T., Lawrence, T. S., & Rosenberg, S. A. (2018). *DeVita, Hellman, and Rosenberg's cancer: Principles & practice of oncology.* Alphen aan den Rijn: Wolters Kluwer.

Gallamini, A., & Juweid, M. (Eds.). (2021). *Lymphoma [Internet].* Brisbane: Exon Publications. Available from:. https://www.ncbi.nlm.nih.gov/books/NBK578253/. http://doi.org/10.36255/exon-publications.lymphoma.2021.

Kaseb, H., & Babiker, H. M. (2022). Hodgkin lymphoma. [Updated 2022 Mar 19]. In: *StatPearls [Internet].* Treasure Island, FL: StatPearls Publishing. Available from: https://www.ncbi.nlm.nih.gov/books/NBK499969/.

Kumar, E., Pickard, L., & Okosun, J. (2021). Pathogenesis of follicular lymphoma: Genetics to the microenvironment to clinical translation. *British Journal of Haematology, 194*(5), 810–821. https://doi.org/10.1111/bjh.17383.

Leukemia and Lymphoma Society (LLS). (2022). *NHL subtypes.* https://www.lls.org/lymphoma/non-hodgkin-lymphoma/nhl-subtypes. Retrieved 02.04.22.

Martig, D. S., & Fromm, J. R. (2022). A comparison and review of the flow cytometric findings in classic Hodgkin lymphoma, nodular lymphocyte predominant Hodgkin lymphoma, T cell/histiocyte rich large B cell lymphoma, and primary mediastinal large B cell lymphoma. *Cytometry Part B: Clinical Cytometry, 102*(1), 14–25. https://doi.org/10.1002/cyto.b.22045.

National Cancer Institute (NCI). (2022a). *Hodgkin lymphoma – Cancer stat facts. SEER.* https://seer.cancer.gov/statfacts/html/hodg.html. Retrieved 02.04.22.

National Cancer Institute (NCI). (2022b). *Non-Hodgkin lymphoma – cancer stat facts. SEER.* https://seer.cancer.gov/statfacts/html/nhl.html. Retrieved 02.04.22.

National Comprehensive Cancer Network (NCCN). (2022a). *NCCN clinical practice guidelines in oncology (NCCN Guidelines®) B-cell lymphomas, version 3.2022—April 25, 2022.* NCCN. https://www.nccn.org/professionals/physician_gls/pdf/b-cell.pdf Retrieved 08.02.23.

National Comprehensive Cancer Network (NCCN). (2022b). *NCCN Guidelines® insights: Hodgkin lymphoma, version 2.2022* .

https://jnccn.org/view/journals/jnccn/20/4/article-p322.xml. Retrieved 07.05.22.

O'Malley, D. P., Dogan, A., Fedoriw, Y., Medeiros, L. J., Ok, C. Y., & Salama, M. E. (2019). American Registry of Pathology expert opinions: Immunohistochemical evaluation of classic Hodgkin lymphoma. *Annals of Diagnostic Pathology, 39*, 105–110. https://doi.org/10.1016/j.anndiagpath.2019.02.001.

Sapkota, S., & Shaikh, H. (2022). Non-Hodgkin lymphoma. [Updated 2022 May 1]. In: *StatPearls [Internet].* Treasure Island, FL: StatPearls Publishing. Available from https://www.ncbi.nlm.nih.gov/books/NBK559328/.

Swerdlow, S. H., Campo, E., Pileri, S. A., Harris, N. L., Stein, H., Siebert, R., et al. (2016). The 2016 revision of the World Health Organization classification of lymphoid neoplasms. *Blood, 127*(20), 2375–2390. https://doi.org/10.1182/blood-2016-01-643569.

21

Multiple Myeloma

Laura B. LaRose

OVERVIEW

I. Definition
   A. Multiple myeloma (MM) is a malignancy of plasma cells that ultimately results in damage to the bone marrow and renal failure (Padala et al., 2021).

II. Epidemiology
   A. In the United States, an estimated 34,470 new cases diagnosed and 12,640 deaths from MM in 2022 (Siegel, Miller, Fuchs, & Jemal, 2022)
      1. Highest incidence among men, Blacks, and older adults (National Cancer Institute, 2021)
   B. Second most common hematologic malignancy in the United States; constitutes approximately 1.8% of all new cancers (National Cancer Institute, 2021; Siegel et al., 2022)
      1. Incidence has increased globally by 126% and by 40% in the United States since 1990 (Padala et al., 2021).
   C. Risk factors
      1. Older age—most are diagnosed between 65 and 74 with fewer than 14% of cases being diagnosed before age 55 (National Cancer Institute, 2021).
      2. Race—MM is twice as common among Blacks (Padala et al., 2021).
         a. MM is the leading hematologic malignancy among Blacks (Pierre & Williams, 2020).
      3. Sex—globally, MM is 1.5× more common among men (Padala et al., 2021).
      4. Environmental exposures have been linked to MM (Cordas dos Santos, Erickson, Gerland, Jundt, & Theurich, 2020; Korde, Mailankody, Kazandjian, & Landgren, 2019).
      5. Family history, though germline pathogenic variants have yet to be identified (Padala et al., 2021).
      6. Obesity (American Cancer Society [ACS], 2022; Cordas dos Santos et al., 2020)
      7. History of monoclonal gammopathy of undetermined significance (MGUS)
         a. MGUS is present in about 3%–7% of the population over age 50 (Padala et al., 2021; Rajkumar, 2020).

III. Pathophysiology
   A. MM is a malignancy of the plasma cells (terminally differentiated B cells) that results in the production of a complete or partial monoclonal immunoglobulin protein, resulting in osteolytic bone lesions, renal disease, anemia, hypercalcemia, and immunodeficiency (Lichtman et al., 2017).
      1. The accumulation of Bence-Jones proteins in the urine can lead to kidney damage and ultimately kidney failure (Padala et al., 2021)
      2. Osteoclasts are activated by MM through *receptor activator of NF-κβ ligand* resulting in bone destruction (Padala et al., 2021).
   B. MM develops over time from many complex genetic acts (Noonan, 2021).
   C. MM is nearly always preceded by MGUS.
      1. The risk for transformation from MGUS to MM increases by about 1% every year (Korde et al., 2019).
   D. Smoldering MM (SMM) is a clinical stage between MGUS and symptomatic MM.
      1. The risk of transforming to active MM is about 10% per year during the first 5 years after diagnosis with a median time to progression of about 5 years (Bolli et al., 2021).
   E. Hypercalcemia, renal impairment, anemia, and osteolytic bone lesions, a constellation known as CRAB symptoms, are common presentations of MM (Noonan, 2021).
   F. While MM is referred to as a single disease, it is a collection of many different cytogenetically unique plasma cell malignancies (Rajkumar, 2020).

IV. Primary Prevention (Cordas dos Santos et al., 2020)
   A. Maintain a healthy weight
      1. Being overweight or obese increases the risk for MM by 12%–21%.
   B. Limit occupational exposure to certain chemicals (asbestos, benzene, pesticides, and other chemicals used in rubber manufacturing) or ionizing radiation.
   C. Consume a diet rich in fruits and whole grains.
   D. No proven link between MM and tobacco use or alcohol consumption.
   E. Physical activity not shown to be preventative for MM, but can help with symptom management of those with the disease.

V. Diagnosis
   A. Diagnosis is based on clinical, radiologic, and biologic findings (Noonan, 2021).

B. Initial diagnostic workup to include (Korde et al., 2019; National Comprehensive Cancer Network [NCCN], 2022)

1. History and physical exam
2. Complete blood count with differential
3. Serum BUN/creatinine, electrolytes, liver function tests, uric acid, creatinine clearance
4. Serum lactate dehydrogenase (LDH), albumin, and beta-2 microglobulin (all essential for staging)
5. Serum quantitative immunoglobulins, serum protein electrophoresis, serum immunofixation electrophoresis, and free light chain assay
6. 24-hour urine for total protein, urine protein electrophoresis, and urine immunofixation electrophoresis
7. Whole-body low-dose CT or FDG PET/CT
   a. Skeletal survey is less sensitive but is acceptable in certain circumstances.
   b. If CT or PET/CT negative, consider whole-body MRI to discern smoldering myeloma from MM.
8. Unilateral bone marrow aspirate and biopsy including immunohistochemistry, cytogenetics, and fluorescence in situ hybridization (FISH)
   a. Evaluate for t(11;14), t(4;14), t(14;16), t(6;14), t(14;20), trisomies, del(17p) (Rajkumar, 2020).

C. Major and minor criteria needed to confirm the diagnosis of MM, determine staging, and differentiate from SMM, MGUS, and other plasma cell disorders (Kehrer, Koob, Strauss, Wirtz, & Schmolders, 2017)

1. MGUS (Noonan, 2021)
   a. Diagnosis of exclusion after SMM and MM ruled out
   b. Serum monoclonal protein <3 g/dL
   c. Urinary protein (Bence-Jones protein) <500 mg/24 h
   d. Bone marrow plasma cells <10%
   e. Absence of myeloma-defining events (MDE)
2. SMM (asymptomatic) (Rajkumar et al., 2014)
   a. Serum monoclonal protein ≥3 g/dL OR
   b. Urinary protein (Bence-Jones protein) ≥500 mg/24 h AND/OR
   c. Clonal bone marrow plasma cells 10%–59% AND
   d. Absence of amyloidosis MDE
3. MM (Rajkumar et al., 2014)
   a. Clonal bone marrow plasma cells ≥10% or extramedullary plasmacytoma
   b. At least one MDE
4. Differential could also include solitary plasmacytoma, POEMS syndrome, and systemic amyloidosis

D. MDE (Rajkumar et al., 2014)

1. Evidence of end organ damage attributable to underlying plasma cell disorder (CRAB features):
   a. Hypercalcemia—>1 mg/dL higher than upper limit of normal or >11 mg/dL
   b. Renal insufficiency—creatinine >2 mg/dL or creatinine clearance <40 mL/min

c. Anemia—hemoglobin <10 g/dL or >2 g/dL below the lower limit of normal
d. Osteolytic bone lesions

2. Biomarkers of malignancy
   a. Clonal bone marrow plasma cell percentage ≥60%
   b. Involved: uninvolved serum-free light-chain ratio ≥100
   c. >1 focal lesion on MRI of at least 5 mm

VI. Histopathology

A. Several signaling pathways lead to myeloma progression which are complex, interdependent, and overlapping (Noonan, 2021).
B. Translocation involving immunoglobulin heavy chain gene locus or hyperdiploidy gain drives the development of MM (van de Donk, Pawlyn, & Yong, 2021).
C. Myeloma cells classified into four types (Fujino, 2018):
   1. Mature—nearly identical to normal cells
   2. Immature—irregular nucleus, prominent nucleoli
   3. Pleomorphic—increased nuclear polymorphism, prominent nucleoli
   4. Plasmablastic—resemble diffuse large B-cell lymphoma
D. Patterns in which myeloma infiltrates bone marrow (Fujino, 2018)
   1. Nodular—displace cells forming nodular lesion in marrow
   2. Interstitial—form in a cluster and infiltrate individual spaces between normal cells
   3. Diffuse—large number of cells diffusely infiltrate marrow
E. Multiple gene abnormalities are responsible for the development and progression of MM (Fujino, 2018).

VII. Staging

A. Previous staging systems include Durie–Salmon Staging System (DSS) and International Staging System (ISS), both of which measure tumor burden, but neither take into account chromosomal abnormalities which can ultimately determine overall survival (OS) (Noonan, 2021; Padala et al., 2021).

1. DSS (stages I–III)—quantifies tumor volume on the basis of the amount of M proteins in urine and blood, along with clinical parameters, hemoglobin, serum calcium level, and presence of bone lesions (Durie & Salmon, 1975).
   a. More subjective, so reproducibility can be problematic (Noonan, 2021)
2. ISS (stages I–III) is based on laboratory values—serum beta-2 microglobulin and albumin (Greipp et al., 2005):
   a. Stage I—serum beta-2 microglobulin <3.5 mg/L, albumin ≥3.5 g/dL
   b. Stage II—not stage I or III
   c. Stage III—serum beta-2 microglobulin ≥5.5 mg/L
   d. Can be confounded by other health problems not specific to MM (Noonan, 2021)

B. In 2015 the International Myeloma Working Group developed the Revised ISS (R-ISS), combining both tumor burden and biomarkers to better reflect prognosis and response to treatment (Palumbo et al., 2015).

1. Stage I—ISS stage I and standard-risk chromosomal abnormalities by FISH and normal LDH
2. Stage II—not R-ISS stage I or III
3. Stage III—ISS stage III and either high-risk chromosomal abnormalities by FISH or high LDH
   a. LDH
      (1) Normal—serum LDH<the upper limit of normal
      (2) High—serum LDH>the upper limit of normal
   b. Chromosomal abnormalities by FISH
      (1) High risk—presence of del(17p) and/or translocations t(4;14) and/or t(14;16)
      (2) Standard risk—no high-risk chromosomal abnormalities

C. R-ISS is a more complete and objective way to stage newly diagnosed MM (Noonan, 2021).

VIII. Prognosis and survival

A. Survival has improved significantly over the last two decades, with an overall 5-year survival in the United States of 55.6% (National Cancer Institute, 2021).

B. No cure currently exists for MM, but increases in OS are due to the ongoing development of new therapies and a better understanding of the disease (Noonan, 2021).

C. R-ISS staging uses prognostic factors to help predict patient survival (Palumbo et al., 2015).

1. R-ISS stage I—82% 5-year OS rate
2. R-ISS stage II—62%
3. R-ISS stage III—40%

D. MM has one of the highest number of prognostic factors of any malignancy including factors related to patient, tumor load, cytogenetics (Corre, Munshi, & Avet-Loiseau, 2021).

1. Response to treatment is a significant prognostic factor—early relapse after intensive first-line therapy negatively affects survival (Corre et al., 2021).
2. Specific gene abnormalities are important indicators of prognosis (Fujino, 2018).
   a. Cytogenetics associated with shorter survival included del(17p), del(1p32), gain 1q, t(4;14), and trisomy 21 (Corre et al., 2021).
3. Age, comorbidities, and performance status are important prognostic factors that are not included in R-ISS staging system (Palumbo et al., 2015).
4. High-risk patients have an OS of less than 3 years (Noonan, 2021).

E. While race plays a large factor in one's risk of developing MM, studies have not shown race to make a difference in OS (Padala et al., 2021).

1. Disparities in care and outcomes do exist among racial subgroups likely due to unequal access to treatment (Ailawadhi et al., 2018).

MANAGEMENT

(NCCN, 2022)

I. Medical Management

A. Solitary plasmacytoma—treated with radiation therapy (RT) ± surgical removal
B. SMM—consider lenalidomide in certain patients with high-risk disease; otherwise strongly consider clinical trial or observation
C. Treatment options are based on patient's eligibility for stem cell transplant (SCT) (NCCN, 2022; Table 21.1).
   1. Standard therapy remains using two drugs+steroid (triplet regimen) unless performance status prohibits.

TABLE 21.1 Chemotherapy Agents for Multiple Myeloma (NCCN, 2022)

Population/ Treatment Phase	Preferred	Other recommended Options
Primary therapy for transplant candidates (avoid myelotoxic agents including alkylating agents and nitrosoureas which compromise stem cell reserve)	Bortezomib/ lenalidomide/ dexamethasone (category 1) Carfilzomib/ lenalidomide/ dexamethasone	Daratumumab/lenalidomide/ bortezomib/dexamethasone
Maintenance therapy for transplant candidates	Lenalidomide (category 1)	Bortezomib Daratumumab Ixazomib (category 2B)
Primary therapy for non-transplant candidates	Bortezomib/ lenalidomide/ dexamethasone (category 1) Daratumumab/ lenalidomide/ dexamethasone (category 1)	Daratumumab/bortezomib/ melphalan/prednisone (category 1) Carfilzomib/lenalidomide/ dexamethasone Daratumumab/ cyclophosphamide/ bortezomib/dexamethasone Ixazomib/lenalidomide/ dexamethasone
Maintenance therapy for non-transplant candidates	Lenalidomide (category 1)	Bortezomib Ixazomib (category 2B)

a. First-line setting usually includes immunomodulatory drugs (IMiDs) and proteasome inhibitors.

b. Lenalidomide, bortezomib, and dexamethasone are the most recommended regimen.

2. Consider dose modifications based on age and performance status.

D. High-dose chemotherapy followed by autologous SCT remains the standard treatment for newly diagnosed MM in eligible patients (Attal et al., 2017).

1. Tandem SCT—planned second course of high-dose therapy and SCT within 6 months of the first course. May be an option as salvage therapy for relapse or progressive disease (Koniarczyk, Ferraro, & Miceli, 2017)

a. Allogeneic SCT—an option as part of a clinical trial or salvage therapy in patients with progressive disease

E. Maintenance therapies with lenalidomide (Pulte et al., 2018) or bortezomib are being evaluated; maintenance therapy is beneficial for improving progression-free survival and OS (Chakraborty et al., 2018).

F. Treatment for relapsed or refractory MM are complex, and providers should consider both disease- and patient-related factors (Cook, Zweegman, Mateos, Suzan, & Moreau, 2018).

1. For relapses that occur greater than 6 months, the same regimen may be repeated; otherwise a new triplet therapy should include drugs or drug classes to which the patient is naïve.

2. Drug classes in this setting include histone deacetylase inhibitor, monoclonal antibodies, and second-generation IMiDs (Cook et al., 2018).

3. Allogeneic SCT may be an option as part of a clinical trial or salvage therapy in patients with relapsed or refractory disease.

G. Supportive care

1. Bone disease

a. Bisphosphonates or denosumab for 2 years

(1) Baseline dental exam and monitor for osteonecrosis of the jaw

(2) Closely monitor renal function on bisphosphonates

b. RT for painful lesions or spinal cord compression (SCC); SCC is a structural oncologic emergency

c. Orthopedic consultation for cord compression, vertebral instability, fractures (impending or actual)

2. Hypercalcemia

a. Hydration, bisphosphonates or denosumab, steroids, calcitonin

3. Anemia

a. Erythropoietin-stimulating agents

4. Infection

a. Pneumococcal vaccination

b. Intravenous immunoglobulin

c. Prophylaxis for opportunistic infections related to high-dose steroids, including *Pneumocystis jiroveci* pneumonia, herpes zoster, and fungal infections

5. Venous thromboembolism (VTE)

a. Consider patient's risk for VTE based on factors pertaining to individual risk (previous VTE, pelvic fractures), risk related to patient's disease and treatment (IMiD, high-dose dexamethasone).

b. Patients at highest risk for VTE in first 6 months following new MM diagnosis.

c. Consider aspirin for low-risk patients, and prophylactic anticoagulation for patients at high risk for VTE.

6. Renal dysfunction

a. Provide hydration and monitor fluid status.

b. Treat metabolic abnormalities (hypercalcemia, hyperuricemia).

c. Discontinue nephrotoxic medications and renally dose other medications.

II. Nursing considerations (Brigle et al., 2017; Faiman et al., 2017; Rome, Noonan, Bertolotti, Tariman, & Miceli, 2017)

A. Individualized, holistic, and evidence-based plan of care for patients with lymphoid malignancy

B. Develop and implement the plan of care with the patient, family, and multidisciplinary team

C. Interventions related to physical, emotional, psychological, social, and spiritual distress during extensive diagnostic testing and treatment regimen

1. Encourage patient to verbalize feelings about disease and treatment.

2. Explore coping options with the patient and family and validate effective mechanisms.

3. Refer to mental health specialists, community resources, support groups (Leukemia and Lymphoma Society, American Cancer Society, International Myeloma Foundation), as needed.

4. Teach patient and family to identify, manage, and report symptoms.

5. Provide pharmacologic and nonpharmacologic interventions to manage the side effect.

D. Interventions related to the prevention of complication

1. Ongoing assessment for potential disease and treatment-related complications: tumor lysis syndrome, superior vena cava syndrome, hypercalcemia, hyperviscosity, renal impairment, skeleton-related events, anemia, infection, cardiac toxicity, and coagulation disorders

REFERENCES

Ailawadhi, S., Jacobus, S., Sexton, R., Stewart, A. K., Dispenzieri, A., Hussein, M. A., et al. (2018). Disease and outcome disparities in multiple myeloma: Exploring the role of race/ethnicity in the Cooperative Group clinical trials. *Blood Cancer Journal*, 8(7), 67. https://doi.org/10.1038/s41408-018-0102-7.

American Cancer Society. (2022). *Cancer facts & figures 2022*. Atlanta, GA: Author. Retrieved from https://www.cancer.org/content/dam/cancer-org/research/cancer-facts-and-statistics/annual-cancer-facts-and-figures/2022/2022-cancer-facts-and-figures.pdf.

Attal, M., Lauwers-Cances, V., Hulin, C., Leleu, X., Caillot, D., Escoffre, M., et al. (2017). Lenalidomide, bortezomib, and dexamethasone with transplantation for myeloma. *New England Journal of Medicine, 376*(14), 1311–1320. https://doi.org/10.1056/NEJMoa1611750.

Bolli, N., Sgherza, N., Curci, P., Rizzi, R., Strafella, V., Delia, M., et al. (2021). What is new in the treatment of smoldering multiple myeloma? *Journal of Clinical Medicine, 10*(3), 421. https://doi.org/10.3390/jcm10030421.

Brigle, K., Pierre, A., Finley-Oliver, E., Faiman, B., Tariman, J. D., & Miceli, T. (2017). Myelosuppression, bone disease, and acute renal failure: Evidence-based recommendations for oncologic emergencies. *Clinical Journal of Oncology Nursing, 21*(5), 60–76. https://doi.org/10.1188/17.CJON.S5.60-76.

Chakraborty, R., Muchtar, E., Kumar, S. K., Buadi, F. K., Dingli, D., Dispenzieri, A., et al. (2018). Outcomes of maintenance therapy with lenalidomide or bortezomib in multiple myeloma in the setting of early autologous stem cell transplantation. *Leukemia, 32*(3), 712–718. https://doi.org/10.1038/leu.2017.256.

Cook, G., Zweegman, S., Mateos, M.-V., Suzan, F., & Moreau, P. (2018). A question of class: Treatment options for patients with relapsed and/or refractory multiple myeloma. *Critical Reviews in Oncology/Hematology, 121*, 74–89. https://doi.org/10.1016/j.critrevonc.2017.11.016.

Cordas dos Santos, D., Erickson, N., Gerland, L., Jundt, F., & Theurich, S. (2020). Primär- und sekundärprävention des multiplen myeloms – Lebensstilfaktoren und supportivmaßnahmen [Primary and secondary prevention of multiple myeloma – Lifestyle factors and supportive measures]. *Deutsche medizinische wochenschrift [German Medical Weekly], 145*(12), 836–842. https://doi.org/10.1055/a-1221-3527.

Corre, J., Munshi, N. C., & Avet-Loiseau, H. (2021). Risk factors in multiple myeloma: Is it time for a revision? *Blood, 137*(1), 16–19. https://doi.org/10.1182/blood.2019004309.

Durie, B. G., & Salmon, S. E. (1975). A clinical staging system for multiple myeloma. Correlation of measured myeloma cell mass with presenting clinical features, response to treatment, and survival. *Cancer, 36*(3), 842–854.

Faiman, B., Doss, D., Colson, K., Mangan, P., King, T., & Tariman, J. D. (2017). Renal, GI, and peripheral nerves: Evidence-based recommendations for the management of symptoms and care for patients with multiple myeloma. *Clinical Journal of Oncology Nursing, 21*(5), 19–36. https://doi.org/10.1188/17.CJON.S5.19-36.

Fujino, M. (2018). The histopathology of myeloma in the bone marrow. *Journal of Clinical and Experimental Hematopathology, 58*(2), 61–67. https://doi.org/10.3960/jslrt.18014.

Greipp, P. R., San Miguel, J., Durie, B. G. M., Crowley, J. J., Barlogie, B., Bladé, J., et al. (2005). International staging system for multiple myeloma. *Journal of Clinical Oncology, 23*(15), 3412–3420. https://doi.org/10.1200/JCO.2005.04.242.

Kehrer, M., Koob, S., Strauss, A., Wirtz, D. C., & Schmolders, J. (2017). Multiples myelom – Aktuelle standards in diagnostik und therapie [Multiple myeloma – Current status in diagnostic testing and therapy]. *Zeitschrift für orthopädie und unfallchirurgie, 155*(5), 575–586. https://doi.org/10.1055/s-0043-110224.

Koniarczyk, H. L., Ferraro, C., & Miceli, T. (2017). Hematopoietic stem cell transplantation for multiple myeloma. *Seminars in Oncology Nursing, 33*(3), 265–278. https://doi.org/10.1016/j.soncn.2017.05.004.

Korde, N., Mailankody, S., Kazandjian, D., & Landgren, O. (2019). Multiple myeloma. In G. P. Rodgers & N. S. Young (Eds.), *The Bethesda handbook of clinical hematology* (4th ed., pp. 252–267). Alphen aan den Rijn: Wolters Kluwer.

Lichtman, M. A., Kaushansky, K., Prchal, J. T., Levi, M. M., Burns, L. J., & Armitage, J. O. (2017). In K. Edmonson & H. Liebowitz (Eds.), *Williams manual of hematology* (9th ed.). New York: McGraw-Hill Education.

National Cancer Institute. (2021). *SEER cancer stat facts: Myeloma.* Bethesda, MD: National Cancer Institute. https://seer.cancer.gov/statfacts/html/mulmy.html.

National Comprehensive Cancer Network (NCCN). (2022). NCCN clinical practice guidelines in oncology: Multiple myeloma, version 5.2022 February 9, 2022. https://www.nccn.org/professionals/physician_gls/pdf/myeloma.pdf.

Noonan, K. (2021). Pathobiology, epidemiology, and diagnosis of multiple myeloma. In B. Faiman & J. D. Tariman (Eds.), *Multiple myeloma: A textbook for nurses* (pp. 9–37). Pittsburgh, PA: Oncology Nursing Society.

Padala, S. A., Barsouk, A., Barsouk, A., Rawla, P., Vakiti, A., Kolhe, R., et al. (2021). Epidemiology, staging, and management of multiple myeloma. *Medical Sciences, 9*(1), 3. https://doi.org/10.3390/medsci9010003.

Palumbo, A., Avet-Loiseau, H., Oliva, S., Lokhorst, H. M., Goldschmidt, H., Rosinol, L., et al. (2015). Revised international staging system for multiple myeloma: A report from International Myeloma Working Group. *Journal of Clinical Oncology, 33*(26), 2863–2869. https://doi.org/10.1200/JCO.2015.61.2267.

Pierre, A., & Williams, T. H. (2020). African American patients with multiple myeloma: Optimizing care to decrease racial disparities. *Clinical Journal of Oncology Nursing, 24*(4), 439–443. https://doi.org/10.1188/20.CJON.439-443.

Pulte, E. D., Dmytrijuk, A., Nie, L., Goldberg, K. B., McKee, A. E., Farrell, A. T., et al. (2018). FDA approval summary: Lenalidomide as maintenance therapy after autologous stem cell transplant in newly diagnosed multiple myeloma. *Oncologist, 23*(6), 734–739. https://doi.org/10.1634/theoncologist.2017-0440.

Rajkumar, S. V. (2020). Multiple myeloma: 2020 update on diagnosis, risk-stratification and management. *American Journal of Hematology, 95*(5), 548–567. https://doi.org/10.1002/ajh.25791.

Rajkumar, S. V., Dimopoulos, M. A., Palumbo, A., Blade, J., Merlini, G., Mateos, M.-V., et al. (2014). International Myeloma Working Group updated criteria for the diagnosis of multiple myeloma. *The Lancet, 15*(12), e538–e548. https://doi.org/10.1016/S1470-2045(14)70442-5.

Rome, S., Noonan, K. A., Bertolotti, P. A., Tariman, J. D., & Miceli, T. (2017). Bone health, pain, and mobility: Evidence-based recommendations for patients with multiple myeloma. *Clinical Journal of Oncology Nursing, 21*(5), 47–59. https://doi.org/10.1188/17.CJON.S5.47-59.

Siegel, R. L., Miller, K. D., Fuchs, H. E., & Jemal, A. (2022). Cancer statistics, 2022. *CA: A Cancer Journal for Clinicians, 72*(1), 7–33. https://doi.org/10.3322/caac.21708.

van de Donk, N. W. C. J., Pawlyn, C., & Yong, K. L. (2021). Multiple myeloma. *The Lancet, 397*(10272), 410–427. https://doi.org/10.1016/S0140-6736(21)00135-5.

22

Myelofibrosis

Kathryn Johnson

OVERVIEW

I. Definition
   A. Myelofibrosis (MF) is a rare, chronic, and progressive blood cancer. The World Health Organization classifies MF as a BCR-ABL negative myeloproliferative neoplasm (MPN), and MF is often grouped together with essential thrombocythemia (ET) and polycythemia vera (PV) and referred to as JAK2 MPNs (Tefferi, 2021, p. 146).
   B. MF can occur as a primary disease type or secondary to ET and/or PV referred to as post-ET MF and post-PV MF, respectively (Mascarenhas, Najfeld, Kremyanskaya, & Keyzner, 2018, p. 1125; Tefferi, 2021, pp. 145–146).
   C. Primary MF is characterized by clonal proliferation of myeloid stem cells, abnormal megakaryocyte production, fibrosis or scarring of the bone marrow, hepatosplenomegaly, anemia, thrombocytopenia, presence or acquisition of driver mutations, and constitutional symptoms (Mascarenhas et al., 2018, p. 1125; Tefferi, 2021, pp. 145–146).
   D. On an average, MF progresses over several years, though the clinical course may vary widely depending upon individual patient presentation.
II. Epidemiology
   A. Primary MF is estimated to occur in an average of 1 in 100,000 persons in the United States annually, with some studies suggesting a range of up to 1.3 in 100,000 persons (Mascarenhas et al., 2018; Mehta, Wang, Iqbal, & Mesa, 2014).
   B. Post-ET MF and post-PV MF may affect up to 15% of patients with a primary diagnosis of ET or PV in their lifetime (Tefferi, 2021).
      1. Incidence of post-ET MF is estimated to be similar to that of Primary MF with up to 1.1 in 100,000 persons annually (Mehta et al., 2014).
      2. Post-PV MF has a slightly lower incidence at up 0.7 cases per 100,000 annually (Mehta et al., 2014).
   C. Risk factors:
      1. MF is most often diagnosed in persons older than 50 years, with an average age at diagnosis of about 65–67 years (Leukemia and Lymphoma Society, 2021; National Organization for Rare Disorders [NORD], 2018).

      2. There are no known additional risks based on lifestyle or environmental factors, gender, race, or ethnicity (NORD, 2018).
III. Pathophysiology
   A. Mutations in DNA alter normal cell development and function of multiple cell types deriving from myeloid stem cells including red blood cells, white blood cells, and platelets.
      1. There are three primary or driver mutations including JAK2, CALR, and MPL which contribute to pathologic function of MF for a majority of patients (Gangat & Tefferi, 2020). Additional mutations including ASXL1, IDH1/2, EZH2, and SRSF2 are considered high-risk and may factor into patient prognosis (Guglielmelli et al., 2018).
   B. Abnormal megakaryocyte production, referred to as megakaryocyte hyperplasia, is a hallmark of MF and leads to the overactivation of inflammatory cytokines and the development of bone marrow fibrosis (Gangat & Tefferi, 2020).
      1. Bone marrow fibrosis, or scarring, progressively disrupts normal marrow function and further alters the bone marrow's production of myeloid cells.
   C. Spleen and liver biopsy results may demonstrate evidence of extramedullary hematopoiesis (Mascarenhas et al., 2018).
IV. Histopathology
   A. Biopsy pathology results may show alterations in cellularity, possibly hypercellular or hypocellular (Mascarenhas et al., 2018).
   B. Marrow fibrosis is scored on a scale of 0, 1, 2, or 3 in ascending order of density. A score of 0 represents the absence of fibrosis, and a score of 3 represents a maximum density of fibrotic tissue (Mascarenhas et al., 2018).
   C. Blasts in either the bone marrow or peripheral blood smear should not exceed 10% in chronic phase and may be between 10% and 19% in blast or accelerated phase MF (Marcellino & Mascarenhas, 2019).
V. Clinical presentation (Mascarenhas et al., 2018)
   A. MF has a heterogenous presentation
      1. Symptoms may include the following:
         a. Fatigue
         b. Bone pain

c. Early satiety

d. General abdominal discomfort

e. Pain localized to the left upper quadrant of the abdomen

f. Itching

g. Night sweats

h. Neuropathy

i. Difficulty concentrating

2. Physical exam

a. Cachexia

b. Hepatosplenomegaly

c. Pallor

d. Ecchymoses, petechiae, and/or purpura

B. Laboratory

1. Complete blood count (CBC)

a. Anemia

b. Thrombocytopenia

c. Leukocytosis

d. Leukopenia

e. Neutropenia

2. Elevated lactate dehydrogenase (LDH)

3. Elevated uric acid

4. Elevated or decreased erythropoietin (EPO)

VI. Diagnosis and staging

A. Diagnostic evaluation for MF should include the following components (Tefferi, 2021):

1. Laboratory:

a. CBC with differential

b. LDH

c. EPO

d. Peripheral blood smear

e. Bone marrow biopsy

f. If and when available, genetic testing includes the following:

(1) Cytogenetics

(2) Neogenomics

(3) Flow cytometry

2. Physical exam including measurement of palpable spleen and liver size if hepatosplenomegaly present

3. Radiographic imaging including ultrasound, computed tomography, and/or magnetic resonance imaging as indicated for hepatosplenomegaly

VII. Prognosis and survival

A. Allogeneic hematopoietic stem cell transplant (HSCT) is the only known curative treatment for MF (Tefferi, 2021).

B. Overall survival for patients with primary MF is estimated to be about 7 years from diagnosis (Mascarenhas et al., 2018, p. 1139).

C. Median overall survival for patients with post-ET and post-PV MF is dependent upon karyotype and ranges from 2 to 6 years (Passamonti, Mora, Barraco, & Maffioli, 2018, p. 177).

MANAGEMENT

I. Medical Management

Etc.

II. Nursing Considerations

A. Management of MF is often driven by and adapted to each patient's clinical presentation and risk category as determined by prognostic scoring systems including International Prognostic Scoring System (IPSS), Dynamic International Prognostic Scoring System (DIPSS), and Mutation-enhanced International Prognostic Scoring System (MIPSS) (Gangat & Tefferi, 2020; Tefferi, 2021).

B. Treatment strategies may include:

1. Low-risk patients may follow "watch-and-wait" treatment strategy with diligent clinical observation in favor of systemic therapy (National Cancer Comprehensive Network [NCCN], 2022).

2. HSCT is the only curative treatment available for MF and should be considered for high-risk patients. However, not all patients are candidates for transplant, and there is significant morbidity and mortality associated with HSCT. Posttransplant survival may be as low as 50% (Tefferi, 2021, pp. 149–151).

3. Janus kinase (JAK) inhibitors are the first-line therapy for intermediate and high-risk MF, and some low-risk MF patients (NCCN, 2022).

a. Ruxolitinib

b. Fedratinib

c. Pacritinib

4. Clinical trials

a. As curative treatments are not available, clinical trials with potentially disease-modifying agents are recommended for patients with MF, especially for those patients who are refractory to treatment with JAK inhibitors (NCCN, 2022; Tremblay & Mascarenhas, 2021).

5. Other systemic therapy (NCCN, 2022; Tefferi, 2021)

a. Corticosteroids

b. Androgen therapies (NCCN, 2022; Tefferi, 2021)

(1) Danazol

c. Cytoreductive therapy (NCCN, 2022; Tefferi, 2021)

(1) Hydroxyurea

(2) Pegylated interferon alfa 2a

d. Immunomodulators (NCCN, 2022; Tefferi, 2021)

(1) Thalidomide

(2) Lenalidomide

(3) Pomalidomide

6. Supportive care for anemia and thrombocytopenia

a. Red blood cell and platelet transfusion (NCCN, 2022; Tefferi, 2021)

b. Corticosteroids (NCCN, 2022; Mascarenhas et al., 2018)

      c. Clinical trial (NCCN, 2022)

      d. EPO stimulating agents

         (1) Darbepoetin alfa

         (2) EPO

    7. Splenectomy and splenic radiation may be considered for some patients (Tefferi, 2021)

IX. Nursing considerations

    A. Assess for anemia, thrombocytopenia, and subjective symptoms burden.

    B. Educate patient on disease signs and symptoms versus therapy side effects.

    C. Assess for treatment adherence and educational needs.

REFERENCES

Gangat, N., & Tefferi, A. (2020). Myelofibrosis biology and contemporary management. *British Journal of Haematology*, *191*(2), 152–170. https://doi.org/10.1111/bjh.16576.

Guglielmelli, P., Lasho, T. L., Rotunno, G., Mudireddy, M., Mannarelli, C., Nicolosi, M., et al. (2018). MIPSS70: Mutation-enhanced international prognostic score system for transplantation-age patients with primary myelofibrosis. *Journal of Clinical Oncology*, *36*(4), 310–318. https://doi.org/10.1200/jco.2017.76.4886.

Leukemia & Lymphoma Society. (2021). *Myelofibrosis (MF)*. Retrieved 25.02.22 from https://www.lls.org/myeloproliferative-neoplasms/myelofibrosis.

Marcellino, B., & Mascarenhas, J. (2019). Management of advanced phase myeloproliferative neoplasms. *Clinical Advances in Hematology & Oncology*, *17*(7), 405–411.

Mascarenhas, J., Najfeld, V., Kremyanskaya, M., & Keyzner, A. (2018). Primary myelofibrosis: *Hematology: Basic principles and practice* (pp. 1125–1150). Amsterdam: Elsevier.

Mehta, J., Wang, H., Iqbal, S. U., & Mesa, R. (2014). Epidemiology of myeloproliferative neoplasms in the United States. *Leukemia & Lymphoma*, *55*(3), 595–600. https://doi.org/10.3109/10428194.2013.813500.

National Cancer Comprehensive Network (NCCN). (2022). *Myeloproliferative neoplasms*. https://www.nccn.org/professionals/physician_gls/pdf/mpn.pdf.

National Organization for Rare Disorders (NORD). (2018). *Primary myelofibrosis*. https://rarediseases.org/rare-diseases/primary-myelofibrosis/.

Passamonti, F., Mora, B., Barraco, D., & Maffioli, M. (2018). Post-ET and post-PV myelofibrosis: Updates on a distinct prognosis from primary myelofibrosis. *Current Hematologic Malignancy Reports*, *13*(3), 173–182. https://doi.org/10.1007/s11899-018-0453-y.

Tefferi, A. (2021). Primary myelofibrosis: 2021 update on diagnosis, risk-stratification and management. *American Journal of Hematology*, *96*(1), 145–162. https://doi.org/10.1002/ajh.26050.

Tremblay, D., & Mascarenhas, J. (2021). Next generation therapeutics for the treatment of myelofibrosis. *Cells*, *10*(5), 1034. https://doi.org/10.3390/cells10051034.

23

Neurologic System Cancers

Jaya Mini Gill

OVERVIEW

I. Physiology and pathophysiology
  A. Brain anatomy and physiology (National Brain Tumor Society, 2019; Fig. 23.1)
  B. Pathophysiology of central nervous system (CNS) cancers
    1. Primary CNS tumors
      a. Benign—"benign" may suggest a nonmalignant process but has the potential to cause significant morbidity/mortality depending on the location, size, and affected structures
        (1) Benign primary brain tumors (PBTs)
        (2) Benign primary spinal tumors—more likely to occur inside the dura but outside the spinal cord (extramedullary); the most common types of intradural extramedullary (IDEM) spinal tumors are meningiomas and nerve sheath tumors. IDEMs develop in the spinal cord's arachnoid membrane (meningiomas), in the nerve roots that extend out from the spinal cord (schwannomas and neurofibromas), or at the spinal cord base (filum terminale ependymomas). Less common include solitary fibrous tumor/hemangiopericytoma and malignant peripheral nerve sheath tumor.
      b. Malignant
        (1) Malignant PBT—arise from any cell in the CNS
          (a) Rare for PBT to metastasize outside of CNS
          (b) PBT may invade dura and adjacent structures
          (c) PBT may have drop metastases to spine
        (2) Malignant primary spine tumors
          (a) Frequently arise from intramedullary (within the spinal cord) support cells
          (b) Symptoms determined by tumor location, size, compression of nearby structures (including cerebrospinal fluid [CSF] flow, spinal nerves, or blood vessels)
    2. Metastatic CNS tumors
      a. Spread through hematogenous seeding, direct extension, or invasion to the CNS
II. Epidemiology
  A. CNS tumors—pediatric

1. Brain and spinal cord tumors are the second most common cancers in children (after leukemia) (American Cancer Society [ACS], 2022).
  a. Prevalence of CNS tumors (Ostrom, Cioffi, Waite, Kruchko, & Barnholtz-Sloan, 2021)
    (1) Pilocytic astrocytoma
      (a) World Health Organization (WHO) grade I glioma
      (b) The most common glioma in children; accounts for up to 40% of all glioma diagnoses among those under age 20 (Knight & De Jesus, 2021)
    (2) Malignant glioma
    (3) Medulloblastoma
    (4) Neuronal and mixed neuronal-glial tumors
    (5) Ependymoma
    (6) Embryonal tumors
    (7) Brainstem gliomas
    (8) Optic nerve gliomas
  b. Pediatric brain tumors are the leading cause of cancer-related death among children and adolescents aged 0–19, surpassing leukemia.
2. More than 4000 primary CNS tumors are diagnosed in children and teens each year.
3. 75% of children/teens survive more than 5 years after their CNS tumor diagnosis.
4. Tumors most frequently associated with CNS metastases are germ cell tumors and sarcomas (Ostrom, Francis, & Barnholtz-Sloan, 2021).
  B. CNS tumors—adult (ACS, 2022)
    1. Primary CNS tumors
      a. About 25,050 (14,170 males; 10,880 females) primary brain or spinal cord tumors diagnosed in adults each year
        (1) Incidence higher if benign (noncancer) tumors were also included
        (2) About 18,280 people (10,710 males; 7570 females) die annually
      b. PBTs (PDQ Adult Treatment Editorial Board, 2021)
        (1) Incidence in decreasing order of frequency
          (a) Glioblastoma and anaplastic astrocytomas (38% of PBT)

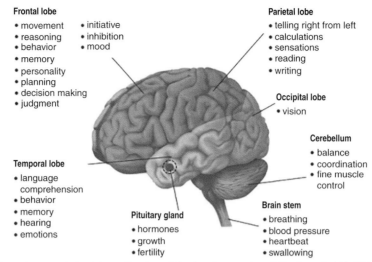

Frontal lobe
- movement
- reasoning
- behavior
- memory
- personality
- planning
- decision making
- judgment

- initiative
- inhibition
- mood

Parietal lobe
- telling right from left
- calculations
- sensations
- reading
- writing

Occipital lobe
- vision

Cerebellum
- balance
- coordination
- fine muscle control

Temporal lobe
- language comprehension
- behavior
- memory
- hearing
- emotions

Pituitary gland
- hormones
- growth
- fertility

Brain stem
- breathing
- blood pressure
- heartbeat
- swallowing

Fig. 23.1 Brain anatomy and physiology. Courtesy Schering Corporation, & Kenilworth, NJ. (2004). In Vassall, E. (Ed.), *The essential guide to brain tumors*. National Brain Tumor Foundation.

(b) Meningiomas and other mesenchymal tumors (27% of PBT)
(c) Pituitary tumors
(d) Schwannomas
(e) Primary CNS lymphoma
(f) Oligodendroglioma
(g) Ependymoma
(h) Low-grade astrocytoma
(i) Medulloblastoma

c. Prevalence (Ostrom et al., 2021)
   (1) Meningiomas make up 37% of all PBT.
   (2) Gliomas (such as glioblastoma, ependymomas, astrocytomas, and oligodendrogliomas) make up 74.6% of malignant brain tumors.
   (3) An estimated 700,000 Americans are living with a brain tumor.
       (a) 70.9% are benign
       (b) 29.1% are malignant

d. Primary spine tumors (PDQ Adult Treatment Editorial Board, 2021)
   (1) Incidence in decreasing order of frequency
       (a) Schwannomas, meningiomas, and ependymomas (comprise 79%)
       (b) Sarcomas
       (c) Astrocytomas
       (d) Vascular tumors
       (e) Chordomas

2. CNS metastatic disease
   a. Site of CNS metastatic presentation (Nolan & DeAngelis, 2018)
      (1) Brain 10%–35%
      (2) Skull 15%–20%
      (3) Spine 20%
      (4) Leptomeningeal 4%–15%
      (5) Dura 9%–10%

b. Brain metastases (BM) (Ostrom et al., 2021; Janavicius, Lachej, Anglickiene, Vincerzevskiene, & Brasiuniene, 2020)
   (1) Incidence (PDQ Adult Treatment Editorial Board, 2021)
       (a) 72.2% of individuals across all histologies have solitary BM.
       (b) Nearly 37% of individuals across all histologies have at least three BM.
   (2) Most common metastatic histologies to brain
       (a) Lung (18%–64%), breast (2%–21%), melanoma (20%), cancer of unknown primary (1%–18%), colorectal (2%–12%), and kidney (1%–8%)
       (b) Lung
           i. Non–small cell lung cancer (NSCLC) accounts for 85% of lung cancer diagnoses; the most common primary tumor metastasizing to brain; about 9% of patients with NSCLC develop BM.
           ii. About 50%–60% of those newly diagnosed with SCLC will develop BM within 2 years.
           iii. More likely to present with multiple BMs
           iv. Younger age, larger tumor size, hilar node involvement, lymphovascular space invasion associated with increased risk of BM.
           v. 5-year risk of developing BM ≈10% in those who received surgical treatment for stage I–II NSCLC; 24%–55% in those with stage III.
       (c) Breast
           i. Most common type of BM in women

ii. Likely to present with a single metastasis

iii. Risks for BM: age <35 years old at the time of primary breast cancer diagnosis, high histologic grade, tumor size >2 cm, node positive

iv. Higher odds of developing BM in HER2-positive breast cancers compared with other subtypes

(d) Melanoma

i. Of all tumors, melanoma has the strongest affinity to metastasize to CNS.

ii. Likely to present with multiple BMs

iii. High incidence of hemorrhagic BM

(e) Renal—likely to present with a single metastasis

(f) Colorectal

i. Likely to present with a single metastasis

ii. Survival after diagnosis with BM from gastrointestinal tumors is significantly decreased compared with breast, lung, and renal cancers.

(g) Leukemia and lymphoma (American Society of Clinical Oncology [ASCO] Cancer.Net, 2021) also commonly metastasize to the CNS.

(h) Biomarker predictors of BM

i. HER2 in breast cancer

ii. Anaplastic lymphoma kinase gene rearrangement in NSCLC

iii. BRAF pathogenic variants in melanoma

c. Spinal metastases

(1) Leptomeningeal carcinomatosis (Batool & Kasi, 2022; PDQ Adult Treatment Editorial Board, 2021; Schubert & Bell, 2022)

(a) Occurs in 5%–8% of all cancer patients

(b) Median overall survival (OS) is ≈12 weeks

(c) Breast tumors (22%), lung tumors (15%), and prostate (10%); lymphoma (10%); kidney (7%); gastrointestinal tract (5%); melanoma (4%); unknown (4%); and others (24%)

(2) Site of spinal metastatic presentation

(a) Epidural 94%

(b) IDEM 5%

(c) Intramedullary 1%

(3) Vertebral body metastases (Ziu et al., 2022)

(a) Breast (21%), lung (19%), and prostate (7.5%) most common

(b) 40% of tumors that originate outside CNS will metastasize to spine: thoracic 70%, lumbar 20%, and cervical 10%.

III. Risk factors (Table 23.1)

IV. Diagnostics

A. Neurologic examination (Alpert, 2019)

1. A detailed and accurate history

2. Mental status testing

3. Cranial nerve testing

4. Motor strength testing

5. Sensation testing: light touch, pain, temperature, vibration, proprioception, and dermatomal sensory patterns

6. Reflexes

7. Balance and gait

8. Coordination testing

a. Rapid alternating movement tests

b. Rhomberg

c. Finger-to-nose

d. Finger-to-finger

e. Tandem walking

f. Heel-to-shin

B. Diagnostic imaging examinations (Stupp, Brada, van den Bent, Tonn, & Pentheroudakis, 2014; Zaccagna et al., 2021)

1. X-rays

a. Useful in assessing the bones of the skull and spine. X-rays of the spine can be used to evaluate fractures or misalignment. X-rays are also particularly useful in determining the stability of the spine.

2. Computed tomography (CT) of brain and spine

a. Without contrast—helpful at initial presentation to evaluate stroke versus intracranial lesions in persons with new-onset neurologic symptoms

b. With intravenous radiocontrast—surgical and radiation planning or for surveillance of patients not able to get magnetic resonance imaging (MRI)

c. Malignant tumors best visualized with contrast-enhanced scans

(1) CT is a test of choice for evaluating spinal bony metastases

(a) Superior for detecting hemorrhage and calcification

(b) Less expensive than MRI

(2) Conventional MRI of brain and spine

(a) Without gadolinium—helpful in evaluating edema, nonenhancing tumors, radiation-induced leukoencephalopathy, or acute blood products

(b) With intravenous gadolinium—test of choice for visualizing brain and spine lesions and for ongoing disease surveillance

(c) Diagnostic choice in persons with symptoms of brain tumor, soft tissue tumors involving the spine

(d) High-grade tumors best visualized with contrast

(e) Superior contrast resolution and multiplanar capability

TABLE 23.1	Central Nervous System Tumor Risk Factors	
Type of Risk Factor	**Risk Factors**	**References**
Known intrinsic risk factors	• Age—children and older adults • Gender—men, glioma; women, meningioma • Race/ethnicity—Caucasian northern European; meningioma more common in African American populations	• ACS (2022) • ASCO Cancer.net (2021)
Known situational risk factors	• Epstein–Barr virus increases risk of CNS lymphoma • Exposure to vinyl chloride • Immunocompromised—HIV/AIDS, immunosuppressive medical therapies, congenital immunodeficiency • Injury—history of head trauma associated with meningiomas • Personal history of cancer	• ASCO Cancer.net (2021) • PDQ Adult Treatment Editorial Board (2021)
Known extrinsic risk factors	• IR—causal relationship between therapeutic irradiation of doses >2500 cGy and development of brain tumors; risk higher for nerve sheath tumors and meningiomas than gliomas • Children with leukemia—risk highest if treated before age 5 years • Panorex radiography before age 10 associated with increased risk of meningioma • Prior radiation for treatment of *Tinea capitis*—common in the 1950s	• ASCO Cancer.net (2021)
Genetic/inherited risk factors (5%–17% of primary brain tumors associated with genetic disorders)	• Neurofibromatosis 1 (*NF1* gene, 17q11) • Neurofibromatosis 2 (*NF2* gene, 22q12) • Turcot syndrome type 1 (*APC* gene, 3p21, 7p22) • Turcot syndrome type 2 (*APC* gene, 5q21) • Gorlin syndrome (*PTCH* gene) • Tuberous sclerosis (*TSC1*, 9q34, and *TSC2*, 16p13, genes) • Li–Fraumeni syndrome (*TP53* gene, 17p13) • von-Hippel–Lindau disease (*VHL* gene, 3p25–26) • *BRCA1*, *BRCA2*, and *PALB2* germline pathogenic variants • *P14 (ARF)* germline pathogenic variants • Nevoid basal cell carcinoma syndrome (9q22.3) • Brain cancer "clusters" in families without known genetic cause	• ACS (2022) • ASCO Cancer.net (2021) • Kyritsis, Bondy, Rao, and Sioka (2010) • Zhang et al. (2015) • PDQ Adult Treatment Editorial Board (2021)
Unproven risk factors currently under investigation	• Late menarche in females • Obesity • Exposures—pesticides, vinyl chloride, petrochemicals, electromagnetic fields, inks and solvents, dietary N-nitroso compounds, long-term use of black or brown hair dyes, cell phones, aspartame, and certain viral exposures	• ACS (2022) • ASCO Cancer.net (2021)

CNS, Central nervous system; *IR*, ionizing radiation.

(f) MRI CSF flow study for evaluating the flow of CSF around the brain, brainstem, and spinal cord when concern about obstruction exists

(g) Functional MRI—for identifying areas of eloquent brain preoperatively

(h) MR spectroscopy—to differentiate normal versus abnormal tissues

(3) Nuclear medicine studies—provide physiologic as opposed to structural picture

(a) Positron emission tomography—high sensitivity to high-grade malignancies and radiation necrosis but low specificity

(b) Octreotide scan—may be useful in evaluating malignant meningioma or primitive neuroectodermal tumors (PNET)

(c) Bone scan—indicated for staging medulloblastoma

(4) Radiography (spine)

(5) Myelography—aids in finding the source of spinal compression

(6) Electromyography—detects muscular innervation dysfunctions peripherally

(7) Points of care where neuroimaging is indicated (Stupp et al., 2014)

(a) Preoperatively—identify patterns of cerebral edema or location of lesions

(b) Postoperative imaging with CT or MRI recommended within 24 hours of surgical resection to assess residual tumor volume and establish a new baseline to measure treatment effect

(c) Follow-up examinations—every 3–4 months is typical standard practice outside of clinical trials unless clinically indicated

C. Diagnostic lumbar puncture

1. Laboratory and pathology evaluations

a. Cell count and differential, glucose level, and protein concentration

b. Gram stain, culture, and sensitivity

c. Tumor markers, cytopathology

D. Diagnostic blood tests

1. Serum tests—vary according to primary disease diagnosis; no serum evaluation for the diagnosis of gliomas

2. Tumor markers—may include beta-human chorionic gonadotropin, alpha-fetoprotein, and placental isoenzyme of alkaline phosphatase for germinoma tumors or teratomas

E. Bone marrow biopsy—workup with CNS lymphoma

F. Neuro-ophthalmology examination—evaluate for intraocular CNS lymphoma

V. Staging, histopathology, genetic, and molecular classification of CNS tumors

A. Brain and spine tumor staging

1. Metastatic CNS malignancies

a. A non-CNS primary tumor metastasizing to brain or spine is a stage IV according to classic tumor–node–metastasis (TNM) staging

2. Primary CNS malignancy staging (PDQ Adult Treatment Editorial Board, 2021)

a. TNM classification not used because two of three indicators are not applicable (no nodes and extracranial metastases extraordinarily rare)

b. WHO classification of CNS that is universally applicable and prognostically valid

(1) WHO grade I—lesions with low proliferative potential, frequently discrete nature, possibility of cure after surgical resection alone.

(2) WHO grade II—lesions generally infiltrating, low in mitotic activity, recur more frequently than grade I, some progress to higher grades.

(3) WHO grade III—lesions with histologic evidence of malignancy, for example, nuclear atypia and increased mitotic activity, anaplastic histology, and infiltrative capacity. They are usually treated with aggressive adjuvant therapy.

(4) WHO grade IV—lesions mitotically active, necrosis prone, generally associated with a rapid preoperative/postoperative progression and fatal outcomes. Lesions are usually treated with aggressive adjuvant therapy.

c. See Table 23.2 for biomarkers with diagnostic/prognostic value in PBT.

VI. Prognosis and survival

A. Primary brain and spine tumors

1. Gliomas

a. Extent of tumor resection, patient age, tumor histology, performance status, molecular markers (1p19q codeletion, isocitrate dehydrogenase status, O6-methylguanine-DNA methyltransferase [MGMT] promoter methylation status, Alpha thalassemia/mental retardation syndrome X-linked [ATRX] pathogenic variant) predictive of outcome (Nadeem et al., 2020)

b. Expected median survival with glioma (Stupp et al., 2014)

(1) Grade II

(a) Astrocytoma—7–10 years

(b) Oligodendroglioma with 1p/19q codeletion—>10–15 years

(2) Grade III

(a) Anaplastic astrocytoma—3.5 years

(b) Anaplastic oligodendroglioma with 1p/19q codeletion—>10 years

(3) Grade IV—glioblastoma—15 months, 2-year survival 27%

(a) MGMT methylated—23 months, 2-year survival 49%

(b) MGMT unmethylated—13 months, 2-year survival 12%

c. Malignant transformation of low-grade (WHO II) to high-grade (WHO III) gliomas ranges from 25% to 72% and occurs within 5 years (Satar, Hotton, & Samandouras, 2021)

B. Metastatic brain and spine tumors

1. BMs (Nolan & DeAngelis, 2018)

a. Prognostic factors vary according to the cancer type and include the number of BM, age, Karnofsky Performance Score, and extent of systemic disease.

b. Survival for patients with BM is poor, typically in the range of 3–6 months.

c. Age <65 years, Karnofsky Performance Score >70, and controlled systemic disease are predictors of better OS, with median OS of 7.1 months versus an OS of 2.3 months if all factors were poor.

2. Spine metastases (SM)

a. Only 10%–20% of patients with SM will be alive 2 years after initial diagnosis.

b. Poor performance status at diagnosis strongest predictor of poor OS; low systemic disease load and favorable tumor histology are associated with increased OS.

3. Leptomeningeal carcinomatosis

a. Median OS 10–12 weeks

MANAGEMENT

I. Surgery, radiation, chemo/biotherapy, clinical trials, and active surveillance

A. Surgery

1. Brain tumor surgical management (Rivera, Norman, Sehgal, & Juthani, 2021)

a. Goals of brain surgery

(1) Symptom relief (i.e., reduction in mass effect)

(2) Obtaining a diagnosis (initial or restaging)

(3) Cytoreduction

b. Brain surgical intervention—provides tissue diagnosis and may improve outcomes (survival and global functioning)

TABLE 23.2   Biomarkers in Primary Brain Tumors

Biomarker/Description	Clinical Significance	Source
1p19q Codeletion • 1p and 19q chromosome arms	• 1p/19q codeletion has predictive value for response to chemotherapy in surgically diagnosed anaplastic oligodendrogliomas with nearly a doubling of survival in those treated with procarbazine–lomustine–vincristine plus radiotherapy compared with those being treated with radiotherapy alone • 1p/19q codeletion is a strong independent prognostic biomarker associated with improved survival in both diffuse low-grade and anaplastic brain tumors • With very few exceptions, 1p/19q codeletion is mutually exclusive with *TP53* and *ATRX* pathogenic variant	Li et al. (2022) Cairncross, Wang, and Shaw (2013) van den Bent et al. (2013)
ATRX • ATRX gene • A telomere maintenance–related gene	• 90% of IDH-mutant diffuse gliomas have pathogenic variants in ATRX and/or TERT • IDH wild-type glioblastomas, ATRX alterations are associated with favorable outcomes	Carlos-Escalante, Calderón, and Wegman-Ostrosky (2021)
BRAF • Human gene that encodes a protein belonging to the RAF family of serine/threonine protein kinases • Plays a role in regulating the MAP kinase/ERK signaling pathway, which affects cell division, differentiation, and secretion • Pathogenic variant of valine 600 to glutamic acid (V600E) is the most prevalent BRAF pathogenic variant	• Tandem duplication at 7q34 leading to a fusion between KIAA1549 and BRAF is found in approximately 70% of pilocytic astrocytomas • An activating point pathogenic variant in BRAF (V600E) is found in an additional 5%–9% of these tumors, and in general, RAF alterations occur in approximately 80% of pilocytic astrocytomas • BRAF V600E pathogenic variants are observed (in about 60%) of other benign glioma variants, including pleomorphic xanthoastrocytoma and ganglioglioma, whereas BRAF tandem duplications are not found in these variant glioma tumors	PDQ Adult Treatment Editorial Board (2021)
EGFR • EGFR • Tyrosine kinase ligand • Exists on the cell surface • Activated by various growth factors, which leads to cell proliferation	• EGFR expression • Amplified ≈50% of primary glioblastoma • Associated with poor prognosis • Coexpression of *EGFR* deletion mutant variant III (*EGFRvIII*) with PTEN poor prognostic indicator • *EGFRvIII* expression associated with a worse prognosis than wild-type EGFR expression (amplification) alone	Abdullah, Adamson, and Brem (2016)
IDH • IDH1 • IDH2 • Enzyme pathogenic variants found in multiple human cancers	• *IDH1* and *IDH2* pathogenic variants occur in a mutually exclusive manner in nearly 80% of grades II and III oligodendrogliomas and astrocytomas and secondary glioblastomas • IDH-mutant tumors frequently have other molecular alterations, including 1p/19q codeletion, *CIC*, *FUBP*, and *TERT* promoter pathogenic variants • The presence of IDH2 pathogenic variant predicts improved sensitivity of glioma to radiation	Carlos-Escalante et al. (2021)
INI₁ • A member of the SWI/SNF chromatin remodeling complex located on chromosome 22q11.2, hSNF5/ SMARCB1 • *INI₁* gene deletion or pathogenic variant	• Deletion or pathogenic variant in atypical teratoid/rhabdoid tumors	Abdullah et al. (2016)
PTEN • Phosphatase and tensin homolog • Protein encoded by PTEN gene • Plays a role in cancer suppression	• PTEN loss pathogenic variant associated with the proliferation of glioblastoma	Abdullah et al. (2016)

TABLE 23.2 Biomarkers in Primary Brain Tumors—cont'd

Biomarker/Description	Clinical Significance	Source
TERT • Telomerase reverse transcriptase gene promoter pathogenic variant • A telomere maintenance–related gene	• In IDH-mutant 1p/19q-codeleted oligodendrogliomas, those tumors with TERT wild type have significantly worse overall survival than those with TERT pathogenic variant • In IDH wild-type astrocytomas, TERT wild type has significantly better overall survival than the TERT pathogenic variant group	Pekmezci et al. (2017)
MGMT • *MGMT* gene • The protein encoded by MGMT is a DNA repair protein that is involved in cellular defense against mutagenesis and toxicity from alkylating agents. The protein catalyzes the transfer of methyl groups from O(6)-alkylguanine and other methylated moieties of the DNA to its own molecule, which repairs the toxic lesions.	• Methylation of the MGMT promoter has been associated with several cancer types, including colorectal cancer, lung cancer, lymphoma, and glioblastoma • MGMT promoter methylation is associated with a more favorable response to alkylating agents	Stupp et al. (2014)

ATRX, Alpha thalassemia/mental retardation syndrome X-linked; *EGFR*, epidermal growth factor receptor; *IDH*, isocitrate dehydrogenase; *MGMT*, methylguanine methyltransferase; *PTEN*, phosphatase and tensin homolog; *TERT*, telomerase reverse transcriptase.

(1) Gross total—removal of all measurable tumor tissue; may improve response to therapy due to smaller residual tumor volume

(2) Subtotal resection—removal of measurable tumor volume; preferred resection type if tumor near eloquent areas, and aggressive surgical approach could result in worse neurologic deficits

(3) Stereotactic brain biopsy—goal is to obtain a tissue diagnosis

    (a) Preferred method if tumor near eloquent areas, location difficult to access, or very poor surgical candidate

    (b) Risk for sampling error due to small volume obtained with needle sample; may result in underdiagnosis

2. Spine tumor surgical management (Wagner, Haag, & Joerger, 2021)

  a. Goals for spinal surgery

    (1) Obtain tissue diagnosis: biopsy, surgical resection

    (2) Symptom relief

      (a) Preservation or restoration of neurologic function and ambulation

      (b) Maintain spinal stability

      (c) Durable local tumor control

      (d) Improved quality of life (e.g., pain control, neurologic preservation)

  b. Indications for spinal surgery

    (1) Neurologic status is deteriorating

    (2) Unknown tumor type

    (3) Tumor is not radiosensitive

B. Radiation (see Chapter 27)

  1. PBT radiation (PDQ Adult Treatment Editorial Board, 2021)

  a. High-grade gliomas (WHO grade III or IV) or other high-grade PBT

    (1) External beam radiation therapy (EBRT)

      (a) Conformal or intensity-modulated RT

      (b) Thirty fractions over 6 weeks totaling 60 Gy

      (c) Treat tumor plus 2- to 3-cm margins on the MRI-based volumes

      (d) EBRT is the standard first-line adjuvant therapy with or without concurrent adjuvant chemotherapy after surgical diagnosis

      (e) Provides a significant survival advantage compared with no EBRT

    (2) No survival or quality-of-life benefit has been demonstrated with alternative RT strategies (i.e., radiosurgery with or without EBRT, hypofractionated RT, brachytherapy).

  b. Low-grade gliomas (WHO I or II) or other low-grade PBT

    (1) Although there is a delayed time to progression in low-grade tumors treated with EBRT up front, there is no difference in OS compared with waiting until the progression of disease to treat with EBRT.

    (2) Treatment plan would be the same as with high-grade gliomas.

  c. Maximum tolerable dose to normal brain is considered 60 Gy.

2. Primary spine tumor radiation (National Comprehensive Cancer Center Network [NCCN], 2021)

  a. Intradural intramedullary tumor well defined/well circumscribed

    (1) EBRT only if symptomatic

b. Intradural intramedullary tumor poorly defined/infiltrative
  (1) EBRT depends on tumor histology, presentation, and symptoms
c. IDEM
  (1) Single versus multiple lesions
  (2) RT decision depends on surgical candidacy, symptoms, and goals of therapy
d. Multidisciplinary input for treatment planning
3. Metastatic CNS malignancy radiation
  a. BMs (Nolan & DeAngelis, 2018)
    (1) Single BM—radiosurgery±surgical resection
    (2) Multiple BMs
      (a) Whole-brain RT (WBRT) is the mainstay of treatment.
      (b) Radiation is palliative.
      (c) If one to three BM, consider stereotactic radiosurgery (SRS) alone (16–24 Gy); more than four BM, consider WBRT.
      (d) Hypofractionated radiosurgery (21–25 Gy over three to five fractions) recommended for BM >3 cm due to the high risk of radiation necrosis.
  b. Spinal metastases (Dohm, Oliver, Yu, Hsiang-Hsuan, & Ahmed, 2022)
    (1) Neurologic, oncologic, mechanical instability, and systemic disease framework for principled assessments in treatment decision-making for SM
    (2) Location of disease in the spine (L), mechanical instability (M), neurology (N), oncology (O), patient fitness, prognosis and response to prior therapy (P) framework is intended to provide general guidance based on key principles to radiation oncologists and spine surgeons (Spratt et al., 2017).
    (3) Surgery and radiation are the mainstays of treatment for SM.
    (4) Conventional EBRT (cEBRT)
      (a) Typically 30 Gy over 10 fractions
      (b) Tumor histology is the most important predictor for response to cEBRT.
    (5) SRS—single (16–24 Gy) or hypofractionated (24–30 Gy over two to three fractions)
C. Chemotherapy/biotherapy (NCCN, 2021; PDQ Adult Treatment Editorial Board, 2021; Stupp et al., 2014)
  1. PBT
    a. Gliomas
      (1) Low-grade gliomas
        (a) Temozolomide (TMZ) depending on disease burden or progression status
        (b) Consider lomustine or carmustine, procarbazine with lomustine and vincristine (PCV), or platinum-based therapy after TMZ failure
      (2) High-grade gliomas
        (a) Anaplastic gliomas and glioblastoma
          i. TMZ is the standard of care for adjuvant treatment of anaplastic astrocytoma after surgery and radiation and in glioblastoma concurrently with RT, then adjuvant.
          ii. Other cytotoxic treatments after TMZ have failed to provide benefit and include lomustine or carmustine, PCV, or platinum-based therapy
          iii. Implanted carmustine-impregnated wafers—Food and Drug Administration–approved therapy; used more at second or third craniotomy resecting recurrent or progressive high-grade gliomas in heavily treated individuals
          iv. Bevacizumab—for progressive glioblastoma
            • Generally, well tolerated; risks include hypertension, proteinuria, vascular events such as stroke and intracranial bleed, and gastrointestinal perforation
            • To manage radiation necrosis–related cerebral edema (Levin et al., 2011)
        (b) Anaplastic oligodendrogliomas
          i. Patients with 1p/19q-codeleted tumors should be treated with PCV after RT, depending on the ability to tolerate therapy.
          ii. At progression, TMZ and nitrosoureas should be considered.
          iii. Other regimens include cyclophosphamide, platinum-based regimens, irinotecan, or etoposide.
    b. Medulloblastoma and supratentorial PNET
      (1) Optimal use of adjuvant chemotherapy for adults is unclear.
      (2) At recurrence, drugs used include etoposide, TMZ, and high-dose chemotherapy with autologous stem cell transplant.
    c. CNS lymphoma
      (1) High-dose methotrexate (MTX)–based regimens (3.5 g/m^2 or higher)
      (2) If CSF or spinal MRI positive, intra-CNS chemotherapy considered
      (3) If eye examination positive, intraocular chemotherapy considered
      (4) Other agents used in combination with MTX include dexamethasone, vincristine, procarbazine, cytarabine, rituximab, and ifosfamide.
  2. Ependymoma
    a. The role of chemotherapy is poorly defined.
    b. Sometimes considered palliative after RT has failed to control the disease with drugs such as carboplatin or cisplatin, etoposide, lomustine or carmustine, bevacizumab, and TMZ.
  3. Meningiomas

a. Cytotoxic therapies generally not efficacious

b. Refractory meningiomas may benefit from somatostatin analogs or α interferon

4. Metastatic brain and spine tumors

a. Systemic chemo/biotherapy not routine treatment for brain/spine metastasis due to

(1) Poor penetration through blood–brain barrier

(2) Heavily pretreated tumors are less chemosensitive

b. Breast cancer

(1) MTX may be an option

(2) Platinum plus etoposide

(3) Capecitabine with or without lapatinib

c. Melanoma

(1) Ipilimumab and BRAF inhibitors (dabrafenib and vemurafenib)

(2) TMZ may be useful in some patients

d. Leptomeningeal metastases (LM)

(1) Intrathecal chemotherapy

(a) MTX for breast cancer, lymphoma, and leukemia

(b) Cytarabine and liposomal cytarabine for lymphoma and leukemia

(c) Thiotepa

(d) Rituximab for lymphoma

(e) Topotecan

(f) Etoposide

(g) Trastuzumab for breast cancer

(h) Interferon alpha

(2) High-dose MTX for breast LM

(3) Weekly pulse erlotinib for NSCLC with epidermal growth factor receptor exon 19 or exon 21 deletions

e. Corticosteroids to manage spinal cord compression

D. Tumor-treating fields (TTFields) (Liu et al., 2021)

1. Optune is a portable, battery-operated device that generates TTFields and is designed to be worn continuously for the treatment of supratentorial glioblastoma.

2. TTFields produce antimitotic effects by physically interacting with highly charged macromolecules and organelles in rapidly dividing cancer cells to disrupt their proper alignment during different stages of mitosis.

3. TTFields plus TMZ compared with TMZ alone after concomitant TMZ and radiotherapy in newly diagnosed glioblastoma patients demonstrated statistically significant improvement in survival (Liu et al., 2021; Stupp et al., 2015).

4. TTFields approved as monotherapy in patients with recurrent glioblastoma; approved treatment option without systemic side effects for patients with recurrent glioblastoma who did not have TTFields plus TMZ as the first-line therapy.

E. Blood and marrow transplantation—used for the treatment of recurrent medulloblastoma

F. Clinical trials—experimental treatment regimens should be considered at all stages of disease as appropriate based upon availability, functional status, and desire

G. Medical interventions for symptom management

1. Glucocorticoids

a. High dose to manage acute cerebral edema

b. High dose to manage extradural spinal lesions causing compression of spinal cord

c. Dosed 16 mg or more per day; use the lowest possible dose for the shortest time possible to reduce serious steroid-related complications such as myopathy, diabetes, infections, and other comorbid conditions

2. Mannitol

a. Generally used only in emergency situations to capitalize on the osmotic properties of mannitol effects on brain edema resulting from leakage of plasma into the brain parenchyma through dysfunctional cerebral capillaries

b. Only administered in intensive care unit setting

c. Often last effort for cerebral edema management if bevacizumab is not an option

3. Ventricular interventions

a. Ventriculoperitoneal (VP) shunt—placed for management of hydrocephalus

(1) Programmable VP shunt—may be affected by magnetic fields during MRI; patient will require plain film within 4 hours of MRI to assess valve settings

(2) Nonprogrammable VP shunt

b. Ommaya reservoir—placed for delivery of intrathecal chemotherapy

c. Ventriculostomy—performed to relieve pressure within the CNS

II. Nursing implications

A. Assessment and management of symptoms—symptoms are related to the tumor or related to the treatment, as there is frequent overlap

1. Fatigue (Cahill, LoBiondo-Wood, Bergstrom, & Armstrong, 2012; Stupp et al., 2014)—most frequent and severe symptom reported by persons with PBT

2. Headache

a. Head pain or headache in PBT is the strongest independent predictor of BM.

b. Less prevalent in survivors of PBT

3. Nausea and vomiting (N/V)—common at diagnosis in 30%–40% PBT

4. Neurologic/mental status symptoms

a. Sensory changes with vision, hearing, or smelling are common at presentation for all BT types; numbness and tingling may be present in 15% of PBT.

b. Dizziness, weakness, gait instability, coordination, and balance symptoms are broadly associated with BM from all tumor types.

5. Seizures

a. Presenting symptom in 15% of PBT, in 20% of BM

b. Risk highest with cortical tumors; temporal tumors tend to be most epileptogenic

c. Antiepileptic drug (AED) therapy indicated in those with seizures and during the perioperative craniotomy setting; prophylactic use of anticonvulsants not indicated otherwise

    (1) First-line agents: lamotrigine, levetiracetam, pregabalin, or valproic acid

    (2) First-generation AEDs are strong inducers of hepatic metabolism and are not preferred (i.e., phenytoin, carbamazepine, phenobarbital, and their derivatives) due to numerous drug interactions

6. Venous thrombotic events, for example, deep vein thrombosis (DVT), pulmonary embolism (PE)

  a. Glioma patients at increased risk due to tumor-induced hypercoagulable state, neurologic deficits, immobility, steroid use, and chemotherapy treatments

  b. 20%–30% of glioma patients will have a DVT or PE

  c. Standard anticoagulant treatment not contraindicated in patients with brain tumor

7. Corticosteroid use and associated complications

  a. Dexamethasone to manage tumor-associated cerebral edema and improve clinical symptoms

  b. Monitor blood glucose

  c. Long-term therapy complications: hyperglycemia, myopathy, weakness, lymphopenia, increased risk of infection, osteoporosis, insomnia, agitation, Cushing syndrome

8. Toxicities of treatment

  a. Radiation complications

    (1) Acute effects (during and immediately after RT)

      (a) Global—headaches, neurocognitive changes, seizures, and somnolence

      (b) Focal—specific neurologic deficits based on tumor location

    (2) Subacute effects (within weeks to 4–6 months after radiation)

      (a) Somnolence, exacerbation of tumor-related symptoms

    (3) Late radiation effects (occurring >6 months to several years after RT)

      (a) Radiation necrosis

      (b) Diffuse white matter changes

      (c) Neurocognitive effects

      (d) Cerebrovascular events

      (e) Optic nerve toxicities

      (f) Endocrine toxicities

      (g) Secondary malignancies

        i. Most common—meningiomas, gliomas, and nerve sheath tumors

        ii. Risk greatest with cranial radiation given to young children

B. Oncologic emergencies (see Chapters 52 and 53)

C. Caregiver burden (Saría et al., 2017; see Chapter 48)

REFERENCES

Abdullah, K. G., Adamson, C., & Brem, S. (2016). The molecular pathogenesis of glioblastoma. In *Glioblastoma* (pp. 21–31). Elsevier Inc. https://doi.org/10.1016/B978-0-323-47660-7.00003-3.

American Cancer Society (ACS). (2022a). *Cancer facts and figures 2022.* https://www.cancer.org/content/dam/cancer-org/research/cancer-facts-and-statistics/annual-cancer-facts-and-figures/2022/2022-cancer-facts-and-figures.pdf.

American Cancer Society (ACS). (2022b). *Key statistics for brain and spinal cord tumors in children.* https://www.cancer.org/cancer/brain-spinal-cord-tumors-children/about/key-statistics.html. Retrieved 12.03.22.

American Society of Clinical Oncology (ASCO). (2021). Cancer.net. *Brain tumor: Risk factors.* https://www.cancer.net/cancer-types/brain-tumor/risk-factors. Retrieved 13.03.22.

Alpert, J. N. (2019). Neurologic examination: *The neurologic diagnosis.* Cham: Springer. https://doi.org/10.1007/978-3-319-95951-1_4.

Batool, A., & Kasi, A. (2022). Leptomeningeal carcinomatosis. [Updated 2021 Mar 25]. In: *StatPearls [Internet].* Treasure Island, FL: StatPearls Publishing. Available from https://www.ncbi.nlm.nih.gov/books/NBK499862/.

Cahill, J., LoBiondo-Wood, G., Bergstrom, N., & Armstrong, T. (2012). Brain tumor symptoms as antecedents to uncertainty: An integrative review. *Journal of Nursing Scholarship, 44*(2), 145–155. https://doi.org/10.1111/j.1547-5069.2012.01445.x.

Cairncross, G., Wang, M., Shaw, E., et al. (2013). Phase III trial of chemoradiotherapy for anaplastic oligodendroglioma: Long-term results of RTOG 9402. *Journal of Clinical Oncology, 31*(3), 337–343.

Carlos-Escalante, J. A., Calderón, J. P., & Wegman-Ostrosky, T. (2021). Diagnostic, prognostic and predictive biomarkers in gliomas. In A. Monroy-Sosa, S. S. Chakravarthi, J. G. de la Garza-Salazar, A. M. Garcia, & A. B. Kassam (Eds.), *Principles of neuro-oncology.* Cham: Springer. https://doi.org/10.1007/978-3-030-54879-7_4.

Dohm, A. E., Oliver, D. E., Yu, H.-H. M., & Ahmed, K.A. (2022). Commentary: From postoperative to preoperative: A case series of hypofractionated and single-fraction neoadjuvant stereotactic radiosurgery for brain metastases. *Operative Neurosurgery, 22*(6), e283–e284. https://doi.org/10.1227/ons.0000000000000187.

Janavicius, M., Lachej, N., Anglickiene, G., Vincerzevskiene, I., & Brasiuniene, B. (2020). Outcomes of treatment for melanoma brain metastases. *Journal of Skin Cancer, 2020,* 7520924. https://doi.org/10.1155/2020/7520924.

Kyritsis, A. P., Bondy, M. L., Rao, J. S., & Sioka, C. (2010). Inherited predisposition to glioma. *Neuro-Oncology, 12*(1), 104–113. https://doi.org/10.1093/neuonc/nop011.

Levin, V. A., Bidaut, L., Hou, P., Kumar, A. J., Wefel, J. S., Bekele, B. N., et al. (2011). Randomized double-blind placebo-controlled trial of bevacizumab therapy for radiation necrosis of the central nervous system. *International Journal of Radiation Oncology, Biology, and Physics, 79*(5), 1487–1495. https://doi.org/10.1016/j.ijrobp.2009.12.061.

Li, Y., Ammari, S., Lawrance, L., Quillent, A., Assi, T., Lassau, N., et al. (2022). Radiomics-based method for predicting the glioma subtype as defined by tumor grade, IDH mutation, and 1p/19q codeletion. *Cancers, 14*(7), 1778. https://doi.org/10.3390/cancers14071778.

Liu, S., Shi, W., Zhao, Q., Zheng, Z., Liu, Z., Meng, L., et al. (2021). Progress and prospect in tumor treating fields treatment of glioblastoma. *Biomedicine & Pharmacotherapy, 141*, 111810. https://doi.org/10.1016/j.biopha.2021.111810.

Nadeem, M. W., Ghamdi, M. A. A., Hussain, M., Khan, M. A., Khan, K. M., Almotiri, S. H., et al. (2020). Brain tumor analysis empowered with deep learning: A review, taxonomy, and future challenges. *Brain Sciences, 10*(2), 118. https://doi.org/10.3390/brainsci10020118.

National Brain Tumor Society. (2019). *Brain tumor facts.* https://braintumor.org/brain-tumors/about-brain-tumors/brain-tumor-facts/.

National Comprehensive Cancer Center Network (NCCN). (2021). NCCN guidelines version 2.2021. In: *Central nervous system cancers.* https://www.nccn.org/professionals/physician_gls/pdf/cns.pdf. Date is V.2.2022-September 29, 2022.

Nolan, C., & Deangelis, L. M. (2018). Overview of metastatic disease of the central nervous system. *Handbook of Clinical Neurology, 149*, 3–23. https://doi.org/10.1016/B978-0-12-811161-1.00001-3.

Ostrom, Q. T., Cioffi, G., Waite, K., Kruchko, C., & Barnholtz-Sloan, J. S. (2021). CBTRUS statistical report: Primary brain and other central nervous system tumors diagnosed in the United States in 2014–2018. *Neuro-Oncology, 23*(3), iii1–iii105. https://doi.org/10.1093/neuonc/noab200.

Ostrom, Q. T., Francis, S. S., & Barnholtz-Sloan, J. S. (2021). Epidemiology of brain and other CNS tumors. *Current Neurology and Neuroscience Reports, 21*(12), 68. https://doi.org/10.1007/s11910-021-01152-9.

PDQ Adult Treatment Editorial Board. (2002). Adult central nervous system tumors treatment (PDQ®): Patient version. 2021 Aug 6. In: *PDQ cancer information summaries [Internet].* Bethesda, MD: National Cancer Institute (US). Available from: https://www.ncbi.nlm.nih.gov/books/NBK66023/

Pekmezci, M., Rice, T., Molinaro, A. M., Walsh, K. M., Decker, P. A., Hansen, H., et al. (2017). Adult infiltrating gliomas with WHO 2016 integrated diagnosis: Additional prognostic roles of ATRX and *TERT. Acta Neuropathologica, 133*(6), 1001–1016. https://doi.org/10.1007/s00401-017-1690-1.

Rivera, M., Norman, S., Sehgal, R., & Juthani, R. (2021). Updates on surgical management and advances for brain tumors. *Current Oncology Reports, 23*(3), 35. https://doi.org/10.1007/s11912-020-01005-7.

Saría, M. G., Nyamathi, A., Philips, L. R., Stanton, A. L., Evangelista, L., Kesari, S., et al. (2017). The hidden morbidity of cancer: Burden in caregivers of patients with brain metastases. *Nursing Clinics of North America, 52*(1), 159–178. https://doi.org/10.1016/j.cnur.2016.10.002.

Satar, Z., Hotton, G., & Samandouras, G. (2021). Systematic review—Time to malignant transformation in low-grade gliomas: Predicting a catastrophic event with clinical, neuroimaging, and molecular markers. *Neuro-Oncology Advances, 3*(1), vdab101. https://doi.org/10.1093/noajnl/vdab101.

Schubert, R., Bell, D., Deng F, et al. *Spinal metastases.* Reference article, Radiopaedia.org. https://doi.org/10.53347/rID-13677 Accessed 14.02.23.

Spratt, D. E., Beeler, W. H., de Moraes, F. Y., Rhines, L. D., Gemmete, J. J., Chaudhary, N., et al. (2017). An integrated multidisciplinary algorithm for the management of spinal metastases: An International Spine Oncology Consortium report. *The Lancet, 18*(12), e720–e730. https://doi.org/10.1016/S1470-2045(17)30612-5.

Stupp, R., Brada, M., van den Bent, M. J., Tonn, J.-C., & Pentheroudakis, G. (2014). High-grade glioma: ESMO clinical practice guidelines for diagnosis, treatment and follow-up. *Annals of Oncology, 25*(S3), iii93–iii101. https://doi.org/10.1093/annonc/mdu050.

Stupp, R., Taillibert, S., Kanner, A. A., Kesari, S., Steinberg, D. M., Toms, S. A., et al. (2015). Maintenance therapy with tumor-treating fields plus temozolomide vs temozolomide alone for glioblastoma: A randomized clinical trial. *Journal of the American Medical Association, 314*(23), 2535–2543. https://doi.org/10.1001/jama.2015.16669.

van den Bent, M. J., Brandes, A. A., Taphoorn, M. J. B., et al. (2013). Adjuvant procarbazine, lomustine, and vincristine chemotherapy in newly diagnosed anaplastic oligodendroglioma: Long-term follow-up of EORTC brain tumor group study 26951. *Journal of Clinical Oncology, 31*(3), 344–350.

Wagner, A., Haag, E., Joerger, A.-K., et al. (2021). Comprehensive surgical treatment strategy for spinal metastases. *Scientific Reports, 11*(1), 7988. https://doi.org/10.1038/s41598-021-87121-1.

Knight, J., & De Jesus, O. (2021). Pilocytic astrocytoma. In: *StatPearls.* Treasure Island, FL: StatPearls Publishing. PMID: 32809449.

Zaccagna, F., Grist, J. T., Quartuccio, N., Riemer, F., Fraioli, F., Caracò, C., et al. (2021). Imaging and treatment of brain tumors through molecular targeting: Recent clinical advances. *European Journal of Radiology, 142*, 109842. https://doi.org/10.1016/j.ejrad.2021.109842.

Zhang, J., Walsh, M. F., Wu, G., Edmonson, M. N., Gruber, T. A., Easton, J., et al. (2015). Germline mutations in predisposition genes in pediatric cancer. *New England Journal of Medicine, 373*, 2336–2346. https://doi.org/10.1056/NEJMoa1508054.

Ziu, E., Viswanathan, V. K., & Mesfin, F. B. (2022). Spinal metastasis. [Updated 2021 Aug 27]. In: *StatPearls [Internet].* Treasure Island, FL: StatPearls Publishing. Available from https://www.ncbi.nlm.nih.gov/books/NBK441950/.

24

Reproductive System Cancers

Deborah L. Bolton and Laura B. LaRose

CERVICAL CANCER

Overview

I. Definition
   A. Cervical cancer forms in the lowermost part of the uterus and is highly preventable with vaccination and appropriate screening.
II. Epidemiology
   A. Cervical cancer is the fourth most common cancer worldwide, with an estimated 604,000 new cases in 2020 (Sung et al., 2021).
   B. In the United States it is rare, accounting for less than 1% of all new cancer cases (National Cancer Institute [NCI], 2022b).
   C. Worldwide it is the fourth leading cause of cancer death in women, though an overwhelming majority occur in underdeveloped or developing countries (Sung et al., 2021).
      1. Most cervical cancer cases occur in developing countries where there exists a lack of framework for screening and treatment (Oleszewski, 2018).
      2. Even within the United States, the poorest counties had a cervical cancer mortality rate that was twice as high as their wealthier counterparts (Siegel, Miller, & Jemal, 2019).
   D. Death rates have decreased since the implementation of Papanicolaou (Pap) test screening for preinvasive disease (Oleszewski, 2018).
   E. Most frequently diagnosed among women aged 35–44 with a median age at time of diagnosis of 50 (NCI, 2022b).
   F. Black, American Indian/Alaska Native, and Hispanic women are more likely to not only be diagnosed with cervical cancer but also to die from it compared to their White counterparts (NCI, 2022b).
III. Pathophysiology (Okunade, 2020; Oleszewski, 2018)
   A. The cervix is the narrow lower end of the uterus that forms a canal between the uterine cavity and vaginal canal.
   B. The exocervix (squamous epithelial cells) and the endocervix (columnar glandular epithelial cells) meet at the squamocolumnar junction (transition zone), which is the site of most pathologic changes.
   C. Preinvasive intraepithelial neoplasia typically precedes cervical cancer.

D. More than 99% of cervical cancer cases are caused by persistent infection with a high-risk strain of human papillomavirus (HPV).
   1. When HPV infects the mucocutaneous epithelium and virus particles are produced in mature epithelial cells, it disrupts normal cell-cycle control.
   2. Uncontrolled cell division leads to buildup of genetic damage.
   3. There are 12 high-risk strains of HPV including 16, which is responsible for squamous cell carcinoma (SCC) and is the most carcinogenic, and 18, which is responsible for adenocarcinoma.
   E. The process by which HPV infections lead to precancerous cells and eventually cancer usually takes years.
IV. Primary Prevention
   A. HPV vaccination
      1. 9-valent HPV vaccine (Gardasil 9) is the only vaccine recommended in the United States by the Centers for Disease Control and Prevention (CDC); protects against types 6, 11, 16, 18, 31, 33, 45, 52, and 58 (Wilkes & Barton-Burke, 2020)
         a. HPV types 16 and 18 account for 70% of all cervical cancers (Oleszewski, 2018).
   B. Smoking can damage the DNA of cervical cells and lower the immune system's ability to fight off HPV infection (Oleszewski, 2018).
   C. Large number of sexual partners and infection with other STIs such as HIV and chlamydia have been shown to increase the risk for cervical cancer (Oleszewski, 2018).
   D. Condom use can lower the risk of contracting HPV (NCI, 2021).
   E. Long-term oral contraceptive use and teenage pregnancy are also associated with higher rates of cervical cancer (Oleszewski, 2018).
V. Diagnosis
   A. Initial diagnostic workup should include (National Comprehensive Cancer Network [NCCN], 2021a):
      1. History and physical
         a. Watery vaginal discharge, intermittent vaginal spotting, postcoital bleeding, but preliminary stages may be asymptomatic

b. Pelvic exam allows for the examination of reproductive organs and lymph nodes for enlargement (Oleszewski, 2018).

2. Blood work including complete blood count, liver function test, renal function studies, and HIV testing

3. HPV testing

4. Colposcopy

5. Cervical biopsy
   a. Cone biopsy if cervical biopsy is inadequate

6. Pelvic magnetic resonance imaging (MRI) and positron emission tomography (PET)/computerized tomography (CT) to rule out metastatic disease

7. Cystoscopy and proctoscopy if bladder or rectal invasion suspected

VI. Histopathology

A. Two main histology types include SCCs (80%–90% of cases) and adenocarcinoma (10% of cases) (Oleszewski, 2018).
   1. Cytology is less able to offer early detection of adenocarcinoma compared with SCC (Siegel, Miller, Fuchs, & Jemal, 2022).

B. Histologic grade
   1. Precancerous changes include cervical intraepithelial neoplasia (CIN grades 1, 2, and 3), atypical squamous cells, and adenocarcinoma in situ (Jeronimo et al., 2017).
   2. Grading by degree of differentiation: unable to assess (GX), well (G1), moderately (G2), or poorly/undifferentiated (G3) (Olawaiye et al., 2020)
      a. Grading encouraged but not a basis for modifying stage assignment and is not a strong prognostic factor (Olawaiye et al., 2020)

VII. Staging

A. Two staging symptoms used in staging most types of cervical cancer
   1. International Federation of Gynecology and Obstetrics (FIGO) system (Bhatla, Aoki, Sharma, & Sankaranarayanan, 2018)
      a. Most used staging method
      b. Newest revision now allows for imaging to be used in addition to clinical exam and accounts for nodal involvement.
   2. American Joint Committee on Cancer (AJCC) TNM staging (Olawaiye et al., 2020)

B. FIGO and AJCC staging are aligned and both use I–IV staging for cervical cancer.
   1. Stage I—Carcinoma confined to the cervix
   2. Stage II—Carcinoma invades beyond the uterus, but has not extended into the lower third of the vagina or to the pelvic wall
   3. Stage III—Carcinoma involves the lower third of the vagina and/or extends to the pelvic wall and/or causes hydronephrosis or nonfunctioning kidney and/or involves pelvic and/or para-aortic lymph nodes
   4. Stage IV—Carcinoma extended beyond the true pelvis or involves the bladder or rectum

VIII. Prognosis and survival

A. Prognosis is related to how extensive disease is at diagnosis (Oleszewski, 2018).

B. In the United States, the 5-year survival rate for localized cervical cancer is nearly 92%, while it is less than 60% for disease that has spread to local lymph nodes, and only about 17% for metastatic disease (NCI, 2022b).

Management

I. Management (NCCN, 2021a)

A. Preinvasive disease (CIN1–3) may be treated by diagnostic modality (Loop electrosurgical excision procedure [LEEP], cone biopsy), local cauterization or cryotherapy, or hysterectomy if fertility sparing is not desired.

B. For invasive disease treatment generally includes surgery, radiation therapy (RT), chemotherapy, or some combination.

C. Treatments for early-stage disease (IA1–IA2)
   1. Fertility sparing: conization with cold knife or LEEP procedure, lymph node evaluation if lymphovascular space invasion (LVSI) is present, radical trachelectomy
   2. Non–fertility sparing: simple or modified radical hysterectomy with or without lymph node evaluation
   3. Consider pelvic external beam RT (EBRT) or brachytherapy in patients for whom surgery is not an option.

D. Treatments for more advanced stages
   1. Radical hysterectomy+lymphadenectomy
   2. Pelvic EBRT+brachytherapy±concurrent platinum-based chemotherapy
   3. Systemic therapy±individualized RT for distant metastases
      a. Systemic regimens include
         (1) Cisplatin/paclitaxel±bevacizumab
         (2) Carboplatin if cisplastin not an option
         (3) Add pembrolizumab for PD-L1-positive disease

E. Recurrent disease: RT, systemic therapy, local ablation, surgical resection

F. Metastatic disease: RT with or without chemotherapy, palliative systemic agents, best supportive care

G. Nursing management (Falardeau, 2020)
   1. Manage treatment- and cancer-related symptoms
      a. Cancer-related symptoms can include significant bleeding, pain, urinary or bowel obstruction/invasion, and complications of metastatic sites of local structures, lymph nodes, and distant sites.
      b. Abdominal/pelvic surgery: alterations in urinary, bowel, and vaginal function. Management of catheterization, urinary tract infection, constipation, bowel obstruction, and shortening of the vagina.
      c. Preoperative and postoperative care, including risks for bleeding, infection, deep vein thrombosis, lymphedema after lymph node dissection (LND). See Chapter 25.

d. Abdominal/pelvic RT: changes in bowel and urinary function may include loose stools, obstructions, fistula formation, ulceration, pain, radiation cystitis, and urinary frequency or retention. Changes in vaginal function may involve stenosis, dryness, and atrophy. See Chapter 27.

e. Systemic agents and toxicities: cisplatin, fluorouracil, carboplatin, paclitaxel, topotecan, and bevacizumab. Particular attention to renal and hepatic function, CINV, hypersensitivity reactions, myelosuppression, and neuropathy. See Chapter 28 for more information on chemotherapies.

2. Assess for signs of recurrent disease: pain, changes in bowel/bladder, vaginal bleeding, leg swelling, groin mass/changes, abnormal follow-up examination.

3. Sexual and reproductive function
   a. Even with fertility-sparing treatment, changes in vaginal function may still affect sexual function.
      (1) Encourage open communication with the patient, provider, and sexual partner.
      (2) Vaginal dilators and lubricants, certain sexual positions may be helpful.
   b. Contraception should be used during and for a period after active treatment, depending on treatment type.
   c. Discuss infertility with patient prior to treatment start in non-fertility sparing treatment.

UTERINE CANCER

Overview

I. Definition
   A. A collection of cancers arising from either the endometrial lining of the uterine walls (referred to as endometrial cancer or uterine corpus cancer) or the stromal and muscle of the uterus (uterine sarcomas)

II. Epidemiology
   A. Sixth most common cancer diagnosed in women worldwide (Sung et al., 2021)
      1. Highest rates are in North America and Europe, with incidence rates increasing in many other regions globally (Sung et al., 2021)
   B. United States and trends. Most common cancer of the female genital tract in the United States with incidence increasing steadily since the early 2000s (NCI, 2022e).
      1. Most common cancer of the female genital tract in the United States with stable incidence but increasing mortality annually from 2005 to 2014. Most cases are diagnosed in postmenopausal women aged 55–74, with incidence rates fairly evenly distributed among racial and ethnic groups (NCI, 2022e; Redlin-Frazier, 2018).
      2. Incidence is highest in women aged 55–64, mortality highest aged 65–74, and disproportionately represented in African American women. Black women are twice as likely to die from uterine

cancer compared to women of other racial and ethnic groups (NCI, 2022e).

III. Pathophysiology
   A. The uterus is a fibromuscular, pear-shaped, hollow female reproductive organ consisting of the endometrium (innermost layer of the uterus), myometrium (muscle wall of uterus), and perimetrium (Crosbie et al., 2022; Falardeau, 2020).
      1. Most uterine cancers arise from the endometrium and are referred to as endometrial cancers; those arising from the myometrium are uterine sarcomas (Koskas, Amant, Mirza, & Creutzberg, 2021).
   B. The endometrium is hormonally driven for vascular proliferation to support the fetus (Falardeau, 2020).
   C. Estrogen stimulates endometrium to proliferate, and unopposed estrogen results in unbalanced proliferation (Crosbie et al., 2022).
      1. Conditions that create increased estrogen largely contribute to increased risk factors for uterine cancer, which include obesity, type 2 diabetes, early menarche, late menopause, advanced age, tamoxifen use, nulliparity, polycystic ovary syndrome.
   D. Endometrial adenocarcinomas progress through a premalignant phase of intraepithelial endometrial neoplasia (Koskas et al., 2021).
   E. Endometrial carcinomas arise from a series of somatic DNA pathogenic variants (Koskas et al., 2021).
   F. Nonendometrioid tumors have a hormone-inde-pendent pathogenesis and lack any precursor lesions (Lu & Broaddus, 2020).

IV. Primary prevention
   A. Maintain a healthy weight.
      1. Uterine cancer is strongly associated with obesity.
   B. Physical activity reduces the risk for endometrial cancer (Koskas et al., 2021).
   C. Avoid unopposed estrogen therapy (Crosbie et al., 2022).
      1. Combination oral contraceptive and progestin-releasing intrauterine device use is protective and can offer long-term risk reduction (Crosbie et al., 2022; Karlsson, Johansson, Höglund, Ek, & Johansson, 2021; Koskas et al., 2021).
      2. Cigarette smoking reduces estrogen stimulation to the endometrium, providing a protective benefit from endometrial cancer (though risk of lung cancer with smoking negates the benefit) (Redlin-Frazier, 2018).
   D. Women at high risk (e.g., Lynch syndrome, atypical hyperplasia) for whom fertility preservation is not desired can undergo prophylactic hysterectomy (Redlin-Frazier, 2018).
   E. Aspirin is recommended for women with Lynch syndrome (Crosbie et al., 2022).

V. Diagnosis
   A. History and physical
      1. Clinical presentation commonly includes postmenopausal bleeding (Crosbie et al., 2022).

2. In premenopausal women, look for prolonged, heavy, intermenstrual bleeding (Crosbie et al., 2022).

B. Transvaginal ultrasound showing thickened endometrium (Crosbie et al., 2022)

1. Endometrial thickness ≥5 mm warrants endometrial biopsy, and hysteroscopy should be added in the presence of irregularities or polyps (Crosbie et al., 2022).

C. Pelvic MRI allows for the assessment of tumor origin and local disease spread including lymph node involvement and myometrial invasion (Crosbie et al., 2022; NCCN, 2021c).

D. PET/CT if metastatic disease is suspected (NCCN, 2021c)

1. Most common sites for metastases include lung, vagina, and ovaries (Koskas et al., 2021).

2. Chest x-ray is a reasonable low-cost method for ruling out lung metastases, especially in early-stage disease when it is less likely (Koskas et al., 2021; NCCN, 2021c).

E. Laboratory tests: complete blood count (CBC), renal and liver function, CA-125 (Koskas et al., 2021; NCCN, 2021c)

F. Proctoscopy and/or cystoscopy are helpful in assessing direct extension to the rectum or bladder (Koskas et al., 2021).

G. Genetic evaluation of tumor and inherited cancer risk (NCCN, 2021c)

VI. Histopathology (Koskas et al., 2021; NCCN, 2021c)

A. Atypical hyperplasia is not malignant but is a precursor to endometrial cancer with a 45-fold increased risk for progression to malignancy.

B. Uterine cancer can be divided by whether the malignant cell arises from the endometrium or the stromal and muscle cells of the uterus.

1. Malignant epithelial (carcinoma): pure endometrioid cancer, serous carcinoma, clear cell carcinoma, carcinosarcoma (i.e., malignant mixed mesodermal/Mullerian tumor), and undifferentiated carcinoma

a. Endometrioid cancers make up the majority of endometrial cancers and usually present at an early stage, are often hormone dependent, and have a very favorable prognosis.

b. Nonendometrioid cancers are more aggressive and carry a greater risk of early distant spread and often present at a more advanced stage.

(1) Carcinosarcomas are treated as aggressive, high-grade endometrial cancer.

2. Malignant mesenchymal (sarcoma): uterine leiomyosarcoma, undifferentiated uterine sarcoma, low-grade endometrial stromal sarcoma (ESS) or adenocarcinoma, high-grade ESS

a. Account for about 3%–7% of all uterine cancers (Mbatani, Olawaiye, & Prat, 2018)

C. Molecular analysis

1. Estrogen receptor testing should be done for advanced or recurrent disease.

2. HER2 immunohistochemistry for advanced-stage or recurrent serous endometrial carcinoma or carcinosarcoma

3. Testing for molecular subgroups (POLE pathogenic variant, microsatellite instability, high somatic copy-number alterations, and copy-number low group without a specific driver pathogenic variant) is important for prognostication.

VII. Staging

A. Uterine cancer is staged surgically; histological confirmation of the type, grade, and extent of involvement is critical for staging (Crosbie et al., 2022).

B. FIGO and TNM staging systems are used (and are essentially the same) for both endometrial carcinomas and uterine sarcomas.

1. FIGO/TNM staging for endometrial carcinomas (Amin et al., 2017; Koskas et al., 2021)

a. Stage I—Tumor confined to corpus uteri

b. Stage II—Tumor invades cervical stroma but does not extend beyond the uterus

c. Stage III—Local and/or regional tumor spread

d. Stage IV—Tumor invades bladder and/or bowel mucosa, or distant metastases

2. FIGO/TNM staging of uterine sarcomas (Amin et al., 2017; Mbatani et al., 2018)

a. Stage I—Tumor limited to uterus

b. Stage II—Tumor extends to pelvis

c. Stage III—Tumor invades abdominal tissues

d. Stage IV—Tumor invades bladder and/or rectum or distant metastases

C. Grading of endometrioid carcinomas is dependent on the percentage of glandular and solid-tumor components—Grades 1 (<6%) and 2 (6%–50%) are considered low grade and grade 3 (>50%) are high grade (Lu & Broaddus, 2020).

VIII. Prognosis and survival

A. Uterine cancer has a good prognosis with an overall 5-year relative survival rate of over 80%, but prognosis is very much dependent on tumor type and stage at diagnosis (NCI, 2022e)

1. Localized disease has a 95% 5-year survival rate while that rate falls to 70% for regional involvement, and 18% for distant metastases (NCI, 2022e).

2. Prognosis favorable in younger patients with early-stage, low-grade disease (NCCN, 2021c)

3. Prognosis less favorable with increased age, positive lymph nodes (LNs), larger tumor, LVSI, involvement of the lower uterine segment, and nonendometrioid histology (Koskas et al., 2021; NCCN, 2021c)

a. Leiomyosarcomas, even when diagnosed at an early stage, are associated with a poor prognosis (Mbatani et al., 2018).

b. Carcinosarcoma carries a 5-year survival of 30% and compared to other high-grade endometrial cancers carries a worse prognosis even while diagnosed at an early stage (Lu & Broaddus, 2020; Mbatani et al., 2018).

4. Molecular subgroups are becoming increasingly important to prognosis (e.g., POLE mutated tumors have a favorable prognosis, while p53 abnormal is unfavorable) (Crosbie et al., 2022).

B. Unlike other common cancer types, survival rates have been declining and death rates increasing for uterine cancers (Siegel et al., 2022).

Management

I. Treatment Overview (Crosbie et al., 2022; Koskas et al., 2021; NCCN, 2021c)

A. The backbone of treatment for uterine cancer is total hysterectomy (TH) and bilateral salpingo-oophorectomy (BSO).

   1. Minimally invasive surgery is preferred for early-stage disease.
   2. Consider ovarian conservation in premenopausal women with early-stage disease.
   3. Surgical options for patients with extrauterine disease depend on patient suitability, location of metastatic disease, and likelihood of complete cytoreduction.

B. Lymphadenectomy should be performed only for staging, and sentinel lymph node biopsy is the preferred method.

C. Adjuvant treatment options for endometrioid cancers include observation (Stage I only), vaginal brachytherapy, EBRT, and systemic therapy.

D. Adjuvant chemoradiation or chemotherapy alone should be considered in patients with advanced disease.

   1. Primary preferred regimen is carboplatin/paclitaxel in endometrioid carcinoma.
   2. Doxorubicin and docetaxel/gemcitabine are preferred in uterine sarcomas.

E. Fertility-sparing treatment using continuous progestin therapy can be considered for low-grade, early-stage endometrial adenosarcoma; however, TH is recommended after completion of childbearing.

F. If not a surgical candidate: EBRT and/or brachytherapy, systemic therapy, or hormonal therapy for ER/PR-positive endometrioid histology

G. Recurrent disease

   1. Local/confined recurrence or isolated metastasis: second-line systemic therapy, RT, and/or secondary surgery (if complete cytoreduction is likely)
   2. Low-grade, disseminated disease: hormonal or systemic chemotherapy
   3. High-grade, disseminated disease: systemic therapy with or without palliative RT
   4. Biomarker-directed systemic therapy in the second line includes pembrolizumab ± Lenvatinib depending on microsatellite instability and tumor pathogenic variant burden.

H. Nursing implications (Falardeau, 2020)

   1. Promote healthy lifestyle behaviors and risk reduction: weight and dietary management, identify high-risk populations due to genetic, socioeconomic, and reproductive risk factors and screen for abnormal bleeding and report to provider.
   2. Manage treatment- and cancer-related symptoms.
      a. Cancer-related symptoms may include pain, abnormal bleeding, vaginal discharge, changes in urinary function.
      b. Surgery and RT of the abdomen/pelvis and associated pretreatment and posttreatment care, including hypoestrogenism after BSO, which may induce hot flashes, mood changes, vaginal dryness, pelvic tissue atrophy, osteoporosis, and increased cardiovascular disease (CVD) risk (NCCN, 2021c).
      c. Management of systemic therapies and toxicities: common agents include cisplatin, carboplatin, doxorubicin, docetaxel, gemcitabine, paclitaxel, ifosfamide, everolimus, and aromatase inhibitors (Chapter 28).
   3. Assess for recurrent disease: typically, within 3 years of initial diagnosis, presenting with vaginal bleeding, poor appetite, weight loss, pain, cough, abdominal or leg swelling (NCCN, 2021c)
   4. Sexual and reproductive functioning
      a. Appropriate use of lubricants, changes in sexual position, and teaching
      b. Encourage communication with patient and sexual partner regarding fertility concerns and sexual function before, during, and after treatment.
   5. Genetic risk factors may have implications for extended family members.

OVARIAN CANCER

Overview

I. Definition
   A. Cancer that forms in tissues of the ovary

II. Epidemiology
   A. Eighth most common cancer in women worldwide (Sung et al., 2021)
   B. Rates are highest in developing countries, except for Japan (Berek, Renz, Kehoe, Kumar, & Friedlander, 2021).
   C. Ovarian cancer is relatively rare, accounting for about 1% of all new cancer cases in the United States, and incidence rates have been declining in recent years (NCI, 2022c).
   D. Ovarian cancer incidence increases with age, and most women are diagnosed after age 55 (NCI, 2022c).
   E. Only about 23% of gynecologic cancers are ovarian in origin, but they account for 47% of all gynecologic cancer deaths (Berek et al., 2021).

III. Pathophysiology (Falardeau, 2020; Martin & Stewart, 2018)
   A. Ovaries are the female reproductive glands located deep in the pelvis, lateral to the uterus and posterior to the fallopian tubes, providing ova and reproductive hormone regulation and production.
   B. Ovarian cancer originates from tissue of the ovary or fallopian tube and may seed the peritoneal cavity and adjacent pelvic and lymphatic structures.

C. Hormonal, genetic, and environmental factors play a role in the development of ovarian cancer.
   1. BRCA1/BRCA2 pathogenic variants, Lynch syndrome increase the risk for ovarian cancer, and as many as 20% of all ovarian cancer cases are due to hereditary factors.
D. Cell division and regeneration of the epithelium in the ovaries during ovulation provide an opportunity for malignant transformation.
   1. There is a 6% increase in a woman's ovarian cancer risk with each year of ovulation.

IV. Primary prevention
A. Reducing ovulation cycles is protective against ovarian cancer, so the increased number of pregnancies and lactation can reduce the risk of developing ovarian cancer (Martin & Stewart, 2018).
B. Oral contraceptive use can offer long-term risk reduction in ovarian cancer (Karlsson et al., 2021).
C. Prophylactic BSO in high-risk patients with *BRCA1* or *BRCA2* pathogenic variants (NCCN, 2022a)
D. Smoking increases the risk for mucinous carcinomas (NCCN, 2022a).
E. Practice safe sex, limiting the number of partners and using barrier protection.
   1. Pelvic inflammatory disease is associated with an increased risk of borderline ovarian tumors (Rasmussen et al., 2017).
   2. *Chlamydia trachomatis* infections are associated with a higher risk for ovarian cancer (Fortner et al., 2019).

V. Diagnosis (Berek et al., 2021; NCCN, 2022a)
A. Complete history and physical
   1. Clinical presentation with bloating, pain, early satiety, dyspepsia, urinary urgency or frequency, especially if symptoms are new or frequent
   2. Obtain a careful family history given genetic component of disease.
   3. Evaluate the performance and nutritional status.
   4. Pelvic exam to search for ovarian mass
      a. Masses are most suspicious if they are painless, immobile, irregular, or there is bilateral ovarian involvement (Martin & Stewart, 2018).
B. Imaging can include ultrasound, abdominal/pelvic CT or MRI, chest CT or x-ray (screening for pleural effusions or concern for metastatic disease), or PET/CT for indeterminate lesions.
C. Laboratory should include CBC, comprehensive metabolic panel (CMP), and CA-125.
   1. Other tumor markers could include inhibin, β-human chorionic gonadotrophin (hCG), alphafetoprotein, LDH, CEA, and CA19-9.
D. Patient should be referred to a gynecologic oncologist for suspicious lesions.

VI. Histopathology (Berek et al., 2021; NCCN, 2022a)
A. Epithelial ovarian cancer makes up about 90% of all ovarian malignancies, and the main types include serous (most common), endometrioid, clear cell, and mucinous.
   1. Arise from cells that cover the outer surface of the ovary
   2. Low-grade serous cancers make up about 8% of all ovarian cancers and tend to have more indolent behavior and are resistant to chemotherapy.
B. Sex-cord stromal tumors arise from tissues that produce estrogen and progesterone and hold the ovary together.
   1. Granulosa cell tumors most common form of sex-cord stromal tumors and about 5% of all ovarian cancers
      a. Can present as juvenile or adult
C. Germ cell tumors arise from the primitive germ cells of the embryonic gonad and are classified as dysgerminoma, embryonal carcinoma, teratoma, or extraembryonal differentiation.
D. Ovarian sarcomas include malignant mixed Müllerian tumors or carcinosarcomas.
E. Grading is more important than histologic subtype from a prognostic standpoint (Martin & Stewart, 2018).
   1. Serous tumors are either low grade (grade 1) or high grade (grades 2 and 3).
   2. Endometrioid and mucinous carcinomas and stage 1C tumors are graded G1 to G3.

VII. Staging
A. Ovarian, fallopian tube, and peritoneal cancers should be staged surgically, and a staging laparotomy is an important part of early disease management (Berek et al., 2021).
B. FIGO and AJCC TNM staging used for ovarian cancer (Amin et al., 2017; Berek et al., 2021)
   1. Stage I—Tumor limited to ovaries (one or both) or fallopian tubes
   2. Stage II—Tumor involves one or both ovaries or fallopian tubes with pelvic extension below pelvic brim or primary peritoneal cancer
   3. Stage III—Tumor involves one or both ovaries or fallopian tubes, or primary peritoneal cancer, with microscopically confirmed peritoneal metastases outside the pelvis and/or metastatic disease to the retroperitoneal lymph nodes
   4. Stage IV—Distant metastasis including positive cytology from pleural effusion

VIII. Prognosis and survival (NCI, 2022c)
A. Most ovarian cancers are diagnosed in advanced stages, carrying a poor prognosis with a 5-year relative survival rate less than 50%.
B. However, death rates are decreasing, and 5-year survival has increased in recent years.
C. Survival varies greatly by stage, with localized disease carrying a 93% survival rate, compared to less than 31% for metastatic disease.
   1. Only 17% of ovarian cancers are diagnosed before disease has spread.
D. Prognosis determined not only by stage at diagnosis but also histologic type and grade, and maximum diameter of residual disease after cytoreductive surgery (Berek et al., 2021).

E. Age and performance status are important patient-related prognostic indicators (Martin & Stewart, 2018).

Management

I. Management (Berek et al., 2021; NCCN, 2022a)
   A. Fertility-sparing unilateral salpingo-oophorectomy may be adequate for unilateral stage I tumors. For stage IB tumors, a BSO with preservation of the uterus may be an option.
   B. Surgical staging with total abdominal hysterectomy/BSO and LND as indicated, debulking, and adjuvant chemotherapy (platinum/taxane)
      1. Aside from women with stage I, grade 1 tumors, most will require treatment after surgical staging.
      2. Consider neoadjuvant chemotherapy for bulky disease/poor surgical candidates (evaluation should be done by a gynecological oncologist).
      3. Hyperthermic intraperitoneal chemotherapy with cisplatin can be considered at time of an interval debulking surgery for stage III disease.
      4. Intraperitoneal chemotherapy if stage III disease is optimally debulked
   C. Maintenance therapy with a PARP inhibitor, bevacizumab, or a combination of the two depending on BRCA and homologous recombination deficient status
   D. Relapsed ovarian cancer
      1. Most women will experience a disease relapse, and one objective of follow-ups should be for the earliest detection of signs or symptoms of recurrence.
      2. Most studies have shown that treating an elevated CA-125 in asymptomatic patients, with no radiologic evidence of progression, did not improve overall survival and only had a negative impact on quality of life.
      3. For those with poor response to chemotherapy or short interval from completion of platinum-based chemotherapy to relapse (<6m) (i.e., platinum-resistant disease): clinical trials, supportive care, second-line systemic chemotherapy (non-platinum based), and targeted therapy (PARP inhibitors, bevacizumab, and hormone therapy)
      4. If complete remission and relapse >6 months after primary platinum-based chemotherapy (i.e., platinum-sensitive disease): surgery, clinical trials, best supportive care, platinum-based systemic chemotherapy, and PARP inhibitors
   E. Indications for hormonal therapy or treatment of less common ovarian histopathologies according to diagnosis
   F. Nursing implications (Falardeau, 2020)
      1. Risk mitigation depends on early identification of risk factors, referral for genetic risk evaluation, and addressing of modifiable risk factors such as tobacco cessation and prevention of PID/sexually transmitted infections.
      2. Manage treatment- and cancer-related symptoms
         a. Cancer-related symptoms commonly include gastrointestinal dysfunction, ascites, and abdominal pain.
         b. Surgery and RT of the abdomen/pelvis and associated pretreatment and posttreatment care as described previously
         c. Management of systemic toxicities for common agents such as carboplatin, cisplatin, paclitaxel, docetaxel, bevacizumab, gemcitabine, pegylated liposomal doxorubicin, PARP inhibitors; patients will generally go through multiple lines of therapy
            (1) Almost 80% of women with advanced disease relapse after a response to first-line therapy with a median time to recurrence of 16 months (Berek et al., 2021).
         d. Be prepared for hypersensitivity reactions as it is a common possibility with many of the drugs used to treat ovarian cancer (NCCN, 2022a).
         e. Address fertility and surgically/chemotherapy-induced menopause for patients who were previously premenopausal.
      3. Recurrent disease is frequent due to later stages of diagnosis.
         a. Assess for abdominal bloating, bowel/bladder changes, weight loss, early satiety, nausea, vomiting, ascites.
         b. CA-125 and imaging surveillance per guidelines

GESTATIONAL TROPHOBLASTIC NEOPLASIA

Overview

I. Definitions: Gestational trophoblastic neoplasia (GTN) refers to lesions that have the potential for local and metastatic invasion.
   A. GTN includes a number of interrelated diseases that originate from the placenta and malignant neoplasms. The most important change has been the curing and preservation of reproductive function. However, these advances are based upon the early and appropriate management and timely follow-up.
   B. Hydatidiform moles (HMs): Benign placental tumors with malignant potential (Wang et al., 2017)
      1. Complete
      2. Partial
   C. GTN: placental tumors with malignant behavior
      1. Post molar GTN
      2. Invasive mole
   D. Gestational choriocarcinoma
      1. Placental site trophoblastic tumor (PSTT)
      2. Epithelioid trophoblastic tumor (ETT)
II. Epidemiology and risk factors:
   A. Epidemiology: relatively uncommon overall and is more common in Asia than Europe or North America (Berkowitz, Horowitz, & Elias, 2022)
   B. Risk factors (Berkowitz et al., 2022; Soper, 2021)
      1. Very young or geriatric pregnancy (under 16 or over 45)
      2. Autosomal-recessive familial recurrent HM
      3. Some evidence for menarche after age 12, history of light menses, OCP use

III. Physiology and pathophysiology (Soper, 2021)
   A. Arise from components of the placenta
   B. Malignant GTN: malignant invasive mole, choriocarcinoma, PSTT/ETT
   C. Result of abnormal conception leading to molar pregnancy: HM
IV. Primary prevention (Soper, 2021)
   A. Early detection with hCG level monitoring after molar pregnancies facilitates earlier treatment and better outcomes
V. Diagnosis (NCCN, 2021b; Soper, 2021)
   A. Clinical presentation (see Table 24.1)
      1. HM presents with vaginal bleeding in the first trimester (Berkowitz et al., 2022).
      2. Diagnosed and staged by suction D&C and histologic examination, hCG monitoring, pelvic ultrasound, and chest x-ray with or without CT and brain MRI
   B. Choriocarcinoma (CC), placental site trophoblastic tumour (PSTT)/, epithelioid trophoblastic tumors (ETT): may also include lumbar puncture to determine occult central nervous system disease.

C. PSTT/ETT: occurs after any pregnancy; diagnosis commonly delayed. hCG monitoring indicated for metastatic disease in women of childbearing potential.
D. Differential diagnosis will include the addition of immunohistochemical markers such as GATA-3 that is sensitive for both benign and malignant GTN.
E. Diagnostic tests will include:
   1. Labs
      a. hCG
      b. Thyroid function tests
      c. Liver function tests
      d. Renal function tests
      e. CBC with differential
      f. Testosterone levels in the presence of virilization
   2. Imaging studies
      a. Pelvic ultrasound
      b. Chest imaging
      c. With evidence of metastatic disease or initial evaluation:
         (1) CT of abdomen and pelvis or PET
         (2) MRI/CT of brain
VI. Histopathology (NCCN, 2021b; Soper, 2021)

TABLE 24.1 Clinical Presentation of Gestational Trophoblastic Neoplasia (GTN)

Type of GTN	Onset of Symptoms	Symptoms	Symptoms Associated With elevated hCG

Invasive mole	Follows molar pregnancy	Elevated hCG >1,000,000 mill-IU/mL
		Bilateral ovarian enlargement
		Previous cesarean section
		AUB or amenorrhea
		Pelvic pain or pressure related to enlarged uterus or ovarian cysts
		Symptoms of metastases related to involved organs:
		  Pulmonary (80%): dyspnea, chest pain, cough hyptosis. Trophoblastic emboli can cause pulmonary artery occlusion and pulmonary hypertension.
		  Vaginal (30%): vaginal bleeding or purulent vaginal discharge
		  Central nervous system (10%): initially as asymptomatic. Progression to ICP: headache, neuropathy, dizziness, nausea, slurred speech, visual disturbances, and/or hemiparesis; high association with brain metastases
		Liver: jaundice, epigastric or back pain
		Nephrotic syndrome (rare)
		Virilization: hCG overstimulation of the ovary leading to the cell hyperplasia with elevated testosterone
			Endocrine symptoms: hyperthyroidism, ovarian theca lutein cysts, hyper emesis (rare) or preeclampsia (rare)

Choriocarcinoma	Follows any type of pregnancy with or without molar type	Bleeding from metastatic site(s)	Low level hCG
PSTT	Months or years postpartum	Localized uterine symptoms with masses in the myometrium; irregular bleeding or amenorrhea	Low levels
ETT	Slow growing	Hemorrhagic, solid and cystic lesions in the fundus, lower uterine segment or endocervix; irregular bleeding or amenorrhea	Low or absent hCG levels
GTN	Postmolar or any pregnancy event	Following evacuation of HM, enlarged uterine size, elevated hCG, bilateral ovarian enlargement, AUB	
GTN	Following PHM	Enlarged uterus	
GTN	Following term or preterm	Amenorrhea, AUB with invasion of uterine tumor	

AUB, Abnormal uterine bleeding; *ETT*, epithelioid trophoblastic tumor; *ICP*, increased intracranial pressure; *PHM*, partial hydatidiform mole; *PSTT*, placental site trophoblastic tumor.

A. Villous trophoblast: complete or partial HM (CHM/PHM)

B. Epithelial tumor: choriocarcinoma (CC)

C. PSTT: lower hemorrhage risk, lower hCG levels. ETT behaves similarly.

VII. Staging (Berkowitz et al., 2022; NCCN, 2021b)

A. Both the FIGO staging system and the WHO Prognostic Risk Scoring System is used in combination. A report may show a stage (II) with a PSS score of 3 that would be reported as II:3. The WHO PSS includes the following variables: age, antecedent pregnancy, interval from last pregnancy, pretreatment hCG, largest tumor, site of metastases, number of metastases, and prior chemotherapy treatment.

  1. WHO PSS Scoring: Note primarily used for FIGO stages II and III.

    a. 0–6: low-risk resistance to single-agent chemotherapy.

    b. >7: high-risk resistance to monotherapy and requires combination chemotherapy.

    c. >12: ultra-high risk and associated with non-molar pregnancy, brain metastases. Multidrug regimens are recommended.

  2. Note: WHO PSS is not used for FIGO Stage 1 GTN who are at low risk.

  3. For CHM/PHM, CC: patient age, pregnancy history, hCG, metastases, largest tumor, and history of prior chemotherapy to determine overall prognostic score as low (0–6) or high (≥7) risk.

  4. PSTT/ETT is staged I, II, III, or IV depending on the spread of disease.

VIII. Prognosis and survival (NCCN, 2021b; Soper, 2021)

A. Prognostic factors: interval from pregnancy to diagnosis, stage at presentation, and high mitotic index (poor prognosis for PSTT) (NCCN, 2021b; Soper, 2021).

B. Five-year survival: approximately 100% for low-risk and 90% for high-risk groups.

Management

I. Management (NCCN, 2021b; Soper, 2021)

A. GTN after HM, CC: single-agent chemotherapy for low risk and multiagent therapy for high risk. Treatment continues until hCG normalized 6–8 weeks.

B. PSTT/ETT: stage I recommended for hysterectomy with lymph node sampling, chemotherapy, and secondary surgical resection of residual masses. Advanced stages recommended for combination/high-dose chemotherapy.

C. Recurrent disease: 3% overall relapse rate, most common within 1 year of treatment. For GTN after HM, second-line and salvage chemotherapy with or without resection has excellent cure rates.

D. Risk factors and prevention: review family/personal history of molar pregnancies, encourage regular prenatal and OB/GYN care.

E. Cancer- and treatment-related symptoms (NCCN, 2021b; Soper, 2021).

  1. Due to rise in hCG, many cancer-related symptoms are similar, but more severe, than those in pregnancy, bleeding.

  2. Chemotherapy regimens for more advanced or recurrent disease have many significant side effects, and toxicities should be managed closely. Common agents for GTN include methotrexate, etoposide, cyclophosphamide, vincristine, actinomycin-D (NCCN, 2021b).

    a. High-risk protocols may also include cisplatin, paclitaxel, and bleomycin.

    b. For chemotherapy-resistant GTN the following protocols include:

      (1) PD-1/PD-L1 inhibitors such as pembrolizumab, nivolumab, and avelumab

      (2) Capecitabine-based regimens

      (3) Gemcitabine with or without cisplatin

      (4) Peripheral stem cell transplant protocols

  3. Postsurgical care after hysterectomy and/or surgical resections

F. Assess for recurrent disease; will include timely follow-up even beyond the first year of hCG surveillance (NCCN, 2021b; Soper, 2021).

G. Sexual and reproductive function (Soper, 2021)

  1. No obvious increase in the risk of congenital malformations or decrease in fertility after treatment but avoid pregnancy for at least 1 year after completion of therapy.

  2. Infertility in case of hysterectomy (with or without surgical menopause).

  3. Involve sexual partners and patient in discussion surrounding fertility issues, contraception recommendations before, during, and after treatment.

  • Hyperthyroidism (rare): There is growing evidence that hyperthyroidism is associated with GTN. It coincides with rising HCG levels following GTN treatment. Monitoring of the thyroid post therapy should be included with the hCG (Pereira & Lim, 2021).

VULVAR CANCER

Overview

I. Definition

A. A type of cancer that occurs on the outer surface of the female genitals (i.e., labia majora, labia minora, clitoris, and Bartholin glands) (NCI, 2022f).

B. Fourth most common gynecologic malignancy in the United States following uterine, ovarian, and cervical cancers (Siegel et al., 2022).

II. Epidemiology (Berek & Karam, 2022; Siegel et al., 2022)

A. Relatively rare worldwide and in the United States; most commonly diagnosed in women aged 55–75 years, with most associated deaths occurring over 84 years. Average age in the United States is 68 years.

B. Associated deaths have increased over the past 10 years when diagnosed early.

III. Pathophysiology (Berek & Karam, 2022; NCI, 2022f)

A. External female genitalia from mons pubis to perineum, including labia majora and minora, with smooth internal mucosal membranes that are continuous with the female urogenital tract.

B. Premalignant and malignant changes may involve only the vulva; malignant changes may extend to lymph nodes, local structures, distant sites (Berek & Karam, 2022).

C. Risk factors: oncogenic HPV infection, cigarette smoking, inflammatory conditions of the vulva, immunodeficiency (Berek & Karam, 2022; Siegel et al., 2022).
   1. High number of sexual partners
   2. Initiation of early-age sexual intercourse
   3. History of abnormal Pap smears
   4. Previous history of cervical cancer
   5. Northern European ancestry

IV. Primary Prevention (NCCN, 2021d; Rogers & Cuello, 2018)
   A. Vaccination for HPV subtypes 16 and 18
   B. Identification and early treatment of preinvasive disease

V. Diagnosis (Berek & Karam, 2022; NCCN, 2021d)
   A. Clinical presentation
      1. Vulvar lesion that may be asymptomatic but some present with vulvar pruritus or bleeding, and complaints of a groin mass, urinary or lower GI symptoms that are associated with more advanced disease.
   B. Diagnosis includes:
      1. History of risk factors or symptoms associated with vulvar cancers.
      2. Visual inspection looking at the quality of the lesions (e.g., firm, white, red, or skin-colored papules, nodules, plaques, degree of erosion or ulceration, and possible friable surface).
      3. Determined by vulvar biopsy, EUA cystoscopy, or proctoscopy as indicated.
         a. Possible colposcopy for identification of subclinical lesions.

VI. Histopathology (Berek & Karam, 2022; NCCN, 2021d)
   A. The most common histology is squamous (75%).
      1. Noninvasive vulvar intraepithelial neoplasia (VINs) and VINs related to HPV infection are classified as squamous intraepithelial lesions (SILs).
      2. SCC
   B. Less common histology: melanoma, extramammary Paget disease, Bartholin gland adenocarcinoma, verrucous carcinoma, basal cell carcinoma, and sarcoma
   C. Histologic grade (Berek & Karam, 2022; NCI, 2022f)
      1. VIN1/low-grade SIL (LSIL): considered nonneoplastic
      2. VIN2/VIN3/high-grade SIL (HSIL): neoplastic with chance of carcinogenesis

VII. Staging (NCCN, 2021d)
   A. Staging involves biopsy, lymph node evaluation, imaging, and/or cystoscopy.

VIII. Prognosis and survival (NCCN, 2021d; NCI, 2022f)
   A. Prognosis is most influenced by the involvement of lymph nodes and biomarkers.
   B. Poorer prognosis with larger primary tumor, greater depth of invasion, and LVSI.

C. Post surgically influenced by status of the tumor margin after primary resection.

D. Overall, 5-year survival in the United States is 72.1% (NCI, 2022f) and by stage is localized (86.4%), regional (56.9%), distant (17.4%), and unstaged (56.2%).

Management

I. Management (Berek & Karam, 2022; NCI, 2022f)
   A. Early stage (I/II): conservative tumor excision and lymph node evaluation
   B. Locally advanced (stage III/IVA): concurrent chemoradiation, surgical resection (modified or radical vulvectomy), and lymph node evaluation
   C. Distant metastatic (IVB—extra pelvic disease): EBRT for local control and/or chemotherapy, treatments extrapolated from cervical cancer
   D. RT may be used if not a surgical candidate and for nodal involvement.
   E. Local recurrence: re-excision, EBRT with or without concurrent chemotherapy, brachytherapy
      1. Chemoradiation regimens may include cisplatin, 5-FU, and mitomycin C.
         a. Distant/nodal recurrence or metastatic disease: dependent on prior treatments and recurrence site(s). RT, chemotherapy, rarely resection, and may involve the best supportive care. Advanced or recurrent metastatic regimens may include cisplatin, carboplatin, paclitaxel, bevacizumab, vinorelbine, erlotinib, and gemcitabine.
         b. TMB-H, PD-L1+, and MSI-high/MMR deficient tumors: nivolumab.
         c. NTRK gene fusion-positive tumors: Larotrectinib.
   F. Client safety and risk reduction: early detection of history of vulvar chronic inflammation, lesions, or HPV infection; encourage HPV vaccination, tobacco cessation, regular pelvic examinations, and posttreatment surveillance
   G. Cancer- and treatment-related symptoms
      1. Cancer-related symptoms may involve local site irritation, mass, pain, or complications of LN involvement or metastases.
      2. Local care of excision and/or biopsy sites and nursing care after abdominal/pelvic surgery or RT.
      3. Management of chemotherapy/immunotherapy and systemic toxicities.
   H. Patient education and counseling related to:
      1. Smoking cessation
      2. Reduction in sexual partners

VAGINAL CANCER

Overview

I. Definition: Cancer that forms in the tissues of the vagina. The vagina leads from the cervix to the outside of the body. The most common type is squamous cell.

II. Epidemiology (National Cancer Institute [NCI], 2022a)

A. Occurrence is rare in the United States: less than 1 of every 1000 women (American Cancer Society, 2022; Karam, Berek, & Kidd, 2022).

B. Elderly women are more commonly affected (Karam et al., 2022).

C. Risk factors (Karam et al., 2022)
  1. Oncogenic HPV infection (in 80% of vaginal cancer SCCs)
  2. Similar risk factors as cervical cancer: multiple sexual partners, early age of first intercourse, and current smoker
  3. Older age >60 years of age
  4. Diethylstilbestrol (DES) exposure in utero increases the risk of clear cell adenocarcinoma.

III. Pathophysiology
  A. The vaginal canal consists of connective, muscular, and erectile tissue covered with mucosal membrane with many rugae, extending from the vulvar opening to the uterine cervix, in proximity with lymphatics and blood vessels.
  B. Preinvasive and invasive changes of the vagina may be similar to those found in cervical cancers or an extension of a cervical cancer.
  C. Highly mediated by HPV infection subtypes 16 or 18.

IV. Primary prevention: HPV vaccination and early detection of preinvasive lesions

V. Diagnosis:
  A. Clinical presentation: Commonly asymptomatic and found with cytologic screening and pelvic exam.
    1. Vaginal bleeding post coital or postmenopausal. The discharge may be watery. Blood tinged or malodorous.
    2. Symptoms may be associated with the local extension of the disease:
    3. Presence of a vaginal mass.
      a. Urinary: frequency, dysuria, hematuria
      b. GI: Tenesmus, constipation, melena
      c. Pelvic pain
  B. Diagnostic workup: History to include DES exposure, exam to include vaginal inspection with rectovaginal exam, vaginal cytology, and biopsy.
  C. Imaging studies: Chest and further exams based on the extent of the disease and staging recommendations.

VI. Histopathology (Karam et al., 2022; PDQ, 2022)
  A. Most commonly SCC or VIN, which involves squamous epithelial cells but not underlying tissue
  B. Less common: adenocarcinoma, clear cell carcinoma, and vaginal melanoma
  C. Histologic grade
    1. VIN associated with HPV infection stratified by LSIL or HSIL
    2. VIN1 is considered LSIL; VIN2/VIN3 are considered HSIL

VII. Staging: FIGO and AJCC TNM stages (PDQ, 2022)

VIII. Prognosis and survival (Karam et al., 2022; PDQ, 2022)
  A. Prognostic factors influenced by histologic type and extent of disease
    1. SCC and adenocarcinoma (highest 5-year survival rates—about 50%)
    2. Vaginal melanoma (poor survival, about 13% at 5 years)
  B. Five-year relative survival by stage at diagnosis in the United States: stage I (84%), stage II (75%), and stage III/IV (57%)

Management

I. Management (Karam et al., 2022; PDQ, 2022)
  A. Treatments are dependent on the degree of invasion and LN status and may include the following:
    1. Stages I and II: surgery and/or radiation
    2. Stages III and IV: chemoradiation with fluorouracil and/or cisplatin
  B. Preinvasive disease may be treated with local agents, excision, or brachytherapy.
  C. The mainstay of invasive disease involves surgical excision, RT, brachytherapy, chemotherapy, or a combination of modalities.
  D. Surgical: partial or total vaginectomy (high morbidity) or pelvic exenteration.
  E. Recurrent disease is retreated dependent on site and extent of recurrence.
  F. Nursing implications
    1. Client safety and risk reduction involve early detection for the development of lesions, HPV vaccination, screen patients for congenital abnormalities, and/or DES exposure in utero.
    2. Cancer- and treatment-related symptoms
      a. Beyond abdominal/pelvic surgery/RT, reproductive and sexual function affected by the significant surgical loss of vaginal length and changes secondary to chemotherapy or radiotherapy modalities (may include stenosis, dryness)
      b. Use of dilators and/or lubricants as indicated
      c. Management of chemotherapy-induced toxicities
      d. Management of complications from distant metastatic sites
    3. Patient education and smoking cessation

TESTICULAR CANCER

Overview

I. Definition
  A. Cancer that forms in the tissue of one or both testicles. The cancer starts in the germ cells. Germ cells are found in the sperm.
  B. Most common solid malignancy affecting males from 15 to 35 years and the most curable (NCI, 2022d).

II. Epidemiology
  A. Rare in the United States overall with most cases of diagnosis or death in males aged 20–43 and less common in African American or Asian/Pacific Islander males (NCI, 2022d).
  B. Over 10 years the incidence has risen; death rates are stable (NCCN, 2022c).

C. Risk factors include personal or male family history of germ cell tumor (GCT), cryptorchidism, testicular dysgenesis, and Klinefelter syndrome (NCCN, 2022c).

III. Pathophysiology

A. Male ovoid reproductive glands descending from the inguinal canal during gestation into the scrotal sac, producing testosterone and spermatogenesis.

B. Testicular cancer is usually unilateral, arising from the germinal epithelium.

IV. Primary prevention

A. Early screening, detection, and treatment for excellent options of cure. Surgical correction of undescended testicles before puberty lowers the risk of testicular cancer.

V. Diagnosis (NCCN, 2022c)

A. Clinical presentation: Usually a painless unilateral mass, confirmed on ultrasound. May initially be suspected as epididymitis or orchitis if pain or swelling is present. Extragonadal disease confirmed on biopsy, and possible diagnostic orchiectomy for gonadal tumors may also be therapeutic.

B. Tumor markers: Seminoma will have elevated beta-hCG and lactate dehydrogenase (LDH). Nonseminomas indicated with elevated AFP levels.

VI. Histopathology (NCCN, 2022c)

A. Most tumors in testes are GCTs (95%).

B. Nonseminomatous GCTs, mixed seminoma/nonseminomas, seminomas with elevated AFP: more clinically aggressive.

C. Pure seminomas are less aggressive and spread more slowly.

VII. Staging

A. CT, MRI as indicated and TNM staging based on post-orchiectomy values of beta-hCG, LDH, and AFP.

B. Prognostic groupings combine TNM (clinical and pathologic) with serum tumor markers (AFP, LDH, beta-hCG) and report as SX, S0, S1, S2, and S3 per AJCC guidelines (Amin et al., 2017; NCCN, 2022c).

C. Risk classifications are based on primary tumor location, presence/absence of nonpulmonary visceral metastases, and tumor marker status.

1. Nonseminoma: good, intermediate, or poor risk status

2. Seminoma: good or intermediate risk status (none are poor risk status)

VIII. Prognosis and survival

A. Initial prognosis by tumor marker status and disease bulk (NCCN, 2022c)

B. Prognostic factors at relapse (NCCN, 2022c)

1. Favorable: complete response to first-line therapy, low postorchiectomy tumor markers, low-volume disease

2. Unfavorable: incomplete first-line response, high tumor markers, high-volume disease, extra testicular primary

C. Five-year relative survival by stage at diagnosis in the United States: localized (99.2%), regional (96.1%), distant (73.2%), unstaged (76.7%), and with an overall 50-year survival of 95.1% (NCI, 2022d)

Management

I. Management (NCCN, 2022c)

A. Treatments

1. Radical inguinal orchiectomy with or without an open inguinal biopsy of contralateral testis.

2. Fertility preservation: consider sperm banking before surgery, RT, or chemotherapy.

3. Seminoma: orchiectomy is followed by surveillance, RT, and/or chemotherapy.

4. Nonseminoma: orchiectomy is followed by surveillance, chemotherapy, and retroperitoneal LND (RLND).

B. Recurrent disease

1. Favorable: standard second-line chemotherapy. Possible surgical salvage if solitary resectable relapse site

2. Unfavorable: clinical trial chemotherapy, second-line or high-dose chemotherapy, palliative chemotherapy, salvage surgery

3. Chemotherapy regimens may include BEP, VIP, TIP, EP, and VeIP. Additional protocols may include carboplatin, gemcitabine, oxaliplatin, paclitaxel, and pembrolizumab (NCCN, 2022c).

C. Nursing implications

1. Client safety and risk reduction centers around early detection (testicular self-examination and clinical examination), detection of recurrent cancer, patient education, and family history or presence of other risk factors.

2. Cancer- and treatment-related symptoms

a. Surgical issues may involve local pain and discomfort or more extensive postoperative care for RLND.

b. Chemotherapy toxicity management should be aggressive due to intensive GCT.

c. RT may cause local irritation and affect fertility.

d. Metastatic symptoms of advanced disease/palliation.

3. Sexual and reproductive function should be discussed with client and sexual partner at the time of diagnosis (NCCN, 2022c).

a. Esthetic changes may be mitigated by a testicular implant, which may be placed at the time of initial surgery (NCCN, 2022c).

b. Sperm banking may be done before or after surgery, but ideally before any RT or chemotherapy.

c. Retrograde ejaculation after bilateral RLND, infertility.

PENILE CANCER

Overview

I. Definition

A. An external cancer that forms on the skin on the outer skin surface of the penis.

B. Overview: Cancers of the penis are rare in the industrialized countries of the United States and Europe. There is a much higher incidence in parts of South America, Africa, and Asia.

II. Epidemiology
- A. Usual presentation at 50–70 years (NCCN, 2022b; Steele, Richie, & Michaelson, 2022)
- B. Risk factors (NCCN, 2022b; Pettaway & Pagliaro, 2022)
- C. HIV/HPV infection (positive in 60%–80% of penile cancers, type 16 and 18)
  1. Phimosis, balanitis, chronic inflammation, penile trauma, lack of circumcision, lichen sclerosis, tobacco use, poor hygiene, and low socioeconomic status
  2. History of psoriasis treatment with psoralen and ultraviolet light

III. Pathophysiology (Steele et al., 2022)
- A. Penile root and shaft terminate at the glans and urinary meatus. In uncircumcised males the glans is covered with the prepuce (foreskin).
- B. Composed of fascia, nerves, lymphatics, sebaceous glands, and vascular erectile tissue. The glans is the most common site of penile cancers.
- C. Functions: excretion of urinary waste, internal fertilization, and reproduction.

IV. Primary prevention: control of modifiable risk factors such as vaccination for HPV, prevention of HIV infection, avoiding tobacco use, and early detection of lesions.

V. Diagnosis
- A. Clinical presentation of palpable/visible lesion (foreskin of uncircumcised men, on the penis tip or the shaft, with or without pain, discharge, or bleeding, or constitutional symptoms of cancer and diagnosed on biopsy)
  1. Changes in skin thickness or color, rash, bluish-brown growths, swelling at the penis, lumps in the groin
- B. Physical exam, biopsy, and imaging (chest, CT scans, ultrasound, and MRI)

VI. Histopathology (NCCN, 2022b; Pettaway & Pagliaro, 2022)
- A. Premalignant penile intraepithelial neoplasia
- B. SCC (95% of penile cancers) subtypes: verrucous (low malignant potential), papillary squamous, warty, and basaloid
- C. Histologic grade: degree of differentiation Gx, G1, G2, and G3 (NCCN, 2022b)

VII. Staging (NCCN, 2022b)
- A. TNM staging criteria; can involve MRI and/or ultrasound evaluation of primary lesion, depth of invasion and of lymph nodes that are otherwise difficult to assess.

VIII. Prognosis and survival
- A. Prognostic factors (Pettaway & Pagliaro, 2022)
  1. Inguinal LN metastasis is most prognostic factor.
  2. Earlier stage at diagnosis and treatment is favorable, up to 80% cure rate.
- B. Overall 5-year survival is 50%, with 5-year relative survival affected by LN status: negative nodes (>85%), positive nodes (29%–40%), pelvic lymph node involvement (0%).

Management

I. Management (Diorio, Leone, & Spiess, 2016; NCCN, 2022b)
- A. Treatments (NCCN, 2022b; Pettaway & Pagliaro, 2022)
  1. Penile organ–sparing approaches are available for Tis, ta, some T1 lesions, which include topical treatments, laser therapy, wide or local excision, glansectomy, and Mohs surgery, and are often followed by surveillance.
  2. To preserve functional anatomy and control primary tumor, radiation/brachytherapy or concurrent chemoradiation may be recommended.
  3. Treating penile cancer with higher grades or deeper invasion may involve partial or total penectomy, with inguinal LN dissection/lymphadenectomy for high-risk penile cancers.
  4. Neoadjuvant chemotherapy, chemoradiation, or adjuvant chemotherapy may be recommended based on LN status.
- B. Treatment for recurrent disease varies based on prior surgery, radiation, systemic treatment/chemotherapy, and LN status at recurrence. May involve retreatment or best supportive care.
- C. Nursing implications (NCCN, 2022b; Pettaway & Pagilaro, 2022)
  1. Encourage modification of risk factors: HPV vaccination, prevent HIV infection, circumcision before puberty, maintain good hygiene (retraction of foreskin and cleansing of the glans regularly), smoking cessation.
  2. Cancer- and treatment-related (radiation and/or chemotherapy) symptoms
     - a. Care related to treatment involves teaching and safety of topical treatments (imiquimod, 5-FU) and site care/wound care after minor and major surgical resection (including risks for sexual dysfunction and lymphedema) and during RT.
       (1) The role of neoadjuvant chemotherapy may include paclitaxel, ifosfamide, and cisplatin or 5-FU and cisplatin.
       (2) For recurrent/metastatic disease with and/or without radiation may include pembrolizumab, cetuximab, mitomycin C, or capecitabine (NCCN, 2022b).
     - b. Manage toxicities such as myelosuppression, renal or liver dysfunction, and neuropathy of agents such as cisplatin, ifosfamide, and paclitaxel.
     - c. Advanced disease requires supportive care.
  3. Assess for recurrent disease after topical treatment for early stages; may involve teaching for weekly self-checks in reliable patients.
  4. Sexual and reproductive function should be discussed at diagnosis with client and sexual partner.
     - a. Sexual function is best preserved with topical, less invasive, or RT treatments, and is significantly affected by partial or full penectomy.
     - b. Prosthetics and alternative ways to express sexual intimacy may be explored.

REFERENCES

American Cancer Society. (2022). *Survival rates for vaginal cancer.* https://www.cancer.org/cancer/vaginal-cancer/detection-diagnosis-staging/survival-rates.html. Retrieved 01.05.22.

Amin, M. B., Edge, S. B., Greene, F. L., Byrd, D. R., Brookland, R. K., Washington, M. K., et al. (Eds.). (2017). *AJCC cancer staging manual* (8th ed.). Berlin: Springer.

Berek, J. S., & Karam, A. (2022). In A. Chakrabarti (Ed.), *Vulvar cancer: Epidemiology, diagnosis, histopathology, and treatment.* Waltham, MA: UpToDate. Retrieved 25.05.22 from https://www.uptodate.com/contents/vulvar-cancer-epidemiology-diagnosis-histopathology-and-treatment.

Berek, J. S., Renz, M., Kehoe, S., Kumar, L., & Friedlander, M. (2021). Cancer of the ovary, fallopian tube, and peritoneum: 2021 update. *International Journal of Gynecology & Obstetrics, 155*(S1), 61–85. https://doi.org/10.1002/ijgo.13878.

Berkowitz, R. S., Horowitz, N. S., & Elias, K. M. (2022). In A. Chakrabarti & S. R. Vora (Eds.), *Gestational trophoblastic neoplasia: Epidemiology, clinical features, diagnosis, staging, and risk stratification.* Waltham, MA: UpToDate. Retrieved 25.05.22 from https://www.uptodate.com/contents/gestational-trophoblastic-neoplasia-epidemiology-clinical-features-diagnosis-staging-and-risk-stratification.

Bhatla, N., Aoki, D., Sharma, D. N., & Sankaranarayanan, R. (2018). Cancer of the cervix uteri. *International Journal of Gynecology & Obstetrics, 143*(Suppl. 2), 22–36. https://doi.org/10.1002/ijgo.12611.

Crosbie, E. J., Kitson, S. J., McAlpine, J. N., Mukhopadhyay, A., Powell, M. E., & Singh, N. (2022). Endometrial cancer. *The Lancet, 399*(10333), 1412–1428. https://doi.org/10.1016/S0140-6736(22)00323-3.

Diorio, G. J., Leone, A. R., & Spiess, P. E. (2016). Management of penile cancer. *Urology, 96*, 15–21. https://doi.org/10.1016/j.urology.2015.12.041.

Falardeau, D. (2020). Reproductive cancers. In J. Brant (Ed.), *Core curriculum for oncology nursing* (6th ed.). Pittsburgh, PA: Oncology Nursing Society.

Fortner, R. T., Terry, K. L., Bender, N., Brenner, N., Hufnagel, K., Butt, J., et al. (2019). Sexually transmitted infections and risk of epithelial ovarian cancer: Results from the Nurses' Health Studies. *British Journal of Cancer, 120*(8), 855–860. https://doi.org/10.1038/s41416-019-0422-9.

Jeronimo, J., Castle, P. E., Temin, S., Denny, L., Gupta, V., Kim, J. J., et al. (2016). Secondary prevention of cervical cancer: ASCO resource-stratified clinical practice guideline. *Journal of Global Oncology, 3*(5), 635–657. https://doi.org/10.1200/JGO.2016.006577.

Karam, A., Berek, J. S., & Kidd, E.A. (2022). In S. R. Vora & A. Chakrabarti (Eds.), *Vaginal cancer.* Waltham, MA: UpToDate. Retrieved 25.05.22 from https://www.uptodate.com/contents/vaginal-cancer.

Karlsson, T., Johansson, T., Höglund, J., Ek, W. E., & Johansson, Å. (2021). Time-dependent effects of oral contraceptive use on breast, ovarian, and endometrial cancers. *Cancer Research, 81*(4), 1153–1162. https://doi.org/10.1158/0008-5472.CAN-20-2476.

Koskas, M., Amant, F., Mirza, M. R., & Creutzberg, C. L. (2021). Cancer of the corpus uteri: 2021 update. *International Journal of Gynecology & Obstetrics, 155*(S1), 45–60. https://doi.org/10.1002/ijgo.13866.

Lu, K. H., & Broaddus, R. R. (2020). Endometrial cancer. *The New England Journal of Medicine, 383*(21), 2053–2064. https://doi.org/10.1056/NEJMra1514010.

Martin, V. R., & Stewart, L. (2018). Ovarian cancer. In C. H. Yarbro, D. Wujcik, & B. H. Gobel (Eds.), *Cancer nursing: Principles and practice* (8th ed.). Burlington, MA: Jones and Bartlett Learning.

Mbatani, N., Olawaiye, A. B., & Prat, J. (2018). Uterine sarcomas. *International Journal of Gynecology and Obstetrics, 143*(S2), 51–58. https://doi.org/10.1002/ijgo.12613.

National Cancer Institute (NCI). (2021). *HPV and cancer.* https://www.cancer.gov/about-cancer/causes-prevention/risk/infectious-agents/hpv-and-cancer.

National Cancer Institute (NCI). (2022a). *Vaginal cancer treatment (PDQ®) – Health professional version.* National Cancer Institute. https://www.cancer.gov/types/vaginal/hp/vaginal-treatment-pdq. Updated 24.02.22.

National Cancer Institute (NCI). (2022b). *SEER cancer stat fact sheets: Cervical cancer.* Surveillance, Epidemiology, and End Results (SEER) Program. http://seer.cancer.gov/statfacts/html/cervix.html.

National Cancer Institute (NCI). (2022c). *SEER cancer stat fact sheets: Ovarian cancer.* Surveillance, Epidemiology, and End Results (SEER) Program. http://seer.cancer.gov/statfacts/html/ovary.html.

National Cancer Institute (NCI). (2022d). *SEER cancer stat fact sheets: Testicular cancer.* Surveillance, Epidemiology, and End Results (SEER) Program. http://seer.cancer.gov/statfacts/html/testis.html.

National Cancer Institute (NCI). (2022e). *SEER cancer stat fact sheets: Uterine cancer.* Surveillance, Epidemiology, and End Results (SEER) Program. http://seer.cancer.gov/statfacts/html/corp.html.

National Cancer Institute (NCI). (2022f). *SEER cancer stat fact sheets: Vulvar cancer.* Surveillance, Epidemiology, and End Results (SEER) Program. http://seer.cancer.gov/statfacts/html/vulva.html.

National Comprehensive Cancer Network (NCCN). (2021a). *NCCN clinical practice guidelines in oncology (NCCN Guidelines®): Cervical cancer [v.1.2022].* https://www.nccn.org/professionals/physician_gls/pdf/cervical.pdf.

National Comprehensive Cancer Network (NCCN). (2021b). *NCCN clinical practice guidelines in oncology (NCCN guidelines®): Gestational trophoblastic neoplasia [v.1.2022].* https://www.nccn.org/professionals/physician_gls/pdf/gtn.pdf.

National Comprehensive Cancer Network (NCCN). (2021c). *NCCN clinical practice guidelines in oncology (NCCN guidelines®): Uterine neoplasms [v.1.2022].* https://www.nccn.org/professionals/physician_gls/pdf/uterine.pdf.

National Comprehensive Cancer Network (NCCN). (2021d). *NCCN clinical practice guidelines in oncology (NCCN Guidelines®): Vulvar cancer (squamous cell carcinoma) [v.1.2022].* https://www.nccn.org/professionals/physician_gls/pdf/vulvar.pdf.

National Comprehensive Cancer Network (NCCN). (2022a). *NCCN clinical practice guidelines in oncology (NCCN guidelines®): Ovarian cancer including fallopian tube cancer and primary peritoneal cancer [v.1.2022].* https://www.nccn.org/professionals/physician_gls/pdf/ovarian.pdf.

National Comprehensive Cancer Network (NCCN). (2022b). *NCCN clinical practice guidelines in oncology (NCCN guidelines®): Penile cancer [v.2.2022].* https://www.nccn.org/professionals/physician_gls/pdf/penile.pdf.

National Comprehensive Cancer Network (NCCN). (2022c). *NCCN clinical practice guidelines in oncology (NCCN guidelines®): Testicular cancer [v.2.2022].* https://www.nccn.org/professionals/physician_gls/pdf/testicular.pdf.

Okunade, K. S. (2020). Human papillomavirus and cervical cancer. *Journal of Obstetrics and Gynaecology, 40*(5), 602–608. https://doi.org/10.1080/01443615.2019.1634030.

Olawaiye, A. B., Hagemann, I., Otis, C., Gress, D. M., Bhosale, P., Vandenberg, J., et al. (2020). *AJCC cancer staging system: Cervix uteri (Version 9)*. Chicago, IL: American College of Surgeons.

Oleszewski, K. (2018). Cervical cancer. In C. H. Yarbro, D. Wujcik, & B. H. Gobel (Eds.), *Cancer nursing: Principles and practice* (8th ed.). Burlington, MA: Jones and Bartlett Learning.

Pereira, J. V.-B., & Lim, T. (2021). Hyperthyroidism in gestational trophoblastic disease – A literature review. *Thyroid Research, 14*(1), 1. https://doi.org/10.1186/s13044-021-00092-3.

Pettaway, C. A., & Pagliaro, L. C. (2022). In S. Shah (Ed.), *Carcinoma of the penis: Surgical and medical treatment*. Waltham, MA: UpToDate. Retrieved 25.05.22 from https://www.uptodate.com/contents/carcinoma-of-the-penis-surgical-and-medical-treatment.

Rasmussen, C. B., Kjaer, S. K., Albieri, V., Bandera, E. V., Doherty, J. A., Høgdall, E., et al. (2017). Pelvic inflammatory disease and the risk of ovarian cancer and borderline ovarian tumors: A pooled analysis of 13 case-control studies. *American Journal of Epidemiology, 185*(1), 8–20. https://doi.org/10.1093/aje/kww161.

Redlin-Frazier, S. (2018). Endometrial cancer. In C. H. Yarbro, D. Wujcik, & B. H. Gobel (Eds.), *Cancer nursing: Principles and practice* (8th ed.). Burlington, MA: Jones and Bartlett Learning.

Rogers, L. J., & Cuello, M. A. (2018). Cancer of the vulva. *International Journal of Gynecology & Obstetrics, 143*(S2), 4–13. https://doi.org/10.1002/ijgo.12609.

Siegel, R. L., Miller, K. D., Fuchs, H. E., & Jemal, A. (2022). Cancer statistics, 2022. *CA: A Cancer Journal for Clinicians, 72*(1), 7–33. https://acsjournals.onlinelibrary.wiley.com/doi/10.3322/caac.21708.

Siegel, R. L., Miller, K. D., & Jemal, A. (2019). Cancer statistics, 2019. *CA: A Cancer Journal for Clinicians, 69*(1), 7–34. https://acsjournals.onlinelibrary.wiley.com/doi/10.3322/caac.21551.

Soper, J. T. (2021). Gestational trophoblastic disease: Current evaluation and management. *Obstetrics and Gynecology, 137*(2), 355–370. https://doi.org/10.1097/AOG.0000000000004240.

Steele, G. S., Richie, J. P., & Michaelson, M. D. (2022). In S. Shah (Ed.), *Clinical manifestations, diagnosis, and staging of testicular germ cell tumors*. Waltham, MA: UpToDate. Retrieved 25.05.22 from https://www.uptodate.com/contents/clinical-manifestations-diagnosis-and-staging-of-testicular-germ-cell-tumors.

Sung, H., Ferlay, J., Siegel, R. L., Laversanne, M., Soerjomataram, I., Jemal, A., et al. (2021). Global cancer statistics 2020: GLOBOCAN estimates of incidence and mortality worldwide for 36 cancers in 185 countries. *CA: A Cancer Journal for Clinicians, 71*(3), 209–249. https://doi.org/10.3322/caac.21660.

Wang, Q., Fu, J., Hu, L., Fang, F., Xie, L., Chen, H., et al. (2017). Prophylactic chemotherapy for hydatidiform mole to prevent gestational trophoblastic neoplasia. *The Cochrane Database of Systematic Reviews, 9*(9), CD007289. https://doi.org/10.1002/14651858.CD007289.pub3.

Wilkes, G. M., & Barton-Burke, M. (2020). *2020–2021 oncology nursing drug handbook*. Burlington, MA: Jones and Bartlett Learning.

25

Skin Cancer

Krista M. Rubin

OVERVIEW

I. Definition
   A. Nonmelanoma skin cancers (NMSC)
      1. Also known as *keratinocyte carcinomas*, which are becoming the preferred term for basal cell carcinoma (BCC) and cutaneous squamous cell carcinoma (cSCC) to differentiate from other skin cancers more accurately (Nehal & Bichakjian, 2018; Nasr, 2021)
         a. BCC: a neoplasm arising from basal cells in the epidermis
         b. cSCC: a neoplasm arising from squamous cells in the epidermis
      2. Merkel cell carcinoma (MCC; Akaike & Nghiem, 2022)
         a. Merkel cells are thought to be a type of skin neuroendocrine cell because they share some features with nerve cells and hormone-making cells; however, *normal Merkel cells are no longer deemed to be the cell of origin of MCC. The cell of origin is not known.*
   B. Melanoma (American Cancer Society [ACS], 2019a; Mohamed & Hargest, 2022)
      1. A neoplasm arising from melanocytes, pigment-producing cells located in the epidermis.
         a. Melanocytes originate from the neural crest and migrate to the skin, meninges, mucous membranes, upper esophagus, and eyes.
      2. Most melanomas are located on the skin, but may occur anywhere melanocytes are found.
II. Epidemiology (ACS, 2019a, 2022a, 2022b)
   A. Skin cancer is the most common cancer in the United States and worldwide (Skin Cancer Foundation [SCF], 2022).
      1. BCC—most common skin cancer: ~3.6 million cases/year in the United States
      2. cSCC—second most common: ~1.8 million cases/year in the United States; number of cases has increased 200% in the last three decades
      3. MCC—rare: ~3000 cases/year in the United States; incidence has been rising rapidly over the past two decades
      4. Melanoma—99,780 cases/year in the United States estimated in 2022

III. Pathogenesis
   A. Skin carcinogenesis is a multistep process of progressive and accumulating genetic and epigenetic alterations in key signaling pathways that regulate cell survival, cell cycle, and genome maintenance (Lim & Asgari, 2021).
   B. Primary cause—ultraviolet radiation (UVR; both solar and artificial); two main types (Lopez, Liu, & Geskin, 2018; McKnight, Shah, & Hargest, 2022)
      1. UVA—longer rays that penetrate deep into the dermis causing *indirect* DNA damage resulting in actinic damage and skin aging
      2. UVB—shorter rays that penetrate mostly into the epidermis causing direct DNA damage resulting in erythema, sunburn, and increasing the risk for malignancy
   C. Genomics
      1. BCC—The majority of BCCs are associated with pathogenic variants in the PTCH1 and SMO genes in the hedgehog signaling pathway and the TP53 gene (Cameron et al., 2019; Nasr, 2021)
      2. cSCC—associated with p53 gene pathogenic variant and NOTCH signaling pathway genes
      3. MCC—in MCPyV-negative disease, associated pathogenic variant include RB and p53 (Akaike & Nghiem, 2022; Walsh & Cerroni, 2021)
      4. Melanoma—over 80% of melanomas possess genetic abnormalities in at least one key node in the MAPK signaling pathway, most commonly BRAF, (~50%) and most commonly found in the 600th codon (V600), followed by pathogenic variants in NRAS (Jenkins & Fisher, 2021)
   D. Hereditary syndromes (Cameron et al., 2019; Nasr, 2021; Walker & Hardwicke, 2022)
      1. Xeroderma pigmentosum: inability to repair UV-induced DNA damage resulting in multiple skin cancers at an early age
      2. Oculocutaneous albinism: autosomal recessive disorders in which there is a partial or total absence of melanin
      3. Basal cell nevus syndrome (Gorlin syndrome): a rare autosomal dominant disorder characterized by abnormal facial features and the development of numerous BCCs at an early age

4. Familial atypical multiple mole and melanoma syndrome (FAMMM): a familial melanoma variant frequently associated with germline CDKN2A pathogenic variant characterized by numerous (hundreds) of atypical nevi and increased risk of melanoma and pancreatic cancer (Rashid & Tsao, 2021)

5. BAP1 tumor syndrome: rare but important cause of hereditary melanoma, both cutaneous and ocular melanoma due to pathogenic variant in the tumor suppressor gene, BAP 1 (Swetter et al., 2019)

E. Risk factors (Tables 25.1 and 25.2)

F. Fitzpatrick skin phototypes (Table 25.3)

1. Used to help predict a person's overall risk of skin cancer.

IV. Prevention and early identification measures (Box 25.1)

V. Diagnosis

A. NMSC (Nasr, 2021)

1. Presumptive diagnosis and biopsy type are based on the clinician's interpretation of clinical information, including appearance and morphology, anatomic location, genetic risk factors, and patient-reported history.

2. Biopsy types: shave (saucerization or scoop technique to penetrate to deep dermis) punch, incisional, excisional. Shave most commonly for nonpigmented lesions.

B. Melanoma (Vakharia, 2021)

1. Signs and symptoms

a. ABCDEs of mole/melanoma recognition (Table 25.4)

b. The choice of biopsy technique depends on lesion size, location, and shape, but should provide enough tissue to assess the full thickness of the lesion.

TABLE 25.1 Risk Factors for Keratinocyte Carcinomas (Basal Cell Carcinoma [BCC] and Squamous Cell Carcinoma [SCC])

Extrinsic	Intrinsic

• Main risk factor is UV exposure, particularly in fair-skinned individuals
  • BCC—intense, intermittent exposure
  • cSCC—cumulative exposure
  • Increased risk—outdoor workers or who have a history of childhood or adolescent sunburn
• Tanning bed use
  • Risk of BCC—dose-dependent increase when exposed during adolescence
  • Risk of cSCC—when exposed during young adulthood (25–35 years of age)
• Prior PUVA[a] therapy for psoriasis or other skin conditions
• Chronic immunosuppression—solid organ transplant, those with CLL or HIV (higher risk for cSCC)
• Exposure to ionizing radiation—particularly for the treatment of childhood cancer
• Exposure to manufacturing chemicals
• Exposure to arsenic
• Chronic skin ulcers, nonhealing wounds, or burn scars
	• Male>females
	• Increasing age
	• Immunosuppression
	• Family history of skin cancer
	• Fitzpatrick skin types I/II
	• Inherited disorders

CLL, Chronic lymphocytic leukemia; *cSCC,* cutaneous squamous cell carcinoma; *UV,* ultraviolet.
[a]*PUVA,* Psoralen and UVA radiation.
Adapted from Nasr (2021), Walker and Hardwicke (2022), Cameron et al. (2019), Nehal and Bichakjian (2018), ACS (2022a), and SCF (2022).

TABLE 25.2 Risk Factors for Merkel Cell Carcinoma (MCC) and Melanoma

Risk Factors for MCC	Risk Factors for Melanoma

Extrinsic
  Chronic UV exposure
  Chronic immunosuppression, especially solid organ transplant, CLL, HIV
  MCPyV infection
Intrinsic
  Personal history of melanoma and NMSC
  Fitzpatrick skin type I/II
  Advanced age: >75 years
  M>F
	Extrinsic
	  UV exposure: intense, intermittent exposure
	  Tanning bed use
	  Geographically: increases with altitude and decrease with latitude
	Intrinsic
	  Personal history of melanoma and NMSC
	  Number of moles (typical and atypical)
	  Fitzpatrick skin type I/II
	  Immunosuppression
	  Age: Females>males before age 50; after age 50 the risk is higher in men
	  Hereditary disorders

CLL, Chronic lymphocytic leukemia; *NMSC,* nonmelanoma skin cancers; *UV,* ultraviolet.
Risk factors for MCC: Adapted from Akaike & Neighm, 2022; SCF, 2022, Babadzhanov et al., 2021.
Risk factors for melanoma: Adapted from Rashid & Tsao, 2021; ACS 2019b.

TABLE 25.3   Fitzpatrick Skin Types

Skin Type	Skin Color	Features	Ability to Tan
I	White	Very light complexion, blue or green eye color, and blond or red hair	Always burns, never tans
II	White	Fair complexion, light eye color	Burns easily, rarely tans
III	Beige	Darker light complexion, light brown or dark hair	Sometimes burns, sometimes tans
IV	Brown	Olive or light brown skin, dark hair	Rarely burns, tans easily
V	Dark brown	Olive or dark complexion	Very rarely burns, tans very easily
VI	Black	Black skin, dark hair	Never burns, tans very easily

Adapted from Walker and Hardwicke (2022), Rashid and Tsao (2021), and SCF (2022).

BOX 25.1   Skin Cancer Prevention/Early Identification Measures

- Avoid excess exposure to UVR, particularly prolonged midday sunlight exposure
- UVR penetrates even on cloudy or hazy days; UVR reflects off surfaces like water, sand, cement, and snow
- Seek shade
- Do not burn
- Avoid tanning and never use tanning beds
- Use clothing whenever possible: long-sleeved shirts, long pants, and long skirts offer protection from UVR
- Tightly woven fabric offers the most protection
- UV protective clothing
- Wear a wide-brim hat or shade cap
- Use a broad-spectrum (UVA/UVB), water-resistant sunscreen with an SPF of 30+ and reapply every 2 h, and/or after swimming or sweating
- Use lip protection
- Wear UV-blocking sunglasses that protect against UVA/UVB
- Keep babies <6 months out of direct sunlight; use a hat and protective clothing, use sunscreen on babies >6 months
- Perform skin self-exam monthly; see a dermatologist at least once yearly for a professional skin exam

Adapted from ACS (2022a) and SCF (2022).

TABLE 25.4   ABCDEs of Mole/Melanoma Recognition

A	Asymmetry	Normal moles are symmetrical in appearance (1/2 of the lesion is a mirror image of the other half), while melanomas tend to be asymmetrical
B	Border	Normal moles tend to have even, regular borders, while melanomas tend to have irregular, jagged borders
C	Color	Normal moles are uniformly one color, while melanomas tend to have color variegation
D	Diameter	Normal moles tend to be ≤6 mm in size, while melanomas tend to be larger than 6 mm
E	Evolving	Normal moles should not change (evolve) in size, shape, or color; while melanoma may possess features such as evolving size, shape, and color, or concerning symptoms such as itching or bleeding

Adapted from SCF (2022), ACS (2019a, 2019b), Vakharia (2021), and Rashid and Tsao (2021).

VI. Histopathology
  A. NMSC
    1. BCC
      a. No precursor or premalignant states
      b. Diagnosed histologically if (Nasr, 2021):
        (1) The tumor cells resemble basal cells of the epidermis with large hyperchromatic, oval nuclei, and little cytoplasm
        (2) The tumor cells are aggregated together in one large mass
        (3) The tumor cells in the periphery of the tumor align in a palisading pattern (parallel arrangement, like picket fencing)
      c. Subtypes (Table 25.5) have distinct histopathologic findings; many lesions demonstrate >1 histopathologic pattern (Cameron et al., 2019)
      d. Clinical characteristics (Table 25.5)
    2. cSCC (Fania et al., 2021; Walker & Hardwicke, 2022)
      a. Precursors and premalignant states
        (1) Actinic keratoses
        (2) cSCC in situ (Bowen disease)
      b. Clinical features depend largely on the degree of differentiation (Box 25.2)
      c. Several histologic variants (subtypes) exist and can be associated with metastatic disease
      d. Prognostic factors (Table 25.6)
    3. MCC
      a. Majority of MCCs in the northern hemisphere are associated with MCPyV (~80%); the remainder are attributed to UVR exposure (Akaike & Nghiem, 2022)
      b. Clinical characteristics (Table 25.7)
      c. Histopathology (Table 25.7)
  B. Melanoma
    1. Precursors and premalignant states
      a. Atypical nevi
      b. Melanoma in situ (MIS)—confined to the epidermis
    2. Subtypes (Table 25.8)
    3. Histologic features of primary melanoma included in pathology report (Table 25.9)
VII. Staging
  A. BCC
    1. The eighth edition of the American Joint Committee on Cancer (AJCC) staging system now includes BCC.

TABLE 25.5 Subtypes and Features of Basal Cell Carcinoma (BCC)

Subtype	Clinical Characteristics	Risk
Nodular	• Most common subtype; 50%–80% • Typically located on the head and neck • Often present as a shiny, pearly papule or nodule with smooth surface and rolled borders • Often see telangiectasias within the lesion • May or may not be crusted, ulcerated, or bleeding • Pigmented BCCs are a variant of the subtype	Low
Superficial	• 10%–30% • Most commonly found on the trunk, but can often be seen on the legs, and less so on the head and neck • Typically presents as a well-circumscribed, erythematous, thin patch or plaque with scale, central clearing, and thin-rolled borders • Lesions are slowly progressive	Low
Micronodular	• Aggressive subtype • May appear as an erythematous macule or thin papule or plaque that turns yellow to white when stretched • Firm to touch	High
Infiltrative	• 5%; develops primarily in the head and neck region of older individuals • Poorly defined, indurated, flat, or depressed plaque with white, yellow, or pale pink color often with overlying crust or ulceration	High
Morphoeic/sclerosing	• 3%–6% • A high-risk subtype, commonly found on the head and neck • Infiltrated plaque with poorly defined borders and shiny surface; may be flat or depressed, with white, yellow, or pale pink color • Firm to touch	High
Basosquamous	• Rare, <2% • Often highly aggressive and difficult to treat • Some are the result of a BCC colliding with an adjacent SCC • Vast majority found on the head and neck	High

SCC, Squamous cell carcinoma.
Adapted from Nasr, I. (2021). Basal cell carcinoma: A review and summary of the British Association of Dermatologists guidelines for its management in adults (2021). *Dermatological Nursing, 20*(3),10–23; Cameron, M. C., Lee, E., Hibler, B. P., Barker, C. A., Mori, S., Cordova, M., et al. (2019). Basal cell carcinoma: Epidemiology; pathophysiology; clinical and histological subtypes; and disease associations. *Journal of the American Academy of Dermatology, 80*(2), 303–317. https://doi.org/10.1016/j.jaad.2018.03.060.

BOX 25.2 Clinical Features of cSCC

• Typically arise in sun-exposed areas
• Head and neck locations
• Dorsum of hands and forearms
• Well-differentiated cSCC manifests as scaly nodes or plaques
• Poorly differentiated cSCC presents mostly as soft, ulcerated, or hemorrhagic lesions
• Typically slow growing; however, those arising in non-sun exposed sites (e.g., lips, genitalia, and perianal areas) are more aggressive with a higher risk of metastases
• The most common type of skin cancer that occurs in African Americans and Asian Indians

PUVA: psoralen and ultraviolet A radiation.
Adapted from Walker and Hardwicke (2022) and Stanganelli et al. (2022).

TABLE 25.6 Prognostic Factors Associated With Poor Prognosis in Cutaneous Squamous Cell Carcinoma

Intrinsic	Extrinsic
• Tumor size >2 cm • Location: ear, temples, and lips (vermillion) • Tumor depth: >6 mm or invasion beyond subcutaneous fat • Perineural invasion • Poorly differentiated histology • Desmoplasia • Rapidly growing	• Positive surgical margin (incomplete resection) • Recurrent disease • Site of prior radiation or chronic inflammatory process (e.g., leg ulcer, burn scar, and radiation dermatitis) • Immunosuppression • Comorbid conditions • Neglected lesions

Adapted from Brancaccio G., Briatico, G., Pellegrini, C., Rocco, T., Moscarella, E., & Fargnoli, M. C. (2021). Risk factors and diagnosis of advanced cutaneous squamous cell carcinoma. *Dermatology Practical & Conceptual, 11*(Suppl. 2), e2021166S. https://doi.org/10.5826/dpc.11s2a166s; Dessinioti, C., & Stratigos, A. J. (2022). Overview of guideline recommendations for the management of high-risk and advanced cutaneous squamous cell carcinoma. *Journal of the European Academy of Dermatology and Venereology, 36*(S1), 11–18. https://doi.org/10.1111/jdv.17531.

2. National Comprehensive Cancer Network (NCCN) guidelines are favored for clinical practice, as it stratifies localized tumors into low or high risk.
B. cSCC
   1. Multiple staging systems exist; no one system is universally accepted.

TABLE 25.7   Characteristics and Histopathology of MCC

Characteristics	Histopathology
• Most commonly found on sun-damaged skin on the head/neck of an elderly Caucasian patient • Lesions can be located anywhere: limbs, trunk, or other sites • Usually appears as a firm, nontender, red, or skin-colored nodule or plaque • Most lesions are <2 cm in diameter at the time of diagnosis; rapid growth is common • 4% of cases present with no known primary • The mnemonic "AEIOU" is used to describe common clinical features • Asymptomatic • Expanding rapidly • Immunosuppression • Older than 50 years • Ultraviolet exposed/fair skin	• Characterized by dense blue round cells in the dermis and/or subcutis • Involvement of the epidermis is uncommon • Tumor cells form sheets, nests, and rarely ribbons • There are numerous mitoses; may be necrosis • Involvement of intratumoral or peritumor lymphatics is common

Adapted from Akaike, T., & Nghiem, P. (2022). Scientific and clinical developments in Merkel cell carcinoma: A polyomavirus-driven, often-lethal skin cancer. *Journal of Dermatological Science*, *105*(1), 2–10. https://doi.org/10.1016/j.jdermsci.2021.10.004; Walsh, N. M., & Cerroni, L. (2021). Merkel cell carcinoma: A review. *Journal of Cutaneous Pathology*, *48*(3), 411–421. https://doi.org/10.1111/cup.13910.

TABLE 25.8   Subtypes and Features of Melanoma

Type	Frequency (%)	Features
SSM	60–75	• Most common subtype • Arise from a preexisting mole, or de novo • Can be found anywhere on the body, but more likely to occur on the trunk in men and lower legs in women • Often have color variation and irregular borders • More likely to harbor BRAF pathogenic variant than other subtypes
NM	15–30	• Often appear as a smooth, dark polypoid nodule, but may also be red or flesh-colored (amelanotic) • Preferentially located in truncal locations, also head and neck • Most aggressive and more likely to metastasize • Distinct from other subtypes; frequently do not meet ABCDE criteria
LMM	4–15	• Most commonly found in chronically sun-damaged skin in the middle aged and elderly • Usually presents as a tan or brown macule (lentigo) that progressively enlarges over time • About 5% of LMs will progress to LMM
ALM	<5	• Typically appears as a black or brown discoloration under the nails or on the soles of the feet or palms of the hands and occasionally on mucosal surfaces • Most common subtype among those with Asian or African descent • Associated with advanced stage and poor prognosis; often misdiagnosed

ALM, Acral lentiginous; *LMM*, lentigo maligna; *NM*, nodular; *SSM*, superficial spreading.
Adapted from Rashid and Tsao (2021), Vakharia (2021), and SCF (2022).

TABLE 25.9   Histologic Features of Primary Melanoma Included in Pathology Report

Recommended Features to be Reported in the Pathology Report	Optional Histopathological Features in the Pathology Report
Size of specimen	Histologic subtype
Tumor thickness/depth (Breslow)[a] reported to the nearest 0.1 mm	Cell type
	Amount of pigmentation
Ulceration[a]	Clark level
Mitotic rate[a]	Tumor growth phase
Microscopic satellites	Tumor infiltrating lymphocytes
Status of surgical margins (peripheral and deep)	LVI
	perineural invasion
	Regression
	Associated nevus

[a]Important prognostic feature.
Adapted from Wilson, M. L. (2021). Histopathologic and molecular diagnosis of melanoma. *Clinics in Plastic Surgery*, *48*(4), 587–598. https://doi.org/10.1016/j.cps.2021.05.003; Swetter et al. (2019), and NCCN (2022b).

2. Consensus recommendations for risk stratification (Rabinowits et al., 2021)
   a. AJCC—N staging—to identify patients at increased risk of regional treatment failure after surgery with or without radiation therapy (RT), which (only) includes tumor staging for cSCC arising from the head and neck region
   b. Brigham and Women's classification—T staging—used to estimate the risk of recurrence and metastasis and identify patients who may benefit from radiologic nodal staging or increased surveillance for recurrence
   c. NCCN guideline framework establishes low- and high-risk features (National Comprehensive Cancer Network [NCCN], 2022a).
C. MCC (Akaike & Nghiem, 2022; Babadzhanov et al., 2021; Walsh & Cerroni, 2021)
   1. AJCC staging system most commonly applied; encompasses prognostic markers for overall survival

2. Clinical stage is the main determinant of prognosis
3. Sentinel lymph node biopsy (SLNB) should be considered for all patients with early disease, as one-third will have occult lymph node involvement

D. Melanoma
   1. AJCC staging system is most often used; employs both pathologic and clinical stages

VIII. Prognosis and survival
   A. NMSC—When detected and managed early, most have an excellent prognosis
      1. BCC rarely metastasize; if untreated can result in significant morbidity and cosmetic disfigurement (Nasr, 2021)
      2. cSCC (Brancaccio et al., 2021; Rabinowits et al., 2021)
         a. Most patients have low-risk (localized) disease with 5-year survival rates ≥90%; ~35% of patients will have locally advanced disease with 5- and 10-year survival of 60% and <20% respectively.
         b. Distant metastatic disease has <10% 10-year survival.
      3. MCC (Akaike & Nghiem, 2022; Walsh & Cerroni, 2021)
         a. Considered an aggressive disease with high recurrence and metastatic potential
         b. MCPyV-positive tumors have a better prognosis than virus-negative tumors.
         c. 5-year survival rates of 51% for local disease, 35% for nodal disease, and 14% for distant disease
   B. Melanoma
      1. General estimate of 5-year survival rates (based on data from 2011 to 2017) (ACS, 2022b)
         a. Localized disease 99%
         b. Regional disease 68%
         c. Metastatic disease 30%
      2. Significant clinical advances in the past decade have dramatically improved outcomes for patients with advanced melanoma. Five-year overall survival rates have increased from <10% to up to 40%–50% (Comito et al., 2022).

MANAGEMENT

Clinical trials should be considered for the following:
I. BCC (Walker & Hardwicke, 2022)
   A. Surgical—treatment of choice for majority of lesions
      1. Electrodessication and curettage (ED+C)—uses a curette to remove the lesion, then cautery or electrodessication destroys the remainder of the tissue
      2. Excision—removal of the tumor and a margin of clinically uninvolved tissue
      3. Mohs micrographic surgery (MMS)—combines surgical excision with immediate microscopic analysis in order to completely excise a lesion with minimal surgical margins

a. Indicated for high-risk BCC in areas where peripheral margins would result in unacceptable morbidity such as periorbital, nasal oral lesions

B. Topical—primarily for low-risk lesions
   1. Cryotherapy—destroys tissue by exposing it to sub-zero temperatures, causing tissue damage and subsequent cell death
   2. Imiquimod—immune modulator
   3. 5-Fluorouracil (5-FU)—chemotherapy
   4. Photodynamic therapy—combines photosensitizing medications with light or lasers to generate free radicals which lead to cell death
      a. Used for superficial and nodular BCC or those that are poor surgical candidates
   5. RT therapy—may be considered for high-risk primary or recurrent tumors, particularly if the risk of surgery is unacceptably high

C. Systemic therapy (Table 25.10)
   1. Vismodegib for locally advanced/metastatic disease and sonidegib for locally advanced disease
   2. Cemiplimab for locally advanced disease

II. cSCC (Walker & Hardwicke, 2022)
   A. Surgical—treatment of choice for resectable primary tumors
      1. Excision
         a. Goal is to eradicate the primary tumor and any metastases if present, considering the possibility of in-transit disease
         b. Minimal surgical margins (Box 25.3)
      2. MMS

TABLE 25.10 **Currently Approved Immunotherapy (Immune Checkpoint Inhibitors) and Targeted Therapy Regimens for Nonmelanoma Skin Cancers and Melanoma**	
Immunotherapy	**Targeted Therapy**
Immune checkpoint inhibitors Anti-PD-1 Antibody	**Agents directed against the MAPK pathway, specifically BRAF and MEK**
• Pembrolizumab	*BRAF inhibitors, MEK inhibitors*
• Nivolumab	Vemurafenib+cobimetinib
• Cemiplimab	Dabrafenib+trametinib
Anti-PD-L1	Encorafenib+binimetinib
Antibody	**Agents directed against the**
• Avelumab	**sonic hedgehog pathway (HH**
• Atezolizumab	**inhibitors)**
Anti-CTLA-4 antibody	Vismodegib, sonidegib
• Ipilimumab	**Combination immunotherapy/**
Anti-LAG-3 antibody	**targeted therapy:** atezolizumab+
• Relatlimab	vemurafenib+cobimetinib

Anti-CTLA-4, Anti-cytotoxic lymphocyte 4; *anti-PD-1*, anti-programmed death-1; *anti-PD-L1*, anti-programmed death ligand-1.
Adapted from Comito et al. (2022), Jenkins and Fisher (2021), NCCN (2022a, 2022b, 2022c), Walker and Hardwicke (2022), Rabinowits et al. (2021), Dessinioti and Stratigos (2021), and Akaike and Nghiem (2022).

BOX 25.3 Minimum Surgical Margins for cSCC

Low-Risk Lesion (mm)	High-Risk Lesion (mm)	Very-High-Risk Lesion (mm)
4	6	10

Note: A clearance margin of at least 1 mm in all margins should be obtained.
Adapted from Walker and Hardwicke (2022).

TABLE 25.11 Recommended Surgical Margins for Primary Melanoma Excision (Swetter et al., 2019)

T Category	Tumor Thickness (mm)	Recommended Margin (cm)[a]
T0	In situ	0.5–1
T1	≤1.0	1.0
T2	1.0–2	1–2
T3	2.0–4	2.0
T4	>4	2.0

[a]Margins may be modified to accommodate individual anatomic or functional considerations.
Adapted from Swetter, S. M., Tsao, H., Bichakjian, C. K., Curiel-Lewandrowski, C., Elder, D. E., Gershenwald, J. E., et al. (2019). Guidelines of care for the management of primary cutaneous melanoma. *Journal of the American Academy of Dermatology, 80*(1), 208–250. https://doi.org/10.1016/j.jaad.2018.08.055.

      a. Used for certain tumors where a large margin would cause functional issues

    3. ED+C

      a. May be used for small, low-risk lesions in certain instances only

  B. RT

    1. May be considered for primary or recurrent tumors, particularly if the risk of surgery is unacceptably high, or patient-specific contraindications for surgery

    2. May be used as adjuvant therapy for close excision margins or

    3. Recommended for lesions with perineural invasion, recurrent or incompletely excised tumors, or for other high-risk diseases

  C. Systemic therapy—advanced disease (Rabinowits, et al., 2021)

    1. Immunotherapy: considered the standard first-line therapy (Table 25.10)

      a. Cemiplimab, pembrolizumab

    2. Chemotherapy or targeted therapy may be considered in patients who are not candidates for immunotherapy, have progressed on immunotherapy, or cannot tolerate it due to toxicity. Response rates are low and of short duration.

III. MCC (Akaike & Nghiem, 2022; Babadzhanov et al., 2021; NCCN, 2022c)

  A. Surgery—localized disease

    1. Wide excision of the primary site; SLNB should be considered in all cases

  B. RT—MCC is a radiosensitive tumor and therefore used as both adjuvant and definitive treatments

  C. Systemic therapy

    1. Regional disease, recurrent

      a. Consider pembrolizumab if curative surgery and RT are not feasible.

    2. Immunotherapy—considered the standard first-line therapy for advanced disease (Table 25.10)

      a. Avelumab, pembrolizumab, and nivolumab

    3. Neoadjuvant immunotherapy may be considered in certain cases.

    4. Chemotherapy: chemotherapy-sensitive tumor, but no survival benefit. Reserved for palliative treatment. If used, typically platinum+etoposide.

IV. Melanoma

  A. Surgery for primary tumor (Swetter et al., 2019)

    1. Wide local excision is the preferred treatment

      a. Tumor thickness determines appropriate surgical margins (Table 25.11)

    2. SLNB: recommended for lesions of at least 1 mm, considered for lesions 0.8–1 mm with or without ulceration, or for lesions <0.8 mm with adverse histologic features (ulceration, LVI, and/or high mitotic rate)

      a. Tumor thickness most reliable predictor of positive SLNB, which also predicts overall survival

      b. Completion lymph node dissection (LND) is no longer performed as standard after positive SLNB due to the lack of survival benefit.

        (1) Patients may be monitored with ultrasound of involved nodal basin; completion LND considered in the setting of multiple involved sentinel nodes and/or high-risk histologic features of the primary tumor

  B. Surgery for advanced melanoma (Enomoto, Levine, Shen, & Votanopoulos, 2020; O'Neill, McMasters, & Egger, 2020; NCCN, 2022b)

    1. Nodal disease (see above)

    2. Metastasectomy improves overall survival for select subset of patients

      a. Consider for patients with a stable or responding oligometastatic disease or isolated progressive lesions with stable disease elsewhere when complete macroscopic resection can be achieved

    3. Palliative—for example, resection of tumors causing a wound, bleeding, or intestinal obstruction

    4. Isolated limb perfusion and infusion for in-transit (locally metastatic) disease not suitable for local or topical therapy

  C. RT (NCCN, 2022b; Swetter et al., 2019)

    1. Rarely, RT may be used as primary therapy for MIS, LM type when complete excision is not possible.

    2. Adjuvant—may be used in certain instances to increase regional control

3. Distant metastatic disease
   a. Palliative—for symptomatic lesions (e.g., pain or bleeding)
   b. Brain metastases
      (1) Stereotactic radiosurgery (SRS) (favored)—delivers a high dose of radiation to a specific target while delivering a minimal dose to surrounding tissues
      (2) Whole brain RT—palliative purposes when SRS is not feasible
D. Adjuvant therapy for high-risk resected, or recurrent disease (Stage IIIa/b/c, Stage IV resected) (Jenkins & Fisher, 2021; NCCN, 2022b; Table 25.10)
   1. Immunotherapy (generally for Stage IIIb/c)
      a. pembrolizumab
      b. nivolumab
      c. ipilimumab
   2. Targeted therapy (for patients with BRAF V600 pathogenic variant) (Stage IIIa/b/c)
      a. dabrafenib+trametinib
E. Systemic therapy for metastatic or unresectable disease (Jenkins and Fisher, 2021; NCCN, 2022b; Table 25.10):
   1. Immunotherapy (preferred the first-line treatment)
      a. Pembrolizumab
      b. Nivolumab
      c. Combination ipilimumab+anti-PD-1 (nivolu-mab or pembrolizumab)
      d. Combination nivolumab+relatlimub (approved 3/18/22)
   2. Other immunotherapies used in certain subsets of patients in certain clinical situations (NCCN, 2022b)
      a. T-VEC—modified, intralesional oncolytic herpes virus for in-transit or localized disease
      b. High-dose interleukin-2: second-line as it can provide a durable long-term survival benefit, but for a small number of patients
   3. Combination targeted therapy (for patient with BRAF V600 pathogenic variant and unable to tolerate immunotherapy) (Table 25.10)
      a. dabrafenib+trametinib
      b. vemurafenib+cobimetinib
      c. encorafenib+binimetinib
   4. Combination immunotherapy+targeted (for patients with BRAF V600 pathogenic variant)
      a. atezolizumab+vemurafenib+cobimetinib
   5. Chemotherapy—generally used for salvage therapy, often for disease control or to reduce tumor load
      a. Dacarbazine or temozolomide (oral analog of dacarbazine) and paclitaxel with or without carboplatin
   6. Best supportive/palliative care—generally reserved for those with very poor performance status, who have progressed despite multiple lines of therapy

REFERENCES

Akaike, T., & Nghiem, P. (2022). Scientific and clinical developments in Merkel cell carcinoma: A polyomavirus-driven, often-lethal skin cancer. *Journal of Dermatological Science, 105*(1), 2–10. https://doi.org/10.1016/j.jdermsci.2021.10.004.

American Cancer Society (ACS). (2019a). *What is melanoma skin cancer?* https://www.cancer.org/cancer/melanoma-skin-cancer/about/what-is-melanoma.html. Retrieved 13.03.22.

American Cancer Society (ACS). (2019b). *Risk factors for melanoma skin cancer.* https://www.cancer.org/cancer/melanoma-skin-cancer/causes-risks-prevention/risk-factors.html. Retrieved 13.03.22.

American Cancer Society (ACS). (2022a). *Key statistics for basal and squamous cell skin cancers.* https://www.cancer.org/cancer/basal-and-squamous-cell-skin-cancer/about/key-statistics.html. Retrieved 13.03.22.

American Cancer Society (ACS). (2022b). *Cancer facts and figures.* https://www.cancer.org/content/dam/cancer-org/research/cancer-facts-and-statistics/annual-cancer-facts-and-figures/2022/2022-cancer-facts-and-figures.pdf. Retrieved 13.03.22.

Babadzhanov, M., Doudican, N., Wilken, R., Stevenson, M., Pavlick, A., & Carucci, J. (2021). Current concepts and approaches to merkel cell carcinoma. *Archives of Dermatological Research, 313*(3), 129–138. https://doi.org/10.1007/s00403-020-02107-9.

Brancaccio, G., Briatico, G., Pellegrini, C., Rocco, T., Moscarella, E., & Fargnoli, M. C. (2021). Risk factors and diagnosis of advanced cutaneous squamous cell carcinoma. *Dermatology Practical & Conceptual, 11*(Suppl. 2), e2021166S. https://doi.org/10.5826/dpc.11s2a166s.

Cameron, M. C., Lee, E., Hibler, B. P., Barker, C. A., Mori, S., Cordova, M., et al. (2019). Basal cell carcinoma: Epidemiology; pathophysiology; clinical and histological subtypes; and disease associations. *Journal of the American Academy of Dermatology, 80*(2), 303–317. https://doi.org/10.1016/j.jaad.2018.03.060.

Comito, F., Pagani, R., Grilli, G., Sperandi, F., Ardizzoni, A., & Melotti, B. (2022). Emerging novel therapeutic approaches for treatment of advanced cutaneous melanoma. *Cancers, 14*(2), 271. https://doi.org/10.3390/cancers14020271.

Dessinioti, C., & Stratigos, A. J. (2022). Overview of guideline recommendations for the management of high-risk and advanced cutaneous squamous cell carcinoma. *Journal of the European Academy of Dermatology and Venereology, 36*(S1), 11–18. https://doi.org/10.1111/jdv.17531.

Enomoto, L. M., Levine, E. A., Shen, P., & Votanopoulos, K. I. (2020). Role of surgery for metastatic melanoma. *Surgical Clinics of North America, 100*(1), 127–139. https://doi.org/10.1016/j.suc.2019.09.011.

Fania, L., Didona, D., Di Pietro, F. R., Verkhovskaia, S., Morese, R., Paolino, G., et al. (2021). Cutaneous squamous cell carcinoma: From pathophysiology to novel therapeutic approaches. *Biomedicines, 9*(2), 171. https://doi.org/10.3390/biomedicines9020171.

Jenkins, R. W., & Fisher, D. E. (2021). Treatment of advanced melanoma in 2020 and beyond. *Journal of Investigative Dermatology, 141*(1), 23–31. https://doi.org/10.1016/j.jid.2020.03.943.

Lim, J. L., & Asgari, M. (2021). *Cutaneous squamous cell carcinoma: Epidemiology and risk factors.* Waltham, MA: UpToDate. Retrieved 13.03.22 from https://www.uptodate.com/contents/cutaneous-squamous-cell-carcinoma-epidemiology-risk-factors-and-molecular-pathogenesis?search=skin%20 carcinogenesis&source=search_result&selectedTitle=2~150&usa ge_type=default&display_rank=2#H959077544.

Lopez, A. T., Liu, L., & Geskin, L. (2018). Molecular mechanisms and biomarkers of skin photocarcinogenesis. In M. Blumenberg (Ed.), *Human skin cancers – Pathways, mechanisms, targets and treatments* (pp. 175–200). London: IntechOpen. https://doi.org/10.5772/intechopen.70879.

McKnight, G., Shah, J., & Hargest, R. (2022). Physiology of the skin. *Surgery (Oxford), 40*(1), 8–12. https://doi.org/10.1016/j.mpsur.2021.11.005.

Mohamed, S. A., & Hargest, R. (2022). Surgical anatomy of the skin. *Surgery (Oxford), 40*(1), 1–7. https://doi.org/10.1016/j.mpsur.2021.11.021.

Nasr, I. (2021). Basal cell carcinoma: A review and summary of the British Association of Dermatologists guidelines for its management in adults (2021). *Dermatological Nursing, 20*(3), 10–23.

National Comprehensive Cancer Network (NCCN). (2022a). *Squamous cell skin cancer.* https://www.nccn.org/professionals/physician_gls/pdf/squamous_blocks.pdf. Retrieved 13.03.22.

National Comprehensive Cancer Network (NCCN). (2022b). *Melanoma: Cutaneous (version 2.022).* https://www.nccn.org/login?ReturnURL=https://www.nccn.org/professionals/physician_gls/pdf/cutaneous_melanoma.pdf. Retrieved 13.03.22.

National Comprehensive Cancer Network (NCCN). (2022c). *Merkel cell carcinoma (version 2.022).* https://www.nccn.org/professionals/physician_gls/pdf/mcc.pdf. Retrieved 13.03.22.

Nehal, K. S., & Bichakjian, C. K. (2018). Update on keratinocyte carcinomas. *New England Journal of Medicine, 379*(4), 363–374. https://doi.org/10.1056/NEJMra1708701.

O'Neill, C. H., McMasters, K. M., & Egger, M. E. (2020). Role of surgery in stage IV melanoma. *Surgical Oncology Clinics of North America, 29*(3), 485–495. https://doi.org/10.1016/j.soc.2020.02.010.

Rabinowits, G., Migden, M. R., Schlesinger, T. E., Ferris, R. L., Freeman, M., Guild, V., et al. (2021). Evidence-based consensus recommendations for the evolving treatment of patients with high-risk and advanced cutaneous squamous cell carcinoma. *JID Innovations, 1*(4), 100045. https://doi.org/10.1016/j.xjidi.2021.100045.

Rashid, S., & Tsao, H. (2021). Recognition, staging, and management of melanoma. *Medical Clinics of North America, 105*(4), 643–661. https://doi.org/10.1016/j.mcna.2021.04.005.

Skin Cancer Foundation. (2022). *Skin cancer facts & statistics.* https://www.skincancer.org/skin-cancer-information/skin-cancer-facts/. Retrieved 13.03.22.

Stanganelli, I., Spagnolo, F., Argenziano, G., Ascierto, P. A., Bassetto, F., Bossi, P., et al. (2022). The multidisciplinary management of cutaneous squamous cell carcinoma: A comprehensive review and clinical recommendations by a panel of experts. *Cancers, 14*(2), 377. https://doi.org/10.3390/cancers14020377.

Swetter, S. M., Tsao, H., Bichakjian, C. K., Curiel-Lewandrowski, C., Elder, D. E., Gershenwald, J. E., et al. (2019). Guidelines of care for the management of primary cutaneous melanoma. *Journal of the American Academy of Dermatology, 80*(1), 208–250. https://doi.org/10.1016/j.jaad.2018.08.055.

Vakharia, K. T. (2021). Clinical diagnosis and classification: Including biopsy techniques and noninvasive imaging. *Clinics in Plastic Surgery, 48*(4), 577–585. https://doi.org/10.1016/j.cps.2021.06.006.

Walker, H. S., & Hardwicke, J. (2022). Non-melanoma skin cancer. *Surgery (Oxford), 40*(1), 39–45. https://doi.org/10.1016/j.mpsur.2021.11.004.

Walsh, N. M., & Cerroni, L. (2021). Merkel cell carcinoma: A review. *Journal of Cutaneous Pathology, 48*(3), 411–421. https://doi.org/10.1111/cup.13910.

26

Surgery

Gail W. Davidson

OVERVIEW

I. Principles of cancer surgery
  A. Surgical oncology is an essential part of cancer care delivery; the surgical oncologist is a dual specialist as a surgeon and oncologist (Balch & Morita, 2018).
  B. Cancer treatment involves a multidisciplinary approach with surgery for staging and treatment for local control (Balch & Morita, 2018).
  C. Before surgery, it is important to define:
    1. Goal of surgery (e.g., disease prevention, disease control, and symptom palliation)
    2. Functional importance of the involved organ or structure
    3. Ability to reconstruct or restore function if needed
    4. Patient's physical condition to undergo procedure, risk assessment (Zaydfudim, Hu, & Adams, 2022)
      a. "Operable" describes the patient's physiologic condition.
      b. "Resectable" describes the ability to safely remove cancer with appropriate outcomes.
II. Role of surgery in the oncology patient (Table 26.1 lists surgical approaches).
  A. Diagnosis and staging—histologic examination of tissue is necessary to determine the diagnosis and treatment of most cancers (Samuels, Bardelli, Wolf, & López-Otin, 2019). Tissue sampling methods are included in Table 26.2.
  B. Curative surgery—achieve "R0" microscopic complete resection (Winter, Brody, Abrams, Posey, & Yeo, 2019): remove primary tumor, lymph nodes, adjacent affected organs with negative margins attained via the least invasive means
    1. Local excision—removal of cancer and a small margin of surrounding tissue
    2. Wide excision—removal of cancer and adjacent tissue±regional lymph nodes
    3. En-bloc resection—removal of bulky cancer with contiguous tissues, lymph nodes, and vascular structures required to attain safe margins

  C. Surgery for cancer prevention—prophylactic risk-reducing surgery (e.g., mastectomy, oophorectomy, and total colectomy) when found to have a genetic link/mutation such as *BRCA1*, *BRCA2*, *TP53*, *PTEN*, *STK11*, *CDH1*, and Lynch syndrome (Guillem et al., 2019)
  D. Palliative cancer surgery—to improve comfort when curative resection is not possible; includes surgical debulking, decompression, or diversion via stent or ostomy (e.g., gastrojejunostomy, colostomy) (Davis, Ripley, & Hernandez, 2019)
  E. Restorative "oncoplastic" surgery—to improve the function or appearance of a surgical defect improving the quality of life (e.g., breast reconstruction, sarcoma defect repair) (Gilmore et al., 2021; Sama et al., 2021)
  F. Surgery for oncologic emergencies such as hemorrhage, organ ischemia or perforation, drainage/washout for abscess or infection, cord compression

ASSESSMENT

I. Principles of patient selection (Zaydfudim et al., 2022)
  A. Select patient based on appropriate indication and benefit outweighs risk
    1. Use objective tools for risk stratification, for example, the American College of Surgeons National Surgical Quality Improvement Program (NSQIP) risk calculator (American College of Surgeons [ACS], 2022),
    2. Evaluate functional assessment with standardized tools (e.g., Karnofsky scale).
    3. Cardiopulmonary clearance and American Society of Anesthesiologists class for anesthesia preparation
    4. Patient preoperative assessment and education
  B. History
    1. Preexisting conditions, allergies, recent infections, and recent vaccinations including COVID-19 (National Comprehensive Cancer Network [NCCN], 2021a)
    2. Previous surgery, reaction to anesthesia and blood products

TABLE 26.1 Glossary of Types of Cancer Surgeries and Surgical Approaches

Surgical Term	Description
Biopsy	• A fine needle sample or tissue sample removed to diagnose the cancer • Application: breast biopsy
Cryosurgery	• The use of liquid nitrogen to freeze the cancer • Application: cervical cancer
Debulking	• Surgery conducted to remove as much of the tumor as possible to help shrink the tumor burden • Application: ovarian cancer
Endoscopic Surgery	• A technique used to biopsy and/or remove tissues of the colon, bladder, or other nearby organs without an external incision or scar • Application: transvaginal cholecystectomy
Laparoscopic Surgery	• Multiple small incisions are made to apply cameras and other tools into the area to allow tissue removal and manipulation • Application: laparoscopic hysterectomy
Laser Surgery	• Precise beams apply photosensitive agents into the tumor bed to cause damage at the cellular level • Example: photodynamic therapy for lung cancer
Mohs Surgery	• Removes a thin layer of the skin, one at a time, until normal cells are revealed • Example: skin cancer
Palliative Surgery	• Used to relieve pain or pressure caused by a tumor, to remove gastrointestinal obstruction, to stop bleeding, place a port or tube for medication support, and to prevent fractures. • Example: stent placement to alleviate urinary obstruction
Reconstructive Surgery	• Reconstruct body parts affected by cancer surgery or treatment • Example: breast reconstruction following mastectomy
Robotic Surgery	• Remote controlled instruments are used for finer control and improved optics within the surgical environment, lessening tissue manipulation • Example: colon resection

Data from Johns Hopkins Medicine. What are the different methods of surgery? The Johns Hopkins University, The Johns Hopkins Hospital, and Johns Hopkins Health System, 2023. https://www.hopkinsmedicine.org/health/treatment-tests-and-therapies/methods-of-surgery; American Cancer Society. Less invasive cancer surgery techniques. American Cancer Society, Inc., 2023. https://www.cancer.org/treatment/treatments-and-side-effects/treatment-types/surgery/special-surgical-techniques.html; National Cancer Institute: Surgery to Treat Cancer. National Cancer Institute at the National Institutes of Health. https://www.cancer.gov/about-cancer/treatment/types/surgery

TABLE 26.2 Tissue Sampling Methods

Tissue Sampling Procedure	Description
Fine needle aspiration	Percutaneous fine needle guided to mass to remove tissue fragments
Core or needle biopsy	Larger needle used to sample tissue via percutaneous stick
Incisional biopsy	Small incision over mass to remove tissue sample
Excisional biopsy	Removal of entire mass through an incision
Sentinel lymph node biopsy	Intradermal injection of isosulfan blue (dye) for lymphatic mapping to identify primary (sentinel) node(s) for histopathic examination for metastatic disease; spares regional node dissection and associated morbidity
Endoscopic/laparoscopic biopsy	Direct visualization of mass, adjacent lymph nodes through scopes, cameras for tissue samples or washings for cytology

3. Previous chemotherapy or radiation and effects that could influence surgical selection and outcomes (Lorusso et al., 2018)
4. Current medications (beta-blockers, anticoagulants), herbal and vitamin supplements
5. Social history (smoking, alcohol, and illicit drug use), social support for after-care

C. Physical examination
1. Cardiovascular changes—increased risk of cardiac event if previous injury (e.g., myocardial infarction/ischemia, stroke), anemia, and venous thromboembolism (VTE)
2. Pulmonary function alterations related to anemia, obstructive sleep apnea, aerodigestive cancers with increased aspiration risk, pleural effusions, or pneumonia
3. Hematologic—assess for anemia, coagulopathy, and bone marrow suppression related to chemotherapy, immunotherapy, and radiation
4. Gastrointestinal, hepatic—assess for malnutrition, malabsorption, cachexia, coagulopathy, fluid balance, vomiting, diarrhea, and constipation, which can affect surgery readiness and recovery
5. Renal—evaluate function and fluid and electrolyte balance, renal dose medications and dialysis the day before surgical procedures if end-stage renal disease exists
6. Endocrine—glycemic control before surgery is optimal; metabolic stress from surgery leads to insulin resistance and hyperglycemia invoking volume depletion, electrolyte imbalance, osmotic diuresis, diabetic ketoacidosis, increased surgical site infections, and poor wound healing (Holder-Murray, Esper, Wang, Cui, & Wang, 2019)

D. Psychosocial evaluation, patient and caregiver education
1. Assess for psychosocial support, stressors, and coping mechanisms
2. Plan for postdischarge care and recovery site
3. Caregiver readiness, access to services/supplies

4. Advance directive discussion and access
5. Preoperative directions—report in time/place, home medication instructions, and expectations related to surgery and discharge
6. Enhanced recovery after surgery (ERAS) instruction as prescribed—includes smoking cessation, pre/post habilitation plan, skin care, nutrition, hydration, anesthesia and pain management, and VTE prevention (Holder-Murray et al., 2019)

MANAGEMENT

I. Surgery as part of the multimodal cancer treatment plan
A. Chemotherapy or radiation may be delivered before surgery (neoadjuvant) to downsize disease or improve margins—can affect wound healing
B. Intraoperative chemotherapy delivered directly to tissue or vasculature (e.g., hyperthermic intraperitoneal chemotherapy, isolated limb perfusion)
C. Intraoperative radiation—a single dose of radiation delivered directly to tissue via open incision typically to deep margins that cannot be resected without significant morbidity; or via brachytherapy—surgically implanted device is sourced with a radioactive agent (Pilar, Gupta, Ghosh Laskar, & Laskar, 2017)
D. Postoperative chemotherapy (adjuvant) may be given if cancer was node positive, incompletely resected or if cytoreduction/debulking surgery was planned to improve chemotherapy delivery to active tumors (Bresalier, 2021), or via a surgically implanted chemotherapy pump (hepatic arterial infusion pump)
E. Postoperative radiation (adjuvant) to treat potential microscopic disease when conservative surgery performed (e.g., radiation after lumpectomy)

II. Interventional radiology as part of the interdisciplinary team
A. Before surgery, may perform biopsy, tissue sampling, and central line placement
B. Instead of surgery may perform minimally invasive procedures such as percutaneous ablation, vascular embolization
C. Postoperative and supportive care—drain or stent placement

III. ERAS (Table 26.3)
A. A multimodal integrated evidenced-based care pathway to optimize patient care

TABLE 26.3 Enhanced Recovery After Surgery Interventions and Outcomes

Intervention	Outcome
Preop anesthesia evaluation—identifies respiratory risk, addresses multimodal anesthesia options (spinal, blocks, general, avoid opioids)	• Reduce cancellations/delays (88%) • Decrease length of stay • Cost reduction • Decrease in-hospital mortality
Preop exercise and prehabilitation	• Enhance functional capacity to withstand surgery stress • Awareness of postop expectations/activity
Preop smoking cessation	• Decrease postop mortality • Decrease prolonged ventilation • Decrease DVT risk • Decrease wound infection risk • Improve wound healing • Improve bone fusion
Preop nutrition/carbohydrate loading 100 g CHO clear liquid drink prior night, 50 g CHO clear liquid drink 2- to 3-h preop	• Decrease nausea • Decrease fasting discomfort • Stabilize glucose and protein metabolism • Decrease length of stay
Preop skin care—betadine or chlorhexidine showers and scrubs, no shaving surgical areas	• Decrease surgical wound infections
Intra-op—minimally invasive procedure	• Decrease length of stay and complications • Decrease use of catheters and drains
Peri-op venous thromboembolism prophylaxis (avoid DVT or PE) with early ambulation, compression stockings, intermittent pneumatic compression, meds (low dose fractionated heparin, low molecular weight heparin, factor Xa inhibitors)	• Avoid #1 cause of preventable death
Peri-op fluid management—goal directed—maintain perfusion without overload	• Decrease complication risks (i.e., cardiopulmonary congestion vs. hypotension, renal perfusion, bowel edema, wound healing) • Decrease length of stay
Peri-op pain management—multimodal analgesia avoiding opioids, encourage NSAIDs, acetaminophen	• Decrease complications—constipation, abuse
Postoperative nausea—avoid general anesthesia, nitrous, opioids, ensure hydration, antiemetics, steroids, anticholinergics	• Decrease complications—hypovolemia, electrolyte disorders
Postop early nutrition and mobilization to avoid postop ileus—the most common reason for prolonged hospitalization and readmission	• Improve well-being • Decrease length of stay

Compiled from Holder-Murray, J., Esper S., Wang, Z., Cui, Z., & Wang, X. (2019). Optimizing perioperative care: Enhanced recovery and Chinese medicine. In F. Brunicardi, D. K. Andersen, T. R. Billiar, D. L. Dunn, L. S. Kao, J. G. Hunter, J. B. Matthews, & R. E. Pollock (Eds.), *Schwartz's principles of surgery* (11e). New York: McGraw Hill. https://accessmedicine-mhmedical-com.proxy.lib.ohio-state.edu/content.aspx?bookid=2576&sectionid=216218692.

B. Accelerates functional recovery, improves patient outcomes

C. Improves quality care and cost metrics (Holder-Murray et al., 2019)

IV. Safety and management of the perioperative/procedural patient

A. Multiple agencies have collaborated to develop safety goals, procedures, and tools to improve safe caregiving, including:

1. Association of periOperative Registered Nurses (Association of periOperative Registered Nurses, 2019) comprehensive tool includes aspects from each of the following agencies:

a. World Health Organization checklist (World Health Organization, 2009)—ensures patient confirmation, consent, site marking, safe environment, and team collaboration through all perioperative phases

b. The Joint Commission National Patient Safety Goals (The Joint Commission, 2018) ensures patient, team, and equipment preparation, site marking, "universal protocol" and "time out" safety goals.

c. The Surgical Care Improvement Project embellished by The Joint Commission—developed from the Centers for Medicare and Medicaid, the Centers for Disease Control, and the Institute of Healthcare Improvement to evaluate and publically report surgical site infection data through the timing of the preop antibiotic use, glucose control, maintenance of normothermia, beta-blockers, removing urinary catheters, and VTE prophylaxis to decrease complications, cost, and length of stay (Sandberg, Dmochowski, & Beauchamp, 2022).

2. The Centers for Disease Control, Surgical Site Infection Guideline (Berrios-Torres et al., 2017)

3. American College of Surgeons National Surgical Quality Improvement Program (NSQIP) (ACS, 2022)

B. Postoperative recovery

1. Close monitoring until discharge/transition criteria met

2. Postoperative report handoff communication includes patient name, diagnosis, history, reason for surgery, type of surgery and anesthesia, patient condition, vital signs, oxygenation, level of consciousness, counts correct, length of time in operating room, venous thromboembolic prophylaxis, specimens sent, pain level, last medication and time due, location of incision, bandage, drains, urinary catheter/urine output, intravenous fluid, amount, location, medications given and due, specific care, any complications, and estimated blood loss and replacement if planned (Njambi, Rawson, & Redley, 2021).

3. Employ mobilization and pulmonary toilet to prevent atelectasis, pneumonia, aspiration with cough and deep breathing, incentive spirometry, early ambulation, oral hygiene, and elevate head of bed (Miskovic & Lumb, 2017).

4. Venous thromboembolic prophylaxis (sequential compression, early ambulation/return to preoperative activity level, antithrombotic therapy) to avoid DVT, pulmonary embolism (NCCN, 2023)

REFERENCES

American College of Surgeons (ACS). (2022). *ACS NSQIP surgical risk calculator.* https://riskcalculator.facs.org/RiskCalculator/. Retrieved 02.03.22.

Association of periOperative Registered Nurses. (2019). *AORN comprehensive surgical checklist.* https://www.aorn.org/-/media/aorn/guidelines/tool-kits/correct-site-surgery/aorn-comprehensive-surgical-checklist-2019.docx?la=en&hash=03A11CDC0388572BB2CAEEBC3A9D0866.

Balch, C. M., & Morita, S. Y. (2018). Defining the specialty of surgical oncology. In S. Y. Morita, C. M. Balch, V. Klimaberg, T. M. Pawlik, M. C. Posner, & K. K. Tanabe (Eds.), *Textbook of complex general surgical oncology.* New York, NY: McGraw Hill. https://accesssurgery-mhmedical-com.proxy.lib.ohio-state.edu/content.aspx?bookid=2209&sectionid=168936625.

Berríos-Torres, S. I., Umscheid, C. A., Bratzler, D. W., Leas, B., Stone, E. C., Kelz, R. R., et al., Healthcare Infection Control Practices Advisory Committee. (2017). Centers for Disease Control and Prevention Guideline for the prevention of surgical site infection, 2017. *JAMA Surgery, 152*(8), 784–791. https://doi.org/10.1001/jamasurg.2017.0904.

Bresalier, R. S. (2021). Colorectal cancer. In M. H. Sleisenger & J. S. Fordtran (Eds.), *Sleisenger and Fordtran's gastrointestinal and liver disease* (11th ed., pp. 2108–2152). Amsterdam: Elsevier.

Davis, J. L., Ripley, R. T., & Hernandez, J. M. (2019). Endoscopic and robotic surgery. In V. T. DeVita, T. S. Lawrence, & S. A. Rosenberg (Eds.), *DeVita, Hellman, and Rosenberg's cancer: Principles & practice of oncology* (11th ed., pp. 519–527). Philadelphia, PA: Lippincott Williams & Wilkins.

Gilmour, A., Cutress, R., Gandhi, A., Harcourt, D., Little, K., Mansell, J., et al. (2021). Oncoplastic breast surgery: A guide to good practice. *European Journal of Surgical Oncology, 47*(9), 2272–2285. https://doi.org/10.1016/j.ejso.2021.05.006. Epub 2021 May 11. PMID: 34001384.

Guillem, J. G., Berchuck, A., Norton, J. A., Subhedar, P., Seastedt, K. P., & Untch, B. R. (2019). Role of surgery in cancer prevention. In V. T. DeVita, T. S. Lawrence, & S. A. Rosenberg (Eds.), *DeVita, Hellman, and Rosenberg's cancer: Principles & practice of oncology* (11th ed., pp. 401–419). Philadelphia, PA: Lippincott Williams & Wilkins.

Holder-Murray, J., Esper, S., Wang, Z., Cui, Z., & Wang, X. (2019). Optimizing perioperative care: Enhanced recovery and Chinese medicine. In F. Brunicardi, D. K. Andersen, T. R. Billiar, D. L. Dunn, L. S. Kao, J. G. Hunter, J. B. Matthews, & R. E. Pollock (Eds.), *Schwartz's principles of surgery* (11e). New York: McGraw Hill. https://accessmedicine-mhmedical-com.proxy.lib.ohio-state.edu/content.aspx?bookid=2576&sectionid=216218692.

The Joint Commission. (2018). *National Patient Safety Goals.* https://www.jointcommission.org/standards/national-patient-safety-goals/.

Lorusso, R., Vizzardi, E., Johnson, D. M., Mariscalco, G., Sciatti, E., Maessen, J., et al. (2018). Cardiac surgery in adult patients with remitted or active malignancies: A review of preoperative screening, surgical management and short- and long-term postoperative results. *European Journal of Cardio-Thoracic Surgery, 54*(1), 10–18. https://doi.org/10.1093/ejcts/ezy019.

Miskovic, A., & Lumb, A. B. (2017). Postoperative pulmonary complications. *British Journal of Anaesthesia, 118*(3), 317–334. https://doi.org/10.1093/bja/aex002.

National Comprehensive Cancer Network (NCCN). (2021). *NCCN clinical practice guidelines in perioperative management of anticoagulation and antithrombotic therapy [v.3.2021].* https://www.nccn.org/professionals/physician_gls/pdf/vte.pdf.

National Comprehensive Cancer Network (NCCN). (2023). *Cancer and COVID-19 vaccination [v.8.0].* https://www.nccn.org/docs/default-source/covid-19/2021_covid-19_vaccination_guidance_v8-0.pdf?sfvrsn=b483da2b_126.

Njambi, M., Rawson, H., & Redley, B. (2021). A brief intervention to standardize postanesthetic clinical handoff. *Nursing & Health Sciences, 23*(1), 219–226. https://doi.org/10.1111/nhs.12803.

Pilar, A., Gupta, M., Ghosh Laskar, S., & Laskar, S. (2017). Intraoperative radiotherapy: Review of techniques and results. *Ecancermedicalscience, 11*, 750. https://doi.org/10.3332/ecancer.2017.750. PMID: 28717396; PMCID: PMC5493441.

Samà, L., Binder, J. P., Darrigues, L., Couturaud, B., Boura, B., Helfre, S., et al. (2021). Safe-margin surgery by plastic reconstruction in extremities or parietal trunk soft tissue sarcoma: A tertiary single centre experience. *European Journal of Surgical Oncology, 48*(3),
526–532. https://doi.org/10.1016/j.ejso.2021.10.010. Epub ahead of print. PMID: 34702592.

Samuels, Y., Bardelli, A., Wolf, Y., & López-Otin, C. (2019). The cancer genome. In V. T. DeVita, T. S. Lawrence, & S. A. Rosenberg (Eds.), *DeVita, Hellman, and Rosenberg's cancer: Principles & practice of oncology* (11th ed., pp. 2–25). Philadelphia, PA: Lippincott Williams & Wilkins.

Sandberg, W., Dmochowski, R., & Beauchamp, R. D. (2022). Safety in the surgical environment. In C. M. Townsend (Ed.), *Sabiston textbook of surgery* (21st ed., pp. 187–200). Amsterdam: Elsevier, Inc.

Winter, J. M., Brody, J. R., Abrams, R. A., Posey, J. A., & Yeo, C. J. (2019). Cancer of the pancreas. In V. T. DeVita, T. S. Lawrence, & S. A. Rosenberg (Eds.), *DeVita, Hellman, and Rosenberg's cancer: Principles & practice of oncology* (11th ed., pp. 804–836). Philadelphia, PA: Lippincott Williams & Wilkins.

World Health Organization. (2009). *Surgical safety checklist.* https://apps.who.int/iris/bitstream/handle/10665/44186/9789241598590_eng_Checklist.pdf.

Zaydfudim, V. M., Hu, Y., & Adams, R. B. (2022). Principles of preoperative and operative surgery. In C. M. Townsend (Ed.), *Sabiston textbook of surgery* (21st ed., pp. 187–222). Amsterdam: Elsevier, Inc.

27

Hematopoietic Stem Cell Transplantation and CAR-T-Cell Therapy

Jennifer Peterson and Terry Wikle Shapiro

HEMATOPOIETIC STEM CELL TRANSPLANT

Overview

I. Principles of hematopoietic stem cell transplant (HSCT) (Brown, 2018; Forman, Negrin, Antin, & Appelbaum, 2016; Wikle Shapiro, 2023)

A. A dose-related response to chemotherapy or radiation therapy (RT) is exhibited by many malignancies.
1. Increasing the dose raises the number of cells destroyed.
2. Chemotherapy or RT dose delivered is limited by the degree of marrow toxicity.
3. High-dose chemotherapy or RT may be administered to treat more aggressive, higher-risk diseases.
4. A potent antitumor effect can be immunologically derived from donor T lymphocytes known as the *graft-versus-tumor* (GVT) *effect* in allogeneic HSCT.

B. Process of HSCT (Brown, 2018; Forman et al., 2016; Wikle Shapiro, 2023) (Fig. 27.1)
1. HSC source is identified. Bone marrow or stem cells from either the patient (autograft) or a donor (allograft) are infused and engraft to "rescue" the patient's hematopoietic function from the toxic effects of antineoplastic therapy or RT. Box 27.1 outlines sources of autografts and allografts.
2. Stem cell source
   a. Allogeneic patient receives bone marrow, peripheral blood stem cells (PBSCs), or umbilical cord blood (UCB) from a healthy related or unrelated donor.
   b. Autologous patient receives own bone marrow or PBSCs harvested or collected before pretransplant conditioning.
3. Factors affecting the source of donor stem cells
   a. Primary disease to be treated
   b. Availability of a histocompatible donor
   c. Age and size of the patient

C. Allografting
1. Involves transplanting marrow, PBSCs, or UCB to a genetically different recipient.
   a. The human leukocyte antigen (HLA) system is used to determine the best possible stem cell donor for transplant.
   b. HLA is a protein or marker found on most cells in the body, including white blood cells (WBCs).
   c. The immune system uses HLA markers to recognize "self" versus "non-self."
   d. Half of the HLA antigens (HLA type) are inherited from each parent.
   e. Eight HLA antigens are used in HLA typing allogeneic transplant recipients.
   f. The most preferred situation is for HSCs to be donated by a 10-out-of-10 (10/10) antigen, HLA-matched sibling.
   g. Partially matched family members or matched unrelated donors from a volunteer pool may also be used as donors (e.g., 6/10 match).
   h. Within certain limitations, UCB may be used as a source of allogeneic stem cells in the related matched sibling and unrelated donor situations.
   i. Allografts are indicated for some congenital abnormalities of bone marrow function or in disease involving marrow that is not amenable to cure with standard treatment (e.g., leukemias). Box 27.2 shows diseases treated with allogeneic transplant.
   j. Reduced intensity or nonmyeloablative HSCTs are used in the allogeneic transplant setting when the patient is older, has preexisting comorbidities, and has a disease that will benefit from the GVT immunologic effect (Brown, 2018).
      (1) The patient receives lower doses of chemotherapy plus immunotherapy often followed by a small dose of total-body irradiation (TBI) prior to allogeneic transplant of marrow or PBSCs.
      (2) The objective is to induce an immunologic response known as the *GVT effect*, whereby the donor stem cells recognize the malignant cells and destroy them.
      (3) This treatment is usually reserved for older patients (>60 years) or those with comorbidities (limited organ function) and reduces the risk of acute toxicities from the lowered doses of chemotherapy and radiotherapy.
2. Allografting requires the use of posttransplant immunosuppression to prevent overwhelming graft-versus-host disease (GVHD), a condition in which

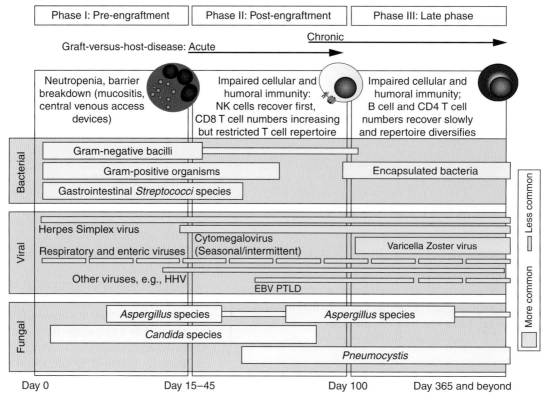

Fig. 27.1 Hematopoietic stem cell transplantation. From Tomblyn, M., Chiller, T., Einsele, H., Gress, R., Sepkowitz, K., Storek, J., et al. (2009). Guidelines for preventing infectious complications among hematopoietic cell transplantation recipients: A global perspective. *Biology of Blood and Marrow Transplantation, 15*(10), 1143–1238. https://doi.org/10.1016/j.bbmt.2009.06.019.

BOX 27.1   Sources of Marrow or Stem Cells

Allografts
- Matched sibling donor
- Bone marrow
- Peripheral blood stem cells
- Umbilical cord blood
- Identical twin donor
- Partially matched family member
- Peripheral blood stem cells
- Matched unrelated donor

Autografts
- Autologous bone marrow
- Autologous peripheral blood stem cells
- Autologous umbilical cord blood (rare)

---

donor T lymphocytes mount an immune response against the patient.

D. Autografting (Forman et al., 2016; Wikle Shapiro, 2023)

1. Autografting involves transplanting marrow or PBSCs back into the person from whom the blood cells originated.

2. Autologous bone marrow or PBSC transplant is used as a method for treating several malignant disorders.

3. Using autologous marrow or PBSCs is not feasible in patients who have a deficiency of their functional bone marrow, as is the case with aplastic anemia, inborn errors of metabolism, and immunodeficiency states.

4. Autografting may be preferable to using an allogeneic source of stem cells (e.g., to avoid GVHD, in situations in which marrow contamination with malignant cells is unlikely, and when no evidence of an immunologic antitumor effect [GVT] with allogeneic transplant exists).

5. Autologous stem cell transplant (ASCT) is most frequently used for the treatment of multiple myeloma and lymphoma. ASCT is also utilized in the treatment of other malignancies such as lymphoma, neuroblastoma, and brain tumors that have a relatively low chance for cure with standard or conventional doses of chemotherapy. In this case ASCT is considered a marrow or stem cell "rescue." Box 27.3 illustrates diseases treated with autologous transplant.

6. In some autografting situations, it is debated whether a low (undetectable) level of tumor cells persisting in the infused cells may promote relapse. However, routine purging, even in diseases that involve bone marrow, is unproven. Using PBSCs instead of bone marrow is known to lower the risk of tumor infusion.

7. PBSCs are almost exclusively used as an autografting source.

BOX 27.2 Diseases Treated With Allografting of Hematopoietic Stem Cells

Leukemias—Syndromes
Acute myelogenous leukemia
Acute lymphoblastic leukemia
Chronic myelogenous leukemia
Myelodysplastic syndromes

Myelofibrosis Immunodeficiencies
Severe combined immunodeficiency
Wiskott–Aldrich syndrome
Miscellaneous immunodeficiencies

Hematologic Disorders
β-Thalassemia
Sickle cell anemia
Congenital neutropenia
Osteopetrosis

Bone Marrow Failure
Severe aplastic anemia
Fanconi anemia
Reticular dysgenesis

Nonhematologic Genetic Disorders
Inclusion cell (I-cell) disease
Mucopolysaccharidosis
Adrenal leukodystrophy
Glycogen storage diseases
Miscellaneous metabolic storage disorders

Lymphoproliferative Disorders
Hodgkin disease
Non-Hodgkin lymphoma
Multiple myeloma
Chronic lymphocytic leukemia

BOX 27.3 Diseases Treated With Autografting of Hematopoietic Stem Cells

Lymphoproliferative Disorders
Hodgkin disease
Non-Hodgkin lymphoma
Multiple myeloma

Solid Tumors
Neuroblastoma
Ewing sarcoma
Hepatoblastoma
Testicular cancer
Osteosarcoma
Central nervous system tumors

Others
Autoimmune diseases
Systemic lupus erythematosus
Rheumatoid arthritis
Juvenile-onset diabetes

8. Autologous PBSC collection is generally performed after several cycles of chemotherapy.
9. Autologous HSCT can be effective in treating some autoimmune diseases because it allows for high doses of immunosuppressive therapy to be administered (de Silva & Seneviratne, 2019).
10. Optimally, transplant is performed when the patient has achieved complete remission, when the disease is "chemo responsive," the patient has "minimal residual disease," or both (Wikle Shapiro, 2023).

E. In the patient receiving an allogeneic transplant, histocompatibility testing must be done to determine whether the patient and donor are genetically compatible (Kapadia & Greiner, 2018; National Marrow Donor Program [NMDP], 2018).
1. HLA testing—major histocompatibility complex encoded by genes (one pair from each parent) present on chromosome 6
   a. Major loci of importance when using allogeneic marrow or PBSC donors are HLA-A, -B, -C, DRB1, and DQB1 (10 antigens). Only HLA-A, HLA-B, and DRB1 antigens (six antigens) are tested when using a UCB unit (Kapadia & Greiner, 2018).
   b. The success of allogeneic transplant is related to the degree of histocompatibility between the donor and recipient.
   c. Patients have a one in four chance of having a 10/10 antigen–matched donor among their full siblings.
   d. Patients without an HLA-matched sibling donor have approximately a 66%–70% chance (depending on race or ethnicity) of finding an HLA-matched unrelated volunteer donor or donated UCB donor from the National Marrow Donor Registry. Ethnic minority patients are less likely to find an HLA-compatible donor. Use of matched unrelated donors carries more risk because of higher incidence of GVHD and delay in immune reconstitution.
2. Further DNA testing of HLA-DR—performed to determine the degree of histocompatibility between donor and recipient
F. HSC recipient is prepared with dose-intense (marrow-ablative) therapy (Wikle Shapiro, 2023).
1. The conditioning protocol is established based on the primary disease, patient's functional status, and type of transplant.
2. The goals of a pretransplant conditioning regimen are as follows:
   a. To eradicate the remaining malignancy in the recipient
   b. To suppress the immune system of the recipient to allow for marrow engraftment (allografts only)
   c. To open space within the marrow compartment for newly infused PBSCs or marrow to engraft

3. The conditioning regimen may include high-dose chemotherapy alone or in combination with total lymph node irradiation or TBI.
4. Immunosuppressive therapy may also be used as part of the conditioning regimen in the allogeneic transplant setting.
5. Conditioning regimen is usually completed before HSC infusion.

G. Marrow, PBSCs, or UCB from the donor (allogeneic) or the patient (autologous) is harvested and processed (Kitko, Gatwood, & Connelly, 2018).
1. Bone marrow harvesting is performed with the patient under general or regional anesthesia; most used in pediatric transplant.
   a. Two to four punctures are made in the posterior iliac crests bilaterally.
   b. Approximately 10 mL/kg of the recipient's body weight is aspirated from the donor.
   c. Marrow is then filtered to remove bone and fat particles.
   d. If a major ABO incompatibility exists between recipient and donor, the red blood cells (RBCs) are removed before infusion.
   e. Processed marrow is placed in a blood administration bag for cryopreservation (autologous) or immediate infusion (allogeneic).
   f. Matched, unrelated donor marrow or PBSCs are generally collected at the donor's closest NMDP collection center and then transported to the recipient's transplant center for infusion. Further processing is generally performed at the recipient center.
2. PBSCs are generally collected after stem cell mobilization with hematopoietic growth factors and/or chemotherapy (autologous only). Immunomodulators such as plerixafor may be used before stem cell collection.
   a. Cells are collected, usually via a large-bore intravenous catheter or a centrally placed pheresis catheter, using a special cell separator. After processing, autologous PBSCs are cryopreserved in small aliquots for future infusion.
   b. A minimum of 2.0×10^6 CD34+ cells are required to ensure successful engraftment.
   c. With UCB, lower cell doses may be utilized.
   d. Patients undergo the conditioning regimen. Next, previously collected cells are thawed and reinfused. Fresh allogeneic PBSCs are infused as soon as possible, often not sooner than 24 hours after high-dose therapy is completed.
3. Stem cells from an umbilical cord may be used as a source, although UCB is generally reserved for patients weighing less than 60 kg. Studies are currently underway using multiple (>1) matched cord blood units for larger patients (Dehn et al., 2019).
   a. Related and unrelated UCB cells are harvested at birth from volunteer maternal donors and are cryopreserved at a designated cord blood bank. Donated cord blood is accessible via the NMDP's Cord Blood Registry (Krishnamurti, 2021; NMDP, 2018).
   b. The cells are transported to the recipient's transplant center, thawed, and infused on the day of transplant.
4. Some centers are using a variety of experimental techniques to purge autologous marrow of possible tumor contaminants.
   a. Purging may be performed using monoclonal antibodies, chemotherapy, or physical means (centrifugation).
   b. Purging may damage the stem cells, thus increasing the risk of delayed engraftment or rejection.

H. Marrow HSCs are infused through a central venous catheter.
1. Autologous HSCs are thawed at the patient's bedside and reinfused via a central venous catheter.
2. Freshly harvested HSCs are brought to the patient's room and infused in a similar fashion to a unit of packed RBCs.
3. If allogeneic cord blood is used, cells are thawed at the bedside and reinfused.

I. The patient is supported through the period of marrow aplasia (10–30 days). Preventive measures are instituted to decrease potential complications (e.g., infection, GVHD, sinusoidal obstructive syndrome [SOS]/veno-occlusive disease [VOD]). See Table 27.1 for preventive measures for HSC transplant–associated complication control practices (Ladha, Mannis, & Muffly, 2021). See Table 27.2 for infectious complications that occur following HSCT.

II. Role of HSC transplant
A. Cure—each patient is evaluated with curative intent.
B. Disease control (palliation)—in some patients, notably those with multiple myeloma and mantle cell lymphoma, autologous transplant is used to increase the patient's progression-free survival.

Assessment

I. Pertinent medical history
A. Diagnosis (see Boxes 27.2 and 27.3 for conditions commonly treated with HSCT) (Schmit-Pokorny & Eisenberg, 2020; Wikle Shapiro, 2023).
B. Potential candidates for HSC transplant—patients with malignancies at high risk for recurrence after standard therapy; malignancies must demonstrate a response to either antineoplastic therapy or RT.
C. Factors that may increase the incidence of complications of HSC transplant (Duque-Afonso et al., 2021; Estey, 2020; Toenges et al., 2021).
1. Amount of previous cancer therapy, length of time since last therapy, response to past therapy, and length of disease-free interval
2. Underlying kidney, lung, liver, or cardiac dysfunction
3. Previous pretransplant or active infections and response to therapy

TABLE 27.1 Preventive Measures for Hematopoietic Stem Cell Transplant–Associated Complications

Complication	Infection	Preventive and Treatment Measures	Nursing Implications
GVHD, acute and chronic	• Results from engraftment of immunocompetent donor T lymphocytes reacting against immunocompetent recipient tissues (skin, GI tract, and liver) • Occurs in 30%–60% of all allogeneic HSC transplant recipients • Risk is increased when donor is not a 6/6 HLA antigen match or when a matched unrelated donor is used • May be either acute or chronic	• Depletion of T cells from marrow • Preventive immunosuppressive agents • Cyclosporine A (Gengraf, Sandimmune oral: Neoral) • FK-506 (tacrolimus) • High-dose steroids • Antithymocyte globulin • Alemtuzumab (Campath) • Muromonab-CD3 (OKT-3/Ontak) • Thalidomide (Thalomid) • Monoclonal antibodies • Polyclonal antibodies • MMF (Cellcept) • Methotrexate (Mexate) • Sirolimus (Rapamune) • Mesenchymal stem cells	• Monitor for delayed marrow engraftment • Monitor for prolonged lymphopenia and neutropenia • Evaluate the cyclosporine or tacrolimus levels, and notify the practitioner of significant abnormalities • Monitor the side effects of immunosuppressive agents • Monitor for signs of infection • Monitor weekly infection markers (viral PCRs, galactomannan) • Maintain skin integrity • Maintain patient's functional capacity • Monitor for signs of hemolytic–uremic syndrome
Idiopathic pulmonary interstitial pneumonitis (infectious and noninfectious)	• Occurs most frequently in patients >30 years with a history of chest irradiation or previous bleomycin therapy; allogeneic transplantation, and CMV-positive with CMV-negative donor • Causative agents infectious • Cytomegalovirus • *Aspergillus* species • *Pneumocystis jiroveci* • Other infections 15% • Noninfectious cause • DAH • Chemotherapy-related • GVHD • Radiation therapy	• Use of CMV-seronegative blood products • Use of filtered air system high-efficiency particulate absorbing filter • Antimicrobial therapy • Ganciclovir (Cytovene) • Foscarnet (Foscavir) • Intravenous immunoglobulin • Trimethoprim and sulfamethoxazole • Aerosolized or IV pentamidine (NebuPent, Pentacarinat, Pentam 300) • Azoles (voriconazole, posaconazole) • Amphotericin B (Abelcet, AmBisome)	• Monitor for side effects of antimicrobial therapy • Implement turning, coughing, and deep-breathing routine • Encourage activity • Provide transfusion therapy (DAH)
Hepatic sinusoidal obstruction syndrome	• Damage to the small sinusoids of the liver from pretransplantation conditioning regimen • Occurs in 5%–54% of patients; most common in patients undergoing matched, unrelated donor transplants and those with pretransplantation liver enzyme elevations or previous radiation to abdomen	• Defibrotide • Ursodiol (Actigall) • Heparin • Diuretics • Renal dose of dopamine • Strict fluid management	• Monitor liver function studies • Monitor for weight gain • Evaluate abdominal pain • Use caution when administering drugs that are cleared via hepatic system because increased toxicity may occur • Monitor renal function

CMV, Cytomegalovirus; *DAH*, diffuse alveolar hemorrhage; *GI*, gastrointestinal; *GVHD*, Graft-versus-host disease; *HLA*, human leukocyte antigen; *HSC*, hematopoietic stem cell; *IV*, intravenous; *MMF*, mycophenolate mofetil; *PCRs*, polymerase chain reactions.
Adapted from Becze, E. (2012). Veno-occlusive disease is the most common hepatic complication in stem cell transplants. *ONS Connect*, *27*(11), 16–17; Schmit-Pokorny, K., & Eisenberg, S. (Eds.). (2020). *Hematopoietic stem cell transplantation: A manual for nursing practice* (3rd ed.). Pittsburgh, PA: Oncology Nursing Society.

4. Age—older patients (>17 years) more likely to develop complications
5. Patients who are overweight or experiencing malnutrition at the time of transplant
6. Psychosocial dysfunction

II. Physical examination

A. Pulmonary—respiratory rate, depth, and rhythm; lung expansion; adventitious breath sounds; oxygen saturation

B. Renal—color and odor of urine and urinary output, edema, and weight gain

C. Mobility—muscle strength and endurance, range of motion, gait, and activity level

D. Nutrition—weight; skin turgor; amount, content, and patterns of nutritional intake

E. Comfort level—pain rating, anxiety, and ability to rest or engage

TABLE 27.2   Infectious Complications and Sites of Occurrence in Hematopoietic Stem Cell Transplantation Recipients

Type	Organism, Disease	Common Site
First Month After Transplantation		
Viral	HSV	Oral, esophageal, skin, GI tract, and genital
	RSV	Sinopulmonary
	EBV	Oral, esophageal, skin, GI tract
	HHV6	Pulmonary, CNS, GI tract
Bacterial	Gram-positive organisms (*Staphylococcus epidermidis, Staphylococcus aureus*, streptococci)	Skin, blood, sinopulmonary
	Gram-negative organisms (*Escherichia coli, Pseudomonas aeruginosa, Klebsiella*)	GI tract, blood, oral, perirectal
Fungal	*Candida* (*C. albicans, C. glabrata, C. krusei*)	Oral, esophageal, skin
	Aspergillus fumigatus, A. flavus	Sinopulmonary, skin
1–4 Months After Transplantation		
Viral	CMV	Pulmonary, hepatic, GI tract
	Enteric viruses (rotavirus, coxsackie virus, adenovirus)	Pulmonary, urinary, GI tract, hepatic
	RSV	Sinopulmonary
	Parainfluenza virus	Pulmonary
	BK human polyoma virus	Genitourinary
Bacterial	Gram-positive organisms	Sinopulmonary, skin, venous access devices
Fungal	*Candida* species	Oral, hepatosplenic, integument, venous access devices
	Aspergillus species	Sinopulmonary, CNS, skin
	Mucormycosis	Sinopulmonary
	Coccidioidomycosis	Sinopulmonary
	Cryptococcus neoformans	Pulmonary, CNS
Protozoa	*Pneumocystis jiroveci* (*carinii*)	Pulmonary
	Toxoplasma gondii	Pulmonary, CNS
4–12 Months After Transplantation		
Viral	CMV, echoviruses, RSV, VZV, human polyoma virus	Integument, pulmonary, hepatic, genitourinary
Bacterial	Gram-positive organisms (*Streptococcus pneumoniae*)	Sinopulmonary, blood
	Haemophilus influenzae (pneumococci)	Sinopulmonary
Fungal	Aspergillosis	Sinopulmonary
	Coccidioidomycosis	Sinopulmonary
Protozoa	*P. jiroveci* (*carinii*)	Pulmonary
	T. gondii	Pulmonary, CNS
12 Months After Transplantation		
Viral	VZV	Integument
	CMV	Pulmonary, hepatic
Bacterial	Gram-positive organisms (streptococci, *H. influenzae*, encapsulated bacteria)	Sinopulmonary, blood

CMV, Cytomegalovirus; *CNS*, central nervous system; *EBV*, Epstein–Barr virus; *GI*, gastrointestinal; *HHV6*, human herpesvirus type 6; *HSV*, herpes simplex virus; *RSV*, respiratory syncytial virus; *VZV*, varicella zoster virus.
Data from Schmit-Pokorny, K. & Eisenberg, S. (Eds.). (2020). *Hematopoietic stem cell transplantation: A manual for nursing practice* (3rd ed., pp. 125–128). Pittsburgh, PA: Oncology Nursing Society.

F. Cardiovascular—heart rate and rhythm, heart sounds, blood pressure, and perfusion

G. Gastrointestinal—volume, color, consistency, and caliber of stool; abdominal pain; distention; bowel sounds

H. Genitourinary—color of urine, suppleness of bladder, condition of perineum

I. Integumentary—color and intactness of skin, condition of oral mucous membranes, dental evaluation, and condition of perineum and rectum

J. Neurologic—mental status, orientation, sensation, and reflexes

III. Psychosocial examination

A. Psychological evaluation

1. Feelings on the decision to undergo HSC transplant

2. Understanding of treatment aggressiveness, goals of therapy, and chances of survival

3. Number, type, and effectiveness of coping mechanisms used in past stressful situations (before transplant therapy) by patient and family members

TABLE 27.3 Grading of Acute Graft-Versus-Host Disease (GVHD) Extent of Organ Involvement

Organ	Stage		Parameters	
Rash[a]				
Skin	I		<25% BSA	
	II		25%–50% BSA	
	III		Rash on >50% BSA	
	IV		Generalized erythroderma with bullous formation	
Total Bilirubin				
Liver	I		2–3 mg/dL	
	II		3–6 mg/dL	
	III		6–15 mg/dL	
	IV		>15 mg/dL	
Volume of Diarrhea		Adult		Pediatric
Gut	I	>500 mL/day		10–15 mL/kg/day
	II	>1000 mL/day		15–20 mL/kg/day
	III	>1500 mL/day		20–30 mL/kg/day
	IV	Adult and pediatric: severe abdominal pain with or without an ileus		
Overall Clinical Grade				
Grade	Description			
I	Stage I and II clinical skin GVHD			
II	Stage III clinical skin GVHD *or*			
	Stage I liver and/or stage I gut GVHD			
	Only one system stage III or greater			
III	Stage II and III liver and/or stage II–IV gut GVHD			
	Only one system stage III or greater			
IV	Stage IV clinical skin GVHD (with grade 2 or higher histology) *and*			
	Stage IV clinical liver and/or gut GVHD			

BSA, Body surface area.
[a]Use the rule of nines or burn chart to determine the extent of rash.

Adapted from Dignan, F. L., Clark, A., Amrolia, P., et al. Haemato-oncology Task Force of British Committee for Standards in Haematology, & British Society for Blood and Marrow Transplantation. (2012). Diagnosis and management of acute graft-versus-host disease. *British Journal of Haematology 158*(1), 30–45. https://doi.org/10.1111/j.1365-2141.2012.09129.x; Schmit-Pokorny, K., & Eisenberg, S. (Eds.). (2020). *Hematopoietic stem cell transplantation: A manual for nursing practice* (3rd ed., pp. 141). Pittsburgh, PA: Oncology Nursing Society.

Corbacioglu, S., Jabbour, E. J., & Mohty, M. (2019). Risk factors for development of and progression of hepatic veno-occlusive disease/sinusoidal obstruction syndrome. *Biology of Blood and Marrow Transplantation: Journal of the American Society for Blood and Marrow Transplantation, 25*(7), 1271–1280. https://doi.org/10.1016/j.bbmt.2019.02.018.

Dehn, J., Spellman, S., Hurley, C. K., Shaw, B. E., Barker, J. N., Burns, L. J., et al. (2019). Selection of unrelated donors and cord blood units for hematopoietic cell transplantation: Guidelines from the NMDP/CIBMTR. *Blood, 134*(12), 924–934. https://doi.org/10.1182/blood.2019001212.

Duque-Afonso, J., Ihorst, G., Waterhouse, M., Zeiser, R., Wäsch, R., Bertz, H., et al. (2021). Comparison of reduced-toxicity conditioning protocols using fludarabine, melphalan combined with thiotepa or carmustine in allogeneic hematopoietic cell transplantation. *Bone Marrow Transplant, 56*(1), 110–120. https://doi.org/10.1038/s41409-020-0986-2.

Hill, J. A., & Seo, S. K. (2020). How I prevent infections in patients receiving CD19-targeted chimeric antigen receptor T cells for B-cell malignancies. *Blood, 136*(8), 925–935. https://doi.org/10.1182/blood.2019004000.

Krishnamurti, L. (2021). Hematopoietic cell transplantation for sickle cell disease: Updates and future directions. *Hematology. American Society of Hematology. Education Program, 2021*(1), 181–189. https://doi.org/10.1182/hematology.2021000251.

Mellgren, K., Nierop, A. F. M., & Abrahamsson, J. (2019). Use of multivariate immune reconstitution patterns to describe immune reconstitution after allogeneic stem cell transplantation in children. *Biology of Blood and Marrow Transplantation: Journal of the American Society for Blood and Marrow Transplantation, 25*(10), 2045–2053. https://doi.org/10.1016/j.bbmt.2019.06.018.

Ramachandran, V., Kolli, S. S., & Strowd, L. C. (2019). Review of graft-versus-host disease. *Dermatologic Clinics, 37*(4), 569–582. doi:10.1016/j.det.2019.05.014.

Rautenberg, C., Germing, U., Haas, R., Kobbe, G., & Schroeder, T. (2019). Relapse of acute myeloid leukemia after allogeneic stem cell transplantation: Prevention, detection, and treatment. *International Journal of Molecular Sciences, 20*(1), 228. https://doi.org/10.3390/ijms20010228.

Schmit-Pokorny, K., & Eisenberg, S. (2020). *Hematopoietic stem cell transplantation: A manual for nursing practice* (3rd ed.). Pittsburgh, PA: Oncology Nursing Society.

Toenges, R., Greinix, H., Lawitschka, A., Halter, J., Baumgartner, A., Simon, A., et al. (2021). Current practice in nutrition after allogeneic hematopoietic stem cell transplantation – Results from a survey among hematopoietic stem cell transplant centers. *Clinical Nutrition (Edinburgh, Scotland), 40*(4), 1571–1577. https://doi.org/10.1016/j.clnu.2021.02.030.

Webster, J. A., Luznik, L., & Gojo, I. (2021). Treatment of AML relapse after Allo-HCT. *Frontiers in Oncology, 11,* 812207. https://doi.org/10.3389/fonc.2021.812207.

Zuanelli Brambilla, C., Lobaugh, S. M., Ruiz, J. D., Dahi, P. B., Goldberg, A. D., Young, J. W., et al. (2021). Relapse after allogeneic stem cell transplantation of acute myelogenous leukemia and myelodysplastic syndrome and the importance of second cellular therapy. *Transplantation and Cellular Therapy, 27*(9), 771.e1–771.e10. https://doi.org/10.1016/j.jtct.2021.05.011.

4. Perceptions of patient and family about isolation, prolonged hospitalization, living will, use of life support technology, and potential death or survival

5. Caregiver's availability and ability to comprehend the role

B. Social evaluation

1. Previous roles and responsibilities in the family and community

2. Type, number, and history of use of support systems in the family and community

3. Financial status—employment, insurance coverage, and resources for daily living

4. Eligibility for community resources

IV. Critical laboratory and diagnostic data unique to HSC transplant (Schmit-Pokorny & Eisenberg, 2020)

A. Hematologic—complete blood cell count, differential, platelet count, coagulation studies, type/crossmatch with HSC donor, donor chimerism, minimal residual disease markers, T-cell subsets with enumeration, and mitogen stimulation studies (Mellgren, Nierop, & Abrahamsson, 2019; Schmit-Pokorny & Eisenberg, 2020; Talekar & Olsen, 2018)

B. Hepatic—liver transaminases (aspartate aminotransferase and alanine aminotransferase), lactic acid dehydrogenase, bilirubin, and coagulation studies; and liver duplex ultrasonography (Brown, 2018)

C. Renal—electrolytes, blood urea nitrogen, serum creatinine, and creatinine clearance; cyclosporine A, tacrolimus (FK-506), aminoglycoside, and vancomycin levels; viral urine cultures, BK virus polymerase chain reaction (PCR), electron microscopy, and renal ultrasonography (Kapadia & Wikle Shapiro, 2018)

D. Cardiovascular—electrocardiography, echocardiogram (echo) with cardiac ejection fraction or shorting fractions (in children), and venography

E. Pulmonary—chest radiography, computed tomography of chest or sinuses, pulmonary function tests (e.g., diffusing capacity of the lungs for carbon monoxide [DLCO]), arterial blood gases, and oxygen saturation (pulse oximetry)

F. Immune—antibody titers for cytomegalovirus (CMV) and herpesviruses (pretransplant), Epstein–Barr virus by quantitative PCR, hepatitis B surface antigen, immunoglobulin levels, HIV antibody, hepatitis C PCR, T-cell subsets (enumeration), CD45 RA/RO

G. Infectious disease (Pereira, Pouch, & Scully, 2019)—blood cultures for bacteria and fungi; urine and stool cultures for bacteria, fungi, and viruses; CMV quantitative PCR studies, adenovirus quantitative PCR studies, human herpesvirus type 6 (RNA) studies, herpesvirus titers and cultures, toxoplasmosis antigenemia studies, respiratory and sputum cultures for bacteria, fungi, viruses, *Legionella* antigen (urine), acid-fast bacilli; stool and urine for electron microscopy cultures, stool for *Clostridium difficile* toxin, stains for *Pneumocystis carinii* pneumonia (PCP), multiviral respiratory panel, galactomannan, beta D glucan

V. Assess for unique complications after HSC transplant

A. GVHD (Table 27.3; Bride, Patel, & Freedman, 2018; Ramachandran, Kolli, & Strowd, 2019; Wikle Shapiro, 2023)

1. Monitor condition of skin (erythema, rash), especially the face, palms of hands, and soles of feet.

2. Evaluate changes in liver function study results.

3. Monitor of amount, consistency, frequency, and color of stool.

a. Monitor viral and fungal infection.

4. Monitor cyclosporin or tacrolimus levels.

B. Hepatic sinusoidal obstruction syndrome or hepatic VOD (Box 27.4; Brown, 2018; Corbacioglu, Jabbour, & Mohty, 2019; Wikle Shapiro, 2023)

1. Weigh the patient daily; notify the medical practitioner of weight gain more than 5% of pretransplant weight.

2. Monitor the location of pain (right upper quadrant).

3. Evaluate for elevation in serum bilirubin level.

4. Evaluate for bleeding, poor response to platelet transfusions, and abnormal coagulation factors.

5. Evaluate for changes in mental status.

6. Measure abdominal girth daily if possible VOD.

7. Provide skin care for patients with hyperbilirubinemia.

8. Evaluate the level of abdominal pain.

C. Idiopathic pulmonary interstitial pneumonitis—infectious and noninfectious (Kapadia & Wikle Shapiro, 2018)

1. Monitor temperature.

2. Assess for cough, chest pain, adventitious breath sounds, diminished oxygen saturation.

3. Evaluate activity tolerance.

Management

I. Implement conditioning regimen ordered by the physician or other provider.

II. Administer prophylactic antimicrobial therapy as ordered (Centers for Disease Control, 2000).

A. Antibacterial prophylaxis with fluoroquinolones, third-generation cephalosporins

---

BOX 27.4   Risk Factors for the Development of Hepatic Sinusoidal Obstruction Syndrome

- Pretransplant chemotherapy (conditioning regimens containing cyclophosphamide, with or without busulfan)
- Abdominal radiation
- Pretransplant hepatotoxic drug therapy (e.g., gemtuzumab ozogamicin [Mylotarg], inotuzumab ozogamicin [Besponsa])
- Elevated transaminases before conditioning regimen
- Human leukocyte antigen-mismatched or unrelated allogeneic transplant
- Viral hepatitis
- Metastatic liver disease
- Karnofsky score <90% before transplant
- Second transplant
- Older age recipient
- Female gender

B. Antifungal prophylaxis with amphotericin B by nebulation, fluconazole (Diflucan), posaconazole, voriconazole (Vfend), isavuconazole (Cresemba), and micafungin (Mycamine) (Neofytos, 2019)

C. Monitor therapeutic drugs' levels of posaconazole and voriconazole.

D. Trimethoprim–sulfamethoxazole (Septra, Bactrim), intravenously (IV) or inhaled pentamidine (NebuPent, Pentacarinat, Pentam 300), or dapsone for prevention of PCP

E. Acyclovir (Zovirax) for prevention of herpesvirus infection, ganciclovir (Cytovene), foscarnet (Foscavir), or cidofovir for prevention and treatment of CMV and other viral infections

F. Intravenous immunoglobulin G (IVIg) for the prevention and treatment of CMV and other viral infections.

III. Administer hematopoietic growth factors as ordered.

IV. Administer immunosuppressive therapy to prevent and treat GVHD with cyclosporine, tacrolimus, sirolimus, mycophenolate, and antithymocyte globulin, systemic steroids, alemtuzumab (Campath), or others.

V. Administer ursodeoxycholic acid (Actigall), defibrotide, analgesics, vitamin K, fresh frozen plasma, and other blood products for patients with VOD/SOS.

VI. Employ measures to prevent bladder toxicity—for patients receiving high-dose cyclophosphamide (Cytoxan), hemorrhagic cystitis is a potential complication (Kapadia & Wikle Shapiro, 2018).

A. Administer mesna (Mesnex), a uroprotectant, with high-dose cyclophosphamide.

B. Provide IV hyperhydration.

Nonpharmacologic Management

I. Maximize safety for the patient and family.

A. Maintain aseptic techniques and the level of protective isolation identified by the HSCT program (see Table 27.1 for general guidelines).

B. Teach the patient and family strategies to decrease the risk of infection, bleeding, and injury during period of aplasia after HSC infusion.

II. Minimize the incidence and severity of complications unique to HSC transplant.

A. Anxiety

1. Provide a thorough orientation to the inpatient and outpatient HSC transplant units and procedures.

2. Implement strategies to encourage the patient and family to express concerns about HSC transplant demands.

3. Consult with an occupational therapist for diversional activities during isolation.

4. Teach new anxiety-relieving strategies as desired or needed by patient and family.

5. Assess caregiver's ability to implement care demands.

B. Risk for infection—Fig. 27.1 displays common opportunistic infections and time of occurrence after transplant (Bride et al., 2018; Wikle Shapiro, 2023)

1. Notify the provider of initial temperature greater than 101°F (38.3°C) or other symptoms indicative of infection.

2. Teach the patient and family strategies to decrease the risk of endogenous infections.

   a. Meticulous hand washing
   b. Routine oral and perineal care
   c. Skin care, including frequent baths for patients receiving thiotepa

3. Teach the patient and family strategies to decrease the risk of exogenous infections.

   a. Restrict visitors with suspected or known infections.
   b. Limit visits by children (especially school-age children).
   c. Avoid invasive procedures (e.g., peripheral IV catheter, intramuscular injections, urinary catheterization, rectal examinations, rectal temperatures).
   d. Recommend influenza vaccination for all close-contact individuals.
   e. Proper care of central venous catheter
   f. Collect routine surveillance cultures for bacteria, fungi, and viruses, antigenemia/PCR studies, and *Aspergillus* antigen study.

4. Transfuse irradiated, CMV-seronegative blood products or leukocyte-poor filtered blood products for all patients.

C. Risk for injury

1. Encourage frequent voiding, accurate urine output, necessary after high-dose cyclophosphamide.

2. If mesna is not used with cyclophosphamide administration, provide continuous bladder irrigation as ordered, administration of antispasmodics and analgesics for bladder spasms.

3. Check urine specific gravity with each void on days of high-dose cyclophosphamide and 24 hours after the last dose as ordered.

4. Monitor for cyclophosphamide-induced hyponatremia caused by syndrome of inappropriate antidiuretic hormone secretion.

D. Alteration in oral mucous membranes

1. Encourage cryotherapy (ice chips) for patients receiving melphalan.

2. Encourage good oral hygiene.

E. Alteration in skin integrity

1. Instruct patient to bathe four times daily while receiving thiotepa because drug is excreted via the integumentary system and may lead to skin problems

2. Apply barrier creams to prevent perianal breakdown

F. Alteration in cardiovascular status

1. Monitor blood pressure and heart rate frequently with high-dose etoposide.

2. Assess orthostatic hypotension with cyclophosphamide and high-dose etoposide.

3. Assess the decreased level of consciousness related to alcohol content in high-dose etoposide.

G. Altered oral mucous membranes (see Chapter 41)

H. Nausea and vomiting (see Chapter 38)

III. Interventions to enhance adaptation and rehabilitation

A. Implement a program of range-of-motion and isometric exercises during the isolation period, especially if the patient is taking high-dose steroids.

B. Discuss potential changes in lifestyle and social interaction required immediately after discharge from the hospital.

C. Provide long-term follow-up (Dandekar, 2018).

1. Educate patient and family members on common outpatient problems after HSCT—fatigue, weight loss, sexual dysfunction, cataracts, chronic GVHD, chronic lung disease, herpes zoster virus, endocrinopathies, depression, isolation.

2. Ensure survivorship issues are addressed through long-term follow-up program.

a. Lifelong evaluation of allogeneic recipient for chronic GVHD

b. Posttransplant vaccinations

c. Fertility issues

d. Reentry into community and work

e. Delayed organ dysfunction (pulmonary, cardiac, renal, adrenal dysfunction)

D. Posttransplant relapse

1. Currently, there is no standard treatment for relapsed disease post HSCT. Potential post relapse treatment options include disease-directed maintenance therapy, donor lymphocyte infusion (DLI), reduce/withdraw immunosuppression (allogeneic), second transplant, or clinical trial enrollment. Palliative care should also be considered (Schmit-Pokorny & Eisenberg, 2020).

2. Maintenance therapy (Schmit-Pokorny & Eisenberg, 2020)

a. Standard disease-directed treatments including:

i. Immunomodulatory agents or proteasome inhibitors for multiple myeloma

ii. Antibody–drug conjugate for Hodgkin lymphoma

iii. Anti-CD20 monoclonal antibody for mantle cell lymphoma

iv. Tyrosine kinase inhibitors for Philadelphia chromosome-positive acute lymphoblastic leukemia (ALL)

3. Reduce/withdraw immunosuppression (Schmit-Pokorny & Eisenberg, 2020; Webster, Luznik, & Gojo, 2021).

a. Uses the GVT effect where donor immune cells eliminate malignant cells

b. Avoid active GVHD.

c. Increased the risk of developing GVHD with this approach

4. DLI for allogeneic HSCT recipients (Rautenberg, Germing, Haas, Kobbe, & Schroeder, 2019; Zuanelli Brambilla et al., 2021)

a. Lymphocytes from the HSCT donor are infused to promote GVT.

b. Patient may receive more than one DLI infusion dependent on their response.

c. DLI increases the risk of developing GVHD.

5. Second transplant (Rautenberg et al., 2019; Zuanelli Brambilla et al., 2021)

a. Multiple myeloma patients may receive a second autologous HSCT or an allogeneic HSCT if donor is available.

b. Second allogeneic HSCT may use the same donor or different donors.

6. Clinical trial/immunotherapy (Schmit-Pokorny & Eisenberg, 2020)

a. Eligibility for clinical trial participation

b. Immunotherapy with chimeric antigen receptor (CAR) T cells, checkpoint inhibitors, targeted therapies, or monoclonal antibodies

7. Palliative care (Schmit-Pokorny & Eisenberg, 2020)

a. Patients may choose to forego further therapy.

b. Treatment goals shift to supportive care/end-of-life care.

CHIMERIC ANTIGEN RECEPTOR T-CELL THERAPY

Overview

I. Definition:

A. CAR-T-cell therapy is immunotherapy that utilizes a patient's modified autologous lymphocytes to recognize an antigen expressed by the targeted malignant cells.

B. CAR-T cells can identify the malignant cell that had previously evaded T-cell destruction (Lamprecht & Dansereau, 2019; Schmit-Pokorny & Eisenberg, 2020). WBC are collected from the patient via apheresis, and the lymphocytes are isolated.

1. The lymphocytes are sent to a manufacturing facility where the T cells are modified using a viral vector to create the CAR on the surface of the T cells.

2. The CAR-T cells are expanded to ensure an adequate number of cells are infused for effective treatment, evaluated to ensure quality standards are met, cryopreserved and shipped back to the treatment facility (Lamprecht & Dansereau, 2019; Schmit-Pokorny & Eisenberg, 2020).

II. Target antigens for CAR-T cells:

A. CAR-T-cell therapy approved to treat B-cell malignancies (leukemia and lymphoma target CD 19); an antigen expressed on all B cells, healthy and malignant, at all stages of maturation (Brudno & Kochenderfer, 2019; Schmit-Pokorny & Eisenberg, 2020)

1. CD 19–directed CAR-T cells used to treat ALL and B-cell lymphomas:

a. Tisagenlecleucel (Kymriah)

b. Axicabtagene ciloleucel (Yescarta)

c. Lisocabtagene maraleucel (Breyanzi)

d. Brexucabtagene autoleucel (Tecartus)

B. CAR-T therapy approved to treat multiple myeloma target B-cell maturation antigen (BCMA), expressed on healthy plasma cells and multiple myeloma cells (Schmit-Pokorny & Eisenberg, 2020).
  1. BCMA-directed CAR-T cells to treat multiple myeloma include:
    a. Idecabtagene vicleucel (Abecma)
    b. Ciltacabtagene autoleucel (Carvykti)

III. Administration regulatory requirements:
  A. The FDA requires individuals who prescribe, dispense, and administer CAR-T-cell therapy to complete the Risk Evaluation and Mitigation Strategy (REMS) program for approved CAR-T-cell therapies.
  B. REMS is a safety program to ensure providers are aware of serious side effects and understand the risks and how to mitigate side effects safely Food and Drug Administration [FDA], 2021.
  C. Staff education and training are required prior to the administration of CAR-T-cell therapy to ensure safe patient care is provided (Anderson & Latchford, 2019).
  D. Patient and caregiver education must include providing a wallet card listing: date of infusion, provider contact information and symptoms of cytokine release syndrome (CRS) and immune effector cell associated neurotoxicity syndrome (ICANS) to monitor and report to the treating provider (Anderson & Latchford, 2019; Schmit-Pokorny & Eisenberg, 2020).

Assessment

I. Patient selection (Maziarz & Slater, 2021)
  A. Performance status and comorbidities
  B. Relapsed/refractory disease without active infection
  C. Sufficient absolute lymphocyte count for collection and manufacturing of cells
  D. Washout period for lymphotoxic therapies

II. Assess for potential CRS.
  A. CRS: An inflammatory response caused by the release of inflammatory cytokines and other immune cells in response to CAR-T-cell therapy (Brudno & Kochenderfer, 2019).
    1. Symptoms include fever, hypotension, hypoxia, tachycardia, and organ dysfunction. Fever is the hallmark sign of CRS.
    2. C-reactive protein and serum ferritin levels:
      a. often elevated
      b. can be used to assist with diagnosis of CRS (Anderson & Latchford, 2019; Schmit-Pokorny & Eisenberg, 2020)

III. Assess for neurotoxicity/ICANS (Brudno & Kochenderfer, 2019).
  1. The pathophysiology of ICANS is not completely understood. Inflammation and CAR-T-cell activity in the central nervous system may play a role.
  2. The three timepoints when ICANS may occur are:
    a. concurrently with CRS
    b. after CRS has resolved
    c. independent of CRS

  3. Signs and symptoms include:
    a. altered level of consciousness/mental status
    b. confusion/agitation
    c. headache
    d. changes in handwriting
    e. tremors
    f. aphasia
    g. seizures
    h. cerebral edema
    i. hemorrhage
  4. Neurotoxicity symptoms are usually transient and resolve (Anderson & Latchford, 2019; Schmit-Pokorny & Eisenberg, 2020).

Management

I. Administration of cells
  A. Patients receive lymphodepleting chemotherapy approximately one week prior to infusion of CAR-T cells.
  B. Fludarabine and cyclophosphamide are the commonly used regimen for lymphodepletion to reduce lymphocytes allowing for the expansion and proliferation of CAR-T cells (Schmit-Pokorny & Eisenberg, 2020).
  C. Premedication includes acetaminophen and diphenhydramine 30–60 minutes prior to cell infusion.
  D. Identification and product verification are required prior to thawing and infusing CAR-T cells.
  E. CAR-T cells are infused IV, without a filter, approximately 2 days following the completion of lymphodepleting chemotherapy (Lamprecht & Dansereau, 2019; Lee & Shah, 2020; Schmit-Pokorny & Eisenberg, 2020).
  F. CAR-T cells proliferate the post infusion, and persistence of CAR-T cells assists with durable remission (Lamprecht & Dansereau, 2019).

II. Manage serious and potentially life-threatening side effects that may occur after CAR-T-cell therapy (Brudno & Kochenderfer, 2019).
  A. The onset of side effects varies, and nurses play a key role in the assessment, identification, and management of side effects.
  B. Treatment is based on the grade and severity of side effects (Anderson & Latchford, 2019; Schmit-Pokorny & Eisenberg, 2020).
  C. Manage CRS
    1. Supportive care including antipyretics, oxygen therapy, and hydration/vasopressors to mitigate symptoms
    2. Tocilizumab (Actemra), a humanized monoclonal antibody approved to treat CRS (Anderson & Latchford, 2019; Lee & Shah, 2020; Schmit-Pokorny & Eisenberg, 2020)
  D. Manage neurotoxicity/ICANS
    1. Imaging to rule out other causes of neuro symptoms is recommended.
    2. In the absence of CRS, neurotoxicity is treated with antiepileptics and corticosteroids.
    3. Patients are prohibited from driving or operating heavy machinery for 8 weeks.

E. Manage prolonged cytopenia ("on-target, off-tumor").

1. Prolonged cytopenia increases the risk of infection while CAR-T cells persist and eliminate targeted cells.

2. Cytopenia after lymphodepleting chemotherapy increases the risk for infection.

3. Full workup to rule out an infectious etiology for fever should be completed, including initiation of antimicrobial therapy.

4. CRS and sepsis present with similar signs and symptoms; both must be considered with CAR-T-cell therapy.

5. Antiviral and antifungal prophylaxis is recommended along with broad-spectrum antibiotic coverage.

F. Manage hypogammaglobulinemia.

1. B-cell aplasia occurs due to the expression of CD 19 on healthy B cells.

2. Immunoglobulin levels should be monitored post CAR-T-cell therapy and replaced as indicated by treatment center protocol (Hill & Seo, 2020).

G. Manage infections.

1. Monoclonal antibody and/or corticosteroid use for the treatment of CRS also increases the risk of infection.

2. Treat with appropriate antibiotics.

H. Manage tumor lysis syndrome (TLS).

1. Preventative measures should include IV hydration and allopurinol prophylaxis.

2. Monitoring electrolytes, uric acid, and renal function is essential to identify TLS and intervene promptly (Anderson & Latchford, 2019).

REFERENCES

Anderson, K., & Latchford, T. (2019). Associated toxicities: Assessment and management related to CAR T-Cell therapy. Clinical Journal of Oncology Nursing, 23(2), 13–19. https://doi.org/10.1188/19.CJON.S1.13-19.

Bride, K. L., Levy, E., Wohlschlaeger, A., & Freedman, J. L. (2018). Infectious complications and HSCT. In V. Brown (Ed.), Hematopoietic stem cell transplantation for the pediatric hematologist/oncologist (pp. 241–255). Cham: Springer. https://doi.org/10.1007/978-3-319-63146-2_17.

Brown, V. (Ed.). (2018). Hematopoietic stem cell transplantation for the pediatric hematologist/oncologist. Cham: Springer.

Brudno, J. N., & Kochenderfer, J. N. (2019). Recent advances in CAR T-cell toxicity: Mechanisms, manifestations and management. Blood Reviews, 34, 45–55. https://doi.org/10.1016/j.blre.2018.11.002.

Centers for Disease Control. (2000). Guidelines for Preventing Opportunistic Infections Among Hematopoietic Stem Cell Transplant Recipients. https://www.cdc.gov/mmwr/preview/mmwrhtml/rr4910a1.htm

Corbacioglu, S., Jabbour, E. J., & Mohty, M. (2019). Risk factors for development of and progression of hepatic veno-occlusive disease/sinusoidal obstruction syndrome. Biology of Blood and Marrow Transplantation: Journal of the American Society for Blood and Marrow Transplantation, 25(7), 1271–1280. https://doi.org/10.1016/j.bbmt.2019.02.018.

Dandekar, S. (2018). Life after HSCT: Survivorship and long-term issues. In V. Brown (Ed.), Hematopoietic stem cell transplantation for the pediatric hematologist/oncologist (pp. 385–4012). Cham: Springer.

Dehn, J., Spellman, S., Hurley, C. K., Shaw, B. E., Barker, J. N., Burns, L. J., et al. (2019). Selection of unrelated donors and cord blood units for hematopoietic cell transplantation: Guidelines from the NMDP/CIBMTR. Blood, 134(12), 924–934. https://doi.org/10.1182/blood.2019001212.

de Silva, N. L., & Seneviratne, S. L. (2019). Haemopoietic stem cell transplantation in systemic lupus erythematosus: A systematic review. Allergy, Asthma & Clinical Immunology, 15(59), 1–12. https://doi.org/10.1186/s13223-019-0373-y.

Duque-Afonso, J., Ihorst, G., Waterhouse, M., Zeiser, R., Wäsch, R., Bertz, H., et al. (2021). Comparison of reduced-toxicity conditioning protocols using fludarabine, melphalan combined with thiotepa or carmustine in allogeneic hematopoietic cell transplantation. Bone Marrow Transplantation, 56(1), 110–120. https://doi.org/10.1038/s41409-020-0986-2.

Estey, E. H. (2020). Acute myeloid leukemia: 2021 update on risk-stratification and management. American Journal of Hematology, 95(11), 1368–1398.

Food and Drug Administration (FDA). (2021). FDA Updates REMS for CAR T-Cell Therapies. https://www.formularywatch.com/view/fda-updates-rems-for-car-t-cell-therapies.

Forman, S., Negrin, R. S., Antin, J. H., & Appelbaum, F. (Eds.). (2016). Thomas' hematopoietic cell transplantation (5th ed.). Malden, MA: Wiley-Blackwell.

Hill, J. A., & Seo, S. K. (2020). How I prevent infections in patients receiving CD19-targeted chimeric antigen receptor T cells for B-cell malignancies. Blood, 136(8), 925–935. https://doi.org/10.1182/blood.2019004000.

Kapadia, M., & Greiner, R. (2018). How to select a donor and hematopoietic stem cell source: Related versus unrelated donors for allogeneic HSCT. In V. Brown (Ed.), Hematopoietic stem cell transplantation for the pediatric hematologist/oncologist (pp. 97–110). Cham: Springer.

Kapadia, M., & Wikle Shapiro, T. (2018). Pulmonary complications associated with HSCT. In V. Brown (Ed.), Hematopoietic stem cell transplantation for the pediatric hematologist/oncologist (pp. 301–325). Cham: Springer.

Kitko, C.-L., Gatwood, K., & Connelly, J. (2018). Preparing the patient for HSCT: Conditioning regimens and their scientific rationale. In V. Brown (Ed.), Hematopoietic stem cell transplantation for the pediatric hematologist/oncologist (pp. 139–174). Cham: Springer.

Krishnamurti, L. (2021). Hematopoietic cell transplantation for sickle cell disease: Updates and future directions. Hematology. American Society of Hematology. Education Program, 2021(1), 181–189. https://doi.org/10.1182/hematology.2021000251.

Ladha, A., Mannis, G., & Muffly, L. (2021). Hepatic veno-occlusive disease in allogeneic stem cell transplant recipients with prior exposure to gemtuzumab ozogamicin or inotuzumab ozogamicin. Leukemia & Lymphoma, 62(2), 257–263. https://doi.org/10.1080/10428194.2020.1827247.

Lamprecht, M., & Dansereau, C. (2019). CAR T-Cell therapy: Update on the state of the science. Clinical Journal of Oncology Nursing, 23(2), 6–12. https://doi.org/10.1188/19.CJON.S1.6-12.

Lee, D. W., & Shah, N. N. (2020). Chimeric antigen receptor T-cell therapies for cancer: A practical guide. Amsterdam; Cambridge, MA: Elsevier.

Maziarz, R. T., & Slater, S. S. (2021). Blood and marrow transplant handbook: Comprehensive guide for patient care. Cham: Springer.

Mellgren, K., Nierop, A. F. M., & Abrahamsson, J. (2019). Use of multivariate immune reconstitution patterns to describe immune reconstitution after allogeneic stem cell transplantation in children. *Biology of Blood and Marrow Transplantation: Journal of the American Society for Blood and Marrow Transplantation*, 25(10), 2045–2053. https://doi.org/10.1016/j.bbmt.2019.06.018.

National Marrow Donor Program (NMDP). *(2018). Be the match.* https://bethematch.org. Accessed 26.02.19.

Neofytos, D. (2019). Antimicrobial prophylaxis and preemptive approaches for the prevention of infections in the stem cell transplant recipient, with analogies to the hematologic malignancy patient. *Infectious Disease Clinics of North America*, 33(2), 361–380. https://doi.org/10.1016/j.idc.2019.02.002.

Pereira, M. R., Pouch, S. M., & Scully, B. (2019). Infections in allogeneic stem cell transplantation. In A. Safdar (Ed.), *Principles and practice of transplant infectious diseases*. New York: Springer. Available at https://doi.org/10.1007/978-1-4939-9034-4_11.

Ramachandran, V., Kolli, S. S., & Strowd, L. C. (2019). Review of graft-versus-host disease. *Dermatologic Clinics*, 37(4), 569–582. https://doi.org/10.1016/j.det.2019.05.014.

Rautenberg, C., Germing, U., Haas, R., Kobbe, G., & Schroeder, T. (2019). Relapse of acute myeloid leukemia after allogeneic stem cell transplantation: Prevention, detection, and treatment. *International Journal of Molecular Sciences*, 20(1), 228. https://doi.org/10.3390/ijms20010228.

Schmit-Pokorny, K., & Eisenberg, S. (Eds.). (2020). *Hematopoietic stem cell transplantation: A manual for nursing practice* (3rd ed.). Pittsburgh, PA: Oncology Nursing Society.

Talekar, M. K., & Olson, T. (2018). Immune reconstitution after hematopoietic stem cell transplantation. In V. Brown (Ed.), *Hematopoietic stem cell transplantation for the pediatric hematologist/oncologist* (pp. 371-383). Cham: Springer. https://doi.org/10.1007/978-3-319-63146-2_26.

Toenges, R., Greinix, H., Lawitschka, A., Halter, J., Baumgartner, A., Simon, A., et al. (2021). Current practice in nutrition after allogeneic hematopoietic stem cell transplantation – Results from a survey among hematopoietic stem cell transplant centers. *Clinical Nutrition (Edinburgh, Scotland)*, 40(4), 1571–1577. https://doi.org/10.1016/j.clnu.2021.02.030.

Webster, J. A., Luznik, L., & Gojo, I. (2021). Treatment of AML relapse after Allo-HCT. *Frontiers in Oncology*, 11, 812207. https://doi.org/10.3389/fonc.2021.812207.

Wikle Shapiro, T. (2023). Hematopoietic stem cell transplantation. In S. Newton, M. Hickey, & J. M. Brant (Eds.), *Mosby's oncology nursing advisor: A comprehensive guide to clinical practice* (pp. 179–205). St. Louis, MO: Elsevier.

Zuanelli Brambilla, C., Lobaugh, S. M., Ruiz, J. D., Dahi, P. B., Goldberg, A. D., Young, J. W., et al. (2021). Relapse after allogeneic stem cell transplantation of acute myelogenous leukemia and myelodysplastic syndrome and the importance of second cellular therapy. *Transplantation and Cellular Therapy*, 27(9), 771.e1–771.e10. https://doi.org/10.1016/j.jtct.2021.05.011.

28

Radiation Therapy

Lorraine Drapek

OVERVIEW

I. Background
   A. One of the oldest cancer treatments, at over 100 years old (Gianfaldoni et al., 2017)
   B. Radiation therapy is the use of high energy-rays or other radiation particles to treat malignant and some benign conditions (Gibbons, 2020; Perevalova, 2021).
   C. Types of ionizing radiation used in treatment
      1. External beam radiation: of electromagnetic radiation from a machine such as a linear accelerator and includes photons or x-rays. External beam radiation also includes particulate radiation such as protons: positively charged particles; neutrons: large uncharged particles; and electrons: small negatively charged particles, which can be delivered by a cyclotron or linear accelerator.
      2. Gamma rays: photons emitted from a radioactive source such as cobalt-60, cesium-137, and iridium-192 (Gibbons, 2020). These are often used in brachytherapy with the placement of a radioactive source directly into or adjacent to tumors (Perevalova, 2021).
   D. The Radiation Oncology Team
      1. The radiation oncology nurse is a registered nurse who functions interdependently within a radiation oncology team to support patients undergoing radiation therapy (Altman, Butler, & Shern, 2016; Thomas, 2021).
      2. Radiation oncology nurses span the continuum of care from screening and cancer risk reduction and includes diagnosis, treatment, survivorship, palliative care, and end of life (Thomas, 2021). Advanced Practice Nurses team with Radiation Oncologists as patient providers within radiation therapy, across the continuum of care, from screening and cancer risk reduction, through diagnosis, treatment, survivorship, palliative care, and end of life (Thomas, 2021).
      3. Radiation therapists have a college degree, certification, and license to administer the radiation for patients, following the plan of care under the supervision of radiation oncologists (Radiological Society of North America, 2022).
      4. Therapeutic Medical Physicists are medical physicists who work directly with radiation oncologists in treatment planning and delivery (Radiological Society of North America, 2022).
      5. Dosimetrists use treatment planning software to assist radiation oncologists to develop a plan of care that includes contouring normal tissues and organs at risk (OAR).
      6. Radiation oncologists are licensed physicians who are certified by the American Board of Radiology to oversee the cancer treatment of patients receiving radiation therapy (Radiological Society of North America, 2022).
      7. Social workers help coordinate patient care and provide supportive services during radiation treatment.
      8. Mold and cast technicians create custom devices or blocks for patient immobilization to maintain consistent, safe positioning.

II. Radiation therapy purpose
   A. Purpose of radiation: Used to treat local or regional disease; rarely used to treat systemic disease. The goal of radiation therapy is to destroy malignant cells within the treatment area while minimizing damage to healthy tissue (Perevalova, 2021).
      1. Definitive treatment: Primary treatment of the cancer with or without chemotherapy. Examples: head and neck cancer, anal cancer, prostate, lung, bladder, as well as Hodgkin lymphoma.
      2. Neoadjuvant treatment: Radiation is given prior to definitive treatment—usually surgery. The goal is to improve the chances of successful resection. Examples are colorectal or esophageal cancers.
      3. Adjuvant treatment: Radiation therapy is given following definitive treatment which includes surgery, chemotherapy, or immunotherapy. The goal is to improve local control. Examples include breast or lung cancers.
      4. Prophylactic treatment: Radiation therapy is delivered to high-risk, asymptomatic areas to prevent cancer growth. Examples are prophylactic cranial radiation in some lung cancers.
      5. Benign conditions: Radiation therapy can also be given prophylactically to treat keloids or other nonmalignant conditions.
      6. Palliation: Used for symptom management. Examples include pain, bleeding, neurologic complications, or

life-threatening problems in patients with incurable disease (Perevalova, 2021).

III. Modern radiation techniques
   A. Hypo fractionization: shorter courses of treatment.
   B. Hyper fractionization: multiple daily fractions (usually two/day).
   C. VMAT (volumetric modulated arc therapy): treatment can be focused on the tumor, while protecting normal tissue in a faster period.
   D. Image-guided radiation therapy (IGRT) is the use of image guidance to localize the target both before and during treatment.
   E. Combined treatment of immunotherapy with radiation therapy.
   F. More clinical trials that include combined therapy modalities.
   G. Stereotactic body radiation therapy (SBRT) is a highly effective local therapy that requires accurate targeting, immobilization, and tumor motion management to deliver a large dose of radiation therapy in fewer fractions (Perevalova, 2021).

IV. Five Rs of radiobiology—the rationale for fractionization of radiation (Choi, Yu, Blakely, & Murnane, 2018)
   A. *Repair:* Refers to DNA repair lethal radiation damage. Treatment fractionization allows for repair of normal tissue.
   B. *Reassortment:* Following a fraction of radiation, there is redistribution of cells into a radiosensitive phase of the cell cycle.
   C. *Repopulation:* During radiation, tumor cell proliferation can occur. During the prolonged duration of radiation therapy treatment, this can be problematic.
   D. *Reoxygenation:* Tumors consist of both oxygenated and hypoxic cells. Oxygenation of hypoxic cells following a radiation treatment refers to the process of reoxygenation. Oxygenation of hypoxic cells increases the sensitivity of tumor cells to radiation therapy.
   E. *Radiosensitivity:* Refers to the differences in cell metabolism, maturity, and microenvironment of cells. This explains the differences in sensitivities of different tissues (Choi et al., 2018).

V. Treatment planning and delivery
   A. Consultation and radiation treatment consent process
   B. Comprehensive treatment planning
      1. Simulation—CT scanner used to plan radiation—including patient positioning and immobilization.
      2. Data acquisition: data from diagnostic CT scans, MRI, or PET to assist with radiation planning.
      3. Digital treatment planning system using patient data from CT simulation and data acquisition.
      4. Treatment design.
      5. Plan implementation.
      6. Evaluation and review of the plan and finding optimal dosing to tumor with sparing healthy tissue.
      7. Quality assurance process.
      8. Verification simulation: reviews actual patient treatment, including radiation beam arrangements, and

can address any issues and changes for patient setup during treatment (Perevalova, 2021).
   C. Radiation therapy treatment prescriptions
      1. A method of prescription documentation based on three separate boundaries as defined by the International Commission on Radiation Units and Measurements:
         a. Visible tumor
         b. Areas of predicted microscopic tumor spread
         c. Area to account for uncertainties of positioning
      2. Prescription terminology
         a. Gross target volume (GTV) outlines the gross tumor based on imaging studies.
         b. Clinical target volume (CTV) contains the GTV and any microscopic clinical disease.
         c. Internal target volume considers variations in size, position, or shape of the CTV within the patient, such as breathing.
         d. Planning target volume is a margin that is added to the CTV to allow for any physiologic variations such as patient position or beam position.
         e. OAR are healthy radiosensitive organs that can influence treatment planning or dose prescription if located close to or within the treatment field, such as the spinal cord (Jones, 1994; Khan, Gibbons, & Sperduto, 2016; Perevalova, 2021).
   D. Radiation dose
      1. Medical dosimetry includes the calculation of absorbed radiation dose and treatment optimization in radiation dose delivery (radiation-dosimetry.org).
      2. Dosimetry takes tissue composition into consideration along with any target variations.
      3. Measurement
         a. Gray (Gy) is the unit of absorbed energy per unit mass, based on the International System.
         b. Centigray (cGy) is often used, as this is equivalent to the former terminology of radiation absorbed dose (previously known as rad).
         c. 1 Gy is equal to 100 cGy or 100 rad (Gibbons, 2020; Perevalova, 2021).
      4. Radiation treatment dosing is dependent on the following:
         a. Size of the field on the skin surface
         b. Depth below the point of beam entry
         c. Tissue density
         d. Distance from the source of radiation to the skin
         e. Energy and penetration of the radiation beam
   E. Treatment delivery
      1. Three-dimensional conformal radiation therapy (3DCRT) conforms the distribution of radiation dose as closely as possible to the volume of the target, with minimizing dose to healthy tissue surrounding the target.
         a. 3DCRT is delivered with photon and electron beams and involves the use of multileaf collimators or blocks to shape the treatment field. This

helps to achieve uniform dosing at the prescribed treatment depth (Cashell, 2021).

2. Intensity-modulated radiation therapy (IMRT) is an updated, complex form of 3DCRT that uses beamlets or beams of various intensities.
   a. Radiation ray intensity within each beam can be altered to allow for the radiation dose to conform to irregularly shaped targets (Behrend, 2018).
   b. VMAT is a newer advanced form of IMRT that changes the intensity and shape of the radiation beams (Cashell, 2021).

3. IGRT uses imaging to assess and modify problems that arise from treatment variations in patient setup as well as anatomy.
   a. IGRT allows for two- to three-dimensional imaging to correlate the radiation treatment plan with the position of the tumor, which enables accurate radiation dose delivery (Perevalova, 2021).
   b. Examples of IGRT: Cone beam CT, fiducial markers, and linear accelerators that incorporate imaging to verify treatment plans, make corrections, and synchronize and target treatment with patient movement (Cashell, 2021).

4. Stereotactic radiosurgery is a single fraction of radiation used primarily to treat brain lesions using multiple beams (Perevalova, 2021).

5. SBRT can be used to treat a variety of tumors such as spine, liver, pancreas, lung, prostate, and kidney.
   a. Immobilization must be precise to enable accurate treatment of the target, as well as management of tumor motion. Breath-hold techniques are also used to track tumor motion.
   b. Requires fewer fractions (Perevalova, 2021).

6. Brachytherapy is a radiation therapy approach where a radioactive source is either placed within a cavity (cervical, endometrial cancer) or very near the area of the tumor (interstitial—head and neck, ocular) (DeBaun, 2021; Skowronek, 2017).
   a. Can be part of a treatment course along with external beam radiation therapy (e.g., gynecologic cancers).
   b. Advantage is providing a high dose of radiation directly to the tumor target while sparing surrounding healthy tissue.
   c. Radionuclides are used in brachytherapy procedures. These can consist of Cesium-137, Iridium-192, Gold-198, Radium-226, and Tantalum-182.
   d. Because of their complexity, brachytherapy requires a radiation safety officer along with the radiation treatment team to implement a very individualized treatment plan (Debaun, 2021; Orio, 2019).

F. Radiation therapy treatment machines (Table 28.1)
   1. Megavoltage machines deliver external beam radiation therapy.

TABLE 28.1	External Beam Radiation	
Treatment	**Type**	**Delivery**
Photons	X-rays	Linear accelerator
Protons	Positive charged particles	Cyclotron or linear accelerator
Neutrons	Uncharged particles	Cyclotron or linear accelerator
Electrons	Small negatively charged particles	Cyclotron or linear accelerator

   a. Megavolts (MV) is the unit of energy for therapeutic x-rays.
   b. Megaelectron volts (MeV) is expressed as the energy of therapeutic electrons.
   c. Linear accelerators are megavoltage machines that produce x-rays and electrons with various energy ranges that can range from 4 to 25 MeV and treat various treatment depths.
   d. High-energy electrons are used to treat more superficial tumors.
   e. X-rays are used to treat intermediate to deep-depth tumors and give low-to-moderate doses to the skin (Gibbons, 2020; Perevalova, 2021).

   2. Cyclotrons are large machines that produce protons or neutrons.
      a. High doses can be delivered to tumors while limiting the dose to healthy tissue, achieved by a rapid fall of the dose deposited beyond the target. There is no exit dose with protons.
      b. The rapid decrease in the energy of protons as they travel through tissue is called the Bragg peak (Cashell, 2021).

   3. Cyberknife consists of a robotic arm with a linear accelerator that delivers multiple-beam treatment. It provides continual image guidance to track target motion (Alexander et al., 2019; Cashell, 2021).

G. Radiation safety
   1. The guiding principle of radiation safety is "ALARA." ALARA stands for "as low as reasonably achievable." Therefore, the goal is to keep radiation exposure as low as possible in health care professionals as well as the public and to prevent detrimental health problems that can occur when there is exposure to ionizing radiation (Pierce, 2021).
      a. A radiation safety officer is responsible for monitoring and reporting radiation exposure (Domenech, 2017; Pierce, 2021).

   2. The principles of radiation safety include time, distance, and shielding (Table 28.2).
      a. The amount of radiation exposure is directly related to the time spent near a radioactive source.
      b. The amount of radiation exposure is inversely related to the distance from the radioactive source.

TABLE 28.2	**Radiation Safety Principles**	
Time	**Distance**	**Shielding**
Decrease the time of exposure to penetrating ionizing radiation.	Increase the distance from the radiation source to decrease the amount of radiation exposure.	Shielding absorbs radiation exposure. The correct shielding needs to be selected to stop the type of radiation being used.

From https://www.epa.gov/radtown.

   c. The amount of radiation exposure can be decreased using shielding material that is placed between the person receiving the exposure and the radioactive source (Domenech, 2017; Pierce, 2021).

3. Radiation treatment machines are inside vaults that are sealed with concrete, lead, cast iron, or steel to prevent radiation exposure outside the treatment room.

4. There are alarms and safety measures in place so that the machine cannot operate if the treatment room is not secure.

5. There is electronic signage and lighting indicating when a treatment machine is in operation.

6. Personal monitoring devices measure the amount of radiation exposure received by staff (Garcia-Sanchez, Garcia Angosto, Moreno Riquelme, Serna Berna, & Ramos-Amores, 2018; Pierce, 2021).

7. Radiation protection warning signs to recognize radiation-restricted areas are mandated by federal and state governments and should be posted in areas where there is a risk of potential radiation exposure (Pierce, 2021).

8. Nursing implications:
   a. Gather specific information needed to avoid radiation exposure and alleviate possible fears and misconceptions (Fencl, 2015; Jones, 2016; Pierce, 2021).
   b. Focus on the balance of meeting the needs of patients receiving radionuclides while maintaining time, distance, and shielding (Behrend, 2018).

ASSESSMENT

I. Pretreatment
  A. Assess the health literacy and understanding of radiation therapy and provide individualized patient education (Papadakos et al., 2018; Sandstrom, 2021).
  B. Assess gaps in knowledge or attitudes (Sandstrom, 2021).
  C. Assess risk factors for side effects.
    1. Patient risk factors: comorbidities, performance status, concurrent treatment with chemotherapy or immunotherapy, nutrition status, and skin integrity
    2. Treatment-related effects: site of treatment, size of treatment field, dose and number of treatments, type of treatment, and radiosensitivity

II. During and following treatment—General radiation treatment effects
  A. Radiation skin changes (radiation dermatitis) (see Chapter 41)
    1. Radiation dermatitis is common in patients receiving radiation, with up to 95% of patients experiencing skin changes (Backler, Bruce, Suarez, & Ginex, 2020).
    2. Radiation skin changes can vary from very little change, or mild skin dryness, to blisters, peeling, and moist desquamation that can impact the quality of life. Modern techniques such as IMRT are often skin sparing and have decreased the severity of radiation dermatitis.
    3. Skin changes are dose dependent and usually occur within 90 days of radiation treatment exposure (Benc, 2021; Bray, Simmons, Wolfson, & Nouri, 2016).
    4. Skin changes can affect all layers of the skin (epidermis and dermis) (Benc, 2021).
    5. Treatment risk factors for increased skin reaction:
     a. Type of energy (photons, electrons, protons)
     b. Type of treatment field (tangential—higher doses within thinner areas)
     c. Skin bolus (gel-like sheets placed over skin to increase the skin dose)
     d. Size of the treatment field
     e. Radiation dose
     f. Use of a concurrent radiosensitizer
     g. Previous radiation exposure to the treatment field (Benc, 2021; Chao, Perez, & Wang, 2018)
    6. Nontreatment-related risk factors
     a. General skin condition
     b. Moist areas of the body within the treatment field (inframammary, groin, and perineum)
     c. Skin folds or bony prominences
     d. Age, hydration status, and nutrition status
     e. Prior exposure to chemotherapy or immunotherapy (radiation recall)
     f. Comorbidities that delay wound healing (diabetes, smoking) (Benc, 2021; Chao et al., 2018)
    7. Acute skin reactions typically occur at different dosages:
     a. Erythema usually occurs 2–4 weeks into treatment
     b. Dry desquamation usually occurs after 3 weeks into treatment
     c. Moist desquamation can occur at about 4 weeks of treatment
     d. These acute skin changes can overall occur within 90 days of radiation exposure (Benc, 2021; Bray et al., 2016)
    8. Healing
     a. Typically starts 1–2 weeks following the completion of treatment.
     b. Changes in the healing process can result in post-radiation fibrosis, which is considered a late effect of treatment (Borrelli, 2019).

B. Fatigue in patients receiving radiation can include cognitive, emotional, psychosocial, and somatic factors (Baumgartner, 2021; O'Higgins, Brady, O'Connor, Walsh, & Reilly, 2018).

1. Estimates of fatigue in patients receiving radiation therapy are 80% (Baumgartner, 2021; NCCN, 2020).

2. Risk factors for fatigue include anemia, nutritional deficits or disturbances, emotional distress, sleep disorders, cancer therapies (received prior to radiation therapy), comorbidities, and site of radiation therapy (Baumgartner, 2021; Mahtani, 2017; O'Higgins et al., 2018).

3. Fatigue can begin within 2–3 weeks after the start of radiation treatment and can worsen throughout the course of treatment and completion. Fatigue can continue for 1–4 months post treatment, depending on other comorbid factors.

4. Assess fatigue regularly during and following treatment.

C. Assess for other radiation therapy-associated effects based on the radiation treatment field, patient comorbidities, and risk factors.

MANAGEMENT

I. Provide a holistic approach to assisting patients through the radiation treatment process.

A. Fully inform patients about treatment, including risks, benefits, and alternatives so that shared decision-making can occur (Bonin et al., 2018; Sandstrom, 2021).

B. Ongoing assessment is imperative as patients need information according to what they are experiencing over the course of cancer care (Sandstrom, 2021).

C. Include caregivers in the patient education process.

D. Patient and caregiver education begins at the radiation treatment planning process; provide information about treatment processes, potential side effects, and managing toxicities.

E. Consider inviting patients and caregivers to view a radiation treatment room prior to the initiation of treatment (Behrend, 2018).

F. Provide reassurance that safety measures are in place and followed (Cashel, 2021; Obinata, Yamada, & Sasai, 2019).

G. Manage radiation-related toxicities.

1. Provide skin care interventions based on evidence-based practice.
Current evidence-based practice includes:

a. Hygiene—washing the treatment area daily with mild, fragrance-free soap and gently drying, avoiding friction. No further therapy is recommended in patients without radiation dermatitis (Backler et al., 2020; Benc, 2021).

b. Deodorant/antiperspirant may be used in the truncal area during radiation (Backler et al., 2020).

c. Topical steroids to intact skin may be used to minimize the effects, as well as symptomatic

TABLE 28.3 Grading of Radiation Dermatitis According to the Common Terminology Criteria for Adverse Events—Version 5

Grade	Characteristics
Grade 1	Faint erythema or dry desquamation
Grade 2	Moderate to brisk erythema, patchy moist desquamation, confined to skin folds and creases, and moderate edema
Grade 3	Moist desquamation in areas other than skin folds and creases; bleeding induced by minor trauma or abrasion
Grade 4	Life-threatening consequences; skin necrosis or ulceration of the full thickness dermis; spontaneous bleeding from the affected site; skin graft is indicated
Grade 5	Death

Adapted from U.S. Department of Health and Human Services. (2017). Common terminology criteria for adverse events (CTCAE) version 5.0. *Cancer Therapy Evaluation Program (CTEP)*. https://ctep.cancer.gov/protocolDevelopment/electronic_applications/ctc.htm Retrieved 29.08.22.

relief of radiation dermatitis (Backler et al., 2020; Benc, 2021).

d. Semipermeable dressings may minimize the development of radiation dermatitis (Backler et al., 2020; Benc, 2021).

e. There are many creams and lotions that can be recommended.

f. See Table 28.3 for grading of radiation dermatitis.

g. Posttreatment interventions for radiation dermatitis include keeping the skin supple by using moisturizing lotions, protection from sunlight as skin is more sensitive following radiation and has an increased risk of skin cancer (Benc, 2021; Bolderston et al., 2018).

h. Late effects of radiation can include telangiectasia, fibrosis, and necrosis. These can occur following recovery due to physiologic changes in the treated tissue during the wound-healing process (Benc, 2021).

2. Provide site-specific interventions for radiation-induced toxicities (Table 28.4).

3. Reevaluate toxicities on an ongoing basis. Measure the severity of side effects based on a grading system such as Freites-Martinez, Santana, Arias-Santiago, & Viera, (2017) or RTOG (Cox, Stetz, & Pajak, 1995).

H. Discharge teaching regarding self-care measures, all possible side effects and symptoms, and contact information for questions or concerns.

II. Specific procedures: Provide additional patient education for specific procedures (Bastable & Kitchie, 2020).

A. IGRT-specific information should be completed and include the following:

1. Purpose of IGRT

2. Time involved to complete IGRT

3. Specific equipment being used

4. Involvement of medical physicist and dosimetrist (Behrend, 2018)

TABLE 28.4 Common Site-Specific Radiation Toxicities and General Interventions

Toxicity	Symptoms	Late Effects	Intervention
Cerebral edema (cranial radiation)	Headache, seizure, nausea, vomiting, change in mental status, tingling/weakness of extremities, changes in speech	Irreversible neurologic deficits Brain radionecrosis	Steroid therapy. Dexamethasone is often used. Dose adjustment is often necessary as symptoms improve (Allen & Allen, 2021). Neurological assessment. Assess for oral thrush.
Mucositis (head and neck radiation)	Xerostomia, dry mouth, thick secretions, hearing changes	Xerostomia, dry mouth, possible permanent loss of taste, dental cavities, soft tissue or bone changes in the jaw, hypothyroidism	Dental evaluation prior to radiation therapy. Early nutrition referral and speech/swallowing therapy, topical and systemic pain management (Cecil, 2021).
Anorexia	Decreased appetite, early satiety	Malnutrition, decrease in quality of life	Nutrition referral, high protein diet, small frequent meals, pharmacologic interventions can be considered.
Radiation-induced nausea and vomiting	Nausea—subjective symptom that can be accompanied by vomiting—a neurophysiologic reaction (Cerillo, 2021)	May require hospitalization, nonoral forms of nutrition	Pharmacologic management including antiemetic prophylaxis, with serotonin receptor antagonists (ondansetron), Corticosteroids (dexamethasone), Dopamine receptor antagonists (prochlorperazine) (Cerillo, 2021).
Diarrhea	Radiation-induced diarrhea occurring within 6 weeks of radiation and resolving within 2–6 months (Cerillo, 2021)	Chronic ulcers, bleeding, intestinal stenosis, intestinal fistula (Cerillo, 2021)	Dietary modification: options are lactose free, low fat, low fiber. Small frequent meals, foods high in soluble fiber. Pharmacologic management can include loperamide, diphenoxylate and atropine, octreotide, and probiotics (Cerillo, 2021).
Sexual dysfunction	Loss of sexual desire Lack of sexual enjoyment Orgasmic dysfunction Premature ovarian insufficiency Decreased testicular function (Bruner, 2021)	Vaginal dryness Vaginal stenosis Erectile dysfunction	Sexual health counseling, vaginal lubricants and moisturizers, vaginal dilators. Pelvic floor physical therapy. Penile implants, injectable medications, vacuum devices, PDE5 inhibitors (Bruner, 2021; Carter, Lacchetti, & Rowland, 2018).

B. Brachytherapy
1. Pretreatment assessment and evaluation of patient
2. Coordination of nursing care before, during, and following brachytherapy
3. Patient education regarding the brachytherapy procedure
4. Administer premedication as ordered
5. Assist with brachytherapy procedure as needed
6. Assess patient post treatment and provide discharge instructions

REFERENCES

Alexander, R., Schwartz, C., Ladisich, B., Hitzl, W., Heidorn, S.-C., Winkler, P. A., et al. (2019). Cyberknife radiosurgery in recurrent brain metastases: Do the benefits outweigh the risks? *Cureus.* https://doi.org/10.7759/cureus.c18.

Allen, K., & Allen, D. H. (2021). Brain and central nervous system. In M. McQuestion, L. C. Drapek, & M. E. Witt (Eds.), *Manual for radiation oncology nursing practice and education* (pp. 159–180). Pittsburgh, PA: Oncology Nursing Society.

Altman, S. H., Butler, A. S., & Shern, L. (2016). *Assessing progress on the Institute of Medicine Report the Future of Nursing.* Washington, D.C.: The National Academies Press. https://doi.org/10.17226/21838.

Backler, C., Bruce, S., Suarez, L., & Ginex, P. (2020). Radiodermatitis: Clinical summary of the ONS guidelines™ for cancer treatment-related radiodermatitis. *Clinical Journal of Oncology Nursing, 24*(6), 681–684. https://doi.org/10.1188/20.cjon.681-684.

Bastable, S., & Kitchie, S. (2020). Determinants of learning: *Nurse as educator: Principles of teaching and learning for nursing practice* (pp. 119–162). Burlington, MA: Jones & Bartlett Learning. Essay.

Baumgartner, S. (2021). Fatigue. In M. McQuestion, L. C. Drapek, & M. E. Witt (Eds.), *Manual for radiation oncology nursing practice and education* (pp. 37–45). Pittsburgh, PA: Oncology Nursing Society.

Behrend, Susan, W. (2018). Radiation treatment planning. In C. H. Yarbro, D. Wujcik, & B. H. Gobel (Eds.), *Cancer nursing: Principles and practice* (pp. 286–328). Burlington, MA: Jones & Bartlett Learning.

Benc, R. (2021). Skin reactions. In M. McQuestion, L. C. Drapek, & M. E. Witt (Eds.), *Manual for radiation oncology nursing practice and education* (pp. 45–58). Pittsburgh, PA: Oncology Nursing Society.

Bolderston, A., Cashell, A., McQuestion, M., Cardoso, M., Summers, C., & Harris, R. (2018). A Canadian survey of the management of radiation-induced skin reactions. *Journal of Medical Imaging and Radiation Sciences, 49*(2), 164–172. https://doi.org/10.1016/j.jmir.2018.01.003.

Bonin, K., McGuffin, M., Lechtman, E., Cumal, A., Harth, T., Calabrese, E., et al. (2018). Evaluation of an online education resource on radiation therapy created for patients with postprostatectomy prostate cancer and their caregivers. *Journal of Medical Imaging and Radiation Sciences, 49*(4), 365–370. https://doi.org/10.1016/j.jmir.2018.07.007.

Borrelli, M. R., Shen, A. H., Lee, G. K., Momeni, A., Longaker, M. T., & Wan, D. C. (2019). Radiation-Induced Skin Fibrosis: Pathogenesis, Current Treatment Options, and Emerging Therapeutics. Annals of plastic surgery, 83(4S Suppl 1), S59–S64. https://doi.org/10.1097/SAP.0000000000002098.

Bray, F. N., Simmons, B. J., Wolfson, A. H., & Nouri, K. (2016). Acute and chronic cutaneous reactions to ionizing radiation therapy. *Dermatology and Therapy*, 6(2), 185–206. https://doi.org/10.1007/s13555-016-0120-y.

Bruner, D. (2021). Sexual function and dysfunction. In M. McQuestion, L. C. Drapek, & M. E. Witt (Eds.), *Manual for radiation oncology nursing practice and education* (pp. 68–80). Pittsburgh, PA: Oncology Nursing Society.

Carter, J., Lacchetti, C., & Rowland, J. H. (2018). Interventions to address sexual problems in people with cancer: American Society of Clinical Oncology clinical practice guideline adaptation summary. *Journal of Oncology Practice*, 14(3), 173–179. https://doi.org/10.1200/jop.2017.028134.

Cashell, A. (2021). External beam radiation therapy. In M. McQuestion, L. C. Drapek, & M. E. Witt (Eds.), *Manual for radiation oncology nursing practice and education* (pp. 299–304). Pittsburgh, PA: Oncology Nursing Society.

Cecil, E. (2021). Head and neck cancer. In M. McQuestion, L. C. Drapek, & M. E. Witt (Eds.), *Manual for radiation oncology nursing practice and education* (pp. 180–202). Pittsburgh, PA: Oncology Nursing Society.

Cerillo, R. (2021). Gastrointestinal tract and abdomen. In M. McQuestion, L. C. Drapek, & M. E. Witt (Eds.), *Manual for radiation oncology nursing practice and education* (pp. 229–240). Pittsburgh, PA: Oncology Nursing Society.

Chao, K., Perez, C. A., & Wang, T. J. (2018). *Radiation oncology management decisions*. Philadelphia, PA: Lippincott Williams & Wilkins.

Choi, S., Yu, Y., Blakely, E. A., & Murnane, J. (2018). Clinical Radiobiology and physics: *Handbook of evidence-based radiation oncology*. New York: Springer International Publishing. Essay.

Cox, J. D., Stetz, J., & Pajak, T. F. (1995). Toxicity criteria of the radiation therapy oncology group (RTOG) and the European Organization for Research and Treatment of Cancer (EORTC). *International Journal of Radiation Oncology, Biology, Physics, 31*(5), 1341–1346. https://doi.org/10.1016/0360-3016(95)00060-C.

DeBaun, K. (2021). Low dose and high dose rate brachytherapy. In M. McQuestion, L. C. Drapek, & M. E. Witt (Eds.), *Manual for radiation oncology nursing practice and education* (pp. 304–310). Pittsburgh, PA: Oncology Nursing Society.

Domenech, H. (2017). *Radiation safety: Management and programs*. Cham: Springer. https://doi.org/10.1007/978-3-319-42671-6.

Fencl, J. L. (2015). Guideline implementation: Radiation safety. *AORN Journal, 102*(6), 629–639. https://doi.org/10.1016/j.aorn.2015.10.010.

Freites-Martinez, A., Santana, N., Arias-Santiago, S., & Viera, A. (2021). Using the Common Terminology Criteria for Adverse Events (CTCAE - Version 5.0) to Evaluate the Severity of Adverse Events of Anticancer Therapies. CTCAE versión 5.0. Evaluación de la gravedad de los eventos adversos dermatológicos de las terapias antineoplásicas. *Actas dermo-sifiliográficas, 112*(1), 90–92. https://doi.org/10.1016/j.ad.2019.05.009.

Garcia-Sanchez, A.-J., Garcia Angosto, E., Moreno Riquelme, P., Serna Berna, A., & Ramos-Amores, D. (2018). Ionizing radiation measurement solution in a hospital environment. *Sensors, 18*(2), 510. https://doi.org/10.3390/s18020510.

Gianfaldoni, S., Tchernev, G., Wollina, U., Roccia, M. G., Fioranelli, M., Gianfaldoni, R., et al. (2017). History of the baths and thermal medicine. *Open Access Macedonian Journal of Medical Sciences, 5*(4), 566–568. https://doi.org/10.3889/oamjms.2017.126.

Gibbons, J. P. (2020). *Khan's the physics of radiation therapy*. Alphen aan den Rijn: Wolters Kluwer.

Jones, D. (1994). ICRU Report 50—Prescribing, recording and reporting photon beam therapy. *Medical Physics, 21*(6), 833–834. https://doi.org/10.1118/1.597396.

Jones, E., & Mathieson, K. (2016). Radiation safety among workers in health services. *Health Physics, 110*(5), 52–58. https://doi.org/10.1097/hp.0000000000000485.

Khan, F. M., Gibbons, J. P., & Sperduto, P. W. (2016). *Khan's treatment planning in radiation oncology*. Philadelphia, PA: Lippincott Williams & Wilkins.

Mahtani, R. L. (2017). Insomnia in the cancer patient: A complex problem. *The Breast Journal, 23*(4), 385–386. https://doi.org/10.1111/tbj.12761.

Mock, V., Atkinson, A., Barsevick, A., Cella, D., Cimprich, B., Cleeland, C., et al. (2000). NCCN practice guidelines for cancer-related fatigue. *Oncology (Williston Park, N.Y.), 14*(11A), 151–161. https://pubmed.ncbi.nlm.nih.gov/11195408/.

Obinata, M., Yamada, K., & Sasai, K. (2019). Unusual olfactory perception during radiation sessions for primary brain tumors: A retrospective study. *Journal of Radiation Research, 60*(6), 812–817. https://doi.org/10.1093/jrr/rrz060.

O'Higgins, C. M., Brady, B., O'Connor, B., Walsh, D., & Reilly, R. B. (2018). The pathophysiology of cancer-related fatigue: Current controversies. *Supportive Care in Cancer, 26*(10), 3353–3364. https://doi.org/10.1007/s00520-018-4318-7.

Orio, P.F., & Viswanathan, A.N. (2019). *Sustaining the art and outcomes of brachytherapy*.

Papadakos, J. K., Hasan, S. M., Barnsley, J., Berta, W., Fazelzad, R., Papadakos, C. J., et al. (2018). Health literacy and cancer self-management behaviors: A scoping review. *Cancer, 124*(21), 4202–4210. https://doi.org/10.1002/cncr.31733.

Perevalova, E. (2021). Practice of radiation oncology. In M. McQuestion, L. C. Drapek, & M. E. Witt (Eds.), *Manual for radiation oncology nursing practice and education* (pp. 8–15). Pittsburgh, PA: Oncology Nursing Society.

Pierce, D. (2021). Radiation protection and safety. In M. McQuestion, L. C. Drapek, & M. E. Witt (Eds.), *Manual for radiation oncology nursing practice and education* (pp. 17–32). Pittsburgh, PA: Oncology Nursing Society.

Radiological Society of North America. (2022). *Professions in radiation therapy*. https://www.radiologyinfo.org/en/info/professions-radiation-therapy.

Sandstrom, S. (2021). Patient, caregiver, and family education. In M. McQuestion, L. C. Drapek, & M. E. Witt (Eds.), *Manual for radiation oncology nursing practice and education* (pp. 461–468). Pittsburgh, PA: Oncology Nursing Society.

Skowronek, J. (2017). Current status of brachytherapy in cancer treatment – Short overview. *Journal of Contemporary Brachytherapy, 9*(6), 581–589. https://doi.org/10.5114/jcb.2017.72607.

Thomas, N. (2021). Scope of practice for the registered nurse. In M. McQuestion, L. C. Drapek, & M. E. Witt (Eds.), *Manual for radiation oncology nursing practice and education* (pp. 1–3). Pittsburgh, PA: Oncology Nursing Society.

29

Chemotherapy, Hormonal Therapy, and Oral Adherence

Anna Howard, Chrystal Martin, and Patti Davis

CHEMOTHERAPY AND HORMONAL THERAPY

Overview

I. Principles of cancer chemotherapy (Wellstein, 2018)
  A. Cancer chemotherapy remains an integral component of systemic therapy in both hematologic and solid tumors.
  B. The use of chemotherapy is based on concepts of cellular kinetics, which includes the cell-cycle phases, cell-cycle time, growth fraction, and tumor burden.
    1. Cell cycle—a highly regulated five-stage process of reproduction that occurs in both normal and malignant cells (Malumbres, 2020; Olsen, LeFebvre, & Brassil, 2019; Wellstein, 2018)
      a. Gap 0 (G0), or resting phase
        (1) Cells are not dividing and are only susceptible to cell cycle–nonspecific chemotherapy; cellular activity continues but with a reduced rate of protein synthesis.
        (2) Entry into and out of the resting phase is influenced by growth factors and mitogen interaction with cell surface receptors.
      b. Gap 1 (G1): postmitotic phase, or interphase
        (1) Cells are activated to proliferate.
        (2) Enzymes for DNA synthesis are produced.
        (3) Protein and RNA synthesis occur.
      c. Synthesis (S)
        (1) Cellular DNA is replicated in preparation for DNA division.
      d. Gap 2 (G2), or premitotic phase
        (1) Further protein and RNA synthesis occurs.
        (2) Precursors of the mitotic spindle apparatus are produced.
        (3) Cells are ready for division or mitosis.
      e. Mitosis (M)—the shortest phase of the cell cycle in which cellular division occurs in five phases: prophase, prometaphase, metaphase, anaphase, and telophase. Some chemotherapies target microtubules during prophase.
      f. Cyclin complexes with cyclin-dependent kinases (CDKs) signal the cell to move through each phase of the cell cycle (Malumbres, 2020; Olsen et al., 2019).
        (1) CDK mutations can cause tumor development.
        (2) Anti-CDK/cyclin inhibitors are a new class of antineoplastic agents; the first approved agent was in 2015.
    2. Cell-cycle time—the amount of time required for a cell to move from one mitosis to the next mitosis (Wellstein, 2018)
      a. The length of the total cell cycle varies with the specific type of cell. A shorter cell-cycle time results in higher cell kill with exposure to cell cycle–specific agents.
    3. Growth fraction of tumor—the percentage of cells actively dividing at a given point in time
      a. A higher growth fraction results in a higher cell kill with exposure to cell cycle–specific agents.
      b. Tumors with a greater fraction of cells in G0 are more sensitive to cell cycle–nonspecific agents.
    4. Tumor burden—volume of cancer present
      a. Smaller: more sensitive to antineoplastic therapy.
      b. As the tumor burden increases, the growth rate slows and the number of cells actively dividing decreases.
      c. The higher the tumor burden, the greater heterogeneity of tumor cells, which in turn increases the likelihood of drug-resistant clone development.
  C. Approaches to chemotherapy (Doroshow, 2020; Olsen et al., 2019; Wellstein, 2018)
    1. Single-agent chemotherapy
      a. Most common application is in the recurrent setting
      b. May be sequential based on regimen, toxicity, or response to therapy
        (1) Sequential—single chemotherapy agents administered one after the other (e.g., drug A until disease progression followed by drug B).
        (2) Persistent use of single-agent chemotherapy increases the probability that drug-resistant clones will emerge.
    2. Combination chemotherapy—use of two or more antineoplastic agents to produce additive or synergistic results against tumor cells
      a. Increases the number of cells exposed to cytotoxic effects if cells are in different cell-cycle phases.

b. One agent modulates the toxicity of another agent.

c. Effective in large tumors containing a small number of proliferating cells; agents kill a high proportion of tumor cells and stimulate (recruit) remaining tumor cells to enter the proliferative phase; additional agents kill newly proliferating cells.

d. Emergence of drug resistance forestalled by combining agents.

e. May be given with target-specific agents (e.g., monoclonal antibodies)

f. Criteria for selection of antineoplastic agents for combination therapy
   (1) Cytotoxic activity when used alone to treat a specific cancer
   (2) Different, nonoverlapping toxicities
   (3) Toxicities that occur at different points of time from the treatment
   (4) Biological effects that result in enhanced cytotoxicity

3. Adjuvant chemotherapy—chemotherapy is delivered after the known cancer has been surgically removed or radiated

4. Neoadjuvant chemotherapy—chemotherapy delivered before surgery to provide optimal surgical removal or cosmesis

5. Concurrent chemotherapy and radiation—chemotherapy sensitizes tumor cells to radiation
   a. Useful in locally advanced cancers of esophagus, stomach, pancreas, cervix, anus, and head and neck
   b. Common chemotherapies used as radiosensitizers: 5-fluorouracil, cetuximab, cisplatin, mitomycin C, and temozolomide

6. Systemic chemotherapy—chemotherapy doses absorbed and distributed via the bloodstream to exert effects widely throughout the body. May be administered as oral or intravenous (IV) therapy.

7. Regional chemotherapy—method of delivering doses of chemotherapy to the specific site of the tumor—for example, the liver, bladder, peritoneal cavity, central nervous system, and pleural space—while reducing the intensity of systemic toxicity.

8. High-dose chemotherapy—higher dose administered with supportive therapy or with an antidote to diminish toxicity (e.g., high-dose methotrexate with leucovorin rescue, ifosfamide with mesna).

9. Dose-dense chemotherapy—able to administer at more frequent intervals due to the use of supportive therapy (e.g., colony-stimulating factors).

D. Factors influencing treatment response (Olsen et al., 2019)
   1. Characteristics of the tumor—location, size or tumor burden, growth rate or fraction, resistance (inherent or acquired), ratio of sensitivity of malignant cells and normal affected cells, genotype (e.g., molecular characteristics or hormone receptor status), or adequate blood supply with adequate drug uptake
   2. Characteristics of the patient—physical status, performance status, age, comorbidities, physiologic deficits, prior therapies, psychosocial status, and body mass index
   3. Administration or schedule—may influence efficacy or toxicity; best to deliver planned doses of chemotherapy on time if possible (Lehman, Howard, & Mancini, 2019; Morales, Joy, & Zbona, 2020)
   4. Routes (Imlygic, 2021; Wilkes & Barton-Burke, 2020)—see Table 29.1

II. Role of chemotherapy in cancer care
   A. Cure—to have the same life expectancy as if not diagnosed with cancer
   B. Control—to extend the length and quality of life when cure is not realistic
   C. Palliation—improve comfort when neither cure nor control is possible; relief of tumor-related symptoms

III. Types and classifications of chemotherapy (Table 29.2)—antineoplastic agents classified according to the phase of action during the cell cycle, mechanism of action (MOA), biochemical structure, or physiologic action (Collins, 2020; Doroshow, 2020; Wellstein, Giaccone, Atkins, & Sausville, 2018)

TABLE 29.1   Routes of Administration of Antineoplastic Agents

Route	Advantages	Disadvantages	Complications	Nursing Considerations
Oral (see Chapter 30 for more information on oral adherence).	Ease of administration. Gives patient sense of control and independence. Decreases time in health care facility and infusion center.	Inconsistency of absorption. Potential for drug–drug, food–drug, or herbal–drug interactions. Compliance (over or under). Expensive. Complex dosing and schedules. Difficult to swallow.	Drug-specific complications.	Monitor patient response via laboratory tests and follow-up via phone or appointment. Teach adherence with medication schedule. Teach patient techniques for handling drugs. Caregivers should use gloves for handling chemotherapy; wash hands after handling (even when gloves used); bring unused oral chemotherapy back to the facility for disposal unless otherwise directed (e.g., lenalidomide/thalidomide/pomalidomide must be sent to Celgene for disposal). Do not crush tablets or open capsules unless specified in package insert.

TABLE 29.1   Routes of Administration of Antineoplastic Agents—cont'd

Route	Advantages	Disadvantages	Complications	Nursing Considerations
Subcutaneous or intramuscular	Ease of administration. Intramuscular = rapid absorption.	Requires adequate muscle mass and tissue for absorption. Inconsistent absorption.	Infection Bleeding/bruising Pain or localized reaction at injection site Nerve damage Tissue necrosis	Evaluate platelet count before administration as needed. Use smallest gauge needle possible. Prepare injection site with an antiseptic solution. Assess injection site for signs and symptoms of infection. Wear PPE. Rotate injection sites. Do not massage; use heat or ice packs on injection site.
Intravenous	Consistent absorption; most common method of chemotherapy administration. Required for vesicants (central access preferred for vesicants).	Sclerosing of veins over time.	Infection Phlebitis Infiltration/ extravasation Pain Thrombosis	Use smallest catheter available. Always use a closed-system transfer device. Observe for signs and symptoms of infiltration. Avoid areas of flexion, lower extremities, and arms where lymph nodes have been removed. Peripheral IV site should not be older than 24 h. Assess the potential risk for extravasation. Utilize infusion pump and verify programming unless IV push medication.
Intra-arterial	Increased doses to tumor with decreased systemic side effects. Common sites: liver, head and neck, bone. Able to avoid extensive surgeries. Patients with liver metastases may be surgical candidates after treatment.	Requires surgical procedure or special radiography for catheter, port placement, or pump. Not all patients are candidates. Patients require specialized nursing care.	Bleeding Embolism Pain Infection Catheter issues (migration or dislodgement) Occlusion Clots Device failure	Monitor for signs and symptoms of bleeding or occlusion. Monitor catheter site and affected limb. Clearly label lines for intra-arterial use to prevent accidental IV administration.
Intrathecal or intraventricular	Delivers drug directly into cerebrospinal fluid.	Requires lumbar puncture or surgical placement of reservoir or implanted pump. Pump occlusion or malfunction. Requires additional education for nurse, patient, family. Each state Board of Nursing may vary for intrathecal or intraventricular chemotherapy administration rules for nurse administration. Preservative-free medications used with epidural and intraspinal may be difficult to obtain.	Increased intracranial pressure Headaches Confusion Lethargy Nausea or vomiting Seizures Infection Malposition/ migration of catheter	Observe site for signs of infection. Monitor reservoir or pump functioning. Assess patient for headache or signs of increased intracranial pressure. Evaluate platelet count before procedure. Vinca alkaloids are NEVER given IT because of the potential for lethal neurotoxicity or necrosis. They should always be in an IV bag and never in a syringe to prevent accidental IT administration. Time-out should be performed before procedure.
Intraperitoneal	Direct exposure of intraabdominal surfaces to drug. Higher and prolonged concentration in peritoneal cavity.	Requires placement of Tenckhoff catheter or intraperitoneal port. Only patients with minimal disease are candidates. May have more severe side effects.	Abdominal pain, distention Bleeding Ileus Intestinal perforation Infection Nausea Increased bladder irritation Dyspnea	Administer chemotherapy at room temperature (unless using heated intraperitoneal chemotherapy "Hyperthermic Intraperitoneal Chemoperfusion (HIPEC)" which is administered in operating room). Clearly label lines for intraperitoneal use only. Place patient in semi-Fowler's position Access with 19-g noncoring needle, 1–1.5 in. long. Check the patency of catheter. (Note: There will not be blood return.) Instill drug or solution according to protocol—infuse, dwell, and drain. Rotate patient side to side every 15 min for 1 h postinfusion.

Continued

TABLE 29.1   Routes of Administration of Antineoplastic Agents—cont'd

Route	Advantages	Disadvantages	Complications	Nursing Considerations
Intravesicular	Direct exposure of bladder surfaces to drug.	Requires insertion of indwelling catheter.	Urinary tract infection Cystitis Bladder contracture Urinary urgency Allergic drug reactions	Maintain sterile technique when inserting indwelling catheter. Follow provider's orders for positioning of patient and draining of agent.
Intrapleural	Sclerosing of pleural lining. May prevent the recurrence of malignant pleural effusion.	Requires the insertion of a thoracotomy tube. State Board of Nursing may not allow nurse to administer drug via intrapleural route. Physicians may administer instead.	Pain Infection Pneumothorax	Monitor for complete drainage from pleural space before instillation of drug. Allow agent to remain for entire dwell time. Assess patient for pain, respiratory distress, and anxiety.
Intraureteral	Direct exposure of ureter surfaces to drug. Nonsurgical alternative for the treatment of low-grade upper tract urothelial cancer.	Requires insertion of retrograde ureteral catheter with each treatment.	Ureteric obstruction Flank pain Hematuria Urinary tract infection	Advise patient they will potentially see a change in urine color due to the violet color of the medication. Urinate seated to avoid splashing and avoid contact with urine for at least 6 h, flush toilet multiple times with the lid down. Wash hands thoroughly after urination with soap and water. Instruct patients to immediately contact their provider if experiencing flank pain or fever, as they could be experiencing ureteric obstruction.
Intratumoral (viral immunotherapy)	Genetically modified virus replicates in cancer cells to promote oncolysis, which aids in local control. May cause antitumor immune response in some noninjected lesions (visceral and nonvisceral).	Must have a low burden of disease and injectable lesions.	Herpetic infection	If pregnant or immunocompromised—do not administer and avoid contact with patient. Utilize proper PPE and ensure injection site is covered post administration and PPE is used in the handling of the dressing. Instruct patient to keep site covered for at least one week, using gloves and washing hands well if needing to change the dressing. Place dressing in sealed baggie for disposal. If family members are pregnant or immunocompromised, they should not change dressings or clean the injection site.

IT, Intrathecally; *IV*, intravenous; *PPE*, personal protective equipment.
Data from Olsen, M., LeFebvre, K., Brassil, K. (2019). *Chemotherapy and immunotherapy guidelines and recommendations for practice*. Pittsburgh, PA: ONS Press; Wellstein, A. (2018). General principles in the pharmacotherapy of cancer. In L. L. Brunton, R. Hilal-Dandan, & B. C. Knollmann (Eds.), *Goodman and Gilman's the pharmacological basis of therapeutics* (13th ed.). New York: McGraw-Hill. eBook (chap. 65); Wilkes, G. M., & Barton-Burke, M. (2020). *2020–2021 Oncology nursing drug handbook* (23rd ed.). Burlington, MA: Jones and Bartlett Learning; Jelmyto. (2021). *Package insert*. Princeton, NJ: Urogen Pharma, Inc.; Kleinmann, N., Matin, S. F., Pierorazio, P. M., Gore, J. L., Shabsigh, A., Hu, B., et al. (2020). Primary chemoablation of low-grade upper tract urothelial carcinoma using UGN-101, a mitomycin-containing reverse thermal gel (OLYMPUS): An open-label, single-arm, phase 3 trial. *The Lancet Oncology, 21*(6), 776–785. https://doi.org/10.1016/S1470-2045(20)30147-9; Imlygic. (2021). *Package insert*. Thousand Oaks, CA: Amgen, Inc.; Adambekov, S., Lopa, S., Edwards, R. P., Lemon, L., Wang, S., Taylor, S. E., et al. (2020). Survival and recurrence after intraperitoneal chemotherapy use: Retrospective review of ovarian cancer hospital registry data. *Cancer Medicine, 9*(20), 7388–7397. https://doi.org/10.1002/cam4.3340; van Driel, W. J., Koole, S. N., Sikorska, K., Schagen van Leeuwen, J. H., Schreuder, H. W. R., Hermans, R. H. M., et al. (2018). Hyperthermic intraperitoneal chemotherapy in ovarian cancer. *The New England journal of medicine, 378*(3), 230–240; OCE. (2021). *Safe handling of oral chemotherapy*. https://www.oralchemoedsheets.com/index.php/supplement-library/27-supplemental-available/493-safe handlingoforalchemotherapy. Retrieved 13.03.22.

A. Phase of action during the cell cycle
1. Cell cycle–specific agents
   a. Major cytotoxic effects are exerted on actively dividing cells at specific phases throughout the cell cycle.
   b. Agents are not active against cells in the resting phase (G0).
   c. Agents are schedule dependent and most effective if administered in divided doses or by continuous infusion.
   d. Cytotoxic effects occur during the cell cycle and are expressed when cell repair or division is attempted.
   e. Continuous infusion and multiple frequent doses of cell cycle–specific agents result in exposure of

TABLE 29.2   Classifications of Cancer Therapy Drugs

Alkylating Agents

<u>Alkyl sulfonates</u>
Busulfan (Myleran [PO]); Busulfex (IV)

<u>Nitrogen mustards</u>
Bendamustine (Treanda)
Chlorambucil (Leukeran)
Cyclophosphamide (Cytoxan)
Ifosfamide (Ifex)
Melphalan (Alkeran)
Melphalan flufenamide (Pepaxto)
Mechlorethamine (Mustargen)

<u>Aziridines</u>
Altretamine (Hexalen)
Thiotepa (Thioplex)

<u>Nitrosoureas</u>
Carmustine (BCNU)
Lomustine (CNU)
Streptozocin (Zanosar)

<u>Triazenes and hydrazine</u>
Dacarbazine (DTIC-DOME)
Procarbazine (Matulane)
Temozolomide (Temodar)
Platinum analogs
Carboplatin (Paraplatin)
Cisplatin (Platinol)
Oxaliplatin (Eloxatin)

Antimetabolites

<u>Pyrimidine analogs</u>
Azacitidine (Vidaza, Onureg)
Capecitabine (Xeloda)
Cytarabine (Cytosar)
Cytarabine, liposomal (DepoCyt)
Decitabine (Dacogen)
Floxuridine (FUDR)
5-Fluorouracil (Adrucil)
Gemcitabine (Gemzar)

<u>Folate antagonists</u>
Methotrexate (Folex)
Pemetrexed (Alimta)
Pralatrexate (Folotyn)

<u>Purine analogs</u>
Cladribine (Leustatin)
Clofarabine (Clolar)
Fludarabine (Fludara)
Mercaptopurine (Purinethol)
Nelarabine (Arranon)
Pentostatin (Nipent)
Thioguanine (6-TG)

Antimicrotubule Agents

<u>Epothilones</u>
Ixabepilone (Ixempra)

<u>Taxanes</u>
Cabazitaxel (Jevtana)
Docetaxel (Taxotere)
Paclitaxel (Taxol)
Paclitaxel, protein bound (Abraxane)

<u>Miscellaneous</u>
Eribulin mesylate (Halaven)

Vinca Alkaloids
Vinblastine (Velban)

Vincristine (Oncovin)
Vincristine, liposomal (Marqibo)

Vindesine (Eldisine)
Vinorelbine (Navelbine)

Miscellaneous
Asparaginase (Elspar, Erwinase, Rylaze)
Bexarotene (Targretin)

Dactinomycin (Actinomycin-D)
Hydroxyurea (Hydrea)
Lurbinectedin (Zepzelca)
Mitotane (Lysodren)

Omacetaxine (Synribo)
Trabectedin (Yondelis)
Tretinoin (Vesanoid)
Pegaspargase (Oncospar)
Pomalidomide (Pomalyst)
Lenalidomide (Revlimid)

Topoisomerase I Inhibitors (Camptothecins)
Topotecan (Hycamtin)

Irinotecan (Camptosar)

Topoisomerase II Inhibitors

<u>Anthracyclines</u>
Daunorubicin (Cerubidine)
Daunorubicin, liposomal (DaunoXome)
Daunorubicin/Cytarabine liposomal (Vyxeos)
Doxorubicin (Adriamycin)
Doxorubicin, liposomal (Doxil)
Epirubicin (Ellence)
Idarubicin (Idamycin)
Valrubicin (Valstar)

<u>Anthracenedione</u>
Bleomycin sulfate (Blenoxane)
Mitomycin (Mutamycin, Jelmyto)
Mitoxantrone (Novantrone)

<u>Epipodophyllotoxins</u>
Etoposide (VePesid)
Etoposide phosphate
  (Etopophos)
Teniposide (Vumon)

Continued

TABLE 29.2 Classifications of Cancer Therapy Drugs—cont'd

Miscellaneous

Histone deacetylase inhibitors
Belinostat (Beleodaq)
Panobinostat (Farydak)
Romidepsin (Istodax)

Proteosome inhibitors
Bortezomib (Velcade)
Carfilzomib (Kyprolis)
Ixazomib (Ninlaro)

Differentiating agents
All-Trans Retinoic Acid (ATRA; Tretinoin)
Arsenic trioxide (Trisenox)
Enasidenib (IDHIFA)
Ivosidenib (Tibsovo)

Antibody Drug Conjugates

Ado-trastuzumab emtansine (Kadcyla)
Belantamab mafodotin-blmf (Blenrep)
Brentuximab vedotin (Adcetris)
Enfortumab vedotin-ejfv (Padcev)

Fam-trastuzumab deruxtecan-nxki (Enhertu)
Gemtuzumab ozogamicin (Mylotarg)
Inotuzumab ozogamicin (Besponsa)
Loncastuximab tesirine-lpyl (Zynlonta)

Moxetumomab pasudotox-tdfk (Lumoxiti)
Polatuzumab vedotin-piiq (Polivy)
Sacituzumab govitecan-hziy (Trodelvy)
Tisotumab vedotin-tftv (Tivdak)

Hormones

Antiestrogens
Fluvestrant (Faslodex)
Megestrol acetate (Megace)
Tamoxifen citrate (Nolvadex)
Toremifene (Fareston)

Miscellaneous hormonal agents
Abiraterone acetate (Zytiga, Yonsa)
Enzalutamide (Xtandi)
Estramustine (Emcyt)

Aromatase inhibitors
Anastrazole (Arimidex)
Exemestane (Aromasin)
Letrazole (Femara)

Antiandrogens
Bicalutamide (Casodex)
Flutamide (Eulexin)
Nilutamide (Nilandron)

LHRH analogs and antagonists
Goserelin (Zoladex)
Leuprolide (Lupron)
Degarelix (Firmagon)

Data from Olsen, M., LeFebvre, K., Brassil, K. (2019). *Chemotherapy and immunotherapy guidelines and recommendations for practice* Pittsburgh, PA: ONS Press; Wellstein, A. (2018). General principles in the pharmacotherapy of cancer. In L. L. Brunton, R. Hilal-Dandan, & B. C. Knollmann (Eds.), *Goodman and Gilman's the pharmacological basis of therapeutics* (13th ed.). New York: McGraw-Hill. eBook (chap. 65); Wilkes, G. M., & Barton-Burke, M. (2020). *2020–2021 Oncology nursing drug handbook* (23rd ed.). Burlington, MA: Jones and Bartlett Learning; Collins, J. M. (2020). Cancer pharmacology. In J. E. Niederhuber, J. O. Armitage, J. H. Doroshow, M. B. Kastan, & J. E. Tepper (Eds.), *Abeloff's clinical oncology* (6th edition). Philadelphia, PA: Elsevier (chap. 25); Doroshow, J. H. (2020). Approach to the patient with cancer. In L. Goldman, A. I. Schafer, & R. L. Cecil (Eds.), *Goldman-Cecil medicine* (26th ed.). Philadelphia, PA: Elsevier (chap. 169); Oncopeptides AB (2021). *Pepaxto (melphalan flufenamide) [package insert]*. Stockholm; ADC Therapeutics SA. (2021). *Zynlonta (loncastuximab tesirine-lpyl) [package insert]*. Epalinges: ADC Therapeutics SA.

a greater number of cells and in a higher cell kill in tumors with short cell-cycle times.

   f. Cell cycle–specific drugs include antimetabolites and plant alkaloids.

2. Cell cycle–nonspecific agents
   a. Major cytotoxic effects are exerted on cells at any phase in the cell cycle, including G0.
   b. Agents are dose dependent; most effective if administered by bolus doses, as the number of cells affected is proportional to the amount of drug given.
   c. Cytotoxic effects occur during the cell cycle and are expressed when cell division is attempted.
   d. Effective in treating tumors with slowly dividing cells.
   e. Cell cycle–nonspecific agents include alkylating agents, antitumor antibiotics, hormonal therapies, and nitrosoureas.

B. Biochemical structure, MOA, or derivation
   1. Alkylating agents (Wellstein et al., 2018)
      a. Among the first antineoplastic drugs developed
      b. MOAs—interfere with DNA replication through cross-linking of DNA strands, DNA strand breakage, and abnormal base pairing of proteins, all interfering with normal DNA replication
      c. Most are cell cycle–nonspecific agents

   d. Major toxicities often directly related to the administered dose; pancytopenia, nausea and vomiting, mucosal/gastrointestinal (GI) toxicity, and neurotoxicity
   (1) General: peripheral granulocyte nadir approximately 6–10 days after administration with recovery about 14–21 days.
   (2) Nitrosoureas: peripheral granulocyte nadir is delayed; may appear about 4–6 weeks after dose.
   e. Seven major subgroups—nitrogen mustards, aziridines, alkyl sulfonates, DNA methylating agents, nitrosoureas, platinum compounds, and triazine compounds
   f. Special dosing considerations: carboplatin dose calculation using the Calvert equation is based on the area under the curve (AUC), a measure of drug exposure, and the patient's renal function (NCCN, 2020; Olsen et al., 2019)

2. Antimetabolites (Wellstein et al., 2018)
   a. Includes antifolates, pyrimidine analogs, and purine analogs
   b. MOA—inhibit protein synthesis, substitute erroneous metabolites or structural analogs during DNA synthesis, and inhibit DNA synthesis

c. Most agents cell cycle specific (S phase)

d. Major toxicities in the hematopoietic and GI systems

3. Topoisomerase-targeting agents (Wellstein et al., 2018)

a. Topoisomerase I–directed agents—include the camptothecins
   (1) MOA: prevent realignment of DNA strands, maintain single-strand DNA breaks
   (2) Major toxicities affecting the hematopoietic and GI systems

b. Topoisomerase II–targeting agents—anthracyclines, anthracenediones, actinomycins, and epipodophyllotoxins
   (1) MOA: prevent realigning of DNA strands, maintain double-strand DNA breaks
   (2) Major toxicities: hematopoietic, GI, cardiac (anthracyclines) systems

4. Microtubule-targeting agents (Wellstein et al., 2018)

a. MOA: prevents microtubule polymerization so the mitotic spindle cannot form; the cell cycle is stopped in metaphase; cells undergo apoptosis

b. Include taxanes and vinca alkaloids, epothilone analogs

c. Most agents cell cycle specific, primarily late G2 and M phases

d. Major toxicities: hematopoietic, integumentary, neurologic, and reproductive systems

5. Differentiating agents (Gasparovic, Weiler, Higi, & Burden, 2020; Pollyea et al., 2019; Roboz et al., 2020; Wellstein et al., 2018)

a. Used in the treatment of acute myeloid leukemia with certain mutations or in treatment of acute promyelocytic leukemia

b. Tretinoin, also known as *all-trans retinoic acid*; oral agent
   (1) Produces maturation of primitive promyelocytes
   (2) Major toxicities: hepatotoxicity, differentiation syndrome (massive cytokine release from promyelocyte maturation may cause fever, dyspnea, pulmonary infiltrates, pericardial infiltrates)

c. Arsenic trioxide, IV
   (1) MOA not well understood
   (2) Major toxicities: hepatotoxicity, QT prolongation, differentiation syndrome (although less common than tretinoin)

d. Ivosidenib, PO
   (1) Inhibits IDH1 preventing an increase in metabolites that impair hematopoietic differentiation in patients with mutation in this enzyme
   (2) Major toxicities: differentiation syndrome (black box warning; may occur 1–90 days after therapy start date), diarrhea, leukocytosis, QT prolongation, mucositis, nausea, myalgia/arthralgia, and anemia

e. Enasidenib, PO
   (1) Inhibits IDH2 preventing an increase in metabolites that impair hematopoietic differentiation in patients with mutation in this enzyme (Pollyea et al., 2019)
   (2) Major toxicities: differentiation syndrome (black box warning; may occur 1 day to 5 months after therapy start date), nausea, vomiting, diarrhea, elevated bilirubin, and decreased appetite

f. Differentiation syndrome is prevented/treated with corticosteroids

6. Antibody–drug conjugates

a. A form of targeted immunotherapy

b. A monoclonal antibody is combined with a chemotherapy agent via a chemical linker

c. The monoclonal antibody directs the agent to the specific cancer cell where it unloads the chemotherapy, known as the payload

IV. Hormonal therapy (Table 29.3)

A. Overview
1. First targeted therapy ever developed
2. Used to treat breast, prostate, endometrial, ovarian cancers, and adrenal
3. Suppressing select hormones may inhibit cancerous cell growth of hormone-sensitive cancers
4. May also lead to side effects that may decrease patient's quality of life

Assessment

(Neuss et al., 2017; Olsen et al., 2019)

I. Pretreatment

A. Cancer diagnosis information
1. Pathology: cell type, cytogenetic findings (when relevant)
2. Stage and grade of disease
3. Risks and benefits of treatment

B. Laboratory results
1. Complete blood cell count with differential
2. Comprehensive metabolic panel
3. Electrolytes—including magnesium, potassium, and phosphorus
4. Genetic/genomic considerations (e.g., HER2, KRAS, BRAF, EGFR, and Alk rearrangement)

C. Patient-related information
1. Family and personal medical histories
2. Comorbidities and preexisting conditions
3. Thorough review of cardiac (including ejection fraction as indicated), pulmonary, GI, renal, reproductive, and neurologic functioning
4. Behavioral and cognitive functioning
5. Performance status
6. Venous access—peripheral versus central
7. Patient and family experience of prior therapies
   a. Side effects experienced and their severity
   b. Self-care measures and effectiveness in reducing side effects
8. Understanding of the goal of therapy

TABLE 29.3 Hormonal Therapy

Hormone Category	Mechanism of Action	Uses	Side Effects
Adrenocorticoids	Lead to cell death—exact mechanism unknown	Lymphoma, acute lymphoblastic leukemia, chronic lymphocytic leukemia, and multiple myeloma	Hyperglycemia, insomnia, hypersensitivity, hypertension, osteoporosis, diabetes, and immune suppression
Adrenolytics		Adrenal cancer	Decreased appetite, GI upset, increased glucocorticoid and cholesterol, hypothyroid
Androgens	Inhibit androgen binding to AR; inhibit AR binding to DNA	Metastatic breast cancer, hypogonadism	Gynecomastia, headache, decreased libido
Antiandrogens	Block testosterone and dihydrotestosterone	Castration-resistant prostate cancer, typically used in combination therapies	Hot flashes, loss of libido, impotence, weight gain, nausea, diarrhea, decreased bone density
Antiestrogens Pure antiestrogens	Function as an estrogen antagonist with no estrogen-agonist effects	Postmenopausal women with advanced breast cancer who had relapsed or progressed on prior endocrine therapy	Hot flashes, headache, dyspepsia, facial swelling, and vaginal discharge
AIs	Inhibits synthesis of estrogen by preventing the conversion of estrogen precursors to estrogen	Postmenopausal and premenopausal breast cancer with ovarian suppression or ablation	Osteoporosis, hot flashes, elevated cholesterol, arthralgias, decreased libido, decreased vaginal lubrication
CYP17 inhibitors	Blocks androgen production	Prostate cancer	Hypokalemia, hypertension, fatigue, dizziness (ketoconazole can cause severe hepatoxicity)
GnRH agonists also known as LHRH agonists	Bind to specific receptors on pituitary gonadotrophs responsible for gonadotropin secretion and synthesis. Suppress ovarian production of estrogen in women. Decrease testosterone production in males	Metastatic breast cancer; premenopausal; can be used with AI	Hot flashes, mood changes, weight gain, injection site reaction
GnRH antagonists also known as LHRH antagonists	Compete with GnRH for receptors on gonadotroph cell membranes; inhibit GnRH-induced signal transduction and gonadotrophin secretion	Metastatic breast cancer, adjuvant therapy	Hot flashes, decreased libido, injection site reaction
Progestins	Exact mechanism unknown. Thought to block the synthesis of luteinizing hormone in the pituitary gland without affecting ovarian sensitivity to gonadotrophins	Estrogen receptor positive, progesterone receptor positive metastatic breast cancer. May be used as appetite stimulants due to side effects	Increased appetite, weight gain, diarrhea, rash
SERMs	Block estrogen activity (i.e., serve as estrogen antagonists) in some tissues (e.g., breast tissue) but also mimic estrogen effects (i.e., serve as estrogen agonists) in other tissues (e.g., endometrium)	Premenopausal and postmenopausal women with hormone-positive breast cancer	Hot flash, stroke, thromboembolic risk, uterine cancer, vaginal discharge, menstrual irregularities

AIs, Aromatase inhibitors; *AR*, androgen receptors; *GI*, gastrointestinal; *LHRH*, luteinizing hormone-releasing hormone; *SERMs*, selective estrogen receptor modulators.

From Wilkes, G. M., & Barton-Burke, M. (2020). *2020–2021 Oncology nursing drug handbook* (23rd ed.). Burlington, MA: Jones and Bartlett Learning; Olsen, M., LeFebvre, K., & Brassil, K. (2019). Chemotherapy and immunotherapy guidelines: Recommendations for practice. Pittsburgh, PA: Oncology Nursing Press.

II. Ongoing
   A. Performance status
   B. Vital signs
   C. Weight and height at least weekly when patient is in the health care setting
   D. Medication reconciliation
   E. Dietary intake, unintentional weight loss, use of nutraceuticals, supplements, and complementary therapies that could interact with treatment
   F. Allergies or history of hypersensitivity or infusion reactions (note cycle of therapy)
      1. Taxane reactions occur most often in first or second infusion.
      2. Reactions to platinum agents occur most often during the fifth (oxaliplatin), sixth, or later infusion (carboplatin).
   G. Knowledge of, rationale for, and goals of treatment; schedule of agents to be given; potential side effects

H. Psychosocial examination
   1. Previous responses to stressors and effective coping mechanisms
   2. Level of independence and responsibility, ability for self-care
   3. Support systems and personnel available to the patient and family
   4. Cultural, spiritual, and financial considerations
III. Management
   A. Interventions to maximize the safe administration of chemotherapy (Neuss et al., 2017; Olsen et al., 2019)
      1. Review of orders
         a. Compare orders with drug protocol or reference source, ensuring accuracy and completeness
         b. Orders to be regimen specific, preprinted, or electronic with a list of all agents and calculations in the regimen
         c. Verbal orders not allowed except to hold or stop chemotherapy administration
         d. Complete orders for IV treatment to include the patient's full name and a second identifier; date order is written; date medication is administered; diagnosis; regimen or protocol name, number, cycle number, and day when applicable; criteria to treat; number of cycles order is valid; allergies; full generic names of the agents; doses are written after abbreviation; trailing zeros and leading zero standards; dose calculation methodology; parameters for holding or modifying the treatment; route and rate of administration; supportive care agents or treatments; sequence; and time specifications (Neuss et al., 2017)
      2. Determination of drug dosage
         a. Verification of actual height and weight on day of administration
         b. Calculation of body surface area or appropriate dose calculation (e.g., AUC)
         c. Recalculation of drug dosage and checking against order
      3. Review drugs to be administered and potential side effects and toxicities.
      4. Review and obtain orders for other medications: prehydration and posthydration IV fluids, antiemetics, premedications, if indicated, for hypersensitivity reactions.
      5. Verification of previous and current laboratory test values or need for dosage adjustment, if indicated.
      6. Verification that informed consent is documented according to practice or institution policies and procedures.
      7. Patient and caregiver teaching (e.g., chemotherapy administration procedures, antiemetic schedule, and self-care measures for potential side effects).
      8. Prepare drugs, as appropriate, following safe handling policies and procedures (Connor, MacKenzie, DeBord, Trout, & O'Callaghan, 2016; Olsen et al., 2019; Power & Coyne, 2018; USP, 2020, 2021).
         a. Chemotherapies are hazardous drugs and may evidence one or more of the following characteristics:
            (1) Carcinogenic (cancer causing)
            (2) Teratogenic (fetal malformation or defects)
            (3) Associated with adverse reproductive outcomes
            (4) Genotoxic (damage genetic material)
            (5) Potential for other organ or system evidence of exposure or toxicity
         b. Employ safe handling of agents to minimize potential risks for occupational exposure to hazardous drugs:
            (1) Increased risk for malignancies
            (2) Embryofetal toxicities
            (3) Chromosomal damage
            (4) Other evidence of exposures (e.g., skin injury, alopecia, and dermatitis)
         c. Mixing or compounding chemotherapy
            (1) Adhere to guidelines and recommendations from the Oncology Nursing Society (ONS), the Occupational Safety and Health Administration, and the American Society of Health-Systems Pharmacists (ASHP)
               (a) ONS guidelines for safe handling of chemotherapy or hazardous drugs (ONS, 2018)
               (b) National Institute for Occupational Safety and Health (NIOSH) Alert on Preventing Occupational Exposure to Antineoplastic and Other Hazardous Drugs in Health Care Settings, 2016
               (c) US Pharmacopeia (USP), General Chapter 797 "Pharmaceutical Compounding – Sterile Preparations," 2008
               (d) ASHP Guidelines on Handling Hazardous Drugs, 2018
         d. USP, General Chapter 800 "Hazardous Drugs – Handling in Healthcare Settings," 2020; potentially high risk for exposure if proper procedures and guidelines are not followed.
         e. Correct use of personal protective equipment (PPE) can significantly reduce exposure to hazardous drugs.
         f. All chemotherapy preparations, including opening capsules and crushing agents that can be administered as a powder, should take place in a primary engineering control (C-PEC) setting—biologic safety cabinet or a compounding aseptic containment isolator.
            (1) Use vertical unidirectional air flow.
            (2) Preparation area is vented to the outside (optimal) with exhaust emitted through a high-efficiency particulate air filter.

(3) Fan is operating continuously.

(4) Preparation area is housed in an area with negative pressure.

(5) C-PEC is inspected and serviced per manufacturer's recommendations; recertified if moved or repaired; filter should be replaced every 6 months.

(6) Training essential to use techniques that minimize interference with air flow.

g. Wash hands and don PPE appropriate for use with chemotherapy.

h. Gather necessary supplies for compounding; limit items housed in the PEC to reduce both the contamination of items and the interference with air flow.

i. Use closed-system transfer devices (CSTDs) to reduce environmental contamination during drug preparation.

j. Use double gloves for all handling; change every 30 minutes and whenever contamination occurs.

k. Use CSTDs.

l. Avoid overfilling syringes.

m. IV fluid (IVF)—spike and prime tubing before chemotherapy are added to minimize exposure.

n. Damp-wipe outside of product (i.e., syringe, IVF) before placing in transport container; container should be identified as hazardous according to policy and procedures.

o. Transport containers or bags—label to ensure awareness of contents; avoid contamination of the outside of the transport container or bags.

p. Dispose contaminated compounding materials in a sealed container within the PEC; place into a puncture-proof container located adjacent to the PEC.

q. Remove and discard outer gloves, followed by the gown and the inner gloves, taking care not to contaminate self.

r. Wash hands with soap and water.

9. Label drugs with the patient's full name and a second identifier (e.g., date of birth), generic drug name, route of administration, total dose, total volume, date of administration, sequence of drug administration (when applicable); drugs in divided doses need the total number of doses (i.e., 1 of 2), date and time of preparation and expiration, warning sticker for handling requirements (Neuss et al., 2017).

10. Oral drugs to be labeled with patient's name and a second identifier, date and time of preparation and expiration, full generic drug name, dosage form and strength, quantity dispensed, number of pills per dose, administration schedule including how many times per day and any days off if applicable, instructions relating to food and other medication interactions, warning sticker for hazardous drug and for handling and/or storage requirements, and prescriber name (Neuss et al., 2017).

11. Before each chemotherapy administration, at least two practitioners approved by the health care setting to administer or prepare chemotherapy, verify and document the following: drug name, drug dose, infusion volume, or volume in syringe; rate of administration; expiration dates and/or times; appearance of drug; rate set on infusion pump, when applicable (ASCO, 2020; Neuss et al., 2017).

12. Ensure appropriate supplies or pump is available.

a. Emergency equipment

b. Agents for management of extravasation and/or anaphylaxis, as indicated

c. Spill kit

d. PPE

13. Don PPE or apply principles of safe handling throughout chemotherapy administration.

a. Potential routes of exposure: absorption, inhalation, ingestion, and injection

b. Guidelines regarding PPE

(1) Gloves—powder-free disposable gloves tested for use with hazardous drugs.

(a) Double-glove for drug preparation, administration, and handling of contaminated waste.

(b) Inspect for defects before use; remove and discard immediately after use, damage, drug spill, or 30 minutes of wear.

(c) Do not reuse.

(2) Gowns—should be disposable, lint free, low permeability, with a solid front, long sleeves, tight cuffs, and back closure.

(a) Discard if visibly contaminated, after handling hazardous drugs, or after leaving the area.

(b) Do not reuse.

(3) Respirators—NIOSH-approved protective respirator when aerosolization, if possible.

(a) Check the material safety data sheet for appropriate respiratory protection.

(b) Surgical masks are not respirators; do not protect against vapors or aerosols.

(4) Eye and face protection—plastic face shield to be worn when splashing is possible; surgical masks do not provide protection for eye and face exposures.

(5) Chemotherapy precautions for handling body fluids and soiled linens.

(a) Precautions remain in effect for 48 hours after chemotherapy administration is complete.

(b) Laundry handling in the home setting: patients will wear gloves when handling soiled linen. Patients are to place their soiled clothes in a pillow case, washing twice in hot water using regular detergent. It is important to keep soiled clothing separate from other laundry.

(c) Skin exposure: remove soiled garment and wash the skin thoroughly with soap and water.

(d) Flush the toilet twice with the lid down to prevent particles from splashing; when a lid is not present, cover the toilet bowl with a plastic-backed pad (Polovich & Olsen, 2018).

(e) The following chemotherapies may have metabolites present in urine or feces for up to a week and require personal protection for this time period: carmustine, cisplatin, docetaxel, doxorubicin, etoposide, gemcitabine, methotrexate, mitoxantrone, teniposide, vincristine, and vinorelbine.

14. Venipuncture site selection criteria (Gorski et al., 2021)

a. Select the distal sites before proximal sites.

b. Evaluate the general condition of veins.

c. Note the type of medications to be infused.

d. Avoid sites where damage to underlying tendons or nerves is more likely to occur—for example, antecubital region, wrist, dorsal surface of the hand; areas with recent venipuncture sites, sclerosed veins; or areas of previous surgery such as skin grafts, side of mastectomy, lumpectomy, node dissection, or partial amputation.

15. Monitor the central or peripheral IV administration for the presence of blood return before, during, and after the administration of therapy.

16. Administer prechemotherapy hydration, antiemetics, and other medications as ordered.

17. Administer chemotherapy drugs according to agency policy and procedures, following safe handling procedures in accordance with ASCO/ONS chemotherapy administration standards.

18. Administer agents designed to protect against specific toxic effects of chemotherapy (Collins, 2020; Olsen et al., 2019).

a. Dexrazoxane (Zinecard)—to protect against cardiotoxicity in patients who require more than 300 mg/m^2 of doxorubicin (Pfizer, 2016)

b. Amifostine (Ethyol)—to protect against renal toxicity from cisplatin therapy or xerostomia from radiation to the head and neck

c. Mesna (Mesnex)—to protect against bladder toxicity from ifosfamide or high-dose cyclophosphamide

d. Leucovorin—used as a rescue agent with methotrexate to prevent mucositis and other toxicities related to impaired methotrexate elimination

19. Assess the patient for signs of infiltration (burning, pain, swelling, and redness).

20. Flush the IV tubing with appropriate solution after administering each agent and at completion of the infusion.

21. After drug administration, remove intact administration setup; the spike from the IVF containers should not be removed or tubing reused.

22. Remove the needle or IV catheter.

a. Apply gauze to the peripheral IV site.

b. Apply gentle pressure to the site to reduce local bleeding.

23. Wash potentially contaminated surfaces; may include multiple steps depending on institution guidelines.

a. Deactivate chemotherapy (bleach, peroxide, etc.).

b. Decontaminate to remove chemotherapy residue (e.g., alcohol, water, bleach, or peroxide).

c. Cleanse and disinfect with germicidal agents and disinfectants.

24. Discard contaminated materials in the appropriate hazardous waste container.

25. Document medication administration, infusion site, patient education, and outcomes or response according to agency policy.

IV. Interventions to minimize the risk of extravasation (Jackson-Rose, Del Monte, & Groman, 2017; Karius & Colvin, 2021; Olsen et al., 2019)

A. Prevention is the best approach for avoiding extravasation injury.

1. Chemotherapy administration should be limited to knowledgeable, clinically competent staff as defined per institutional policy. Competence is based on didactic education and clinical experience.

2. Risk for extravasation should be assessed before treatment administration. Vigilance is always required during administration.

3. Policies and procedures in the management of extravasations should be clearly delineated, readily accessible in all sites where vesicants may be administered, and periodically reviewed.

B. If extravasation is suspected, appropriate materials and antidotes should be obtained for the management of extravasation.

1. Extravasation—infiltration or leakage of an IV antineoplastic agent into local tissues

a. Irritants—agents that cause a local inflammatory reaction but do not cause tissue necrosis

b. Vesicants—agents that have the potential to cause cellular damage or tissue destruction, or are inadvertently administered into the tissue; see Table 29.4 for a list of agents associated with extravasation and tissue injury

(1) Observe for swelling, redness, lack of blood return, IV that slows or stops infusing, leaking around needle or catheter.

(2) Instruct the patient to report pain, burning, or changes in sensations during chemotherapy administration.

(3) Administer vesicants in larger veins of the arm, above the wrist, and below the elbow. Avoid areas of flexion or areas with minimal overlying tissue.

TABLE 29.4   Agents Associated With Extravasation or Tissue Injury

Vesicant	Irritant	Vesicant or Irritant
Amsacrine: none	Carboplatin: none	Bendamustine: none
Cisplatin: sodium thiosulfate	Carmustine: none	Bleomycin: none
Dacarbazine: none	Cyclophosphamide: none	Cabazitaxel: cold
Dactinomycin: cold	Gemcitabine: none	Dacarbazine
Daunorubicin: dexrazoxane, cold	Ifosfamide: none	Etoposide: none
Docetaxel: cold	Irinotecan: none	Fluorouracil: none
Doxorubicin: dexrazoxane, cold	Liposomal doxorubicin: none	Paclitaxel: cold
Epirubicin: dexrazoxane, cold	Methotrexate: none	Paclitaxel protein bound: none
Idarubicin: dexrazoxane, cold	Plicamycin: none	
Mechlorethamine: sodium thiosulfate, cold	Teniposide: none	
Melphalan: none	Topotecan: none	
Mitomycin: none		
Mitoxantrone: cold		
Oxaliplatin: dexamethasone (limited data), heat		
Streptozocin: none		
Trabectedin: cold		
Vinblastine: hyaluronidase, heat		
Vincristine: hyaluronidase, heat		
Vindesine: hyaluronidase, heat		
Vinorelbine: hyaluronidase, heat		

Medication: Antidote, cold versus heat therapy if indicated.
Data from Wellstein, A. (2018). General principles in the pharmacotherapy of cancer. In L. L. Brunton, R. Hilal-Dandan, & B. C. Knollmann (Eds.), *Goodman and Gilman's the pharmacological basis of therapeutics* (13th ed.). New York: McGraw-Hill. eBook (chap. 65); Wilkes, G. M., & Barton-Burke, M. (2020). *2020–2021 Oncology nursing drug handbook* (23rd ed.). Burlington, MA: Jones and Bartlett Learning; Jackson-Rose, J., Del Monte, J., Groman, A., et al. (2017). Chemotherapy extravasation: Establishing a national benchmark for incidence among cancer centers. *Clinical Journal of Oncology Nursing, 21*(4), 438–445. https://doi.org/10.1188/17.CJON.438-445.

(4) Assess blood return on short-term/minibag infusions before, every 5 minutes during, and after the infusion is complete; limit administration to 30–60 minutes; do not administer through an IV pump; administer via gravity through a free-flowing primary IV line using a CSTD; remain with patient during the entire infusion.

(5) Assess blood return on IV pushes every 2–5 mL when administering IV push and every 5 minutes for piggyback infusion.

(6) Assess blood return on continuous infusions before, during (per health care facility policy), and at completion; always infuse through a central access device.

c. If extravasation occurs or is suspected, do the following:

(1) Immediately discontinue infusion, leaving needle or IV catheter in place.

(2) Aspirate residual medication and blood from the IV tubing.

(3) Remove the IV needle or device.

(4) Assess symptoms or suspected site of extravasation.

(5) For most medications, treatment of extravasation is nonpharmacologic.

(a) Avoid applying pressure to the area to decrease the spread of drug infiltrate.

(b) Administer antidote, if appropriate. Treatment for anthracycline extravasation with dexrazoxane is a 3-day regimen. It should begin as soon as possible but within 6 hours of extravasation (Totect [Dexrazoxane] [package insert]. Nashville, TN) (Cumberland Pharmaceuticals, 2017).

(c) Use heat or cold compresses as indicated for the agent extravasated (see Table 29.4).

(d) Elevate the affected extremity to decrease swelling.

(6) Notify the physician of extravasation; arrange follow-up.

(7) Document the extravasation event to include the date, time, needle size and type, site, method of administration, medications administered, sequence of antineoplastic agents, approximate amount of agent extravasated, patient-reported symptoms, nursing assessment of site, interventions, notification of physician, instructions given to patient, measurements and photographs, and follow-up measures.

V. Interventions to decrease the incidence and severity of complications of chemotherapy (Table 29.5)

TABLE 29.5   Specific Toxicities and Nursing Interventions for Selected Chemotherapeutic Agents

Toxicity	Chemotherapeutic Agents	Nursing Interventions
Hypersensitivity	Asparaginase Paclitaxel Bleomycin Carboplatin Cisplatin Docetaxel Etoposide Liposomal doxorubicin hydrochloride Oxaliplatin	Identify patients at risk—patients with previous allergic reactions to this or other medications; cycle of therapy. Assess for early signs of hypersensitivity—urticaria, pruritus, generalized uneasiness, hypertension, progressing to more severe reactions, including shortness of breath, chest pain, back pain, hypotension, bronchospasm, cyanosis, rigors, and chills. Taxane reactions generally occur at the onset of the first and/or second infusion; platinum reactions generally occur after the fifth infusion and during the infusion. Assess for signs of anaphylaxis-type reactions. Stop infusion if reaction is suspected. Administer oxygen to keep saturation 90% or greater. Administer medications to help resolve reaction (diphenhydramine, dexamethasone, famotidine, and epinephrine).
Pulmonary injury (pulmonary toxicity presenting as pneumonitis that may progress to pulmonary fibrosis)	Bleomycin Mitomycin Cyclophosphamide Methotrexate Cytosine arabinoside Carmustine Procarbazine	Monitor the cumulative dose of bleomycin, which should not exceed 400 units; doses above this limit significantly increase the risk of pulmonary toxicity. Avoid administering drugs with overlapping pulmonary toxicity together. Assess for signs of pulmonary toxicity—dry persistent cough, dyspnea, tachypnea, cyanosis, and basilar rales. Provide pulmonary toilet or adequate exercise. Higher levels of fraction of inspired oxygen (FiO_2) or use of G-CSF agents with bleomycin may increase pulmonary toxicity potential.
Renal toxicity	Cisplatin High-dose methotrexate	Monitor creatinine, BUN, and urinary output. Avoid the use of other nephrotoxic agents. Provide adequate hydration or diuresis.
Ototoxicity	Carboplatin Cisplatin Oxaliplatin	Teach patient to report tinnitus. Monitor dose levels; risk increases with dosage >60–75 mg/m^2. Refer patient for audiography, if indicated.
Ocular toxicity	Belantamab mafodotin Tisotumab vedotin-tftv	Visual acuity and slit lamp testing for corneal damage at baseline, prior to each dose, and more frequent if patient experiencing symptoms. Ocular toxicity may occur without vision changes. Ensure patient uses eye drops per medication-specific recommendations. Patients should avoid wearing contact lenses. Assess for signs of toxicity—dry eyes, blurred vision, and worsening visual acuity.
Hemorrhagic cystitis	Cyclophosphamide Ifosfamide	Ensure adequate fluid intake >3000 mL/day unless contraindicated. Have the patient void every 2–4 h during day and every 4 h at night. Educate patient to report signs of cystitis. Administer mesna as ordered. Oral doses of cyclophosphamide should be given early in the day.
Cardiotoxicity manifested by ECG changes, CHF, cardiomyopathy, angina, dysrhythmias, tachycardia, bradycardia	Doxorubicin Daunorubicin Epirubicin Idarubicin Cyclophosphamide (high dose) 5-Fluorouracil Capecitabine Mitoxantrone Trastuzumab Pertuzumab	Monitor cumulative doses of anthracyclines; maximum cumulative dose is 550 mg/m^2 for doxorubicin—doses above this significantly increase the risk for cardiotoxicity; maximal cumulative dose for doxorubicin is 450 mg/m^2 if patient received or is concurrently receiving radiation to mediastinum or cyclophosphamide. Assess for signs of cardiotoxicity, including ECG changes; weight gain, pedal edema, chest pain, heart rate (irregular, too fast, or too slow), shortness of breath, LVEF, and JVD. Mitoxantrone—risk is not as great as with daunorubicin and doxorubicin; risk is increased with cumulative doses >140 mg/m^2. HER2-targeted agents should not be administered concomitantly with anthracyclines due to increased cardiotoxicity. They should be administered sequentially (e.g., regimen Adriamycin-cyclophosphamide followed by Paclitaxel (taxol) trastuzumab (Herceptin).

Continued

TABLE 29.5   Specific Toxicities and Nursing Interventions for Selected Chemotherapeutic Agents—cont'd

Toxicity	Chemotherapeutic Agents	Nursing Interventions

Diarrhea	Irinotecan
	Panobinostat
	5-Fluorouracil
		Diarrhea may be managed with loperamide or atropine–diphenoxylate (Lomotil).
		Irinotecan:
		   Give atropine prophylactically.
		   Early and late diarrhea can be dose-limiting.
		   Early diarrhea occurs within 24 h of administration and is generally cholinergic; treatment may include atropine.
		   Late diarrhea occurs >24 h after dose and is managed with loperamide.
		   Monitor electrolytes.

Peripheral neuropathy	Paclitaxel Cisplatin Carboplatin Oxaliplatin Bortezomib Vincristine	Monitor for sensory and motor nerve changes and stocking–glove distribution of dysesthesia. Peripheral neuropathy appears in the distal extremities of hands and feet and progresses proximally. Dose modifications or delays may be utilized to minimize neuropathy. Loss of sense includes loss of proprioception, vibration, pain, temperature, and touch.
Hypotension	Etoposide	Rapid infusion may precipitate hypotension; administer over 30–60 min. Monitor the blood pressure.
Neurotoxicity (central)	Ifosfamide Methotrexate Vincristine Cytarabine Intrathecal administration	Monitor creatinine, BUN, and albumin; risk of neurotoxicity increases with decreased renal function and low albumin level. Neurologic checks should be performed every 4 h for patients at risk (e.g., high-dose ARA-C or ifosfamide). Complete a cerebellar toxicity assessment to monitor patient prior to administration of high-dose ARA-C, which should be performed prior to each dose with two nurses. Teach patients and families to report early signs of neurotoxicity.
Neurotoxicity (peripheral)	Paclitaxel Docetaxel Vincristine Vinorelbine Vinblastine Cisplatin Carboplatin Oxaliplatin	Assess for numbness and tingling of hands and feet, foot drop, decreased fine and gross motor abilities. Oxaliplatin—educate patients about cold sensitivity. Monitor for constipation as a potential early sign of neurotoxicity. Teach patient to report symptoms of neurotoxicity.
Nasopharyngitis	Cyclophosphamide	Infuse slowly over 30–60 min to decrease the risk of nasopharyngitis (aka *wasabi nose*).

BUN, Blood urea nitrogen; *CHF*, congestive heart failure; *ECG*, electrocardiography; *G-CSF*, granulocyte-colony-stimulating factor; *JVD*, jugular vein distention; *LVEF*, left ventricular ejection fraction.

Data from Wellstein, A. (2018). General principles in the pharmacotherapy of cancer. In L. L. Brunton, R. Hilal-Dandan, & B. C. Knollmann (Eds.), *Goodman and Gilman's the pharmacological basis of therapeutics* (13th ed.). New York: McGraw-Hill. eBook (chap. 65); Olsen, M., LeFebvre, K., & Brassil, K. (2019). *Chemotherapy and immunotherapy guidelines: Recommendations for practice.* Pittsburgh, PA: Oncology Nursing Press; BLENREP. (2022). *Package insert.* Research Triangle Park, NC: GlaxoSmithKline; Tisotumab vedotin-tftv. (2021). *Package insert.* Bothell, WA: Seagen Inc.; Collins, J. M. (2020). Cancer pharmacology. In J. E. Niederhuber, J. O. Armitage, J. H. Doroshow, M. B. Kastan, & J. E. Tepper. *Abeloff's clinical oncology* (6th ed.). Philadelphia, PA: Elsevier (chap. 25); Doroshow, J. H. (2020). Approach to the patient with cancer. In L. Goldman, A. I. Schafer, & R. L. Cecil. *Goldman-Cecil medicine* (26th ed.). Philadelphia, PA: Elsevier (chap. 169).

ORAL ADHERENCE

Overview

I. Definition of terms
   A. Adherence: The degree to which an individual's behavior corresponds to medical advice (Gonderen, Cakmak, & Kapucu, 2021).
   B. Medication adherence: Extent to which a person follows their health care provider's pharmaceutical recommendations (Skrabal Ross, Gunn, Suppiah, Patterson, & Olver, 2020).

II. Challenges (Skrabal, Ross et al., 2020)
   A. Treatment related
      1. Toxicities/side effects/adverse reactions
         a. Main reason of nonadherence
         b. Patients self-modify dosing to lessen side effects
         c. Vary depending on the agent and individual tolerance
      2. Complicated regimen
         a. Multiple doses per day
         b. Noncontinuous cycles (i.e., 14 days on, 7 off)
      3. Polypharmacy

a. Patients taking 10 or more prescriptions are less likely to get them filled at the pharmacy
b. Taking multiple medications increases the risk of drug–drug and drug–food interactions
4. Refills
a. Patients do not fill their prescriptions 25% of the time and do not take them about 50% of the time
b. Free medications or discounted medications are key to keeping patients adherent (Washburn & Thompson, 2020)
B. Patient related
1. Unintentional disregard to take medication
a. 38%–62% of patients reported forgetting to take their medication
b. Patients forget to pick up their prescriptions
c. Patients forget provider instructions
d. Patients forget the medication schedule
e. Age <50 years old most likely to forget (Skrabal, Ross et al., 2020)
2. Disease education
a. Patients less satisfied with the information doctors provided had lower compliance
b. Difficulty understanding prescription instructions led to lower compliance
c. Drug–food and drug–drug interactions led to lowered compliance
3. Perceived lack of efficacy by the patient
a. Cancer is seen as more of a chronic disease and is treated with oral medications like other chronic illnesses; this may be hard for patients to accept (Fennimore & Ginex, 2017).
b. Improved compliance coincides with the necessity of taking medication (Fennimore & Ginex, 2017).
4. Comorbidities lead to inferior results if patients are nonadherent to medications (Washburn & Thompson, 2020).
5. Expense
a. High medication out-of-pocket expenses lead to nonadherence.
b. Unreasonable copayments lead to decreased compliance and delays in refilling prescriptions.
6. Age—both younger and older are at risk for nonadherence
C. Health care system barriers
1. Lack of continuity of care among specialists
2. Poor patient education and follow-up
3. Limitations of the electronic medical record
4. Poor doctor–patient relationship

Assessment

I. Regimen
A. Over half of all newly approved cancer medications are oral agents (Fennimore & Ginex, 2017)
B. One in four medications used to treat cancer is an oral antineoplastic medication (Gonderen, Cakmak, Kapucu, 2021)

C. Complexity of regimen including multiple medications and dosing schedules
D. Number of pills taken and the patient's ability to open the packages and swallow the pills
E. Management of side effects
F. Food and drug interactions (ONS, 2022)
II. Demographics favorable for nonadherence (ONS, 2022)
A. Age—young and old
B. High school education or lower
C. Low socioeconomic status
D. Drug and alcohol abuse
E. High medication cost
F. Lack of insurance
G. Rural living area/limited access to health care (Konstantinou et al., 2020)
H. Language barriers
I. Regimen does not fit into the patient's lifestyle
J. Inability to safely store medications in the home (ONS, 2022)
III. Literacy
A. The capacity to read educational materials may be limited due to a lack of literacy (Washburn & Thompson, 2020).
B. Poor understanding of prescription instructions and medical terminology is linked to lower education (Konstantinou et al., 2020).
IV. Outcomes
A. Nonadherence leads to reduced drug efficacy including a negative impact on progression-free survival and disease recurrence, leading to poor disease outcomes including higher mortality
B. Overadherence leads to increased toxicities
1. Oral chemotherapy medicines have a narrow therapeutic index; there is little discrepancy between effective and toxic concentrations
2. Rise in hospitalizations, clinical visits, and duration of stay (Gonderen, Cakmak, & Kapucu, 2021)

Management

I. Strategies to improve adherence
A. Patient education (ONS, 2022)
B. Appropriate reading level education including chronic side effects and notifying the provider of any new or uncontrolled symptoms (Fennimore & Ginex, 2017)
C. Telephone follow-up calls at home (Gonderen, Cakmak, & Kapucu, 2021)
D. Text messages including reminders and medication education
E. Reinforcement and motivational messages
F. Patient calendars for easy reference of complicated regimens
G. Patient diaries to track side effects and symptoms
H. Medication assistance programs for financial assistance (ONS, 2022)
I. Pillboxes
J. Motivational interviewing

1. Evidenced-based counseling program to improve adherence and promote positive health behaviors
2. Focuses on the patient's specific needs for change

K. Online forums for support and side effect management (Konstantinou et al., 2020)

REFERENCES

Association for Clinical Oncology (ASCO). (2020). *Quality Oncology Practice Initiative Certification Program standards manual.*

Collins, J. M. (2020). Cancer pharmacology. In J. E. Niederhuber, J. O. Armitage, J. H. Doroshow, M. B. Kastan, & J. E. Tepper (Eds.), *Abeloff's clinical oncology* (6th ed.). Philadelphia, PA: Elsevier (Chap. 25).

Connor, T. H., MacKenzie, B. A., DeBord, D. G., Trout, D. B., & O'Callaghan, J. P. (2016). NIOSH list of antineoplastic and other hazardous dru gs in healthcare settings, 2016. In: *National Institute for Occupational Safety and Health, DHHS (NIOSH) publication number 2016–161 (Supersedes 2014–138).* Cincinnati, OH: U.S. Department of Health and Human Services, Centers for Disease Control and Prevention.

Cumberland, Pharmaceuticals. (2017). *Totectfi (Dexrazoxane) [package insert].* Nashville, TN: Cumberland Pharmaceuticals.

Doroshow, J. H. (2020). Approach to the patient with cancer. In L. Goldman, A. I. Schafer, & R. L. Cecil (Eds.), *Goldman-Cecil medicine* (26th ed.). Philadelphia, PA: Elsevier. chap. 169.

Fennimore, L. A., & Ginex, P. K. (2017). Oral agents for cancer treatment: Effective strategies to assess and enhance medication adherence. *Nursing Clinics of North America, 52*(1), 115–131. https://doi.org/10.1016/j.cnur.2016.10.007.

Gasparovic, L., Weiler, S., Higi, L., & Burden, A. M. (2020). Incidence of differentiation syndrome associated with treatment regimens in acute myeloid leukemia: A systematic review of the literature. *Journal of Clinical Medicine, 9*(10), 3342. https://doi.org/10.3390/jcm9103342. PMID: 33081000; PMCID: PMC7603213.

Gönderen Çakmak, H. S., & Kapucu, S. (2021). The effect of educational follow-up with the motivational interview technique on self-efficacy and drug adherence in ca ncer patients using oral chemotherapy treatment: A randomized controlled trial. *Seminars in Oncology Nursing, 37*(2), 151140. https://doi.org/10.1016/j.soncn.2021.151140.

Gorski, L. A., Hadaway, L., Hagle, M. E., Broadhurst, D., Clare, S., Kleidon, T., et al. (2021). *Infusion therapy standards of practice, 8th edition. Journal of Infusion Nursing, 44*(1S Suppl 1), S1–S224.

Imlygic. (2017). *Package insert.* Thousand Oaks, CA: Amgen, Inc.

Jackson-Rose, J., Del Monte, J., Groman, A., et al. (2017). Chemotherapy extravasation: Establishing a national benchmark for incidence among cancer centers. *Clinical Journal of Oncology Nursing, 21*(4), 438–445. https://doi.org/10.1188/17.CJON.438-445.

Karius, D. L., & Colvin, C. M. (2021). Managing chemotherapy extravasation across transitions of care. *Journal of Infusion Nursing, 44*(1), 14–20. https://doi.org/10.1097/NAN.0000000000000411.

Konstantinou, P., Kassianos, A. P., Georgiou, G., Panayides, A., Papageorgiou, A., Almas, I., et al. (2020). Barriers, facilitators, and interventions for medication adherence across chronic conditions with the highest non-adherence rates: A scoping review with recommendations for intervention development. *Translational Behavioral Medicine, 10*(6), 1390–1398. https://doi.org/10.1093/tbm/ibaa118.

Lehman, A. D., Howard, A., & Mancini, R. (2019). Chemotherapy administration sequencing: An update on the current literature. *Journal of Hematology Oncology Pharmacy, 9*(4), 175–181.

Malumbres, M. (2020). Control of the cell cycle. In J. E. Niederhuber, J. O. Armitage, J. H. Doroshow, M. B. Kastan, & J. E. Tepper (Eds.), *Abeloff's clinical oncology* (6th ed.). Philadelphia, PA: Elsevier (chap. 4).

Morales, A. S. R., Joy, J. K., & Zbona, D. M. (2020). Administration sequence for multi-agent oncolytic regimens. *Journal of Oncology Pharmacy Practice, 26*(4), 933–942. https://doi.org/10.1177/1078155219895070. Epub 2020 Jan 21. PMID: 31964220.

NCCN. (2020). *Chemotherapy order templates (NCCN Templates®) Appendix B.* https://www.nccn.org/professionals/OrderTemplates/PDF/appendix_B.pdf.

Neuss, M. N., Gilmore, T. R., Belderson, K. M., Billett, A. L., Conti-Kalchik, T., Harvey, B. E., et al. (2017). 2016 Updated American Society of Clinical Oncology/Oncology Nursing Society Chemotherapy Administration safety standards, including standards for pediatric oncology. *Oncology Nursing Forum, 44*(1), 31–43. https://doi.org/10.1188/17.ONF.31-43.

Olsen, M., LeFebvre, K., & Brassil, K. (2019). *Chemotherapy and immunotherapy guidelines: Recommendations for practice.* Pittsburgh, PA: Oncology Nursing Press.

Oncology Nursing Society (ONS). (2018). Toolkit for safe handling of hazardous drugs for nurses in oncology. https://www.ons.org/sites/default/files/2018-06/ONS_Safe_Handling_Toolkit_0.pdf. Retrieved 12.03.22.

Oncology Nursing Society (ONS). (2022). Oral anticancer medication toolkit. https://www.ons.org/clinical-practice-resources/oral-adherence-toolkit. Accessed 02.06.22.

Pfizer. (2016). *Zinecardfi (dexrazoxane) [package insert].* New York: Pfizer.

Pollyea, D. A., Tallman, M. S., de Botton, S., Kantarjian, H. M., Collins, R., Stein, A. S., et al. (2019). Enasidenib, an inhibitor of mutant IDH2 proteins, induces durable remissions in older patients with newly diagnosed acute myeloid leukemia. *Leukemia, 33*(11), 2575–2584. https://doi.org/10.1038/s41375-019-0472-2. Epub 2019 Apr 9. PMID: 30967620.

Polovich, M., & Olsen, M. M. (2018). *Safe handling of hazardous drugs* (3rd ed.). Pittsburgh, PA: ONS.

Power, L. A., & Coyne, J. W. (2018). ASHP guidelines on handling hazardous drugs. *American Journal of Health-System Pharmacy, 75*(24), 1996–2031.

Roboz, G. J., DiNardo, C. D., Stein, E. M., de Botton, S., Mims, A. S., Prince, G. T., et al. (2020). Ivosidenib induces deep durable remissions in patients with newly diagnosed IDH1-mutant acute myeloid leukemia. *Blood, 135*(7), 463–471. https://doi.org/10.1182/blood.2019002140. PMID: 31841594; PMCID: PMC7019193.

Skrabal Ross, X., Gunn, K. M., Suppiah, V., Patterson, P., & Olver, I. (2020). A review of factors influencing non-adherence to oral antineoplastic drugs. *Support Care in Cancer, 28*(9), 4043–4050. https://doi.org/10.1007/s00520-020-05469-y.

USP. (2020). USP general chapter 800 "Hazardous drugs – Handling in healthcare settings." http://www.usp.org/compounding/general-chapter-hazardous-drugs-handling-healthcare.

USP. (2021). USP general chapter 797 "Pharmaceutical compounding – Sterile preparations." http://www.uspnf.com/notices/general-chapter-797-proposed-revision.

Washburn, D. J., & Thompson, K. (2020). Medication adherence barriers: Development and retrospective pilot test of an evidence-based screening instrument. *Clinical Journal of Oncology Nursing, 24*(2), E13–E20. https://doi.org/10.1188/20.CJON.E13-E20.

Wellstein, A. (2018). General principles in the pharmacotherapy of cancer. In L. L. Brunton, R. Hilal-Dandan, & B. C. Knollmann (Eds.), *Goodman and Gilman's the pharmacological basis of therapeutics* (13th ed.). New York: McGraw-Hill. eBook (chap. 65).

Wellstein, A., Giaccone, G., Atkins, M. B., & Sausville, E. A. (2018). Cytotoxic drugs. In L. L. Brunton, R. Hilal-Dandan, & B. C. Knollmann (Eds.), *Goodman and Gilman's the pharmacological basis of therapeutics* (13th ed.). New York: McGraw-Hill. eBook (chap. 66).

Wilkes, G. M., & Barton-Burke, M. (2020). *2020–2021 Oncology nursing drug handbook* (23rd ed.). Burlington, MA: Jones and Bartlett Learning.

30

Biotherapies: Targeted Therapies and Immunotherapies

Kristine Deano Abueg and Brenda Keith

BIOTHERAPIES

Overview

I. The terms *biotherapy*, *immunotherapy*, and *targeted therapy* encompass a wide range of modalities, targets, and mechanisms. Sometimes referred to as *molecularly targeted drugs or therapies* or *precision medicines*.
  A. Biotherapy—a broad range of treatments made from living organisms that mimic or augment the signals that normally control cell functions to reverse the deleterious effects of tumor genes. These substances may occur naturally in the body or may be made in the laboratory (National Cancer Institute [NCI], 2022a, 2022b).
  B. For the purpose of this chapter's discussion, biotherapies will be subdivided into two main categories: targeted therapies and immunotherapies.
    1. Biotherapies that **interfere** with specific molecules or pathways involved with tumor growth and progression are referred to as *targeted therapies* (NCI, 2019). Examples include lapatinib and trastuzumab, which both target human epidermal growth factor receptor 2 (HER/EGFR-2) implicated in tumor growth and metastases.
    2. Biotherapies that **use, stimulate, augment, or suppress** the immune system are referred to as *immunotherapy* or *biological response modifier therapy* and include monoclonal antibodies (moAbs), checkpoint inhibitors (CPIs), cytokines, vaccines, and T-cell transfer therapy (American Society of Clinical Oncology [ASCO], 2018; NCI, 2019; Zhang & Chen, 2018; Zhang & Zhang, 2020).
II. Genomic instability encompasses various aspects of mutations resulting in altered protein products, which disrupt the biological processes in which they are involved (Das, Choudhury, Kumar, & Baruah, 2021; Martínez-Jímenez et al., 2020).
  A. Normal cell metabolism, growth, and proliferation are tightly controlled by circulating growth signals, regulatory cytokines, and cell signaling pathways.
  B. Actions of altered gene products include the following:
    1. Activation in the absence of appropriate growth signals
    2. Bypassing cell signaling pathways
    3. Bypassing or resistance to regulatory inhibition

III. Companion diagnostics evaluate molecular, genetic, and chemical characteristics of the tumor for appropriate application of the targeted therapy (Table 30.1; Lin, 2020; Zhong et al., 2021).
  A. Developed in parallel with the drug and have clinical utility after a drug's approval; included in the labeling instructions for both the therapeutic product and the corresponding diagnostic test (Food & Drug Administration [FDA], 2020).
  B. A companion assay is used to identify patients who are:
    1. Most likely to benefit from a therapeutic product
    2. Likely to be at increased risk of serious adverse reactions as a result of treatment with a particular therapeutic product (NCI, 2019)
IV. Biosimilars are Food & Drug Administration (FDA) approved agents that are highly similar and have no clinically meaningful difference in safety, purity, and potency from the FDA reference product (FDA, 2022; Tariman, 2018).

TARGETED THERAPIES

Overview

I. Targeted therapies interfere with molecules associated with cancer cell proliferation, growth, spread, and metabolism (AL-Busairi & Khajah, 2019; Bedard, Hyman, Davids, & Siu, 2020; Zam & Ali, 2021). Specific targeted oncogenic mechanisms are as follows:
  A. Binding and inhibition of excess circulating growth factors: aberrant, excessive cell growth in cancer is often mediated by the interaction of excessive growth signals with overabundant receptors. Binding of growth factors or their receptors effectively "puts the brakes" on these pathways.
  B. Competing with aberrant cancer molecules for binding sites at specific activation points along the cell signaling pathway.
    1. Proliferation, differentiation, migration, metabolism, and apoptotic processes are tightly regulated by intracellular cell signaling pathways.
    2. Deregulation of cell signaling pathways leads to oncogene activation within a cell resulting in aberrant proliferation, invasion, metastases, and vascularization.

TABLE 30.1 Companion Diagnostics

Summary of Selected Agents Whose FDA Indication Requires Expression of Specific Biomarker

Agent	Biomarker
Erlotinib	EGFR exon 19 deletion or exon 21 L858R substitution
Cetuximab	EGFR, KRAS (nonmutated; wild type); BRAF V600E
Panitumumab	KRAS (nonmutated; wild type)
Afatinib	EGFR
Gefitinib	EGFR exon 19 deletion or exon 21 L858R substitution
Dacomitinib	EGFR exon 19 deletion or exon 21 L858R substitution
Osimertinib	EGFR exon 19 deletion or exon L858R substitution EGFR T790M
Imatinib	BCR-ABL C-kit PDGFR-b
Dasatinib	BCR-ABL
Nilotinib	BCR-ABL
Ponatinib	BCR-ABL T315I
Trastuzumab	HER2-neu
Pertuzumab	HER2-neu
Lapatinib	HER2-neu
Neratinib	HER2-neu
Trastuzumab emtansine	HER2-neu
Tucatinib	HER2-neu
Trastuzumab deruxtecan	HER2-neu
Pembrolizumab	PD-L1
Cemiplimab	PD-L1 (non–small-cell lung cancer indication)
Atezolizumab	PD-L1
Olaparib	BRCA
Rucaparib	BRCA
Niraparib	BRCA
Rucaparib	BRCA
Trametinib–dabrafenib	BRAF
Alectinib (Alecensa)	ALK
Ceritinib (Zykadia)	ALK
Crizotinib (Xalkori)	ALK
Brigatinib (Alunbrig)	ALK
Erlotinib	EGFR
Crizotinib	ALK
Vemurafenib	BRAF
Encorafenib	BRAF
Ivosidenib	IDH1
Capmatinib	MET exon 14 skipping
Alpelisib	PIK3CA
Larotrectinib	NTRK
Gilteritinib	FLT3
Midostaurin	FLT3
Lumakras	KRAS G12C mutation
Tazemetostat	EZH2

ALK, Anaplastic lymphoma kinase; *BCR-ABL*, breakpoint cluster region–Abelson murine leukemia; *BRAF*, Braf proto-oncogene, serine/threonine kinase; *EGFR*, epidermal growth factor receptor; *FDA*, Food & Drug Administration; *HER*, human epidermal growth factor receptor; *KRAS*, kirsten rat sarcoma viral oncogene homolog; *NTRK*, neurotrophic tyrosine receptor kinase; *PDGFR*, platelet-derived growth factor receptor.
From *FDA*. (2022). *List of cleared or approved companion diagnostic devices (in vitro and imaging tools).* https://www.fda.gov/medical-devices/in-vitro-diagnostics/list-cleared-or-approved-companion-diagnostic-devices-in-vitro-and-imaging-tools.

3. Deregulation results from excessive production of constituent proteins or production of proteins that are activated independent of ligands.

4. Inhibition or binding of the aberrant protein prevents the transmission of molecular "messages" down the cell signaling pathway. Doing so effectively shuts down the aberrant cell signaling pathway.

C. Affecting regulatory proteins involved with apoptosis and the cell life cycle (AL-Busairi & Khajah, 2019).

II. Targeted therapy differs from standard chemotherapy in several ways. See Chapter 29.

A. Act on specific molecular targets; most standard chemotherapies act on rapidly dividing normal and cancerous cells. Deliberately chosen or designed to interact with their target, whereas many standard chemotherapies were identified because they kill cells.

B. Targeted therapies are cytostatic, meaning they block tumor cell development and metabolism, whereas standard chemotherapy agents are cytotoxic, meaning they destroy already developed tumors (Anttila et al., 2019; NCI, 2022a, 2022b).

C. Targeted therapies are designed to enhance activity towards cancer cells while reducing their systemic toxicity profile (AL-Busairi & Khajah, 2019).

III. The efficacy and specificity of targeted therapy lie heavily on the appropriate identification and selection of target molecules; thus, target molecules are selected on their ability to meet specific criteria (Gerber, Sibener, Lee, & Gee, 2020; Lee, Tan, & Oon, 2018; NCI, 2022a; 2022b):

A. Targeted tumor molecules should be critical to cell growth or survival.

B. Targeted tumor molecules should be disproportionately overexpressed on cancer cells or in tumor environments and with low to minimal expression on normal cells.

1. An example is the human EGFR-2 (HER2), which is present in normal cells but is expressed at high levels on the surface of cancer cells (Oh & Bang, 2020).

2. Therapies targeting the HER2 pathway (trastuzumab, pertuzumab, and ado-trastuzumab emtansine, tucatinib, trastuzumab deruxtecan) are associated with significant survival benefits in HER2-positive breast cancer (Meric-Bernstam et al., 2019).

C. Target molecules may be highly expressed in normal and malignant cells, for example, CD20, which has a role in B-cell maturation and development; also expressed in B-cell lymphomas (Klein, Jamois, & Nielsen, 2021).

D. Proteins produced because of carcinogenic gene mutations are called neoantigens and are common targets (Martinez-Jimenez et al., 2020; Zhang et al., 2021).

1. An example is the cell growth signaling protein BRAF (Braf proto-oncogene, serine/threonine kinase) V600E, which is a mutation found in many melanoma diagnoses. The cell growth signaling protein causes BRAF to keep dividing without stopping, causing a tumor to develop.

2. Vemurafenib targets this mutant form of the BRAF protein.

E. Chromosomal abnormalities may be potential targets (Zhang et al., 2021).

1. Chromosomal abnormalities present in some cancer cells, but not normal cells, may result in the creation of a fusion gene whose product is called a fusion protein.

2. For example, imatinib mesylate targets the breakpoint cluster region–Abelson murine leukemia (BCR-ABL) fusion protein, which is made from pieces of two genes that get joined together in some leukemia cells (Philadelphia chromosome).

3. Another example is anaplastic lymphoma kinase (ALK), which is a rearrangement of the echinoderm microtubule-associated protein-like 4 gene and the ALK gene resulting in a fusion oncogene. ALK-positive non–small-cell lung cancer occurs in approximately 5% of all lung cancer (Eldridge, 2020).

IV. Targeted therapies can be classified according to their targets and their mechanism of action.

A. Targets: target molecules include, but are not limited to, cell surface displayed antigens, circulating growth factors, ligands, and intracellular cell signal molecules.

B. Mechanisms: either *engineered moAbs* that bind with target molecules either outside the cell or on the cell surface as they are relatively large and generally cannot enter cells or *small-molecule inhibitors* that are typically developed for targets located inside of the cell (NCI, 2022a, 2022b). MoAbs can be classified as both a targeted therapy and an immunotherapy and will be discussed under immunotherapy sections (Sadeghalvad & Rezaei, 2021).

V. Target molecules can be classified by their role in cancer cell growth, migration, and metabolism. Major classes of target molecules are described here.

A. Circulating growth factors in serum that stimulate growth (e.g., vascular endothelial growth factor [VEGF]) (Chen et al., 2021).

B. Cluster of differentiation molecules: membrane-bound antigens used for identification and classification for immunophenotyping of cells (e.g., CD20 in lymphoma) (Klein et al., 2021).

C. Extracellular portion of membrane-bound tyrosine kinases (also referred to as *tyrosine kinase receptor* [TKR]): receive and initiate cell signaling pathways either upon binding to a growth factor found in serum or upon interaction (dimerization) with another TKR. Examples include VEGF receptor and endothelial growth factor receptor (Chen et al., 2021; Oh & Bang, 2020).

D. Intracellular protein kinase chains that communicate signals from the membrane-bound TKR to the DNA.

1. The most important protein kinases are the serine/threonine and tyrosine kinases.

2. Examples include the protein kinases such as rat sarcoma virus (RAS), rapidly accelerated fibrosarcoma

(RAF), mesenchymal–epithelial transition (MET), and extracellular signal-related kinase (ERK).

E. Cell cycle kinases that control the mitotic cell cycle (e.g., CDK4, CDK6) (Zhong et al., 2021).

F. Intracellular enzymes that control DNA repair and cellular apoptosis. Main examples include proteasome inhibitors and poly(ADP-ribose) polymerase (PARP) inhibitors.

G. Angiogenesis proteins that promote vascular development in tumor environments.

VI. Major classes of target molecule inhibitors are described here.

A. Signal transduction inhibitors block the activities of molecules that participate in the process by which a cell responds to signals from its environment. Normal cells have overlapping pathways that allow for alternative signal transduction when one is inhibited; cancer cells have hyperactive pathways due to overexpression of certain proteins or mutations (AL-Busairi & Khajah, 2019). Situations where signal transduction inhibitors could be utilized:

1. A cell surface growth factor receptor, known as EGFR1 when bound to a complementary ligand, can activate various downstream signaling molecules inside the cell through tyrosine kinase activity. This type of activity is seen in some non–small-cell lung cancers. Mutations within the receptor kinase portion of EGFR1 can also occur (e.g., L858R point mutation), resulting in cancer cell growth.

2. Overexpression of growth factor receptors (e.g., HER2) can result in the proliferation of cancer cell growth (AL-Busairi & Khajah, 2019).

3. In some cancers, malignant cells are stimulated to divide continuously without being prompted to do so by external growth factors (NCI, 2022a, 2022b).

B. Angiogenesis inhibitors block the growth of new blood vessels and terminate the blood supply to tumor tissues and microenvironment, resulting in widespread hypoxia and necrosis. Some angiogenesis inhibitors interfere with the action of VEGF. Other angiogenesis inhibitors target other molecules that stimulate new blood vessel growth.

C. Apoptosis inducers cause cancer cells to undergo a process of controlled cell death called apoptosis. Cancer cells have strategies to avoid apoptosis. Apoptosis inducers can bypass these strategies to cause the death of cancer cells.

D. Gene expression modulators modify the function of proteins that play a role in controlling gene expression.

E. Immunotherapies trigger the immune system to destroy cancer cells. Some immunotherapies are moAbs that recognize specific molecules on the surface of cancer cells. Other moAbs bind to certain immune cells to help these cells better kill cancer cells. Immunotherapy is discussed later in this chapter (Sadeghalvad & Rezaei, 2021).

F. Cancer vaccines and gene therapy are sometimes considered targets because they interfere with the growth of specific cancer cells (NCI, 2022a, 2022b).

VII. Small-molecule inhibitors (Table 30.2).

A. Generally, orally available, synthetic chemicals of smaller molecular size and weight than moAbs. They are typically developed for targets that are located inside the cell (NCI, 2022a, 2022b).

1. Small molecule–targeted therapies have a higher rate of cell entry relative to moAbs and are designed to interfere with intracellular signaling molecules (AL-Busairi & Khajah, 2019).

2. May interact with multiple targets simultaneously or act on a single target (Bedard et al., 2020). Multiple-target inhibitors increase the risk of toxicity.

B. Unlike moAbs, small-molecule inhibitors do not stimulate immune response.

VIII. Types of small-molecule inhibitors: the targets of small-molecule inhibitors cover a large scope (Zhong et al., 2021).

A. Protein kinase is a kind of enzyme that catalyzes the transfer of a phosphate group from adenosine triphosphate (ATP) to a hydroxyl group and is key for the regulation of cellular processes.

1. It is important in cell growth, proliferation, and differentiation.

2. Protein kinases can be classified as:
   a. tyrosine kinases (both receptor and nonreceptor tyrosine kinases)
   b. serine/threonine kinases
   c. tyrosine kinase-like enzymes

3. Small molecules intended to impede with the enzymatic action of the target protein are enzyme inhibitors. They are classified according to the enzyme they inhibit.

B. Receptor tyrosine kinase inhibitors (TKIs) are agents that target receptor tyrosine kinases.

1. ALK inhibitors. ALK is a single transmembrane tyrosine kinase of the insulin receptor family and can activate multiple downstream signaling pathways. It has an important role in the development of the nervous system. Constitutive activation of ALK through point mutations or chromosomal rearrangements has been identified in multiple human cancers.

2. Cellular-MET factor (c-MET) inhibitors. c-MET is also known as hepatocyte growth factor receptor. Aberrant activation of c-MET has been implicated in the development of various solid tumors.

3. EGFR inhibitors. EGFR is a transmembrane protein implicated in a wide variety of biological processes. First-generation EGFR-TKIs are reversible inhibitors (e.g., gefitinib, erlotinib). Second-generation irreversible EGFR-TKIs (e.g., afatinib, dacomitinib) are designed to conquer mutations in EGFR (e.g., T790M). Osimertinib is the first approved

TABLE 30.2   Small-Molecule Inhibitors

Primary Therapeutic Target	Small-Molecule Inhibitors	Side Effects	Administration Considerations
ALK	Alectinib (Alecensa) RET	Fatigue, edema, constipation	Take with food
	Ceritinib (Zykadia) IGF-1R, InsR, ROS1	Diarrhea, fatigue, abdominal pain	With food
	Crizotinib (Xalkori) HGFR, ROS1	Vision problems, pneumonitis, nausea, diarrhea, vomiting	With food
	Brigatinib (Alunbrig) ROS1, IGF-1R, FLT3, EGFR	Nausea, diarrhea, fatigue, cough	With/without food
BCR-ABL	Bosutinib (Bosulif) Src family	Diarrhea, nausea, myelosuppression, rash,	With food
	Imatinib mesylate (Gleevec) PDGF, SCF, c-Kit (CD117)	Edema, nausea, vomiting, muscle cramps, musculoskeletal pain	With food
	Dasatinib (SPRYCEL SRC family, c-KIT, EPHA2, PDGFR-b)	Myelosuppression, fluid retention, diarrhea, headache, skin rash	With/without food
	Nilotinib (Tasigna)	Myelosuppression, rash, nausea, headache	Without food
BCR-ABL; T3151 (VEGFR, PDGFR, EPH receptors, SRC kinases, Kit, RET, TIE2, FLT3)	Ponatinib (Iclusig)	Myelosuppression, rash, nausea, headache, hypertension	With/without food
BCL-2	Venetoclax (Venclexta)	Myelosuppression, diarrhea, nausea, upper respiratory tract infection, fatigue	With food
BRAF V600E	Dabrafenib (Tafinlar) (administer with trametinib)	Pyrexia, rash, chills, headache, arthralgia, nausea	Without food
	Vemurafenib (Zelboraf)	Arthralgia, rash, alopecia, fatigue, photosensitivity reaction	With/without food
BTK	Acalabrutinib (Calquence)	Anemia, thrombocytopenia, headache, neutropenia, diarrhea, fatigue, myalgia, bruising	With/without food
	Ibrutinib (Imbruvica)	Myelosuppression, diarrhea, muscle pain	With/without food
CDK 4 and 6	Abemaciclib (Verzenio)	Diarrhea, neutropenia, nausea, abdominal pain, infections	With/without food
	Palbociclib (Ibrance)	Neutropenia, infections, leukopenia, fatigue, nausea	With/without food
	Ribociclib (Kisqali)	Neutropenia, nausea, fatigue, diarrhea, leukopenia,	With/without food
EGFR	Erlotinib (Tarceva)	Rash, diarrhea, anorexia, fatigue, dyspnea, cough, nausea, and vomiting	Empty stomach
	Afatinib (Gilotrif) HER2, HER4	Diarrhea, rash/acneiform dermatitis, stomatitis, paronychia, dry skin, decreased appetite, nausea	Empty stomach
	Gefitinib (Iressa) Reversible inhibitor	Skin reactions, diarrhea	With/without food
	Osimertinib (Tagrisso)	Diarrhea, rash, dry skin, fatigue	With/without food
HER1/EGFR and HER2	Lapatinib (Tykerb)	Diarrhea, palmar–plantar erythrodysesthesia, nausea, rash, vomiting, fatigue	At least 1 h before or 1 h after a meal
	Neratinib (Nerlynx) Irreversible inhibitor EGFR, HER4	Diarrhea, nausea, abdominal pain, fatigue, vomiting, rash, stomatitis, decreased appetite, muscle spasms, dyspepsia, AST or ALT increase	With food
Multiple kinases (VEGFR-1, -2, -3; FGFR-1, -2, -3, -4; PDGFR-a, KIT, and RET)	Lenvatinib (Lenvima)	Hypertension, fatigue, diarrhea, arthralgia/myalgia, decreased appetite, weight decreased, nausea, stomatitis, headache	With/without food

TABLE 30.2   Small-Molecule Inhibitors—cont'd

Primary Therapeutic Target	Small-Molecule Inhibitors	Side Effects	Administration Considerations
Multiple tyrosine kinases (EGFR, VEGFR families, RET, BRK, TIE2, members of the EPH receptor and Src kinase families)	Vandetanib (Caprelsa)	Diarrhea/colitis, rash, acneiform dermatitis, hypertension, nausea, headache	With/without food
VEGFR-1, VEGFR-2, VEGFR-3	Axitinib (Inlyta)	Diarrhea, hypertension, fatigue, decreased appetite, nausea, dysphonia, palmar–plantar erythrodysesthesia (hand–foot) syndrome	With/without food
VEGF, EGFR (RET, VEGFR-1, -2, -3, Kit, PDGFR-a and b, FGFR-1, -2, TIE2, DDR2, TrkA, Eph2A, RAF-1, BRAF, BRAF V600E, SAPK2, PTK5, Abl, CSF1R)	Regorafenib (Stivarga)	Pain (including gastrointestinal and abdominal pain), asthenia/fatigue, diarrhea, decreased appetite/food intake, hypertension, infection	Take with a low-fat breakfast
Multiple tyrosine kinases (MET, VEGFR-1, -2, and -3, AXL, RET, ROS1, TYRO3, MER, KIT, TRKB, FLT3, and TIE2)	Cabozantinib (Cabometyx) Tablet form (Cometriq) Capsule form	Diarrhea, fatigue, nausea, decreased appetite, hypertension, palmar–plantar erythrodysesthesia	At least 2 h before and at least 1 h after meals
MEK1 and MEK2	Cobimetinib (Cotellic) Reversible inhibitor	Diarrhea, photosensitivity reaction, nausea, pyrexia, vomiting, elevated liver function tests	With/without food
	Trametinib (Mekinist)	Pyrexia, rash, diarrhea, lymphedema	With/without food
PARP	Niraparib (Zejula)	Myelosuppression, palpitations, nausea, constipation	With/without food
	Olaparib (Lynparza)	Myelosuppression, fatigue, nausea, infection	With/without food
	Rucaparib (Rubraca)	Nausea, fatigue (including asthenia), vomiting, anemia, dysgeusia, AST/ALT elevation, constipation, decreased appetite, diarrhea, thrombocytopenia, neutropenia, stomatitis, nasopharyngitis/URI, rash, abdominal pain/distention, dyspnea	With/without food
PI3K	Copanlisib (Aliqopa)	Hyperglycemia, diarrhea, hypertension, myelosuppression, and nausea	IV
	Idelalisib (Zydelig)	Diarrhea, fatigue, nausea, cough, pyrexia, abdominal pain, pneumonia, and rash	With/without food
Proteasome inhibitor	Bortezomib (Velcade)	Nausea, diarrhea, myelosuppression, peripheral neuropathy, fatigue, neuralgia, constipation, vomiting, rash, pyrexia, and anorexia	IV/SQ
	Carfilzomib (Kyprolis)	Anemia, fatigue, thrombocytopenia, nausea, pyrexia, dyspnea, diarrhea, headache, cough, and edema peripheral	IV
	Ixazomib (Ninlaro)	Diarrhea, constipation, thrombocytopenia, peripheral neuropathy, nausea, peripheral edema, vomiting, and back pain	1 h before or at least 2 h after food
IDH2 enzyme	Enasidenib (Idhifa)	Nausea, vomiting, diarrhea, and elevated bilirubin	With/without food

Continued

TABLE 30.2 Small-Molecule Inhibitors—cont'd

Primary Therapeutic Target	Small-Molecule Inhibitors	Side Effects	Administration Considerations
mTOR	Everolimus (Afinitor)	Stomatitis, infection, rash, and fatigue	With/without food
	Temsirolimus (Torisel)	Rash, asthenia, mucositis, nausea, edema, anorexia, anemia, hyperglycemia, hyperlipidemia, hypertriglyceridemia, and elevated transaminases	IV
Multiple tyrosine kinases (VEGFR-1, -2, -3; PDGFR-a and -b; FGR-1 and -3, Kit, Itk, Lck, c-Fms)	Pazopanib (Votrient)	Diarrhea, hypertension, hair color changes (depigmentation), nausea, anorexia, and vomiting	At least 1 h before or 2 h after a meal
JAK1 and JAK2	Ruxolitinib (Jakafi)	Myelosuppression, bruising, dizziness, and headache	With/without food
Smoothened (a protein involved in hedgehog pathway signal transduction)	Sonidegib (Odomzo)	Muscle spasms, alopecia, dysgeusia, fatigue, nausea, musculoskeletal pain, and diarrhea	Empty stomach, at least 1 h before or 2 h after a meal
	Vismodegib (Erivedge)	Muscle spasms, alopecia, dysgeusia, weight loss, fatigue, nausea, and diarrhea	With/without food
Multiple intracellular (c-CRAF, BRAF, mutant BRAF) and cell surface kinases (KIT, FLT3, RET, RET/PTC, VEGFR-1, -2, -3)	Sorafenib (Nexavar)	Diarrhea, fatigue, infection, alopecia, hand–foot skin reaction, rash, and weight loss	Without food
Multiple tyrosine kinases (PDGFR-a and -b, VEGFR-1, -2, -3, KIT, FLT3, CSF1R, RET)	Sunitinib malate (Sutent)	Fatigue/asthenia, diarrhea, mucositis/stomatitis, nausea, decreased appetite/anorexia, vomiting, and abdominal pain	With/without food

ALK, Anaplastic lymphoma kinase; *BCL-2,* B-cell lymphoma 2; *BCR-ABL,* breakpoint cluster region–Abelson murine leukemia; *BRAF,* Braf proto-oncogene, serine/threonine kinase; *BRK,* breast tumor kinase; *BTK,* Bruton tyrosine kinase; *CD,* clusters of differentiation; *CDK,* cyclin-dependent kinase; *c-Fms,* transmembrane glycoprotein receptor tyrosine kinase; *CLL,* chronic lymphocytic leukemia; *CML,* chronic myelogenous leukemia; *c-CRAF,* Craf proto-oncogene, serine/threonine kinase; *CSF1R,* colony stimulating factor-1 receptor; *EPHA2,* ephrin receptor A2; *FGFR,* fibroblast growth factor receptor; *FLT3,* Fms-like tyrosine kinase 3; *GIST,* gastrointestinal stromal tumor; *GVHD,* graft-versus-host disease; *HER1/EGFR,* human epidermal growth factor receptor 1/epidermal growth factor receptor; *HER2/HER4,* human epidermal growth factor receptor 2 or 4; *HCC,* hepatocellular carcinoma; *HGFR,* hepatocyte growth factor receptor; *IDH2,* isocitrate dehydrogenase 2; *IGF-1R,* insulin-like growth factor-1 receptor; *InsR,* insulin receptor; *Itk,* interleukin-2 receptor-inducible T-cell kinase; *JAK1/JAK2,* Janus-associated kinases; *KIT,* stem cell factor receptor; *Lck,* lymphocyte-specific protein tyrosine kinase; *MEK1/MEK2,* mitogen-activated extracellular signal–regulated kinase 1 or 2; *MET,* mesenchymal–epithelial transition factor receptor; *NSCLC,* non–small-cell lung cancer; *mTOR,* mammalian target of rapamycin; *NHL,* non-Hodgkin lymphoma; *PARP,* poly(ADP-ribose) polymerase; *Ph +,* Philadelphia chromosome-positive; *PDGF,* platelet-derived growth factor; *PDGFR,* platelet-derived growth factor receptor; *PI3K,* phosphatidylinositol 3-kinase; *PNET,* pancreatic neuroendocrine tumor; *PTK5,* protein tyrosine kinase 5; *RCC,* renal cell cancer; *RET,* rearranged during transfection; *RET/PTC,* rearranged in transformation/papillary thyroid carcinomas; *RON,* recepteur d'origine nantais; *ROS1,* c-ros oncogene 1; *SCF,* stem cell factor; *SLL,* small lymphocytic lymphoma; *SAPK2,* stress-activated protein kinase 2; *TRKB,* tropomyosin receptor kinase B; *TYRO3,* tyrosine-protein kinase receptor Byk; *TIE2,* tyrosine kinase with immunoglobulin-like and EGF-like domains 2; *VEGFR,* vascular endothelial growth factor receptor.

third-generation EGFR inhibitor with success in overcoming acquired resistance due to its high potency and selectivity against the EGFR T790M mutation. Lapatinib and neratinib are dual-target inhibitors that inhibit the activities of EGFR and HER2.

4. Fms-like tyrosine kinase 3 (FLT3) inhibitors. FLT3 is widely expressed in hematopoietic stem and progenitor cells and is a transmembrane protein encoded by the proto-oncogene FLT3. FLT3 activates intracellular signaling cascades such as PI3K/AKT/mTOR, RAS/RAF/MAPK, and JAK/STAT (*JAK,* Janus-associated kinase; *MAPK,* mitogen-activated protein kinase; *mTOR,* mammalian target

of rapamycin; *PI3K,* phosphatidylinositol 3-kinase; *STAT,* signal transducer and activator of transcription proteins). Gilteritinib is a second-generation FLT3 inhibitor used in the treatment of acute myelogenous leukemia.

5. Angiogenesis inhibitors. Well-known pro-angiogenic factors involved in blood vessel growth include VEGF, basic fibroblast growth factor, and platelet-derived growth factor, transforming growth factor, insulin-like growth factor, EGF, and angiopoietin. There are numerous multikinase angiogenesis inhibitors available for the treatment of multiple malignancies.

6. Tropomyosin receptor kinase (TRK) inhibitors. There are three members of the TRK family which are encoded by the neurotrophic tyrosine receptor kinase (*NTRK*) genes *NTRK1*, *NTRK2*, and *NTRK3*. *NTRK* gene rearrangements have been identified as oncogenic drivers of various cancers, although they occur in only 1% of all malignancies. Examples of first-generation TRK inhibitors are entrectinib (multikinase inhibitor) and Larotrectinib (selective pan-TRK inhibitor) (Zhong et al., 2021).

C. Nonreceptor TKIs
1. BCR-ABL inhibitors. The Philadelphia chromosome translocation results in the union of *ABL1* gene on chromosome 9 and the BCR of chromosome 22 forming a BCR-ABL fusion that drives uncontrolled proliferation of leukemia cells in almost all cases of chronic myelogenous leukemia (CML) and 20% of acute lymphoblastic leukemia. Imatinib was the first BCR-ABL inhibitor and greatly improved outcomes for CML patients. The increasing recognition of imatinib resistance stimulated the development of second-generation BCR-ABL inhibitors (e.g., dasatinib, nilotinib, bosutinib).
2. Bruton's agammaglobulinemia tyrosine kinase (BTK) inhibitors. The BCR pathway has a key role in the progression of a variety of B-cell malignancies. BTK is a crucial component of the BCR pathway and is abundantly expressed in B-cell leukemias and lymphomas. Inhibiting BTK is an effective therapeutic strategy for some hematologic malignancies. Ibrutinib is a first-generation BTK inhibitor. Acalabrutinib and zanubrutinib are second-generation BTK inhibitors.
3. JAK inhibitors. JAKs transfer extracellular signals to the nucleus and activate STAT proteins. STAT is frequently activated in malignant tumors, especially hematopoietic cancers. Ruxolitinib was the first JAK inhibitor. JAK inhibitors are also used to treat graft-versus-host disease and autoimmune diseases (Zhong et al., 2021).

D. Serine/threonine kinase inhibitors.
1. BRAF/MEK (mitogen-activated extracellular signal–regulated kinase)/ERK inhibitors. Dysregulation of RAS/RAF/MEK (MAP kinase)/ERK signaling can be observed in a large number of cancers, most commonly due to mutations in RAS or BRAF. Examples include vemurafenib, dabrafenib, encorafenib, and cobimetinib.
2. Cyclin-dependent kinase (CDK) inhibitors. CDKs are critical enzymes regulating cell cycle progression. CD4 and CD6 are necessary for regulating growth signaling and the transition of the cell cycle from G1 to S phase. CDK4/6 induces phosphorylation of tumor suppressor retinoblastoma protein 1 (RB1) early in the G1 phase. Dysregulation of the CDK4/6-RB1 pathway is a significant feature of hormone receptor–positive breast cancer. Dual inhibition of CDK4 and CDK6 is essential. Examples include palbociclib, ribociclib, and abemaciclib.
3. PI3K/AKT/mTOR inhibitors. The PI3K/V-AKT murine thymoma viral oncogene homolog (AKT)/mTOR signaling pathway has an important role in cell growth, proliferation, survival, apoptosis, and motility. It is often activated in cancer. PI3Ks can be divided into three classes. Class 1 is the major isoform implicated in cancer and is further divided into PI3Kalpha, PI3Kbeta, and PI3Kdelta encoded by respective genes *PIK3CA*, *PIK3CB*, and *PIK3CD*. *PIK3CA* gene is frequently dysregulated in multiple cancers, both by point mutations and amplification. Hyperactivation of PI3K/AKT/mTOR signaling is not only common in a variety of tumors but also closely related to drug resistance.
   a. Idelalisib was the first approved PI3Kdelta inhibitor. Alpelisib was the first PI3K inhibitor for the treatment of breast cancer.
   b. mTOR inhibitors can be divided into two categories: rapamycin analogs (rapalogs) and ATP-competitive inhibitors. Examples of rapalogs include sirolimus, temsirolimus, and everolimus.
   c. The development of AKT inhibitors has been relatively slow. Ipatasertib, capivasertib, afuresertib, and uprosertib have been studied but not yet approved (Zhong et al., 2021).

E. Epigenetic inhibitors: epigenetics is a branch of genetics that studies the change of gene expression rather than alteration of the genetic code itself. It is strictly regulated by a variety of chemical modifying enzymes and recognition proteins which are referred to as writers, erasers, and readers. Writers refer to enzymes that transfer chemical groups to DNA or histones and are methyltransferases. The erasers remove post-translational modifications and include histone deacetylases (HDACs). The readers are proteins that can recognize the modified histones or DNA. Abnormal epigenetic regulation is closely related to various diseases including cancer and immune diseases.
1. Enhancer of zeste homolog 2 (EZH2) inhibitors: EZH2 is a histone methyltransferase. Dysfunction of EZH2 is closely related to tumorigenesis and progression. An approved EZH2 inhibitor is tazemetostat.
2. HDAC inhibitors: Aberrant upregulation of HDACs has been reported in various types of cancers. Such changes alter the transcription of oncogenes and tumor suppressor genes which contribute to cancer cell proliferation and angiogenesis. Approved agents include vorinostat, belinostat, romidepsin, and panobinostat.
3. DH1/2 inhibitors: Isocitrate dehydrogenases (IDHs) include three subtypes (IDH1, IDH2, and IDH3) and are key enzymes in cellular metabolism and DNA repair. Mutated forms of IDH1 and IDH2 in particular are found in several types of tumors. IDH1/2 inhibitors include enasidenib and ivosidenib.

4. B-cell lymphoma 2 (BCL-2) inhibitors: The BCL-2 family of proteins consists of more than 20 members that regulate the intrinsic apoptosis pathway. Dysregulation of the apoptosis pathway is common in hematological malignancies especially. Venetoclax was the first selective BCL-2 inhibitor (Zhong et al., 2021).

F. Hedgehog (HH) pathway inhibitors: The HH signaling pathway has an important role in embryonic development and tissue regeneration. HH signaling can be abnormally activated through various mechanisms such as HH ligand upregulation, and Patched-1 (PTCH1) or Smoothened (SMO) mutations, resulting in oncogenesis and progression of a variety of tumors. Approved agents include vismodegib, sonidegib, and glasdegib.

G. Proteasome inhibitors block proteasome, which is a large protein complex that breaks down proteins in the cell nucleus when they are no longer needed.
1. The ubiquitin–proteasome system is the major pathway for intracellular protein degradation when proteins are damaged or unassembled. More than 80% of cellular proteins are degraded through this pathway.
2. Defects in the UPP pathway are associated with several diseases, including cancer, particularly multiple myeloma. Approved proteasome inhibitors include bortezomib, carfilzomib (both are injectable agents), and ixazomib (oral agent).

H. PARP inhibitors block the PARP enzyme in cells. Genomic instability is a typical characteristic of tumor cells. To maintain genomic integrity, tumor cells have multiple mechanisms to repair DNA. The repair pathway of DNA double-strand breaks (DSBs) includes homologous recombination (HR) and non-homologous end joining (NHEJ). The repair pathway for single-strand breaks (SSBs) includes base excision repair, nucleotide excision repair, and mismatch repair. When DNA SSBs occur, PARP binds to damaged DNA and catalyzes the repair. Upon repair, PARP dissociates from the site. PARP inhibitors suppress the repair of SSB and the unrepaired SSB is converted to DSB which is toxic to cells (Zhong et al., 2021).
1. Breast cancer susceptibility genes BRCA1 and BRCA2 are two key tumor suppressors that repair DSBs. Mutations in BRCA1 and BRCA2 are susceptible to breast and ovarian cancers. DSBs are not easily repaired in BRCA-mutant tumor cells through HR, and NHEJ is not efficient to repair the DSBs, thus resulting in genomic instability and cell death. Therefore, PARP inhibition in BRCA-mutant cancers can be lethal due to the simultaneous blockade of both DSB and SSB repair pathways (Zhong et al., 2021).
2. PARP inhibitors are used primarily in the management of patients with epithelial ovarian cancer who have known mutations (germline or somatic) in BRCA. Olaparib was the first approved agent. Other approved agents are rucaparib, niraparib, and talazoparib.

IX. Adverse events (AEs) of targeted therapies
A. "On-target, off-tumor" AEs result from drug activity against normal tissue that displays similar or identical molecules as the primary target (NCI, 2019). Examples are listed next.
1. EGFR is highly expressed in normal skin and gastrointestinal cells. Introduction of anti-EGFR therapies will block normal EGFR-based cell signaling in those organs, resulting in dermatologic and gastrointestinal toxicity (Hofheinz, Segaert, Safont, Demonty, & Prenen, 2017).
2. Cardiomyopathy in trastuzumab-treated patients results from on-target, off-tumor attachment on myocytes that express HER2-neu.
B. Selected targeted therapy AEs are biomarkers of efficacy.
1. Examples: Acneiform eruption induced by EGFR inhibitors has been reported to be a surrogate marker of therapeutic response. An association between hand–foot syndrome and reduced risk of death has been noted with sorafenib (Dagher, 2021). Patients who develop hypertension while being treated with bevacizumab generally have had better outcomes (NCI, 2022a, 2022b).
2. Early identification and management are preferable to early dose reduction or treatment discontinuation (Dagher, 2021).

X. AEs of targeted therapy vary according to the mechanism and target. Highlights of key AEs relative to targeted therapies are discussed next.
A. EGFR-targeted therapies are frequently associated with cutaneous reactions such as rash, hair, and nail changes, as well as diarrhea resulting from EGFR therapy's impact on intestinal mucosa (Tables 30.3 and 30.4).
1. Rash can occur with tyrosine kinases inhibitors that target EGFR. Because EGFR is present in epithelial cells lining the skin, inhibition with certain TKIs can produce an acneiform rash. The same is true for MEK inhibitors (MEKIs). In this case the rash presents as papules and pustules on the front torso and the face.
2. The objective for prevention strategies is to prevent dose reductions or discontinuation of the targeted therapy. Patients should be educated on preventive measures such as avoiding alcohol-based lotions and irritating products, using gentle cleansers, regular use of emollients, and sun-protective measures (Dagher, Blom, Chabanol, & Funck-Brentano, 2021).
3. Nail toxicities can occur with many targeted therapies such as EGFR, MEK, and mTOR inhibitors. Paronychia is a type of skin infection surrounding the toenail or fingernail and is characterized by inflammation, swelling, and pain. The development

TABLE 30.3　Management of Acneiform Rash

Description and assessment	• Rash onset within first 2 weeks; median duration 9–10 weeks. • Severity influenced by therapeutic regimen, dose intensity, and certain patient characteristics. • Assess patient's skin prior to initiating EGFR inhibitor therapy and monitor regularly.	
Nonpharmacologic management	Moisturize the entire body at least twice daily	Use thick, alcohol-free, perfume-free moisturizers, (preferably with 5%–10% urea) at least twice daily.
	Culture skin lesions if infection is suspected	To determine the presence of bacteria, virus, and fungus.
	Minimize sun exposure	Use broad-spectrum physical sunscreen (ultraviolet [UV]A/UVB) with SPF of at least 15. Wear protective clothing, including a wide-brimmed hat. Zinc oxide- or titanium dioxide-containing sunscreens preferred.
	Hydrate the skin	Maintain oral hydration. Avoid hot showers and products that dry out the skin (e.g., benzoyl peroxide), as they can aggravate the rash.
	Referral to dermatologist	Recommended for patients who experience severe (grade 3 or 4) skin-related toxicities or who have preexisting skin conditions.

EGFR, Epidermal growth factor receptor; *IV*, intravenous; *MESTT*, Multinational Association for Supportive Care in Cancer Epidermal Growth Factor Receptor Inhibitor Skin Toxicity Tool; *moABs*, monoclonal antibodies; *SPF*, sun protection factor; *TKI*, tyrosine kinase inhibitor.
From Lacouture, M. E., Sibaud, V., Gerber, P. A., van den Hurk, C., Fernández-Peñas, P., Santini, D., Jahn, F., et al. (2021). Prevention and management of dermatological toxicities related to anti-cancer agents: ESMO Clinical Practice Guidelines. *Annals of Oncology, 32*(2), 157–170. https://doi.org/10.1016/j.annonc.2020.11.005.

TABLE 30.4　Other Dermatologic Adverse Events

Toxicity	Causative Agents	Symptoms/Notes
HFSR	Multikinase angiogenesis inhibitors, BRAF inhibitors	Painful sensation in palms and soles, burning, tingling, swelling, redness, hypersensitivity to hot objects.
Xerosis	EGFR inhibitors, multikinase inhibitors, mTOR inhibitors, VEGF inhibitors, MEK inhibitors	Abnormally dry skin, pain, skin fragility; skin fissures and deep cracks in the fingertips, palms, or knuckles can form due to significant xerosis.
Nail changes	EGFR inhibitors, MEK inhibitors, mTOR inhibitors	Nail changes in nail bed (onycholysis), nail fold (paronychia), nail matrix; lesions affect mainly thumbs and toes; develop several weeks or months after treatment onset; preventive strategies include educating patients to avoid friction, wearing gloves or cotton socks to protect nails, wearing comfortable well-fitting shoes, and limiting pressure on the nails. Patient should also avoid cutting nails too short or biting nails. Consideration should be given to seeing a podiatrist to correct lateral nail curvature. Treatments include topical corticosteroids, antibiotics, antimicrobial soaks, and silver nitrate (Phillips et al., 2019).
Skin or hair depigmentation	Selected multikinase angiogenesis inhibitors, c-kit inhibitors, BCR-ABL inhibitors	No specific treatment is available to alleviate the condition; depigmentation is reversible once treatment is stopped.
Pruritus	EGFR inhibitors, VEGFR inhibitors, mTOR inhibitors, CD20 moABs	An intense itching sensation; often associated with xerosis; onset can be concurrent with rash.

BCR-ABL, Breakpoint cluster region–Abelson murine leukemia; *BRAF*, Braf proto-oncogene, serine/threonine kinase; *EGFR*, epidermal growth factor receptor; *HFSR*, hand–foot skin reaction; *MEK*, mitogen-activated extracellular signal–regulated kinase; *moAbs*, monoclonal antibodies; *mTOR*, mammalian target of rapamycin; *VEGF*, vascular endothelial growth factor; *VEGFR*, vascular endothelial growth factor receptor.
Adapted from Dagher, S. H., Blom, A., Chabanol, H., & Funck-Brentano, E. (2021). Cutaneous toxicities from targeted therapies used in oncology: Literature review of clinical presentation and management. *International Journal of Women's Dermatology, 7*(5, Part A), 615–624. https://doi.org/10.1016/j.ijwd.2021.09.009.

of lesions is also common and can lead to brittle nails and onycholysis. See Chapter 41 for additional details on the appropriate management of rash and skin AEs.

B. Cardiac toxicities manifest in multiple fashions, including left ventricular ejection fraction (LVEF) dysfunction, hypertension, and arrhythmias (Tables 30.5 and 30.6).

1. LVEF decreases can result from anti-HER2 therapies' binding of the HER2 protein, which is physiologically expressed on myocytes. The exact mechanism of trastuzumab-induced cardiotoxicity is still unknown (Bouwer et al., 2020).

2. Hypertension is frequently noted with angiogenesis inhibitors. This is primarily due to impaired nitric oxide signaling and reduced prostacyclin production when VEGF is inhibited. The treatment for VEGF-induced hypertension is combination therapy consisting of angiotensin-converting enzyme inhibitors

TABLE 30.5 Assessment and Management of Hypertension in Vascular Endothelial Growth Factor (VEGF)–Treated Patients

Initial assessment	• Prior medical history: age >60, preexisting cardiovascular disease, diabetes mellitus, previously documented left ventricular hypertrophy, elevated body mass index, smoking, obesity, sedentary lifestyle, stress, diet, medications, and family history of cardiovascular disease • Physical examination: blood pressure, large body habitus, headaches, peripheral edema, and evidence of cardiovascular compromise • Labs: serum creatinine, urinalysis with protein, and lipid profile • Assess for signs and symptoms of hypertension (headaches, dizziness, nosebleeds, flushing, peripheral edema, blurred vision, and dyspnea) • Assess vital signs, heart and lung sounds, and presence of JVD • CBC, urine analysis to evaluate for proteinuria, electrolytes, creatinine, and BUN

Ongoing Assessment While on Therapy

• Physical examination: headaches, dizziness, nosebleeds, flushing, peripheral edema, blurred vision, dyspnea, vital signs, heart and lung sounds, and presence of JVD
• CBC, urine analysis to evaluate for proteinuria, electrolytes, creatinine, and BUN

Grading of hypertension	Grade 1	Grade 2	Grade 3	Grade 4
	Adult: Systolic BP 120–139 mm Hg or diastolic BP 80–89 mm Hg	Adult: Systolic BP 140–159 mm Hg or diastolic BP 90–99 mm Hg if previously WNL; change in baseline medical intervention indicated; recurrent or persistent ($\geq$24 h); symptomatic increase by >20 mm Hg (diastolic) or to >140/90 mm Hg; monotherapy initiated	Adult: Systolic BP $\geq$160 mm Hg or diastolic BP $\geq$100 mm Hg; medical intervention indicated; more than one drug or more intensive therapy than previously used indicated	Adult and pediatric: Life-threatening consequences (e.g., malignant hypertension, transient or permanent neurologic deficit, and hypertensive crisis); urgent intervention indicated

Pharmacologic management	• Address preexisting hypertension before initiation of treatment with targeted therapy; for preexisting hypertension, BP target for initiating VEGF inhibitor treatment should be <140/90 mm Hg, or lower if proteinuria present • Antihypertensive agents should be prescribed immediately upon detection of hypertension; • Assess medication adherence and monitor for adverse events • Treatment of VEGF inhibitor–related hypertension (ACE inhibitors, beta-blockers, ARB, calcium channel blockers, thiazide or thiazide-type diuretics)
Nonpharmacologic management	• Monitor BP weekly during the first cycle of treatment followed by routine monitoring every 2–3 weeks for the duration of treatment • Monitor BP after discontinuation of angiogenesis inhibitor therapy and adjust antihypertensive therapy • Educate patients and families in monitoring for symptoms of hypertension and hypotension • Consider collaboration with cardiologist, nephrologist especially if preexisting cardiovascular disease, kidney dysfunction, stroke • Educate patients in healthy lifestyle changes (smoking cessation, regular exercise, limited alcohol intake, weight loss, psychosocial management, diet modifications [low salt, low fat]); consider cardiac rehabilitation

ACE, Angiotensin-converting enzyme; *ARB,* angiotensin II receptor blockers; *BMI,* body mass index; *BP,* blood pressure; *BUN,* blood urea nitrogen; *CBC,* complete blood count; *JVD,* jugular venous distension.

TABLE 30.6 Cardiotoxicity

Assessment	• Assess for risk factors (previous anthracycline exposure, hypertension, low baseline LVEF, age >65, diabetes mellitus, obesity, compromised cardiac function before treatment, short time between anthracycline treatment and anti-HER2 therapy, previous radiation therapy) • Assess for signs and symptoms of cardiac toxicity • Obtain baseline LVEF via echocardiogram or MUGA with periodic testing • CBC, BUN, creatinine, electrolytes, and electrocardiogram	
Grading: left ventricular systolic dysfunction	Grade 3	Grade 4
	Symptomatic due to drop in ejection fraction responsive to intervention	Refractory or poorly controlled heart failure due to drop in ejection fraction; intervention such as ventricular assist device, intravenous vasopressor support, or heart transplant indicated
Pharmacologic management	• Consideration of ACE inhibitors or beta-blockers	
Nonpharmacologic management	• Educate patients to report symptoms promptly • Collaboration with cardiologist • Educate patients in healthy lifestyle changes (smoking cessation, dietary modifications [low salt, low fat], regular exercise, limited alcohol intake, weight loss, stress management)	

ACE, Angiotensin-converting enzyme; *CBC,* complete blood count; *BUN,* blood urea nitrogen; *EF,* ejection fraction; *LVEF,* left ventricular ejection fraction; *MUGA,* multigated acquisition scan.

Data from Bouwer, N. I., Jager, A., Liesting, C., Kofflard, M. J. M., Brugts, J. J., Kitzen, J. J. E. M., et al. (2020). Cardiac monitoring in HER2-positive patients on trastuzumab treatment: A review and implications for clinical practice. *The Breast, 52,* 33–44. https://doi.org/10.1016/j.breast.2020.04.005.

TABLE 30.7	**Oral Mucositis**
Assessment	• Inspect oral mucosa, dentition, surrounding gums. • Assess symptoms (ranging from mild tingling to painful ulcers). • Mucositis-related mTOR inhibitors characterized by distinct ulcers, aphthous in appearance, oval, gray-white center, surrounded by erythematous halo. Lesions appear within 5 days of the start of the first cycle. Lesions are clustered or coalescing, usually <1 cm in diameter. Localized to lips, lateral tongue, soft palate. May be accompanied by mouth pain, dysgeusia, or dysphagia without any evidence of clinically visible oral lesions. Patients with oral lesions are more likely to develop concurrent skin rashes and hand–foot syndrome.
Pharmacologic management	• Steroid-based mouthwashes may be of benefit in patients receiving everolimus based on the hypothesis that stomatitis due to that agent may arise from an inflammatory process. • Preventive care with 10 mL alcohol-free dexamethasone mouthwash (0.5 mg/5 mL oral solution) 4 times a day (swish for 2 min and spit) for 8 weeks significantly minimized or prevented all grades of mucositis in women receiving everolimus for advanced breast cancer. • Treatments for mTOR inhibitor stomatitis: • Topical analgesics for pain • Mucoadhesive gels or viscous solutions that coat the oral cavity (to protect oral mucosa) • Prophylactic antibiotics (to avoid secondary infections) • Steroid-based mouth rinses, topical steroids, topical antiinflammatory agents (to reduce inflammation/immune response) • Systemic analgesics/corticosteroids for moderate to severe stomatitis
Nonpharmacologic management	• Referral to dentist before initiation of therapy and during treatment to prevent serious sequelae. • Education about oral hygiene: frequent brushing with soft bristles every 2–3 h for mild stomatitis; every 1–2 h for more severe symptoms, using mild toothpaste (children's) or toothpaste without sodium lauryl sulfate; flossing and rinsing with saline or sodium bicarbonate after every meal to get rid of food particles; nonalcoholic mouthwashes. • Diet instructions: soft, moist, nonirritating foods; drink fluids. • Lip balms to help reduce mouth and lip dryness.

(ACEIs) and calcium channel blockers. Dose reduction of therapy may be warranted in more severe cases (Phillips et al., 2019).

3. Drug-induced QTc interval prolongation recorded via electrocardiogram is a common risk associated with multiple TKI classes (e.g., BRAF inhibitors, VEGF agents, and BCR-ABL inhibitors).

C. Fluid retention (i.e., peripheral edema, pulmonary edema) observed in patients treated with BCR-ABL agents.

D. Oral mucositis is commonly observed with mTOR, oral EGFR, and oral multikinase inhibitors (Table 30.7).

E. Hypothyroidism can occur with TKIs as they change the blood flow to the thyroid, which causes destructive thyroiditis. Many of the symptoms can be confused with the symptoms of cancer and can include fatigue, muscle weakness, constipation, and hair thinning. Thyroid-stimulating hormone (TSH) should be monitored. Treatment with replacement therapy is warranted in patients who are symptomatic and have severe hypothyroidism (Phillips et al., 2019).

F. Dyslipidemia is seen in many patients on mTOR inhibitors. A lipid profile should be obtained before the start of mTOR inhibitor therapy and repeated every 6 weeks while the patient is on treatment. It may be necessary to interrupt mTOR therapy and dose reduce if grade 3 toxicity occurs. Patients with elevated cholesterol should start treatment with lipid-lowering agents,

although cytochrome P450 3A4 substrate statins (simvastatin and atorvastatin) are associated with drug interactions that must be evaluated prior to first use (Phillips et al., 2019).

G. Diarrhea is commonly observed with anti-EGFR moAbs (Table 30.8).

1. Diarrhea is common in patients treated with an EGFR TKI. EGF is responsible for maintaining mucosal integrity.

2. The underlying mechanism is poorly understood but is believed to be due to excessive chloride secretion, which leads to a secretory form of diarrhea.

3. May involve multiple factors including altered gut motility or changes in intestinal microflora (Li & Gu, 2019).

Assessment

I. Pertinent personal history

A. Assessment of current medications, including prescription and nonprescription, especially those that may be contraindicated with targeted therapies

1. CYP450 substrates, inhibitors, and inducers

2. Drugs that affect gastric pH (proton pump inhibitors, antacids)

3. Warfarin and other coumarin-derived anticoagulants

4. Aspirin, nonsteroidal antiinflammatory drugs

TABLE 30.8   Diarrhea From Epidermal Growth Factor Receptor (EGFR) Therapies

Assessment	• Baseline bowel history beginning 6 weeks before starting EGFR treatment • Complete medication list (prescription, over-the-counter, laxatives and stool softeners, opioids or recent opioid withdrawal, recent antibiotic therapy, herbals, vitamins) • Type of diet • Other clinical and medical conditions • Travel history • Signs and symptoms of dehydration (orthostatic hypotension, dry mouth, excessive thirst, dizziness, feelings of weakness, decreased urination, weight loss) • Abdominal assessment (tenderness, distention) • Frequency and characteristics of stools, nocturnal stools, incontinence, cramping • Nausea/vomiting • Laboratory tests (CBC, stool test for occult blood, metabolic panel, stool cultures for enteric pathogens, *Clostridium difficile*, and ova and parasites)
Pharmacologic management	Loperamide • An opioid that decreases intestinal motility by directly affecting the smooth muscle of the intestine; few, if any, systemic effects due to minimal absorption • As diarrhea from targeted therapies is usually secretory, loperamide is the first drug of choice • Initial dose for grade 1 or 2 diarrhea is 4 mg followed by 2 mg every 4 h or after every unformed stool (maximum daily dose of 16–20 mg) until there have been no episodes of diarrhea for 12 h. If diarrhea persists over 48 h, loperamide may be continued or discontinued, with use of other agents such as octreotide or tincture of opium. Octreotide Decreases the secretion of several hormones, prolongs intestinal transit time, increases absorption of fluid and electrolytes • Given subcutaneously at titrated doses from 100 to 150 µg three times daily up to 500 µg three times a day Deodorized tincture of opium • Contains the equivalent of 10 mg/mL of morphine • Recommended dose is 10–15 drops every 3–4 h Short-term opioid treatment • Codeine 30 mg/day, which can be increased up to 60 mg four times a day, maybe beneficial; although it should be stopped if the EGFR TKI treatment is discontinued Budesonide • Reduces inflammation Colestipol
Nonpharmacologic management	• Instruct patients to report any change in bowel activity, especially if duration >48 h or accompanied by fever or is grade 3 or 4 • Dietary instructions: low fat, low fiber; minimal intake of fruit, red meat, alcohol, spicy food, and caffeine • Dietary modifications: foods that build stool consistency (low in fiber; pectin containing), foods high in potassium, foods at room temperature to minimize peristalsis, increased fluids • Consider referral to dietitian upon initiating EGFR treatment • Consider referral to gastroenterologist if diarrhea does not improve despite discontinuation of EGFR therapy • Isotonic solutions 1–1.5 L/day; limit hypotonic fluids (water, tea, and fruit juice) to 0.5 L/day • Maintain skin integrity: cleanse rectal area after each stool, apply topical skin barrier; sitz baths may help with anal discomfort

ADL, Activities of daily living; *CBC*, complete blood count.

5. Medications that may alter mentation or cognition
6. Immunosuppressants
7. Antihypertensive therapy
8. Herbals, vitamins, and other over-the-counter medications
9. Laxatives, especially those used chronically

B. Other concurrent anticancer therapies (radiation, hormonal, chemotherapy, targeted therapy, biotherapy, and immunotherapy)
  1. Comorbidities may be exacerbated by side effects of targeted therapies

2. Assess for the history of, tolerance of, and response to prior therapies

C. Disease status
  1. Site of cancer, stage of cancer, and histology
  2. Drug-specific companion testing to determine sensitivity to targeted therapy, including single mutation assays and genomic panel assays

D. Knowledge of goals of therapy, line of treatment, and agents to be given

E. Treatment details (e.g., diagnostic, curative, palliative, supportive, or investigational)

1. Treatment plan, including duration and sequencing of therapy
2. Requirements of treatment such as length of hospitalization, follow-up clinic visits, laboratory and diagnostic test requirements, and financial obligations
3. Expected side effects and self-care skills required

II. Assessment of AE-specific risk factors
  A. Rash (see Table 30.3)
    1. Obtain bacterial/viral/fungal cultures if infection is suspected (Lacouture et al., 2021).
    2. Evaluate skin at initial visit and treat any underlying skin conditions. Patients with preexisting eczema should intensify their usual skin care routine, and those with active rosacea, acne, or eczema may need to be immediately referred to dermatology.
    3. Patients who are more susceptible to skin toxicities from EGFR inhibitors include men, obesity, and smoking. Ethnicity may be a risk factor, as the frequency of some skin toxicities is higher in Asian countries (Li et al., 2022). High skin surface lipid levels prior to EGFR inhibitor therapy and oily skin are risk factors for severe acneiform eruptions (Jacobs, 2019).
  B. Hypertension (see Table 30.5)
    1. The risk of developing or exacerbating hypertension differs depending on the clinical situation. Hypertension can be almost two times higher in patients with early stages of disease compared with that of more advanced oncological disease. In addition, the development of hypertension is higher in women (Patel, Dushenkov, Jungsuwadee, Krishnaswami, & Barac, 2020).
    2. Assess for preexisting hypertension and underlying cardiac risk factors. The presence of existing cardiovascular disease (coronary artery disease, heart failure, and history of stroke) or kidney dysfunction at the time of treatment initiation requires referral to corresponding cardiology, neurology, or nephrology to optimize management (Patel et al., 2020).
    3. Time to new onset hypertension or exacerbation of previously well-controlled blood pressure (BP) has been reported within days to months after treatment initiation. The greatest increase in BP is noted within the first 4 weeks of VEGF inhibitor therapy, and the increase gradually declines between 4 and 16 weeks, but BP often remains significantly elevated (Waliany et al., 2019).
    4. Common risk factors identified with cardiovascular toxicities by angiogenesis inhibitors include age over 60, high body mass index (BMI) greater than or equal to $25\,kg/m^2$, and preexisting hypertension (Patel et al., 2020).
  C. Trastuzumab-induced cardiotoxicity
    1. Risk factors for trastuzumab-induced cardiotoxicity include age over 65, obesity (BMI>$30\,kg/m^2$),

previous radiation therapy, short time between anthracycline treatment and anti-HER2 treatment, and compromised cardiac function before treatment (Bouwer et al., 2020; Dent, Morse, Burnette, Guha, & Moore, 2021).
    2. Baseline assessment with echocardiogram or multigated acquisition scan.
  D. Diarrhea (see Table 30.8)
    1. Baseline bowel history before initiation of EGFR inhibitor therapy. Obtain information about the patient's bowel habits for the 6-week period before starting treatment (Li & Gu, 2019).
    2. Assess for signs and symptoms of dehydration: orthostatic hypotension, dry mouth, excessive thirst, dizziness, weakness, decreased urination, and weight loss.

III. Physical examination: thorough physical assessment by body system before initiation of therapy (to serve as baseline for comparison) and at regular intervals during therapy to evaluate tolerance and response. The reader is directed to symptom-specific sections of this book for detailed assessment guidance.
  A. Assess respiratory function, heart rate, respiratory rate, cough, and peripheral edema for evidence of cardiopulmonary compromise with HER2 and MEK therapies.
  B. Monitor BP throughout treatment; more frequently during the first cycle of treatment.
  C. Monitor abdominal pain, ascites, and jaundice as evidence of liver dysfunction.
  D. Monitor weight loss as a potential sign of hypophysitis.
  E. Review skin for evidence of rash as a sign of allergic reaction, baseline and ongoing skin integrity, infection, autoimmune skin toxicity, and loss of skin turgor as a sign of dehydration.
  F. Monitor the level of consciousness, confusion, mental acuity, and evidence of seizures in patients at risk for cytokine release syndrome (CRS).
  G. Assess for the status of preexisting comorbidities with emphasis on diabetes.

IV. Psychosocial examination
  A. Assessment of baseline mental status
  B. Assessment of cultural factors and health-related beliefs
  C. Assessment of current social structure, including support systems, primary caregiver, housing and living arrangements, and employment/work status
  D. Assessment of type, number, and effectiveness of previous coping strategies used by patient and family
  E. Determination of response to illness and emotional state
  F. Assessment for the ability to perform self-care activities
  G. Assessment for patient adherence, especially oral targeted therapies, barriers
  H. Consideration of financial status—need for referral to social worker or access to patient assistance programs (community and/or pharmaceutical sponsored)

Management

I. Pharmacologic
  A. Cardioprotective treatments such as dexrazoxane may be added to address LVEF decline, allowing patients to continue treatment with HER2 inhibitors (see Chapter 34).
  B. ACEIs, beta-blockers, angiotensin II receptor blockers (ARB), thiazide or thiazide-like diuretics, and calcium channel blockers for VEGF inhibitor–related hypertension included, although currently there is no clear evidence of superiority of any specific agent.
    1. Treatment selection should be based on the presence of comorbidities, current drug therapies, contraindications, and special cautions (e.g., proteinuria, diarrhea, and hepatotoxicity) (Patel et al., 2020).
    2. A suggested algorithm for VEGF inhibitor treatment and BP monitoring:
       a. BP <140/90: continue treatment
       b. BP equal to or >140/90 OR diastolic increased by >20 mmHg: start or adjust antihypertensives—calcium channel blockers or ACEI/ARB first-line
       c. BP equal to or >160/100: consider holding or reducing dose of VEGF inhibitor
       d. Hypertensive emergency: discontinue VEGF inhibitor (Ruf, Yarandi, Ortiz-Melo, & Sparks, 2021)
  C. Rash management
    1. Prophylactic treatment modalities for rash include corticosteroids, moisturizers, and sunscreen. Other therapies include dapsone gel and oral doxycycline. When a bacterial skin infection is suspected, clinicians should initiate antibiotics (Phillips et al., 2019).
    2. Rash management should focus on supportive care to alleviate associated symptoms (pruritis, pain), psychosocial coping, and prevention of superinfection (Lacouture et al., 2021).
    3. Topical low/moderate steroids and oral antibiotics for 6 weeks (minocycline, doxycycline, or oxytetracycline).
    4. Reassess after 2 weeks. If reactions worsen or do not improve, add systemic corticosteroids for 7 days with consideration for the addition of isotretinoin at low doses only after discontinuation of tetracyclines to lower the risk of cerebral edema (Dagher et al., 2021; Lacouture et al., 2021).
  D. Loperamide (escalated to octreotide as indicated) with oral hydration with electrolytes at the first episode of watery stool for therapy-induced diarrhea. For grade 1–2 diarrhea, EGFR TKI treatment should be continued at the same dose. If grade 2 diarrhea persists for more than 48 hours despite antidiarrheal treatment, EGFR TKI interruption or dose reduction is recommended. In the event of grade 3–4 diarrhea, consideration should be given to hospitalization with aggressive intravenous fluid replacement initiated with interruption of EGFR TKI therapy (Li & Gu, 2019).
  E. Prophylactic steroids such as dexamethasone mouthwashes are effective at reducing the incidence and severity of mucositis in patients who receive mTOR inhibitor therapy. In extreme cases of refractory mucositis from mTOR inhibitors, systemic treatment with high-dose steroids may be warranted (Brown & Gupta, 2020).
  F. Analgesics (topical and systemic) to ameliorate pain symptoms related to stomatitis.
  G. Antiinfectives (antifungals, antibiotics) to treat or prevent superinfection (Lacouture et al., 2021). Consideration to be given with potential drug–drug interactions and efficacy for oral agents.
  H. Premedication with corticosteroid, acetaminophen, and antihistamine to prevent infusion reactions and hypersensitivity reactions.
  I. For patients experiencing dyspepsia, suggest the use of short-acting antacids or H2 blockers as alternatives to proton pump inhibitors.
II. Nonpharmacologic measures
  A. Early identification and management of side effects are preferred over dose reduction or modifications.
  B. Monitor for tolerance during infusions, assessing for risk of cytokine release especially in initial infusions, and for allergic reaction in subsequent infusions.
  C. Education on adherence, symptoms to report, and healthy habits.
  D. Education to manage and report symptoms.
  E. Patients should record the consistency and frequency of stools, preceding foods, and treatments.
  F. Multidisciplinary collaboration with interprofessional teams (Scott, 2021). Dietitians, dermatologists, gastroenterologists, pulmonologists, ophthalmologists, cardiologists, nephrologists, pharmacists, rheumatologists, and internal medicine practitioners should be consulted for the appropriate management of organ-specific disorders.
  G. Focused education related to oral self-medication starting at initiation of drug therapy, including regularly scheduled assessments to evaluate compliance and tolerance.

IMMUNOTHERAPY

Overview

I. Immunotherapy—use of immunologic cells and pathways to directly attack tumors, or to engage the immune system to fight cancer (ASCO, 2018; Brahmer, Lacchetti, & Schneider, 2018; NCI, n.d.; Zhang & Chen, 2018).
  A. Immunotherapy utilizes antibodies, T cells, cytokines, and engineered viruses to orchestrate immune-mediated cytotoxicity against the tumor.
  B. Immunotherapy capitalizes on the immune system's unique specificity and memory abilities.
    1. Specificity refers to the ability to distinguish between molecules that characterize "self" and "nonself" structures.

2. Memory refers to the ability to recall previous encounters with an antigen. Memory T cells and B cells can more rapidly respond to tumor recurrence, leading to more lasting results.

II. Immunotherapy is used to overcome a variety of tumor escape mechanisms (Friedrich, Jasinski-Bergner, & Lazaridou, 2019; Jiang et al., 2019; Landskron, De la Fuente, Thuwajit, Thuwajit, & Hermoso, 2014; Mortezaee, 2020; Tumeh et al., 2014; Waldman, Fritz, & Lenardo, 2020).

   A. Tumor escape occurs when the immune system fails to recognize an in situ tumor, resulting from either deficient host immunity (from age- or disease-related alterations) or suppressive tumor microenvironments.

   B. The tumor microenvironment suppresses natural immune response by upregulating checkpoint molecules, manipulating T-cell activity, manipulating cytokine control, and increasing pro-tumor vasculature (Zhang et al., 2021).

      1. Tumor cells abnormally overexpress PD-L1 molecules that inhibit T-cell killing capacity.

      2. The balance of cytokines such as tumor necrosis factors, interferons (IFNs), and interleukins (ILs) promotes tumor development rather than tumor suppression.

      3. Tumors produce VEGF that hijacks blood vessel development toward tumor (Chen et al., 2021).

   C. T-cell exhaustion is the fading of cytotoxic and memory functions resulting from prolonged exposure to a specific antigen (Zhang, Liu et al., 2020).

III. Classes of immunotherapy—immunotherapy can be classified by the specific immune system pathway utilized: immunomodulators, vaccine therapy, moAbs, bispecific antibodies (bsAbs), CPIs, and T-cell therapy (Zahavi & Weiner, 2020).

IV. Immunomodulators such as cytokines, IL, and IFN are naturally occurring chemicals that inhibit and suppress immune activity (see Chapter 9) (Berraondo et al., 2019; Conlon, Miljkovic, & Waldmann, 2019; Rallis et al., 2021).

   A. Upon administration, cytokines orchestrate host immune cells communicating inflammatory, stimulatory, or suppressive chemical signals.

   B. Development of cytokine monotherapy has been hampered by high toxicity resulting from widespread immune activation.

   C. Examples of immunomodulators include the cytokines IFN-α and IL-2.

   D. Immune-related AEs (irAEs) are common (80%) and include constitutional symptoms of fever, fatigue, headache, myalgia, and depression.

V. Vaccine therapy is an active form of immunotherapy that conditions the host's immune system to generate its own sustained response to current and future tumor growth (Hemminki, Dos Santos, & Hemminki, 2020).

   A. Oncolytic viral therapy (ex> T-vec) is the injection of an attenuated virus into tumor, resulting in tumor lysis and presentation of tumor-associated antigen (TAA) to circulating T cells and B cells (Larocca, LeBoeuf, Silk, & Kaufman, 2020).

   B. Dendritic cell vaccines (ex> sipuleucel-T) are personalized therapies based on a patient's own extracted antigen-presenting cells (dendritic cells) engineered to recognize TAAs (Sutherland, Ju, Horvath, & Clark, 2021).

   C. Vaccines are associated with injection site pain, localized cellulitis, and flu-like symptoms (fatigue, chills, pyrexia, nausea, and hypotension), and long-term irAEs include vitiligo (Andtbacka et al., 2019; Dandreon Corporation, 2019).

VI. MoAbs are engineered immunoglobulins that bind to tumor-related target antigens, resulting in tumor lysis, reactivation of apoptosis, or recruitment of phagocytic immune cells (American Cancer Society, 2019; Ayati et al., 2020; Balocco, De Sousa Guimaraes Koch, Thorpe, Weisser, & Malan, 2022; Waldman et al., 2020; Zahavi & Weiner, 2020; Table 30.9).

   A. Naturally occurring antibodies recognize "foreign antigens, neutralize them, and elicit a further immune response."

   B. MoAb therapy reduces current tumor burden but does not impart significant immunologic memory for protection against future tumors.

   C. MoAbs can be mass-produced to target tumor antigens theoretically shared by all patients harboring specific tumor markers. Examples include trastuzumab targeting the HER2 protein on HER2-positive cancers and rituximab targeting the CD20 cell surface receptor on lymphoid tumors.

   D. Both naturally occurring and engineered antibodies are constructed of two major regions (Fab and Fc) arranged in a Y shape.

      1. The tips of the Y, the Fab region, target-specific antigens.

      2. The base of the Y, the Fc region, links to immune effector cells (natural killer [NK] cells, neutrophils, monocytes, dendritic cells, and eosinophils) and initiates complement-dependent cytotoxicity (CDC).

   E. MoAbs reduce tumor burden using a variety of mechanisms (Ayati et al., 2020; Waldman et al., 2020; Zahavi & Weiner, 2020).

      1. MoAbs interrupt the binding between tumor-related growth factors in the serum (ligands) and TKRs on the cell surface, thereby restoring apoptosis and halting intracellular proliferation, migration, and invasion signaling pathways.

      2. MoAbs bind to target cells and initiate CDC, triggering the release of chemotactic factors that lyse cell membranes.

      3. In antibody-dependent cellular cytotoxicity (ADCC), moAbs coat target cells, flagging them for destruction by cytotoxic circulating NK cells and dendritic cells.

      4. In antibody-dependent cellular phagocytosis (ADCP), the Fab region of the moAb binds to tumor and the Fc region attracts phagocytic macrophages.

TABLE 30.9   Monoclonal Antibodies

Target	Antibody	Class-Associated Adverse Events
CCR4	Mogamulizumab	Pruritus, rash, skin pain, infusion reaction, fatigue, arthralgias, pancytopenia, hypoalbuminemia, hypocalcemia, hypercalcemia
CD19 and CD3	Blinatumomab (Blincyto) (bispecific antibody)	Infusion reactions Neurologic symptoms
CD20	Obinutuzumab (Gazyva) Ofatumumab (Arzerra) Rituximab (Rituxan) Rituximab and hyaluronidase human (Rituxan Hycela) Ibritumomab tiuxetan (Zevalin)	Infusion reactions, neutropenia, lymphopenia, asthenia, severe mucocutaneous reactions, hepatitis B reactivation
CD22	Inotuzumab ozogamicin (Besponsa)	Pancytopenia, fatigue, pyrexia, nausea
CD30	Brentuximab vedotin (Adcetris)	Pancytopenia, peripheral neuropathy, fatigue, nausea, diarrhea, pyrexia, rash, URI
CD33	Gemtuzumab ozogamicin (Mylotarg)	Pancytopenia, nausea, vomiting, diarrhea, pyrexia, chills, hypokalemia, shortness of breath, asthenia,
CD38	Daratumumab (Darzalex) Isatuximab (Sacrlisa)	Upper respiratory infection, infusion reactions, diarrhea, fatigue, cough, pyrexia
CD52	Alemtuzumab (Campath)	Infusion reactions, opportunistic infections, cytopenia
EGFR/HER1	Necitumumab (Portrazza) Cetuximab (Erbitux) Panitumumab (Vectibix) Cetuximab (Erbitux)	Infusion reactions, rash, nail changes, diarrhea, opportunistic infections
GD2	Dinutuximab (Unituxin)	Pain, pyrexia, thrombocytopenia, lymphopenia, infusion reactions, hypotension, hyponatremia, increased alanine aminotransferase, anemia, vomiting
HER2	Trastuzumab (Herceptin) Pertuzumab (Perjeta) Fam-trastuzumab deruxtecan-nxki (enhertu) Margetuximab (anti-HER2 mAb) Ado-trastuzumab emtansine (Kadcyla)	Rash, diarrhea; alopecia (conjugated antibodies), diarrhea, cytopenias, fatigue; fever, chills, and headache
NECT-4	Enfortumab vedotin	Rash, neuropathy
PDGFR-a	Olaratumab (Lartruvo)	Cytopenias, hyperglycemia, decreased electrolytes, nausea, fatigue, musculoskeletal pain, mucositis, alopecia, vomiting, diarrhea, decreased appetite, abdominal pain, neuropathy, and headache
RANKL	Denosumab (Xgeva)	Musculoskeletal pain after injection, osteonecrosis of the jaw
SLAMF7	Elotuzumab (Empliciti)	Fatigue, diarrhea, pyrexia, constipation, cough, peripheral neuropathy, nasopharyngitis, upper respiratory tract infection, decreased appetite, and pneumonia
VEGF	Bevacizumab (Avastin) Inhibition of VEGF interaction with its receptors	Hypertension, bleeding, and proteinuria
VEGFR-2	Ramucirumab (Cyramza) Inhibition of angiogenesis via binding of VEGFR	Hypertension, diarrhea, and headache
HER2	Ado-trastuzumab emtansine (Kadcyla) Chemotherapy conjugate: maytansine	Thrombocytopenia, neuropathy, and elevated LFTs
	Fam-trastuzumab deruxtecan-nxki (Enhertu) Chemotherapy conjugate: topoisomerase inhibitor	Interstitial lung disease, cytopenias, and elevated LFTs
BCMA	Belantamab mafodotin-blmf (Blenrep) Chemotherapy conjugate: microtubule inhibitor	Vision changes, thrombocytopenia, and infusion-related reactions
CD30	Brentuximab vedotin (Adcetris) Chemotherapy conjugate: monomethyl auristatin E	Cytopenias, neutropenia, and GI
CD33	Gemtuzumab ozogamicin Chemotherapy conjugate: antitumor antibiotic ozogamicin	Hemorrhage, infection, fever, GI, headache, elevated LFTs, rash, and mucositis
CD20	Ibritumomab tiuxetan (Zevalin) Conjugate: radioisotope yttrium-90	Pancytopenia, nausea, infusion reaction, and asthenia

TABLE 30.9 Monoclonal Antibodies—cont'd

Target	Antibody	Class-Associated Adverse Events
CD19	Loncastuximab tesirine-lpyl (Zynlonta) Chemotherapy conjugate: alkylating agent	Effusions, edema, myelosuppression, infections, and cutaneous reactions
CD22	Inotuzumab ozogamicin (Besponsa) Chemotherapy conjugate: antitumor antibiotic ozogamicin	Pancytopenia, increased LFTs, fatigue, pyrexia, and nausea
	Moxetumomab pasudotox-tdfk (Lumoxiti) Conjugate: Pseudomonas exotoxin	Capillary leak syndrome, hemolytic uremic syndrome, infusion-related reactions
CD79b	Polatuzumab vedotin-piiq (Polivy) Chemotherapy conjugate: monomethyl auristatin E	Infusion reactions, peripheral neuropathy, hypocalcemia, diarrhea, pancytopenia, URI, pyrexia
Nect-4	Enfortumab vedotin-ejfv (Padcev) Chemotherapy conjugate: monomethyl auristatin E	Cutaneous effects, hyperglycemia
TF	Tisotumab vedotin-tftv (Tivdak) Chemotherapy conjugate: monomethyl auristatin E	Visual disorders, peripheral neuropathy, and pneumonitis
TROP2	Sacituzumab govitecan-hziy (Trodelvy) Chemotherapy conjugate: topoisomerase inhibitor	Neutropenia, diarrhea, infusion-related reactions, and nausea
CD19 on tumor cells and CD3 on T cells	Blinatumomab (Blincyto)	Cytokine release syndrome, neurotoxicities, infections, tumor lysis syndrome, pyrexia
gp100 protein on tumor cells and CD3 on T cells	Tebentafusp-tebn (Kimmtrak)	Cytokine release syndrome, rash, and pruritis
EGFR and MET on tumor cells	Amivantamab (Rybrevant)	Rash, infusion-related reactions

ADCC, Antibody-dependent cellular cytotoxicity; *ADCP*, antibody-dependent cellular phagocytosis; *BCMA*, B-cell maturation antigen; *CCR4*, chemokine receptor type 4; *CD*, clusters of differentiation; *CDC*, complement-dependent cytotoxicity; *CLL*, chronic lymphocytic leukemia; *EGFR*, epidermal growth factor receptor; *GD2*, glycolipid disialoganglioside; *HER*, humanized epidermal growth factor receptor; *IgG*, immunoglobulin; *IL-6*, interleukin-6; *NHL*, non-Hodgkin lymphoma; *MET*, mesenchymal–epithelial transition; *PDGFR-α*, platelet-derived growth factor receptor alpha; *RANKL*, receptor activator of nuclear factor kappa-B ligand; *SLAMF7*, signaling lymphocytic activation molecule family member 7; *TF*, tissue factor; *TROP2*, trophoblast antigen 2; *VEGF*, vascular endothelial growth factor; *VEGFR-2*, vascular endothelial growth factor receptor 2.
From https://www.fda.gov/drugs/resources-information-approved-drugs/oncology-cancer-hematologic-malignancies-approval-notifications.

5. Antibody–drug conjugates facilitate highly specific delivery of cytotoxic agents to the intended cancer cell target (moABs conjugated to radioisotopes or toxins or chemotherapy) in addition to actions of unconjugated moABs (Dahan, 2022).
6. MoABs classified as either unconjugated or conjugated.
   a. Unconjugated=consists of unbound moAB, primary action due to cell signaling disruption, ADCC, CDC, or ADCP.
   b. Conjugated=moABs carrying radioisotopes or chemotherapy to the intended cancer cell target in addition to actions of unconjugated moABs (Chau, Steeg, & Figg, 2019).
7. AEs of non-CPI moABs are generally on-target, off-tumor AEs with irAEs restricted to hypersensitivity reactions including infusion reactions, CRS, and anaphylaxis.
8. The approval of subcutaneous administration of moABs represents a significant shift in treatment paradigms. The addition of an enzyme,

hyaluronidase, to these preparations results in a change in techniques for administration. The enzyme allows for additional volumes to be given at one injection site A thorough understanding of anatomy and physiology is required (Eisenberg, 2021).

F. Nomenclature of targeted therapies reveals their mechanism, derivation, and components (Table 30.10).

VII. BsAbs combine at least two distinct Fc (antigen binding) regions allowing them to bind to different target molecules simultaneously (Krishnamurthy & Jimeno, 2018; Lejeune et al., 2020; Tian, Liu, Zhang, & Wang, 2021).
   A. Bispecific T-cell engagers (BiTEs) are one type of bsAb that binds to tumor antigen on one binding site and simultaneously binds to effector T cells on the other binding site.
   B. The BiTE connects the tumor and the T cell, (1) bringing the T cell into close proximity with the tumor cell and (2) activating the T cell to release enzymes destroying nearby tumor.

TABLE 30.10 Nomenclature

Small-molecule–targeted therapies nomenclature:
Prefix+substem(s)+stem
Stem=-ib (except HDAC and BCL-2)

Substem	Substem+Stem	Target	Example
-tini-	-tinib	Tyrosine kinase inhibitors	Afatinib, axitinib, bosutinib, dasatinib, erlotinib, gefitinib, and sunitinib
-rafe-	-rafenib	RAF tyrosine kinase RAF/RAS/MEK pathway	Dabrafenib, regorafenib, sorafenib, and vemurafenib
-metin-	-metinib	MEK tyrosine kinase RAF/RAS/MEK pathway	Cobimetinib, trametinib
-den-	-denib	IDH2 enzyme inhibitor	Enasidenib
-par-	-parib	PARP inhibitors of mammalian polyadenosine 5′-diphosphoribose polymerase enzyme	Olaparib, rucaparib
-lis-	-lisib	PI3K	Idelalisib
-deg-	-degib	Sonic hedgehog pathway inhibitors	Sonidegib, vismodegib
-cicl-	-ciclib	CDK 4 and 6	Palbociclib
-zo-	-zomib	Proteosome inhibitors	Bortezomib, carfilzomib, ixazomib
-inostat	NA	HDAC	Vorinostat, belinostat, and panobinostat
-toclax	NA	BCL-2 inhibitors	Venetoclax

Monoclonal antibody targeted therapies nomenclature
Proprietary prefix+substem A target class+substem B monoclonal antibody derivation+conjugated toxin (if applicable)+stem (mab)
Substem A: Target class examples

Substem A	Substem Target Class	Example
-tu- or -ta-	Target located on tumor	Tras**tu**zumab (targeted HER2, a cell surface–bound antigen)
-ci-	Target located in circulatory system	Beva**ci**zumab (targeting VEGF, growth factor found in circulation)
-li-	Target located on immune system	Ip**ili**mumab (targeted CTLA-4, protein found on T cells)

Substem B: the species on which the immunoglobulin sequence of the mAb is based

Substem B	Monoclonal Antibody Derivation	Example
-**xi**mab	Chimeric human-mouse	Cetu**xi**mab Chimeric antibody with a tumor target (EGFR)
-**zu**mab	Humanized mouse	Beva**ci**zumab Humanized mouse antibody with a circulatory system target (VEGF-A)
-(**m**)**u**mab	Fully human	Panitum**u**mab Fully human antibody with a tumor target (EGFR)
-m**o**mab	Mouse (murine)	Ibritum**o**mab Mouse-based antibody targeting CD20

Conjugated MoABs list the bound toxin (chemotherapy or radioisotope)

Substem A Target Class	Substem B: Origin Species	Bound Toxin	Example
-tu-	-zu-	Emtansine	Trastuzumab emtansine (monoclonal antibody) targeting the HER2 cell surface–bound molecule attached to the chemotherapy emtansine
-tu-	-mo-	Tiuxetan	Ibritumomab tiuxetan (monoclonal antibody targeting CD20 on lymphoma cells delivering yttrium-90 radiotherapy)

INN Programme Revised nomenclature System
Infix (mode of action or target class)

-ki-	Cytokine or cytokine receptor
-eni-	Enzyme inhibition
-ta-	Tumor
-sto-	Immunostimulatory
-pru-	Immunosuppressive

TABLE 30.10 **Nomenclature—cont'd**	
The new naming system eliminates the stem "mAb" and replaces it with one of four stems classifying the construction of the immunoglobulin	
-tug	Unmodified monospecific immunoglobulins
-bart	Engineered monospecific immunoglobulins
-mig	Bispecific or multispecific immunoglobulins
-ment	Fragments of immunoglobulins

In 2021 the INN Programme adopted a revised nomenclature system that simplifies naming rules. Substem B (derivation) has been eliminated and the stem -mab has been subdivided into four categories listed below. The new naming scheme is Proprietary prefix+Infix (mode of action or target class)+stem. ADC will adopt this nomenclature scheme. No special suffix is added, as the second word indicates that the substance is a conjugate. *ADC*, Antibody–drug conjugates; *BCL-2*, B-cell lymphoma 2; *CDK*, cyclin-dependent kinase; *EGFR*, epidermal growth factor receptor; *HDAC*, histone deacetylase inhibitors; *HER*, humanized epidermal growth factor receptor; *IDH2*, isocitrate dehydrogenase 2; *INN*, International Nonproprietary Names; *MEK*, mitogen-activated extracellular signal–regulated kinase; *moAbs*, monoclonal antibodies; *PARP*, poly(ADP-ribose) polymerase; *PI3K*, phosphatidylinositol 3-kinase; *RAF*, rapidly accelerated fibrosarcoma; *RAS*, rat sarcoma virus; *VEGF*, vascular endothelial growth factor.

C. Natural occurring antibodies lack the structure required to directly recruit activated T cells into close contact with tumor.

D. CRS leading to neurological events is a potentially serious irAE of bsAbs.

VIII. CPIs are moAbs that target regulatory checkpoint molecules (Waldman et al., 2020; Zam & Ali, 2021; Zhang & Zhang, 2020).

A. In a healthy state, regulatory checkpoint molecules promote "tolerance to self" and prevent autoimmune reactions (Esfahani et al., 2020).

1. Checkpoint regulatory molecules reside on naïve T cells and self-cells.

2. Binding of checkpoint regulatory molecules shuts off cytotoxic and memory T-cell function, thus preventing self-cell destruction.

3. Key examples of target regulatory proteins are CTLA-4 and PD-L1 ligand and its receptor, PD-1.

B. In a cancerous state, malignant tumors cloak themselves in checkpoint molecules and simultaneously induce overexpression on T cells, thus shielding the tumor from immune recognition and allowing unchecked tumor growth (Zam, 2021; Zhang et al., 2021).

C. CPI therapy interrupts regulatory checkpoint molecules from binding with their partner proteins, thus "releasing the brakes" and allowing for T-cell recognition.

1. See Table 30.11 for the summary of CPIs.

2. Ongoing studies combine CPIs with other immunotherapy approaches such as cytokines to further restore T-cell function (Zam, 2021; Zhang & Zhang, 2020).

D. Diagnostic assays measure PD-L1 expression in tumors as a predictive biomarker for sensitivity to CPI therapy (Davis & Patel, 2019).

E. Pseudoprogression occurs in a small subset of patients treated with CPIs.

1. Pseudoprogression is due to infiltrating T cells causing initial growth of tumor size (observed radiologically) followed by shrinkage.

TABLE 30.11 **Checkpoint Inhibitors**	
Name	**Target**
CTLA-4	Ipilimumab (Yervoy)
PD-1	Pembrolizumab (Keytruda)
	Nivolumab (Opdivo)
PD-L1	Atezolizumab (Tecentriq)
	Avelumab (Bavencio)
	Durvalumab (Imfinzi)
	Cemiplimab-rwlc

2. Pseudoprogression is not accompanied by clinical worsening of disease.

F. IrAEs for CPIs result from autoimmune attack on normal cells by activated T cells.

1. Common (>20%) irAEs include skin rash, hepatic toxicity, fatigue, pneumonitis, and gastrointestinal toxicity.

2. Less common (<20%) irAEs include neurologic, endocrine, ocular, pancreatic enzymes, and hematological symptoms.

3. CTLA-4 is generally associated with more severe AEs than PD-1 therapies. See Table 30.12.

IX. Adoptive T-cell therapies are highly individualized treatments wherein the patient's own T cells are extracted, enhanced in a laboratory, then reinfused back to the patient to destroy tumor (June, O'Connor, Kawalekar, Ghassemi, & Milone, 2018; NCI, 2022a, 2022b; Janelle & Delisle, 2021).

A. Adoptive T-cell therapies can overcome the limitations of native, nonmodified T cells.

1. Adoptive T-cell therapies can recognize tumor cells without the interaction of antigen-presenting cells, which is required by native, nonmodified T cells.

2. Adoptive T-cell therapies include "all of the necessary elements for intracellular signaling and activation of helper and cytotoxic T lymphocytes" (Janelle & Delisle, 2021).

3. Adoptive T-cell therapy delivers a larger volume of activated T lymphocytes than the volume naturally produced in situ.

B. Chimeric antigen receptor (CAR) is one form of adoptive T-cell therapy wherein extracted, purified lymphocytes are modified to target a specific known antigen, grown in large quantities, then reinfused back to the patient. Refer to Chapter 27 for a detailed discussion on CAR-T therapy.

C. Tumor-infiltrating lymphocytes (TIL) therapy is a rapidly emerging therapy wherein activated T cells are extracted from a patient's solid tumor, expanded, and modified in a lab (NCI, 2022a, 2022b).

D. CAR-T therapy recognizes one specific antigen, whereas TILs are theoretically able to recognize a wide variety of antigens (Kumar, Watkins, & Vilgelm, 2021).

E. Adoptive T-cell therapy, particularly CAR-T, is associated with CRS, neurotoxicity, and decreased B cells (B-cell aplasia) (Dholaria, Bachmeier, & Locke, 2019; Santomasso et al., 2021).

(ASCO, 2020a; 2020b; Olsen, LeFebvre, & Brassil, 2019).

X. AEs from immunotherapy agents can be classified as "On-target, off-tumor" effects (discussed above), or as irAEs (Schneider et al., 2021).

A. "On-target, off-tumor" AEs result from drug activity against normal tissue that displays similar or identical molecules as the primary target (see discussion above).

B. irAEs are immunotherapy side effects resulting from an excessively activated immune system (T cells) that inadvertently targets self-cells (Brahmer et al., 2018; Dholaria et al., 2019; Johnson, Nebhan, Moslehi, & Balko, 2022).

1. The frequency and type of irAEs depend on the agents used, the length of exposure, the dose, and the patients' preexisting risk factor.

2. irAEs can affect almost any organ with varying frequencies and severities; however, cutaneous, pulmonary, and hepatic irAEs are the most common.

3. Immunotherapy AEs are different from chemotherapy AEs in terms of timing, pathophysiology, and management.

4. Immunotherapies activate the memory function of immune cells; thus AEs may appear and/or persist for the duration of the immune cell lifespan; can occur/recur after therapy cessation.

5. Combining chemotherapy and immunotherapy or combining two or more immunotherapies can increase the risk of AEs and broaden the range of potential AEs.

6. IrAEs are classified as chronic or acute (Johnson et al., 2022)

   a. Chronic irAEs persist for several weeks, or permanent, after treatment discontinuation, affecting approximately 40% of patients. Endocrine irAEs are the most common chronic irAE.

   b. Acute irAEs are generally short-term AEs affecting 80%–90% of patients, and presentation patterns vary according to drug and dose.

7. Data suggest the development of mild irAEs is associated with improved overall survival (Hussaini et al., 2021; Park, Lopes, & Saeed, 2021; Petrelli et al., 2020).

Assessment

I. Pertinent personal and family history (Brahmer et al., 2018; Puzanov et al., 2017)

A. Documentation: family and medical history and comorbidities.

B. Note history of preexisting autoimmune disease such as rheumatoid arthritis, myasthenia gravis, myositis, autoimmune hepatitis, systemic lupus erythematosus, inflammatory bowel disease, Wegener granulomatosis, Sjögren syndrome, Guillain–Barré syndrome, multiple sclerosis, vasculitis, or glomerulonephritis.

C. Record all medications, including prescriptions, over-the-counter medications, homeopathic preparations, herbal supplements, taking particular note of corticosteroids, proton pump inhibitors, antibiotics endocrine replacement therapy (Buti et al., 2021).

D. Assess for tolerance of prior lines of therapy and residual adverse drug reactions.

E. Assess for concomitant conditions that increase the risk for specific irAEs.

   1. Preexisting lung inflammation, radiotherapy, smoking, or lung disease increases the risk for pneumonitis.

   2. Irritable bowel syndrome, chronic use of antiinflammatory agents, and primary colorectal malignancy increase the risk for colitis (Som et al., 2019).

II. Disease history, stage, and molecular characteristics

A. Review molecular assays (e.g., fluorescence in situ hybridization, immunohistochemical) that indicate expression levels of target proteins such as PDL-1 and CD19.

B. Review the extent of disease as discussed in pathology reports, biopsies, and imaging.

C. Higher disease burden is correlated with a higher risk of severe CRS in patients treated with CAR-T-cell therapy (Acharya et al., 2019; Frey & Porter, 2019).

III. Knowledge of, rationale for, and goals of treatment, agent to be given.

A. Assess patient's expectations of efficacy and tumor response.

B. Assess patient's attitude toward tumor response monitoring and pseudoprogression.

C. Assess patient's awareness that immunotherapy AEs may present at any time after drug initiation (i.e., rash may appear months after drug cessation). See Table 30.13.

IV. Laboratory and diagnostic data (Frey & Porter, 2019)

A. Complete blood count with differential with emphasis on long-term trends

B. Liver function tests (aspartate aminotransferase, alanine aminotransferase, and total bilirubin)

C. Endocrine function tests, especially with CPIs (TSH, T4, T3, adrenocorticotropic hormone [ACTH], and cortisol)

D. Amylase and lipase for evidence of pancreatic dysfunction

E. Complete metabolic panel, including electrolytes and kidney function, to check for autoimmune activity and tumor lysis syndrome

F. Inflammatory marker elevation: cytokines including IL-6, lactate dehydrogenase, C-reactive protein, and ferritin

V. Physical examination

A. Complete physical examination in all patients should include the following elements:

1. Assess respiratory function, heart rate, respiratory rate, cough, and peripheral edema for evidence of cardiopulmonary compromise.

2. Monitor abdominal pain, ascites, and jaundice as evidence of liver dysfunction.

3. Monitor weight loss as a potential sign of hypophysitis.

4. Review skin for evidence of rash as a sign of allergic reaction or autoimmune skin toxicity and for loss of skin turgor as sign of dehydration.

5. Monitor lung sounds and cough as evidence of pneumonitis.

B. Specific immunotherapy classes should focus on high-risk, drug-specific assessments.

1. MoAbs: focus on target-specific functions. Examples include the following:

   a. LVEF and evidence of cardiomyopathy in HER2-treated therapies

   b. Maculopapular rash in EGFR-targeted therapies

2. CPIs: colitis, rash, pneumonitis-associated shortness of breath, and endocrinopathy-associated fatigue and malaise (Som et al., 2019; Weingarden, Rubin, & Gubatan, 2021).

3. CAR-T: fever, tachycardia, arrhythmia, and neurologic changes; peripheral edema indicative of CRS. Assess for preexisting comorbidities with emphasis on diabetes and other autoimmune disorders.

VI. Psychosocial examination

A. Assess for coping skills and evidence of coping dysfunction.

B. Assess for stressors brought on by irAEs.

C. Assess for socioeconomic burdens imposed by long-term therapy.

VII. Pathological examination: irAEs that do not respond to symptomatic therapy or short-course steroids should be evaluated microscopically by biopsy sampling to assess for the increased presence of immune inflammatory and phagocytic cells (Martins et al., 2019).

Management

I. Pharmacologic (Tables 30.12 and 30.13)

A. Provide symptomatic relief for irAEs, cytokine release, and infusion reactions (Brahmer et al., 2018; NCCN, 2022).

1. Oral and topical antihistamines can be effective to control skin reactions.

2. Loperamide (Imodium) can be an effective first-line agent for mild diarrhea.

3. IrAEs are primarily treated with short courses of topical or oral corticosteroids until symptoms resolve to baseline or ≤grade 1 (Brahmer et al., 2018; NCCN, 2022) If symptoms do not respond, intensify immunosuppressant therapy with prednisone/methylprednisolone 1–2 mg/kg/day.

4. Corticosteroids should be tapered over 4–6 weeks.

5. Other agents used (depending on specific irAE) include infliximab, vedolizumab, omalizumab, gamma-aminobutyric acid agonists, and mycophenolate (liver dysfunction).

B. Autoimmune endocrine disease is treated with thyroid hormone (levothyroxine) and/or short-course steroids (1 mg/kg prednisone or equivalent) and, if severe, may require indefinite physiologic steroid replacement (Brahmer et al., 2018; NCCN, 2022).

C. CAR-T AEs require intensive supportive care (see Chapter 27).

II. Nonpharmacologic

A. Before starting immunotherapy

1. Providers should familiarize themselves with updated guidelines and recommendations for the care of immunotherapy-related toxicities, including review of the National Comprehensive Cancer Network (NCCN) and ASCO guidelines.

2. Assure patient verbalizes monitoring instructions after infusion, has printed instructions, and has 24/7 contact information for the treatment team.

3. Educate patient on the importance of effective contraception for at least 5 months after the final dose of immunotherapy.

4. Patients should be advised to carry wallet cards that describe specific immunotherapy, expected irAEs, and the health care contact team.

5. Review drug-specific side effect profiles before every administration and assess for those symptoms.

B. Patient education (Brahmer et al., 2018)

1. Patient education should focus on (1) expected patterns of irAEs, (2) self-care of toxicities, and (3) interprofessional collaboration.

2. Educate patients that while evidence suggests a correlation between survival and incidence of irAEs; if unchecked, irAEs can become serious and should be addressed by their oncology team (Hussaini et al., 2021).

3. Educate patients about the immunotherapy component of their therapy, including the normal role of the immune system and mechanism of their immunotherapy agent.

4. Educate patients about the nature of AEs of immunotherapies, emphasizing the following:

   a. Multiple organ systems can be affected simultaneously.

   b. Autoimmune disorders can result from immune system activation from immunotherapy.

TABLE 30.12   Immune-Related Adverse Events Organized by Body System, Associated Immune-Related Condition, and Recommended Mode of Evaluation

Body System	Presenting Symptoms	Interventions
Dermatologic: maculopapular rash	Vitiligo, pruritus, and maculopapular rash	Consider dermatology referral. Skin biopsy if indicated.
Endocrine: hypothyroidism and/or hyperglycemia-related diabetic ketoacidosis	Hyperthyroidism, hypophysitis (alterations in TSH, T4, T3, and ACTH; significant fatigue, decreased appetite, and somnolence)	Consider endocrinology referral. Monitor labs.
Gastrointestinal	Colitis (abdominal pain with endoscopic evidence of inflammation), watery diarrhea (increase in the frequency of stools)	Consider stool evaluation to rule out infectious etiology. Consider holding immunotherapy. Hydration, loperamide, monitoring, and dietary modification.
Hepatic	Liver dysfunction (elevated ALT, AST, and total bilirubin), hepatitis	Rule out viral, drug, or disease-related etiology. Reduce hepatotoxic medications. Abdominal MRI. Hold immunotherapy for worrisome lab value trends.
Pneumonitis	Persistent dry cough, ground-glass opacities on imaging, and fine inspiratory crackles	Pulse oximetry, chest CT with contrast, infectious disease work-up, and consider corticosteroids.
Fatigue	Loss of stamina, shortness of breath, malaise, and muscle weakness	Assess the impact on ADLs. Pause immunotherapy to assess for improvement in fatigue. Consider consultation based on associated abnormalities (endocrine, GI, pulmonary).
Musculoskeletal	Arthralgia, polyarthritis	NSAIDs, corticosteroids, x-ray/ultrasound/MRI of joints. Antinuclear antibodies, C-reactive protein, ESR, and RF.
Pancreas	Elevations on lipase and amylase	Assess for signs of other causes. Abdominal CT with contrast. IV hydration, consider gastroenterology referral, corticosteroids.

ADL, Activities of daily living; *ALT*, alanine aminotransferase; *AST*, aspartate aminotransferase; *ESR*, erythrocyte sedimentation rate; *IV*, intravenous; *NSAIDs*, nonsteroidal antiinflammatory drugs; *RF*, rheumatoid factor.
From Brahmer, J. R., Lacchetti, C., Schneider, B. J., et al. (2018). Management of immune-related adverse events in patients treated with immune checkpoint inhibitor therapy: American Society of Clinical Oncology clinical practice guideline. *Journal of Clinical Oncology*, 36(17), 1714–1768. Available at: http://ascopubs.org/doi/abs/10.1200/JCO.2017.77.6385; Hussaini, S., Chehade, R., Boldt, R. G., Raphael, J., Blanchette, P., Maleki Vareki, S. M., et al. (2021). Association between immune-related side effects and efficacy and benefit of immune checkpoint inhibitors – A systematic review and meta-analysis. *Cancer Treatment Reviews*, 92, 102134. https://doi.org/10.1016/j.ctrv.2020.102134; National Comprehensive Cancer Network. (2022). *Management of immunotherapy-related toxicities. Version 1.2022—February 28, 2022.*

TABLE 30.13   Immune-Related Adverse Events Frequency and Timing

Adverse Event	Typical Onset Timing (Weeks)	Typical Resolution (Weeks)	Key Signs and Symptoms
Colitis	2–4	10	Watery diarrhea, cramping, urgency, abdominal pain, and blood and mucus in the stool
Liver toxicity	6	14	Elevated transaminases
Endocrinopathies	7	12–14	Hypothyroidism (low TSH), hypophysitis (low ACTH, low cortisol), adrenal insufficiency (rare with CPIs), thyrotoxicosis (low TSH with high T4/T3)
Dermatological	2	6	Maculopapular rash, pruritus, vitiligo, Stevens–Johnson syndrome
Nephritis	14	Variable	Acute kidney injury
Pneumonitis	10	>20	Dry cough, interstitial pneumonia, ground-glass opacities on radiological imaging

ACTH, Adrenocorticotropic hormone; *CPI*, checkpoint inhibitors; *TSH*, thyroid-stimulating hormone.
From Martins, F., Sofiya, L., Sykiotis, G. P., Lamine, F., Maillard, M., Fraga, M., et al. (2019). Adverse effects of immune-checkpoint inhibitors: Epidemiology, management and surveillance. *Nature Reviews. Clinical Oncology, 16*(9), 563–580. https://doi.org/10.1038/s41571-019-0218-0; National Comprehensive Cancer Network. (2022). *Management of immunotherapy-related toxicities. V. 1.2022—February 28, 2022.*

c. Organs that share the same antigen as the target may be affected by immunotherapy.
d. Onset of irAEs can occur/recur any time after treatment initiation or after treatment has stopped.
e. Combination therapy increases the risk of AEs.

5. Educate patients that nononcology providers should consult with the oncology team when any new symptoms occur because these may require immune-specific interventions not typical in nononcology patients.

TABLE 30.14	General Principles of Management of Immune-Related Adverse Events (IrAEs)	
General principles	Assume symptoms are immune related unless proven otherwise	
	Patients, caregivers, and families should be provided with timely and updated information about irAEs prior to therapy initiation, throughout treatment and survivorship	
	Specific neurological, hematologic, and cardiac toxicities require interventional care regardless of grade	
Less than grade 1	• Proactively monitor for symptoms and signs of adverse events	
At first appearance of symptoms	• Rule out nonimmune-related causes	
	• Grade symptoms using a standardized assessment scale	
Grade 1 or grade 2	• Increase monitoring	
	• Treat symptoms	
	• Consider holding immunotherapy	
	• Monitor for resolution to ≤grade 1	
Grade 2	• Initiation of corticosteroids	
	• Monitor for resolution to ≤grade 1	
	• Monitor tolerance to corticosteroids	
	• If not responding, intensification of corticosteroids or addition to alternative immunosuppressive therapy according to affected organ	
Grade 3 or grade 4	• Prepare for potential discontinuation of immunotherapy	
	• Consult with interdisciplinary team for management of affected organ/system	
	• Intensify high-dose corticosteroid and consider the addition of alternative immunosuppressive therapy	

From Brahmer, J. R., Lacchetti, C., Schneider, B. J., et al. (2018). Management of immune-related adverse events in patients treated with immune checkpoint inhibitor therapy: American Society of Clinical Oncology clinical practice guideline. *Journal of Clinical Oncology*, 36(17), 1714–1768. Available at: http://ascopubs.org/doi/abs/10.1200/JCO.2017.77.6385; Hussaini, S., Chehade, R., Boldt, R. G., Raphael, J., Blanchette, P., Vareki, S. M., et al. (2021). Association between immune-related side effects and efficacy and benefit of immune checkpoint inhibitors – A systematic review and meta-analysis. *Cancer Treatment Reviews*, 92, 102134. https://doi.org/10.1016/j.ctrv.2020.102134; National Comprehensive Cancer Network. (2022). *Management of immunotherapy-related toxicities. Version 1.2022—February 28, 2022*; Puzanov, I., Diab, A., Abdallah, K., Bingham, C. O., 3rd, Brogdon, C., Dadu, R., et al., Society for Immunotherapy of Cancer Toxicity Management Working Group. (2017). Managing toxicities associated with immune checkpoint inhibitors: Consensus recommendations from the Society for Immunotherapy of Cancer (SITC) Toxicity Management Working Group. *Journal for ImmunoTherapy of Cancer*, 5(1), 95. https://doi.org/10.1186/s40425-017-0300-z.

C. Monitor for safety during therapy.
   1. Assume a high level of suspicion that symptoms are treatment related unless definitive evidence supports an alternative cause.
   2. Monitor laboratory values before each infusion and at all follow-up visits.
   3. Assess symptoms and grade severity using a standardized grading scale such as the Common Terminology Criteria for Adverse Events (Common Terminology Criteria for Adverse Events, 2017).
      a. In general, patients experiencing grade 1 AEs should be carefully monitored during treatment.
      b. Moderate or grade 2 AEs will generally require dose interruption or delay until symptoms resolve.
      c. Severe or grade 3 and higher AEs generally require treatment cessation and intensive long-term management to prevent deleterious autoimmune sequelae.
   4. Monitor for early signs of CRS, including fever, tachycardia, hypotension, respiratory distress, peripheral edema, and altered level of consciousness.
   5. Monitor for infusion reactions: fever/chills/rigors, pruritus, edema, flushing/headache, hyper-/hypotension, shortness of breath, cough, wheezing, change in level of consciousness, diaphoresis, and arthralgia.
   6. Rule out other potential causes for common symptoms.
      a. Assess recent dietary pattern, community sources of infection, and assess for *Clostridium difficile* for patients experiencing diarrhea.
      b. Assess for allergen contact in patients experiencing rash.
      c. Assess community sources of infection, seasonal allergies in patients experiencing cough.
D. Manage emergent AEs appropriately.
   1. Review treatment plan for emergency medication orders before infusion.
   2. Educate patient about worrisome signs of symptoms that require immediate reporting.
   3. Assure availability of safety equipment.
   4. Stop infusion immediately if evidence of infusion reaction.
      a. Infusions may be restarted or slowed with mild reactions.
      b. Infusions may be discontinued permanently with severe reactions.
      c. Monitor for tolerance of corticosteroids and other immunosuppressive agents used for irAEs.

Prepare for possible rechallenge with immuno-therapies if irAEs resolve to ≤grade 1.

E. Collaborate with interprofessional teams.

   1. Dermatologists, gastroenterologists, pulmonologists, ophthalmologists, cardiologists, rheumatologists, and internal medicine practitioners should be consulted for the appropriate management of organ-specific disorders.

   2. Because irAEs can present at any time after initiation of drug and persist after cessation, nurses should assure that primary care providers are aware of long-term risk and associated signs of immune dysfunction.

REFERENCES

Acharya, U. H., Dhawale, T., Yun, S., Jacobson, C. A., Chavez, J. C., Ramos, J. D., et al. (2019). Management of cytokine release syndrome and neurotoxicity in chimeric antigen receptor (CAR) T cell therapy. *Expert Review of Hematology, 12*(3), 195–205. https://doi.org/10.1080/17474086.2019.1585238.

AL-Busairi, W., & Khajah, M. (2019). The principles behind targeted therapy for cancer treatment. In A. Lasfar & K. Cohen-Solal (Eds.), *Tumor progression and metastases.* London: IntechOpen. https://www.intechopen.com/chapters/67515.

American Cancer Society (ACS). (2019). Monoclonal antibodies and their side effects. https://www.cancer.org/treatment/treatments-and-side-effects/treatment-types/immunotherapy/monoclonal-antibodies.html#:~:text=The%20antibody%20delivers%20radioactivity%20directly,known%20as%20radioimmunotherapy%20(RIT).

American Society of Clinical Oncology (ASCO). (2018). *What is Immunotherapy?* https://www.cancer.net/navigating-cancer-care/how-cancer-treated/immunotherapy-and-vaccines/understanding-immunotherapy.

American Society of Clinical Oncology (ASCO). (2020a). *What is Targeted Therapy?* https://www.cancer.net/navigating-cancer-care/how-cancer-treated/personalized-and-targeted-therapies/understanding-targeted-therapy#:~:text=Drugs%20called%20monoclonal%20antibodies%20block,therapy%20reach%20cancer%20cells%20better.

American Society of Clinical Oncology (ASCO). (2020b). What is Immunotherapy? https://www.cancer.net/navigating-cancer-care/how-cancer-treated/immunotherapy-and-vaccines/understanding-immunotherapy Retrieved 19.03.22.

Andtbacka, R. H. I., Collichio, F., Harrington, K. J., Middleton, M. R., Downey, G., Öhrling, K., et al. (2019). Final analyses of OPTiM: A randomized phase III trial of talimogene laherparepvec versus granulocyte-macrophage colony-stimulating factor in unresectable stage III-IV melanoma. *Journal for ImmunoTherapy of Cancer, 7*(1), 145. https://doi.org/10.1186/s40425-019-0623-z.

Anttila, J. V., Shubin, M., Cairns, J., Borse, F., Guo, Q., Mononen, T., et al. (2019) Contrasting the impact of cytotoxic and cytostatic drug therapies on tumour progression. *PLoS Computational Biology,15*(11): e1007493. https://doi.org/10.1371/journal.pcbi.1007493.

Ayati, A., Moghimi, S., Salarinejad, S., Safavi, M., Pouramiri, B., & Foroumadi, A. (2020). A review on progression of epidermal growth factor receptor (EGFR) inhibitors as an efficient approach in cancer targeted therapy. *Bioorganic Chemistry, 99,* 103811. https://doi.org/10.1016/j.bioorg.2020.103811.

Balocco, R., De Sousa Guimaraes Koch, S., Thorpe, R., Weisser, K., & Malan, S. (2022). New INN nomenclature for monoclonal antibodies. *The Lancet (London, England), 399*(10319), 24. https://doi.org/10.1016/S0140-6736(21)02732-X.

Bedard, P. L., Hyman, D. M., Davids, M. S., & Siu, L. L. (2020). Small molecules, big impact: 20 years of targeted therapy in oncology. *Lancet (London, England), 395*(10229), 1078–1088. https://doi.org/10.1016/S0140-6736(20)30164-1.

Berraondo, P., Sanmamed, M. F., Ochoa, M. C., Etxeberria, I., Aznar, M. A., Pérez-Gracia, J. L., et al. (2019). Cytokines in clinical cancer immunotherapy. *British Journal of Cancer, 120*(1), 6–15. https://doi.org/10.1038/s41416-018-0328-y.

Bouwer, N., Jager, A., Liesting, C., Kofflard, M., Brugts, J., Kitzen, J., et al. (2020). Cardiac monitoring in HER2-positive patients on trastuzumab treatment: A review and implications for clinical practice. *The Breast, 52,* 33–44.

Brahmer, J. R., Lacchetti, C., Schneider, B. J., Atkins, M. B., Brassil, K. J., Caterino, J. M., et al. (2018). Management of immune-related adverse events in patients treated with immune checkpoint inhibitor therapy: American Society of Clinical Oncology clinical practice guideline. *Journal of Clinical Oncology, 36*(17), 1714–1768. https://doi.org/10.1200/JCO.2017.77.6385.

Brown, T. J., & Gupta, A. (2020). Management of cancer therapy-associated oral mucositis. *JCO Oncology Practice, 16*(3), 103–109. https://ascopubs.org/doi/abs/10.1200/JOP.19.00652.

Buti, S., Bersanelli, M., Perrone, F., Tiseo, M., Tucci, M., Adamo, V., et al. (2021). Effect of concomitant medications with immune-modulatory properties on the outcomes of patients with advanced cancer treated with immune checkpoint inhibitors: Development and validation of a novel prognostic index. *European Journal of Cancer, 142,* 18–28. https://doi.org/10.1016/j.ejca.2020.09.033.

Chau, C. H., Steeg, P. S., & Figg, W. D. (2019). Antibody-drug conjugates for cancer. *The Lancet (London, England), 394*(10200), 793–804. https://doi.org/10.1016/S0140-6736(19)31774-X.

Chen, W., Shen, L., Jiang, J., Zhang, L., Zhang, Z., Pan, J., et al. (2021). Antiangiogenic therapy reverses the immunosuppressive breast cancer microenvironment. *Biomarker Research, 9*(1), 59. https://doi.org/10.1186/s40364-021-00312-w.

Common Terminology Criteria for Adverse Events. (2017). Version 5.0. https://ctep.cancer.gov/protocoldevelopment/electronic_applications/docs/CTCAE_v5_Quick_Reference_5x7.pdf Accessed 31.03.2022.

Conlon, K. C., Miljkovic, M. D., & Waldmann, T. A. (2019). Cytokines in the treatment of cancer. *Journal of Interferon & Cytokine Research, 39*(1), 6–21. https://doi.org/10.1089/jir.2018.0019.

Dagher, S. H., Blom, A., Chabanol, H., & Funck-Brentano, E. (2021). Cutaneous toxicities from targeted therapies used in oncology: Literature review of clinical presentation and management. *International Journal of Women's Dermatology, 7*(5, Part A), 615–624.

Dahan, R. (2022). *Monoclonal antibodies, antibody drug conjugates, and bispecific antibodies.* New York: Cancer Research Institute. https://www.cancerresearch.org/en-us/immunotherapy/treatment-types/targeted-antibodies.

Dandreon Corporation. (2019). *Provenge.* Seattle, WA.

Das, B., Choudhury, B., Kumar, A., & Baruah, V. J. (2021). Genomic instability and DNA repair in cancer. In P. Behzadi (Ed.), *DNA – Damages and repair mechanisms.* London: IntechOpen. https://doi.org/10.5772/intechopen.95736.

Davis, A. A., & Patel, V. G. (2019). The role of PD-L1 expression as a predictive biomarker: An analysis of all US Food and Drug Administration (FDA) approvals of immune checkpoint inhibitors. *Journal for ImmunoTherapy of Cancer, 7*(1), 278. https://doi.org/10.1186/s40425-019-0768-9.

Dent, S., Morse, A., Burnette, S., Guha, A., & Moore, H. (2021). Cardiovascular toxicity of novel HER2-targeted therapies in the treatment of breast cancer. *Current Oncology Reports, 23*(11), 128. https://doi.org/10.1007/s11912-021-01114-x.

Dholaria, B. R., Bachmeier, C. A., & Locke, F. (2019). Mechanisms and management of chimeric antigen receptor T-cell therapy-related toxicities. *BioDrugs, 33*(1), 45–60. https://doi.org/10.1007/s40259-018-0324-z.

Eisenberg, S. (2021). Subcutaneous administration: Evolution, challenges, and the role of hyaluronidase. *Clinical Journal of Oncology Nursing, 25*(6), 663–671.

Eldridge, L. (2020). What is ALK-positive lung cancer? *Verywell Health.* https://www.verywellhealth.com/alk-positive-lung-cancer-definition-and-treatment-2248944.

Esfahani, K., Roudaia, L., Buhlaiga, N., Del Rincon, S. V., Papneja, N., & Miller, W. H., Jr. (2020). A review of cancer immunotherapy: From the past, to the present, to the future. *Current Oncology (Toronto, Ont.), 27*(Suppl 2), S87–S97. https://doi.org/10.3747/co.27.5223.

Food & Drug Administration (FDA). (2020). *Developing and Labeling in vitro companion diagnostic devices for a specific group of oncology therapeutic products.*

Food & Drug Administration (FDA). (2022) *Biosimilars.*

Frey, N., & Porter, D. (2019). Cytokine release syndrome with chimeric antigen receptor T cell therapy. *Biology of Blood and Marrow Transplantation, 25*(4), e123–e127. https://doi.org/10.1016/j.bbmt.2018.12.756.

Friedrich, M., Jasinski-Bergner, S., Lazaridou, M.-F., Subbarayan, K., Massa, C., Tretbar, S., et al. (2019). Tumor-induced escape mechanisms and their association with resistance to checkpoint inhibitor therapy. *Cancer Immunology, Immunotherapy, 68*, 1689–1700. https://doi.org/10.1007/s00262-019-02373-1.

Gerber, H.-P., Sibener, L. V., Lee, L. J., & Gee, M. H. (2020). Identification of antigenic targets. *Trends in Cancer, 6*(4), 299–318. https://doi.org/10.1016/j.trecan.2020.01.002.

Hemminki, O., Dos Santos, J. M., & Hemminki, A. (2020). Oncolytic viruses for cancer immunotherapy. *Journal of Hematology & Oncology, 13*(1), 84. https://doi.org/10.1186/s13045-020-00922-1.

Hofheinz, R.-D., Segaert, S., Safont, M. J., Demonty, G., & Prenen, H. (2017). Management of adverse events during treatment of gastrointestinal cancers with epidermal growth factor inhibitors. *Critical Reviews in Oncology/Hematology, 114*, 102–113. https://doi.org/10.1016/j.critrevonc.2017.03.032.

Hussaini, S., Chehade, R., Boldt, R. G., Raphael, J., Blanchette, P., Vareki, S. M., et al. (2021). Association between immune-related side effects and efficacy and benefit of immune checkpoint inhibitors – A systematic review and meta-analysis. *Cancer Treatment Reviews, 92*, 102134. https://doi.org/10.1016/j.ctrv.2020.102134.

Jacobs, S. (2019). Skin changes, risk for severe acneiform eruptions seen with EGFR inhibitor therapy. *Dermatology Advisor.* https://www.dermatologyadvisor.com/home/topics/acne/skin-changes-risk-for-severe-acneiform-eruptions-seen-with-egfr-inhibitor-therapy/.

Janelle, V., & Delisle, J. S. (2021). T-Cell Dysfunction as a Limitation of Adoptive Immunotherapy: Current Concepts and Mitigation Strategies. *Cancers, 13*(4), 598. https://doi.org/10.3390/cancers13040598.

Jiang, X., Wang, J., Deng, X., Xiong, F., Ge, J., Xiang, B., et al. (2019). Role of the tumor microenvironment in PD-L1/PD-1-mediated tumor immune escape. *Molecular Cancer, 18*(1), 10. https://doi.org/10.1186/s12943-018-0928-4.

Johnson, D. B., Nebhan, C. A., Moslehi, J. J., & Balko, J. M. (2022). Immune-checkpoint inhibitors: Long-term implications of toxicity. *Nature Reviews Clinical Oncology, 19*, 254–267. https://doi.org/10.1038/s41571-022-00600-w.

June, C. H., O'Connor, R. S., Kawalekar, O. U., Ghassemi, S., & Milone, M. C. (2018). CAR T cell immunotherapy for human cancer. *Science, 359*(6382), 1361–1365. https://doi.org/10.1126/science.aar6711.

Klein, C., Jamois, C., & Nielsen, T. (2021). Anti-CD20 treatment for B-cell malignancies: Current status and future directions. *Expert Opinion on Biological Therapy, 21*(2), 161–181. https://doi.org/10.1080/14712598.2020.1822318.

Krishnamurthy, A., & Jimeno, A. (2018). Bispecific antibodies for cancer therapy: A review. *Pharmacology & Therapeutics, 185*, 122–134. https://doi.org/10.1016/j.pharmthera.2017.12.002.

Kumar, A., Watkins, R., & Vilgelm, A. E. (2021). Cell therapy with TILs: Training and taming T cells to fight cancer. *Frontiers in Immunology, 12*, 690499. https://doi.org/10.3389/fimmu.2021.690499.

Lacouture, M., Sibaud, V., Gerber, P., van den Hurk, C., Fernández-Peñas, P., Santini, D., et al. (2021). Prevention and management of dermatological toxicities related to anticancer agents: ESMO Clinical Practice Guidelines. *Annals of Oncology, 32*(2), 157–170. https://doi.org/10.1016/j.annonc.2020.11.005.

Landskron, G., De la Fuente, M., Thuwajit, P., Thuwajit, C., & Hermoso, M. A. (2014). Chronic inflammation and cytokines in the tumor microenvironment. *Journal of Immunology Research, 2014*, 149185. Seminal work cited 1394 times. https://doi.org/10.1155/2014/149185.

Larocca, C. A., LeBoeuf, N. R., Silk, A. W., & Kaufman, H. L. (2020). An update on the role of talimogene laherparepvec (T-VEC) in the treatment of melanoma: Best practices and future directions. *American Journal of Clinical Dermatology, 21*(6), 821–832. https://doi.org/10.1007/s40257-020-00554-8.

Lee, Y. T., Tan, Y. J., & Oon, C. E. (2018). Molecular targeted therapy: Treating cancer with specificity. *European Journal of Pharmacology, 834*, 188–196. https://doi.org/10.1016/j.ejphar.2018.07.034.

Lejeune, M., Köse, M. C., Duray, E., Einsele, H., Beguin, Y., & Caers, J. (2020). Bispecific, T-cell-recruiting antibodies in B-cell malignancies. *Frontiers in Immunology, 11*, 762. https://doi.org/10.3389/fimmu.2020.00762.

Li, J., & Gu, J. (2019). Diarrhea with epidermal growth factor receptor tyrosine kinase inhibitors in cancer patients: A meta-analysis of randomized controlled trials. *Critical Reviews in Oncology/Hematology, 134*, 31–38. https://doi.org/10.1016/j.critrevonc.2018.12.001.

Li, Y., Fu, R., Jiang, T., Duan, D., Wu, Y., Li, C., et al. (2022). Mechanism of lethal skin toxicities induced by epidermal growth factor receptor inhibitors and related treatment strategies. *Frontiers in Oncology, 12*, 804212. https://doi.org/10.3389/fonc.2022.804212.

Lin, K. (2020). Utilizing companion diagnostics to drive clinical decisions. *Pharmacy Times, 2*(6). https://www.pharmacytimes.com/view/utilizing-companion-diagnostics-to-drive-clinical-decisions.

Martínez-Jiménez, F., Muiños, F., Sentís, I., Deu-Pons, J., Reyes-Salazar, I., Arnedo-Pac, C., et al. (2020). A compendium of mutational cancer driver genes. *Nature Reviews. Cancer, 20*(10), 555–572. https://doi.org/10.1038/s41568-020-0290-x.

Martins, F., Sofiya, L., Sykiotis, G. P., Lamine, F., Maillard, M., Fraga, M., et al. (2019). Adverse effects of immune-checkpoint inhibitors: Epidemiology, management and surveillance. *Nature Reviews. Clinical Oncology, 16*(9), 563–580. https://doi.org/10.1038/s41571-019-0218-0.

Meric-Bernstam, F., Johnson, A. M., Dumbrava, E., Raghav, K., Balaji, K., Bhatt, M., et al. (2019). Advances in HER2-targeted therapy: Novel agents and opportunities beyond breast and gastric cancer. *Clinical Cancer Research, 25*(7), 2033–2041. https://doi.org/10.1158/1078-0432.CCR-18-2275.

Mortezaee, K. (2020). Immune escape: A critical hallmark in solid tumors. *Life Sciences, 258*, 118110. https://doi.org/10.1016/j.lfs.2020.118110.

National Cancer Institute (NCI). (n.d.). NCI dictionary of cancer terms: Immunotherapy. https://www.cancer.gov/publications/dictionaries/cancer-terms/def/immunotherapy. Retrieved 07.02.22.

National Cancer Institute (NCI). (2019). Dictionary of cancer terms. https://www.cancer.gov/publications/dictionaries/cancer-terms/def/biotherapy; https://www.cancer.gov/publications/dictionaries/cancer-terms/def/companion-diagnostic-test.

National Cancer Institute (NCI). (2022a). Targeted therapy to treat cancer. https://www.cancer.gov/about-cancer/treatment/types/targeted-therapies/targeted-therapies-fact-sheet.

National Cancer Institute (NCI). (2022b). Targeted cancer therapies. https://www.cancer.gov/about-cancer/treatment/types/targeted-therapies/targeted-therapies-fact-sheet. Accessed 04.04.23.

National Comprehensive Cancer Network. (2022). Management of immunotherapy-related toxicities. V. 1.2022—February 28, 2022. https://www.cancer.gov/about-cancer/treatment/types/immunotherapy/t-cell-transfer-therapy.

Oh, D.-Y., & Bang, Y.-J. (2020). HER2-targeted therapies – A role beyond breast cancer. *Nature Reviews. Clinical Oncology, 17*(1), 33–48. https://doi.org/10.1038/s41571-019-0268-3.

Olsen, M., LeFebvre, K. B., & Brassil, K. J. (2019). *Chemotherapy and immunotherapy guidelines and recommendations for practice.* Pittsburgh, PA: Oncology Nursing Society.

Park, R., Lopes, L., & Saeed, A. (2021). Anti-PD-1/L1-associated immune-related adverse events as harbinger of favorable clinical outcome: Systematic review and meta-analysis. *Clinical & Translational Oncology, 23*(1), 100–109. https://doi.org/10.1007/s12094-020-02397-5.

Patel, S., Dushenkov, A., Jungsuwadee, P., Krishnaswami, A., & Barac, A. (2020). Team-based approach to management of hypertension associated with angiogenesis inhibitors. *Journal of Cardiovascular Translational Research, 13*, 463–477. https://doi.org/10.1007/s12265-020-10024-5.

Petrelli, F., Grizzi, G., Ghidini, M., Ghidini, A., Ratti, M., Panni, S., et al. (2020). Immune-related adverse events and survival in solid tumors treated with immune checkpoint inhibitors: A systematic review and meta-analysis. *Journal of Immunotherapy, 43*(1), 1–7. https://doi.org/10.1097/CJI.0000000000000300.

Phillips, G. S., Wu, J., Hellmann, M. D., Postow, M. A., Rizvi, N. A., Freites-Martinez, A., et al. (2019). Treatment outcomes of immune-related cutaneous adverse events. *Journal of Clinical Oncology, 37*(30), 2746-2758. https://doi.org/10.1200/JCO.18.02141.

Puzanov, I., Diab, A., Abdallah, K., Bingham, C. O., 3rd, Brogdon, C., Dadu, R., et al. (2017). Managing toxicities associated with immune checkpoint inhibitors: Consensus recommendations from the Society for Immunotherapy of Cancer (SITC) Toxicity Management Working Group. *Journal for ImmunoTherapy of Cancer, 5*(1), 95. https://doi.org/10.1186/s40425-017-0300-z. Seminal guidelines, 694 citations.

Rallis, K. S., Corrigan, A. E., Dadah, H., George, A. M., Keshwara, S. M., Sideris, M., et al. (2021). Cytokine-based cancer immunotherapy: Challenges and opportunities for IL-10. *Anticancer Research, 41*(7), 3247–3252. https://doi.org/10.21873/anticanres.15110.

Ruf, R., Yarandi, N., Ortiz-Melo, D., & Sparks, M. (2021). Onco-hypertension: Overview of hypertension with anti-cancer agents. *Journal of Onco-Nephrology, 5*(1), 57–69. https://doi.org/10.1177/23993693211001374.

Sadeghalvad, M., & Rezaei, N. (2021). Introduction on monoclonal antibodies. In N. Rezaei (Ed.), *Monoclonal antibodies.* London: IntechOpen. https://doi.org/10.5772/intechopen.98378.

Santomasso, B. D., Nastoupil, L. J., Adkins, S., Lacchetti, C., Schneider, B. J., Anadkat, M., et al. (2021). Management of immune-related adverse events in patients treated with chimeric antigen receptor T-cell therapy: ASCO guideline. *Journal of Clinical Oncology, 39*(35), 3978–3992. https://doi.org/10.1200/JCO.21.01992.

Schneider, B. J., Naidoo, J., Santomasso, B. D., Lacchetti, C., Adkins, S., Anadkat, M., et al. (2021). Management of immune-related adverse events in patients treated with immune checkpoint inhibitor therapy: ASCO guideline update. *Journal of Clinical Oncology, 39*(36), 4073–4126. https://doi.org/10.1200/JCO.21.01440.

Scott, B. (2021). Multidisciplinary team approach in cancer care: A review of the latest advancements. *EMJ Oncology,* (9, Suppl), 2–13. https://www.emjreviews.com/oncology/article/multidisciplinary-team-approach-in-cancer-care-a-review-of-the-latest-advancements-s130921/.

Som, A., Mandaliya, R., Alsaadi, D., Farshidpour, M., Charabaty, A., Malhotra, N., et al. (2019). Immune checkpoint inhibitor-induced colitis: A comprehensive review. *World Journal of Clinical Cases, 7*(4), 405–418. https://doi.org/10.12998/wjcc.v7.i4.405.

Sutherland, S. I. M., Ju, X., Horvath, L. G., & Clark, G. J. (2021). Moving on From Sipuleucel-T: New Dendritic Cell Vaccine Strategies for Prostate Cancer. *Frontiers in immunology, 12*, 641307. https://doi.org/10.3389/fimmu.2021.641307.

Tariman, J. D. (2018). Biosimilars: Exploring the history, science, and progress. *Clinical Journal of Oncology Nursing, 22*(5), 5–12. https://doi.org/10.1188/18.CJON.S1.5-12.

Tian, Z., Liu, M., Zhang, Y., & Wang, X. (2021). Bispecific T cell engagers: An emerging therapy for management of hematologic malignancies. *Journal of Hematology & Oncology, 14*(1), 75. https://doi.org/10.1186/s13045-021-01084-4.

Tumeh, P. C., Harview, C. L., Yearley, J. H., Shintaku, I. P., Taylor, E. J., Robert, L., et al. (2014). PD-1 blockade induces responses by inhibiting adaptive immune resistance. *Nature, 515*(7528), 568–571. https://doi.org/10.1038/nature13954.

Waldman, A. D., Fritz, J. M., & Lenardo, M. J. (2020). A guide to cancer immunotherapy: From T cell basic science to clinical practice. *Nature Reviews Immunology, 20*(11), 651–668. https://doi.org/10.1038/s41577-020-0306-5.

Waliany, S., Sainani, K. L., Park, L. S., Zhang, C. A., Srinivas, S., & Witteles, R. M. (2019). Increase in blood pressure associated with tyrosine kinase inhibitors targeting vascular endothelial growth factor. *JACC CardioOncology, 1*(1), 24–36. https://doi.org/10.1016/j.jaccao.2019.08.012.

Weingarden, A. R., Rubin, S., & Gubatan, J. (2021). Immune checkpoint inhibitor-mediated colitis in gastrointestinal malignancies and inflammatory bowel disease. *World Journal of Gastrointestinal Oncology, 13*(8), 772–798. https://doi.org/10.4251/wjgo.v13.i8.772.

Zahavi, D., & Weiner, L. (2020). Monoclonal antibodies in cancer therapy. *Antibodies (Basel, Switzerland)*, *9*(3), 34. https://doi.org/10.3390/antib9030034.

Zam, W., & Ali, L. (2021). Immune checkpoint inhibitors in the treatment of cancer. *Current Clinical Pharmacology*, *17*(2), 103–113. PMID: 33823768. https://doi.org/10.2174/1574884716666210325095022.

Zhang, H., & Chen, J. (2018). Current status and future directions of cancer immunotherapy. *Journal of Cancer*, *9*(10), 1773–1781. https://doi.org/10.7150/jca.24577.

Zhang, Y., & Zhang, Z. (2020). The history and advances in cancer immunotherapy: Understanding the characteristics of tumor-infiltrating immune cells and their therapeutic implications. *Cellular & Molecular Immunology*, *17*(8), 807–821. https://doi.org/10.1038/s41423-020-0488-6.

Zhang, Z., Liu, S., Zhang, B., Qiao, L., Zhang, Y., & Zhang, Y. (2020). T cell dysfunction and exhaustion in cancer. *Frontiers in Cell and Developmental Biology*, *8*, 17. https://doi.org/10.3389/fcell.2020.00017.

Zhang, Z., Lu, M., Qin, Y., Gao, W., Tao, L., Su, W., et al. (2021). Neoantigen: A new breakthrough in tumor immunotherapy. *Frontiers in Immunology*, *12*, 672356. https://doi.org/10.3389/fimmu.2021.672356.

Zhong, L., Li, Y., Xiong, L., Wang, W., Wu, M., Yuan, T., et al. (2021). Small molecules in targeted cancer therapy: Advances, challenges, and future perspectives. *Signal Transduction and Targeted Therapy*, *6*(1), 201. https://doi.org/10.1038/s41392-021-00572-w.

31

Support Therapies and Access Devices

Dawn Camp-Sorrell

BLOOD COMPONENT THERAPY

Overview

I. Use of blood component therapy in cancer care has increased because of the following reasons (Capraru et al., 2021; Leader, Hofstetter, & Spectre, 2021; Mahecic, Dunser, & Meier, 2020; Nair et al., 2020; National Comprehensive Cancer Network [NCCN], 2018; Ngo, Masel, Cahill, Blumberg, & Refaai, 2020; Stephens & Tano, 2021; Wang, Zhou, Han, & Zhang, 2021):
   A. Advancement of surgical oncology techniques
   B. Use of more aggressive single-modality and multimodality cancer therapy and the resulting bone marrow suppression
   C. Development of donor programs, hemapheresis technology, and hematopoietic stem cell transplantation (HSCT) therapies, all of which serve to increase the available range of blood component therapies
   D. Less use of erythropoietin due to the potential for disease progression

II. Types of blood component therapy (Table 31.1)

III. Sources of blood components (Alcaina, 2020; Capraru et al., 2021; Gea-Banacloche, 2017; Leader et al., 2021; Mahecic et al., 2020; Nair et al., 2020; Ngo et al., 2020; Shmookler & Flanagan, 2020; Wang et al., 2021)
   A. Allogeneic blood component—blood collected from screened donors for transfusion to another individual
   B. Autologous blood—blood collected from the intended recipient
      1. Self-donation usually made before elective surgery
      2. Red blood cell (RBC) salvage during surgery by the use of automated "cell saver" device or manual suction equipment
   C. Directly donated blood—blood component collected from a donor designated by the intended recipient
   D. All blood products are stored in a bag containing anticoagulant (citrate) and preservative nutrients such as citric acid, dextrose, and phosphate

IV. Benefits of transfusion (Alcaina, 2020; Capraru et al., 2021; Gea-Banacloche, 2017; Mahecic et al., 2020; Nair et al., 2020; NCCN, 2018 2017; Schiffer et al., 2017; Stephens & Tano, 2021; Wang et al., 2021)
   A. RBCs—correction of anemia
      1. Hemoglobin should increase 1 g/dL or hematocrit by 3% with 1 unit
      2. Improvement of symptoms (e.g., fatigue, weakness, and shortness of breath [SOB])
   B. Platelets—correction of thrombocytopenia
      1. Increase of 35–40 µL with 1 unit of apheresis platelets
         a. Pooled—four to six donors
         b. Apheresis—one donor
         c. Platelet additive solution (PAS)
         d. Human leukocyte antigen (HLA) typing for refractoriness
      2. Decrease in signs of bleeding
   C. Plasma—correct clotting factor deficiencies, expand blood volume, and provide osmotic diuresis
   D. White blood cells (WBCs)—increase of WBCs and prevent and/or treat infections in neutropenic patients
   E. Cryoprecipitate—corrects dilution of clotting factors secondary to massive hemorrhage, extensive transfusion, liver failure, or consumption coagulopathy secondary to disseminated intravascular coagulation (DIC) by raising fibrinogen level by 5–10 mg/dL
   F. Immunoglobulin G (IgG)—maintain antibody levels, prevent infection, confer passive immunity

V. Potential complications of blood component therapy (Alcaina, 2020; Capraru et al., 2021; DeLisle, 2018; Kuldanek, Kelher, & Silliman, 2019; Nair et al., 2020; NCCN, 2018; Savinkina et al., 2020; Schiffer et al., 2017; Shmookler & Flanagan, 2020; Stephens & Tano, 2021)
   A. Acute reactions: occurring with 24 hours of the transfusion
      1. Hemolytic reactions: usually due to ABO blood type incompatibility
      2. Febrile nonhemolytic reactions: often a reaction to passively transfused cytokines
      3. Allergic reactions: hypersensitivity reaction to donor plasma proteins
      4. Anaphylaxis: reaction from antibody to donor plasma proteins (IgA, complement 4, or haptoglobin)
      5. Transfusion-associated circulatory overload: rapid infusion causing fluid to accumulate leading to pulmonary edema
      6. Hypothermia
      7. Bacteremia or sepsis

TABLE 31.1 Types of Blood Component Therapy

Blood Component	Indication	Consideration
Whole blood	Replacement of blood volume Replacement of RBCs	Rarely used, except in extreme loss of volume
RBCs (packed)	Correction of anemia, for replacement of RBCs	Volume overload
Leukocyte-reduced RBCs	Prior febrile reactions to packed RBCs Reduction of alloimmunizations Reduction of immunomodulatory effects	May use a leukocyte filter to further reduce the risk of reaction
Washed or plasma-poor RBCs	Prior urticarial reaction, IgA deficiency	Increased viscosity of blood; thin with normal saline before transfusion
Frozen packed RBCs	Rare blood types, autologous donations	Used in patients with a history of severe RBC reactions
Platelets, pooled	Control or prevent bleeding; platelet count <10,000–20,000/mm^3 or patient is bleeding or preoperative	Few RBCs present; ABO compatibility not required
Single-donor platelets	Reduction of alloimmunization, lower risk of infection, exposure to one donor	Inadequate increase in platelet count consider refractory PAS for history of reaction
Leukocyte-reduced platelets	Prior febrile reaction to platelets Reduction of alloimmunization	Febrile reactions; poor increase in platelet count PAS for history of reaction
HLA-matched platelets	Poor response to prior platelet transfusion because of alloimmunization	Obtain posttransfusion platelet count if HLA-matched platelets are used
Granulocytes	Documented refractory infection from bacteria or fungi not responsive to therapy, with severe neutropenia, not expected to recover for several days to 1 week	Long-term therapeutic effect questionable Transfuse within 24 hours after collection
Fresh frozen plasma	Increase in the level of clotting factors in patient with documented coagulation deficiency; expand blood volume, provide osmotic diuresis	Plasma compatibility preferred with recipient; when thawed, must transfuse within 24 h; watch for fluid overload All coagulation factors present
Cryoprecipitate	Increase in levels of factors VIII and XIII, fibrinogen, fibronectin, and von Willebrand factor due to massive hemorrhage, extensive transfusion liver failure or consumption coagulopathy due to DIC	Plasma compatibility preferred; when thawed, must transfuse within 6 h; if pooled, within 4 h
Factor VIII	Hemophilia A or low AT III levels	In patients with volume overload problems, plasma cannot be used
Factor IX	Hemophilia B deficiency	Need replacement of factor; treated by injection of purified factor IX
Colloid solutions	Expand blood volume	ABO compatibility not required
Plasma substitutes	Chiefly 5% and 25% albumin and PPF	Provide volume expansion and colloid replacement without risk of hepatitis or HIV
Serum immune globulins	To provide passive immunity protection (e.g., against cytomegalovirus) or treat hypogammaglobulinemia	Avoid transfusion for patient with allergic reactions to plasma

AT, Antithrombin; *HIV*, human immunodeficiency virus; *HLA*, human leukocyte antigen; *IgA*, immunoglobulin A; *PPF*, plasma protein fraction; *RBCs*, red blood cells.

8. Coagulation problems in massive transfusion (e.g., with hemorrhage)
9. Metabolic derangement such as hypocalcemia or hyperkalemia
10. Transfusion-related acute lung injury: reaction caused by WBC antibodies in the transfused product reacting with patient's WBCs
11. Urticaria reaction

B. Delayed—develops after 24 hours, months, or (rarely) years later depending on onset relative to the inciting transfusion
   1. Hemolytic reactions causing immune destruction of transfused RBCs, which are attacked by the recipient's antibodies
   2. Iron overload from frequent RBC transfusions
   3. Refractory to blood products
   4. Posttransfusion purpura: antibody destroys transfused and patient's own platelets
   5. Transfusion-associated graft-versus-host disease (GVHD): rare occurrence due to engraftment of viable donor T cells from blood component in a susceptible recipient; blood cells irradiated to prevent
   6. Alloimmunization—patient develops alloantibodies against the donor's antigens
   7. Transmission of virus (e.g., hepatitis, human immunodeficiency virus [HIV], herpes, cytomegalovirus [CMV], West Nile, Zika)

C. Transfusion of the incorrect product to the incorrect patient

Assessment

I. Factors that increase the likelihood for receipt of blood (Alcaina, 2020; Leader et al., 2021; Nair et al., 2020; NCCN, 2018; Schiffer et al., 2017; Wang et al., 2021)
   A. Cancer treatment (e.g., chemotherapy, immunotherapy, radiation, surgery, and stem cell transplantation)
   B. Cancer that has invaded the bone marrow
   C. Drugs that suppress bone marrow production
   D. Chronic bacterial, fungal, or viral infection
   E. Older age
   F. Malnutrition, including deficiencies in folate, vitamin B_{12}, and iron
   G. Chronic immune deficiency
   H. Comorbidities—heart disease, diabetes, renal failure, and liver disease
   I. Acute blood loss
   J. Reversal of vitamin K antagonist treatment
   K. Acquired coagulopathies

II. Evaluation of laboratory data (Alcaina, 2020; Capraru et al., 2021; Gea-Banacloche, 2017; Leader et al., 2021; Mahecic et al., 2020; Nair et al., 2020; NCCN, 2018; Ngo et al., 2020; Schiffer et al., 2017; Shmookler & Flanagan, 2020; Wang et al., 2021)
   A. ABO type and Rh factor
   B. Hemoglobin—transfusion guideline less than 7 g/dL or if symptomatic
   C. Platelet count: transfusion guidelines
      1. Less than 10,000/mm³, with or without bleeding
      2. Less than 20,000/mm³, with active bleeding
      3. Less than 50,000/mm³–75,000/mm³ and scheduled for surgical procedure per institution guidelines
   D. Neutrophils—less than 500/mm³, with an infection unresponsive to antibiotic therapy
   E. International normalized ratio greater than 1.69 and partial thromboplastin time and prothrombin time prolonged
   F. DIC—laboratory assessment, if indicated: fibrinogen less than 150 mg/dL, fibrin/fibrinogen degradation products greater than 40, D-dimer assay elevated
   G. IgG level decreased
   H. Autoantibodies—clinically significant; formed from prior transfusions

Management

I. Medical management
   A. Prevent and manage transfusion reactions (Alcaina, 2020; Capraru et al., 2021; DeLisle, 2018; Kuldanek et al., 2019; Savinkina et al., 2020; Shmookler & Flanagan, 2020; Wang et al., 2021).
      1. Premedicate patient with antipyretics and antihistamines, usually acetaminophen and diphenhydramine, especially for previous reaction. Steroid and H2 antagonist may be added as premedication for severe reactions previously.
      2. If a reaction occurs:
         a. Assess the patient clinically for unstableness, for example, chest pain, dyspnea, and rigors.
         b. Stop infusion and keep intravenous (IV) line open with normal saline (NS) solution.
         c. Report reaction to the provider and the transfusion service or blood bank.
         d. Recheck identifying tags and numbers on the blood component at the bedside.
      3. Treat symptoms as ordered:
         a. Diphenhydramine—administer 25–50 mg intravenously.
         b. Hydrocortisone—have 50–100 mg IV available for severe reactions.
         c. Meperidine (Demerol)—25–50 mg IV for uncontrolled rigors.
         d. Acetaminophen—administer 650–1000 mg by mouth (PO).
         e. Oxygen—administer if indicated.
         f. Diuretic—administer for fluid overload or reduce intravascular volume.
         g. Epinephrine or solumedrol—administer for allergic/anaphylactic reaction.
         h. Vasopressor support—administer if indicated for hypotension.
      4. Send blood bag, attached administration set, and labels to the blood bank or service.
      5. Collect blood and urine samples.
   B. Employ pharmacologic management as indicated (Nair et al., 2020; Ngo et al., 2020).
      1. Recombinant factor VIIa for patients with existing coagulopathy
         a. Activates factor X to factor Xa; activated factor Xa converts prothrombin to thrombin, then acts to convert fibrinogen to fibrin, forming a hemostatic plug
         b. Approved for the treatment of bleeding episodes in hemophilia A or B patients with inhibitors to factor VIII or factor IX
         c. Potential use in those with DIC, liver disease, and thrombocytopenia refractory to HLA-matched platelets
      2. Vitamin K—essential for activating factors II, VII, IX, and X because its deficiency impairs the function of clotting factors
      3. Artificial plasma indicated for the treatment of shock, acute liver failure, acute respiratory distress syndrome, severe hyponatremia, and renal dialysis

II. Nursing management

III. Maximize patient safety (Capraru et al., 2021; Ngo et al., 2020; Savinkina et al., 2020; Shmookler & Flanagan, 2020).
   A. Obtain, store, and administer blood components according to institutional protocol.
   B. Ensure bacterial and viral screening of blood components.
   C. Obtain transfusion informed consent.
   D. Check and/or scan blood component type with medical order, identification numbers with another registered nurse with patient identification information before administration.

E. Examine blood product for clots, bubbles, particulates, and discoloration.

F. Ensure that medications or IV fluids are never added to blood products.

G. Restrict transfusion to those who have clear indications for such therapy, and only transfuse the minimum number of units necessary.

H. Administer CMV-negative products to patients who do not have the virus.

IV. Monitor for complications of blood component therapy (DeLisle, 2018; Gea-Banacloche, 2017; Kuldanek et al., 2019; NCCN, 2018; Shmookler & Flanagan, 2020).

A. General signs/symptoms—fever, chills, muscle aches and pain, back pain, chest pain, headache, and warmth or redness at the site of infusion or along vessel

B. Respiratory—SOB, tachypnea, apnea, cough, wheezing, rales, and air embolism

C. Cardiovascular—bradycardia or tachycardia, hypotension or hypertension, facial flushing, cyanosis of extremities, cool clammy skin, distended neck veins, and edema

D. Integumentary—rash, hives, swelling, urticaria, post-transfusion purpura, and diaphoresis

E. Gastrointestinal (GI)—nausea, vomiting, abdominal cramping, and pain

F. Renal—dark, concentrated, and red- to brown-colored urine

G. Delayed complications—hemolytic transfusion reaction, GVHD (from nonirradiated blood), iron overload, alloimmunization, infections (hepatitis, HIV, CMV, bacterial contamination)

V. Decrease incidence and severity of transfusion reaction (Alcaina, 2020; Capraru et al., 2021; DeLisle, 2018; Gea-Banacloche, 2017; Kuldanek et al., 2019; NCCN, 2018; Shmookler & Flanagan, 2020)

A. Attach appropriate filter, blood component set, or both to the blood product.

1. Use leukocyte reduction filter to reduce the number of leukocytes transfused to the patient in a unit of RBCs and platelets.

2. Administer irradiated blood components to all allogeneic HSCT recipients and others to prevent transfusion of leukocytes.

3. Administer PAS with the history of platelet transfusion reaction.

B. Use 22-gauge (preferably 20-gauge) or larger needle for infusion when transfusing RBCs and platelets peripherally.

C. Infuse component over time, according to institutional guidelines.

1. Packed RBCs—infuse slowly initial 15 minutes, then remainder over 1–3 hours per unit; no longer than 4 hours per unit from the time issued from the blood bank

2. Platelets—infuse random-donor or single-donor platelets over 15–30 minutes or according to volume

3. Granulocytes—infused slowly over 2–4 hours

4. Fresh frozen plasma—each unit administered slowly or as tolerated

5. Cryoprecipitate—infused rapidly over 15 minutes or less

6. Concentrated factor VIII or factor IX—infused rapidly over 15 minutes or less

D. Monitor for transfusion reaction—fever/chills, SOB, dyspnea, hives, wheezing, flank/back pain, hematuria, hypotension, tachycardia, chest pain, and headache.

E. Prevent and manage infusion reactions according to protocol (see earlier).

F. Document transfusion reaction.

1. Date and time noted

2. Signs and symptoms observed

3. Actions taken

G. Monitor patient for approximately 1–2 hours after transfusion to ensure that an acute reaction does not occur.

VI. Educate patient and family.

A. Educate about the purpose of the transfusion or blood component therapy.

B. Review of procedure for administration of blood component therapy.

C. Educate about the signs/symptoms of transfusion reaction that should be reported.

VII. Monitor for response to blood component therapy.

A. Monitor changes in laboratory values.

B. Assess for changes in symptoms (e.g., reduction in fatigue or SOB).

C. Monitor for signs and symptoms of bleeding.

VIII. Patients who refuse blood component therapy (NCCN, 2018)

A. Discuss reasons for refusal, such as religious beliefs that prohibit the use of blood products or personal preference.

B. Techniques for the minimization of blood loss or minimize transfusions

1. Minimize routine blood testing.

2. Use pediatric blood collection tubes.

3. Suppress menstrual cycles in patients with thrombocytopenia.

4. Minimize GI bleeding with proton pump inhibitors and bowel management.

5. Administer iron component therapy for iron deficiency.

6. Erythropoietic therapy may be considered for select patients.

7. Avoid anticoagulation, including heparin flushes or alteplase use.

8. Use vitamin supplementation such as folic acid, vitamin B, and vitamin K.

9. Use antifibrinolytic agents for oral bleeding.

ACCESS DEVICES—VENOUS, ARTERIAL, PERITONEAL, INTRAVENTRICULAR, EPIDURAL OR INTRATHECAL, AND PLEURAL

Overview

I. Access devices are essential in the care of patients with cancer because of the following (Akhtar & Lee, 2021; Camp-Sorrell & Matey, 2017; Hawasli, Barton, & Nabhani-Gebara, 2021; Morrell, 2020; Patel, Patel, Singh, Singh, & Khawaja, 2019):
  A. Combination IV therapy in the treatment of cancer
  B. Administering therapies into multiple body systems
  C. Supportive therapy (nutritional support, antibiotics, and blood component therapy)
  D. Increased laboratory monitoring required with aggressive therapy
  E. Use of pleural, arterial, peritoneal, epidural, intrathecal, and intraventricular therapy

II. Types of venous access devices (Akhtar & Lee, 2021; Gupta et al., 2021; Hawasli et al., 2021; Lescinskas et al., 2020; Marin, Bull, Kinzie, & Andresen, 2021; Mielke, Wittig, & Teichgraber, 2020; Morrell, 2020; Patel et al., 2019)
  A. Short-term or intermediate-term peripheral catheters—to infuse fluids, medications, blood products, and peripheral total parenteral nutrition and to obtain blood specimens (Camp-Sorrell & Matey, 2017; Lescinskas et al., 2020; Morrell, 2020)
    1. Description—single-lumen or multilumen catheters
    2. Insertion—peripherally in forearm or antecubital fossa into the cephalic, basilic, or median cubital vein
    3. Types of short-term catheters
      a. Peripheral catheters—inserted into a peripheral vein; change as indicated
      b. Midline catheters—inserted into peripheral vein terminating in the axillary vein in the upper arm; used for therapy for up to 6 weeks or longer
  B. Nontunneled venous short-term catheters (Camp-Sorrell & Matey, 2017; Karpanen et al., 2019)
    1. Description: immediate access; removal when clinically indicated; available in single or multilumen (up to five-lumen design)
    2. Insertion of nontunneled catheters centrally in jugular vein, subclavian vein, superior vena cava (SVC), or inferior vena cava
  C. Long-term venous catheters—maintained for months to years (Akhtar & Lee, 2021; Blanco-Guzman, 2018; Camp-Sorrell & Matey, 2017; Gupta et al., 2021; Lescinskas et al., 2020; Mielke et al., 2020)
    1. Overview—distal tip lies in the lower third of the SVC
      a. Power-injectable designs available to deliver power injection flow rates required for contrast-enhanced injections; withstand high infusion pressures
      b. Available with pressure-activated safety valve located in the catheter hub; designed to permit fluid infusion and decrease the risk of blood reflux
      c. Catheter tip must be confirmed before initial use—by ultrasound (during placement if used), fluoroscopy, or chest x-ray
      d. Available with open or closed distal tip
    2. Tunneled catheter
      a. Description—single-lumen or multilumen catheters
        (1) Dacron cuff attached to the catheter, becoming embedded into the subcutaneous (SC) tissue after tunneling
          (a) Stabilizes the catheter
          (b) Minimizes the risk of ascending infections up the tunnel
          (c) Securement device can be used on anterior chest to stabilize external portion
        (2) Antimicrobial cuff available at the exit site to prevent ascending microbes; releases antimicrobial activity for approximately 4–6 weeks
      b. Insertion—percutaneous insertion using the internal jugular in the interventional radiology (IR) or surgery under ultrasound or fluoroscopy
        (1) Once vein is cannulated, the guidewire is advanced into the vein.
        (2) Catheter is tunneled through the SC tissue to exit on the anterior chest, typically above the nipple line midway between the sternum and clavicle.
    3. Implanted port
      a. Description—single- or double-port device
        (1) Port body with reservoir inside covered with self-sealing septum
        (2) Port body with an attached or nonattached catheter
        (3) Port is accessed with a straight or angled noncoring needle
      b. Types—anterior chest or peripheral (basilic, cephalic, or median cubital veins)
      c. Insertion in IR or surgery using ultrasound or fluoroscopy guidance
    4. Peripherally inserted central catheters (PICCs)
      a. Description—single, double, or triple lumen
        (1) Approved for use up to 12 months; however, evidence supports longer duration if device is functioning without complication
        (2) Securement device stabilizes external portion at the antecubital fossa or just above the elbow
        (3) Insertion at the bedside or IR typically under ultrasound guidance
        (4) Inserted peripherally into the cephalic, accessory cephalic, basilic, or median cubital

III. Types of nonvenous access devices
  A. Arterial catheters (Camp-Sorrell & Matey, 2017; Italiano, 2018; Laface et al., 2021)
    1. Descriptions—for short- or long-term chemotherapy administration
       a. Smaller internal diameters and thicker walls because of higher vascular arterial pressure
       b. Delivers high concentrations of drug directly to the tumor with decreased systemic exposure
       c. One-way valve to prevent retrograde blood flow
       d. Intraarterial therapies are considered regional treatment, with the arterial catheter directly threaded into the artery that feeds the tumor
    2. Insertion in IR or surgery
       a. Catheter inserted into the artery for perfusion, usually hepatic artery, similar to venous placement; hypogastric, femoral, and brachial arteries used
       b. Port or pump surgically placed in SC pocket over a bony prominence
    3. Types—temporary percutaneous, implanted arterial port, implanted pump
  B. Peritoneal catheters—for the administration of chemotherapy into the peritoneal cavity or for the treatment of ascites (Camp-Sorrell & Matey, 2017; Kaya, Nas, & Erdogan, 2019; Yang et al., 2020)
    1. Descriptions
       a. A single-lumen catheter; may have multiple fenestrated holes to permit increased distribution of chemotherapy
       b. Temporarily or permanently implanted into the peritoneal cavity
    2. Insertion in IR or surgery
       a. Catheter placed through the anterior abdominal wall at the level of the umbilicus with tip directed toward cul-de-sac of the pelvis
       b. Tunnel—catheter tunneled in the SC tissue side of the midline or abdomen
       c. Port—placed in SC pocket over a bony prominence, usually a lower rib
    3. Types—temporary catheter, tunneled catheter, implanted port
  C. Intraventricular reservoir (Ommaya^R reservoir)—for access to the ventricular system as an alternative to repeated lumbar punctures; provides direct access to cerebrospinal fluid (CSF) (Camp-Sorrell & Matey, 2017; Magill, Choy, Nguyen, & McDermott, 2020)
    1. Description—dome-shaped with catheter attached
    2. Insertion—in surgery, reservoir surgically placed under the scalp, and the catheter threaded into the lateral ventricle
  D. Epidural and intrathecal catheters—for the administration of opioid analgesics and anesthetic mediations, chemotherapy, CSF sampling, and antispasmodic agents intrathecally (Camp-Sorrell & Matey, 2017; Capozza et al., 2021; Stearns et al., 2020)
    1. Description
       a. Epidural—catheter placed in the epidural space
       b. Intrathecal—catheter inserted below the dura where CSF circulates
    2. Insertion in IR or surgery; at the bedside for short-term use
       a. Catheter inserted into the epidural space, usually at L2–3, L3–4, or L4–5 or intrathecal space, usually at L2–3, L3–4, or L4–5
       b. Tunneled in the SC tissue; exits the waist or side of the abdomen after catheter inserted into epidural or intrathecal space
       c. Pump implanted into a created SC pocket and placed over a bony prominence with catheter inserted into the epidural or intrathecal space
    3. Types—temporary catheter, tunneled catheter, implanted port, and implanted pump
  E. Intrapleural catheters: for the administration of intrapleural medication and to drain the pleural cavity (Camp-Sorrell & Matey, 2017; Vrtis, DeCesare, & Day, 2021)
    1. Description—single lumen with drainage side holes inserted through the chest wall into the pleural cavity between the visceral and parietal pleura
    2. Insertion: in IR or surgery, exception with temporary short term at bedside
    3. Types—nontunneled for short-term use, tunneled for long-term use
IV. Complications associated with access devices (Table 31.2; Akhtar & Lee, 2021; Blanco-Guzman, 2018; Boll et al., 2021; Buetti et al., 2020; Freire et al., 2018; Gupta et al., 2021; Hawasli et al., 2021; Ilhan, Sormaz, & Turkay, 2018; Karpanen et al., 2019; Lau, Kosteniuk, Macdonald, & Megyesi, 2018; Lescinskas et al., 2020; Machat et al., 2019; Marin et al., 2021; Mielke et al., 2020; Oh et al., 2021; Patel et al., 2019; Sayed et al., 2018)
  A. Infection—presence of redness, pain, swelling, warmth, or drainage at exit site or along tunnel or pocket
    1. Preventive measures
       a. Most infections occur at the insertion or access site, hub of catheter, or both. Catheters coated with chlorhexidine, silver sulfadiazine, or antibiotics are recommended to decrease infection in short-term, nontunneled venous catheters.
       b. Hubs can be coated with antiinfective agents such as chlorhexidine.
       c. Use antiseptic before accessing needleless connectors or hubs.
       d. Removal of catheter based on clinical judgment and need for the device.
    2. Dressing changes (Boll et al., 2021; Buetti et al., 2020; Camp-Sorrell & Matey, 2017)
       a. Gauze—changed every other day or prn (as needed) if soiled or nonocclusive
       b. Transparent—changed every 7 days or prn if soiled or nonocclusive
       c. Exit site cleansed with chlorhexidine solution

TABLE 31.2   Interventions for Mechanical Complications of Access Devices

Complication	Prevention	Restoration of Problem
Occlusion	Maintain flushing routine, flush with pulsatile (push-pause) method to cause swirling action in device Always flush with normal saline before and after drug administration, blood withdrawal, and administration of blood products Avoid incompatible drugs	Change patient position, roll on to right or left side, sit up, lie flat Change intrathoracic pressures: have patient inhale fully and hold breath or exhale fully and hold breath Attempt pulsatile method using normal saline-filled syringe (avoid using high force or high pressure) or administer fibrinolytic agent per provider order If occlusion the result of clotted blood, tPA may be instilled with a provider order If drug precipitate, determine type of drug, check with pharmacist for drug to dissolve precipitate
Pinch-off syndrome	Proper placement by surgeon	Surgical removal is performed, as indicated, to avoid fracture
Catheter dislodgement	Avoid pulling on the catheter Use securement device Teach patient to avoid manipulation of catheter or port and prevent trauma to catheter	If tip of the catheter remains in the vessel, use securement device. Monitor the length of catheter. Remove device, as indicated
Catheter migration	Protect the device from trauma Anchor the device appropriately with securement device Monitor the length of catheter (tunnel, midline, PICC) to ensure placement intact Radiography ordered for long-term catheters to confirm placement	Refer to physician for repositioning catheter using fluoroscopy Remove the device, as indicated
Catheter pinholes, tracks, cuts	Avoid the use of scissors or sharp objects near the catheter Clamp properly over reinforced area on catheter	Repair using an appropriate repair kit
Erosion of port through subcutaneous tissue	Avoid placing port at sites of actual or potential tissue damage (in radiation field) Avoid trauma or pressure over port	Device removal
Port–catheter separation	High-pressure infusions or flushing with 1- or 3-mL syringes when clogged	Remove device
Dislodgement of port access needle	Secure needle in place Avoid tension on the needle or tubing	Remove needle, and reaccess port using a sterile noncoring needle

PICC, Peripherally inserted central catheter; *tPA,* tissue plasminogen activator.

d. Use needleless connectors and protective caps to minimize the risk of infections recommended.
3. Bundle care to include the following:
   a. Frequent hand washing before and after use
   b. Optimal catheter site selection
   c. Maximal sterile barrier precautions on insertion of device
   d. Alcohol hub decontamination before each access
   e. Review line necessity daily with prompt removal of unnecessary lines.
B. Occlusion—inability to infuse fluid, or difficulty infusing, or inability to withdraw blood or fluid from a body cavity—that is, peritoneal fluid (Camp-Sorrell & Matey, 2017; Machat et al., 2019; Marin et al., 2021; Oh et al., 2021; Patel et al., 2019)
   1. Preventive measures
      a. Use device-specific flushing procedures according to current guidelines to prevent occlusion

(Camp-Sorrell & Matey, 2017; Mielke et al., 2020; Oh et al., 2021).
      b. Flush with NS before and after each use, for example, medications, blood products, and blood withdrawals.
2. Occlusion—occurs in up to 40% of patients within 1–2 years of device placement
   a. Fibrin sheath—may form at the catheter tip, causing a one-way valve effect, allowing infusion of IV fluids into the patient but causing withdrawal occlusion. The most common cause of thrombotic occlusion and the most common cause of partial occlusion.
   b. Intraluminal blood clot—may cause complete obstruction by forming around the catheter surface.
   c. Mural thrombus—a clot that adheres to the vessel wall, forming a thrombus, and occludes the tip of the catheter.

d. Deep vein thrombosis (DVT)—occludes the vein, typically in the upper extremity. Most commonly found in the subclavian; can be axillary, brachial, and brachiocephalic veins. Recent infection increases risk.

3. Precipitation—occurs when incompatible medications or solutions are simultaneously infused, or sequentially infused without adequate flushing in between

C. Mechanical withdrawal occlusions
   1. Pinch-off syndrome—catheter becomes pinched between the clavicle and the first rib, with possible catheter fracture (Camp-Sorrell & Matey, 2017; Ilham et al., 2018; Machat et al., 2019; Patel et al., 2019).
   2. When complete fracture occurs, the distal portion of the catheter can travel to the pulmonary artery, right atrium, right ventricle, and SVC.

D. Catheter tip migration—regional discomfort, pain, swelling, or difficulty in using device or catheter fracture or tear (Machat et al., 2019)

E. Air embolism—presence of sudden-onset pallor or cyanosis, SOB, cough, or tachycardia (Machat et al., 2019)

F. Pneumothorax—presence of SOB, chest pain, or tachycardia (Ilhan et al., 2018; Machat et al., 2019)
   1. Follow-up imaging after placement
   2. Close monitoring of patient; chest radiography to assess for pneumothorax

G. Arterial injury—bleeding at exit or entrance site caused by puncture of artery near access site; close monitoring of patient after placement (Machat et al., 2019)

H. Phlebitis—mechanical or chemical irritation that may cause injury to vein; close monitoring of exit site (Morrell, 2020)

I. Extravasation—See Chapter 28

J. Arrhythmia—caused by line placement in right atrium or ventricle; reposition catheter (Machat et al., 2019)

V. Infusion systems are essential in patients with cancer because of need to administer chemotherapy, opioids, antibiotics, antifungals, and nutritional therapy in a variety of settings, including the patient's home. Three basic infusion systems exist (Table 31.3; Camp-Sorrell & Matey, 2017; Fernandez-Rubio et al., 2022; Giuliano, Penoyer, Mahuren, & Bennett, 2021; Hawasli et al., 2021; Kirkendall, Timmons, Huth, Walsh, & Melton, 2020).

Assessment

I. Identify potential candidates for access devices and informed consent obtained (Blanco-Guzman, 2018; Boll et al., 2021; Camp-Sorrell & Matey, 2017; Freire et al., 2018; Gupta et al., 2021; Karpanen et al., 2019; Patel et al., 2019).

II. Physical examination
   A. Evaluate potential device insertion site.
   B. Evaluate the condition of skin over potential insertion site.
   C. Assess the patency of access device.
   D. Evaluate patient for potential infection, because most devices would not be placed in the presence of a bloodstream infection.
   E. Assess for coagulopathies and low platelet, as ordered, to assess for bleeding potential.
   F. Assess current medications, especially for anticoagulants and aspirin.

III. Psychosocial examination
   A. Ability of patient or family to care for the access device when applicable
   B. Knowledge of procedures for the use of access device for therapy
   C. Concerns expressed about the implications of insertion of device
   D. Anxiety related to the procedure

TABLE 31.3 Infusion Systems

Infusion System	Use	Method	Infusion rates/ Volume	Mechanism	Alarms	Comments	Complications
Peristaltic	Blood products; IV medications; TPN, IVF, chemotherapy	C/I	Wide range; low to high rates and volume; dual chamber for simultaneous infusions	Linear/rotary peristaltic to propel fluid forward	Visual and audible	Smart pump technology	Occlusion; kinked tubing; pump malfunction
Syringe	Concentrated drugs or antibiotics; chemotherapy	I	Small volume; rate regulated by the size of syringe	Motor-driven gear mechanism propels fluid by forcing plunger of syringe	Audible	Smart pump technology; lightweight; portable	Kinked tubing; pump malfunction
Elastomeric	Antibiotics, chemotherapy	I	Small volume	Infusion pressure when filled causes membrane to deflate	None	Lightweight; portable	Empty reservoir due to runaway rate

C/I, Continuous and intermittent; *IV*, intravenous; *TPN*, total parenteral nutrition.

Management

I. Medical management
   A. Manage access device infection.
      1. Administer antibiotics, as indicated.
         a. Vancomycin recommended for empiric therapy until organism identified.
         b. Adjustment of antibiotics based on culture results.
         c. Consider the use of antibiotic lock therapy in patients diagnosed with catheter-related infection, or at a high risk of infection, or myelosuppressed.
      2. Remove access device, as indicated.
         a. Complicated infection, tunnel, or port pocket infection
         b. Endocarditis, osteomyelitis, or septic thrombosis
         c. Totally occluded catheter from thrombosis or precipitation
         d. Septic shock
         e. Recurrent line infection despite adequate antibiotic therapy
         f. Therapy completed
   B. Ensure accurate device placement.
      1. Obtain radiographic or ultrasound confirmation before accessing the device initially to ensure correct catheter tip placement just above or in the lower third of the SVC at the cavoatrial junction and if complications occur.
      2. Dye study can be ordered if the device needs to be reassessed because of lack of blood draw or inability to infuse.
   C. Maintain catheter patency.
      1. Administer anticoagulant or fibrinolytic, as indicated.
      2. Upper extremity DVT—anticoagulation therapy while device in place; may need to continue anticoagulation for a time after removal
      3. Tissue plasminogen activator administered, as indicated, to restore patency
      4. Use securement devices and avoid sutures to prevent migration for short-term catheters, PICCs, and tunnel catheters.
   D. Avoid femoral line placement.

Nursing Management

I. Maximize patient safety.
   A. Maintain aseptic technique when entering or manipulating the device.
   B. Teach patient and family emergency procedures if the device is damaged.
   C. Obtain radiographic or ultrasound confirmation of device placement before initial use (radiographic imaging not necessary for peripheral and midlines).
   D. Teach family and patient how to care for and maintain access device according to agency policy and procedure.
      1. Evaluate understanding of care, including return demonstration.
      2. Provide visual aids in the teaching process.

II. Minimize the risks for complications of access devices (Akhtar & Lee, 2021; Boll et al., 2021; Camp-Sorrell & Matey, 2017; Gupta et al., 2021; Machat et al., 2019; Marin et al., 2021; Patel et al., 2019).
   A. Obtain cultures, as indicated.
      1. Blood cultures drawn peripherally and through device
      2. Culture exit or entrance site and body fluid such as urine, peritoneal, or spinal fluid

REFERENCES

Akhtar, N., & Lee, L. (2021). Utilization and complications of central venous access devices in oncology patients. *Current Oncology*, *28*(1), 367–377. https://doi.org/10.3390/curroncol28010039.

Alcaina, P. S. (2020). Platelet transfusion: And update on challenges and outcomes. *Journal of Blood Medicine*, *11*, 19–26. https://doi.org/10.2147/JBM.S234374.

Blanco-Guzman, M. O. (2018). Implanted vascular access device options: A focused review on safety and outcomes. *Transfusion*, *58*(Suppl. 1), 558–568. https://doi.org/10.1111/trf.14503.

Böll, B., Schalk, E., Buchheidt, D., Hasenkamp, J., Kiehl, M., Kiderlen, T. R., et al. (2021). Central venous catheter-related infections in hematology and oncology: 2020 updated guidelines on diagnosis, management, and prevention by the Infectious Diseases Working Party (AGIHO) of the German Society of Hematology and Medical Oncology (DGHO). *Annals of Hematology*, *100*(1), 239–259. https://doi.org/10.1007/s00277-020-04286-x.

Buetti, N., Ruckly, S., Schwebel, C., Mimoz, O., Souweine, B., Lucet, J.-C., et al. (2020). Chlorhexidine-impregnated sponge versus chlorhexidine gel dressing for short-term intravascular catheters: Which one is better? *Critical Care*, *24*(1), 458. https://doi.org/10.1186/s13054-020-03174-0.

Camp-Sorrell, D., & Matey, L. (Eds.). (2017). *Access device standards of practice for oncology nursing*. Pittsburgh, PA: Oncology Nursing Society.

Capozza, M. A., Triarico, S., Mastrangelo, S., Attinà, G., Maurizi, P., & Ruggiero, A. (2021). Narrative review of intrathecal drug delivery (IDD): Indications, devices and potential complications. *Annals of Translational Medicine*, *9*(2), 186. https://doi.org/10.21037/atm-20-3814.

Capraru, A., Jalowiec, K. A., Medri, C., Daskalakis, M., Zeerleder, S. S., & Taleghani, B. M. (2021). Platelet transfusion – Insights from current practice to future development. *Journal of Clinical Medicine*, *10*(9), 1990. https://doi.org/10.3390/jcm10091990.

DeLisle, J. (2018). Is this a blood transfusion reaction? Don't hesitate; check it out. *Journal of Infusion Nursing*, *41*(1), 43–51. https://doi.org/10.1097/NAN.0000000000000261.

Fernández-Rubio, B., del Valle-Moreno, P., Herrera-Hidalgo, L., Gutiérrez-Valencia, A., Luque-Márquez, R., López-Cortés, L. E., et al. (2022). Stability of antimicrobials in elastomeric pumps: A systematic review. *Antibiotics*, *11*(1), 45. https://doi.org/10.3390/antibiotics11010045.

Freire, M. P., Pierrotti, L. C., Zerati, A. E., Benites, L., da Motta-Leal Filho, J. M., Ibrahim, K. Y., et al. (2018). Role of lock therapy for long-term catheter-related infections by multidrug-resistant bacteria. *Antimicrobial Agents and Chemotherapy*, *62*(9), e00569–18. https://doi.org/10.1128/AAC.00569-18.

Gea-Banacloche, J. (2017). Granulocyte transfusions: A concise review for practitioners. *Cytotherapy*, *19*(11), 1256–1269. https://doi.org/10.1016/j.jcyt.2017.08.012.

Giuliano, K. K., Penoyer, D., Mahuren, R. S., & Bennett, M. (2021). Intravenous smart pumps during actual clinical use. *Journal of Infusion Nursing*, 44(3), 128–136. https://doi.org/10.1097/NAN.0000000000000415.

Gupta, N., Gandhi, D., Sharma, S., Goyal, P., Choudhary, G., & Li, S. (2021). Tunneled and routine peripherally inserted central catheters placement in adult and pediatric population: Review, technical feasibility, and troubleshooting. *Quantitative Imaging in Medicine and Surgery*, 11(4), 1619–1627. https://doi.org/10.21037/qims-20-694.

Hawasli, R. S. D., Barton, S., & Nabhani-Gebara, S. (2021). Ambulatory chemotherapy: Past, present, and future. *Journal of Oncology Pharmacy Practice*, 27(4), 962–973. https://doi.org/10.1177/1078155220985916.

Ilhan, B. M., Sormaz, I. C., & Türkay, R. (2018). Pinch-off syndrome, a rare complication of totally implatable venous access device implantation: A case series and literature review. *The Korean Journal of Thoracic Cardiovascular Surgery*, 51(5), 333–337. https://doi.org/10.5090/kjtcs.2018.51.5.333.

Italiano, D. (2018). Hepatic arterial infusion pump: Complications and nursing management regarding use in patients with colorectal cancer. *Clinical Journal of Oncology Nursing*, 22(3), 340–346. https://doi.org/10.1188/18.CJON.340-346.

Karpanen, T. J., Casey, A. L., Whitehouse, T., Timsit, J.-F., Mimoz, O., Palomar, M., et al. (2019). A clinical evaluation of two central venous catheter stabilization systems. *Annals of Intensive Care*, 9, 49. https://doi.org/10.1186/s13613-019-0519-6.

Kaya, A., Nas, O. F., & Erdogan, C. (2019). Tunneled peritoneal catheter placement in palliation of malignant ascites: A study with two different types of catheters. *BioMed Research International*. Article 4132396. https://doi.org/10.1155/2019/4132396.

Kirkendall, E. S., Timmons, K., Huth, H., Walsh, K., & Melton, K. (2020). Human-based errors involving smart infusion pumps: A catalog of error types and prevention strategies. *Drug Safety*, 43(11), 1073–1087. https://doi.org/10.1007/s40264-020-00986-5.

Kuldanek, S. A., Kelher, M., & Silliman, C. C. (2019). Risk factors, management and prevention of transfusion-related acute lung injury: A comprehensive update. *Expert Review of Hematology*, 12(9), 773–785. https://doi.org/10.1080/17474086.2019.1640599.

Laface, C., Laforgia, M., Molinari, P., Ugenti, I., Gadaleta, C. D., Porta, C., et al. (2021). Hepatic arterial infusion of chemotherapy for advanced hepatobiliary cancers: State of the art. *Cancers*, 13(12), 3091. https://doi.org/10.3390/cancers13123091.

Lau, J. C., Kosteniuk, S. E., Macdonald, D. R., & Megyesi, J. F. (2018). Image-guided Ommaya reservoir insertion for intraventricular chemotherapy: A retrospective series. *Acta Neurochirurgica*, 160, 539–544. https://doi.org/10.1007/s00701-017-3454-z.

Leader, A., Hofstetter, L., & Spectre, G. (2021). Challenges and advances in managing thrombocytopenic cancer patients. *Journal of Clinical Medicine*, 10(6), 1169. https://doi.org/10.3390/jcm10061169.

Lescinskas, E. H., Trautner, B. W., Saint, S., Colozzi, J., Evertsz, K., Chopra, V., et al. (2020). Use of and patient-reported complications related to midline catheters and peripherally inserted central catheters. *Infection Control and Hospital Epidemiology*, 41(5), 608–610. https://doi.org/10.1017/ice.2020.34.

Machat, S., Eisenhuber, E., Pfarl, G., Stübler, J., Koelblinger, C., Zacherl, J., et al. (2019). Complications of central venous port systems: A pictorial review. *Insights into Imaging*, 10, 86. https://doi.org/10.1186/s13244-019-0770-2.

Magill, S. T., Choy, W., Nguyen, M. P., & McDermott, M. W. (2020). Ommaya reservoir insertion: A technical note. *Cureus*, 12(4), e7731. https://doi.org/10.7759/cureus.7731.

Mahecic, T. T., Dünser, M., & Meier, J. (2020). RBC transfusion triggers: Is there anything new? *Transfusion Medicine and Hemotherapy*, 47(5), 361–368. https://doi.org/10.1159/000511229.

Marin, A., Bull, L., Kinzie, M., & Andresen, M. (2021). Central catheter-associated deep vein thrombosis in cancer: Clinical course, prophylaxis, treatment. *BMJ Supportive & Palliative Care*, 11(4), 371–380. https://doi.org/10.1136/bmjspcare-2019-002106.

Mielke, D., Wittig, A., & Teichgräber, U. (2020). Peripherally inserted central venous catheter (PICC) in outpatient and inpatient oncological treatment. *Supportive Care in Cancer*, 28(10), 4753–4760. https://doi.org/10.1007/s00520-019-05276-0.

Morrell, E. (2020). Reducing risks and improving vascular access outcomes. *Journal of Infusion Nursing*, 43(4), 222–228. https://doi.org/10.1097/NAN.0000000000000377.

Nair, P. M., Rendo, M. J., Reddoch-Cardenas, K. M., Burris, J. K., Meledeo, M. A., & Cap, A. P. (2020). Recent advances in use of fresh frozen plasma, cryoprecipitate, immunoglobulins, and clotting factors for transfusion support in patients with hematologic disease. *Seminars in Hematology*, 57(2), 73–82. https://doi.org/10.1053/j.seminhematol.2020.07.006.

National Comprehensive Cancer Network (NCCN). (2018). *Cancer and chemotherapy-induced anemia guidelines, version 3* (p. 2018). http://www.nccn.org/professionals/physician_gls/pdf/anemia.pdf.

Ngo, A., Masel, D., Cahill, C., Blumberg, N., & Refaai, M. A. (2020). Blood banking and transfusion medicine challenges during the COVID-19 pandemic. *Clinics in Laboratory Medicine*, 40(4), 587–601. https://doi.org/10.1016/j.cll.2020.08.013.

Oh, S.-B., Park, K., Kim, J.-J., Oh, S.-Y., Jung, K.-S., Park, B.-S., et al. (2021). Safety and feasibility of 3-month interval access and flushing for maintenance of totally implantable central venous port system in colorectal cancer patients after completion of curative intended treatments. *Medicine*, 100(2), e24156. https://doi.org/10.1097/MD.0000000000024156.

Patel, A. R., Patel, A. R., Singh, S., Singh, S., & Khawaja, I. (2019). Central line catheters and associated complications: A review. *Cureus*, 11(5), e4717. https://doi.org/10.7759/cureus.4717.

Savinkina, A. A., Haass, K. A., Sapiano, M. R. P., Henry, R. A., Berger, J. J., Basavaraju, S. V., et al. (2020). Transfusion-associated adverse events and implementation of blood safety measures – Findings from the 2017 National Blood Collection and Utilization Survey. *Transfusion*, 60(Suppl. 2), S10–S16. https://doi.org/10.1111/trf.15654.

Sayed, D., Monroe, F., Orr, W. N., Phadnis, M., Khan, T. W., Braun, E., et al. (2018). Retrospective analysis of intrathecal drug delivery: Outcomes, efficacy, and risk for cancer-related pain at a high volume academic medical center. *Neuromodulation*, 21(7), 660–664. https://doi.org/10.1111/ner.12759.

Schiffer, C. A., Bohlke, K., Delaney, M., Hume, H., Magdalinski, A. J., McCullough, J. J., et al. (2017). Platelet transfusion for patients with cancer: American Society of Clinical Oncology clinical practice guideline update. *Journal of Clinical Oncology*, 36(3), 283–299. https://doi.org/10.1200/JCO.2017.76.1734.

Shmookler, A. D., & Flanagan, M. B. (2020). Educational case: Febrile nonhemolytic transfusion reaction. *Academic Pathology*, 7. https://doi.org/10.1177/2374289520934097.

Stearns, L. M., Abd-Elsayed, A., Perruchoud, C., Spencer, R., Hammond, K., Stromberg, K., et al. (2020). Intrathecal drug delivery systems for cancer pain: An analysis of a prospective, multicenter product surveillance registry. *Anesthesia & Analgesia*, 130(2), 289–297. https://doi.org/10.1213/ANE.0000000000004425.

Stephens, J., & Tano, R. (2021). Hemoglobin matters: Perioperative blood management for oncology patients. *Canadian Oncology Nursing Journal, 31*(4), 399–404. https://doi.org/10.5737/23688076314399404.

Vrtis, M. C., DeCesare, E., & Day, R. S. (2021). Indwelling pleural catheters for malignant pleural effusion. *Home Healthcare Now, 39*(6), 302–309. https://doi.org/10.1097/NHH.0000000000001023.

Wang, J., Zhou, P., Han, Y., & Zhang, H. (2021). Platelet transfusion for cancer secondary thrombocytopenia: Platelet and cancer cell interaction. *Translational Oncology, 14*(4), 101022. https://doi.org/10.1016/j.tranon.2021.101022.

Yang, Z., Li, C., Liu, W., Zheng, Y., Zhu, Z., Hua, Z., et al. (2020). Complications and risk factors for complications of implanted subcutaneous ports for intraperitoneal chemotherapy in gastric cancer with peritoneal metastasis. *Chinese Journal of Cancer Research, 32*(4), 497–507. https://doi.org/10.21147/j.issn.1000-9604.2020.04.07.

32

Pharmacologic Interventions

Savanna J. Gilson and Rowena N. Schwartz

ANTIMICROBIALS

Overview

(National Comprehensive Cancer Network [NCCN], 2022a; Taplitz et al., 2018)

I. Rationale and indications
  A. For the treatment of active infections
    1. Neutropenia, immunodeficiency associated with primary cancer, immune suppression, and mucosal barrier injury increase the risk of infection in cancer patients.
      a. Splenectomy and functional asplenia
      b. Immunosuppressive agents, including but not limited to corticosteroids, purine analog (e.g., cladribine, nelarabine), alemtuzumab, anti-CD20 monoclonal antibodies (e.g., rituximab), and temozolomide
    2. Due to compromised immune function, patients with cancer may not exhibit all of the typical signs and symptoms of infection (e.g., inflammation and redness of infection site).
    3. Prompt treatment of suspected infection is required to prevent sepsis and life-threatening sequelae.
  B. For prophylaxis, antiinfectives are sometimes used to prevent infection in high-risk populations. Select examples are listed but are not comprehensive. Recommendation for antiinfective strategies is determined by the clinical situation (Taplitz et al., 2018).
    1. Antimicrobial prophylaxis is not routinely used in patients with cancer that is considered at low risk of overall infection.
      a. Patients receiving standard chemotherapy for most solid tumors
      b. Patients with anticipated neutropenia <7 days
      c. Antiviral prophylaxis may be warranted in patients with prior herpes simplex virus infections.
    2. Antimicrobial prophylaxis may be recommended for patients at intermediate or high risk of profound, protracted neutropenia, or other risk factors for infections.
      a. Patients with anticipated absolute neutrophil count (ANC) <500 cells/μL for >7 days, including but not limited to:

(1) High-dose chemotherapy followed by hematopoietic stem cell transplantation
(2) Chemotherapy induction and consolidation therapy for acute leukemia
      b. Patients receiving immunosuppressive therapy (see earlier)
      c. Patients with prior infections or active infection at the time of treatment
      d. Patients with moderate to severe graft-versus-host disease
      e. *Pneumocystis jirovecii* prophylaxis is recommended for patients receiving anticancer regimens that are associated with >3.5% risk of pneumonia as a result of this organism.
        (1) Those patients receiving ≥20 mg prednisone equivalent daily for ≥1 month
        (2) Select purine analog usage

II. Types of antimicrobial drugs (Table 32.1)
  A. Agents: antibacterial agents, antifungal agents, antiviral agents, and vaccinations
  B. Initial evaluation
    1. Fever may be the earliest and/or only warning sign of infection.
      a. Antipyretics, including acetaminophen, aspirin, and nonsteroidal antiinflammatory agents, should be avoided in individuals at risk for infection and/or neutropenia, as they may mask fever. Evaluate concurrent medication use (including over-the-counter [OTC] medications and combination OTC medications that can contain an antipyretic) before therapy to assure discontinuation of antipyretics; patient/caregiver education about avoiding all antipyretics during neutropenia is essential.
      b. Temperature threshold for neutropenic patients is defined as a single oral temperature of 38.3°C (101°F) or a sustained temperature of 38°C (100.4°F) over 1 hour. Institutional/practice recommendations may be more stringent.
      c. Assure patient and caregiver have a functional thermometer to measure temperature.
      d. For accurate results, axillary temperatures should be avoided. Rectal temperatures should also be

TABLE 32.1   Antimicrobials Used for the Immunocompromised Patient

Antibacterials: Coverage Gram-Negative Infections

- Penicillins
- Group of antibiotics originally derived from *Penicillium* molds. Many of the penicillins currently used in practice are chemically synthesized from naturally produced penicillins.
- β-Lactam antibiotics structurally and pharmacologically related to other β-lactam antibiotics, including cephalosporins, penicillins, and carbapenems.
- Penicillins are divided into groups, including natural penicillins (e.g., penicillin G), penicillinase-resistant penicillins (e.g., oxacillin), aminopenicillins (e.g., ampicillin), and extended-spectrum penicillins (e.g., piperacillin).
- Extended-spectrum penicillins have wider activity than the other groups of penicillins and are available in the United States only in fixed combinations with β-lactamase inhibitors (e.g., clavulanate or tazobactam).

Drug	Coverage Summary	Common Adult Dose[a]	Comments
Piperacillin-tazobactam (Zosyn)	Gram-positive aerobic bacteria Gram-negative aerobic bacterial Anaerobic bacteria	3.375 g IV every 6 h (mild–moderate infections) or 4.5 g IV every 6 h Consider dose reduction with renal dysfunction Note: some institutions used extended infusions	First-line therapy for neutropenic fever May produce false-positive galactomannan Should not be used for meningitis Common adverse effects: Hypersensitivity/rash, drug fever, diarrhea

- Cephalosporins
- Cephalosporins are semisynthetic β-lactam antibiotics that are pharmacologically related to penicillins.
- Cephalosporins are divided into "generations" based on the spectra of activity. First-generation cephalosporins are usually active against Gram-positive cocci but have limited activity against Gram-negative bacteria (e.g., cefazolin). Second-generation cephalosporins are active against some Gram-positive and -negative bacteria. Maybe be less effective against Gram-positive bacteria as compared to the first-generation cephalosporins. Active against most strains of *Haemophilus influenzae* (e.g., cefaclor). Third-generation cephalosporins are less active against some Gram-positive organisms but have increased activity against Gram-negative bacteria compared with first and second generations (e.g., ceftriaxone). Fourth-generation has expanded the spectrum against Gram-negative bacteria, often including *Pseudomonas aeruginosa* (e.g., cefepime). Fifth-generation cephalosporin has activity against both Gram-positive and -negative bacteria, including activity against MRSA (e.g., ceftaroline fosamil).

Drug	Coverage Summary	Common Adult Dose[a]	Comments
Ceftazidime (Fortaz, Tazicef) (third-generation cephalosporin)	Gram-negative bacteria Poor Gram-positive activity (breakthrough streptococcal infections reported)	2 g IV every 8 h (for febrile neutropenia) Dose adjustment needed for renal dysfunction	Limited activity against Gram-positive bacteria and increasing resistance of Gram-negative bacteria; not routinely used as empiric monotherapy in febrile neutropenia in most institutions. Increased resistance reported. Often considered second-line therapy for neutropenic fever due to limitation in coverage compared with other agents. Ceftazidime/avibactam is a combination product. Avibactam inactivates β-lactamases. Common adverse effects: Hypersensitivity/rash, drug fever, diarrhea.
Cefepime (Maxipime) (fourth-generation cephalosporin)	Gram-positive bacteria Gram-negative bacteria	2 g IV every 8 h (for febrile neutropenia) Dose adjustments needed for renal dysfunction	Option for initial empiric therapy for febrile neutropenic patient. Not active against *Enterococcus* species. Not active against most anaerobes.
Ceftaroline fosamil (Teflaro)	Gram-positive bacteria MRSA Gram-negative bacteria	600 mg IV every 12 h Dose adjustments needed for renal dysfunction	Indicated for acute bacterial skin/skin structure infections and community-acquired pneumonia. To reduce the development of drug-resistant bacteria and maintain the effectiveness of ceftaroline, recommended that this antibiotic be used only in infections that are proven or strongly suspected to be susceptible.

- Carbapenem
- Broad-spectrum beta-lactam antibiotics with activity against many Gram-positive, -negative, and anaerobic organisms.
- Doripenem and ertapenem are not included in current NCCN guidelines.

TABLE 32.1 Antimicrobials Used for the Immunocompromised Patient —cont'd

Drug	Coverage Summary	Common Adult Dose[a]	Comments
Doripenem	Gram-positive bacteria	500 mg IV q 8 h	
Ertapenem	Gram-negative bacteria	1 g daily	
Imipenem/cilastatin sodium	Anaerobic organisms	500 mg IV q 6 h	Increasing resistance seen in many institutions.
	Preferred against extended-spectrum beta-lactamase	Dose adjustment needed for renal dysfunction	Lowers seizure threshold.
Meropenem	and serious Enterobacter infections	1–2 g IV q 8 h or	Effective for meningitis, nosocomial pneumonia, and intraabdominal infections.
		500 mg IV q 6 hrs	Carbapenemase-producing bacteria have been documented.
		Dose adjustment needed for renal dysfunction	

- Fluoroquinolones
- Broad-spectrum antimicrobial agents
  - Coverage is dependent on agent
  - Avoid for empiric therapy if patient treated with fluoroquinolone prophylaxis
    - Fluoroquinolone can cause long-lasting, disabling, and potential permanent side effects involving tendons, muscles, and joints (Alves, Mendes, & Batel Marques, 2019)

Drug	Coverage Summary	Common Adult Dose[a]	Comments
Ciprofloxacin (Cipro)	Gram-negative bacteria, including *P. aeruginosa* Atypical bacteria Limited Gram-positive bacteria	PO 500–750 mg PO every 12 h (with amoxicillin or clavulanic acid for low-risk febrile neutropenia) IV 400 mg IV every 8–12 h Dose adjustments needed for renal dysfunction	Role in prevention of infection in immunocompromised host. Not as effective as others in the class for respiratory infection. Used in combination with amoxicillin/clavulanate for patients with low-risk febrile neutropenia.
Levofloxacin (Levaquin)	Gram-positive bacteria Gram-negative bacteria Atypical bacteria Limited anaerobic bacteria	PO 500–750 mg PO every 24 h (prophylaxis of neutropenic fever) IV 500–750 mg IV every 24 h Dose adjustment needed for renal dysfunction	Use as prophylaxis may increase Gram-negative resistance.
Moxifloxacin (Avelox)	Gram-positive bacteria Limited Gram-negative bacteria (limited activity against *Pseudomonas*) Atypical bacteria Anaerobic bacteria	400 mg PO every 24 h 400 mg IV every 24 h No dose adjustment needed for renal dysfunction	

- Aminoglycosides
- Activity is primarily against Gram-negative organisms.
  - Historically used as initial double coverage with another anti-*Pseudomonas* agent as empiric therapy for a neutropenic febrile patient, although the role has changed.
    - Currently used as double coverage based on sensitivities of identified agent or in patients that are seriously ill or hemodynamically unstable patient with suspected infection.

Drug	Coverage Summary	Common Adult Dose[a]	Comments
Amikacin	Gram-negative bacteria	Weight-based dosing (extended interval)	Nephrotoxicity and ototoxicity limit use.
Gentamicin	Gram-negative bacteria Gram-positive bacteria (synergy with beta-lactams)	Dose modification based on renal dysfunction	Good activity against *Pseudomonas*. Used for double coverage of Gram-negative infections.
Tobramycin	Gram-negative bacteria		Dose is adjusted based on pharmacokinetic parameters. Selection of aminoglycoside is often based on institutional sensitivity patterns.

Antibacterial Agents: Active for Gram-Positive Infection

Drug	Coverage Summary	Common Adult Dose[a]	Comments
Vancomycin	Gram-positive bacteria No activity in vancomycin-resistant enterococci (VRE)	15 mg/kg IV q 12 h PO dosing is used for the treatment of *Clostridium difficile*: 125 mg PO every 6 h Dose modifications required in renal dysfunction (based on drug serum concentrations)	Often added to cover Gram-positive infection in patients with febrile neutropenia, although with increased incidence of resistance, recommend limiting routine use. Doses adjusted based on drug serum trough concentrations.

Continued

TABLE 32.1 Antimicrobials Used for the Immunocompromised Patient—cont'd

Drug	Coverage Summary	Common Adult Dose[a]	Comments
Linezolid (Zyvox)	Gram-positive bacteria, including VRE and MRSA	IV: 600 mg IV every 12 h PO: 600 mg PO every 12 h	Hematologic toxicity (e.g., thrombocytopenia) seen most commonly with use >2 weeks. Serotonin syndrome may occur; use with caution with SSRI. Active against VRE.
Daptomycin (Cubicin)	Gram-positive bacteria	6 mg/kg/d IV Dose adjusted for renal function	Active against vancomycin-resistant enterococci, although not FDA approved for this indication. May cause rhabdomyolysis; monitor CPK weekly. **Not active** against pulmonary infections due to inactivation by pulmonary surfactant.
Miscellaneous Antibacterial Agents			
Trimethoprim/ sulfamethoxazole (TMP/ SMX) (Bactrim, Septra)	Activity against Gram-negative and -positive bacteria Active: *Pneumocystis jirovecii* *Toxoplasma gondii* *Nocardia* Not active for: *Pseudomonas*	PO (prophylaxis for pneumocystis): single-strength tablet once daily, double-strength tablet three times weekly IV (treatment): 15 mg/kg daily in divided doses every 6–8 h based on trimethoprim Dose adjustment required for renal dysfunction	Used as prophylaxis and treatment of *P. jiroveci* (commonly used with temozolomide therapy). Assure adequate kidney function, and maintain hydration throughout therapy (drug can precipitate in tubule). Monitor for myelosuppression.
Metronidazole	Activity against anaerobic organisms	500 mg PO every 8–12 h	Avoid alcohol during therapy and for 72 h post treatment.
Antifungals Agents			
Azoles			
• Drug–drug interactions are common and should be assessed prior to therapy and throughout therapy.			
Fluconazole (Diflucan)	*Candida* (resistance maybe seen with *C. glabrata, C. krusei,* and *C. auris*)	100–400 mg IV/PO daily Dose adjustment required in renal dysfunction	Not active against molds. Prolongation of QTc, monitor other medications. Drug–drug interactions are common. Used as prophylaxis in high-risk patient populations (e.g., transplantation, acute leukemia).
Isavuconazonium (Cresemba)	Invasive aspergillosis and mucormycosis	Loading dose: 372 mg IV/PO q 8 h × 6 doses followed by 372 mg IV/PO daily	Drug–drug interactions are common. Contraindicated in familial short QT syndrome.
Itraconazole (Sporanox)	*Candida* Aspergillosis Rare molds Dimorphic fungi *C. neoformans*	PO: 400 mg PO daily Loading doses used in some clinical situations	The capsule and oral solution formulation are not bioequivalent and therefore not interchangeable. Do not use with gastric acid–lowering agents, as they may inhibit absorption. Contraindicated in patients with significant cardiac systolic dysfunction.
Posaconazole (Noxafil)	*Candida* *Aspergillus* sp. *Zygomycetes* sp. Rare molds Dimorphic fungi *C. neoformans*	Prophylaxis: PO: 300 mg PO BID × 1 day, then 300 mg PO daily IV: 300 mg IV q 12 h × 1 day then 300 mg IV daily Off-label use for treatment is a higher dose	Absorption related to stomach pH; avoid acid suppressants. Take with fatty food, nutritional substitute, or acidic beverage to increase absorption. Effective as prophylaxis in patients with acute myeloid leukemia and chronic graft-versus-host disease
Voriconazole (Vfend)	*Candida* *Aspergillus* Dimorphic fungi *C. neoformans*	IV: 6 mg/kg IV twice daily × two doses; then 4 mg/kg IV twice daily PO: 400 mg PO q 12 h × 2 then dose based on weight q 12 h Dose adjustment for renal function in IV formulation only	Poor activity against *Zygomycetes*. Used as empiric therapy in febrile neutropenia. Evidence suggests dose adjustments by weekly troughs increases efficacy. Target concentration for TDM = 1–5.5 mg/L.

TABLE 32.1 Antimicrobials Used for the Immunocompromised Patient —cont'd

Drug	Coverage Summary	Common Adult Dose[a]	Comments
Amphotericin B Formulations			
Amphotericin B deoxycholate	Candida Aspergillus (not Aspergillus terreus) Zygomycetes Cryptococcus Dimorphic fungi	Dose: 0.5–1.5 mg/kg IV once daily	Nephrotoxicity, electrolyte wasting, and infusion reaction limit use. Alternative formulations have replaced this in clinical practice. Prehydration with normal saline and premedication with acetaminophen and diphenhydramine are necessary.
Liposomal amphotericin B (AmBisome)		3–5 mg/kg IV once daily	Less renal and infusional toxicity than deoxycholate.
Amphotericin B lipid complex (Abelcet)		3–5 mg/kg IV once daily	Less renal and infusional toxicity than deoxycholate.
Echinocandins			
• Echinocandins have poor CNS and eye penetration.			
Anidulafungin (Eraxis) Caspofungin (Cancidas)	Candida; C. auris may be resistant Aspergillus	200 mg IV on day 1, then 100 mg IV daily 70 mg IV once daily × 1 dose; then 50 mg IV once daily Dose reduction for patients with liver dysfunction	First-line therapy for candidemia and invasive candidiasis. Empiric therapy for febrile neutropenia when fungal coverage is needed.
Micafungin (Mycamine)		Prophylaxis: 50–100 mg IV once daily Treatment: 100–150 mg IV once daily	
Select Antivirals			
Acyclovir	HSV VZV	Dose is based on clinical situation. Dosing is based on ideal body weight when weight-based dosing is used.	Effective as prophylaxis for patients who are HSV-positive Fluid hydration is necessary if high doses are used.
Famciclovir	HSV VZV	Prophylaxis: 250 mg PO BID Treatment: dose dependent on virus	
Ganciclovir	HSV VZV CMV	Treatment doses and regimens are dependent on clinical situation	Effective preemptive therapy for CMV in high-risk patients. Myelosuppression. Limited data for HHV-6 and HHV-8.
Valacyclovir	HSV VZV	Prophylaxis: 500 mg PO BID or TID Treatment: 1 g PO TID	Metabolized to acyclovir. Improved bioavailability compared with acyclovir.
Valganciclovir	HSV VZV CMV	Prophylaxis: 900 mg PO once daily Preemptive therapy CMV: 900 mg PO twice daily × 2-week minimum and until negative test; then taper dose for maintenance	Metabolized to ganciclovir. Myelosuppression. Prophylaxis used for patients with previous CMV reactivation. Limited data for HHV-6 and HHV-8.
Baloxavir	Influenza A and B	Treatment: 40 mg or 80 mg PO based on weight	Limited data for use in immunosuppressed patients.
Cidofovir	HSV VZV CMV Adenovirus	Treatment: 5 mg/kg IV every week × two doses; then taper per clinical guidelines	Significant renal toxicity requires aggressive pre- and posthydration. Ocular toxicity. Myelosuppression. Give probenecid to prevent renal reabsorption. Second-line therapy for CMV. First-line therapy for adenovirus.
Foscarnet	HSV VZV CMV	Dose determined by clinical setting	Nephrotoxic.

Continued

TABLE 32.1   Antimicrobials Used for the Immunocompromised Patient—cont'd

Drug	Coverage Summary	Common Adult Dose[a]	Comments
Letermovir	CMV		Primary prophylaxis for CMV seropositive patients who undergo allogeneic HSCT.
Oseltamir	Influenza A and B	Prophylaxis: 75 mg PO daily Treatment: 75 mg BID (typically for 5 days)	Nausea. Take with food.
Zanamivir	Influenza A and B	Prophylaxis: Two oral inhalations daily Treatment: Two oral inhalations BID	May cause bronchospasm.

CMV, Cytomegalovirus; *HHV-6*, human herpes virus 6; *HSV*, herpes simplex virus; *IV*, intravenous; *MRSA*, methicillin-resistant *Staphylococcus aureus*; *PO*, by mouth; *SSRI*, selective serotonin reuptake inhibitors; *TDM*, therapeutic drug monitoring; *VZV*, varicella zoster virus.
[a]Doses listed are common doses used in select clinical situations. Dose regimens should be individualized to the patient and treatment setting.
Adapted from *National Comprehensive Cancer Network (NCCN)*. (2022a). Prevention and treatment of cancer-related infections (v. 1.2022). https://www.nccn.org/professionals/physician_gls/pdf/infections.pdf. From *Lexicomp. (2022). Facts and comparisons*. https://www.wolterskluwer.com/en/solutions/lexicomp. *Lexi-drugs online, and package inserts for agents.*

avoided to prevent potential injury to the rectal mucosa.

e. Fever is only one of the potential signs of infection; patients with symptoms of infection without fever should also be considered to have a potential infection (e.g., productive cough, burning on urination, diarrhea, redness or swelling of the skin or mucosa, and pain).

f. Practice-established guidelines for the management of patient with fever should be followed, if available.

2. History and physical examination.

a. Evaluate the patient and family history of infection.

b. Evaluate the presence of patient risk factors for infection, including comorbidities, concurrent medications, and prior history of exposures (e.g., marijuana use, cigarette smoking) and infections.

(1) Prior documented infection(s) in the last 3 months

(2) Recent antibiotic therapy, including for prophylaxis

c. Assess for signs and symptoms of organ-specific infection or inflammation.

d. Laboratory and radiology evaluation

(1) Complete blood count with differential, blood chemistry, liver function, renal function, lactate dehydrogenase, lactic acid, and urinalysis

(2) Chest x-ray or computed tomography (CT) scan with respiratory signs/symptoms

(3) Ultrasound for abdominal or pelvic infections if suspected

(4) Magnetic resonance imaging (MRI) for suspected joint or neurologic infections if suspected

e. Obtain cultures (gold standard for diagnosis)

(1) Blood cultures

(a) One set should be obtained peripherally and one from central lines if patient has a central venous catheter.

(b) Two peripheral culture sets should be drawn if no central venous catheter is in place.

(c) If this is not a standard practice in the clinical setting to draw blood cultures, consider the use of a phlebotomy team for peripheral blood cultures to reduce possible contamination, false positives.

(d) Central venous catheter blood cultures are required to rule out catheter colonization.

(2) Urine cultures if urinary tract infection is suspected

(a) Practitioners should follow institutional guidelines for obtaining samples from urinary catheters.

(b) If patient has urinary catheter present and the urine sample is drawn from the urinary catheter, it should be clearly indicated that sample was from the catheter, and results should be interpreted accordingly.

(3) Sputum cultures

(4) Stool cultures, if diarrhea is present

(5) Wound and drainage cultures, if appropriate

C. Initiation of empiric antimicrobial therapy

1. Initiation of empiric antibiotics should be started as soon after presentation as possible after cultures are obtained. Empiric antimicrobial therapy should not be delayed to determine therapy based on the results of cultures, although adjustment of empiric therapy may be warranted based on culture results.

2. Selection of antibiotics is based on the following:

a. Patient risk assessment, clinical status, organ dysfunction, comorbidities, identified disruption of mucosal barriers (e.g., mucositis and wounds), medications (e.g., prophylactic antibiotics and anticancer therapies), and allergies
   (1) Risk stratification has been validated in adults.
b. Site(s) of suspected infection (if known)
c. Antimicrobial action (bactericidal preferred to bacteriostatic), coverage, and institutional/local susceptibilities of pathogens
3. Low-risk patients with febrile neutropenia
   a. Individuals considered low risk if the expected duration of neutropenia is <7 days. This risk assessment is based on the chemotherapy regimen (e.g., many standard regimens used to treat solid tumors) and patient-specific factors.
   b. Empiric antimicrobial therapy should be guided by patient factors, institutional/practice guidelines, and established guidelines.
   c. Route of administration is determined by patient-specific factors (e.g., ability to tolerate oral medications) and treatment-specific factors (e.g., availability of an oral formulation that provides appropriate coverage for suspected organisms).
   d. Empiric therapy includes antibiotics that covers Gram-negative organisms, including *Pseudomonas aeruginosa.*
      (1) Intravenous (IV) monotherapy that covers *P. aeruginosa* includes imipenem/cilastatin, meropenem, piperacillin/tazobactam, and cefepime. Local institutional bacterial susceptibilities should be considered.
      (2) Oral therapy that covers *Pseudomonas,* including ciprofloxacin+amoxicillin/clavulanate, ciprofloxacin+clindamycin, moxifloxacin, or levofloxacin. Note, this option is not recommended in patients receiving quinolones for prophylaxis.
4. Intermediate- or high-risk febrile neutropenic patients
   a. Many factors are considered to determine intermediate or high risk, including type of anticancer agent, intensity of therapy, anticipated neutropenia, and patient-specific factors.
   b. Antimicrobial prophylaxis may be considered based on regimen and patient risk factors.
   c. Empiric antimicrobial therapy may include IV monotherapy that covers *P. aeruginosa,* including imipenem/cilastatin, meropenem, piperacillin/tazobactam, and cefepime. Local institutional bacterial susceptibilities should be considered for treatment decisions.
   d. Combination IV antibiotic for empiric therapy not routinely recommended but may be considered in selected patients (e.g., clinically unstable patients or a history of resistant infections). Options to double-coverage Gram-negative

bacteria include the addition of an aminoglycoside agent to those noted earlier.
   e. The use of vancomycin as part of the empiric therapy of a febrile neutropenic patient may be considered in select clinical situations (e.g., clinical instability, clinically apparent, serious IV catheter–related infections). The routine use of vancomycin has led to an increased occurrence of vancomycin-resistant pathogens and should be avoided.
D. Modification of empiric antimicrobial therapy
   1. Antibiotic therapy should be modified based on the results of cultures.
   2. Antibiotic therapy should be modified if patient symptoms do not resolve or worsen.
   3. Duration of antimicrobial therapy is sufficient for the resolution of the fever without exposure to unnecessary antimicrobial side effects.
      a. Recovery of neutrophil count (ANC ≥500 cells/mm^3)
      b. Clinical status (e.g., afebrile for 2–3 days)
      c. Identification of pathogen (e.g., positive culture)
      d. Low-risk patients that are clinically stable with negative cultures but the ANC remains <500, consider discontinuation of antibiotics after a total of 5–7 days
   4. If fever and/or clinical status is unresponsive to initial antibiotic therapy, the risk of a nonbacterial cause(s), bacterial organisms resistant to antimicrobial therapy (e.g., methicillin-resistant *Staphylococcus aureus,* vancomycin-resistant *Enterococcus*), inadequate serum and/or tissue concentrations of antimicrobials, or drug fever should be considered.
   5. Antiviral therapy should be considered if patient has a history of positive titers or positive history of an outbreak during chemotherapy (e.g., herpes simplex and herpes zoster).
   6. Antifungal coverage may be appropriate to add to initial antimicrobial regimen.
      a. Consider in patients at risk for fungal infections (e.g., concurrent corticosteroids, history of fungal infection, exposure, duration of antibiotics including prophylaxis, and uncontrolled diabetes).
      b. One-third of febrile neutropenic patients who do not respond to 1 week of antimicrobial therapy have a systemic fungal infection.
      c. The most common organisms include *Candida* and *Aspergillus.*
   7. Consider consultation with infectious disease specialist for complex situations.
III. Potential adverse effects of antimicrobial therapy (see Table 32.1)
   A. Antimicrobial adverse effects may be class specific (e.g., hypersensitivity with β-lactam antibiotics), agent specific, and/or dose related.

B. Antimicrobial adverse effects may occur more commonly in patients with specific risk factors for the toxicity (e.g., fluoroquinolone tendon injuries appear to occur in older adults and individuals on concomitant corticosteroids)

C. Suprainfection secondary to overgrowth of microorganisms not covered

D. Renal toxicity—acute renal tubular necrosis, nephritis, and electrolyte imbalances

E. Hematologic—thrombocytopenia, neutropenia, and anemia

F. Hepatotoxicity—elevated liver function tests

G. Cardiovascular—phlebitis, hypotension, arrhythmias, and prolonged QTc interval

H. Gastrointestinal (GI)—nausea, vomiting, anorexia, diarrhea, colitis, and *Clostridium difficile* infection

I. Neurotoxicity—seizures, dizziness, ototoxicity

J. Dermatologic—rash, Stevens–Johnson syndrome, thrush, esophagitis, vaginitis

K. Fluid and electrolyte imbalances—hypokalemia, hypernatremia, hypomagnesemia, dehydration, fluid volume overload

L. Hypersensitivity reactions

Assessment

I. Assessment for the presence of risk factors
   A. Disruption of skin and mucosal barriers
   B. Altered immune function
      1. Patients with hematologic malignancies have an 8.7 times higher risk for developing an infection due to bone marrow dysfunction compared with patients with solid tumor malignancies.
      2. Advanced or refractory disease.
      3. Concurrent corticosteroids (including inhaled steroids).
      4. Select chemotherapy (e.g., purine antimetabolites).
   C. Comorbidities
      1. Diabetes
      2. HIV disease
      3. Renal or hepatic disease
      4. GI disease
      5. Pulmonary disease
      6. Graft-versus-host disease
   D. Tumor invasion, necrosis, and/or obstruction
   E. Cancer treatment (chemotherapy, radiation, and surgery)
      1. Surgical disruption of skin
      2. Bone marrow suppression
      3. Invasive procedures (e.g., insertion of central venous catheters, indwelling urinary catheters, and nasogastric tubes)
      4. Immunosuppressive agents, corticosteroids, and T-cell–depleting agents
      5. Stem cell transplantation
      6. Stomatitis or mucositis
      7. Blood transfusion
      8. Neutropenia with ANC less than 1500/mm^3

   9. Previous antibiotic therapy
   F. Patient characteristics
      1. Malnutrition
      2. Age
      3. Frequent hospitalizations
      4. History of infectious disease
      5. Recent travel
II. History of drug allergies or drug reaction or intolerance
III. Physical examination
   A. Oral mucosa
   B. Central line insertion site
   C. Abdomen
   D. Lungs
   E. Cardiovascular
   F. Skin
IV. Medication reconciliation, including use of OTC medications
V. Evaluation of diagnostic and laboratory data
VI. Antimicrobial stewardship tasks and functions performed by nurses (Kirby et al., 2020; Olans, Olans, & Witt, 2017)
   A. Appropriately triage and place patients in appropriate isolation precautions.
   B. Gather information about patient allergies, past medical history, and medication reconciliation.
   C. Obtain cultures before starting antibiotics. Monitor and report results to treating physician in a timely manner. Adjust treatment plan based on laboratory and radiology reports.
   D. Administer antimicrobials and monitor for adverse events. Review patient's response to therapy, and communicate changes in status to physician and pharmacist.
   E. Monitor patient's clinical progress and capacity to transition from IV to oral medications.
   F. Communicate and manage transition to outpatient services, skilled nursing facilities, and/or long-term care facilities.
   G. Educate patients/families, perform discharge teaching, infection prevention practices.
VII. Assessment of patient's and family's adherence to protective measures
   A. Maintain good personal hygiene, including frequent hand washing.
   B. Perform frequent oral care.
   C. Avoid exposure to communicable diseases and environmental contaminates.
   D. COVID-19 vaccines are currently recommended in patients with cancer, although there remain many questions (Desai et al., 2021; Kuderer, Hill, Carpenter, & Lyman, 2021).
   E. Maintain vaccination schedule.
      1. Patients receiving chemotherapy and/or immunosuppressive medications should not receive live vaccines due to the potential risk of infection (Hibberd, 2022).
      2. Inactivated vaccines may be administered >2 weeks before chemotherapy; live virus vaccines should

be given >4 weeks before chemotherapy (Hibberd, 2022).

3. Posttransplant immunization schedule
   a. Inactivated vaccines are administered at least 6 months posttransplant and include pneumococcal, diphtheria/tetanus/pertussis, *Haemophilus influenzae* type B, hepatitis B virus, meningococcus, and influenza.
   b. Live virus vaccines: measles/mumps/rubella and zoster (shingles vaccine) are administered at least 24 months posttransplant.
   c. Live virus vaccines should not be given while the patient is taking immunosuppressant medications for graft-versus-host disease.
   d. CD34 markers may be used as a means of timing vaccine administration posttransplant.

F. Proper food selection, handling, preparation, and storage

Management

I. Nonpharmacologic management
   A. Manage elevated body temperature and prevent infection.
      1. Provide patient and family education.
      2. Risk factors, signs, and symptoms for infection (see the "Assessment" section)
      3. Rationale for antimicrobial drug therapy and taking antimicrobials as scheduled
      4. When and how to notify health care provider
         a. Body temperature greater than 100.4°F
         b. Signs or symptoms of infection
         c. Hypersensitivities to antimicrobial medication
   B. Protective measures
   C. Strategies used for infection prevention (e.g., bathing strategies) may differ in different settings (e.g., use of chlorhexidine gluconate [CHG] bathing may be utilized in some clinical settings).
   D. Prevent and monitor the adverse effects of antimicrobial therapy (see Table 32.1).
   E. Monitor the therapeutic response to antimicrobial therapy.
   F. Monitor the temperature, pulse, respirations, and blood pressure.
      1. Monitor the cultures.
      2. Discussion about rationale for immediate evaluation of fever
      3. Assess the changes in laboratory values or fluid volume status.
      4. Medication reevaluation and adjust to individual patient needs with patient education (e.g., antimicrobial)

ANTIINFLAMMATORY AGENTS

Overview

(Brant & Stringer, 2018; NCCN, 2022b)

I. Rationale and indications
   A. To reduce inflammation, manage fevers, and treat pain
      1. Although the inflammatory process is a protective mechanism, in certain situations it may cause harm and pain to the patient.
      2. Inhibition of cyclooxygenase leads to decreased prostaglandin production, which can decrease the adverse effects of inflammation.
II. Types of nonopioids and antiinflammatory agents
   A. Nonsteroidal antiinflammatory drugs (NSAIDs) and salicylates (Table 32.2)
   B. Corticosteroids (Table 32.3)
   C. Acetaminophen
      1. Acetaminophen is analgesic and antipyretic but does not have antiinflammatory effects.

TABLE 32.2 **Analgesics**		
NSAIDs		
Agent	Adult oral dosages (maximum is per 24 h)	Notable drug information.
Diclofenac (various)	Initial: 25–50 mg PO Usual: 25–50 mg PO q 8 h Maximum: 150 mg PO	GI side effects; take with food. Patch available (q 12 h). Gel available (q 4 h). BBW: Cardiovascular thrombotic events, GI bleeding, ulceration, and perforation.
Etodolac (Lodine, Lodine XL)	Initial: 200–400 mg PO Usual: 200–400 mg PO q 6–8 h Maximum: 1000 mg PO	GI side effects, fluid retention. BBW: Cardiovascular thrombotic events, GI bleeding, ulceration, and perforation.
Fenoprofen (generic)	Initial dose: 200 mg PO Usual: 200 mg PO q 4–6 h (pain), 400–600 mg PO q 4–6 h (osteoarthritis) Maximum: 3200 mg PO	Prescription required; dizziness, GI side effects. BBW: Cardiovascular thrombotic events, GI bleeding, ulceration, and perforation.
Ibuprofen PO (generic)	Initial dose: 200–400 mg PO Usual: 200–400 mg PO q 4–6 h; higher doses of 200–800 mg q 8 h PO Maximum: 3200 mg PO	200 mg available OTC; GI side effects. BBW: Cardiovascular thrombotic events, GI bleeding, ulceration, and perforation.

Continued

TABLE 32.2   Analgesics—cont'd

Drug	Dosing	Notes
Ibuprofen IV (Caldolor) (antipyretic)	Initial dose: 400 mg Usual: 400 mg IV q 4–6 prn Maximum: 3200 mg	Patient should be well hydrated before administration. BBW: Cardiovascular thrombotic events, GI bleeding, ulceration, and perforation.
Indomethacin (generic)	Initial: 25 mg PO Usual: 25 mg PO q 8–12 h Maximum: 200 mg PO	Renal toxicity, GI side effects. Note: Extended-release product available for once-daily dosing, suppository for rectal dosing, intravenous. BBW: Cardiovascular thrombotic events, GI bleeding, ulceration, and perforation.
Ketoprofen (various)	Initial dose: 25 mg PO Usual: 25–75 mg PO q 6–8 h Maximum: 300 mg PO	GI side effects, headache, dizziness. Note: Extended-release product available for once-daily dosing. BBW: Cardiovascular thrombotic events, GI bleeding, ulceration, and perforation.

Ketorolac (Toradol)	Oral:
	   Initial: 10–20 mg PO
	   Usual: 10 mg PO q 4–6 h
	   Maximum: 40 mg PO
	Parenteral:
	   Initial: 30–60 mg IM or 15–30 mg IV (single dose only)
	   Usual: 15–30 mg IV q 6 h
	   Maximum: 60–120 mg IV
		Use lower doses in older adults.
		Maximum of 5 days is recommended.
		A nasal spray of ketorolac is also available.
		BBW: Cardiovascular thrombotic events, GI bleeding, ulceration, perforation, hypersensitivity reactions, contraindicated in advanced renal impairment, and risk of bleeding.

Naproxen (generics) (OTC)	Initial: 500 mg PO Usual dose: 250–500 mg PO q 12 h Maximum: 1250 mg PO	BBW: Cardiovascular thrombotic events, GI bleeding, ulceration, and perforation.
Piroxicam (Feldene)	20 mg daily (max. 40 mg)	Long half-life allows for once-daily dosing; use with caution in older patients; causes fluid retention. Not indicated for pain. Indication for osteoarthritis, rheumatoid arthritis, AS. BBW: Cardiovascular thrombotic events, GI bleeding, ulceration, and perforation.
Sulindac (Clinoril)	Initial: 150 mg PO Usual: 150–200 mg PO q 12 h (for indications) Maximum: 400 mg PO	May be associated with less renal toxicity. Not approved for pain. Indication for arthritis, ankylosing spondylitis, and bursitis/tendinitis of shoulder.
Tolmetin (Tolectin)	Initial: 400 mg PO Frequency: 200–600 mg PO q 8 h (for indications) Maximum: 1800 mg PO	Fewer GI side effects; take on empty stomach. Not indicated for pain. Indication for osteoarthritis and rheumatoid arthritis. BBW: cardiovascular risk, GI risk.
NSAIDs: Cox-2 Selective Agent		
Celecoxib (Celebrex)	Initial: 400 mg PO Usual: 100–200 mg PO q 12 h Maximum: 400 mg PO	GI safety advantages yet to be demonstrated with chronic use. Fewer GI and platelet side effects; mostly hepatic metabolism by CYP-2C9 (drug interactions). BBW: Serious cardiovascular risk, serious GI risk.
Salicylates		
ASA, aspirin	Initial: 325 mg PO Usual: 325–650 mg PO q 4–6 h Maximum: 4000 mg PO Rectal: 300–600 mg prn q 4 h for no more than 10 days	Do not combine with NSAIDs (exception is with low dose for cardiovascular use of 81 mg PO daily); potent antiplatelet effects; tinnitus at high doses.
Choline magnesium trisalicylate (Trilisate)	Initial: 1500 mg PO Usual: 1500 mg PO q 12 h Maximum: 3000 mg PO	Has no antiplatelet effect; tinnitus.
Salsalate (Disalcid; various generics)	Initial: 750 mg PO Usual: 750 mg PO q 8–12 h Maximum: 3000 mg PO	Has no antiplatelet effect. No indication for pain. Indication for osteoarthritis, rheumatoid arthritis, and related rheumatic disorders. BBW: Cardiovascular thrombotic events, GI bleeding, ulceration, and perforation.

AS, Ankylosing spondylitis; *ASA,* acetylsalicylic acid; *BBW,* black box warning; *GI,* gastrointestinal; *NSAIDs,* nonsteroidal antiinflammatory drugs; *OTC,* over the counter.

From Lexi-Comp Online. *Lexi-drugs online,* and package inserts for agents; *National Comprehensive Cancer Network (NCCN).* (2022b). *Adult cancer pain (v.1.2022).* https://www.nccn.org/professionals/physician_gls/pdf/pain.pdf.

Corticosteroids	Equivalent Oral Dose[a]	Duration of Hypothalamic–Pituitary–Adrenal (HPA) Suppression
Short Acting (8–12 h)		
Cortisone	25 mg	1.25–1.5 days
Hydrocortisone	20 mg	1.25–1.5 days
Intermediate Acting (12–36 h)		
Methylprednisone (e.g., Medrol)	4 mg	1.25–1.5 days
Prednisolone	5 mg	1.25–1.5 days
Prednisone	5 mg	1.25–1.5 days
Long Acting		
Dexamethasone (Decadron)	0.75 mg	2.75 days

TABLE 32.3 Corticosteroids (Mager, Lin, Blum, Lates, & Jusko, 2003)

[a]Equivalent dosages are general approximations.
From Mager, D. E., Lin, S. X., Blum, R. A., Lates, C. D., & Jusko, W. J. (2003). Dose equivalence evaluation of major corticosteroids: Pharmacokinetics and cell trafficking and cortisol dynamics. *Journal of Clinical Pharmacology, 43*(11), 1216–1227. https://doi.org/10.1177/0091270003258651.

III. Principles of medical management
   A. Treatment of mild-to-moderate musculoskeletal or surgical pain
   B. Management of bone pain, often in combination with other analgesics
   C. Antipyretic—NSAIDs and acetaminophen
IV. Potential adverse effects of NSAIDs (Table 32.4)
   A. GI effects (e.g., nausea, dyspepsia, and ulceration)
   B. Renal toxicity
   C. Decrease platelet function
   D. Cardiac toxicity
   E. Confusion, especially in older adults
V. Potential adverse effects of corticosteroids (Table 32.4)
   A. Cushing syndrome with long-term use
   B. Electrolyte and metabolic imbalances
   C. Neuromuscular and skeletal
   D. Ocular effects
   E. Suppression of pituitary–adrenal function
   F. Psychiatric disturbances
   G. Insomnia
   H. GI effects
   I. Immunosuppression
VI. Potential adverse effects of acetaminophen
   A. Hepatotoxicity
      1. Educate patients and families about the daily dose limit of 4000 mg/day
   B. GI effects (nausea and stomach pain)

Assessment

I. Indications for patient use and considerations
   A. Musculoskeletal pain
      1. Older age
      2. History of arthritis, neuromuscular disease, or diabetes
      3. Bone metastasis
      4. Treatment with high-dose vinblastine, paclitaxel (>250 mg/m²)
   B. Sepsis with persistent high fever

   C. Patients at risk for toxicities with NSAIDs
      1. Age older than 65 years
      2. History of GI ulcers
      3. Renal insufficiency
      4. Cardiovascular disease
      5. Concurrent aspirin or anticoagulant use
      6. History of ulcerative colitis
II. Physical examination
   A. Vital signs (e.g., fever)
   B. Assessment and reassessment of pain—onset, duration, intensity, description, location, aggravating and relieving factors, and functional or quality-of-life impairment
III. Medication reconciliation
   A. The antiplatelet effects of NSAIDs require caution be taken with any anticoagulants and other antiplatelet medications (e.g., clopidogrel)
   B. Acetaminophen should not be taken with other products containing acetaminophen, including opioid–acetaminophen combination products or other OTC products
IV. Evaluation of diagnostic and laboratory data
   A. Complete blood cell count (e.g., platelet count)
   B. Renal and hepatic function
   C. Erythrocyte sedimentation rate
   D. C-reactive protein
   E. Coagulation studies

Management

I. Nonpharmacologic management
   A. Patient and family education
   B. Rationale and medication schedule for antiinflammatory drug therapy
   C. Adverse effects and strategies to prevent and manage them
   D. Adverse effects to report to health care team
   E. Monitor for adverse effects of antiinflammatory drug therapy (see Table 32.4)

TABLE 32.4   Adverse Effects of Nonsteroidal Antiinflammatory Drugs (NSAIDs) and Corticosteroids

Adverse Effects	Nursing Implications
NSAIDs	
GI	
Ulceration, bleeding, gastritis, dyspepsia, abdominal pain, constipation, PUD Risks increase with age, chronic use, concomitant corticosteroid use, and history of PUD; misoprostol (Cytotec) can be used to prevent NSAID-induced ulcers	Administer with food or milk. Note guaiac stool. Assess for signs and symptoms of GI bleeding.
Pancreas	
Pancreatitis reported with sulindac	Monitor serum amylase and lipase levels and urinary amylase level results. Monitor for signs and symptoms of pancreatitis (e.g., sudden and intense epigastric pain, nausea and vomiting, low-grade fever, and jaundice).
Hepatic	
Increased ALT, AST, bilirubin levels; risks for hepatotoxicity include alcoholism, chronic active hepatitis, history of hepatitis, cirrhosis, and CHF	Monitor liver enzymes, bilirubin laboratory results. Assess health history for risk factors.
CNS	
Dizziness, drowsiness, lightheadedness or vertigo, somnolence, and mental confusion	Neurologic examination for alertness and orientation. Advise clients and families to avoid driving or other hazardous activities that require mental alertness until CNS effects can be determined. Implement measures for client safety as needed (e.g., assist with ambulation, fall precautions).
Malaise, fatigue	Avoid alcohol and other CNS depressants. Assess the level of fatigue. Provide for rest periods.
Headache	Monitor CBC laboratory test results. Assess the level of headache and administer pain medications as needed.
Cardiovascular	
CHF, peripheral edema, fluid retention, and hypertension	Monitor fluid status, lung sounds, pitting edema, vital signs, and daily weights.
Renal	
Acute renal failure, elevated BUN and serum creatinine levels, and proteinuria; risks include age, chronic renal disease, CHF, muscle breakdown (e.g., significant exercise), and dehydration	Maintain hydration during use. Monitor urine intake and output. Monitor BUN, creatinine, urinalysis laboratory test results, and blood pressure. Assess for edema. Monitor weight. Assess health history for risk factors.
Hematologic	
Neutropenia, leukopenia, decrease platelet function, decreased hemoglobin and hematocrit levels; *exception:* choline magnesium trisalicylate (Trilisate)	Monitor CBC results with differentials clinically necessary. Assess and implement measures to manage infection, bleeding, and fatigue (see Chapter 30). Monitor platelet levels. No IM injections. Implement bleeding precautions per institution protocol.
Special Senses	
Visual disturbance, blurred vision, photophobia, ocular cataracts, glaucoma, ear pain, and tinnitus	Stress the importance of regular eye examinations and hearing tests. Educate client about reporting blurred vision, eye pain, ear pain, and tinnitus to health care provider and about darkening room or wearing sunglasses if photophobic.
Hypersensitivity	
Asthma and anaphylaxis	Monitor for hypersensitivity reactions—changes in respiratory status, itching, hives, fever, pain, changes in pulse rate, decrease in blood pressure, decrease in urinary output. Assess breath sounds; elevate HOB to ease breathing. Administer oxygen as needed. Administer bronchodilators, antihistamines, and agents as needed.

TABLE 32.4 Adverse Effects of Nonsteroidal Antiinflammatory Drugs (NSAIDs) and Corticosteroids—cont'd

Adverse Effects	Nursing Implications
Respiratory Dyspnea, hemoptysis, bronchospasm, and shortness of breath	NSAIDs are contraindicated in clients with ASA allergy, nasal polyps, and bronchospastic disease. Perform respiratory assessment; monitor breath sounds. Examine sputum for color and consistency. Elevate HOB to ease breathing. Administer bronchodilators and oxygen, as needed.
Dermatologic and Skeletal Rash, erythema, urticarial, photosensitivity, osteoporosis, poor wound healing, skin thinning, and growth arrest	Monitor for skin rashes, urticaria Educate regarding risk of photo-sensitivity and use of sunscreen. Encourage regular exercise to promote bone development. Implement safety measures to prevent falls and injuries.
Pituitary Adrenal insufficiency caused by prolonged use and rapid withdrawal	Monitor blood glucose and electrolyte laboratory test results. Monitor vital signs and the presence of peripheral edema.
Infectious Disease Immunosuppressive with increased risk of infections—bacterial, fungal, viral; activation of tuberculosis and spread of herpes conjunctivitis	Observe for signs of cortisol insufficiency, such as fever, orthostatic hypotension, syncopal episodes, disorientation, myalgia, and arthralgia. Cultures, dermatologic examination. Administer antimicrobial drugs and antipyretics as needed. Be aware that signs and symptoms of infection may be masked by NSAIDs.
CORTICOSTEROIDS	
Cushing Syndrome With Long-Term Use Central obesity, moon face, buffalo hump, easy bruising, acne, hirsutism, striae, and skin atrophy	Assess patient's body image concerns. Provide an opportunity for client to share concerns and discuss coping strategies. Educate regarding care of skin and safety precautions.
Electrolyte and Metabolic Imbalances Hyperglycemia, hypernatremia, hypokalemia, and hypocalcemia, leading to edema, hypertension, diabetes, and osteoporosis	Monitor laboratory results (blood glucose, electrolytes, and calcium), vital signs, and body weight. Assess for edema.
Neuromuscular and Skeletal Arthralgia, myalgia, fatigue, muscle weakness, myopathy, osteoporosis, muscle wasting, and fractures	Monitor muscle strength. Administer pain medication as needed. Encourage regular exercise to promote bone development. Implement safety measures to prevent falls and injuries.
Ocular Effects Cataracts and glaucoma	Regular eye examinations. Educate client to report any eye pain or blurred vision to health care provider. Those with open-angle glaucoma should avoid corticosteroids.
Suppression of Pituitary–Adrenal Function With long-term use, sudden withdrawal may cause acute adrenal insufficiency and dependence, fever, myalgia, arthralgia, malaise; unable to respond to stress. This may occur with chronic use, or with frequent courses over time (e.g., myeloma).	Monitor blood pressure for hypotension. Monitor electrolytes for hyponatremia. Assess for dehydration, fatigue, diarrhea, anorexia. Monitor vital signs and muscle and joint pain; administer pain medication. Educate regarding stressful situations, both physiologic and emotional, and when to contact a health care professional for assistance.
Psychiatric Disturbances Paranoia, psychosis, and hallucinations	Observe for and report any mental status changes. Suicide precautions if needed. Refer to mental health professional as needed.
Insomnia	Take in morning if clinically appropriate.

Continued

TABLE 32.4   Adverse Effects of Nonsteroidal Antiinflammatory Drugs (NSAIDs) and Corticosteroids—cont'd

Adverse Effects	Nursing Implications
GI Peptic ulcers, GI bleeding	Assess for epigastric pain 1–3h after meals. Assess for nausea or vomiting, and observe for hematemesis. Monitor CBC and guaiac stools or emesis.
Miscellaneous Immunosuppression	Increase risk of infection, including fungal infections, viral infections, and opportunistic infections. Counsel patients about appropriate hygiene to minimize the risk of fungal infections, including mouth care.
Poor wound healing, menstrual irregularities, arrest of growth	Assess any wounds for prolonged healing. Monitor CBC with differential; assess and manage effects of low white blood cell, red blood cell, and platelet counts. Monitor height.

ALT, Alanine aminotransferase; *ASA*, acetylsalicylic acid; *AST*, aspartate aminotransferase; *BUN*, blood urea nitrogen; *CBC*, complete blood cell count; *CHF*, congestive heart failure; *CNS*, central nervous system; *GI*, gastrointestinal; *HOB*, head of bed; *IM*, intramuscular; *PUD*, peptic ulcer disease.

Data from Gunter BR, Butler KA, Wallace RL, Smith SM, Harirforoosh S. Non-steroidal anti-inflammatory drug-induced cardiovascular adverse events: A meta-analysis. *J Clin Pharm Ther.* 2017. doi.10.1111/jcpt.12484; Grosser T, & Ricciotti E, & FitzGerald G.A. (2023). Pharmacotherapy of inflammation, fever, pain, and gout. Brunton L.L., & Knollmann B.C.(Eds.), Goodman & Gilman's: The Pharmacological Basis of Therapeutics, 14e. McGraw Hill. https://www.accesspharmacy-mhmedical-com.uc.idm.oclc.org/content.aspx?bookid=3191§ionid=267338476; Harirforoosh S, Asghar W, Jamali F. wAdverse effects of nonsteroidal anti-inflammatory drugs: an update of gastrointerstinal, cardiovascular and renal complications. *J Pharm Pharm Sci* 203;16(5):821–47; Kapugi, Michelle; Cunningham, Kathleen. Corticosteroids. *Orthopaedic Nursing* 38(5):pp. 336–339, September/October 2019. | DOI: 10.1097/NOR.0000000000000595; Roth SH, Fuller P. Diclofenac topical solution compared with oral diclofenac: A pooled safety analysis. *J Pain Res.* 2011;4:159–167. https://doi.10.2147/JPR.S20965.

F. Decrease the incidence and manage the adverse effects of antiinflammatory drug therapy (see Table 32.4)
   1. Establish patient's allergies before administering NSAIDs.
   2. Review patient's current medications for potential drug interactions.
   3. Counsel patient and caregiver to assure communication of all medication changes during and after therapy, including addition of complementary and/or alternative medication or dietary strategies, or discontinuation of therapies.
   4. Review the use of complementary therapy that may alter the metabolism of NSAIDs and/or potentiate the toxicities associated with NSAIDs (e.g., bleeding).
   5. NSAIDs are contraindicated in patients with aspirin allergy or hypersensitivity to acetylsalicylic acid, nasal polyps, and bronchospastic disease.
   6. NSAIDs' effect on renal blood flow may decrease the clearance of medications eliminated via the kidneys and result in increased drug exposure and toxicities (e.g., decrease clearance of pemetrexed and methotrexate, increase renal toxicity with cisplatin).
   7. NSAIDs are antipyretics; may mask a fever in an individual with infection. Agents should be avoided in patients receiving myelosuppressive therapy when neutropenic.
   8. NSAIDs decrease platelet function; should be avoided when patient is thrombocytopenic.

G. Monitor for therapeutic response to antiinflammatory drug therapy.

   1. Assess patient for adequate symptom relief (e.g., pain).
   2. Assess patient for infection because the antipyretic and antiinflammatory actions of NSAIDs may mask signs and symptoms of infection.
   3. Maintain hydration to protect kidney for patients taking NSAIDs.
   4. Avoid the concomitant use of NSAIDs and medications known to decrease platelets (e.g., chemotherapy) or increase risk of bleeding (e.g., anticoagulants and antiplatelet medications).

ANTIEMETIC AGENTS

Overview

(Gupta, Walton, & Kataria, 2021; Hesketh et al., 2020; Navari, 2020; NCCN, 2022c; Walsh et al., 2017)
   I. For prevention and treatment of chemotherapy-induced nausea and vomiting (CINV)
   II. For potential causes and contributing factors for nausea and vomiting in the individual with cancer
   III. Types of nausea and vomiting in the individual with cancer
      A. Chemotherapy induced (see Chapter 38)
         1. Risk factors
            a. Emetogenic potential of chemotherapy agent
            b. Dose, route, frequency, and cycle of chemotherapy
            c. Radiation field (e.g., whole body, upper abdomen, and craniospinal)
            d. Patient characteristics
               (1) history of motion sickness

(2) history of nausea/vomiting

(3) female sex

(4) younger age

(5) anxiety

(6) history of low alcohol intake

(7) history of morning sickness

B. Anticancer induced nausea and vomiting

   1. Many medications used in the management of cancer have the potential for nausea and/or vomiting, including drugs that target actionable mutational alterations (e.g., targeted drugs).

   2. The mechanism of nausea and/or vomiting with anticancer drugs may be different in some anticancer medication as compared to CINV, and strategies to manage may best be tailored to the patient and the agent.

   3. Many anticancer medications are taken daily as chronic therapy, and the strategies employed for the prevention of single-day chemotherapy-induced nausea and vomiting may not be appropriate for chronic therapy.

C. Radiation-induced nausea

D. Nausea and vomiting in advanced cancer (Navari, 2020; Walsh et al., 2017)

E. Nausea and vomiting associated with complications of cancer treatment (e.g., constipation and gastritis)

F. Nausea and vomiting unrelated to cancer treatment

IV. Types of antiemetic drugs (Table 32.5)

   1. Mechanism of action of antiemetics via interference of neurotransmission of nausea to the vomiting center results in interruption of signaling pathways. Some agents target a single neurotransmitter, whereas some antiemetics block multiple neurotransmitters (e.g., olanzapine).

     a. Major neurotransmitter targets

       (1) Serotonin (5-HT3 antagonists; e.g., ondansetron)

       (2) Neurokinin (NK1 antagonists; e.g., aprepitant)

       (3) Dopamine (D2 antagonists; e.g., pro-chlorperazine)

       (4) Histamine (H1 antagonists; e.g., prome-thazine)

       (5) Acetylcholine (muscarinics; e.g., sco-polamine)

       (6) Cannabinoid (cannabinoid agonists; e.g., dronabinol)

     b. Corticosteroids are effective in preventing acute CINV and management of delayed CINV. The mechanism of this effect is not fully understood.

     c. The use of nonpharmaceutical approaches to prevent and/or manage CINV complements the use of pharmacologic strategies.

V. Principles of prevention of chemotherapy-induced nausea and vomiting

A. Goal—prevention of nausea and vomiting

B. Use the lowest effective antiemetic dose(s) of antiemetics to prevent CINV.

C. Select the appropriate antiemetic(s) (see Table 32.5) for optimal prevention of CINV based on both patient-specific factors and treatment-specific factors (e.g., emetogenic potential of the chemotherapy regimen).

D. Administer the antiemetics prophylactically, when appropriate, to assure adequate duration of prevention of CINV from the time of potential onset and throughout the anticipated duration of CINV.

E. Provide effective antiemetic therapy(s) to manage any breakthrough CINV.

F. Assess patient for risk of delayed emesis and prophylactic therapy, if indicated.

G. Follow-up assessment—48–72 hours after chemotherapy

   1. Modify the plan for the management of CINV that occurs.

   2. Ensure supportive care of patient during and following CINV (e.g., maintaining fluids and oral intake).

   3. Modification of antiemetic strategy for subsequent chemotherapy treatments

VI. Prophylaxis of nausea and vomiting

A. Based on recommendations from the National Comprehensive Cancer Network (NCCN) based on single day or multiple days of chemotherapy regimen.

   1. Duration and selection of antiemetic therapy are based on the entire chemotherapy regimen.

B. The selection of agents used prior to chemotherapy influence the need of select agents following treatment.

C. For single-day chemotherapy regimens:

   1. If long-acting NK1 RA used before chemotherapy, no NK1 RA is required after.

   2. If long-acting 5-HT3 RA is used before chemotherapy, no 5-HT3 RA is needed post therapy. Patients should be counseled about the use of an antiemetic with a different mechanism for the management of CINV.

   3. The selection of antiemetic therapy for the prevention of CINV will have an impact on your selection of antiemetic for breakthrough CINV (e.g., if palonosetron, a long-acting 5-HT3 RA, is used prior to chemotherapy, there is no benefit of using a short-acting 5-HT3 RA for breakthrough CINV for approximately 3 days).

   4. Published guidelines for antiemetic strategies for CINV provide multiple options for the prevention of CINV, allowing individualization for patients.

D. Examples of antiemetic strategies for highly emetogenic IV chemotherapy to help prevent both acute and delayed CINV.

   1. Olanzapine+NK1 RA+5-HT3 RA+dexamethasone before chemotherapy followed by olanzapine ±dexamethasone and NK1 RA if long-acting agent not used prior to chemotherapy.

   2. NK1 RA+5-HT3 RA+dexamethasone before chemotherapy followed by NK1 RA (if needed) and dexamethasone

   3. Olanzapine+palonosetron+dexamethasone before therapy followed by olanzapine

E. Examples of antiemetic strategies for moderately emetogenic IV chemotherapy to help prevent both acute and delayed CINV

TABLE 32.5 Antiemetic Therapy: Select Pharmacologic Agents

Name	Route Dose/Schedule (Adult)	Adverse Effects of Class	Nursing Implications
Serotonin Receptor Antagonists (5-HT3 Antagonists)			
Ondansetron	IV 8–16 mg IV before chemotherapy (daily) PO 16–24 mg PO before chemotherapy (daily) Oral is as effective as parenteral route if dosed appropriately	Headache Hiccups	Assess for headache with higher doses and consider acetaminophen for headache.
	Cardiovascular Constipation	Increase QTc, evaluate potential drug and disease interactions. Assess for the number and consistency of stools. Administer stool softeners (e.g., docusate) and stimulants (e.g., senna) to prevent constipation as appropriate. Increase fluids and fiber in diet. Encourage exercise as tolerated.	
Granisetron	IV Dose: 0.01 mg/kg (maximum 1 mg) before chemotherapy (once daily maximum) PO Dose: 2 mg PO before chemotherapy (once daily maximum) Transdermal patch (Sancuso) Dose: 3.1 mg/24 h applied 24–48 h before the first dose Subcutaneous (Sustol): Extended-release product containing 10 mg/0.4 mL in single dose (administered no more frequently than every 7 days)	Transient increases in serum AST, GPT.	Monitor liver function test results. Administration: Give higher doses over at least 30 min to prevent dizziness, headache, hypotension.
Dolasetron	PO Dose: 100 mg PO before chemotherapy		Consider ECG for tachycardia or new onset of shortness of breath.
Palonosetron	IV Dose: 0.25 mg before chemotherapy PO Available as a fixed combination product with netupitant (see later)		Do not use short-acting 5-HT3 antagonist concurrently in patients receiving palonosetron (within 3–5 days of treatment).
Neurokinin Antagonists			
Aprepitant	PO Dose: 125 mg on day 1 before chemotherapy; then 80 mg daily on days 2 and 3 IV (injectable emulsion) Dose: 130 mg IV once before chemotherapy	Constipation	Assess for the number and consistency of stools. Administer stool softeners (e.g., docusate) and stimulants (e.g., senna) to prevent constipation. Increase fluids and roughage in diet.
Fosaprepitant	IV Dose: 150 mg IV once before chemotherapy	Diarrhea Hiccups Fatigue	Monitor for stool number and consistency. Monitor for hiccups. Likely from chemotherapy administration and not the drug itself.
Fosnetupitant (combined with palonosetron)	IV (Akynzeo) Dose: 235 mg fosnetupitant (available as a combination with 0.25 mg palonosetron IV) once before chemotherapy		Administered over 30 min as infusion.
Netupitant (combined with palonosetron)	PO (Akynzeo) Dose: 300 mg (available as a combination with palonosetron 0.5 mg PO) once before chemotherapy		Headache and fatigue.

TABLE 32.5 Antiemetic Therapy: Select Pharmacologic Agents —cont'd

Name	Route Dose/Schedule (Adult)	Adverse Effects of Class	Nursing Implications
Rolapitant	PO Dose: 180 mg PO once before chemotherapy		Dizziness, decreased appetite.

Dopamine receptor antagonists

- Dopamine antagonists include phenothiazines (e.g., prochlorperazine) and butyrophenones (e.g., droperidol). Agents such as metoclopramide and olanzapine target multiple receptors, including dopamine receptors.
- Class-related side effects include sedation, dystonia, akathisia, and constipation.

Name	Route Dose/Schedule (Adult)	Adverse Effects of Class	Nursing Implications
Droperidol	IV Dose: 0.625 mg every 6 h as needed	Sedation	Assess the level of sedation. Patient should avoid tasks that require alertness until drug response is established. Patient should avoid alcohol and other CNS depressants.
Haloperidol		Dystonia Akathisia	Monitor for and be prepared to treat EPSs with diphenhydramine 25 mg IV or PO.
Metoclopramide (mechanism includes combination of dopamine receptor antagonist, serotonin receptor antagonist and enhances response to acetylcholine in GI tract)	PO Dose: 10 mg as needed q 4–6 h prn Historically, higher doses were used Extrapyramidal symptoms (EPSs) (e.g., akathisia, acute dystonic reactions); increased incidence in patients <40 years Diarrhea (high doses)	Hypotension Prolongation of QT interval Monitor ECG If patient complains of shortness of breath or skipped heartbeats, notify health care provider. Black box warning or sudden death due to prolonged QT interval. Assess for EPS reactions. May use lower doses if EPSs occur. Dystonia: anticholinergic agents (e.g., diphenhydramine) to treat. Akathisia presenting as restlessness: manage with benzodiazepines (e.g., lorazepam). Assess the number and consistency of stools. Administration: Do not administer to patients with prior hypersensitivity to procaine or procainamide, epilepsy or pheochromocytoma, or if stimulation of GI motility is contraindicated (e.g., mechanical obstruction, GI bleeding).	Monitor VS.
Olanzapine (mechanism of action includes antagonist of receptors, including dopamine, serotonin, histamine, and acetylcholine-muscarine)	PO Doses of 5 mg po daily at bedtime are recommended for acute and delayed nausea (set duration). This drug is not used as a prn medication. The dose of olanzapine was initially studied at 10 mg PO daily, but lower doses may be appropriate in many patients. Consider the option of smaller tablet size to allow dose escalation and/or de-escalation based on patient response Caution in elderly patients with dementia-related psychosis. Drug interactions with agents such as benzodiazepines and other antiemetics.	CNS including fatigue, drowsiness, and sleep disturbances. Initiate with lower doses than stated in guidelines. Assess medications before initiation of olanzapine.	Assess other medications that may increase side effects. Provide counseling to patients about the class of these medications (e.g., antipsychotic) to help preemptively address concerns.

Continued

TABLE 32.5 Antiemetic Therapy: Select Pharmacologic Agents—cont'd

Name	Route Dose/Schedule (Adult)	Adverse Effects of Class	Nursing Implications
Prochlorperazine	IV Dose: 10 mg every 4–6 h scheduled or as needed PO Dose: 10 mg every 4–6 h as scheduled or needed PR Dose: 25 mg every 12 h as needed	Sedation.	Have patients avoid tasks that require alertness until drug response is established. Have patients avoid alcohol and other CNS depressants.
	Blurred vision EPSs (e.g., akathisia)	Assess vision and impact on safety. Monitor for and be prepared to treat EPSs with diphenhydramine 25 mg IV or PO.	
Promethazine (in addition to dopamine receptor antagonism, promethazine competes with histamine at the histamine receptor)	IV Dose: 12.5–25 mg every 4 h as scheduled or needed PO Dose: 12.5–25 mg every 4 h as scheduled or needed	Dry mouth.	Have patient suck on ice chips or sugar-free hard candy.
	Orthostatic hypotension	Counsel about care when standing from sitting.	
	Anticholinergic crisis with overuse	Give diphenhydramine for the treatment of anticholinergic crisis.	
	Rash (promethazine)	Monitor for new rash with therapy.	
	Photosensitivity (promethazine)	Patients should avoid sun exposure.	
	Respiratory depression (promethazine)	Particular caution for patients taking concomitant respiratory depressants (e.g., opiates).	
Amisulpride (selective dopamine-2 and dopamine-3 receptor antagonist)	IV: Prevention of PONV—5 mg IV over 1–2 min at the time of induction of anesthesia. Treatment of PONV—10 mg IV over 1–2 min in the event of nausea or vomiting after a surgical procedure.	Dose-related increase in AT interval.	
Corticosteroids			
Dexamethasone	Dose: 4–20 mg PO have been used, dependent in part on the combination of antiemetic.	Dyspepsia.	Take with food. Monitor weight.
	Hiccups	Assess for prolonged hiccups.	
	Euphoria and insomnia	Assess emotional status and ability to sleep. Counsel to take doses before noon if possible.	
	Fluid retention	Monitor intake and output and weight. Assess for edema. Monitor blood pressure in at-risk patients.	
	Hyperglycemia	Monitor blood sugar and electrolyte results.	
	Hypokalemia	Assess for effects of low potassium.	
Methylprednisolone	IV	125 mg before chemotherapy	Burning with infusion (see class adverse effects listed under dexamethasone).	Slow IV infusion to prevent perineal itching/burning. Similar side effects as seen with dexamethasone.
Cannabinoid			
Dronabinol	PO 5–10 mg every 3 or 6 h	Sedation and dizziness.	

TABLE 32.5	Antiemetic Therapy: Select Pharmacologic Agents—cont'd		
Name	**Route Dose/Schedule (Adult)**	**Adverse Effects of Class**	**Nursing Implications**
		Dry mouth.	Patient should suck on ice chips or hard candy. Encourage frequent intake of fluids.
	Euphoria or dysphoria	Assess emotional status (more common in older adult patients).	
	Orthostatic hypotension	Monitor VS and BP lying and sitting or standing for orthostatic changes. Educate patient to rise slowly from lying or sitting position.	
Benzodiazepine Lorazepam	IV 0.5–2.0 mg every 4–6 h PO 0.5–2.0 mg every 4–6 h	CNS side effects (sedation, disorientation, dizziness, weakness).	Assess the patient's level of consciousness and risk for oversedation. Patient should avoid tasks that require alertness until drug response is established. Patient should avoid alcohol and other CNS depressants. Implement measures for patient safety, such as fall precautions.
	Autograde amnesia	Assess memory. Minimize patient education while patients are taking benzodiazepines unless caregiver present.	
		Hypotension.	Monitor VS.

AST, Aspartate transaminase; *BP*, blood pressure; *CNS*, central nervous system; *ECG*, electrocardiography; *GI*, gastrointestinal; *GPT*, glutamic-pyruvic transaminase; *IV*, intravenous; *PO*, by mouth; *PR*, per rectum; *prn*, as needed; *VS*, vital signs.
From Lexi-Comp Online. *Lexi-drugs online, and package inserts for agents*; *National Comprehensive Cancer Network (NCCN)*. (2022c). Antiemesis (v. 2.2022). https://www.nccn.org/professionals/physician_gls/pdf/antiemesis.pdf.

1. 5-HT3 RA+dexamethasone chemotherapy followed by dexamethasone or 5-HT3 RA monotherapy
2. Olanzapine+palonosetron+dexamethasone before therapy followed by olanzapine
3. NK1 RA+5-HT3 RA+dexamethasone before therapy followed by NK1 RA (if needed) ±dexamethasone

F. Low-emetogenic agents: treatment options include dexamethasone or metoclopramide or prochlorperazine, or single-agent short-acting 5-HT3 antagonist.
   1. The antiemetic regimen should be developed based on patient factors.
   2. The antiemetic regimen may be modified based on the patient response.
G. No emetogenic risk: no routine prophylaxis is recommended. Antiemetics are appropriate based on patient response and/or risk factors.
VII. Agents for management of breakthrough CINV
   A. The decision for appropriate antiemetics for the management of any breakthrough CINV is determined, in part, by the agent(s) given to prevent CINV. For example, if palonosetron is given before chemotherapy, the use of another 5-HT3 antagonist is not warranted for the management of breakthrough CINV for the initial few days after palonosetron (a long-acting 5-HT3 RA).
   B. Agents used for the management of breakthrough CINV may include:

1. Dopamine receptor (D2) antagonists: prochlorperazine, droperidol, and promethazine
2. Ondansetron
3. Metoclopramide
4. Cannabinoids
   a. Dronabinol
   b. Nabilone
5. Cannabis (medical marijuana) may be legal in some locations and has been used for the management of symptoms, including CINV.
6. Dexamethasone
7. Benzodiazepines have been used historically in select patients.
VIII. Potential adverse effects (see Table 32.5)

Assessment

I. Patient history
   A. Identify the risk factors for CINV.
   B. Concomitant medications including assessment for potential drug–drug interactions
   C. Comorbidities including the assessment for potential drug–disease interactions
   D. Planned chemotherapy and/or anticancer treatment
      1. Nonchemotherapy anticancer therapy
      2. Radiation therapy
   E. Fluid status and dietary intake
   F. Onset of symptoms, accompanying symptoms, and relieving factors

G. Symptom effects on functional status and quality of life

II. Physical examination
   A. Examination of the oral cavity, abdomen, and skin
   B. Number, volume, and characteristics of emetic episodes
   C. Intake and output
      1. Fluid balance (assess for signs of dehydration)
      2. Weight
      3. Concentrated urine or low urine output
      4. Dietary intake and ability to drink fluids
   D. Hematemesis
   E. Orthostatic hypotension
   F. Distress associated with symptoms

III. Effectiveness of prescribed antiemetic regimen

IV. Evaluation of diagnostic and laboratory data
   A. Serum electrolyte values
   B. Renal and hepatic function
   C. Abdomen radiograph (kidney, ureter, and bladder) if obstruction suspected

Management

I. Pharmacologic management
   A. Interventions to manage nausea and vomiting
      1. Follow recommended guidelines for antiemetic chemotherapy prophylaxis.

II. Nonpharmacologic management
   A. Assess patient's nausea and vomiting status during and after chemotherapy administration; telephone follow-up in outpatient setting on days 2 and 3 of cycle.
      1. Education to patient and caregiver to contact health care team with issues including nausea and vomiting
   B. Ensure patient understands the rationale for medication adherence and administration schedule for nausea management at home.
   C. Interventions to manage fluid deficit
      1. Encourage adequate oral (PO) intake.
      2. Provide IV hydration if patient is unable to maintain adequate oral intake.
      3. Monitor weight.
   D. Patient and caregiver education
      1. Rationale for antiemetic drug therapy
      2. Rationale for scheduled antiemetic therapy to prevent CINV
      3. Rationale for as-needed antiemetic therapy to manage nausea and/or nausea
   E. Manage adverse effects of antiemetic regimen, refractory nausea, and vomiting.
      1. Constipation
      2. Hiccups
      3. Dehydration
      4. Agent-specific adverse effects
   F. Adverse effects to report to health care team
      1. Weight loss
      2. Unable to keep down fluids or antiemetic medications
      3. Concentrated urine
   G. Dietary interventions

1. Importance of maintaining calories
2. Optimization of fluid intake
3. Food selections to minimize nausea/vomiting

H. Interventions to decrease the incidence of CINV, monitor response of antiemetic therapy, and manage antiemetic drug therapy adverse effects (see Table 32.5)
   1. Implement strategies to maximize patient safety.

I. Monitor for response to antiemetic therapy after chemotherapy and before each consecutive treatment.
   1. Assess for mental status changes, dizziness, sedation; implementing safety measures (e.g., fall precautions) as needed.
   2. Modify antiemetic strategy as needed for delayed CINV.

ANALGESICS

Overview

(NCCN, 2022b)

I. Rationale and indications (see Chapter 45)
   A. >50% of patients will experience pain during their disease trajectory.
      1. Pain can be related to the disease, cancer treatment, or both.
      2. Patients may also suffer from chronic nonmalignant pain (e.g., back injury).
   B. Analgesics are used to manage both nociceptive and neuropathic pain.
   C. Types of cancer-related pain (see Chapter 45)
      1. Acute: self-limiting pain
      2. Chronic: pain lasts longer than 3 months
      3. Refractory: pain that is resistant to prescribed interventions
      4. Breakthrough: pain occurs despite adequate control of background pain; commonly associated with chronic pain

II. Types of analgesics
   A. Opioids
   B. Nonopioid analgesics (see the "Antiinflammatory Agents" section)
   C. Adjuvants (see the "Psychotropic Drugs: Anxiolytics and Sedative-Hypnotics" section)

III. Principles of medical management
   A. Selection of appropriate analgesia is based on pharmacokinetic factors and patient's physical needs, age, history of analgesia usage, and organ function.
   B. The most appropriate dose is the one that controls pain through a 24-hour period.
   C. If opioids are used, patients should have long-acting and breakthrough options available when pain is constant.
   D. As doses are titrated to effective levels, long-acting and breakthrough doses should be increased; breakthrough dose should be 10%–20% of the 24-hour long-acting dose.
   E. Prophylaxis for constipation with a stool softener and bowel stimulant should be considered for all patients started on opioid analgesics, and the regimen should be optimized to assure regular bowel movements.

F. The effectiveness and the side effect profile should be reassessed (see Chapter 45).

G. Tolerance occurs in patients who take opioids regularly; that is, they require higher doses to achieve the same amount of analgesia.

H. Physical dependence occurs in all patients who take opioids regularly; a withdrawal syndrome will occur if the opioid is abruptly stopped.

I. Psychological dependence is addiction that occurs when patients crave the opioid, use the drug compulsively, and continue use despite harm.

IV. Routes of administration

A. Oral
  1. Often the most convenient and preferred route
  2. Immediate- and extended-release dosing available

B. Transdermal

C. Parenteral: IV, subcutaneous, and intrathecal

D. Topical

E. Buccal, transmucosal, or nasal for rapid-onset opioids

F. Rectal

V. Potential adverse effects

A. Adverse effect profile of opioid analgesics (Table 32.6)

B. Drug interactions with multidrug regimens

C. Dependence
  1. Physical dependence is universal; it is physiologic.
  2. Opioid withdrawal
    a. Doses of opioids should not be abruptly discontinued to avoid opioid withdrawal. A sign of physical dependence, not psychological addiction.
    b. Symptoms of withdrawal
      (1) Nausea and vomiting
      (2) Diarrhea
      (3) Perspiration
      (4) Tachycardia
      (5) Chills
      (6) Restless legs syndrome
      (7) Dysphoria
      (8) Anxiety or paranoia
      (9) Insomnia

D. Other sedative or hypnotic drugs—potentiate sedative properties of opioids and combination opiate substances

E. Adverse drug interactions
  1. Drugs that lower seizure threshold—increased risk of seizures with concomitant administration
  2. Concomitant drugs that alter mental status equilibrium
  3. Drugs that alter hepatic metabolism, renal excretion
  4. Drugs that alter the bioavailability, absorption, or pharmacokinetics of the administered drug

F. Organ alterations
  1. Surgical resections, including gastrectomy, jejunectomy, and duodenectomy, may increase transit time, decrease absorption, or both.
  2. Feeding tubes inserted at various points in the GI tract may not be the appropriate point of absorption of an individual drug.

3. Pharmacologically induced changes in gut motility.
  a. Tube feedings or fluids administered through tubes may increase transit time and decrease absorption
  b. Laxatives
  c. Muscarinics (e.g., atropine)
  d. Prokinetic agents (e.g., metoclopramide)

4. Renal insufficiency—may slow the rate of elimination of drug, metabolites, or both, leading to increased potential for toxicities.

5. Hepatic insufficiency—may increase the amount of drug available to body because of decreased first-pass effect, altered enzyme pathways, and other metabolic pathways.

6. Central nervous system (CNS)—brain metastases, underlying seizure disorders may predispose to CNS toxicity.

7. Urinary—benign prostatic hypertrophy may contribute to urinary retention.

8. Respiratory—underlying restrictive or obstructive disease may potentiate respiratory compromise from opioids.

9. Cardiovascular—coronary artery disease, congestive heart failure.

10. Opioid considerations
  a. Codeine—a prodrug metabolized by p450; some patients lack the enzyme to convert it to the active analgesic form and it is ineffective; others may experience drug accumulation
  b. Meperidine—retention of normeperidine, the active metabolite, may cause seizures
  c. Hydromorphone (metabolites exist but clinical significance is unknown)
  d. Tramadol—risk of serotonin syndrome with antidepressants
  e. Morphine—metabolites can accumulate and cause oversedation

G. Transdermal considerations
  1. Occlusive dressings increase absorption; moisture content can affect skin adherence
  2. Avoid heat
  3. Ulcerations
  4. Fat-to-lean body ratio—transdermal preparations not recommended in cachectic patients; longer time to onset in obese patients

Assessment

I. Identify patients at risk for pain.

A. Assess and reassess pain—onset, duration, intensity, description, location, aggravating and relieving factors.
  1. Reassessment after pharmacologic intervention should occur 1 hour after oral analgesic administration and 15 minutes after parenteral analgesic administration.

B. History of past and current analgesia regimens and their effectiveness

C. Psychological manifestations

TABLE 32.6   Side Effects of Opioid Analgesics (Pathan & Williams, 2012)

Side Effects	Nursing Implications
GI	
Nausea, vomiting	Consider changing to another opioid, as some agents are associated with less nausea (e.g., hydromorphone). Monitor nausea and number of vomiting episodes and effect on comfort and fluid balance; administer antiemetic drug therapy as needed. Assure nausea and vomiting not related to constipation.
Constipation	Assess bowel elimination patterns and compare with patient's normal pattern; administer stool softeners and/or stimulant cathartics prophylactically.
Narcotized bowel	Increase fluid and dietary fiber intake; abdominal assessment; report decreased or absent bowel sounds and increased abdominal pain.
Cardiovascular	
Arteriolar vasodilation and reduced peripheral resistance; decrease in blood pressure; tachycardia, bradycardia	Monitor vital signs, blood pressure for orthostatic hypotension. Provide for patient safety if blood pressure is low.
Respiratory	
Depressant effect on brainstem reduces respiratory rate, minute volume, tidal exchange; irregular and periodic breathing; respiratory arrest	Monitor the level of sedation; respiratory rate and depth; arterial blood gases; vital signs, O_2 saturations; have available narcotic antagonist and measures for respiratory assistance as appropriate for clinical setting.
Decreased cough reflex	Monitor coughing ability postoperatively; use aspiration precautions.
Central Nervous System	
Drowsiness, alteration in mood and mental clouding; visual and auditory hallucinations, euphoria, dizziness, disorientation, and paranoia; lethargy, inability to concentrate, and apathy; seizures, uncontrollable twitching, and myoclonus	Neurologic assessment at baseline to facilitate ongoing assessment. Optimize sleep hygiene, including management of pain during night. Provide for patient safety. Institute fall precautions, as needed. Avoid meperidine use. Monitor closely for any preseizure activity for individuals taking meperidine; monitor for twitching. Level of sedation may indicate degree of respiratory depression. Methylphenidate (Ritalin), 5–10 mg, PO BID or TID, may be helpful for somnolence or mental clouding from opioids.
Pupil	
Miosis	Monitor pupil size and response to light (contraction).
Smooth Muscle	
Contraction of gallbladder, bile duct, and sphincter of Oddi	Monitor for signs of gastric upset; if present, evaluate liver and pancreatic function tests.
Genitourinary	
Urinary retention	Monitor urine output, palpate bladder, catheterize (straight or indwelling), as needed. This is often a transitory side effect seen with initiation and increasing of dose.
Dermatologic	
Skin rash, cutaneous vasodilation	Monitor skin integrity. Administer antihistamines for allergic reactions. Consider change in opioid. Educate patient to avoid scratching. Provide cool environment.

BID, Twice daily; *PO,* by mouth; *TID,* three times daily.

National Comprehensive Cancer Network (NCCN). (2022b). Adult cancer pain (v.1.2022). https://www.nccn.org/professionals/physician_gls/pdf/pain.pdf New version V1.2023 - March 7, 2023 Pathan, H., & Williams, J. (2012). Basic opioid pharmacology: An update. *British Journal of Pain, 6*(1), 11–16. https://doi.org/10.1177/2049463712438493f.

1. Anxiety and/or depression
2. Cognitive behavioral changes
3. Social isolation
   D. Patient and caregiver history: history of addiction or opioid use disorder
   E. Assessment of patient's and caregiver's spiritual and cultural beliefs
II. Physical examination
   A. Presence of inflammation or infection
   B. Sensory examination
   C. Musculoskeletal examination
   D. Psychological examination
   E. Patient safety
      1. Respiratory depression
      2. Sedation
      3. Potential for addiction or opioid use disorder
III. Medication reconciliation
IV. Evaluation of diagnostic and laboratory studies
   A. Radiographic studies (e.g., bone scan, CT, and MRI)
   B. Nerve blocks and nerve conduction studies
   C. Toxicology screen

Management

I. Nonpharmacologic management
   A. Manage the pain effectively and safely.
   B. Provide patient and caregiver education.
      1. Rationale for taking analgesic medications, including schedule of administration—long-acting and breakthrough agents; scheduled and as-needed agents
      2. Adverse effects and strategies for management
         a. Reinforce the need for bowel regimen (e.g., stool softener, stimulant laxative) when taking opioids to prevent constipation.
            (1) Stimulant laxatives are often used in combination with stool softeners to help mitigate opioid-induced constipation. It is important to tailor the bowel regimen to the individual patient.
         b. Take medications with food to prevent GI upset.
         c. Antihistamines for pruritus.
   C. Adverse effects to report to health care team
      1. Respiratory depression or sedation
      2. Analgesics not effective in managing pain
      3. Constipation not relieved with current bowel regimen (e.g., stool softeners and stimulant laxatives)
   D. Signs of physical dependence, addiction, and opioid withdrawal
   E. Prevent/manage adverse effects of medication regimen (see Table 32.6).
      1. Review of patient's medications for possible drug interactions
      2. Presence of comorbidities (e.g., renal, cardiac, respiratory, or hepatic disease)
   F. Patient response to analgesia
      1. Assessment of pain control

2. Assessment for adverse effects, toxicity, and drug interactions
3. Assessment of patient safety and medication tolerance
   G. Reevaluate pharmaceutical plan and adjust according to individual patient needs.

PSYCHOTROPIC DRUGS: ANXIOLYTICS AND SEDATIVE-HYPNOTICS

Overview

(NCCN, 2022d; Zhang, Wan, & Liu, 2020)
I. Rationale and indications
   A. Psychosocial care is a standard of quality cancer care and should be included as routine for treatment of the individual with cancer, including survivorship.
   B. Anxiety (see Chapter 54)
      1. Commonly referred to as *distress*, as it is a less stigmatizing, more acceptable term.
      2. Individuals with cancer have been found to have a significant level of distress at some time throughout their cancer trajectory. The prevalence of distress varies greatly in individuals and may occur at any time during and/or following treatment (Herschbach et al., 2020).
      3. Distress in individuals with cancer often extends beyond psychological stressors and may include social factors and/or physical factors (Johnson, Schreier, Swanson, & Ridner, 2020).
      4. Risk factors for distress
         a. History of anxiety disorder or traumatic experience
         b. Medical factors: cancer site and stage, type of treatment, and concurrent symptoms, including pain
         c. Psychological factors: coping ability, emotional maturity, and diagnosis
         d. Social factors: younger patients, patients without strong familial support, and less educated patients have a higher incidence of distress and anxiety
         e. Stimulants: caffeine and steroids
         f. Medication withdrawal: barbiturates and benzodiazepines
      5. Goal of anxiolytics in patients with cancer
         a. To reduce anxiety associated with cancer and its management
         b. To eliminate functional impairment
         c. To manage comorbid anxiety
         d. To reduce pain associated with anxiety
         e. To manage alcohol or narcotic withdrawal
         f. To prevent or manage anticipatory nausea or vomiting or treat CINV
   C. Sleep disturbance (see Chapter 47)
      1. An estimated one-third to one-half of cancer survivors experience some degree of sleep disturbance.

2. Pharmacologic risk factors for sleep disturbances
   a. Cancer treatment and side effects, medications used to treat side effects (e.g., opioids, antiemetics, anxiolytics, and steroids for symptom management)
   b. Caffeine, alcohol, or other stimulant consumption
   c. Drug therapy impact on physical activity
D. Management of anxiety (Pitman, Suleman, Hyde, & Hodgkiss, 2018)
   1. Identification and management of medical conditions with similar symptoms
   2. Manage symptoms that may be contributing to anxiety (e.g., pain, shortness of breath, and drug-induced anxiety).
   3. Optimization of nonpharmacologic strategies (e.g., relaxation, meditation, yoga, and physical activity)
E. Pharmacologic therapy
   1. Selective serotonin reuptake inhibitors (SSRIs):
      a. Start at low dose and increase to optimal dose.
      b. May induce anxiety symptoms early in therapy
      c. Abrupt discontinuation may precipitate withdrawal syndrome; ensure patients are counseled to communicate with the health care team prior to discontinuation.
      d. Effect may not be seen for the first 2–4 weeks.
      e. Caution in frail elderly patients due to the risk of hyponatremia
      f. Assess for drug–drug interactions prior and throughout therapy (e.g., fluoxetine and paroxetine may inhibit the conversion of tamoxifen to the active metabolite impacting the potential effectiveness of the medication).
   2. Serotonin-norepinephrine reuptake inhibitors (SNRIs)
      a. Start at low dose and increase to optimal dose.
      b. May induce anxiety symptoms early in therapy
      c. Abrupt discontinuation may precipitate withdrawal syndrome; ensure patients are counseled to communicate with the health care team prior to discontinuation.
      d. Effect seen in 2–4 weeks
   3. Benzodiazepines (Table 32.7)
      a. Considered the second line for anxiety but may be useful for short-term mitigation.
      b. Does not treat cognitive symptoms of anxiety (e.g., worry).
      c. Concerns for use include physical dependence and withdrawal effects. It is important to gradually decrease dose over time to avoid discontinuation syndrome.
      d. Abrupt discontinuation may precipitate withdrawal symptoms; ensure patients are counseled to communicate with the health care team prior to discontinuation.
      e. Assess for drug–drug interactions prior to and throughout therapy.
   4. Tricyclic antidepressants (TCAs)

a. Caution with patients with a history of, or at risk for seizures, as some TCAs can lower seizure threshold.
   5. Other agents, including buspirone, mirtazapine, gabapentin, and atypical antipsychotics (e.g., risperidone and olanzapine)
      a. Gabapentin and pregabalin are not Food and Drug Administration (FDA) approved for anxiety disorders.
      b. Atypical antipsychotics have been used in the treatment of anxiety disorders.
   6. Many of the psychotropic agents have the potential to prolong QTc and should be monitored closely in patients receiving other medications known to increase QTc interval (e.g., 5-HT3 RA including ondansetron, antifungals including Diflucan, and beta-blockers).
II. Management of sleep disorders (Matthews, 2018)
   A. Pharmacologic options for sleep disorders
      1. Antihistamines (e.g., diphenhydramine and doxylamine)
         a. Tolerance to the sedative effects may develop within 10 days of frequent use.
         b. Paradoxical excitation may occur in some individuals.
      2. Antidepressants (e.g., trazadone, mirtazapine, and doxepin)
      3. Melatonin
         a. OTC products are not standardized.
         b. Common dose ranges from 3 to 5 mg, although higher doses are frequently used.
      4. Ramelteon (Rozerem)
         a. Receptor agonist (RA) with high affinity for two melatonin receptors
         b. Treatment for sleep latency
      5. Benzodiazepines (see Table 32.7)
         a. Reduce time to sleep onset and prolong the first two stages of sleep
         b. Reduce time in deep sleep and rapid eye movement sleep
         c. Can produce rebound insomnia when discontinued
      6. Nonbenzodiazepines—RAs with effects similar to benzodiazepines
         a. Zolpidem (Ambien) indicated for sleep latency, maintenance, and middle-of-the-night awakenings (dependent on product)
         b. Zaleplon (Sonata) indicated for sleep latency
         c. Zopiclone (Imovane)
         d. Eszopiclone (Lunesta) indicated for sleep latency and maintenance
      7. Suvorexant (Belsomra)
III. Principles of medical management of anxiety and sleep disturbances (Balachandran, Miller, Faiz, Yennurajalingam, & Innominato, 2021; NCCN, 2022d)
   A. Selection of therapy
      1. Assessment of sleep disturbances

a. Manifestations of sleep disturbances (e.g., difficulty falling asleep, difficulty staying asleep, and waking up too early)
b. Duration of sleep disturbances
c. Impact of physical symptoms and/or psychosocial issues on sleep
d. Sleep hygiene

2. Multicomponent approach to management of sleep disturbances
   a. Behavioral and cognitive strategies
   b. Physical activity
   c. Pharmacologic

3. Pharmacologic interventions (see Table 32.7)
   a. Half-life
   b. Sedative properties
   c. Psychomotor and memory impairment
   d. Dose–response profiles
   e. Duration of therapy
   f. Routes of administration
   g. Compromised organ function
   h. Age-related alterations
   i. Cost

IV. Potential adverse effects
   A. CNS effects
   B. Potential for addiction, dependency, and abuse
   C. Rebound insomnia for short-acting agents
   D. Complex sleep-related behaviors (e.g., sleepwalking)
   E. Motor incoordination
   F. Behavioral changes, delirium
   G. Respiratory suppression

1. Sedation
2. Dizziness
3. Lightheadedness
4. Cognitive impairment
5. Particularly in older adults
6. Caution should be used in patients with pulmonary disease (e.g., chronic obstructive pulmonary disease [COPD])

V. Drug interactions
   A. Alcohol
      1. Concomitant consumption of alcohol and these medications should be avoided.
   B. Inhibitors or inducers of hepatic enzymes
   C. Medications for comorbidities and or symptoms

Assessment

I. Identify patients at risk for distress or sleep disturbances.
   A. Assess for signs and symptoms of anxiety and sleep disorders.
   B. Patient screening tools
      1. NCCN Distress Thermometer (scores of 4 or higher are associated with higher levels of distress)
      2. Sleep diaries or questionnaires; Insomnia Severity Index
   C. Patient and family history

II. Physical examination
   A. Alterations in functional performance
   B. Concurrent medication or cancer-related symptoms

III. Medication reconciliation

TABLE 32.7	Comparison of Benzodiazepines		
Drug	**Comparative Oral Dose (mg)**	**Metabolic Pathway**	**Half-Life of Parent Drug (h)**
Short Acting			
Midazolam (Versed)	None		0.5–1
Triazolam (Halcion)	0.25–0.5 mg	CYP3A4 (no active metabolite)	1–4
Intermediate Acting			
Alprazolam (Xanax)	0.5	CYP3A4 (active metabolite)	6–20
Clonazepam (Klonopin)	0.25	CYP3A4 (no active metabolite)	20–40
Lorazepam (Ativan)	1	Glucuronidation (no active metabolite)	10–20
Oxazepam (Serax)	15 mg	(no active metabolite)	10–20
Temazepam (Restoril)	30 mg	Glucuronidation, CYP2C19, and CYP3A4 (no active metabolite)	10–20
Long Acting			
Chlordiazepoxide (Librium)	10 mg	(active metabolite)	5–30
Diazepam (Valium)	5	CYP2C19 and CYP3A4 (active metabolite)	20–50

CYP pathway: Knowledge of the particular enzymes involved in the metabolism of medications is important to assess potential drug–drug interactions and to modify the dose(s) or agents appropriately. If a medication is metabolized by one or multiple CYP enzymes extensively, any modification of those enzymes may result in a change of the exposure to the medication. For example, drugs that inhibit an enzyme important in the metabolism of other medications may result in decreased metabolism and increased exposure of the medication. A drug that induces an enzyme important in the metabolism of other medications may result in increased metabolism and decreased exposure of the medication. A drug that is identified as a substrate for an enzyme is potentially vulnerable to changes in enzyme activity. If you have questions or concerns about the potential for drug–drug interactions while caring for a patient, consider collaboration with a pharmacist.
Data from Lexi-Comp Online. *Lexi-drugs online, and package inserts for agents.*

A. Sudden withdrawal from sedatives can lead to an increase in anxiety.

B. Medications used to treat cancer-treatment side effects can lead to sleep disturbance (e.g., opioids, antiemetics, and steroids).

C. Medication interactions can increase adverse side effects of anxiolytics and sedative-hypnotics.

IV. Evaluate diagnostic and laboratory data
   A. Hepatic and renal function
   B. Toxicology screen

V. Patient safety
   A. Assess for signs of psychomotor or cognitive impairment.
   B. Assess for signs of dependency or abuse.

Management

I. Nonpharmacologic management
   A. Manage sleep disturbances, pain, and emotional distress.
   B. Patient and caregiver education
      1. Rationale for use of sedative-hypnotic or anxiolytic drug therapy and taking them as scheduled or only when needed
      2. Adverse effects of anxiolytics and sedative-hypnotic medications and strategies to manage them
         a. Pharmacologic interventions for sleep disturbances classified by the Oncology Nursing Society as "benefit balanced with harm" due to potentially harmful side effects and medication interactions
         b. Safety considerations due to decreased motor coordination, excessive drowsiness
         c. Potential for addiction, dependency, or abuse
         d. Avoid concurrent use with opioids or alcohol
         e. Side effects more pronounced in older patients
   C. Adverse effects to report to health care team
      1. Signs of medication withdrawal, addiction, tolerance, or dependence
      2. Cognitive impairment
   D. Monitor for adverse effects of sedative-hypnotic or anxiolytic drugs.
   E. Decrease the incidence and manage the adverse effects of sedative-hypnotic or anxiolytic drugs.
      1. Assess baseline data (e.g., vital signs; CNS—orientation, alertness, affect; respiratory effort, rate, and depth).
      2. Review patient's medical history for existing or previous conditions.
      3. Review patient's medications for potential drug interactions.
   F. Monitor for response to psychotropic drugs.
      1. Psychiatry or psychology consultation as needed
      2. Assess the level of anxiety and amount of restful sleep.
   G. Reevaluate pharmaceutical plan and adjust according to individual patient needs.
   H. Refer to psychosocial services (e.g., social work, mental health professional, and counseling) or chaplain as needed.

ANTIDEPRESSANTS

Overview

(NCCN, 2022d)

I. Rationale and indications
   A. For treatment of pain (adjuvant therapy)
   B. For treatment of depression
   C. Definition and incidence of depression (see Chapter 54)
      1. Sad, empty, and irritable mood accompanied by somatic or cognitive changes that affect daily functioning
      2. Major depressive disorder—depressive symptoms lasting most of the day, every day, and for at least 2 weeks; may have suicidal thoughts, recurrent thoughts of dying
      3. Often difficult to identify in cancer patients because symptoms can mimic treatment side effects (e.g., fatigue, weight loss, and changes in appetite)
      4. Occurs in about 25% of patients with cancer, leading to poor quality of life and functional status, higher use of health care services, and nonadherence with treatment
   D. Pharmacologic risk factors for depression
      1. Poor pain control
      2. Medications used in cancer treatment
   E. Purposes of antidepressants
      1. To treat clinical unipolar or bipolar depression or anxiety
      2. To treat depression associated with chronic pain
      3. As adjuvant pharmacologic pain management in pain conditions, including postherpetic neuralgia, migraine and chronic tension headaches, and sundowner syndrome
      4. To treat insomnia

II. Types of antidepressants (Table 32.8)
   A. SSRIs
      1. Toxicities include nausea, constipation, diarrhea, dry mouth, dizziness, nervousness and insomnia, and sexual dysfunction.
      2. Frequency of adverse effects is agent specific.
   B. SNRIs
      1. Toxicities include anxiety, nausea/vomiting, dizziness, constipation, insomnia, diaphoresis and increased blood pressure (agent specific), sexual dysfunction, and discontinuation syndrome.
   C. TCAs
      1. Often used later in therapy (second and third lines) secondary to side effects and risk with overdosage. Overdosages may be lethal; contraindicated in older adults.
      2. Common side effects include anticholinergic effects of blurred vision, dry mouth, constipation, antihistamine effects (including sedation and weight gain), and alpha-adrenergic inhibition (including postural hypotension, reflex tachycardia, and priapism).
   D. Monoamine oxidase inhibitors

TABLE 32.8 Antidepressants

Medication	Classification	Indications
Amitriptyline	TCA	Depression
Amoxapine	TCA	Depression
Bupropion	NDRI	Major depressive disorder
		Seasonal affective disorder
		Smoking cessation (bupropion SR [Zyban])
Citalopram	SSRI	Depression
Clomipramine	TCA	OCD
Desipramine	TCA	Depression
Desvenlafaxine	SSNI	Major depressive disorder
Doxepin	TCA	Depression
		Insomnia
Duloxetine	SSNI	Major depressive disorder
		General anxiety disorder
		Diabetic peripheral neuropathy
		Chronic musculoskeletal pain
Escitalopram	SSRI	Major depressive disorder
		General anxiety disorder
Fluoxetine	SSRI	Major depressive disorder
		OCD
		Bulimia nervosa
		Panic disorder
		Depressive episodes associated with bipolar I disorders (with olanzapine)
Fluvoxamine	SSRI	OCD
		Not first line for treatment of depression
Imipramine	TCA	Depression
Isocarboxazid	MAOI	Depression
Levomilnacipran	SNRI	Major depressive disorder
Milnacipran	SNRI	Fibromyalgia
Mirtazapine	Postsynaptic 5HT and presynaptic α2-adrenergic antagonist	Depression
Nefazodone	Mixed 5HT and norepinephrine uptake	Depression
Nortriptyline	TCA	Depression
Paroxetine	SSRI	General anxiety disorder
		Posttraumatic stress disorder
		Major depression disorder
		OCD
		Panic disorder
		Social anxiety disorders
		Premenstrual dysphoric disorder
Phenelzine	MAOI	Depression
Protriptyline	TCA	Depression
Selegiline	MAOI	Major depressive disorder
Sertraline	SSRI	Panic disorder
		Posttraumatic stress disorder
		Social anxiety disorder
		Premenstrual dysphoric disorder
Tranylcypromine	MAOI	Major depressive disorder
Trazodone	SSRI and 5HT2 receptor antagonist	Depression
		Major depressive disorder
Trimipramine	TCA	Depression
Venlafaxine	SSNI	Major depressive disorder
		General anxiety disorder
		Panic disorder
		Social anxiety disorder
Vilazodone	SPARI	Major depressive disorder
Vortioxetine	SSRI with 5HT1A agonism and 5-HT3 receptor antagonism	Major depressive disorder

5-HT, Serotonin; MAOI, monoamine oxidase inhibitor; NDRI, norepinephrine and dopamine reuptake inhibitor; OCD, obsessive–compulsive disorder; NRI, serotonin-norepinephrine reuptake inhibitors; SPARI, serotonin partial agonist reuptake inhibitor; SSRI, selective serotonin reuptake inhibition; TCA, tricyclic and tetracyclic antidepressants.
Data from Lexi-Comp Online. Lexi-drugs online, and package inserts for agents.

1. Dietary modifications to avoid tyramine.
2. Drug–drug interactions can result in hypertensive crisis. A required washout period for the drug is dependent on the drug's half-life.
3. Toxicity includes hypertensive crisis and serotonin syndrome.
   E. Bupropion
   F. Nefazodone
   G. Trazodone—may also be used as a sleep aid
   H. Mirtazapine—may increase appetite
   I. Vilazodone
   J. Levomilnacipran
   K. Vortioxetine
   L. Lithium
III. Principles of medical management
   A. Selection of therapy
     1. Efficacy (prior history)
     2. Comorbidities
     3. Side effect profile of patient
     4. Concern with the risk of overdose
     5. Optimizing side effects for efficacy (e.g., increasing appetite with weight loss)
     6. Patient preference
IV. Potential adverse effects (Table 32.9)
   A. Drug–drug interactions
   B. Dietary restrictions

Assessment

I. Identification of patients at risk for depression
   A. Patient screening tools
     1. Patient Health Questionnaire
     2. NCCN Distress Thermometer (scores of 4 or higher have clinical significance)
     3. Suicide Risk Assessment
     4. Hospital Anxiety and Depression Scale
   B. Alcohol or substance abuse
   C. Assessment of unrelieved or chronic pain and fatigue
II. Physical examination
III. Medication reconciliation
   A. Several interactions between antidepressant and cancer-treatment medications exist (e.g., antidepressants and tamoxifen).
   B. Antidepressant therapeutic effect can take up to 3 weeks; ensure patient adherence.
   C. Withdrawal symptoms can occur with abrupt discontinuation.
IV. Evaluate the diagnostic and laboratory data.
V. Assess patient's and family's understanding of depression as an illness.

Management

I. Nonpharmacologic management
   A. Manage effects of depression, pain, and fatigue.
   B. Patient and caregiver education
     1. Rationale for use of antidepressant drug therapy and taking antidepressants as scheduled; time necessary for therapeutic response to agent; potential for

withdrawal effects with abrupt cessation; continue therapy for 6 months after improvement in symptoms to avoid relapse of depression; gradually taper dose at discontinuation
     2. Adverse effects to report to health care team
       a. Suicidal ideation and worsening symptoms
       b. Presence of unwanted side effects with prescribed antidepressant therapy (weight gain, dizziness, sedative effects, and palpitations)
       c. Serotonin syndrome (hyperreflexia, tremors, tachycardia, nausea, diarrhea, agitation, and confusion)
   C. Monitor for adverse effects of antidepressants.
     1. Decrease the incidence and manage the adverse effects of antidepressants.
     2. Monitor for therapeutic response to antidepressants.
   D. Monitor the patient for emotional changes, suicidal ideation.
   E. Obtain psychiatric or psychological consultation as needed.
   F. Monitor patient for response to pain management interventions
   G. Assess for adverse effects, toxicity, and drug–drug interactions.
   H. Reevaluate the pharmaceutical plan and adjust according to individual patient needs.
   I. Refer to psychosocial services or chaplain as needed.

ANTICONVULSANTS

Overview

(Gonzalez Castro & Milligan, 2020; Olsen, LeFebvre, & Brassil, 2019; Santomasso et al., 2018)
I. Rationale and indications
   A. Epilepsy
     1. Disturbance of electrical activity in the brain
     2. Classified by where they occur in the brain (the focus), the patient's level of awareness, and the presence of motor movements
   B. For prophylaxis and treatment of seizure activity
     1. Intracranial causes—primary brain tumors, primary CNS lymphoma, or metastatic cancer
     2. Drug-induced causes (treatments that lower the seizure threshold)
       a. Chemotherapy: asparaginase, busulfan, carmustine, cisplatin, cyclophosphamide, dacarbazine, docetaxel, etoposide, 5-FU, gemcitabine ifosfamide, thalidomide, and vinca alkaloids
       b. Antibiotics
       c. Antidepressants
       d. Opioids
       e. Chimeric antigen receptor T-cell therapies
       f. Intrathecal chemotherapy
     3. Metabolic abnormalities
       a. Electrolyte imbalance (hypernatremia, hyponatremia, hypercalcemia, and syndrome of inappropriate antidiuretic hormone secretion)

TABLE 32.9 Antidepressants Toxicity Comparison

Drug	Initial Dose	Anticholinergic	Sedation	Orthostatic Hypotension	Conduction Abnormalities	GI Distress	Weight Gain	Comments
Tricyclic Antidepressants								
Amitriptyline (generic)	25–50 mg q HS	4+	4+	3+	3+	1+	4+	Higher doses are used in the management of depression.
Desipramine (generic)	25–75 mg q HS	1+	2+	2+	2+	–	1+	Dose increases should be made in 25-mg increments.
Imipramine (generic)	25–75 mg q HS	3+	3+	4+	3+	1+	4+	Also used for chronic pain.
Nortriptyline (generic)	25–50 mg q HS	2+	2+	1+	2+	0	2+	Lower doses recommended for older patients.
Selective Serotonin Reuptake Inhibitors								
Citalopram	20 mg q AM	0	0	0	0	3+	1+	Significant sexual dysfunction.
Escitalopram	10 mg q AM	0	0	0	0	3+	1+	Significant sexual dysfunction.
Fluoxetine	10–20 mg q AM	0	0	0	0	3+	1+	CYP2B6 and 2D6 inhibitor (do not use with tamoxifen); significant sexual dysfunction.
Fluvoxamine	50 mg q day	0	1+	0	0	3+	–	
Paroxetine	10–20 mg q AM	1+	1+	0	0	3+	2+	CYP2B6 and 2D6 inhibitor (do not use with tamoxifen); significant sexual dysfunction.
Sertraline	20–50 mg once daily	0	0	0	0	3+	1+	CYP2B6 and 2D6 inhibitor (do not use with tamoxifen); significant sexual dysfunction.
Mixed-Action Agents								
Bupropion	150 mg q AM; BID (SR tab)	0	0	0	1+	1+	0	Contraindicated with seizures, bulimia, or anorexia; low incidence of sexual dysfunction.
Duloxetine	40–60 mg once daily	1+	1+	0	1+	3+	0	Also used for neuropathy.
Venlafaxine	37.5 mg once daily (XR tab)	1+	1+	0	1+	3+	0	Frequency of hypertension increases with dose; often used for hot flashes from tamoxifen.
Desvenlafaxine	50 mg once daily	0	1+	1+	0	3+	0	–
Mirtazapine	15 mg q HS	1+	3+	1+	1+	0	3+	Doses >15 mg/day less sedating; low incidence of sexual dysfunction; reported to increase appetite.
Trazodone	50 mg TID	0	4+	3+	1+	1+	2+	Often used for insomnia (50–150 mg q HS).

AM, Morning; BID, twice daily; HS, at bedtime; q, every; SR, sustained-release; TID, three times a day; XR, extended-release.
Data from Lacy, C. F., Armstrong, L. L., Goldman, M. P., Lance, L. L. (2011). Drug information handbook (20th ed., pp. 1143–1147). Lexi-Comp Online. Lexi-drugs online, and package inserts for agents.

b. Hyperglycemia or hypoglycemia

4. Other causes of seizures in patients with cancer
   a. Cerebral edema (e.g., increased intracranial pressure)
   b. Stroke (e.g., hemorrhage)
   c. CNS infections (e.g., meningitis)
   d. Posterior reversible encephalopathy syndrome
   e. Radiation toxicity

C. As adjuvant pharmacologic therapy for neuropathic pain (e.g., peripheral neuropathy)

II. Types of anticonvulsants (Table 32.10)
   A. Diagnose appropriate seizure activity
   B. Diagnose appropriate pain syndrome
   C. Selection of appropriate pharmacologic therapy (see Table 32.10)
      1. Neurology consultation should be considered.
      2. Determine the etiology of seizure to best manage long term, if needed.
         a. Seizure should not be presumed to be from tumor.
         b. Evaluation of other causes should be undertaken.
      3. No substantial differences between the efficacy of medications.
         a. Agent selection is determined by comorbidities, adverse effects, drug–drug interactions, cost, etc.
      4. Therapeutic selection is based on drug interactions and tolerance.

III. Potential adverse effects (see Table 32.10)

Assessment

I. Identify patients at risk for seizure activity—older adults and pediatric patients at higher risk.

II. Identify patients at risk for neuropathic pain.

III. Physical examination
   A. Neurologic examination
      1. Mental status—general appearance, level of consciousness, mood and affect, thought content and intellectual capacity, behavior
      2. Cranial nerve assessment
      3. Sensory and motor function, gait
      4. Assessment of reflexes
      5. Presence of aura with seizure onset

IV. Medication reconciliation
   A. Medications that lower the seizure threshold
   B. Benzodiazepine withdrawal
   C. Some anticonvulsants are enzyme inducers, which can accelerate the metabolism of other drugs and reduce serum levels.

V. Evaluation of diagnostic and laboratory data
   A. Anticonvulsant serum levels
   B. Serum electrolyte values
   C. Cerebrospinal fluid (CSF) culture
   D. Electroencephalogram, CT, and MRI

Management

I. Nonpharmacologic management
   A. Ensure patient safety in the event of a seizure.
      1. Institute seizure precautions.
      2. Padded side rails, bed in lowest position
      3. Suction setup to maintain airway
      4. Safe environment free of physical hazards
   B. Assess for injuries after completion of the seizure activity.
      1. Vital signs
      2. Neurologic examination
   C. Patient and caregiver education
      1. Rationale for use of anticonvulsant drug therapy and taking as scheduled
      2. Adverse effects and strategies to manage adverse effects
      3. Adverse effects to report to health care team
      4. Emphasize patient safety.
         a. Do not restrain patient during seizure.
         b. Turn patient's head to side if vomiting.
         c. Avoid putting anything in patient's mouth during seizure.
         d. Patients should not drive or operate machinery.
         e. High-risk patients should wear a medical alert bracelet at all times.
   D. Monitor for adverse effects of anticonvulsants.
   E. Decrease the incidence and manage the adverse effects of anticonvulsants.
      1. Assessment of baseline data (e.g., neurologic status)
      2. Review of patient's medical history for existing or previous conditions
      3. Review of patient's medications for potential drug–drug interactions
      4. Conducting patient and family teaching (e.g., good oral hygiene, avoiding driving, or other potentially hazardous activity that requires mental alertness)
   F. Monitor for a therapeutic response to anticonvulsant drug therapy.
      1. Assessment of neurologic status and pain level
      2. Assessment for adverse effects, toxicity, and drug interactions

MYELOID GROWTH FACTORS

Overview

(Camp-Sorrell, 2018; NCCN, 2022e)

I. Rationale and indications
   A. Myeloid growth factors (MGFs)—biological agents that stimulate the proliferation and activation of mature myeloid cells (e.g., neutrophils, erythrocytes, and platelets)
   B. Mature myeloid cells are often destroyed by chemotherapy and radiation treatment.
      1. Nearly all chemotherapy treatments will cause a degree of myelosuppression, which can be a dose-limiting toxicity.
      2. MGF use is supported in high-risk patients: previous chemotherapy regimen, presence of comorbidities (e.g., diabetes, cardiac or kidney disease), poor

TABLE 32.10   Anticonvulsant Medications (Nguyen, Dergalust, & Chang, 2020)

Drug (common brand name)	Dose	Target Serum Concentrations	Side Effects
Brivaracetam (Briviact)	Dose: 50–100 mg BID	0.2–2.0 µg/mL	Fatigue, hypersomnia, and weakness
Carbamazepine (Tegretol)	Adults: 400 mg PO daily	4–12 µg/mL	Dose related: Diplopia, drowsiness, and nausea Others: Hyponatremia, Aplastic anemia, Leukopenia, Rash
Clonazepam (Klonopin)	Initiate at 0.25 mg PO 1–3 times daily, titrate to effectiveness	Not established	Dose related: Ataxia, Memory impairment, Sedation
Eslicarbazepine (Aptiom)	Initial: 400 mg PO daily Dose: 1200 mg PO daily (maximum dose)		Dizziness, drowsiness, nausea, vomiting, headache, diplopia, fatigue, ataxia, and tremor
Ezogabine (Potiga)	Initial: 100 mg PO TID Dose: 600–1200 mg PO daily in divided doses		Urinary retention, dizziness, fatigue, confusion, disorientation, hallucinations, and diplopia Chronic use: Bluish pigmentation of skin, nails, and retina
Felbamate (Felbatol)	Initial: 1200 mg PO Dose: 1200–3600 mg/day in three or four divided doses	30–60 µg/mL	Dose related: Anxiety, Insomnia, Nausea, Anorexia Others: Aplastic anemia (monitor CBC), Liver dysfunction (monitor LFT)
Gabapentin (Neurotin)	Initial: 300 mg PO (may start lower in select patients, or higher in select situations) Dose: 900–3600 mg/day PO in 3–4 divided doses	2–20 µg/mL	Dose related: Sedation, Dizziness, Ataxia Others: Weight gain, Peripheral edema
Lacosamide (Vimpat)	Initial: 100 mg PO per day in divided doses and titrate Dose: 200–400 mg/day PO	Not established	Dose related: Ataxia, Dizziness, Diplopia, Nausea, Headache Others: PR interval prolongation (baseline ECG and monitor as needed), Increase LFT
Lamotrigine (Lamictal)	Dose: 150–500 mg/day PO in 2–3 divided doses. Dose may be lower if used in combination with valproic acid. Note: Initiated at lower dose and titrated based on overall therapy.	4–20 µg/mL	Dose related: Ataxia, Drowsiness, Headache, Insomnia, Sedation, Diplopia Other: Rash

Continued

TABLE 32.10   Anticonvulsant Medications (Nguyen, Dergalust, & Chang, 2020)—cont'd

Drug (common brand name)	Dose	Target Serum Concentrations	Side Effects

Levetiracetam (Keppra)	Initiate at 500–1000 mg/day PO and titrate as needed (divided dose)
	Dose: 1000–3000 mg/day PO
		12–46 µg/mL	Dose related:
			  Somnolence
			  Dizziness
			Others:
			  Depression
			  Rash
			  Psychosis (rare, more common in elderly)

Oxcarbazepine (Trileptal)	Initial: 300 mg PO twice daily and titrate
	Dose: 600–1200 mg/day PO
		3–35 µg/mL	Dose related:
			  Dizziness
			  Somnolence
			  Ataxia
			  Nausea
			Others:
			  Hyponatremia (chronic side effect)
			  Rash
			  23%–30% cross-sensitivity to carbamazepine

Perampanel (Fycompa) CIII	Initial: 2 mg PO q HS Dose: 4–12 mg PO daily		Dizziness, somnolence, headache, and fatigue

Phenobarbital (generic)	Maintenance dose: 1–4 mg/kg/day PO as a single or divided daily dose	15–40 µg/mL	Dose related:
			  Ataxia, drowsiness, and sedation
			Others:
			  Attention deficit, cognitive impairment, and hyperactivity

Phenytoin (Dilantin)
Fosphenytoin (Cerebyx)
Note: Phenytoin prodrug only available IV
	Initial: 3–5 mg/kg
	Loading dose of 15–20 mg/kg may be used
	Dose: 300–600 mg PO daily (based on serum level)
		10–20 µg/mL (total)
		Unbound phenytoin: 0.5–3 µg/mL
			Dose related:
			  Ataxia, nystagmus, dizziness, headache, sedation, lethargy
			Others:
			  Rash
			  Blood dyscrasia
			  Folate deficiency
			  Hirsutism
			  Allergy
			  Hepatotoxicity

Pregabalin (Lyrica)	Initial: 150 mg PO
	Dose: 300 mg PO/day (split doses)
		Not established	Dose related:
			  Dizziness, somnolence, dry mouth, and vision changes
			Others:
			  Pedal edema
			  Increase CPK
			  Thrombocytopenia
			  Weight gain

Rufinamide (Banzel)	Approved as adjunctive treatment of seizures with Lennox–Gastaut syndrome in adults Initial: 400–800 mg PO/day Dose: 3200 mg PO/day (two divided doses)		Somnolence, dizziness, gait disturbances, ataxia QT shortening (up to 20 ms)

Tiagabine (Gabitril)	Initial:
	4–8 mg/day
	Dose: 80 mg
		0.02–0.2 µg/mL	Dose related:
			  Dizziness, fatigue, difficulty concentrating, and nervousness
			  Depression

Topiramate (Topamax)	Initial: 25–50 mg PO daily
	Dose: 200–1000 mg PO per day
		5–20 µg/mL	Dose related:
			  Difficulty concentrating, psychomotor slowing, speech and language problems.
			Others:
			  Metabolic acidosis, acute angle glaucoma, and kidney stones

Drug (common brand name)	Dose	Target Serum Concentrations	Side Effects

Valproic acid	Initial: 15 mg/kg
	Dose: 60 mg/kg (3000–5000 mg)
		50–100 µg/mL	Dose related:
			  GI upset, sedation, unsteadiness, tremor, thrombocytopenia
			Other:
			  Liver dysfunction (monitor LFT)
			  Pancreatitis
			  Alopecia

Vigabatrin (Sabril)	Initial: 500 mg PO twice daily
	Dose: 1500 mg PO twice daily
		0.8–36 µg/mL	Dose related:
			  Visual field defects, fatigue, sedation, tremor, blurred vision, weight gain
			Others:
			  Peripheral neuropathy
			  Anemia

Zonisamide (Zonegran)	Initial: 100 mg PO daily
	Dose: 300–400 mg PO per day
		10–40 µg/mL	Dose related:
			  Sedation, dizziness, cognitive impairment, and nausea
			Others:
			  Rash (sulfa drug)
			  Metabolic acidosis

TABLE 32.10 Anticonvulsant Medications (Nguyen, Dergalust, & Chang, 2020)—cont'd

Note: Phenytoin is highly protein bound, and unbound phenytoin should be measured in patients with low serum albumin.
From, Lexi-Comp Online. *Lexi-drugs online, and package inserts for agents*; Nguyen, V. V., Dergalust, S., & Chang, E. (2020). Epilepsy. In J. T. DiPiro, G. C. Yee, L. M. Posey, S. T. Haines, T. D. Nolin, & V. Ellingrod (Eds.), *Pharmacotherapy: A pathophysiologic approach* (11th ed.). New York: McGraw-Hill.

nutritional status, advanced disease, tumor-related bone marrow involvement.

C. Cancer-related indications
  1. Reduce incidence, length, and severity of neutropenia (ANC less than 500/mm³) and febrile neutropenia (neutropenia plus a temperature of more than 38.5°C) in high-risk patients.
     a. Febrile neutropenia is a serious side effect of treatment and is associated with significant morbidity and mortality.
     b. High-risk cancer types: bladder, breast, esophageal, lymphoma, kidney, melanoma, multiple myeloma, ovarian/testicular, sarcoma, myelodysplastic syndromes, and leukemia
  2. Mobilization of hematopoietic stem cells before stem cell collection and for supportive care after transplant
     a. Granulocyte colony-stimulating factor (G-CSF) is routinely used after autologous and cord blood transplantation to support neutrophil engraftment.
  3. Treatment of malignancy and treatment-related anemia

D. Trilaciclib is a transient inhibitor of cyclin-dependent kinase 4 and 6 that is administered prior to chemotherapy for extensive-stage small cell lung cancer to decrease the incidence of chemotherapy-induced myelosuppression. It is NOT an MGF.

II. Types of growth factors in clinical use:
  A. White blood cell growth factors (WBC-GFs)

  1. G-CSF (filgrastim, pegfilgrastim, Tbo-filgrastim, and biosimilar products)
     a. Filgrastim
     b. Tbo-filgrastim is not licensed as a biosimilar in the United States and does have different FDA-approved clinical indications from filgrastim.
     c. Filgrastim-sndz is licensed in the United States as biosimilar (reference product: filgrastim).
     d. Pegfilgrastim
     e. Pegfilgrastim-jmdb is licensed as a biosimilar (reference product: pegfilgrastim).
  2. Granulocyte-macrophage colony-stimulating factor (GM-CSF) (sargramostim)
     a. Receptors exist on myeloid cell lines.
     b. Major effect stimulates the proliferation and differentiation of the cells destined for the neutrophil and macrophage lines.
     c. GM-CSF enhances the functional activities of neutrophils and monocytes or macrophages and leads to enhanced activity in clearing bacterial and fungal organisms.
     d. GM-CSF stimulates the production of secondary cytokines such as tumor necrosis factor, interleukin-1, and macrophage colony-stimulating factor (M-CSF).
  B. Red blood cell (RBC) growth factors
     1. Erythropoietin (EPO) (epoetin alfa and darbepoetin alfa)
  C. Platelet growth factors
     1. Thrombopoietin RA as part of clinical trial

III. Principles of medical management
   A. G-CSF and GM-CSF
      1. Prevention of febrile neutropenia with G-CSF or GM-CSF is more effective than treatment of febrile neutropenia with G-CSF or GM-CSF.
      2. Prevention of neutropenia by using G-CSF or GM-CSF is indicated in patients with a 20% or greater risk of febrile neutropenia as determined by chemotherapy regimen or patient-specific factors.
      3. Risk of neutropenia determined primarily by chemotherapeutic regimen (review NCCN guidelines for a list of regimens with ≥20% risk of febrile neutropenia).
      4. The intent of treatment may be a consideration for the use of WBC-GF; dose modification may be an appropriate option for individuals that are not receiving treatment for curative intent.
      5. Risk is increased in select patients, including:
         a. Prior chemotherapy or radiation therapy
         b. Persistent neutropenia
         c. Bone marrow involvement of the tumor
         d. Recent surgery or open wounds
         e. Liver dysfunction
         f. Renal dysfunction
         g. Age (>56 years)
      6. G-CSF shown to decrease days on antibiotics and hospital stay by 1 day, but it does not decrease mortality.
      7. Pegfilgrastim at least as effective as filgrastim in the prevention of febrile neutropenia.
      8. Filgrastim is used to mobilize stem cells from the bone marrow to be collected peripherally before allogeneic or autologous stem cell transplantation.
      9. Pegfilgrastim has limited use in stem cell mobilization at this time.
         a. Increased age (>65 years)
         b. Extensive previous treatments (chemotherapy and radiation therapy)
         c. Hematologic malignancy
         d. Multiple comorbidities (e.g., diabetes and COPD)
         e. Some data suggest it may be a more effective agent, but this has not been shown in randomized controlled trials.
   B. Erythropoiesis-stimulating agents (ESAs) or EPO (epoetin alfa, epoetin alfa-epbx, darbepoetin)
      1. EPO causes an increase in hemoglobin (>2 g/dL) more effectively than placebo in patients with anemia caused by chemotherapy.
      2. Concern has been raised by multiple clinical trials suggesting a decrease in progression-free and overall survival in patients receiving EPO during chemotherapy, radiotherapy, or no active treatment. EPO is not recommended for treatment of chemotherapy-induced anemia in the curative setting.
      3. ESA shortened overall survival and/or increased the risk of tumor progression in studies of patients with breast, non–small cell lung cancer, head and neck cancer, lymphoid, and cervical cancers.
      4. EPO should not be given to patients with hemoglobin greater than 10 g/dL.
      5. Treatment goals.
      6. Important to evaluate iron stores before use
         a. EPO also decreases the number of RBC transfusions required to treat anemia.
         b. The FDA eliminated the need for a risk evaluation and migration strategy before the administration of ESAs.
         c. EPO is not recommended in select patient populations.
         d. EPO shown to increase the risk of venous thromboembolism as well.
            (1) Cancer patients not receiving active treatment
            (2) Cancer patients receiving chemotherapy with a curative intent
         e. To prevent RBC transfusions
         f. To ensure that the starting dose and maintenance dose are lowest to prevent RBC transfusion
         g. Iron is an important component of RBCs.
         h. Patients who are iron-deficient will not respond to EPO.
IV. Potential adverse effects
   A. Side effects (Table 32.11)

Assessment

I. Identify patients at risk for the following:
   A. Neutropenia—ANC less than 500/mm³
      1. Patients older than 65 years old
      2. Female gender
      3. Poor nutritional status
      4. Comorbidities (COPD, diabetes, and cardiovascular disease)
      5. Prior chemotherapy and/or radiation
      6. Tumor involvement in the bone marrow
      7. Presence of open sores or unhealed wounds
   B. Anemia—hemoglobin level less than 10 g/dL
   C. Thrombocytopenia—platelet count less than 75,000 cells/mm³
II. Physical examination
   A. Neutropenia—assess for signs of infection or inflammation of the lungs, skin, oral cavity, venous access devices, and GI tract
   B. Anemia—assess for signs of irritability, fatigue, pallor, headaches, and hypotension
   C. Thrombocytopenia—assess for signs of easy bruising, nosebleeds, bleeding gums, blood in the urine or stool, petechiae, headaches, and changes in mental status
III. Medication reconciliation
   A. Date of last chemotherapy cycle
   B. Cell nadir occurs 7–14 days after chemotherapy treatment
IV. Evaluation of diagnostic and laboratory data
   A. Complete blood count with differential

Management

I. Nonpharmacologic management
   A. Manage neutropenia or infection, thrombocytopenia or bleeding, and anemia or fatigue.
   B. Patient and family education
      1. Rationale for medication indication and schedule
      2. High-risk patients need to return to clinic 24–72 hours after the completion of chemotherapy for G-CSF administration.
      3. Subcutaneous injection route and potential for multiple injections (e.g., stem cell mobilization)
   C. Adverse effects and strategies to manage them
      1. Common side effects include bone pain, mild fever, pain at injection site, and changes in blood pressure
      2. Patients should take NSAIDs or nonopioid analgesics to control pain.
   D. Adverse effects to report to health care team
      1. Changes in respiratory status (e.g., dyspnea)
      2. Swelling or redness in lower extremities, which may indicate a blood clot

   3. Pain not relieved by NSAIDs or nonopioid analgesics
   E. Monitor for adverse effects of MGFs (see Table 32.11).
   F. Decrease the incidence and manage the adverse effects of MGFs (see Table 32.11).
      1. Assess baseline data (e.g., vital signs, neurologic status).
      2. Review patient's medical history for existing or previous conditions.
      3. Review patient's medications for potential drug interactions.
      4. Conduct patient and family teaching (e.g., on side effects and self-management; medication administration).
   G. Monitor for response to MGFs.
      1. Monitor laboratory results (e.g., complete blood count).
      2. Assess activity level, presence of infection, and/or bleeding.
      3. Assess for adverse effects, toxicity, and drug interactions.

TABLE 32.11 Hematopoetic Growth Factors

Drug	Indications	Toxicities	Management
White Blood Cell Growth Factors			
Filgrastim (Neupogen)	Use to decrease the risk of infection, as manifested by febrile neutropenia, in patients with nonmyeloid malignancies receiving myelosuppressive chemotherapy. Myeloid recovery after induction or consolidation chemotherapy in AML. Myeloid recovery in patients with nonmyeloid malignancies undergoing myeloablative chemotherapy followed by marrow transplantation. Mobilization of hematopoietic progenitor cells into the peripheral blood for collection by leukapheresis. Patients with severe chronic neutropenia.	Bone pain	Monitor the level of pain; administer acetaminophen for bone pain. Monitor CBC for increase in neutrophils. *Precautions:* Contraindicated in patients with known hypersensitivity to *Escherichia coli*–derived products; do not shake vial vigorously if giving subcutaneous injection.
Filgrastim-sndz (Zarxio) (biosimilar)	Use to decrease the risk of infection, as manifested by febrile neutropenia, in patients with nonmyeloid malignancies receiving myelosuppressive chemotherapy. Myeloid recovery after induction or consolidation chemotherapy in AML. Myeloid recovery in patients with nonmyeloid malignancies undergoing myeloablative chemotherapy followed by marrow transplantation. Mobilization of hematopoietic progenitor cells into the peripheral blood for collection by leukapheresis. Patients with severe chronic neutropenia.	See filgrastim.	See filgrastim.

Continued

TABLE 32.11 Hematopoetic Growth Factors—cont'd

Drug	Indications	Toxicities	Management
Pegfilgrastim (Neulasta)		Bone pain	Monitor the level of pain; administer acetaminophen for bone pain. See "Filgrastim."
		Adult respiratory distress syndrome (rare)	Assess respiratory status (breath sounds, rate, pattern and depth of respirations, oxygen saturation); notify physician of worsening symptoms.
		Splenic rupture	Abdominal assessment and pain; notify physician. Monitor CBC laboratory test results for return of neutrophils. *Precautions:* Contraindicated in patients with known hypersensitivity to *E. coli*–derived proteins; do not administer sooner than 24 h after chemotherapy, and in the case of pegfilgrastim must be no sooner than 14 days before chemotherapy.
Sargramostim (Leukine) GM-CSF	AML after induction chemotherapy. Autologous peripheral blood progenitor cell mobilization and collection. Autologous peripheral blood progenitor cell and bone marrow transplantation. Allogeneic bone marrow transplantation. Allogeneic or autologous bone marrow transplantation: treatment of delayed neutrophil recovery or graft failure. Acute exposure to myelosuppressive doses of radiation.	Low dose: bone pain, local skin reaction, fever, flulike syndrome, headache, arthralgias, and myalgias. High dose: capillary leak syndrome, pericardial effusions, and third spacing of fluids. Phlebitis with peripheral IV administration.	Monitor the level of pain. Management of flulike symptoms with antipyretics if appropriate based on ANC, fluids, rest, comfort measures for symptoms. High dose: closely monitor VS, fluid, edema, I&O, electrolytes, and CBC. Monitor the injection site for pain, redness, or induration.
Tbo-filgrastim (Granix) Not a biosimilar in the United States	Reduce the duration of severe neutropenia in patients with nonmyeloid malignancies receiving myelosuppressive anticancer drugs.	See "Filgrastim."	See "Filgrastim."

Red Blood Cell Growth Factors

Drug	Indications	Toxicities	Management
Erythropoietin (Epogen, Procrit)	Anemia due to chronic kidney disease. Anemia due to zidovudine in patients with HIV infection. Anemia due to chemotherapy in patients with cancer (nonmyeloid malignancies). Reduction of allogeneic red blood cell transfusions in patients undergoing elective, noncardiac, nonvascular surgery. LIMITATIONS: Not indicated in cancer patients who are not receiving myelosuppressive chemotherapy. Not indicated in cancer patient when the anticipated outcome is cure. Not indicated in patients with cancer receiving myelosuppressive chemotherapy in whom the anemia can be managed by transfusion. Not indicated in patients scheduled for surgery who are willing to donate autologous blood. Not indicated in patients undergoing cardiac or vascular surgery. Not indicated as a substitute for RBC transfusions in patients who require immediate correction of anemia.	Hypertension Thrombotic events Seizures Headaches Skin rashes, urticaria; transient rash at injection site.	Monitor blood pressure. Assess for possible emboli in lower extremities or lungs. Assess for seizure activity; implement seizure precautions as needed. Assess the level of headache; administer pain medication as needed. Assess skin before the start of treatment and during treatment; rotate injection sites. Monitor CBC laboratory test results for increase in red blood cell count.

TABLE 32.11 Hematopoetic Growth Factors—cont'd

Drug	Indications	Toxicities	Management
Darbepoetin, (Aranesp)	Anemia due to chronic kidney disease. Anemia due to chemotherapy in patients with cancer. LIMITATIONS: Not indicated in cancer patients who are not receiving myelosuppressive chemotherapy. Not indicated in cancer patient when the anticipated outcome is cure. Not indicated in patients with cancer receiving myelosuppressive chemotherapy in whom the anemia can be managed by transfusion. Not indicated as a substitute for RBC transfusions in patients who require immediate correction of anemia.	Hypertension	Contraindicated in patients with uncontrolled hypertension; closely monitor the blood pressure of all patients; rotate injection sites; monitor blood counts.
		Fatigue	Assess the level of fatigue; provide for periods of rest between activities; educate about energy-conserving strategies.
		Edema	Assess skin for edema; elevate lower extremities; protect skin from damage; intake and output; assess breath sounds.
		Vascular access thrombosis and thrombotic events.	Assess for possible emboli in lower extremities or lungs and in vascular access devices; report positive evidence to physician.
		Fever, pneumonia, dyspnea, sepsis.	Monitor VS; monitor respiratory status (e.g., breath sounds; rate, depth, ease, and pattern of respirations; dyspnea, shortness of breath; oxygen saturation); administer antipyretics and antimicrobials as needed.
		Seizures	Assess for seizure activity; implement seizure precautions as needed.
		Nausea, vomiting, diarrhea, and dehydration.	GI assessment and effect of nausea, vomiting, and diarrhea on comfort, fluid balance, perineal skin; intake and output; administer antiemetic and antidiarrheal drugs as needed; encourage fluids if tolerated; monitor signs of dehydration (dry skin and mucous membranes, concentrated urine, thirst, fever). Monitor CBC laboratory test results for increase in red blood cell count.

CBC, Complete blood cell count; *GI*, gastrointestinal; *GM-CSF*, granulocyte-macrophage colony-stimulating factor; *HIV*, human immunodeficiency virus, *IV*, intravenous; *VS*, vital signs.
Data from Lexi-Comp Online. *Lexi-drugs online, and package inserts for agents.*

REFERENCES

Alves, C., Mendes, D., & Batel Marques, F. (2019). Fluoroquinolones and the risk of tendon injury: A systematic review and meta-analysis. *European Journal of Clinical Pharmacology, 75*(10), 1431–1443. https://doi.org/10.1007/s00228-019-02713-1.

Balachandran, D. D., Miller, M. A., Faiz, S. A., Yennurajalingam, S., & Innominato, P. F. (2021). Evaluation and management of sleep and circadian rhythm disturbance in cancer. *Current Treatment Options in Oncology, 22*(9), 81. https://doi.org/10.1007/s11864-021-00872-x.

Brant, J. M., & Stringer, L. H. (2018). Cancer pain. In C. H. Yarbro, D. Wujcik, & B. H. Gobel (Eds.), *Cancer nursing: Principles and practice* (pp. 781–816). Burlington, MA: Jones & Bartlett.

Camp-Sorrell, D. (2018). Chemotherapy toxicities and management. In C. H. Yarbro, D. Wujcik, & B. H. Gobel (Eds.), *Cancer nursing: Principles & practice* (pp. 497–554). Burlington, MA: Jones & Bartlett.

Desai, A., Gainor, J. F., Hegde, A., Schram, A. M., Curigliano, G., Pal, S., et al. (2021). COVID-19 vaccine guidance for patients with cancer participating in oncology clinical trials. *Nature Reviews Clinical Oncology, 18*(5), 313–319. https://doi.org/10.1038/s41571-021-00487-z.

Gonzalez Castro, L. N., & Milligan, T. A. (2020). Seizures in patients with cancer. *Cancer, 126*(7), 1379–1389. https://doi.org/10.1002/cncr.32708.

Gupta, K., Walton, R., & Kataria, S. P. (2021). Chemotherapy-induced nausea and vomiting: Pathogenesis, recommendations, and new trends. *Cancer Treatment and Research Communications, 26,* 100278. https://doi.org/10.1016/j.ctarc.2020.100278.

Herschbach, P., Britzelmeir, I., Dinkel, A., Giesler, J. M., Herkommer, K., Nest, A., et al. (2020). Distress in cancer patients: Who are the main groups at risk? *Psycho-Oncology, 29*(4), 703–710. https://doi.org/10.1002/pon.5321.

Hesketh, P. J., Kris, M. G., Basche, E., Bohlke, K., Barbour, S. Y., Clark-Snow, R., et al. (2020). Antiemetics: ASCO guideline update. *Journal of Clinical Oncology, 38*(24), 2782–2797. https://doi.org/10.1200/JCO.20.01296.

Hibberd, P. L. (2022). *Immunizations in adults with cancer.* Waltham, MA: UpToDate. Topic 3899, version 26.0. Retrieved from https://www.uptodate.com/contents/immunizations-in-adults-with-cancer.

Johnson, L. A., Schreier, A. M., Swanson, M., & Ridner, S. H. (2020). Dimensions of distress in lung cancer. *Oncology Nursing Forum, 47*(6), 732–738. https://doi.org/10.1188/20.ONF.732-738.

Kirby, E., Broom, A., Overton, K., Kenney, K., Post, J. J., & Broom, J. (2020). Reconsidering the nursing role in antimicrobial stewardship: A multisite qualitative interview study. *British Medical Journal Open, 10*, e042321. https://doi.org/10.1136/bmjopen-2020-042321.

Kuderer, N. M., Hill, J. A., Carpenter, P. A., & Lyman, G. H. (2021). Challenges and opportunities for COVID-19 vaccines in patients with cancer. *Cancer Investigation, 39*(3), 205–213. https://doi.org/10.1080/07357907.2021.1885596.

Mager, D. E., Lin, S. X., Blum, R. A., Lates, C. D., & Jusko, W. J. (2003). Dose equivalency evaluation of major corticosteroids: Pharmacokinetics and cell trafficking and cortisol dynamics. *Journal of Clinical Pharmacology, 43*(11), 1216–1227. https://doi.org/10.1177/0091270003258651.

Matthews, E. E. (2018). Sleep disorders. In C. H. Yarbro, D. Wujcik, & B. H. Gobel (Eds.), *Cancer nursing: Principles & practice* (pp. 1051–1072). Burlington, MA: Jones & Bartlett Learning.

National Comprehensive Cancer Network (NCCN). (2022a). Prevention and treatment of cancer-related infections. (v. 1.2022). https://www.nccn.org/professionals/physician_gls/pdf/infections.pdf.

National Comprehensive Cancer Network (NCCN). (2022b). Adult cancer pain (v. 1.2022). https://www.nccn.org/professionals/physician_gls/pdf/pain.pdf.

National Comprehensive Cancer Network (NCCN). (2022c). Antiemesis. (v. 2.2022). https://www.nccn.org/professionals/physician_gls/pdf/antiemesis.pdf.

National Comprehensive Cancer Network (NCCN). (2022d). Survivorship. (v. 1.2022). https://www.nccn.org/professionals/physician_gls/pdf/survivorship.pdf.

National Comprehensive Cancer Network (NCCN). (2022e). Hematopoietic growth factors. (v. 1.2022). https://www.nccn.org/professionals/physician_gls/pdf/growthfactors.pdf.

Navari, R. M. (2020). Nausea and vomiting in advanced cancer. *Current Treatment Options in Oncology, 21*(2), 14. https://doi.org/10.1007/s11864-020-0704-8.

Nguyen, V. V., Dergalust, S., & Chang, E. (2020). Epilepsy. In J. T. DiPiro, G. C. Yee, L. M. Posey, S. T. Haines, T. D. Nolin, & V. Ellingrod (Eds.), *Pharmacotherapy: A pathophysiologic approach* (11th ed.). New York: McGraw-Hill.

Olans, R. D., Olans, R. N., & Witt, D. J. (2017). Good nursing is good antibiotic stewardship. *American Journal of Nursing, 117*(8), 58–63. https://doi.org/10.1097/01.NAJ.0000521974.76835.e0.

Olsen, M., LeFebvre, K. B., & Brassil, K. (2019). *Chemotherapy and immunotherapy guidelines and recommendations for practice.* Pittsburgh, PA: Oncology Nursing Society.

Pathan, H., & Williams, J. (2012). Basic opioid pharmacology: An update. *British Journal of Pain, 6*(1), 11–16. https://doi.org/10.1177/2049463712438493.

Pitman, A., Suleman, S., Hyde, N., & Hodgkiss, A. (2018). Depression and anxiety in patients with cancer. *British Medical Journal, 361*, k1415 https://doi.org/10.1136/bmj.k1415.

Santomasso, B. D., Park, J. H., Salloum, D., Riviere, I., Flynn, J., Mead, E., et al. (2018). Clinical and biological correlates of neurotoxicity associated with CAR T-cell therapy in patients with B-cell acute lymphoblastic leukemia. *Cancer Discovery, 8*(8), 958–971. https://doi.org/10.1158/2159-8290.CD-17-1319.

Taplitz, R. A., Kennedy, E. B., Bow, E. J., Crews, J., Gleason, C., Hawley, D. K., et al. (2018). Antimicrobial prophylaxis for adult patients with cancer-related immunosuppression: ASCO and IDSA clinical practice guideline update. *Journal of Clinical Oncology, 36*(30), 3043–3054. https://doi.org/10.1200/JCO.18.00374.

Walsh, D., Davis, M., Ripamonti, C., Bruera, E., Davies, A., & Molassiotis, A. (2017). 2016 Updated MASCC/ESMO consensus recommendations: Management of nausea and vomiting in advanced cancer. *Supportive Care in Cancer, 25*(1), 333–340. https://doi.org/10.1007/s00520-016-3371-3.

Zhang, Q., Wan, R., & Liu, C. (2020). The impact of intense nursing care in improving anxiety, depression, and quality of life in patients with liver cancer: A systematic review and meta-analysis. *Medicine, 99*(34), e21677. https://doi.org/10.1097/MD.0000000000021677.

33

Complementary and Integrative Modalities

Tahani Al Dweikat

OVERVIEW

I. Definitions: therapies that may be used to enhance the efficacy of conventional (allopathic, biologic, scientific, orthodox, and Western) medicine therapy, alleviate side effects of conventional treatment, and improve the patient's sense of well-being and quality of life or both (National Center for Complementary and Integrative Health [NCCIH], 2021)

A. Complementary: therapies that fall outside of conventional medicine, such as acupuncture, herbal/botanical medicine, mind–body therapies, nutraceuticals, and energy medicine.

B. Alternative: nonconventional therapies used in place of what is offered conventionally. Patients may choose these therapies if there is nothing offered conventionally, if they have exhausted the conventional treatment options, and/or if what is offered conventionally is not within their belief system or culture.

C. Integrative medicine, integrative health care, and integrative oncology: refer to combining evidence-based complementary therapies with conventional treatment regimens.

D. Complementary and alternative medicine (CAM): describes the entire domain of therapies that fall outside of conventional medicine.

E. Other complementary and integrative modality definitions are listed in Box 33.1.

II. Current trends in the United States

A. CAM use is prevalent among cancer patients—an estimated 62.5% had used CAM with regard to their cancer (Hammersen, Pursche, Fischer, Katalinic, & Waldmann, 2020).

B. CAM use was significantly higher in women with higher educational levels, higher employment status, and statutory health insurance, respectively (Hammersen et al., 2020).

C. A growing number of conventional medicine providers are offering complementary therapies, which has resulted in the increasing utilization of integrative oncology approaches.

1. In palliative care and hospice settings, mind and body practices, including massage therapy, aromatherapy, music therapy, and acupuncture, are common therapies used to treat pain and anxiety (Zeng, Wang, Ward, & Hume, 2018).

2. Many academic and private cancer treatment centers offer a range of complementary services with the establishment of the Society for Integrative Oncology to advance evidence-based, comprehensive, integrative health care to improve the lives of people dealing with cancer (http://www.integrativeonc.org).

III. National Cancer Institute (NCI)—designated cancer centers

A. Located in 36 states, 71 NCI-designated cancer centers are funded by NCI to deliver cancer treatments to patients.

1. Websites have not been evaluated regarding CAM therapies.

2. Websites offer information to patients regarding integrative medicine and CAM services with acupuncture, massage, mediation, yoga, and consultations regarding nutrition, dietary supplements, and herbs being the most commonly offered (NCI, 2019).

IV. Classification of CAM therapies

A. The National Center for Complementary and Integrative Health (NCCIH) lists two subgroups of complementary health approaches (NCCIH, 2021).

1. Natural products, including herbs, vitamins, minerals, and probiotics.

2. Mind and body practices, including yoga, chiropractic and osteopathic manipulation, meditation, massage therapy, acupuncture, relaxation techniques, tai chi, qi gong, healing touch, hypnotherapy, and movement therapies.

B. Other complementary therapies include whole medical systems health approaches and biologically based practices.

C. CAM approaches

1. The NCCIH (2021) describes the main categories of complementary approaches including nutritional, psychological, physical, and combination approaches:

a. Nutritional approach/natural product (e.g., special diets, dietary supplements, herbs, probiotics, and microbial-based therapies)

b. Psychological approach (e.g., meditation, hypnosis, music therapies, relaxation, guided imagery, aromatherapy, and reflexology therapies)

BOX 33.1 Complementary, Alternative, and Integrative Modality Definitions (NCI [Office of Cancer Complementary and Alternative Medicine], 2022)

Alternative medical systems are therapies based upon complete systems of theory and practice that have evolved apart from, and in many cases pre-date, conventional medical approaches used in the United States. Examples of such systems are Ayurveda, traditional Chinese medicine, homeopathy, the traditional medicine of indigenous cultures, naturopathy, and Tibetan medicine, to name a few.

Energy therapies are defined as therapies that use energy fields. Two such therapies are commonly used: (1) biofield therapies, which are aimed at affecting the energy fields that surround and penetrate the human body to restore health. The existence of such energy fields has not been scientifically verified. Examples of such therapies include reiki, qi gong, and therapeutic touch; (2) electromagnetic-based therapies, which use electromagnetic fields such as pulsed fields, magnetic fields, or alternating or direct current fields to affect changes in the body. Examples include magnet therapy and pulsed magnetic fields.

Exercise therapies utilize health-enhancing systems of movement and exercise and include practices such as yoga asanas and tai chi.

Manipulative and body-based methods involve the movement and/or manipulation of one or more parts of the body to influence the health of the whole body. These therapies include chiropractic, therapeutic massage, osteopathy, and reflexology.

Mind–body interventions employ a variety of techniques to enhance the mind's ability to affect the body, its overall function, and its perception of symptoms. These therapies include meditation, hypnosis, art therapy, music therapy, biofeedback, guided imagery, relaxation techniques, cognitive behavioral therapy, support groups, and aromatherapy.

Nutritional therapeutics include the use of nutrients, nonnutrients, bioactive food components used as chemopreventive agents, and specific foods or diets used as cancer prevention of treatment strategies. These therapies include the macrobiotic diet, Gerson therapy, ketogenic diet, vitamins, and minerals.

Pharmacologic and biologic treatments include the off-label use of certain drugs, hormones, complex natural products, vaccines, and other biological interventions not yet accepted in mainstream medicine. Examples include metformin, intravenous vitamin C, low-dose naltrexone, laetrile, antineoplastons, 714X, hydrazine sulfate, alpha-lipoic acid, Dichloroacetate (DCA), and melatonin.

Subcategory: Complex natural products are an assortment of plant samples (botanicals), extracts of crude natural substances, and unfractionated extracts from marine organisms used for the healing and treatment of disease. Examples include herbs and herbal extracts (mistletoe or *Viscum album*, mixtures of tea polyphenols, and mushroom extracts).

Spiritual therapies are therapies that focus on deep, often religious, beliefs and feelings, including a person's sense of peace, purpose, connection to others, and beliefs about the meaning of life. Examples include intercessory prayer and spiritual healing.

Adapted from *NCI (Office of Cancer Complementary and Alternative Medicine)*. (2022). Categories of CAM therapies. https://cam.cancer.gov/health_information/categories_of_cam_therapies.htm.

c. Physical approach (e.g., acupuncture, massage, and spinal manipulation)
d. Combination's approach such as psychological and physical (e.g., yoga, tai chi, dance therapies, and some forms of art therapy) or psychological and nutritional (e.g., mindful eating)

2. NCCIH categorized nutritional approaches as natural products, whereas psychological and/or physical approaches as mind and body practices (NCCIH, 2021).
3. Nutritional approaches include "natural products" or substances produced by plants, microbes, and other living organisms, whereas "dietary supplements" have ingredients that include vitamins, minerals, amino acids, and herbs or other substances that can be used to supplement the diet.
4. Nutritional approaches or natural products are the most widely used complementary therapy by both adults and children (NCCIH, 2021). A National Health Interview survey revealed almost 18% of American adults used a dietary supplement other than vitamins and minerals (e.g., special diets, dietary supplements, herbs, probiotics, and microbial-based therapies).

V. Natural products (Table 33.1)
   A. Herbal/botanical medicine
      1. Supplement use is estimated in over 50% of cancer patients, and one-third do not disclose this use to the health care team (Du et al., 2020).
      2. These substances are usually safe but can pose a significant risk to the patient due to interactions with conventionally prescribed medications.
      3. Many conventional chemotherapeutic agents used today have their roots in botanical medicine (e.g., taxanes: Pacific yew [*Taxus brevifolia*]), vinca alkaloids: periwinkle (*Catharanthus roseus*), camptothecin: xi shu (*Camptotheca acuminata*), and podophyllotoxin (etoposide): mayapple or wild mandrake (*Podophyllum peltatum*).
      4. Herbal/botanical medicine and dietary supplements are not Food and Drug Administration approved or well-regulated in the United States as in other countries; access to safe and effective herbal/botanical medicine is not guaranteed.

VI. Mind–body modalities (Eaton & Hulett, 2019)
   A. Include art and color therapy, eye movement desensitization and reprocessing, guided imagery, meditation, music therapy, neurolinguistics programming, tai chi, and yoga (Eaton & Hulett, 2019) (Table 33.2).

VII. Manipulative and body-based practices (Eaton & Hulett, 2019)
   A. Modalities include acupuncture, acupressure, Alexander technique, cranial osteopathy, dance therapy, Feldenkrais method, lymphatic therapy, and traditional Chinese medicine (Table 33.3).

VIII. Whole medical systems (Mühlenpfordt, Stritter, Bertram, Ben-Arye, & Seifert, 2019)
   A. Therapeutic approaches include Ayurveda, chiropractic medicine, homeopathy, and osteopathic medicine (Table 33.4).

TABLE 33.1 Natural Products

Botanical/Supplement	CyP Isoform Affected	Effects on CYP450	Specific Effects Relevant to Oncology
Allium sativum (garlic)	2E1, 2C9, 2C19, and 3A4	Inhibition	Docetaxel.
Andrographis paniculata (andrographis)	3A4, 2D6	Inhibition	
Angelica sinensis (dong quai)	1A2, 2D6, 2C9, 2E1, and 3A4	Inhibition	
Arctium lappa (burdock)	3A4, 2C19	Inhibition	
Arctostaphylos uva ursi (uva ursi)	3A4	Inhibition	
Boswellia serrata (frankincense)	1A2, 2D6, 2C8, 2C9, 2C19, and 3A4	Inhibition	
Camellia sinensis (green tea)	3A4 (considered minor)	Inhibition	Use with bortezomib (directly blocked the apoptotic effect). In vivo human trials failed to demonstrate effects on 2D6, 1A2, 2C9, and 3A4 at recommended doses.
Centella asiatica (gotu kola)	2C9, 2D6, and 3A4	Inhibition	
Cimicifuga racemosa (black cohosh)	3A4, 2D6	Inhibition	Human data failed to show inhibition or induction of 3A4. It was a potent modulator of 2D6 in in vivo (human) studies; however, failed to demonstrate effect when coadministered with tamoxifen.
Cinnamomum burmannii (cinnamon)	2D6	Inhibition	
Cucruma longa (turmeric)	2C9, 2C19, 2D6, and 3A4	Inhibition	
Echinacea purpurea (echinacea)	2C19, 2D6, and 3A4	Inhibition	Docetaxel.
Ginkgo biloba (ginkgo)	2C9, 2C19, 2E1, and 3A4	Inhibition	
Glycyrrhiza glabra (licorice)	3A4, 2D6	Inhibition	
Hypericum perforatum (St. John's wort)	3A4, 2E1, and 2C19 1A2, 2C9	Inhibition	Irinotecan. Imatinib. Docetaxel.
Hydrastis canadensis (goldenseal)	2C9, 2D6, and 3A4	Inhibition	
Matricaria recutita (chamomile)	1A2, 2C9, 2C19, 2D6, 3A4, 4A9/11, and 2E1	Inhibition	
Mentha piperita (peppermint)	3A4	Inhibition	
Panax quinquefolius (American ginseng)	2C9, 2C19, 2D6, and 3A4	Inhibition	Human trials at recommended doses did not demonstrate induction of 3A4 by Panax ginseng.
Piper methysticum (kava kava)	3A4, 2E1, and 1A2	Inhibition	Human data confirm that kava is a potent inhibitor of 2E1 but does not seem to inhibit 3A4 or 2D6 at recommended doses.
Rhodiola rosea (rhodiola)	2D6, 3A4	Inhibition	
Schisandra chinensis/sphenantherea (schizandra)	3A4	Inhibition	Impact on drugs transported by P-glycoprotein.
Silybum marianum (milk thistle)	3A4, 2C8, 2C9, 2C19, 2D6, and 2E1	Inhibition	Human data did not support the effects in vitro at daily recommended doses and in fact failed to show clinically relevant effects on 3A4, 1A2, 2D6, and 2E1.
Uncaria tomentosa (cat's claw)	3A4	Inhibition	
Tanacetum parthenium (feverfew)	2C9, 2C19, 2D6, and 3A4	Inhibition	
Valeriana officinalis (valerian root)	3A4	Inhibition	
Zingiber aromaticum (ginger)	2C9, 2C19, 2D6, and 3A4	Inhibition	

Data from *National Center for Complementary and Integrative Health (NCCIH). (2021). Complementary, alternative, or integrative health: What's in a name?.* https://nccih.nih.gov/health/integrative-health#types.

IX. Biologically based practices (Knecht, Kinder, & Stockert, 2020)
   A. Therapies that use substances found in nature to treat illness and promote wellness, including biofeedback; herbal therapy; hydrotherapy; nutritional counseling; and energy work, energy therapy, and biofield therapy (Table 33.5).

ASSESSMENT

I. Use of CAM—may negatively interfere or interact with conventional cancer treatment; nursing assessment to include questions directed at determining patient use of CAM and discussion regarding the risks and benefits, as needed (Balneaves, 2018; Knecht et al., 2020)
II. Relevant patient demographics and clinical information

TABLE 33.2 Mind–Body Modalities

Art therapy—different art mediums (drawing, coloring, painting, sculpting, and multimedia) to assist the patient in restoring, maintaining, or improving physical, mental, emotional, and spiritual well-being.	• Based on the concept that the creative process helps people resolve inner conflict and process issues, reduce stress, increase self-esteem and self-awareness, and achieve insight. • Requires a master's degree in art therapy; may require licensure, credentials, or both, depending on the state.
Color therapy (chromotherapy)—uses electronic instrumentation and color receptivity to integrate nervous system and body–mind.	• Based on premise that color conveys energy at different frequencies and the human body responds to these vibrational frequencies. • May be used to increase well-being and is used to treat acute and chronic ailments.
EMDR—a psychotherapy technique based on the concept that distressing events are associated with specific rapid eye movements.	• The therapist helps the patient recall distressing events, eliciting the associated rapid eye movements, and then redirects the eye movements through stimulation or distraction, thereby breaking the connection that is causing distressing thoughts and feelings to persist.
Guided imagery—a structured process that uses live or recorded scripts describing different scenarios or detailed images to guide the patient through a process.	• May lead the patient through progressive muscle relaxation or visualization of a treatment process (e.g., visualization of chemotherapy entering the body and seeking out cancer cells to remove them from the body). • Techniques—use of a coach who narrates the imagery, an audio recording, or a video recording. • Studies have shown that a relaxed state of mind may decrease perceived stress, relieve muscle tension, enhance the sense of well-being, boost immune response.
Meditation—a method of quieting the mind to facilitate inner peace; numerous forms of meditation, ranging from simple focused breathing to transcendental meditation; practices share characteristics and often involve focused breathing and a relaxed yet alert state that promotes control over thoughts and feelings.	• MBSR is a technique whereby patients are trained to develop awareness of experiences moment by moment and in the context of all senses. • Yoga nidra meditation teaches patients to explore sensations, emotions, and thoughts, and then to dissociate from them. • Transcendental meditation uses a *mantra* (a word, sound, and phrase) to direct focus, prevent distraction. • Some states require therapists to have a master's degree, certification, or both.
Music therapy—an applied psychotherapy that uses making or listening to music to explore behavioral, emotional, or spiritual disruption and to assist the patient in resolving these issues.	• Music interventions may have beneficial effects on anxiety, pain, fatigue, and quality of life in people with cancer.
NLP—a systematic approach to changing thought patterns, thereby changing perceptions.	• One example is the use of a "gratitude journal." The patient is instructed to record daily entries in a journal, specifically recalling positive aspects of his or her life to promote a positive outlook over time. The concept is that one gets more of whatever one focuses on.
Tai chi—an ancient Chinese practice of movements coordinated with breathing techniques. Qi gong and tai chi have been found to have positive effects on cancer-specific quality of life, fatigue, immune function, and cortisol levels in patients with cancer.	• Derived from martial art form. • Enhances coordination and balance, and promotes physical, emotional, and spiritual well-being. • Contraindications: none have been reported, but clearance from a provider to engage in exercise/physical activity is recommended.
Yoga—strength and flexibility achieved using specific postures and controlled breathing; found to improve psychological outcomes (e.g., depression, anxiety, and distress), quality-of-life measures, sleep issues, fatigue, gastrointestinal symptoms, and overall health-related quality-of-life measures in patients with cancer.	• Has evolved into mainstream practice with multiple variations, ranging from restorative (gentle) yoga to promote well-being in frail patients to power yoga, which uses a vigorous, fitness-based approach. • Has a meditative component that brings harmony to body, mind, and spirit. • Contraindications: patients with glaucoma, hypertension, those with sciatica, those with movement restrictions, and those currently pregnant need to be cautious while practicing yoga and should modify or avoid certain poses. The risk for injury due to strain/sprain is possible if one is not cautious.

EMDR, Eye movement desensitization and reprocessing; *MBSR*, mindfulness-based stress reduction; *NLP*, neurolinguistic programming.
Data from Eaton, L. H., & Hulett, J. M. (2019). Mind–body interventions in the management of chronic cancer pain. *Seminars in Oncology Nursing*, *35*(3), 241–252. https://doi.org/10.1016/j.soncn.2019.04.005.

A. Demographics—age, gender, education, residence, economic status, and ethnic and cultural identity
B. Clinical information—should include comorbidities, allergies, medications (including CAM), and cancer disease information: type, stage, and cancer treatments
III. Initial and ongoing patient assessment of CAM—should include a comprehensive assessment
 A. Disturbances or imbalances in the following areas:
  1. Physical well-being
  2. Nutritional status, functional performance status
  3. Psychosocial status, emotional and mental well-being
  4. Sexual functioning
  5. Age-related developmental issues
  6. Spiritual well-being
  7. Energy field disturbances
 B. Identification of risk in the areas of the following:
  1. Environmental factors

TABLE 33.3 Manipulative and Body-Based Practices

Acupuncture—an ancient Oriental technique associated with TCM, used to restore or promote health and well-being using fine-gauge needles inserted into specific points on the body to stimulate or disperse the flow of energy.

Acupuncture shown to have therapeutic benefit for the management of cancer-related fatigue, chemotherapy-induced nausea and vomiting, and leukopenia in cancer patients.

- Used in conjunction with methods such as massage, herbal remedies, and nutritional counseling.
- May be a safe and effective treatment for chronic lymphedema related to breast cancer treatment.
- Used for pain and chemotherapy-related nausea and vomiting with mostly favorable results.
- Avoid at the site of tumor or metastasis, at the site of tumor nodules or skin ulcerations, on broken skin, or a site of active infection or radiation burn.
- Avoid acupuncture over any open surgical wound, in limbs with lymphedema, over areas of instability of the spine (e.g., multiple myeloma), or in any areas with considerable anatomic distortion from surgery.
- Contraindicated in patients who are neutropenic or severely thrombocytopenic.

Acupressure—the use of finger or hand pressure over specific points on the body to relieve symptoms or to influence specific organ function.

- May be used to release tension, reestablish the natural flow of energy, or both.
- Contraindicated in patients with bleeding disorders or thrombocytopenia and in those taking anticoagulant medications such as warfarin (Coumadin).
- Should not be done over body areas with tumor, lymphadenopathy, or both.

Alexander technique.

- Uses movement and touch to restore balance in the body and neuromuscular function, thus allowing the body to regain a relaxed, healthy posture.

Aromatherapy—uses essential oils extracted from herbs and other plants.

- Treats physical imbalances and restores psychological and spiritual well-being.
- Essential oils are inhaled, applied topically, or ingested.
- Currently no standardization of practice; a wide range of quality in essential oils, as processing is not regulated.
- Topical application of essential oils to be avoided unless they are prepared by a trained specialist.

Cranial osteopathy—uses gentle manipulation of the skull to reestablish natural configuration and movement.

- Disorders manifested throughout the body can be improved by realigning the skull.

Dance therapy—dance and music combined to facilitate the uplifting of the mind, body, and spirit through natural body movement.

Feldenkrais method—a somatic education system that teaches movement and gentle manipulation to increase body awareness and improve body function.

- Used to improve posture and promote flexibility and freedom of movement.

Lymphatic therapy—the use of vigorous massage to stimulate flow of lymphatic fluid.

- Intended to move lymph fluid and release toxins stored in the lymphatic system; refreshes the immune system.
- Manual, gentle lymphatic drainage used to prevent and treat lymphedema after breast cancer surgery.

Massage—the use of manual pressure and strokes on muscle tissue.

Conflicting results exist for the effectiveness of massage therapy in patients with cancer.

- Used to reduce emotional and physical tension, increase circulation, and relieve muscular pain.
- Can provide comfort and increased body awareness.
- Contraindicated in or near areas of infection, tumors, incisions or indwelling devices, or in presence of contagious disease, contagious rashes, or open sores; patients who are thrombocytopenic (platelet count less than 50,000).
- Patients with peripheral neuropathy (grade 3 or greater) should not receive massage over the affected areas.
- Patients with suspected/known bone metastasis should not receive pressure or jostling over the areas of concern.
- Patients who have received radiation therapy to lymph nodes in the armpit, groin, neck, or jaw, or those who have had removal of these nodes; excessive pressure on the limb or area being drained by those lymph nodes is to be avoided except for those trained in lymphatic drainage.
- Neutropenic precautions (including gloves and a mask) should be used with any patients who are neutropenic. Patients with severe neutropenia (WBC<1500) should not receive massage.
- Massage therapists should wear gloves when massaging patients receiving high-dose methotrexate, cytarabine (Ara-C) and cyclophosphamide, as agents are eliminated through skin.
- Massage should not be performed on patients receiving anthracyclines (or other agents) to avoid increasing peripheral circulation and worsening the risk of hand/foot syndrome.
- Avoid massage in affected limb with the presence of a known DVT and on medications that potentially increase risks of clotting or are at increased risk of clotting due to their disease process.

Continued

TABLE 33.3   Manipulative and Body-Based Practices—cont'd

Neuromuscular therapy—massage therapy that uses moderate pressure on muscles, nerves, and trigger points to decrease pain and tension.

Physical therapy—used to correct mechanical body ailments and restore normal musculoskeletal functioning.

- Procedures designed to relieve pain, reduce swelling, strengthen muscles, and restore range of motion.
- Includes a combination of massage, electrostimulation, ultrasonography, and prescribed exercises.

Qi gong—Chinese meditative practice that combines physical postures with focused intention and breathing techniques to release, cleanse, strengthen, and circulate energy.

- Used for stress reduction and to enhance the body's natural healing abilities.
- May increase vitality and awareness of internal energy that furthers the mind–body connection.
- Can be performed in a standing or sitting position.

Shiatsu—a Japanese form of body work like acupressure.

- Uses finger and palm pressure to manipulate energetic pathways to improve the flow of energy.
- Pressure applied to specific points in a continuous rhythmic sequence.
- Used to calm an overactive sympathetic nervous system, improve circulation, relieve muscle tension, and alleviate stress.
- Patient is fully clothed during treatment, unlike other massage techniques, and no oil is applied to the body.
- May not be safe in cancer patients, who are at increased risk of blood clots, because the type of manipulations may dislodge a blood clot.

Trigger point therapy—a method of compression of specific points in muscle tissue to relieve pain and tension.

- May be used with therapeutic massage and passive stretching.
- Treatment goals aimed at decreasing swelling and stiffness and increasing range of motion.
- Like physical therapy, exercises assigned to be performed at home between treatment sessions.

DVT, Deep vein thrombosis; *TCM*, traditional Chinese medicine; *WBC*, white blood cell.
Data from Eaton, L. H., & Hulett, J. M. (2019). Mind-body interventions in the management of chronic cancer pain. *Seminars in Oncology Nursing*, *35*(3), 241–252. https://doi.org/10.1016/j.soncn.2019.04.005.

TABLE 33.4   Whole Medical Systems

Ayurveda—taken from the Sanskrit, *ayus*, which means "life or lifespan," and *veda*, which means "knowledge."

- Ayurveda—based on the principle that maintaining balance in the body, mind, and consciousness is used to preserve health and treat illness.
- Specific interventions—driven by the individual's *prakriti* (nature), which is determined by the three *gunas* (ways of being: *tamas, rajas, sattva*); human physiology believed to be the result of the combination of the three *doshas* (*pitta, kapha,* and *vatta*) in each individual; energy (or *prana*) flows through the body through channels or *nadis*; disruption in the flow of energy results in disease.
- Interventions—aimed at rebalancing the *doshas* and restoring the flow of energy; may include proper diet, hydration, and lifestyle (e.g., following a set sleep–wake routine, detoxification or cleansing techniques, specific massage techniques [*marma* therapy], specific movements, or spoken words [*mantras*]).

Chiropractic medicine—emphasizes structural alignment of the spine.

- Adjustments made through manipulation of the spine and joints to reestablish normal CNS functioning.
- Interventions include massage, nutrition, and specialized kinesiology.
- Chiropractic medicine contraindicated in patients with bone metastasis, spinal cord compression, thrombocytopenia, or venous thrombosis.

Homeopathy—based on the precept of healing through the administration of specific substances.

- Substances are chosen according to the following beliefs:
  - Like cures like.
  - The more a remedy is diluted, the greater is the potency.
  - Illness is specific to the individual.
  - This form of medicine is based on the belief that symptoms are an indication that the body is attempting to rid itself of disease.
- Treatment based on the whole person as opposed to focusing on symptoms.
- No known interactions with drugs, herbs, foods, laboratory tests, diseases, or conditions.

TABLE 33.4 Whole Medical Systems—cont'd

Osteopathic medicine—focuses on the relationship between the structure and the function of the body; osteopaths are fully licensed to diagnose, treat, and prescribe in conventional medicine.
 	
TCM—originated in China and evolved over thousands of years.
	• Recognizes that structure and function are subject to a range of disorders.
	• Uses physical manipulation to facilitate self-healing in the individual, as well as conventional medical therapies.
	• Includes key concepts:
	  • Yin-yang—concept of two opposing complementary forces that are brought into balance to maintain a healthy body and mind.
	  • Meridians—pathways or channels that run throughout the body through which *qi* (energy, pronounced "chee") or energy flows; disruption in flow of qi results in disease; acupuncture and other techniques used to direct, redirect, or unblock the flow of qi.
	  • Five elements—fire, earth, metal, water, and wood, which correspond to various organs and tissues in the body.
	  • Eight principles—used in TCM to analyze symptoms; principles include cold–heat, interior–exterior, excess-deficiency, and yin-yang.
	  • Interventions—include the use of herbs, acupuncture, and other methods [e.g., moxibustion, cupping, mind–body therapy] to enhance health and treat illness.

CNS, Central nervous system; *TCM*, traditional Chinese medicine.
Data from Mühlenpfordt, I., Stritter, W., Bertram, M., Ben-Arye, E., & Seifert, G. (2019). The power of touch: External applications from whole medical systems in the care of cancer patients (literature review). *Supportive Care in Cancer, 28*(2), 461–471. https://doi.org/10.1007/s00520-019-05172-7.

TABLE 33.5 Biologically Based Practices

Biofeedback—a technique for teaching the patient to recognize, observe, and learn to control biological responses to stress	• Monitors are used to give feedback to the patient about vital signs (blood pressure, heart rate, and respiratory rate), and the patient is taught to relax through visualization and focused breathing, among other methods. • By conscious effort, patients learn to bring about change in vital functions.
Herbal therapy—the use of herbs and their chemical properties to treat specific conditions or to improve general health and well-being	• Herbal preparations are used in alcohol extractions, liquid extractions, salves, teas, capsules, oils, liquids, or in their raw forms and are taken internally, inhaled, or applied directly to the body. Therapeutic aims restoration of health, supporting the body's mechanisms of immunity, elimination, detoxification, and homeostasis. • The use of herbal medicines should be monitored by a knowledgeable provider, members of the health care team, or both. Caution should be used with herbs that are known to affect the CYP3A4267 pathway because of the potential for herb–drug interactions (e.g., St. John's wort).
Hydrotherapy—the application of water to the body in its various forms (ice, water, steam) and at an extreme temperature (hot or cold) to restore and maintain health	• Treatments include water baths, steam baths, saunas, and application of hot or cold compresses. • Contrast hydrotherapy (alternating application of hot and cold).
Nutritional counseling—the use of diet, nutritional supplements, or both to prevent and manage illness or to enhance and maintain health	• Registered dieticians often involved in care of patients going through cancer treatment, but many different practitioners make dietary recommendations. Important to know who is making recommendations and for what therapeutic goal. • Diet therapies may or may not be appropriate. • The recommendation of dietary supplements is like that with herbal medications. It is important to know who is making the recommendations and with what educational background. The health care team (nurses, physicians, pharmacists, etc.) needs to be aware of what someone is taking, and someone knowledgeable in how these supplements interplay with conventional therapies should be monitoring their use.
Energy work, energy therapy, biofield therapy—a broad category of work aimed at influencing the major energy centers (*chakras*) of the body and the flow of a patient's internal and external energy; energy work can be used to treat physical symptoms and emotional or spiritual distress or enhance well-being	• Reiki—an energy healing modality whereby the practitioner uses his or her hands to direct the flow of energy to various parts of the body to facilitate healing and relaxation; hands are placed on the body in specific patterns without deep pressure to redirect or restore energy flow. • Therapeutic touch—a technique for balancing the flow of energy in the body through the transfer of human energy, based on the concept that disruption in energy flow leads to disease and restoring that flow can lead to health, growth, order, and wholeness. • Healing touch—an energy healing technique that uses the nursing process. • Magnetic therapy—use of magnets to influence magnetic fields to positively affect the nervous system, organs, and tissues to stimulate healing.

Data from Knecht, K., Kinder, D., & Stockert, A. (2020). Biologically-based complementary and alternative medicine (CAM) use in cancer patients: The good, the bad, the misunderstood. *Frontiers in Nutrition, 6*, 196. https://doi.org/10.3389/fnut.2019.00196.

2. Cultural practices
3. Family dynamics
4. Socioeconomic status
5. Health behaviors
C. Patient values and preferences
1. Meaning of health and well-being
2. Religious and spiritual practices
3. Cultural practices
4. Lifestyle patterns

MANAGEMENT

I. Nonpharmacologic (Balneaves, 2018; Drozdoff et al., 2019; Latte-Naor & Mao, 2019; Lawrence, 2021; Wolf et al., 2022)
A. Interventions to increase patient knowledge about CAM and its effects on conventional therapy.
1. Encourage open communication about conventional therapy options and CAM.
2. Support informal dialog initiated by nurses, patients, and their caregivers.
a. Success depends on building rapport, ensuring a culturally sensitive and nonjudgmental social and professional environment.
b. Nurses must recognize quick dismissals of CAM may shut down further communication.
c. CAM therapies used by patient, who is guiding the use of the therapies, if known, should be documented.
d. Disclosure of CAM use is an ongoing process shaped by patient's health concerns and rapport with the health care team.
3. Explain conventional therapies in a way that patients can understand.
4. Review and discuss chemotherapeutic agents and potential effects of CAM therapy. Suggest avoidance of all herbs/supplements with the newer classes of drugs (PD-1 inhibitors, PDL-inhibitors, CAR-T cell, PARP inhibitors, Bruton's tyrosine kinase inhibitors, etc.) until more information is available.
5. Try to comprehend why conventional medicine may not satisfy patient (e.g., lack of psychosocial support, poor symptom control, inconvenience, and lack of understanding).
6. Explore patient rationales for using CAM or contemplating CAM use (e.g., accessibility, fear of side effects, social pressure, agency, and empowerment).
7. Emphasize and support the patient's right to choose among therapeutic options.
a. Therapeutic objectives for patient may not be the same as the health care team.
8. Ability to differentiate CAM practices that interfere with conventional medicine from those that complement it.
a. Validate the appropriate use of CAM and explain how some CAM practices may interfere with conventional medicine (e.g., cause antagonistic or other undesirable biophysical results, delay in or termination of conventional treatment) (Table 33.6).

TABLE 33.6   Potential Complementary and Alternative Medicine (CAM) Drug Interactions With Chemotherapeutic Agents

Chemotherapeutic Agent	Cytochrome Enzymes Utilized for Metabolism	Expected Effect on the Drug
Cyclophosphamide	2C8, 2B6, 3A4, 2C9, and 2C19	Increased
Ifosfamide	3A4, 3A5	Decreased
Dacarbazine	1A2	Increased
Paclitaxel	2C8, 3A4	Decreased
Docetaxel	3A4	Decreased
Vinblastine	3A4	Decreased
Vincristine	3A4	Decreased
Navelbine	3A4	Decreased
Etoposide	3A4	Decreased
Irinotecan	3A4, 3A5	Decreased
Topotecan	3A4	Decreased
Tamoxifen	3A4, 1A2	Decreased
Arimidex	3A4, 1A2, 2C8–9, and 2C19	Decreased
Aromasin	3A4, 1A2, 2C8–9, and 2C19	Decreased
Femara	3A4, 1A2, 2C8–9, and 2C19	Decreased
Iressa	3A4	Decreased

Data from Drozdoff, L., Klein, E., Kalder, M., Brambs, C., Kiechle, M., & Paepke, D. (2019). Potential interactions of biologically based complementary medicine in gynecological oncology. *Integrative Cancer Therapies, 18*, 1534735419846392. https://doi.org/10.1177/1534735419846392; Wolf, C. P. J. G., Rachow, T., Ernst, T., Hochhaus, A., Zomorodbakhsch, B., Foller, S., et al. (2022). Complementary and alternative medicine (CAM) supplements in cancer outpatients: Analyses of usage and of interaction risks with cancer treatment. *Journal of Cancer Research and Clinical Oncology, 148*, 1123–1135. https://doi.org/10.1007/s00432-021-03675-7.

B. Incorporation of compatible CAM practices into conventional interventions to increase health care provider's knowledge about CAM, its effects on conventional therapy, and resources
1. Support the need for a well-informed health care team.
a. Familiarity with CAM resources available in the institution, community, and Internet
b. Knowledge about CAM sources (including health food vendors)
c. Recognition that patients are important sources of information about CAM
d. Awareness that CAM may reflect cultural preferences and is an integral component of a patient's family and social identity
e. Ability to effectively discuss CAM from a scientific, evidence-based perspective
(1) Recognition that failure to offer objective information about safety and efficacy compromises patient-initiated dialog about CAM
(2) Offer appropriate referrals to trusted trained professionals, as indicated

REFERENCES

Balneaves, L. G. (2018). The integrative oncology nurse: New role for a new era in cancer care. *ONS Voice*. Retrieved from https://voice.ons.org/news-and-views/the-integrative-oncology-nurse-new-role-for-a-new-era-in-cancer-care.

Du, M., Luo, H., Blumberg, J. B., Rogers, G., Chen, F., Ruan, M., et al. (2020). Dietary supplement use among adult cancer survivors in the United States. *The Journal of Nutrition, 150*(6), 1499–1508. https://doi.org/10.1093/jn/nxaa040.

Drozdoff, L., Klein, E., Kalder, M., Brambs, C., Kiechle, M., & Paepke, D. (2019). Potential interactions of biologically based complementary medicine in gynecological oncology. *Integrative Cancer Therapies, 18*. https://doi.org/10.1177/1534735419846392. 1534735419846392.

Eaton, L. H., & Hulett, J. M. (2019). Mind-body interventions in the management of chronic cancer pain. *Seminars in Oncology Nursing, 35*(3), 241–252. https://doi.org/10.1016/j.soncn.2019.04.005.

Hammersen, F., Pursche, T., Fischer, D., Katalinic, A., & Waldmann, A. (2020). Use of complementary and alternative medicine among young patients with breast cancer. *Breast Care (Basel), 15*(2), 163–170. https://doi.org/10.1159/000501193.

Knecht, K., Kinder, D., & Stockert, A. (2020). Biologically-based complementary and alternative medicine (CAM) use in cancer patients: The good, the bad, the misunderstood. *Frontiers in Nutrition, 6*, 196. https://doi.org/10.3389/fnut.2019.00196.

Latte-Naor, S., & Mao, J. J. (2019). Putting integrative oncology into practice: Concepts and approaches. *Journal of Oncology Practice, 15*(1), 7–14. https://doi.org/10.1200/JOP.18.00554.

Lawrence, L. (2021). Open discussions help nurses introduce integrative services. *Oncology Nursing News, 15*(1). Retrieved from https://www.oncnursingnews.com/view/open-discussions-help-nurses-introduce-integrative-services.

Mühlenpfordt, I., Stritter, W., Bertram, M., Ben-Arye, E., & Seifert, G. (2019). The power of touch: External applications from whole medical systems in the care of cancer patients (literature review). *Supportive Care in Cancer, 28*(2), 461–471. https://doi.org/10.1007/s00520-019-05172-7.

National Cancer Institute (NCI). (2019). NCI-designated cancer centers. https://www.cancer.gov/research/infrastructure/cancer-centers.

National Center for Complementary and Integrative Health (NCCIH). (2021). Complementary, alternative, or integrative health: What's in a name? https://nccih.nih.gov/health/integrative-health#types.

Wolf, C. P. J. G., Rachow, T., Ernst, T., Hochhaus, A., Zomorodbakhsch, B., Foller, S., et al. (2022). Complementary and alternative medicine (CAM) supplements in cancer outpatients: Analyses of usage and of interaction risks with cancer treatment. *Journal of Cancer Research and Clinical Oncology, 148*(5), 1123–1135. https://doi.org/10.1007/s00432-021-03675-7.

Zeng, Y. S., Wang, C., Ward, K. E., & Hume, A. L. (2018). Complementary and alternative medicine in hospice and palliative care: A systematic review. *Journal of Pain and Symptom Management, 56*(5), 781–794.e4. https://doi.org/10.1016/j.jpainsymman.2018.07.016.

34

Cardiovascular Symptoms

Deborah Kirk and Amanda Towell-Barnard

LYMPHEDEMA

Overview

I. Definition—obstruction of the lymphatic system that causes accumulation of lymph fluid in interstitial spaces.

II. Pathophysiology—occlusion or damage to the venous side of capillaries, decreases reabsorption of lymphatic fluid made up of protein, water, fats, and wastes from cells, thereby causing swelling or lymphedema (Azhar, Lim, Tan, & Angeli, 2020; Martin-Almedina, Mortimer, & Ostergaard, 2021).
   A. Primary lymphedema—genetic or familial abnormalities present at birth.
   B. Secondary lymphedema—damage or destruction of the lymphatic system.

III. Incidence
   A. Varies per cancer diagnosis, increased with lymph node dissection and disease involvement of the lymph system.
   B. May occur within days of a traumatic event and last a lifetime if the event is permanent (lymph node dissection).

IV. Risk factors (National Cancer Institute, 2019; Woods, 2019)
   A. Noncancer related
      1. Poor nutrition
      2. Genetics (Martin-Almedina et al., 2021)
      3. Thrombophlebitis
      4. Skin inflammation or chronic disorders of the skin
      5. Obesity/elevated body mass index (BMI)
   B. Cancer diagnosis related
      1. Tumor invasion and/or advanced disease
      2. Infection—affected extremity, concurrent illness
      3. Air travel with suboptimal cabin pressure, long-distance travel, and prolonged immobilization in patients with an altered lymph system
      4. Traumatic injury to affected extremity
      5. Excessive physical use of affected extremity; prolonged standing (lower extremity)
   C. Treatment related
      1. Surgical lymph node dissection, number of lymph nodes removed, type of surgery, seroma formation after surgery, or delayed wound healing
      2. Radiation therapy (RT)—location and formation of scars or fibrosis

Assessment

(Dean et al., 2020; Greene & Goss, 2018)
   I. History
      A. Past medical history—illnesses, type of cancer, and history of thrombus
      B. Current medications
      C. Past surgical history
      D. Treatment history
         1. Attributes of each symptom—onset, location, duration, characteristics, aggravating symptoms, relieving factors, and treatment
            a. Cause, location, and duration of swelling
   II. Physical examination
      A. Tightness of clothing, shoes, wristwatch, and jewelry
      B. Visible puffiness (unilateral vs. bilateral)
      C. Pain, stiffness, weakness, numbness, and paresthesia of affected extremity
      D. Redness, warmth of affected extremity
      E. Tends to occur distal to proximal
      F. Thickening, pitting, and erythema of skin; peau d'orange changes
      G. Increased pigmentation/superficial veins, stasis dermatitis
      H. Induration with nonpitting edema
      I. Secondary cellulitis
      J. Decreased range of motion, feeling of heaviness of affected extremity
   III. Psychosocial assessment
      A. Interventions to assess the quality of life, psychosocial distress, and disability (Bowman, Piedalue, Baydoun, & Carlson, 2020; Leitao et al., 2020)
   IV. Assessment tools (Azhar et al., 2020; Dean et al., 2020; Qin, Bowen, & Chen, 2018; Spinelli et al., 2019)
      A. Objective screening tools
         1. Circumference measurements
         2. Arm measured 5 and 10 cm above and below the olecranon process and compared with the other extremity
         3. Leg measured at the level of the mid-calf
      B. Water displacement method to measure limb volume
         1. Limitations due to difficulty using in clinic setting and does not indicate lymphedema location.

2. Perometer, using infrared light to measure fluid volume of the limb.

3. Bioelectrical impedance uses electrical currents through the regions to determine volume.

C. Subjective screening tools

1. Selected based on the goal of assessment (i.e., screening, referrals, response to treatment)

2. Examples of selected tools—the Functional Assessment of Cancer Therapy questionnaire with breast cancer and arm function subscales (FACT B+4), the Lymphedema and Breast Cancer Questionnaire, and the Morbidity Screening Tool

V. Clinical staging/grading

A. Staging of lymphedema by examination evaluates the progression of the disease. Grading evaluates the severity of signs and symptoms (Table 34.1; National Cancer Institute, 2019, 2021).

B. Imaging and laboratory tests (Jayaraj, Raju, May, & Pace, 2019; Martin-Almedina et al., 2021; Qin et al., 2018).

1. Lymphoscintigraphy—radioactive mapping of lymphatic vessels.

2. Ultrasound (US) for evaluation of tissue and fluid.

3. Computed tomography (CT), magnetic resonance imaging (MRI), or positron emission tomography scan are not approved for evaluation of lymphedema but can be used to evaluate soft tissue or a possible mass.

Management

(National Cancer Institute, 2019; O'Donnell, Allison, & Iafrati, 2020; Streiff et al., 2021)

I. Pharmacologic management

A. Treat suspected infections with early antibiotic treatment

B. Manage acute and chronic pain

C. Axillary reverse mapping

II. Nonpharmacologic management

A. Complete decongestive therapy

B. Compression bandaging, compression garment

C. Exercise

D. Weight management

E. Avoid prolonged standing

F. Elevate affected extremity

G. Avoid extreme heat—may worsen the swelling (e.g., hot tubs)

H. Skin care program with proper bathing, drying, and lubrication

I. Compression garments when flying

J. Patient education

1. Signs and symptoms to report (e.g., high risk for infection)

2. Need for lifelong follow-up

3. Low-sodium, high-fiber, weight-controlled diet

4. Importance of skin care to maintain skin integrity and prevent infections

5. Education to eliminate safety hazards to prevent injury

6. Maintain healthy weight

7. Limit time in extreme temperatures

8. Wear loose-fitting clothes

EDEMA

Overview

I. Definition—fluid accumulation in interstitial spaces.

II. Pathophysiology (Dyadyk, Kugler, Schukina, Zborovskyy, & Suliman, 2018; Itkin, Rockson, & Burkhoff, 2021; Kamel & Blebea, 2020)—the movement of fluid from the vascular space into the interstitial space by an alteration in one or more of the following:

A. Increased capillary pressure—when volume of blood is expanded or with obstruction; extrinsic sodium and water retention by the kidneys caused by renal failure, reduction of cardiac output, or systemic vascular resistance can cause edema. Stimulation of the renin–angiotensin system causes an increase in pressure in the vascular bed (forcing fluid into interstitial spaces) (i.e., heart disease, renal disease, cirrhosis, deep venous thrombosis [DVT]).

B. Increased capillary permeability—from vascular injury (i.e., burns, radiation, drug reactions, infection); treatment with interleukin-2 (IL-2) or vascular endothelial growth factors.

C. Obstruction of lymph system—see "Lymphedema."

D. Decreased plasma oncotic pressure—results in increased fluid in the tissues; albumin causes retention of fluid in the vascular bed. When albumin is decreased,

TABLE 34.1	Staging and Grading of Lymphedema
Stage 1	Mild, spontaneously reversible. Slight heaviness of extremity; skin smooth textured with pitting edema; may have pain and erythema.
Stage 2	Moderate, irreversible. May have tissue fibrosis; skin stretched, shiny, with nonpitting edema.
Stage 3	Severe, lymphostatic elephantiasis, and irreversible. Skin discolored, stretched, and firm; rare in breast cancer.
Grade 1	Swelling, pitting edema; 5%–10% difference in size at greatest point or mass of limbs.
Grade 2	Obvious obstruction, taut skin; 10%–30% difference in size at greatest point or mass of limbs.
Grade 3	Limb starts to look disfigured; interferes with ADLs; more than 30% difference in size at greatest point or mass of limbs.
Grade 4	Often progresses to malignancy; disabling and may need removal of affected extremity; 5%–10% difference in size or mass of limbs.

ADLs, Activities of daily living.
From National Cancer Institute. (2019). Lymphedema (PDQ®)–Health professional version. https://www.cancer.gov/about-cancer/treatment/side-effects/lymphedema/lymphedema-hp-pdq; National Cancer Institute. (2021). Lymphedema (PDQ®)—Patient version. https://www.cancer.gov/about-cancer/treatment/side-effects/lymphedema/lymphedema-pdq.

fluid leaks into interstitial spaces (i.e., proteinuria, hepatic failure, malabsorption, protein malnutrition).

E. Raised hydrostatic pressure—fluid driven from the capillaries into the interstitial spaces (i.e., venous obstruction, fluid retention, prolonged standing).

F. May be associated with the following (Dyadyk et al., 2018; Itkin et al., 2021; Kamel & Blebea, 2020).
   1. Lymphatic obstruction by tumor or DVT.
   2. Cancer—common with kidney, liver, and ovarian.
      a. Malignant ascites
   3. Systemic conditions—heart failure, nephrotic syndrome, liver failure, thyroid disease, and obstructive sleep apnea.
   4. Medications may include hormones, nonsteroidal antiinflammatory drugs, calcium channel blockers, tricyclic antidepressants, steroids, IL-2 therapy, corticosteroids, and beta-blockers.
   5. Chemotherapy (i.e., cisplatin, docetaxel, and gemcitabine).
   6. Monoclonal antibodies (i.e., bevacizumab).
   7. Targeted therapies (i.e., imatinib mesylate).
   8. Antiangiogenesis agents (i.e., thalidomide).

G. Allergic response or septic shock, which leads to histamine release.
   1. Poor nutrition, hypoproteinemia, hypoalbuminemia
   2. Iatrogenic causes—plasma expanders, intravenous (IV) fluid overload, and blood component therapy
   3. Burns, trauma, and sepsis
   4. Allergic reactions

III. Incidence
   A. Unknown because the problem is underreported.
   B. May be increasing because of longer survival rates.

IV. Risk factors (Kamel & Blebea, 2020; Lo-Cao, Hall, Parsell, Dandie, & Fahlström, 2021)
   A. Preexisting cardiac, renal, liver disease, thyroid disease.
   B. Cancer (i.e., kidney, liver, or ovarian cancers).
   C. Cancer treatments (i.e., cisplatin, docetaxel).
   D. Decreased mobility.
   E. Long-distance travel.
   F. Prior history of edema.
   G. Certain medications.
   H. DVT.
   I. Hypertension (HTN).

Assessment

(Assaad, Kratzert, Shelley, Friedman, & Perrino, 2018; Kamel & Blebea, 2020; Lo-Cao et al., 2021; Streiff et al., 2021)
   I. History
   A. Past medical history—cardiac, renal, liver disease, thyroid disease, DVT, popliteal cyst, and trauma
   B. Past surgical history
   C. Treatment history
   D. Medication history
   E. Attributes of each symptom—onset, location, duration, characteristics, aggravating symptoms, relieving factors, and treatment

   1. Timing of edema
   2. Does it change with position
   3. Unilateral/bilateral

II. Physical examination
   A. Tightness of clothing, shoes, jewelry, and watch.
   B. Pain or stiffness.
   C. Weight gain.
   D. Shortness of breath, dyspnea on exertion, orthopnea, paroxysmal nocturnal dyspnea, and rales.
   E. Frequent or decreased urination.
   F. Presence of S_3 or S_4 heart sound.
   G. Increased jugular venous pressure.
   H. Increased blood pressure and tachycardia.
   I. Ascites, hepatomegaly.
   J. Dependent edema (extremities, sacrum).
   K. Skin thickening/skin tightness.
   L. Decreased peripheral pulses.
   M. Changes in skin integrity, temperature, color, texture, and signs of infection or trauma.

III. Psychosocial
   A. Interventions to relieve symptoms and improve quality of life

IV. Laboratory and diagnostic tests
   A. Serum albumin and protein may be decreased.
   B. Creatinine, blood urea nitrogen (BUN) may be increased with kidney disease.
   C. Liver function tests may be increased with cirrhosis.
   D. Thyroid studies should be performed to rule out thyroid disease.
   E. Urinalysis for protein.
   F. Brain natriuretic peptide (BNP) will be elevated with edema that may be caused by heart failure.
   G. Chest x-ray (CXR)—evidence of fluid overload, increased size of heart shadow.
   H. Echocardiogram—decreased ejection fraction (EF) in heart failure.
   I. US to rule out a DVT or thrombophlebitis if edema is unilateral.

Management

(Assaad et al., 2018)
   I. Pharmacologic management
   A. Treat the underlying cause (i.e., congestive heart failure, nephrotic syndrome, liver failure/cirrhosis, thrombophlebitis, lymphedema, and DVT).
   B. Diuretics.
   C. Angiotensin-converting enzyme (ACE) inhibitors or, if not tolerated, angiotensin receptor blockers (ARBs).
   D. Beta-blockers.
   E. Analgesics as needed.
   II. Nonpharmacologic management
   A. Elevate extremities above the level of heart.
   B. Compression stockings.
   C. Maintain lubrication of skin.
   D. Bed rest to promote diuresis; reposition every 2 hours.
   E. Fluid restriction.
      1. Treatment of underlying cause.

2. Monitor intake and output, electrolytes, and serum albumin.

F. Protect extremity from injury.

G. Walk or other exercises.

H. Protect from extreme temperatures.

I. Provide patient education.
   1. Low-sodium, well-balanced diet, and protein in the diet for those with hypoalbuminemia.
   2. Employ appropriate skin care strategies.
   3. Avoid prolonged standing or sitting with legs crossed.
   4. Avoid hepatotoxic drugs and alcohol.
   5. Fluid restriction may be warranted.
   6. Walk or exercise to maintain muscle strength and joint range of motion.
   7. Perform daily weights and report greater than a 3- to 4-pound gain.
   8. Educate patient and family regarding risks for electrolyte disturbance and possible interventions if symptoms occur.
   9. Wear support hoses with instruction on how to apply them appropriately.

MALIGNANT PERICARDIAL EFFUSION

Overview

I. Definition—accumulation of fluid in the pericardial sac that affects cardiac function, resulting in decreased cardiac output.

II. Pathophysiology (Neves et al., 2021; Wang, Zhao, Wang, & Zhang, 2021).
   A. Malignant pericardial effusions may develop from:
      1. Metastatic disease that has moved into the cardiac space through local advancement, spread by blood or lymph systems or obstruction from adenopathy (i.e., most common lung or breast cancer; can occur in lymphoma, renal cell, angiosarcoma, clear cell sarcoma, melanoma, mesothelioma, gastric cancer, ovarian cancer, primary cardiac myxoma, prostate cancer, squamous cell carcinoma of the head and neck, or multiple myeloma)
      2. Treatment complications from radiation fibrosis causing damage to structure; chemotherapy causing damage to endothelial cells or cardiomyocytes, or both
      3. Infection in an immunocompromised patient

III. May be associated with the following (Connolly, Bamford, & Hiriyanna Gowda, 2018):
   A. Primary tumors of the pericardium; mesothelioma most common.
   B. Direct tumor invasion of the myocardium; more common with lung tumors, thymoma, esophageal tumors, and lymphoma.
   C. Obstruction of mediastinal lymph nodes by tumor.
   D. Infection (bacterial, viral, and fungal).
   E. Fibrosis secondary to RT.

F. Drug induced.

G. Autoimmune disease.

IV. Incidence (Neves et al., 2021).
   A. Once diagnosed, prognosis is poor.
   B. Varies by malignant process involved.

V. Risk factors (Connolly et al., 2018; Puwanant et al., 2021).
   A. Coexisting cardiac disease, systemic lupus erythematosus, bacterial endocarditis.
   B. RT of 3000 cGy to more than 33% of heart or fraction sizes of more than 300 cGy/day.
   C. High-dose chemotherapy or biotherapy agents that cause capillary permeability.
      1. Chemotherapy (i.e., cytosine arabinoside, cyclophosphamide, busulfan, doxorubicin, and gemcitabine)
      2. Biological agents (i.e., interferon, IL-2, IL-11, and granulocyte–macrophage colony-stimulating factor)
      3. Targeted agents (i.e., imatinib, dasatinib)
      4. Arsenic trioxide
      5. All-trans retinoic acid
   D. Rare causes include hemorrhagic tamponade from direct injury or infectious etiology.
   E. Malignancies (i.e., lung cancer, breast cancer, melanoma, lymphoma, and leukemia).
   F. Thoracic lymphatic obstruction (i.e., from lymphadenopathy related to HIV disease or malignancies of the lymphatic system, hematologic malignancies, lymphangioleiomyomatosis, extramedullary multiple myeloma, or thymic cancer).

Assessment

(Connolly et al., 2018; Khoshpouri et al., 2021; Neves et al., 2021; Wang et al., 2021)

I. History
   A. Past medical history—cardiac, renal, liver disease, and trauma
   B. Past surgical history
   C. Medication and treatment history
   D. Attributes of each symptom—onset, location, duration, characteristics, aggravating symptoms, relieving factors, and treatment
      1. Sudden onset, location of discomfort, nonproductive cough.
      2. Slowly developing effusions compensate for a progressive reduction in cardiac output as the effusion occurs. May not demonstrate symptoms until more than 1000 mL of fluid is in the pericardial sac.
      3. Most common symptom with malignancy-related pericardial disease is dyspnea.
      4. Excessive yawning has been associated with pericardial effusion.

II. Physical examination
   A. Symptoms reflect chronicity.
      1. Slowly developing effusions may have little or no symptoms.
      2. Rapidly developing effusions may be symptomatic at 50–80 mL (normal pericardial fluid volume = 15–50 mL).

B. Fatigue, malaise, and weakness.

C. Dyspnea at rest and with exertion.

D. Dull, nonpositional chest pain and distant, muffled heart sounds are a late finding.

E. Nonproductive cough.

F. Tachycardia, hypotension, jugular vein distention, and decreased peripheral pulses.

G. Anxiousness, restlessness.

H. Nausea and vomiting.

I. Pericardial friction rub more likely to occur with radiation-induced or nonmalignant effusions.

J. Point of maximal impulse shifted to left.

K. Moderately increased central venous pressure (15–18 cm of H_2O or 8–12 mm Hg).

L. 2 to 3+ pedal edema with slowly developing effusions; may be absent with rapid development of effusion.

M. Narrowing pulse pressure, pulsus paradoxus greater than 13 mm Hg.

N. Cool, clammy extremities.

O. Hepatomegaly/splenomegaly.

III. Imaging and laboratory tests (Khoshpouri et al., 2021; Oyakawa et al., 2018; Wang et al., 2021)

A. CXR indicating cardiac enlargement, widened mediastinum, "water bottle" shape of heart, pulmonary infiltrates.

B. Electrocardiogram (ECG) changes including low-voltage QRS, tachycardia, and nonspecific ST-T changes; electrical alternans is a rare finding.

C. Echocardiogram is a definitive test for effusion and cardiac function.

D. CT of chest especially helpful with large tumor burden.

E. May evaluate pericardial fluid for lactate dehydrogenase, protein, and tumor markers.

F. Cardiac catheterization may be indicated if the diagnosis is in question.

G. Troponins may be elevated.

H. White blood cell count will be elevated with infection.

I. C-reactive protein elevated with inflammation.

J. BNP elevated with fluid overload.

Management

(Besnard et al., 2019; Connolly et al., 2018; Eapen & Firstenberg, 2018; Khoshpouri et al., 2021)

I. Pharmacologic management

A. Chemotherapy may be indicated if tumor responsive (i.e., lymphoma, leukemia, and breast cancer).

B. Administer sclerosing agents into pericardial space as indicated (e.g., talc, bleomycin).

C. Oxygen therapy.

D. Diuretics probably not beneficial.

E. Pain management.

F. Drain of pericardial fluid such as percutaneous pericardiocentesis.

G. Radiation may be indicated, but not common.

H. May consider consulting palliative care.

II. Nonpharmacologic management

A. Elevate the head of bed to relieve dyspnea.

B. Minimize activities to conserve energy.

C. May elect no treatment with close follow-up if asymptomatic.

D. Patient education.

1. Preparation for pericardial drainage.

2. Energy conservation methods.

3. Relaxation techniques.

4. Activity modification to conserve energy.

CARDIOVASCULAR TOXICITY RELATED TO CANCER THERAPY

Overview

I. Definition—damage to the cardiac muscle, conduction system, coronary arteries, valves, and/or pericardium related to cancer therapies that may cause alterations in cardiac function (Alexandre et al., 2020).

II. Types of cardiovascular toxicities (CVT) associated with cancer therapies (Herrmann, 2020a; Herrmann, 2020b).

A. Left ventricular dysfunction (LVD)

B. Heart failure (HF)

C. HTN treatment induced

D. Ischemia

E. Rhythm disturbances

1. Conduction damage

2. QT prolongation

F. Venous thromboembolism (VTE) with or without arterial thromboembolism

G. Myopericarditis

III. Drug classes associated with CVT (Alexandre et al., 2020; Herrmann, 2020a; Russell, 2018; Upshaw, 2020).

A. Alkylating agents—associated with acute myopericarditis, pericardial effusions, arrhythmias, HTN, thromboembolism, and heart failure (i.e., cyclophosphamide)

B. Angiogenesis inhibitors—bradycardia, thromboembolism, and HTN may be seen (i.e., thalidomide, lenalidomide, and pomalidomide)

C. Anthracyclines—may cause toxicity from injury of free radicals that result in myocardial cell loss, fibrosis, and loss of contractility resulting in LVD, HF, and myopericarditis (i.e., doxorubicin, daunorubicin, epirubicin, idarubicin, and mitoxantrone)

D. Antiandrogens—can cause hyperlipidemia, thromboembolism, and QT prolongation

E. Antiangiogenic antibodies—may cause HTN, ischemia (i.e., bevacizumab)

F. Antiestrogens—can cause thromboembolism, HTN

G. Antimetabolites—can cause coronary artery spasm resulting in angina, arrhythmia, myocardial infarction, cardiac arrest, and sudden death; coronary artery thrombosis and apoptosis of myocardial cells (i.e., 5-FU, capecitabine, and gemcitabine).

H. Antimicrotubule agents—may cause early HF, arrhythmias, ischemia (i.e., paclitaxel, docetaxel, etoposide, vincristine, and vinblastine).

I. Checkpoint inhibitors—myopericarditis, atrial fibrillation, ventricular arrhythmias, and HF (i.e., nivolumab, pembrolizumab, and ipilimumab)

J. HER2/neu blockers—inhibit certain pathways critical to cardiac function, which may increase the risk for HF (i.e., trastuzumab, pertuzumab)

K. Histone deacetylase inhibitors—may cause QT prolongation or thromboembolism (i.e., vorinostat)

L. Miscellaneous drugs—such as arsenic trioxide (QT prolongation), tretinoin (HF, hypotension), and bleomycin (myopericarditis)

M. mTOR inhibitors—HTN, angina, DVT/pulmonary embolism (PE) (i.e., everolimus, temsirolimus)

N. Platinum agents—HTN, hypotension, dyslipidemia, early atherosclerosis, coronary artery disease, Raynaud syndrome, thromboembolic events, HF, angina, acute myocardial infarction, autonomic cardiovascular dysfunction, myocarditis, pericarditis, cardiomyopathy, arrhythmias, atrial fibrillation, and complete atrioventricular block

O. Proteasome inhibitors—may cause HF and ischemia (i.e., bortezomib, carfilzomib)

P. Tyrosine kinase inhibitors—may cause HF, QT prolongation, HTN, ischemia, and thromboembolism (i.e., dasatinib, lapatinib, imatinib, and sunitinib)

IV. Incidence (Alexandre et al., 2020; Clark et al., 2019; Ravi & Gang, 2019).

A. Acute reactions—infrequent; reversible.
   1. Occur within 24 hours of drug administration.
   2. Usually self-limiting and cease when the drug is stopped.
   3. May not require discontinuation of the drug.

B. Early onset within 1 year after treatment—infrequent.

C. Late onset after 1 year of completing therapy.
   1. Occurs with cumulative doses of drugs.
   2. Dilated cardiomyopathy can occur.

V. Risk factors (Alexandre et al., 2020; Clark et al., 2019; Polonsky & DeCara, 2019).

A. Preexisting heart disease, HTN, hyperlipidemia.

B. History of smoking.

C. Age younger than 15 years or advanced age > 65.

D. Certain cardiotoxic drugs.
   1. Doses that place patient at risk:
      a. Doxorubicin >550 mg/m^2
      b. Liposomal doxorubicin >900 mg/m^2
      c. Epirubicin >720 mg/m^2
      d. Mitoxantrone >120 mg/m^2
      e. Idarubicin >90 mg/m^2

E. Exceeding recommended total doses of chemotherapy or high dose in short period.

F. Radiation treatment field which includes the heart.

G. Acute cardiac event during treatment.

H. Combination chest radiation with anthracycline.

I. Others: female, obesity, comorbid disease, and previous cancer treatment that had cardiotoxicity.

Assessment

(Alexandre et al., 2020; Clark et al., 2019; Herrmann, 2020a, 2020b; Oikonomou et al., 2018; Ravi & Gang, 2019)

I. History

A. Past medical history—preexisting cardiac disease, electrolyte imbalances, renal or liver disease, dyslipidemia, and diabetes

B. Past surgical history

C. Medication history

D. Treatment history—prior chemotherapy and radiation

E. Attributes of each symptom—onset, location, duration, characteristics, aggravating symptoms, relieving factors, and treatment
   1. Palpitations, chest pain

II. Physical examination

A. Orthostatic symptoms, arrhythmias, jugular vein distention, bilateral pedal edema, presence of S_3 or S_4, murmurs with valvular abnormalities, and decreased cardiac EF
   1. Tachycardia—early sign in anthracycline toxicity.

B. Shortness of breath, dyspnea, orthopnea, and nonproductive cough

C. Exercise intolerance, fatigue

D. Weight gain

E. Syncope

III. Psychosocial assessment

A. Interventions used to relieve symptoms and improve the quality of life

IV. Imaging and laboratory tests (Alexandre et al., 2020; Oikonomou et al., 2018)

A. ECG changes.
   1. Premature atrial contractions, premature ventricular contractions.
   2. Nonspecific ST-T wave changes.

B. Echocardiogram or multigated acquisition (MUGA) scan.
   1. Monitor left ventricular function—usually decreased EF.
      a. Decreased EF to less than 45% or decrease of more than 5% over baseline requires consideration for discontinuing the drug or holding treatment and monitoring the EF until improvement. Resuming drug is individualized.
   2. Pericardial effusion.
   3. Left ventricular hypertrophy.

C. Cardiac MRI—gold standard for evaluation of left ventricular volumes, mass, and function; however, it is cost prohibitive.

D. BMI/waist circumference.

E. Laboratory changes that may affect cardiac function
   1. Laboratory tests affecting cardiac function—potassium, magnesium, calcium, renal function, thyroid, and lipid levels
      a. Electrolytes should be monitored, especially with drugs that may prolong the QT interval.

2. Cardiac biomarkers of early myocardial damage—troponins, BNP

Management

(Alexandre et al., 2020; Herrmann, 2020a, 2020b; Ravi & Gang, 2019; Upshaw, 2020)

I. Pharmacologic management
   A. Interventions to treat cardiotoxicity with pharmacologic methods are based on underlying event.
   B. Lipid-lowering agents if indicated for hyperlipidemia.
   C. Beta-blockers and ACE inhibitors.
      1. Can be used for LVD.
   D. ARBs concurrent with anthracyclines help prevent cardiac damage.
   E. ACE inhibitors and calcium channel blockers to treat HTN.
   F. Minimize risk of QT prolongation.
      1. Avoid drug-to-drug interactions.
      2. Monitor and treat electrolyte disturbances.
   G. Administer cardiac protective iron chelating agents, such as dexrazoxane (Zinecard), to prevent doxorubicin-induced cardiotoxicity in patients with metastatic breast cancer who require more than 300 mg/m^2 of drug; liposomal doxorubicin to decrease cardiotoxicity.
   H. Anticoagulate patients at risk for VTE.
   I. Valvular surgery may be indicated with radiation-induced valvular disease.
   J. Management of underlying disease—both cancer and cardiac.
   K. Radiation management to reduce exposure to cardiac structure.
II. Nonpharmacologic management (Clark et al., 2019; Sheilds, 2018)
   A. Cardiovascular risk assessment before treatment starts.
   B. Screening of cardiovascular function at appropriate intervals.
   C. Prevent cardiotoxicity.
      1. Document the total cumulative dose of drug; discontinue when maximum dose is achieved.
         a. Doxorubicin: 550 mg/m^2
         b. Daunorubicin (Cerubidine, DaunoXome): 600 mg/m^2
         c. Mitoxantrone (Novantrone): 160 mg/m^2
         d. High-dose cyclophosphamide: 144 mg/kg for 4 days
   D. Monitor baseline and interval ECG or MUGA scan.
   E. Monitor vital signs and weight.
   F. Monitor exposure of RT to minimize cardiac toxicity.
   G. Patient education.
      1. Signs and symptoms to report.
      2. Well-balanced diet, with a focus on any restrictions.
      3. Importance for medically approved exercise program.

THROMBOTIC EVENTS

Overview

I. Definition—venous thrombus or arterial embolus interfering with venous drainage or obstructing arterial blood flow.

II. Pathophysiology (Fernandes et al., 2019; Musgrave et al., 2022; Shellack, Modau, & Shellack, 2020).
   A. A thrombus may form in the setting of stasis, endothelial injury, and/or a hypercoagulable state (Virchow triad).
      1. The thrombus is composed of red blood cells, fibrin, and platelets; fills the vessel lumen, causing partial or complete obstruction of blood flow; or may shed emboli, causing PE or cerebrovascular accident.
      2. The thrombus may float freely in the blood vessel, leading to embolization where it lodges in a blood vessel, causing partial or complete obstruction of blood flow.
   B. Tumor cells may be associated with procoagulant activities.
      1. Tumor cells deposit fibrin in tissues, acting late in clotting cascade, providing a surface for prothrombinase assembly.
      2. Microvasculature becomes hyperpermeable, allowing clotting proteins to leak into extravascular space.
      3. Procoagulants released from cancer cells initiate the clotting cascade.
III. Risk factors (Fernandes et al., 2019; Musgrave et al., 2022; Streiff et al., 2021).
   A. Active cancer
      1. Some sites are higher risk (i.e., stomach, brain, and pancreas)
      2. Advanced stage higher risk
   B. Lymphadenopathy
   C. Presence of venous access device
   D. Comorbidities (i.e., infections, HF, and renal disease)
   E. Poor performance status; prolonged immobilization
   F. Older age
   G. Cancer treatments
      1. Cytotoxic agents
      2. Hormonal therapies (i.e., tamoxifen)
      3. Antiangiogenic agents—thalidomide
      4. Erythropoietic-stimulating agents
   H. Smoking
   I. Obesity
   J. Surgery
   K. Hospitalizations—especially prolonged
   L. Prior personal history of VTE; familial/acquired hypercoagulability/thrombophilia
   M. Laboratory abnormalities
      1. Prechemotherapy platelet count >350,000/mcL
      2. Prechemotherapy white blood cell count >11,000/mcL
      3. Hgb <10 g/dL
   N. Blood transfusions
IV. Incidence rates vary in persons with cancer by disease. Ranging from 8% to 19% depending on tumor type (Streiff et al., 2021).
   A. High risk: cancers of the lung, gastrointestinal tract, pancreatic, and prostate, ovary.

B. Leukemias, multiple myeloma, and Hodgkin and non-Hodgkin lymphomas.

C. Advanced disease or metastatic disease.

Assessment

(Streiff et al., 2021)

I. History
  A. Past medical history—including history of VTE
  B. Family history of any blood disorders, thrombus
  C. Past surgical history
  D. Medication history
  E. Treatment history—prior chemotherapy and radiation
  F. Attributes of each symptom—onset, location, duration, characteristics, aggravating symptoms, relieving factors, and treatment
  G. Pain in calf with walking, dull ache, and tight feeling
II. Physical examination
  A. Venous occlusion.
    1. Tenderness over involved vein, palpable venous cord.
    2. Unilateral edema of involved extremity.
    3. Distention of superficial collateral veins.
  B. Arterial embolus.
    1. Severe pain in the involved extremity.
    2. Extremity coolness, pallor.
    3. Absent or decreased pulse.
  C. Pulmonary embolus.
    1. Chest pain.
    2. Dyspnea, shallow respirations, and tachypnea.
    3. Sudden onset of anxiety.
    4. Cardiopulmonary arrest.
    5. Decreased pulse oximetry.
    6. Decreased breath sounds with pleural friction rub.
  D. Clotting abnormalities.
    1. Easy bruising.
    2. Bleeding from mucous membranes, in urine or stool.
III. Imaging and laboratory tests (Streiff et al., 2021)
  A. Complete blood count and platelet count—thrombocytosis.
  B. Abnormal venous US or venogram with VTE.
  C. Liver function tests, BUN, and creatinine.
  D. Abnormal arteriogram with arterial embolus.
  E. Abnormal spiral CT or ventilation–perfusion (V–Q) scan with PE.
  F. Prothrombin time (PT), partial thrombin time (PTT), international normalized ratio (INR), abnormal clotting factors, and D-dimer.
  G. Consider evaluation for hypercoagulable states such as protein C, protein S, antithrombin III, factor V Leiden, prothrombin gene mutation, homocysteine, and antiphospholipid antibodies.
  H. Magnetic resonance venography for pelvic and iliac veins and vena cava—can be cost prohibitive.

Management

(Musgrave et al., 2022; Streiff et al., 2021; Xiong, 2021)

I. Pharmacologic management
  A. Anticoagulation prophylaxis is not recommended in patients receiving standard chemotherapy.
  B. Consider prophylaxis in patients with high risk.
    1. Low-molecular-weight heparin (LMWH)
    2. Unfractionated heparin
    3. Acetylsalicylic acid (ASA) (aspirin), 81 mg
    4. Anticoagulants: warfarin (adjust INR 2–3), rivaroxaban, and apixaban
  C. Treat acute emboli.
    1. LMWH.
      a. Unfractionated heparin IV/subcutaneous.
      b. Direct oral anticoagulation if LMWH is contraindicated.
  D. Treatment of acute embolus.
    1. Place inferior vena cava filter if pharmacologic management is contraindicated.
    2. Arterial embolectomy.
    3. Thrombolytic therapy consideration on case-by-case basis.
  E. Oxygen for PE.
  F. Pain management.
II. Nonpharmacologic management
  A. Ambulate frequently, leg exercises if bedridden.
  B. Elevate foot with knee flexed.
  C. Employ intermittent pneumatic compression device (contraindicated in patients with acute embolus in extremity).
  D. Refer to physical therapy and/or occupational therapy.
  E. Monitor laboratory parameters—PT, PTT, and INR.
  F. Provide patient education.
    1. Medication administration.
    2. Preventive measures.
    3. Bleeding precautions if patient taking anticoagulant.
    4. Dietary restrictions—avoid foods high in vitamin K.
    5. Smoking cessation.
    6. Activity restrictions.

REFERENCES

Alexandre, J., Cautela, J., Ederhy, S., Damaj, G. L., Salem, J.-E., Barlesi, F., et al. (2020). Cardiovascular toxicity related to cancer treatment: A pragmatic approach to the American and European cardio-oncology guidelines. *Journal of the American Heart Association*, 9(18), e018403. https://doi.org/10.1161/JAHA.120.018403.

Assaad, S., Kratzert, W. B., Shelley, B., Friedman, M. B., & Perrino, A., Jr. (2018). Assessment of pulmonary edema: Principles and practice. *Journal of Cardiothoracic and Vascular Anesthesia*, 32(2), 901–914. https://doi.org/10.1053/j.jvca.2017.08.028.

Azhar, S. H., Lim, H. Y., Tan, B.-K., & Angeli, V. (2020). The unresolved pathophysiology of lymphedema. *Frontiers in Physiology*, 11, 137. https://doi.org/10.3389/fphys.2020.00137.

Besnard, A., Raoux, F., Khelil, N., Monin, J.-L., Saal, J. P., Veugeois, A., et al. (2019). Current management of symptomatic pericardial effusions in cancer patients. *Journal of the American College of CardioOncology*, 1(1), 137–140. https://doi.org/10.1016/j.jaccao.2019.07.001.

Bowman, C., Piedalue, K.-A., Baydoun, M., & Carlson, L. E. (2020). The quality of life and psychosocial implications of cancer-related lower-extremity lymphedema: A systematic review of the literature. *Journal of Clinical Medicine, 9*(10), 3200. https://doi.org/10.3390/jcm9103200.

Clark, R. A., Marin, T. S., McCarthy, A. L., Bradley, J., Grover, S., Peters, R., et al. (2019). Cardiotoxicity after cancer treatment: A process map of the patient treatment journey. *Cardio-Oncology, 5*, 14. https://doi.org/10.1186/s40959-019-0046-5.

Connolly, E. A., Bamford, P. A., & Hiriyanna Gowda, G. M. (2018). Malignant pericardial effusions: Single centre retrospective review. *Journal of Clinical Oncology, 36*(15_suppl), e13580. https://doi.org/10.1200/JCO.2018.36.15_suppl.e13580.

Dean, S. M., Valenti, E., Hock, K., Leffler, J., Compston, A., & Abraham, W. T. (2020). The clinical characteristics of lower extremity lymphedema in 440 patients. *Journal of Vascular Surgery: Venous and Lymphatic Disorders, 8*(5), 851–859. https://doi.org/10.1016/j.jvsv.2019.11.014.

Dyadyk, A. I., Kugler, T. E., Schukina, E. V., Zborovskyy, S. R., & Suliman, Y. V. (2018). The pathophysiology of systemic edema. *Nephrology and Dialysis, 19*(4), 438–448. https://doi.org/10.28996/1680-4422-2017-4-438-448.

Eapen, S., & Firstenberg, M. (2018). Standardized approach to pericardial effusion management. *International Journal of Academic Medicine, 4*(2), 160–168. https://doi.org/10.4103/IJAM.IJAM_91_17.

Fernandes, C. J., Morinaga, L. T. K., Alves, J. L., Jr., Castro, M. A., Calderaro, D., Jardim, C. V. P., et al. (2019). Cancer-associated thrombosis: The when, how and why. *European Respiratory Review, 28*(151). https://doi.org/10.1183/16000617.0119-2018.

Greene, A. K., & Goss, J. A. (2018). Diagnosis and staging of lymphedema. *Seminars in Plastic Surgery, 32*(1), 12–16. https://doi.org/10.1055/s-0038-1635117.

Herrmann, J. (2020a). Adverse cardiac effects of cancer therapies: Cardiotoxicity and arrhythmia. *Nature Reviews Cardiology, 17*(8), 474–502. https://doi.org/10.1038/s41569-020-0348-1.

Herrmann, J. (2020b). Vascular toxic effects of cancer therapies. *Nature Reviews Cardiology, 17*(8), 503–522. https://doi.org/10.1038/s41569-020-0347-2.

Itkin, M., Rockson, S. G., & Burkhoff, D. (2021). Pathophysiology of the lymphatic system in patients with heart failure: JACC state-of-the-art review. *Journal of the American College of Cardiology, 78*(3), 278–290. https://doi.org/10.1016/j.jacc.2021.05.021.

Jayaraj, A., Raju, S., May, C., & Pace, N. (2019). The diagnostic unreliability of classic physical signs of lymphedema. *Journal of Vascular Surgery: Venous and Lymphatic Disorders, 7*(6), 890–897. https://doi.org/10.1016/j.jvsv.2019.04.013.

Kamel, M. K., & Blebea, J. (2020). Pathophysiology of edema in patients with chronic venous insufficiency. *Phlebolymphology, 27*(1), 3–10. https://www.phlebolymphology.org/pathophysiology-of-edema-in-patients-with-chronic-venous-insufficiency/.

Khoshpouri, P., Hosseini, M., Iranmanesh, A., Mansoori, B., Bedayat, A., McAdams, H., et al. (2021). Acquired pericardial pathologies: Imaging features, clinical significance, and management. *Applied Radiology, 50*(2), 10–15. https://appliedradiology.com/articles/acquired-pericardial-pathologies-imaging-features-clinical-significance-and-management.

Leitao, M. M., Jr., Zhou, Q. C., Gomez-Hidalgo, N. R., Iasonos, A., Baser, R., Mezzancello, M., et al. (2020). Patient-reported outcomes after surgery for endometrial carcinoma: Prevalence of lower-extremity lymphedema after sentinel lymph node mapping versus lymphadenectomy. *Gynecologic Oncology, 156*(1), 147–153. https://doi.org/10.1016/j.ygyno.2019.11.003.

Lo-Cao, E., Hall, S., Parsell, R., Dandie, G., & Fahlström, A. (2021). Neurogenic pulmonary edema. *The American Journal of Emergency Medicine, 45*, 678.e3–678.e5. https://doi.org/10.1016/j.ajem.2020.11.052.

Martin-Almedina, S., Mortimer, P. S., & Ostergaard, P. (2021). Development and physiological functions of the lymphatic system: Insights from human genetic studies of primary lymphedema. *Physiological Reviews, 101*(4), 1809–1871. https://doi.org/10.1152/physrev.00006.2020.

Musgrave, K. M., Power, K., Laffan, M., O'Donnell, J. S., Thachil, J., & Maraveyas, A. (2022). Practical treatment guidance for cancer-associated thrombosis – Managing the challenging patient: A consensus statement. *Critical Reviews in Oncology/Hematology, 171*, 103599. https://doi.org/10.1016/j.critrevonc.2022.103599.

National Cancer Institute. (2019). Lymphedema (PDQ®)–Health professional version. https://www.cancer.gov/about-cancer/treatment/side-effects/lymphedema/lymphedema-hp-pdq.

National Cancer Institute. (2021). *Lymphedema (PDQ®)–Patient version*. https://www.cancer.gov/about-cancer/treatment/side-effects/lymphedema/lymphedema-pdq.

Neves, M. B. M., Stival, M. V., Neves, Y. C. S., da Silva, J. G. P., da Rocha Macedo, D. B., Carnevalli, B. M., et al. (2021). Malignant pericardial effusion as a primary manifestation of metastatic colon cancer: A case report. *Journal of Medical Case Reports, 15*(1), 543. https://doi.org/10.1186/s13256-021-03085-w. Retrieved from https://www.ncbi.nlm.nih.gov/pubmed/34711280.

O'Donnell, T. F., Jr., Allison, G. M., & Iafrati, M. D. (2020). A systematic review of guidelines for lymphedema and the need for contemporary intersocietal guidelines for the management of lymphedema. *Journal of Vascular Surgery: Venous and Lymphatic Disorders, 8*(4), 676–684. https://doi.org/10.1016/j.jvsv.2020.03.006.

Oikonomou, E., Anastasiou, M, Siasos, G., Androulakis, E., Psyrri, A., Toutouzas, K., et al. (2018). Cancer therapeutics-related cardiovascular complications. Mechanisms, diagnosis and treatment. *Current Pharmaceutical Design, 24*(37), 4424–4435. https://doi.org/10.2174/1381612825666190111101459.

Oyakawa, T., Muraoka, N., Iida, K., Kusuhara, M., Naito, T., & Omae, K. (2018). Characteristics of cellular composition in malignant pericardial effusion and its association with the clinical course of carcinomatous pericarditis. *Japanese Journal of Clinical Oncology, 48*(3), 291–294. https://doi.org/10.1093/jjco/hyx187.

Polonsky, T. S., & DeCara, J. M. (2019). Risk factors for chemotherapy-related cardiac toxicity. *Current Opinion in Cardiology, 34*(3), 283–288. https://doi.org/10.1097/hco.0000000000000619.

Puwanant, S., Kittipibul, V., Songsirisuk, N., Santisukwongchote, S., Sitticharoenchai, P., Chattranukulchai, P., et al. (2022). Idiopathic pericardial effusion in patients with hypertrophic cardiomyopathy. *The International Journal of Cardiovascular Imaging, 38*, 331–337. https://doi.org/10.1007/s10554-021-02424-8.

Qin, E. S., Bowen, M. J., & Chen, W. F. (2018). Diagnostic accuracy of bioimpedance spectroscopy in patients with lymphedema: A retrospective cohort analysis. *Journal of Plastic, Reconstructive & Aesthetic Surgery, 71*(7), 1041–1050. https://doi.org/10.1016/j.bjps.2018.02.012.

Ravi, C., & Gang, M. (2019). Managing complications of new-age cancer therapy. *Emergency Medicine Reports, 40*(7), 31.

Russell, R., 3rd (2018). Cardio-oncology: Understanding cardiotoxicity to guide patient focused imaging. *Journal of Nuclear Cardiology, 25*(6), 2159–2167. https://doi.org/10.1007/s12350-018-01470-5.

Shields, B. (2018). Cardiotoxic effects of cancer therapy. *American Nurse Today*, 13(12), 3.

Schellack, G., Modau, T., & Schellack, N. (2020). Clinical overview of venous thromboembolism. *South African Pharmaceutical Journal*, 87(6). Retrieved from https://hdl.handle.net/10520/ejc-mp_sapj-v87-n6-a5.

Spinelli, B., Kallan, M. J., Zhang, X., Cheville, A., Troxel, A., Cohn, J., et al. (2019). Intra- and interrater reliability and concurrent validity of a new tool for assessment of breast cancer-related lymphedema of the upper extremity. *Archives of Physical Medicine and Rehabilitation*, 100(2), 315–326. https://doi.org/10.1016/j.apmr.2018.08.185.

Streiff, M. B., Holmstrom, B., Angelini, D., Ashrani, A., Elshoury, A., Fanikos, J., et al. (2021). Cancer-associated venous thromboembolic disease, v. 2.2021, NCCN Clinical Practice Guidelines in Oncology. *Journal of the National Comprehensive Cancer Network*, 19(10), 1181–1201. https://doi.org/10.6004/jnccn.2021.0047.

Upshaw, J. N. (2020). Cardioprotective strategies to prevent cancer treatment-related cardiovascular toxicity: A review. *Current Oncology Reports*, 22(7), 72. https://doi.org/10.1007/s11912-020-00923-w.

Wang, S., Zhao, J., Wang, C., & Zhang, N. (2021). Prognosis and role of clinical and imaging features in patients with malignant pericardial effusion: A single-center study in China. *BMC Cardiovascular Disorders*, 21(1), 565. https://doi.org/10.1186/s12872-021-02331-9.

Woods, M. (2019). Risk factors for the development of oedema and lymphoedema. *British Journal of Nursing*, 28(4), 219–222. https://doi.org/10.12968/bjon.2019.28.4.219.

Xiong, W. (2021). Current status of treatment of cancer-associated venous thromboembolism. *Thrombosis Journal*, 19(1), 21. https://doi.org/10.1186/s12959-021-00274-x.

35

Cognitive Symptoms

Catherine E. Jansen

CANCER AND CANCER TREATMENT–RELATED COGNITIVE IMPAIRMENT

Overview

I. Definition—functional decline in one or more cognitive domains (e.g., attention and concentration, executive function, information processing speed, language, motor function, visuospatial skill, learning, and memory) and may represent a single highly specific deficit or a cluster of related deficits (Jansen et al., 2019).

II. Pathophysiology (Allen, Myers, Jansen, Merriman, & Von Ah, 2018; Hong et al., 2020; Mayo et al., 2021; Schagen, Tsvetkov, Compter, & Wefel, 2022; Underwood et al., 2018).

A. The pathophysiology of cancer and cancer treatment–related cognitive impairment is not fully understood and likely multifactorial.

B. Direct effects of central nervous system (CNS) tumors, surgical removal of CNS tumors, and cranial irradiation, which can result in structural and functional damage specific to tumor location (Chang, Mehta, Vogelbaum, Taylor, & Shluwalia, 2019; Constanzo et al., 2020).

C. Proposed underlying mechanisms are related to:
1. Direct injury to neurons and/or other brain structures
2. Disruption of the blood–brain barrier
3. DNA damage
4. Cytokine dysregulation that can impair neural functioning and neurotransmitter metabolism
5. Oxidative stress triggering cell membrane damage and free radical formation
6. Inflammatory responses associated with reduced neurogenesis
7. Changes in hormonal levels (e.g., estrogen, testosterone)

III. Risk factors (Allen et al., 2018; Buskbjerg, Amidi, Demontis, Nissen, & Zachariae, 2019; Mayo et al., 2021).

A. Disease-related factors
1. Primary CNS cancers: prevalence 90%
2. Non-CNS cancers: prevalence variable, estimated up to 40% before treatment
3. Advanced, metastatic, or terminal disease

B. Treatment-related factors:

1. Dose intensity, cumulative effect, and/or multimodality therapy
2. Treatment toxicities (e.g., anemia, fatigue, nausea, and organ dysfunction)
3. Concomitant or supportive medications (e.g., analgesics, anesthesia, anticholinergics, antidepressants, antiemetics, benzodiazepines, corticosteroids, and immunosuppressants)

C. Individual characteristics that may increase the risk for cognitive impairment
1. Age (cognitive decline occurs with aging)
2. Sensory deficits (e.g., hearing, vision)
3. Comorbidities (e.g., cardiovascular disease, hypertension, and diabetes)
4. Genetic polymorphisms (e.g., apolipoprotein E4 allele, brain-derived neurotrophic factor, and catechol-O-methyltransferase val allele); proinflammatory cytokines (e.g., IL-6, TNF-α)
5. Nutritional deficiencies
6. Psychological factors (e.g., anxiety, depression, and stress)

Assessment

(Allen et al., 2018; Mayo et al., 2021; National Comprehensive Cancer Network [NCCN], 2022)

I. History and physical examination

A. Screen for the presence of cognitive complaints with probing questions—difficulties with retaining new information, handling complex tasks, altered perception, and/or impaired communication.

B. Medical history—cancer history (e.g., disease trajectory), current and prior cancer treatments, systemic cancer and/or treatment effects, presence of significant comorbidities, current medications, and symptoms (e.g., pain, fatigue, and sleep disturbance).

C. Neurologic assessment for the presence of any focal deficits and refer for further evaluation and/or neuropsychological testing as indicated.

II. Psychosocial assessment

A. Changes in emotional and behavioral affect (e.g., anxiety, depression, and distress).

B. Lifestyle factors (e.g., alcohol or drug use, diet, and exercise), nutritional deficiencies, and work history.

C. Impact of cognitive impairment on social interactions and ability to function.

III. Imaging and laboratory tests

A. Complete blood cell (CBC) count with differential to rule out anemia.

B. Electrolytes, including calcium, to rule out electrolyte imbalance(s).

C. Liver, renal, and thyroid function tests to determine any organ dysfunction.

D. Vitamin B_1, B_{12}, and folate levels to evaluate for vitamin deficiencies.

E. Computed tomography (CT) or magnetic resonance imaging (MRI) to rule out structural abnormalities in patients with focal neurologic deficits or at high risk for recurrence or metastatic disease to the CNS.

Management

(Jansen et al., 2019; Mayo et al., 2021; NCCN, 2022; Schagen et al., 2022; Von Ah & Crouch, 2020)

I. Pharmacological management has yet to be established as effective.

A. Acetylcholinesterase inhibitors (e.g., donepezil)—effectiveness not established, but NCCN guidelines recommend considering trial use if nonpharmacologic interventions are not effective.

B. Psychostimulants (e.g., dexmethylphenidate, methylphenidate, and modafinil) lack evidence, but NCCN recommends trial use as a second-line intervention.

C. N-Methyl-D-aspartate receptors (e.g., memantine)—effectiveness not established

II. Nonpharmacological management

A. Validate experience and provide patient education.

B. Cognitive training—structured repetitive tasks aimed at improving a specific cognitive skill (e.g., attention, memory).

C. Cognitive behavioral interventions—adaptive strategies aimed at compensating for cognitive impairment.

D. Exercise (e.g., aerobics, resistance training, tai chi, and yoga).

DELIRIUM

Overview

I. Definition—disturbance in the level of attention and awareness, often accompanied by changes in other cognitive domains and characterized by an acute onset (hours to days) with fluctuations in symptom(s) severity throughout the day (Majzoub et al., 2019; Thom, Levy-Carrck, Phil, Bui, & Silbersweig, 2019).

A. Hypoactive delirium: characterized by the presence of psychomotor retardation, sedation, lethargy, and/or decreased awareness of surroundings.

B. Hyperactive delirium: characterized by the presence of restlessness, hypervigilance, agitation, hallucinations, and/or delusions.

C. Mixed delirium: characterized by alternating features of both hypoactive and hyperactive delirium.

II. Pathophysiology (Majzoub et al., 2019; Thom et al., 2019).

A. Indirect effects of cancer, cancer treatment(s), and/or concomitant medications that result in organ failure, metabolic or electrolyte imbalance, infection, inflammation, oxidative stress, and/or paraneoplastic syndromes.

B. Substance intoxication or withdrawal (e.g., alcohol, benzodiazepines).

C. Alteration in neurotransmitter synthesis, function, and/or activity secondary to systemic disturbances.

III. Risk factors (Bush et al., 2018; Jung et al., 2021; Lee, 2020; Majzoub et al., 2019; Thom et al., 2019).

A. Disease related

1. Primary or metastatic CNS disease.

2. Non-CNS cancers: prevalence 25%–40%, most commonly when hospitalized.

3. Advanced or terminal-stage cancers: prevalence 45%–88%, most commonly at end of life.

4. Paraneoplastic syndromes (e.g., syndrome of inappropriate antidiuretic hormone secretion).

B. Treatment related

1. Cancer treatments (e.g., chemotherapy, immunotherapy, radiation to CNS, and surgery [e.g., postoperative effects in elderly]).

2. Concomitant or supportive medications (e.g., analgesics, antidepressants, antiemetics, antihistamines, antiinfectives, antivirals, and corticosteroids).

3. Treatment toxicities (e.g., dehydration, electrolyte, and/or metabolic abnormalities [e.g., calcium, glucose, and sodium], neuropsychiatric complications [e.g., encephalopathy, hallucinations, and delusions]).

C. Other pertinent contributing factors—alcohol or drug (e.g., barbiturates, benzodiazepines, selective serotonin reuptake inhibitors, and opioids) withdrawal, corticosteroids, dehydration, hypoxia, organ dysfunction, systemic infections and sepsis, and unrelieved pain.

D. Individual characteristics—advanced age, baseline dementia, reduced mobility and/or functional performance status, nutritional deficiencies (e.g., B_1, B_9, and B_{12}), sensory impairments (e.g., visual, hearing), and sleep–wake disturbances.

Assessment

(Bush et al., 2018; Lee, 2020; Majzoub et al., 2019; Thom et al., 2019)

I. History and physical examination (involve caregivers)

A. Medical history—cancer history (e.g., disease trajectory), current cancer treatments, recent febrile illness, history of organ failure, and presence of risk factors for delirium.

B. Review current medications and identify those known to cause delirium or that have high anticholinergic potential.

C. Attention to neurologic status (acute change in mental status with a fluctuating course, inattention, disorganized thinking, altered level of consciousness, agitation, restlessness, hallucinations, or delusions).

II. Imaging and laboratory tests targeted to evaluate for suspected etiology
   A. Electrolytes, including calcium, magnesium, and sodium.
   B. CBC with differential.
   C. Urinalysis and culture if indicated.
   D. Arterial blood gas if hypoxic.
   E. Hepatic, renal, and thyroid function tests.
   F. Lumbar puncture can be considered if etiology is not obvious.
   G. Brain imaging (e.g., CT, MRI).

Management

(Bush et al., 2018; Majzoub et al., 2019)

I. Pharmacological management
   A. Identify and treat reversible causes (e.g., dehydration, infection, metabolic imbalance, and pain).
   B. Minimize, taper, or discontinue medications (e.g., anticholinergics, anticonvulsants, benzodiazepines, corticosteroids, and opioids) that may contribute to delirium.
   C. The use of antipsychotic medications is controversial and if utilized, should only be used in a time-limited trial with the lowest effect dose for patients with severe symptoms when nonpharmacological management is not effective.

II. Nonpharmacological management
   A. Minimize sensory deficits (eyeglasses, hearing aid).
   B. Promote uninterrupted sleep.
   C. Encourage ambulation.
   D. Minimize dehydration and/or malnutrition.
   E. Avoid excessive sensory stimulation and/or restraints.
   F. Provide frequent reorientation and reassurance.
   G. Incorporate environmental strategies (e.g., well-lit room with familiar objects, visible clock/calendar, and caregiver continuity).

REFERENCES

Allen, D., Myers, J., Jansen, C., Merriman, J., & Von Ah, D. (2018). Assessment and management of cancer- and cancer treatment related cognitive impairment. *Journal for Nurse Practitioners, 14*(4), 217–224. https://doi.org/10.1016/J.NURPRA.2017.11.026.

Bush, S. H., Lawlor, P. G., Ryan, K., Ceneno, C., Lucchesi, M., Kanji, S., et al. (2018). Delirium in adult cancer patients: ESMO Clinical Practice Guidelines. *Annals of Oncology, 29*(Suppl. 4), iv143–iv165. https://doi.org/10.1093/annonc/mdy147.

Buskbjerg, C. D. R., Amidi, A., Demontis, D., Nissen, E. R., & Zachariae, R. (2019). Genetic risk factors for cancer-related cognitive impairment: A systematic review. *Acta Oncologica, 58*(5), 537–547. https://doi.org/10.1080/0284186X.2019.1578410.

Chang, S. M., Mehta, M. P., Vogelbaum, M. A., Taylor, M. D., & Ahluwalia, M. S. (2019). Neoplasms of the central nervous system. In V. T. DeVita, T. S. Lawrence, & S. A. Rosenberg (Eds.), *DeVita, Hellman, and Rosenberg's cancer: Principles & practice of oncology* (11th ed., pp. 1263–1332). Philadelphia, PA: Lippincott Williams & Wilkins.

Constanzo, J., Midavaine, É., Fouquet, J., Lepage, M., Descoteaux, M., Kirby, K., et al. (2020). Brain irradiation leads to persistent neuroinflammation and long-term neurocognitive dysfunction in a region-specific manner. *Progress in Neuro-Psychopharmacology and Biological Psychiatry, 102*, 109954. https://doi.org/10.1016/j.pnpbp.2020.109954.

Hong, J.-H., Huang, C.-Y., Chang, C.-H., Muo, C.-H., Jaw, F.-S., Lu, Y.-C., et al. (2020). Different androgen deprivation therapies might have a differential impact on cognition – An analysis from a population-based study using time-dependent exposure model. *Cancer Epidemiology, 64*, 101657. https://doi.org/10.1016/j.canep.2019.101657.

Jansen, C. E., Von Ah, D., Allen, D. H., Mayo, S., Merriman, J. D., & Myers, J. S. (2019). *Cognitive impairment*. Pittsburgh, PA: Oncology Nursing Society. https://www.ons.org/pep/cognitive-impairment.

Jung, P., Puts, M., Frankel, N., Syed, A. T., Alam, Z., Yeung, L., et al. (2021). Delirium incidence, risk factors, and treatments in older adults receiving chemotherapy: A systematic review and meta-analysis. *Journal of Geriatric Oncology, 12*(3), 352–360. https://doi.org/10.1016/j.jgo.2020.08.011.

Lee, E. Q. (2020). Neurologic complications in patients with cancer. *Continuum: Lifelong Learning in Neurology, 26*(6), 1629–1645. https://doi.org/10.1212/CON.0000000000000937.

Majzoub, I. E., Abunafeesa, H., Cheaito, R., Cheaito, M. A., & Elsa, A. F. (2019). Management of altered mental status and delirium in cancer patients. *Annals of Palliative Medicine, 8*(5):728–739. https://doi.org/10.21037/apm.2019.09.14.

Mayo, S. J., Lustberg, M., Dhillon, H., Nakamura, Z. M., Allen, D. H., Von Ah, D., et al. (2021). Cancer-related cognitive impairment in patients with non-central nervous system malignancies: An overview for oncology providers from the MASCC Neurological Complications Study Group. *Supportive Care in Cancer, 29*(6), 2821–2840. https://doi.org/10.1007/s00520-020-05860-9.

National Comprehensive Cancer Network (NCCN). (2022). *NCCN clinical practice guidelines in oncology: Survivorship [v.1.2022]*. https://www.nccn.org/professionals/physician_gls/pdf/survivorship.pdf.

Schagen, S. B., Tsvetkov, A. S., Compter, A., & Wefel, J. S. (2022). Cognitive adverse effects of chemotherapy and immunotherapy: Are interventions within reach? *Nature Reviews Neurology, 18*(3), 173–185. https://doi.org/10.1038/s41582-021-00617-2.

Thom, R. P., Levy-Carrick, N. C., Bui, M., & Silbersweig, D. (2019). Delirium. *American Journal of Psychiatry, 176*(10), 785–793.

Underwood, E. A., Rochon, P. A., Moineddin, R., Lee, P. E., Wu, W., Pritchard, K. I., et al. (2018). Cognitive sequelae of endocrine therapy in women treated for breast cancer: A meta-analysis. *Breast Cancer Research and Treatment, 168*(2), 299–310. https://doi.org/10.1007/s10549-017-4627-4.

Von Ah, D., & Crouch, A. (2020). Cognitive rehabilitation for cognitive dysfunction after cancer and cancer treatment: Implications for nursing practice. *Seminars in Oncology Nursing, 36*(1), 150977. https://doi.org/10.1016/j.soncn.2019.150977.

36

Endocrine Symptoms

Deena Centofanti

OVERVIEW

I. Description of the Endocrine System
  A. The endocrine system coordinates body functions through hormones which can affect the organ of origin (paracrine effect), the same cell (autocrine effect), or distant organ (endocrine) (Barnabei et al., 2022; Melmed et al., 2020; Moini, Badolato, & Ahangari, 2021).
  B. Endocrine hormones enter the bloodstream, selectively bind to target cells, and regulate activity.
  C. Cancer and its treatment can cause acute or delayed toxicity of the affected gland or organ.
  D. Endocrine organs are thyroid, parathyroid, adrenal, pituitary gland, hypothalamus, pineal, thymus, pancreas, ovaries, and testes.
    1. Thyroid gland:
      a. Function: secretes triiodothyronine (T_3) and thyroxine (T_4) as a result of the pituitary gland producing and releasing thyroid-stimulating hormone (TSH) into the bloodstream. T_3 and T_4 regulates metabolism, body temperature, and heart rate
      b. Dysfunction: hypothyroidism, hyperthyroidism, thyroiditis, Graves disease, and goiters
    2. Parathyroid gland:
      a. Function: secretes parathyroid hormone (PTH). PHT binds to surface cells in the bone and kidney regulating serum calcium and vitamin D levels.
      b. Dysfunction: hyperparathyroidism, hypoparathyroidism
    3. Adrenal gland:
      a. Function of adrenal cortex (outer part): secretes mineralocorticoids (aldosterone), glucocorticoids (cortisol), and androgens
        (1) Mineralocorticoids help maintain the body's salt and water levels
        (2) Glucocorticoids help regulate body meta-bolism
      b. Function of adrenal medulla (inner part): produces catecholamines during stress (fight or flight response)
      c. Dysfunction: primary or secondary adrenal insufficiency and Cushing syndrome
    4. Pituitary gland:
      a. Function: known as the "master gland" because it produces hormones signaling organs and glands to maintain and regulate function. Secretes adrenocorticotropic hormone, gonadotropic hormones (luteinizing hormone, follicle-stimulating hormone), human growth hormone [ADH], and oxytocin.
      b. Dysfunction: hypopituitarism, hypophysitis, and central diabetes
    5. Pancreas:
      a. Function: the islets of Langerhans help control blood glucose levels by producing insulin and glucagon
      b. Dysfunction: diabetes, hyperinsulinemia, pancreatitis, and benign tumors (insulinoma and glucagonoma)
  E. Etiology and risk factors (Brady, 2019; Chemaitilly et al., 2019; Gebauer, Higham, Langer, Denzer, & Brabant, 2019)
    1. Disease related: cancer of the thyroid, parathyroid, pituitary, adrenal gland, or pancreas as well as multiple endocrine neoplasia
    2. Treatment related:
      a. Surgical resection—thyroid, parathyroid, adrenal, pituitary gland, or pancreas
      b. External radiation—cranial, head and neck (doses of 18 Gy or more), mantle field, total body irradiation, age at time of therapy (children greater risk) (Yu, 2019; Trump, 2020)
      c. Radioiodine (I-131) therapy (Yu, 2019)
      d. System therapy (Brady, 2019; Pandy, Goyal, & Ernstoff, 2022; Trump, 2020; Wood, Moldawer, & Lewis, 2019)
        (1) Chemotherapy: asparaginase, streptozocin, and high-dose cytarabine
        (2) Immune modulatory therapy: immune checkpoint inhibitors (ICIs [pembrolizumab, nivolumab]), interferon-alfa, interleukin-2, lenalidomide, and thalidomide
        (3) Small molecule inhibitors (mTor, TKI): imatinib, sunitinib, and temsirolimus
        (4) High-dose chemotherapy preparative regimens for stem cell transplant: busulfan, cyclophosphamide
        (5) Chimeric antigen receptor therapy

(6) Supportive care medications: bisphosphonates, denosumab, glucocorticoids, granulocyte/macrophage colony-stimulating factor (GM-CSF), and ketoconazole

ASSESSMENT

II. Presentation
(Brahmer et al., 2021; Cooksley et al., 2020; Schneider et al., 2021; Wood et al., 2019)
   A. Initial presentation: may be vague; have a low threshold for clinical suspicion of endocrinopathy (Table 36.1)
      1. Assessment and diagnostic testing should be performed to determine the need for early management.
      2. Undiagnosed and untreated endocrinopathies may lead to life-threatening complications necessitating treatment being temporarily held or discontinued.
      3. Consistent assessment and documentation in the electronic medical record allows health care providers to identify minor changes over the course of treatment.
      4. ICI toxicity:
         a. Grade 2 toxicity: consider holding ICI and resume when symptoms and/or laboratory values reverse to grade 1 or less
         b. Grade 3 toxicity: hold ICI and initiate corticosteroids; rechallenge patient with treatment once symptoms and/or laboratory values resolve
         c. Grade 4 toxicity: discontinuation of ICI unless endocrinopathies are controlled with hormone therapy
   B. Oncology Nursing Society tool kit "Recognize It; Report It": guide for early recognition of adverse effects of treatment and where to report adverse events (Oncology Nursing Society, 2023)
   C. Food and Drug Administration Risk Evaluation and Mitigation Strategy program for medications with endocrine side effects: ipilimumab, lenalidomide, thalidomide (U.S. Food & Drug Administration, 2022)
   D. Identify patients at greater risk of developing endocrinopathies:
      1. Patients with higher BMI and higher baseline TSH with treatment initiation are at increased risk of thyroid dysfunction.
      2. Elderly patients, especially with poor performance status and comorbidities, tend to have increased side effects of treatment.
         a. Diabetes and osteoporosis may worsen with steroid therapy.
         b. Consider prophylactic antibiotics for long-term immunosuppressive therapies (Presley, Gomes, Burd, Kanesvaran, & Wong, 2021).

MANAGEMENT

III. Endocrinopathy Management
(Davies, 2019; National Comprehensive Cancer Network® [NCCN], 2022; Schneider et al., 2021; Trump, 2020; Wood et al., 2019)
   A. Pharmacologic management
      1. Referral to endocrinologist may be required.

   B. Nonpharmacologic management
      1. Provide patient with immunotherapy wallet card or medical alert device so emergency health care providers are aware of treatment and endocrinopathy.
      2. Patient education:
         a. Early identification of treatment side effects
         b. Address patient concerns that treatment will be discontinued as a result of side effects; most side effects can be managed when diagnosed and treated early.
IV. Hyperthyroidism management
   A. Pharmacologic management
      1. Risk factors: women, elderly iodine deficiency/excess, smoking
      2. Secondary to ICIs (NCCN, 2022; Schneider et al., 2021)
         a. Patients at low risk for cardiovascular events: symptomatic treatment with beta-blockers (propranolol 10–20 mg every 4–6 hours for symptoms)
            (1) Assess patient for history of asthma and chronic obstructive airway disease prior to initiating treatment (Fazal-Sanderson, Karavitaki, & Mihai, 2019).
         b. Patients at high risk for cardiovascular events (e.g., history of coronary artery disease, cardiac arrhythmia, and heart failure): methylprednisolone 1–2 mg/kg daily until severity of toxicity is resolved to baseline.
         c. Monitor TSH and free T_4 every 2–3 weeks after diagnosis, as most cases progress to hypothyroidism.
         d. Monitor TSH and T_4 laboratory results, report any abnormalities.
      3. Secondary to other causes (Fazal-Sanderson et al., 2019; Hollenberg et al., 2020)
         a. Antithyroid agents: first-line treatment is methimazole (MMI); propylthiouracil may be indicated but has rare hepatotoxicity
            (1) Monitor for bone marrow suppression: fever, sore throat, stomatitis.
            (2) Patient should be educated to stop medication and call health care team for evaluation and lab work.
         b. Radioactive iodine (I-131)
            (1) Can cause transient exacerbation of hyperthyroidism; consider treatment with beta-blocker or MMI for patients at risk of complications.
            (2) Monitor thyroid function tests 1–2 months after treatment and every 4–6 weeks until patient is euthyroid or hypothyroid.
            (3) Most patients will become hypothyroid after 12 months.
            (4) Educate patients regarding the use of contraception; avoid fathering children for 4 months and pregnancy for 6 months.
         c. Surgery: consider SSKI 2–3 drops twice daily given 7–10 days
   B. Nonpharmacologic management
      1. Promote adequate hydration
      2. Patient education on strategies to manage fatigue (Chapter 37)

TABLE 36.1 Endocrinopathy Assessment

Endocrine Organ Dysfunction	Presentation	Physical Examination	Diagnostic Tests
Hyperthyroidism/ thyrotoxicosis	Anxiety, emotional liability, agitation, weakness, dyspnea, palpitation, heat intolerance, and increased perspiration	Weight loss, tremor, hyperactivity, rapid speech, lid lag, warm and moist skin, hair thinning, tachycardia, irregular pulse, hyperreflexia, and proximal muscle weakness	Low TSH; high (or normal) free T_4 and T_3 concentrations Thyrotoxic storm: rare US, CT scan, or MRI of neck: rarely needed
Hypothyroidism	Fatigue, weakness, depression, dyspnea, constipation, cold intolerance, myalgias, and arthralgias	Weight gain, dry coarse skin, skin thickening, hoarseness, decreased hearing, slow speech, delayed relaxation of tendon reflexes, bradycardia, periorbital edema, enlargement of tongue, and diastolic hypertension	Primary: normal-high TSH; low free T_4 and T_3 concentrations Secondary (due to central dysfunction, i.e., hypophysitis): low or normal TSH; low free T_4
Hyperparathyroidism	"Moans, groans, stones, and bones ... with psychiatric overtones", fatigue, anorexia, weakness, depression, cognitive or neuromuscular dysfunction, bone pain, polyuria, and polydipsia If severe: nausea, emesis, confusion, lethargy, and stupor	Hypertension, bradycardia Renal colic If severe: asymptomatic bone fractures Severe: parathyroid crisis/storm	Hypercalcemia, elevated PTH, normal or elevated 1,25D concentration; hypercalciuric, decreased eGFR, decreased serum phosphate, and magnesium Abdominal US or CT: kidney stones ECG: shortened QT interval If severe: decreased bone density
Hypoparathyroidism	Fatigue, anxiety, depression, and irritability *Acute hypocalcemia:* tetany (perioral numbness, paresthesia of hands and feet, muscle cramps, laryngospasm, imbalance, and seizures) *Chronic hypocalcemia:* coarse hair, dry skin, brittle nails, and pruritis	Acute: hypotension, heart failure Chronic: skeletal abnormalities, dental abnormalities, and cataracts	Hypocalcemia, low PTH level, normal 25[OH]D; normal or low 1,25D concentration Acute hypocalcemia: prolonged QT interval, arrhythmia Skeletal survey to rule out lytic bone lesions
Hypopituitarism, hypophysitis	Fatigue, anorexia, visual changes, headache, myalgias, polyuria, and polydipsia	Hypotension, tachycardia, and weight loss	Secondary adrenal insufficiency: normal or low morning ACTH, low or undetectable cortisol level, hyponatremia Alteration in LH, FSH, and prolactin estradiol (females) and testosterone (males) Central hypothyroidism Type 1 diabetes: hyponatremia MRI of brain with pituitary cuts Electrolyte disturbances
Adrenal insufficiency	Anorexia, nausea, emesis, abdominal pain, fatigue, myalgias, arthralgias, dizziness, syncope, lethargy, impaired memory, irritability, and confusion	Hypotension, postural hypotension Adrenal crisis (life-threatening): hypovolemic shock, coma	Low basal morning serum cortisol (<3 µg/dL [80 nmol/L]), suboptimal response to short ACTH (cosyntropin) stimulation test, low ACTH, hyponatremia, and hypoglycemia (hold opioids for at least 8 h before testing, as opioids can suppress pituitary–adrenal axis) Abdominal CT or MRI: rarely required
Diabetes insipidus	Polyuria, polydipsia		Serum and urine osmolarity after 8–12 h without fluid intake: fluid deprivation test

1,25D, 1,25-Dihydroxyvitamin D; *25[OH]D*, serum 25-hydroxyvitamin D; *ACTH*, adrenocorticotropic hormone; *eGFR*, estimated glomerular filtration rate; *FSH*, follicle-stimulating hormone; *LH*, luteinizing hormone; *PTH*, parathyroid hormone; T_3, total triiodothyronine; T_4, total thyroxine; *TPO*, antithyroid peroxidase; *TSH*, thyroid-stimulating hormone; *US*, ultrasound.
Data from Anderson, B., & Morganstein, D. L. (2021). Endocrine toxicity of cancer immunotherapy: Clinical challenges. *Endocrine Connections*, *10*(3), R116–R124. https://doi.org/10.1530/EC-20-0489; Davies, M. (2019). Acute and long-term adverse events associated with checkpoint blockade. *Seminars in Oncology Nursing*, *35*(5), 150926. https://doi.org/10.1016/j.soncn.2019.08.005.

V. Hypothyroidism (Brent & Weetman, 2020; Trifanescu & Poiana, 2019)
 A. Pharmacologic Management
  1. Monitor TSH and T4 every 4–6 weeks as part of routine care if patient receiving ICI therapy.
  2. Patients will require lifetime repletion (Davies, 2019; Schneider et al., 2021).
   a. Assess for secondary adrenal insufficiency prior to starting levothyroxine to prevent triggering an adrenal crisis.
   b. Asymptomatic/mild hypothyroidism (TSH <10 U/L): monitor TSH, free T_4; consider levothyroxine for TSH >10 U/L
   c. Levothyroxine: 1.6 µg/kg/day, take with water on an empty stomach
   d. Older patients and those with coronary artery disease and patients with comorbidities titrate up from a lower starting dose (25–50 µg/day)
   e. Monitor TSH and T_4 levels. It takes 4–6 weeks to reach steady-state concentration before dose adjustments are made.
    (1) Adjust dosing to patient symptoms and T_4 level; TSH cannot be used to monitor, as it is suppressed in patients taking levothyroxine supplements.
   f. Monitor TSH and T_4 levels every 4–6 weeks until stable, then every 6 months.
   g. Monitor for potential drug interactions that may interfere with the absorption or metabolism of levothyroxine (Table 36.2).
  3. Patients treated with brain, head, and neck irradiation should have TSH and free T_4 measured yearly.
  4. Referral to cardiologist may be required for the management of dyslipidemia and atherosclerosis.
 B. Nonpharmacologic management
  1. Promote rest and hydration
  2. Patient education on strategies to prevent and manage gastrointestinal motility (constipation)
VI. Hyperparathyroidism management (Mundy & Crowley, 2019; Bringhurst, Demay, & Kronenberg, 2020)
 A. Pharmacologic management
  1. Mnemonic "stones, bones, groans, and moans": kidney stone, osteoporosis, gastrointestinal symptoms, and neuropsychiatric symptoms
  2. Assess kidney function for estimated glomerular filtration rate, as at risk for developing kidney stones.
  3. Avoid factors that aggravate hypercalcemia (diuretics, dehydration, and high-calcium diet).
  4. Parathyroidectomy may be necessary.
  5. Medical management for nonsurgical candidate: Cinacalcet initial dose 30 mg twice daily taken with food; monitor for hypocalcemia
 B. Nonpharmacologic management
  1. Encourage adequate hydration to minimize the risk of nephrolithiasis and prevent constipation.
  2. Provide comfort measures to alleviate bone pain.

TABLE 36.2 **Drugs Interfering With Levothyroxine Absorption and Metabolism**	
Mechanism	**Drug**
Decrease levothyroxine (LT_4) absorption	Cholestyramine, colestipol
	Sucralfate
	Aluminum hydroxide
	Ferrous sulfate
	Antiacids, sucralfate, proton pump inhibitors, and H2 receptor antagonists
	Laxatives
	Calcium carbonate (allow at least 3–4 h between LT_4 and calcium tablets)
	Food: Soy protein supplements, coffee, grapefruit juice, dietary fibers
Increase metabolic (nondeiodinative) levothyroxine clearance	Rifampicin carbamazepine, phenobarbital±phenytoin
Block T_4 to T_3 conversion	Amiodarone
	Glucocorticoids
	Beta-blockers
	Selenium deficiency
Increased need for levothyroxine	Estrogens
Precise mechanism unknown	Sertraline, chloroquine tyrosine kinase inhibitors: imatinib, motesanib, and sorafenib

From Trifanescu, R. & Poiana, C. (2019). Diagnosis and management of hypothyroidism in adults. In S. Llahana, C. Follin, C. Yedinak, & A. Grossman (Eds.), *Advanced practice in endocrinology nursing* (pp. 590). Berlin: Springer.

  3. Provide written and verbal information on diet. Consider referral to nutritionist.
   a. Maintain vitamin D intake; stimulates parathormone secretion and bone resorption.
   b. Low-calcium/high-phosphate diet
  4. Promote rest resulting from muscle weakness.
  5. Monitor fluid balance (intake and output) and serum electrolytes (potassium, calcium, phosphates, and magnesium).
VII. Hypoparathyroidism management: treatment depends on severity (Bringhurst et al., 2020; Mundy & Crowley, 2019)
 A. Pharmacologic management
  1. Acute (corrected calcium ≤7.5 mg/dL, tetany, seizures, and prolonged QT interval): will require emergency intervention with intravenous (IV) calcium gluconate
  2. Mild to moderate and chronic (corrected calcium ≥7.5 mg/dL): oral calcium 1 to 2 g calcium carbonate in divided doses and calcitriol 0.25 µg twice daily (vitamin D), titrated weekly to low-normal calcium levels
  3. Monitor serum calcium, albumin, magnesium, and phosphate levels after surgery.
  4. Monitor urine, serum calcium, and phosphate levels weekly after supplementation initiated.

B. Nonpharmacologic management
  1. Educate on diet (increase in calcium-rich foods, lower phosphate intake).
  2. Monitor for side effects from oral calcium supplements.
    a. Calcium supplement should be in divided doses; intestine can only absorb 500 mg at any time.
  3. Educate patients on the use of proton pump inhibitors.
    a. Associated with hypomagnesium, which can reduce PTH release
    b. Increases gastric pH, which interferes with calcium carbonate absorption
  4. Educate patient about how to take phosphate binders.

VIII. Hypophysitis management (Cooksley et al., 2020; Davies, 2019; Follin, 2019)
  A. Pharmacologic management
    1. Risk factors: men, elderly, and dose related
    2. Potentiates the risk for developing secondary hypothyroidism, secondary adrenal insufficiency, and hypogonadism
      a. Secondary hypothyroidism: thyroid repletion after glucocorticoid deficiency is treated to avoid precipitating adrenal crisis
      b. Secondary adrenal insufficiency: glucocorticoid repletion
      c. Secondary hypogonadism: testosterone
    3. ICI-induced thyrotoxicosis generally evolves into hypothyroidism requiring replacement therapy.
    4. Steroid therapy needs to be held prior to AM cortisol evaluation.
    5. Severe hypophysitis; high-dose steroids (methylprednisolone 1.0–2.0 mg/kg/day tapered over 2 weeks)
    6. Central diabetes insipidus: rare water metabolism (rapid water loss) caused by ADH deficiency (Thompson & Verbalis, 2020)
      a. Assessment:
        (1) Monitor serum sodium to prevent hyponatremia.
        (2) Assess for excessive thirst and polyuria.
      b. Treatment:
        (1) Basal-bolus insulin
        (2) Desmopressin acetate (oral, nasal, and subcutaneous) dosed to achieve urine concentrations lasting 8–24 hours and prevent nocturia
  B. Nonpharmacologic management
    1. Fluid management
    2. Assess for altered mental status.
    3. Monitor for risk of decreased cardiac output such as excess fatigue or shortness of breath with exertion.

IX. Adrenal insufficiency management (Llahana, Mitchelhill, Yeoh, & Quinkler, 2019; Llahana, Zopf, Mitchelhill, & Grossman, 2019; Newell-Price & Auchus, 2020)
  A. Pharmacologic management
    1. Glucocorticoid replacement therapy:
      a. Hydrocortisone repletion to mimic normal cortisol secretion; 30 mg/day in divided doses upon wakening and smaller dose late afternoon (15–20 mg in AM and 5–10 mg in PM) or
        (1) Evening hydrocortisone has been associated with insulin resistance
      b. Prednisone 5–10 mg/day
    2. Mineralocorticoid (primary adrenal insufficiency): fludrocortisone 0.1 mg/day
      a. Consider lower dose (0.05 mg/day) if patient is already on hydrocortisone.
    3. Patients should be instructed in "minor sick-day" stress dosing of steroid repletion.
      a. Adjust glucocorticoids dosing; increase two to three times the standard dose during illness.
      b. Instruct patient to call health care provider if illness persists for more than 3 days.

X. Adrenal crisis management (Husebye, Pearce, Krone, & Kämpe, 2021; Llahana, Mitchelhill et al., 2019; Newell-Price & Auchus, 2020)
  A. Pharmacologic management
    1. Risk factors:
      a. Fasting: can lead to dehydration, hypotension, or hypoglycemia
      b. Hyperthyroidism
      c. Shift work or travel across time zones
      d. Illness: gastroenteritis, infection, surgical/dental procedures, hypoglycemia with diabetes
    2. IV hydrocortisone 100 mg every 6–8 hours
    3. Aggressive fluid replacement; assess for fluid overload
  B. Nonpharmacologic management
    1. Patients should carry supplies for emergency stress dosing and should carry a card or bracelet to alert emergency personnel.
    2. Patients should alert health care providers of history, as stress doses of steroids may be necessary for critical illness and surgical procedures.
    3. Assess for medications or foods that may interfere with glucocorticoids and mineralocorticoids (phenytoin, warfarin, erythromycin, oral contraceptive pill, St. John's wort, and grapefruit/grapefruit juice).
    4. Assess for altered nutritional status.
    5. Assess for signs and symptoms related to over- and undertreatment (Prete, Feliciano, Mitchelhill, & Arlt, 2019; Table 36.3).

XI. Hyperglycemia management (Anderson & Morganstein, 2021; Dev, DelFabbro, & Dalal, 2019)
  A. Pharmacologic management
    1. Monitor fasting blood level while on treatment.
    2. Glucocorticoid-induced hyperglycemia increases the risk of infection.
    3. Pre-existing type 2 diabetes may increase the risk of ICI-induced diabetes.
    4. Monitor for insulin resistance resulting for advanced cancer cachexia.
      a. Manage cancer cachexia (Chapter 44).
  B. Nonpharmacologic management
    1. Provide education on treatment, diet, and lifestyle changes.

TABLE 36.3   Signs and Symptoms of Over- and Under-replacement Therapy for Adrenal Crisis

Glucocorticoid treatment: over-replacement	Insomnia, increased appetite, proximal muscle weakness, skin thinning, easy bruising, red stretch marks, weight gain and central obesity, disproportionate supraclavicular and dorsocervical fat pads, facial and upper neck plethora, and facial rounding
Glucocorticoid treatment: under-replacement	Fatigue, weakness, nausea, lack of appetite, dizziness, hypotension, weight loss, and skin hyperpigmentation (due to ACTH excess)
Mineralocorticoid treatment: over-replacement	Hypertension, peripheral edema
Mineralocorticoid treatment: under-replacement	Orthostatic hypotension (e.g., dizziness, lightheadedness, and fainting when standing up); postural blood pressure drop on examination (lying to standing); fatigue, leg cramps, and salt craving

ACTH, Adrenocorticotropic hormone.
From Prete, A., Feliciano, C., Mitchelhill, I., & Arlt, W. (2019). Diagnosis and management of congenital adrenal hyperplasia in children and adults. In S. Llahana, C. Follin, C. Yedinak, & A. Grossman (Eds.), *Advanced practice in endocrinology nursing* (pp. 665). Berlin: Springer.

REFERENCES

Anderson, B., & Morganstein, D. L. (2021). Endocrine toxicity of cancer immunotherapy: Clinical challenges. *Endocrine Connections, 10*(3), R116–R124. https://doi.org/10.1530/EC-20-0489.

Barnabei, A., Corsello, A., Paragliola, R. M., Iannantuono, G. M., Falzone, L., Corsello, S. M., et al. (2022). Immune checkpoint inhibitors as a threat to the hypothalamus–pituitary axis: A completed puzzle. *Cancers, 14*(4), 1057. https://doi.org/10.3390/cancers14041057.

Brady, V. J. (2019). Endocrine toxicities. In M. M. Olsen, K. B. LeFebvre, & K. J. Brassil (Eds.), *Chemotherapy and immunotherapy guidelines and recommendations for practice* (pp. 525–535). Pittsburgh, PA: Oncology Nursing Society.

Brahmer, J. R., Abu-Sbeih, H., Ascierto, P. A., Brufsky, J., Cappelli, L. C., Cortazar, F. B., et al. (2021). Society for Immunotherapy of Cancer (SITC) clinical practice guideline on immune checkpoint inhibitor-related adverse events. *Journal for ImmunoTherapy of Cancer, 9*(6), e002435. https://doi.org/10.1136/jitc-2021-002435.

Brent, G. A., & Weetman, A. P. (2020). Hypothyroidism and thyroiditis. In S. Melmed, R. J. Auchus, A. B. Goldfine, R. J. Koenig, & C. J. Rosen (Eds.), *Williams' textbook of endocrinology* (14th ed., pp. 404–432). Amsterdam: Elsevier.

Bringhurst, F. R., Demay, M. B., & Kronenberg, H. M. (2020). Hormones and disorders of mineral metabolism. In S. Melmed, R. J. Auchus, A. B. Goldfine, R. J. Koenig, & C. J. Rosen (Eds.), *Williams' textbook of endocrinology* (14th ed., pp. 1196–1255). Amsterdam: Elsevier.

Chemaitilly, W., & Sklar, C. A. (2019). Childhood cancer treatments and associated endocrine late effects: A concise guide for the pediatric endocrinologist. *Hormone Research in Paediatrics, 91*(2), 74–82. https://doi.org/10.1159/000493943.

Cooksley, T., Girotra, M., Ginex, P., Gordon, R. A., Anderson, R., Blidner, A., et al. (2020). Multinational Association of Supportive Care in Cancer (MASCC) 2020 clinical practice recommendations for the management of immune checkpoint inhibitor endocrinopathies and the role of advanced practice providers in the management of immune-mediated toxicities. *Supportive Care in Cancer, 28,* 6175–6181. https://doi.org/10.1007/s00520-020-05709-1.

Davies, M. (2019). Acute and long-term adverse events associated with checkpoint blockade. *Seminars in Oncology Nursing, 35*(5), 150926. https://doi.org/10.1016/j.soncn.2019.08.005.

Dev, R., Del Fabbro, E., & Dalal, S. (2019). Endocrinopathies and cancer cachexia. *Current Opinion in Supportive & Palliative Care, 13*(4), 286–291. https://doi.org/10.1097/SPC.0000000000000464.

Fazal-Sanderson, V., Karavitaki, N., & Mihai, R. (2019). Hyperthroidism in adults. In S. Llahana, C. Follin, C. Yedinak, & A. Grossman (Eds.), *Advanced practice in endocrinology nursing* (pp. 521–555). Berlin: Springer.

Follin, C. (2019). Metabolic effects of hypothalamic dysfunction. In S. Llahana, C. Follin, C. Yedinak, & A. Grossman (Eds.), *Advanced practice in endocrinology nursing* (pp. 245–254). Berlin: Springer.

Gebauer, J., Higham, C., Langer, T., Denzer, C., & Brabant, G. (2019). Long-term endocrine and metabolic consequences of cancer treatment: A systematic review. *Endocrine Reviews, 40*(3), 711–767. https://doi.org/10.1210/er.2018-00092. PMID: 30476004.

Hollenberg, A., & Wiersinga, W. M. (2020). Hyperthyroid disorders. In S. Melmed, R. J. Auchus, A. B. Goldfine, R. J. Koenig, & C. J. Rosen (Eds.), *Williams' textbook of endocrinology* (14th ed., pp. 364–403). Amsterdam: Elsevier.

Husebye, E. S., Pearce, S. H., Krone, N. P., & Kämpe, O. (2021). Adrenal insufficiency. *The Lancet (British Edition), 397*(10274), 613–629. https://doi.org/10.1016/S0140-6736(21)00136-7.

Llahana, S., Mitchelhill, I., Yeoh, P., & Quinkler, M. (2019). Diagnosis and management of adrenal insufficiency in children and adults. In S. Llahana, C. Follin, C. Yedinak, & A. Grossman (Eds.), *Advanced practice in endocrinology nursing* (pp. 705–736). Berlin: Springer.

Llahana, S., Zopf, K., Mitchelhill, I., & Grossman, A. (2019). Prevention and management of adrenal crisis in children and adults. In S. Llahana, C. Follin, C. Yedinak, & A. Grossman (Eds.), *Advanced practice in endocrinology nursing* (pp. 1183–1205). Berlin: Springer.

Melmed, S., Auchus, R. J., Goldfine, A. B., Koenig, R. J., Rosen, C. J., Larsen, P. R., et al. (2020). Principles of endocrinology. In S. Melmed, R. J. Auchus, A. B. Goldfine, R. J. Koenig, & C. J. Rosen (Eds.), *Williams' textbook of endocrinology* (14th ed., pp. 2–12). Amsterdam: Elsevier.

Moini, J., Badolato, C., & Ahangari, R. (2021). Endocrine glands: *Epidemiology of endocrine tumors* (pp. 3–28). Amsterdam: Elsevier.

Mundy, A., & Crowley, R. (2019). Hyperparathyroidism and hypoparathyroidism. In S. Llahana, C. Follin, C. Yedinak, & A. Grossman (Eds.), *Advanced practice in endocrinology nursing* (pp. 957–974). Berlin: Springer.

National Comprehensive Cancer Network® (NCCN). (2022). *Management of immunotherapy-related toxicities. Version 1.2022.* National Comprehensive Cancer Network, Inc. https://www.nccn.org/professionals/physician_gls/pdf/immunotherapy.pdf. Retrieved March 22, 2023. Version 1.2023 - March 10, 2023.

Newell-Price, J. D. C., & Auchus, R. J. (2020). The adrenal cortex. In S. Melmed, R. J. Auchus, A. B. Goldfine, R. J. Koenig, & C. J. Rosen (Eds.), *Williams' textbook of endocrinology* (pp. 480–541). Amsterdam: Elsevier.

Oncology Nursing Society. (2023). Recognize it; report it. https://www. ons.org/clinical-practice-resources/recognize-it-report-it.

Pandy, M., Goyal, I., & Ernstoff, M. S. (2022). Endocrine toxicities of immunotherapy. In V. Velcheti & S. R. Punekar (Eds.), *Handbook of cancer treatment-related symptoms and toxicities.* Amsterdam: Elsevier.

Presley, C., Gomes, F., Burd, C., Kanesvaran, R., & Wong, M. (2021). Immunotherapy in older adults with cancer. *Journal of Clinical Oncology, 39*(19), 2115–2127. https://doi.org/10.1200/JCO.21.00138.

Prete, A., Feliciano, C., Mitchelhill, I., & Arlt, W. (2019). Diagnosis and management of congenital adrenal hyperplasia in children and adults. In S. Llahana, C. Follin, C. Yedinak, & A. Grossman (Eds.), *Advanced practice in endocrinology nursing* (pp. 657–678). Berlin: Springer.

Schneider, B. J., Naidoo, J., Santomasso, B. D., Lacchetti, C., Adkins, S., Anadkat, M., et al. (2021). Management of immune-related adverse events in patients treated with immune checkpoint inhibitor therapy: ASCO guideline update. *Journal of Clinical Oncology, 39*(36), 4073–4126. https://doi.org/10.1200/JCO.21.01440.

Thompson, C. J., & Verbalis, J. G. (2020). Posterior pituitary. In S. Melmed, R. J. Auchus, A. B. Goldfine, R. J. Koenig, & C. J. Rosen (Eds.), *Williams' textbook of endocrinology* (14th ed., pp. 303–329). Amsterdam: Elsevier.

Trifanescu, R., & Poiana, C. (2019). Diagnosis and management of hypothyroidism in adults. In S. Llahana, C. Follin, C. Yedinak, & A. Grossman (Eds.), *Advanced practice in endocrinology nursing* (pp. 583–592). Berlin: Springer.

Trump, D. (2020). Endocrine complications: *Abeloff's clinical oncology* (6th ed., pp. 707–714). Philadelphia: Elsevier. https://doi. org/10.1016/B978-0-323-47674-4.00046-3.

U.S. Food & Drug Administration. (2022). Approved risk evaluation and mitigation strategies (REMS). https://www.accessdata.fda.gov/ scripts/cder/rems/index.cfm.

Wood, L. S., Moldawer, N. P., & Lewis, C. (2019). Immune checkpoint inhibitor therapy. *Clinical Journal of Oncology Nursing, 23*(3), 271–280. https://doi.org/10.1188/19.CJON.271-280.

Yu, C. (2019). Endocrine consequences of childhood cancer therapy and transition considerations. *Pediatric Annals, 48*(8), 326–332. https://doi.org/10.3928/19382359-20190729-02.

37

Fatigue

Andrew D. Kass

OVERVIEW

I. Definition—cancer-related fatigue (CRF) is defined as a distressing, persistent, subjective sense of physical, emotional, and/or cognitive tiredness or exhaustion related to cancer or cancer-related treatment that is not proportional to recent activity and interferes with usual functioning (National Cancer Comprehensive Network, 2022a)

II. Physiology (O'Higgins, Brady, O'Connor, Walsh, & Reilly, 2018)
   A. The pathological mechanism of CRF remains unknown.
   B. Common underlying mechanisms may be considered central and/or peripheral in origin.
      1. Central
         a. Cytokine dysregulation
         b. Hypothalamic–pituitary–adrenal axis disruption
         c. Circadian rhythm disruption
         d. Serotonin dysregulation
         e. Vagal afferent nerve
      2. Peripheral
         a. Muscle metabolism
         b. Adenosine triphosphate dysregulation
         c. Contractile properties

III. Risk factors (Raj, Edekar, & Pugh, 2019)
   A. Poor Eastern Cooperative Oncology Group performance status
   B. Greater than 5% weight loss within 6 months
   C. Greater than 10 concurrent medications
   D. Lung cancer
   E. Strong opioid use
   F. History of depression

IV. Medical comorbidities (Raj et al., 2019)
   A. Disturbances in sleep–wake cycles
      1. Poor sleep correlates with high levels of fatigue
      2. Delayed circadian rhythms result in increased daily dysfunction due to fatigue
      3. Other factors leading to insomnia or daytime sleepiness
         a. Disruptions in biologic rhythmicity
         b. Mitotic processes of cancer cells
         c. Oncologic treatments
         d. Pain
         e. Psychiatric disturbances
         f. Radiation
   B. Anemia
      1. Found in 40% of cancer patients and 90% of those receiving chemotherapy

2. Etiology of anemia
   a. Blood loss
   b. Chemotherapy-induced myelosuppression
   c. Erythropoietin deficiencies due to renal disease
   d. Functional iron deficiency
   e. Marrow involvement of tumor
C. Endocrine disorders
   1. Hypothyroidism is a primary factor associated with fatigue
   2. Cytotoxic agents damage thyroid function causing decreased physical activity
   3. Thyroid damage from radioactive iodine agents
   4. Newer immunotherapy agents that affect thyroid function
D. Dietary intake
   1. Poor nutrition may lead to cancer cachexia
   2. Depletion of lean body mass and muscle wasting
E. Influencing factors of CRF (Fig. 37.1)

ASSESSMENT

I. National Comprehensive Cancer Network (NCCN) screening guidelines for fatigue
   A. All patients should be screened using age-appropriate measures for fatigue at their initial visit, at regular intervals during and following cancer treatment, and as clinically indicated.
      1. Patient self-report—the gold standard, 0–10 scale, with 0 being "no tiredness" and 10 being "worst possible tiredness"
      2. Distress Thermometer (DT) (Ownby, 2019)
         a. The DT was developed as a simple tool to effectively screen for symptoms of distress, including symptoms of fatigue.
         b. The NCCN DT is a single-item tool using a 0 (no distress) to 10 (extreme distress)–point Likert scale resembling a thermometer.
         c. In addition to the visual thermometer, a comprehensive list of categories—including practical, family, physical, and emotional problems, as well as spiritual/religious concerns—available to be selected by the patient (Fig. 37.2).
         d. The established cutoff score for further screening evaluation is a "4."

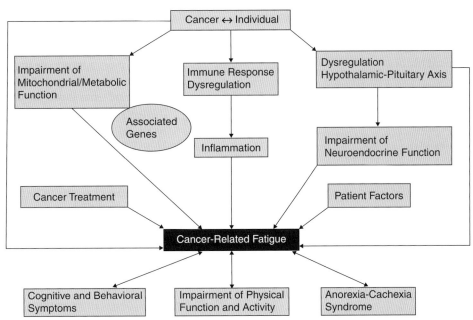

Fig. 37.1 Influencing factors of cancer-related fatigue. From Gebauer, J., Rüffer, J. U., Brabant, G. (2021). Cancer-related fatigue. In J. D. Beck, C. Bokemeyer, & T. Langer (Eds.), *Late treatment effects and cancer survivor care in the young*. Berlin: Springer. https://doi.org/10.1007/978-3-030-49140-6_17.

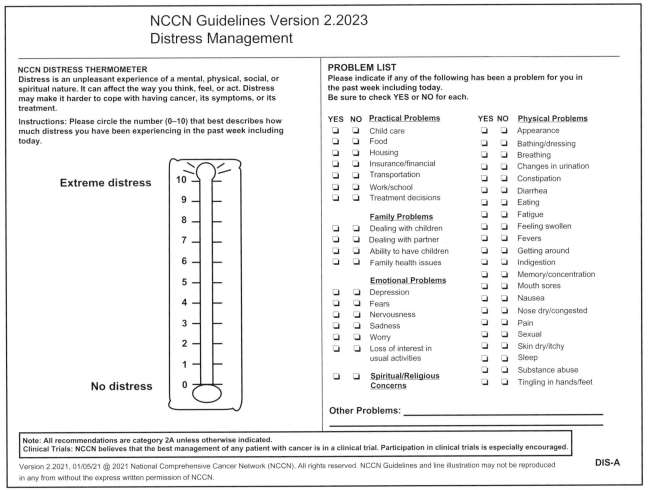

Fig. 37.2 Distress thermometer. Reproduced with permission from the NCCN Clinical Practice Guidelines in Oncology (NCCN Guidelines®) for Distress management V.2.2023. © 2023 National Comprehensive Cancer Network, Inc. All rights reserved. The NCCN Guidelines® and illustrations herein may not be reproduced in any form for any purpose without the express written permission of NCCN. To view the most recent and complete version of the NCCN Guidelines, go online to NCCN.org. The NCCN Guidelines are a work in progress that may be refined as often as new significant data becomes available.

B. Comprehensive assessment for patients with moderate to severe fatigue (National Cancer Comprehensive Network [NCCN], 2022b)
1. Perform a focused history.
   a. Onset
   b. Pattern
   c. Duration
   d. Change over time
   e. Associated factors
   f. Interference
2. Evaluate disease status.
   a. Cancer treatment
   b. Cancer recurrence
   c. Cancer progression
3. Assess treatable contributing factors.
   a. Pain
   b. Depression
   c. Anxiety
   d. Distress
   e. Anemia
   f. Sleep disturbances
   g. Nutritional deficits
   h. Function limitation
   i. Medication adverse effects
   j. Comorbidities
4. Laboratory evaluation based on the presence of other symptoms and onset and severity of fatigue.
   a. Complete blood count with differential
   b. Endocrine evaluation

MANAGEMENT

I. Pharmacological interventions (Klasson, Helde Frankling, Lundh Hagelin, & Björkhem-Bergman, 2021)
   A. Pharmacologic interventions are recommended when other treatments are insufficient.
   B. Treat the malignancy or the underlying cause.
   C. Blood transfusion for severe anemia
   D. Psychostimulants (NCCN, 2022a)
      1. Methylphenidate or dextroamphetamine (used primarily for Attention-deficit/hyperactivity disorder and narcolepsy) may be beneficial.
         a. Both medications are contraindicated for patients with poorly controlled hypertension, underlying coronary heart disease, or tachyarrhythmias.
         b. Black Box Warning indicating high potential for abuse and dependence
   E. Erythropoiesis-stimulating agents (Morga et al., 2021)
      1. Shows improvement
         a. Increase in hemoglobin from baseline
         b. Reduction in need for red blood cell transfusions
      2. Results less consistent
         a. Mortality—may increase mortality
         b. Thromboembolic events
         c. Increased quality of life
      3. Not to be used with myeloid cancers—may stimulate cancer cell growth

F. Low-dose dexamethasone 4 mg twice daily for 2 weeks
   1. Some benefits, but larger trials are lacking
   2. Risks should be carefully weighed with benefits.
   3. May be more appropriate in patients at the end of life
G. Antidepressants (Bhargava & Chasen, 2021)
   1. Paroxetine—has shown no difference in incidence or intensity for CRF treatment but does show improvement in treating depression
   2. Donepezil—placebo-controlled trial showed no difference when studying fatigue and toxicities
H. Testosterone replacement in hypogonadal men with advanced cancer seems to improve fatigue and quality of life in limited trials.
I. Evidence is lacking for the management of fatigue with nutritional supplements and herbal remedies; ginseng has limited evidence.
J. Correction of vitamin D deficiency may have a positive effect on fatigue.

II. Nonpharmacologic interventions (Strasser, 2021)
   A. Education
      1. Counseling of patient and family about fatigue and its natural history
      2. Importance of self-monitoring of severity and impact
   B. Energy conservation and distraction
      1. Set realistic expectations.
      2. Prioritize and pace activities.
      3. Labor-saving techniques.
      4. Delegate less-essential activities.
   C. Physical activity
      1. Counter-intuitive to how "healthy people" deal with fatigue
         a. With cancer, resting and napping do not alleviate fatigue properly.
         b. In the case of CRF, energy creates energy (e.g., walking, lifting light weights weekly will decrease fatigue).
      2. Moderate exercise routines lasting 30 minutes per day, 3 days a week for at least 12 weeks show the greatest benefit.
   D. Nutrition
      1. Intervention is likely to improve muscular weakness and physical fatigue.
      2. Patients should be assessed for malnutrition and associated deficits.
      3. Evaluate for iron deficiency, low vitamin D, vitamin B12, and low levels of zinc.
   E. Creative therapies: art and music
      1. Creative interventions can support patients with CRF to identify, explore, and understand emotions.
      2. Music therapy seems to improve fatigue regardless of whether listening to or performing music.
      3. Art therapy can reduce anxiety, depression, and pain (elements that contribute to fatigue).

III. Integrative strategies (Haylock et al., 2019)
   A. Mind–body medicine
      1. Uses the power of thoughts and emotions to influence physical health

2. Relaxation has the greatest effect on CRF, compared with other interventions (Hilfiker et al., 2018).

3. Yoga includes a mind–body component and has shown promise over other physical activity interventions.

4. Other activities such as biofield therapies (touch therapy), music therapy, relaxation, reiki, and qi gong may offer some benefit but need further research before routinely recommending.

B. Message therapy (Alizadeh et al., 2021)

1. Message is an intervention based on complementary medicine that causes short-term neuro-relaxing effects.

2. Studies have shown decreased fatigue in patients immediately after and 24 hours after receiving chemotherapy.

C. Microbiomes

1. Living within the gastrointestinal tract, it is an array of microorganisms that helps transport and absorb micronutrients and vitamins.

2. During treatment, gut microbiome is assaulted by surgery, chemotherapy, antibiotics, and steroids.

3. Probiotics are one way to promote the restoration of healthy gut (use cautiously with immunocompromised patients).

4. Stool testing may be helpful to determine which bacteria are currently present or absent.

D. Biomarkers

1. A host of biomarkers are being studied in relation to CRF.

2. Some markers—including interleukin-6, C-reactive protein, and tumor necrosis factors—are associated with muscular–skeletal dysfunction, sleep disturbance, and poor nutritional status.

3. All of these contribute to CRF.

4. Biomarkers for CRF could help detect at-risk patients and potentially provide clues towards etiologies and effective therapies.

REFERENCES

Alizadeh, J., Yeganeh, M. R., Pouralizadeh, M., Roushan, Z. A., Gharib, C., & Khoshamouz, S. (2021). The effect of massage therapy on fatigue after chemotherapy in gastrointestinal cancer patients. *Supportive Care in Cancer, 29*(12), 7307–7314. https://doi.org/10.1007/s00520-021-06304-8.

Bhargava, R., & Chasen, M. (2021). Cancer fatigue: *Palliative medicine: A case-based manual.* Oxford: Oxford University Press. https://doi.org/10.1093/oso/9780198837008.003.0011.

Haylock, P. J., & Curtiss, C. P. (Eds.). (2019). *Cancer survivorship: Interprofessional, patient-centered approaches to the seasons of survival.* Pittsburgh, PA: Oncology Nursing Society. Retrieved from https://www.ons.org/books/cancer-survivorship-interprofessional-patient-centered-approaches-seasons-survival.

Hilfiker, R., Meichtry, A., Eicher, M., Balfe, L. N., Knols, R. H., Verra, M. L., et al. (2018). Exercise and other non-pharmaceutical interventions for cancer-related fatigue in patients during or after cancer treatment: A systematic review incorporating an indirect-comparisons meta-analysis. *British Journal of Sports Medicine, 52*(10), 651–658. https://doi.org/10.1136/bjsports-2016-096422.

Klasson, C., Frankling, M. H., Hagelin, C. L., & Björkhem-Bergman, L. (2021). Fatigue in cancer patients in palliative care—A review on pharmacological interventions. *Cancers, 13*(5), 985. https://doi.org/10.3390/cancers13050985.

Morga, A., Atzinger, C., Arber, M., King, S., Phalguni, A., Sanderson, A., et al. (2021). Overview of systematic reviews (SRs) of erythropoiesis-stimulating agents (ESAs) as standards of care for non-myeloid cancer patients with chemotherapy-induced-anemia (CIA). *Blood, 138*(Suppl. 1), 4152. https://doi.org/10.1182/blood-2021-144957.

National Cancer Comprehensive Network (NCCN). (2022a). Cancer-related fatigue, v.2.2022. https://www.nccn.org/professionals/physician_gls/pdf/fatigue.pdf.

National Cancer Comprehensive Network (NCCN). (2022b). Survivorship, version 1.2022. https://www.nccn.org/professionals/physician_gls/pdf/survivorship.pdf.

O'Higgins, C. M., Brady, B., O'Connor, B., Walsh, D., & Reilly, R. B. (2018). The pathophysiology of cancer-related fatigue: Current controversies. *Supportive Care in Cancer, 26*(10), 3353–3364. https://doi.org/10.1007/s00520-018-4318-7.

Ownby, K. K. (2019). Use of the distress thermometer in clinical practice. *Journal of the Advanced Practitioner in Oncology, 10*(2), 175–179. https://doi.org/10.6004/jadpro.2019.10.2.7.

Raj, V. S., Edekar, J., & Pugh, T. M. (2019). Cancer-related fatigue. In A. Cristian (Ed.), *Central nervous system cancer rehabilitation* (pp. 121–131). Amsterdam: Elsevier.

Strasser, F. (2021). Management of cancer-related fatigue. In S. Rauh (Ed.), *Survivorship care for cancer patients.* Berlin: Springer. https://doi-org.proxy.libraries.rutgers.edu/10.1007/978-3-030-78648-9_11.

38

Gastrointestinal Symptoms

Jeanne Held-Warmkessel

XEROSTOMIA

Overview

I. Definition: subjective sensation of mouth dryness, secondary to abnormal salivary gland function (true xerostomia), or without objective signs of hyposalivation. Characterized by decreased or thick saliva (Jensen, Vissink, Limesand, & Reyland, 2019; Mercadante, Al Hamad, Lodi, Porter, & Fedele, 2017; Mercadante et al., 2021; Millsop, Wang, & Fazel, 2017; Strojan et al., 2017; Wolff et al., 2017).
   A. Salivary glands (parotid, submaxillary, sublingual, and others) secrete clear and watery saliva with two major components: ptyalin (digestive enzyme) and mucin (protective, lubricating).
   B. Saliva is antimicrobial, has mechanical cleansing action, controls pH, removes food debris, lubricates oral cavity, protects and maintains oral mucosa, and remineralizes teeth.
   C. Submandibular, sublingual, and minor salivary glands contribute the most whole saliva in the resting phase when not eating.

II. Causes and risk factors for xerostomia are summarized in Table 38.1.
   A. Radiotherapy (RT)±platinum-based chemotherapy (CT) for head and neck cancer (HNC) that includes salivary glands. Effect on salivary function is seen around 40 Gy.
      1. Up to 93% develop salivary gland hypofunction, sticky saliva, and dry mouth.
      2. Reduced saliva flow alters physiologic, biochemical, and antimicrobial functions.
      3. Negatively affects chewing, swallowing, smell, taste, and other oral functions such as difficulty speaking.
      4. May be accompanied by burning or painful mouth, halitosis, glossitis (smooth, erythematous tongue), cracked lips, and dysphagia.
      5. Consequences—oral infections (bacterial, viral, yeast), dental caries, worsened nutritional state, and decreased overall health status and quality of life (QOL).
      6. Transient or prolonged xerostomia related to cumulative RT dose and volume of salivary gland tissue in treatment field. Acute damage to glands begins the first week of RT and worsens during the planned treatment course. Several months later, progressive changes are noted.
      7. Other medications and concomitant diseases.
      8. Lifestyle influences—alterable risk factors.
         a. Alcohol, caffeine, alcohol-based oral rinses
         b. Cigarette smoking, nicotine
         c. Drugs that decrease salivary flow
   B. Prevention
      1. Intensity-modulated RT
      2. Amifostine administered before each RT dose: Food and Drug Administration (FDA) approved for use with RT in the post-operative setting
      3. Reduced dose of RT to the major and minor salivary glands
      4. Acupuncture during RT
      5. Systemic bethanechol during RT (weak evidence)

Assessment

(Carvalho, Medeiros-Filho, & Ferreira, 2018; Millsop et al., 2017)
I. Focused history—ask patient about
   A. Dry mouth—severity, onset, aggravating and alleviating factors
   B. Difficulty chewing or eating (especially crunchy or hard, spicy, or acidic foods)
   C. Difficulty swallowing (observe swallowing)
   D. Altered taste
   E. Change in/difficulty in wearing dentures
   F. Difficulty speaking (note voice quality)
   G. Other medical conditions associated with xerostomia, such as diabetes
   H. Social history (cigarettes, alcohol, and caffeine-containing beverages)
   I. Thoroughly review prescription (Rx) and over-the-counter (OTC) medications/products
   J. Oncology treatment such as RT for head/neck cancer or conditioning regimen for hematopoietic stem cell transplantation (HSCT)
II. Physical examination—use penlight to thoroughly examine mouth for signs of xerostomia
   A. Lips and corner of mouth—dryness, cracking, swelling, or ulceration
   B. Tongue—any lines or fissures, loss of papillae
   C. Mucous membranes/gingiva—are they dry, shiny, and smooth

TABLE 38.1 Some Causes of Xerostomia

Drug Related	Disease Related	Others
Agents with anticholinergic properties	Diabetes mellitus	Radiotherapy to the head and neck
Antihypertensives/antiarrhythmics (e.g., lisinopril, metoprolol, atenolol)	Autoimmune causes:	Stem cell transplantation
Antidepressants (desipramine, fluoxetine, venlafaxine)	• Autoimmune thyroid disease	Chronic GVHD
Antipsychotics (e.g., haloperidol, olanzapine)	• Sjögren syndrome (primary or secondary)	Anxiety or depression
Antiallergy/antipyretics(e.g., azelastine, desloratadine)	• Rheumatoid arthritis	Aging
Anticonvulsants (e.g., pregabalin, sodium valproate)	• Systemic lupus erythematosus	Lifestyle factors:
Antihistamines	• Scleroderma	• Tobacco use
Antiparkinsons	• Primary biliary cirrhosis	• Alcohol use
Antivirals (maraviroc, didanosine, and saquinavir)	Viral infectious causes:	• Caffeinated beverage consumption
Anticholinergic/antimuscarinic agents (hyoscyamine, scopolamine, and atropine)	• Hepatitis C	• Dehydration
Darifenacin (urinary incontinence)	• HIV	• Heavy snoring
Others	• Cytomegalovirus	• Mouth breathing
• Diuretics	• Epstein–Barr virus	• Upper respiratory tract infections
• Opioids	Granulomatosis causes:	
• Nicotine	• Amyloidosis	
• Sedatives	• Sarcoidosis	
• Antineoplastic agents (everolimus, temsirolimus, bevacizumab, sorafenib, immune checkpoint inhibitors, 5-FU- and taxane-based regimens)	• Wegener granulomatosis	

5-FU, 5-Fluorouracil; *GVHD,* graft-versus-host disease; *HIV,* Human immunodeficiency virus.
Data from Mercadante, V., Jensen, S. B., Smith, D. K., Bohlke, K., Bauman, J., Brennan, M.T., et al. (2021). Salivary gland hypofunction and/or xerostomia induced by nonsurgical cancer therapies: ISOO/MASCC/ASCO guideline. *Journal of Clinical Oncology, 39*(25), 2825–2843. https://doi.org/10.1200/JCO.21.01208; Millsop, J. W., Wang, E. A., & Fazel, N. (2017). Etiology, evaluation, and management of xerostomia. *Clinics in Dermatology, 35*(5), 468–476. https://doi.org/10.1016/j.clindermatol.2017.06.010; Wolff, A., Joshi, R. K., Ekström, J., Aframian, D., Pedersen, A. M. L., Proctor, G., et al. (2017). A guide to medications inducing salivary gland dysfunction, xerostomia, and subjective sialorrhea: A systematic review sponsored by the World Workshop on Oral Medicine VI. *Drugs in R&D, 17*(1), 1–28. https://doi.org/10.1007/s40268-016-1053-9.

D. Saliva, consistency/quality—foamy, thick, ropy, and scant saliva; little/none mouth floor
E. Teeth—plaque, detritus, and two or more cavities
F. Mucosal debris on palate
G. Dental mirror or tongue blade may stick to tongue or buccal mucosa

III. Psychosocial assessment
A. Ask about changes in social aspects and enjoyment of eating because of dry mouth
B. Ask about altered taste for sweet, sour, and bitter that decreases pleasure of eating; thick saliva is highly concentrated in sodium that adversely affects tastes
C. Ask about noticeable changes in speaking and discomfort from oral burning or pain

IV. Imaging and laboratory tests
A. Sialometry (measure of saliva flow, evaluated after overnight or after 2-hour fast): with patient sitting upright, normal salivary flow rate stimulated—1.5–2.0 mL/min, unstimulated—0.3–0.4 mL/min; less than 0.12–0.16 mL/min abnormal
B. Other, if indicated by concomitant disease

Management

(Garcia et al., 2019; Jensen et al., 2019; Mercadante et al., 2021; Milsop et al., 2017; Strojan et al., 2017)

I. Pharmacologic management
A. Oral sialogogues—first-line therapy; systemic agents to increase saliva secretion (moderate evidence).

B. Pilocarpine (Salagen) and cevimeline (Evoxac) may increase salivary flow and reduce feeling of dry mouth.
C. Pilocarpine—contraindicated in chronic cardiovascular or pulmonary disease, uncontrolled asthma, narrow-angle glaucoma, or taking beta-blockers.
D. Cevimeline has fewer side effects, is more expensive, and may be better tolerated.
E. Best effect seen after 8 weeks of therapy.
F. Bethanechol has fewer side effects.
G. Topical salivary substitute products temporarily decrease mouth dryness.
H. Mucin-based saliva substitutes (e.g., Aquoral, Biotene Mouthwash, Moi-Stir, NeutraSal, SalivaMAX, Salivart, and Xero-Lube) resemble natural saliva, increase salivary viscosity, and well tolerated.
I. Weak evidence that enzyme-enriched products are better than carboxymethylcellulose products and that more viscous products could be better than thinner products.
J. Gels may be better for night use with severe xerostomia.
K. Trials of different products as one may be more beneficial for a specific patient.

II. Nonpharmacologic management
A. Acupuncture—weak and mixed evidence that it improves salivary flow and requires more research.
B. Fluoride application and routine professional oral hygiene.
C. Teach patients strategies that may decrease oral dryness and associated symptoms.

D. Take frequent sips of water (also helps maintain hydration).

E. Suck ice cubes or sugarless popsicles to help keep the mouth cool and moist.

F. Moisten foods with liquids, milk, or gravy.

G. Avoid crunchy, spicy, acidic, or hard foods. Dietary consultation.

H. Bland mouth rinses (1 teaspoon salt, 1 teaspoon baking soda, and 1 L of water); lessen oral dryness and neutralize pH.

I. Good oral hygiene—toothpastes, mouthwashes, and gels (may be salivary stimulants); regular dental visits with frequent cleaning and topical fluoride application to prevent dental caries.

J. Advise patient to seek prompt medical treatment if infection develops.

K. Chewing sugar-free gum and use sugar-free acidic (but not erosive) candy lozenges and salivary-stimulating lozenges may activate salivary pathway.

L. Lifestyle modifications.
1. Limit alcohol intake. After consuming alcohol, drink a glass of water or brush teeth.
2. Eliminate or limit caffeine-containing beverages.
3. Encourage/support smokers to join smoking cessation program.

DYSPHAGIA (ORAL)

Overview

(Chilukuri, Odufalu, & Hachem, 2018; Clark & Ebersole, 2018; Greco et al., 2018; Lazarescu et al., 2020; Okuni, Otsubo, & Ebihara, 2021; Pezdirec, Strojan, & Boltezar, 2019; Strojan et al., 2017; Zebralla et al., 2021)

I. Definition—impaired or impossible swallowing of ingested food, medications, liquids, or saliva.

II. Swallowing is a highly coordinated, rapid process; food is masticated and combined with saliva, moved from mouth to pharynx, to esophagus, and finally the stomach. Coordinated by voluntary and involuntary central nervous system (CNS) reflexes and coordinated with respirations.

III. Oropharyngeal dysphagia (OD) occurs at start of swallowing and is a symptom of a problem in the mouth or in the pharynx.
A. OD usually causes reflexive coughing and a sense of choking with swallowing.
B. Other possible symptoms are voice change, frequent throat clearing, and earache.

IV. Esophageal dysphagia (ED) caused by esophageal disease is relatively uncommon. Patient feels like food is sticking in their neck or upper chest a few seconds after they start to swallow.

V. Depending on the underlying cause, dysphagia may progress slowly or rapidly and advance from difficulty in swallowing solids, to swallowing liquids, and finally saliva.

VI. Major complications: aspiration, silent aspiration, pneumonia, weight loss and protein-calorie malnutrition, dehydration, and airway obstruction that increases morbidity and mortality.

VII. OD—causes and risk factors.
A. Stroke (most frequent cause of OD)
B. Degenerative neurologic disease (e.g., Parkinson disease, multiple sclerosis, Alzheimer disease, or other dementia), trauma, CNS tumor, and reduced level of consciousness
C. Infections that cause oropharyngeal inflammation and ulceration
D. Cervical spine disorders, congenital skeletal abnormalities, or stenosis
E. Iatrogenic—related to treatment (surgical, drugs, RT, etc.), other medications
F. HNC the most common cancer-related cause of OD
1. Mechanical dysphagia—onset may precede diagnosis of large (T3–T4) base of tongue, supraglottic, or pharyngeal tumors
2. Mechanical dysphagia—may occur postsurgery from resection of tumor and soft tissues, inflammation, and edema
3. OD develops in 30%–50% of HNC patients treated with intensive RT (±CT or targeted agent); ≈33% improve, 50% do not, and 20% worsen over time.
4. Early RT-related damage to base of tongue, pharynx, larynx, or epiglottis causes inflammation, edema, and painful acute OD.
5. RT with concomitant CT/targeted therapy increases incidence and strongly predicts severe (grade 3) acute dysphagia.
6. Late RT-induced OD causes nonspecific fibrosis and/or atrophy and can occur months to years later, even in patients without significant acute dysphagia.
7. 50% of HNC patients with OD have silent aspiration; swallowed substances pass through vocal cords into trachea without inducing cough or other overt OD signs.
8. <50% report symptoms unless a health care professional specifically asks about swallowing problems.
9. High risk for RT-related OD: baseline weight loss, malnutrition, xerostomia, smoking, large local tumor, oropharyngeal or nasopharyngeal tumor, and anticholinergic medications.
10. Has a significant impact on QOL and social functioning

VIII. ED
A. Esophageal drug-related injury (e.g., oral bisphosphonates, nonsteroidal antiinflammatory drugs [NSAIDs], potassium chloride, and theophylline)
B. Gastroesophageal reflux disease, obesity, metabolic syndrome, esophageal obstruction, and mucosal injury
C. Esophageal motility disorder or infection
D. Intrinsic or extrinsic tumor—esophageal carcinoma or hilar lymphadenopathy secondary to lung cancer (both likely advanced disease; treated palliatively)

Assessment

(Bressan et al., 2017; Chilukuri et al., 2018; Clark & Ebersole, 2018; Espitalier et al., 2018; National Cancer Institute [NCI], 2017; Panebianco, Marchese-Ragona, Masiero, & Restivo, 2020; Strojan et al., 2017)

I. Primary assessment goals
   A. Evaluate the patient's ability to swallow without respiratory complications
   B. Determine whether patient is ingesting sufficient calories and water
   C. Collaborative assessment—nurse, physician, speech–language pathologist (SLP), dietician, etc.

II. History—ask patient about
   A. Cancer diagnosis and past/current treatment (RT, CT, and targeted agents)
   B. Other disease states associated with dysphagia
   C. Recent history of recurrent pneumonia
   D. Ask patient if they do not want to eat or if they cannot eat to differentiate anorexia, chronic disease-related malnutrition from dysphagia, starvation-related malnutrition.
   E. Swallowing quality
      1. What happens when you try to swallow? How often does this happen?
      2. Is it difficult for you to swallow solids, liquids, or both?
      3. Cough, choking, throat clearing, or drooling during or after eating, regurgitation or aspiration
      4. How long it takes to eat a meal (compared with usual)?
      5. Estimate severity of dysphagia:
         a. Eating Assessment Tool 10—reliable, valid, and easy to use, patient-reported screen to self-report dysphagia symptoms and aspiration risk and identify the need for further evaluation (http://www.bccancer.bc.ca/managing-symptoms-site/Documents/EAT%2010.pdf)
   F. National Cancer Institute Common Terminology Criteria for Adverse Events (NCI-CTCAE) addresses several gastrointestinal (GI) symptoms, including dysphagia (NCI, 2017).
   G. Patient report of pain or discomfort; weakness of lips, tongue, or jaw; "lump in throat"
   H. Impact of dysphagia on nutrition
   I. OD/ED increases the risk for dehydration, secondary risk for aspiration pneumonia due to lessened oropharyngeal clearing and infection.

III. Physical examination
   A. Observe patient for unilateral facial droop (stroke), drooling, choking or coughing with swallowing, and gurgling voice quality. Ask patient to speak and listen for changes.
   B. Oral examination for associated xerostomia, mucositis, candida, other infections, or abnormalities of tongue, lips, or soft palate.
   C. Observe patient's ability to chew, hold food in mouth, and use tongue to effectively propel food to the back of the mouth and the oropharynx and swallow.
   D. Auscultate lungs because of potential for aspiration.
   E. Weigh patient two to three times a week; follow fluid balance and nutritional status.
   F. SLP or trained nurse can do bedside screens for dysphagia.
      1. Two-step water swallow test
         a. One small (1–5 mL) sip—observe for coughing/choking±voice changes (e.g., wet/gurgly voice quality): rules aspiration in (risk for false negative because of silent aspiration)
         b. Consecutive large (90–100 mL) sips, no clinical signs: rules aspiration out
      2. Cough reflex test useful to identify silent aspiration. Nebulized citric acid, which induces cough, administered by face mask. Coughing or choking signals aspiration (absence of such symptoms does not exclude silent aspiration).

IV. Psychosocial assessment—ask patient about
   A. Changes in mood (e.g., feeling depressed, anxious, embarrassed, frustrated, or angry)
   B. If they eat alone—social isolation is common because of chewing and swallowing difficulties, coughing while eating, taking much longer to finish a meal than others
   C. If they have less or no enjoyment or disinterest in eating

V. Imaging and laboratory tests
   A. "Gold standard" diagnostic tests for OD—either functional endoscopic evaluation of swallowing (FEES) or video fluoroscopy swallowing study (VFSS)
   B. FEES—fiber-optic nasoendoscopic evaluation; easy to do, greater sensitivity
   C. VFSS—dynamic examination; evaluates safety, efficacy, character of swallowing; better quantification of pharyngeal residue; helps assess therapeutic strategies
   D. Fluoroscopic contrast studies such as barium contrast
   E. Esophagram—3D assessment, shows, esophageal strictures, allows for safer endoscopy
   F. Endoscopy
   G. Manometry—useful in the diagnosis of motility disorders

Management

(Beck, Kjaersgaard, Hansen, & Poulsen, 2018; Clark & Ebersole, 20180; Greco et al., 2018; Krisciunas et al., 2017; Panebianco et al., 2020)

I. Pharmacologic management
   A. Antifungal and antibiotic agents, analgesics, or other medications may be indicated for accompanying problems.
   B. Enteral feedings by a nasogastric feeding tube (NGT) or a percutaneous endoscopic gastrostomy are preferred over parenteral nutrition because of cost-effectiveness and lower infection rates. Interventions for ED related to esophageal cancer.
   C. Self-expanding metal stent
   D. RT alternative for some patients

II. Nonpharmacologic management
   A. No evidence that "dysphagia rehabilitation," "swallowing therapy," or "active e-stim" effectively improves symptoms of dysphagia

B. SLP and the dietician/nutritionist—central to formulating OD management plan
   1. Consistency of foods, fluids that can be safely swallowed must be determined before starting nutritional support.
   2. Modifying solids, semisolids may increase palatability and ability to be swallowed.
   3. Low-quality evidence for thickened liquids (e.g., Thick-It, Thick & Easy, nectar) to maintain adequate hydration and prevent aspiration
   4. Therapeutic swallowing maneuvers
   5. Postural modification
   6. Sitting upright
   7. Positioning of head and neck
C. If a patient has been unable to orally consume ≥60% of their estimated daily nutritional need for 1 week, an alternative feeding method should be started.
D. Review patient medications and explore strategies to maintain adherence (e.g., alternative formulations that are easier to swallow, whether pills can be crushed and taken with applesauce, or if they cannot because of slow release).
E. Aspiration precautions
F. SLP program of oral and pharyngeal exercises for jaw range of motion, swallowing function

MUCOSITIS (ORAL)

Overview

(Brown & Gupta, 2020; Correa et al., 2020; Daugėlaitė, Užkuraitytė, Jagelavičiene, & Filipauskas, 2019; Hong et al., 2019; Huang, et al., 2018; Lalla, et al., 2019; Oncology Nursing Society [ONS], 2019a; Pulito, et al., 2020; Saigal & Guerra, 2018; Yu, et al., 2020; Yüce & Yurtsever, 2019)

I. Mucositis—CT- or RT-induced, painful inflammation and ulceration of the mucous membranes lining the GI tract.
II. Oral/oropharyngeal mucositis (OM) affects the keratinized mucosa of the dorsal tongue, gingiva, and/or hard palate; mucositis can also develop in the small intestine (GI mucositis) or the rectal mucosa (proctitis).
   A. OM severity ranges from superficial erythema and soreness to full-thickness mucosal ulcerations with major pain; delayed, interrupted, or discontinued treatment; systemic infection; hospitalization; impaired oral nutrition; and economic burden.
   B. Mucositis is a systemic effect from CT or targeted therapy, and a local effect of RT.
      1. Incidence: 20%–40% of patients receiving standard-dose CT, 60%–100% of those undergoing HSCT, and almost all patients receiving RT for HNC (>50% with grade 3 or 4).
      2. Involves epithelial mucosa, submucosal cells and tissues, and basal membrane.

III. Pathogenesis—time course differs, depending on mucosal location and therapy, and CT or RT. The 5-stage model of oral mucositis:
   A. Initiation—within seconds of injury to highly proliferative, normal cells (mucosa, submucosa, and basal stem) and supporting connective tissues, DNA damage and other cellular responses lead to tissue changes.
   B. Primary damage response—cell injury, activation of p53 and nuclear factor-$_k$B (NF-$_k$B)
   C. Signal amplification—transcription factors such as NF-$_k$B upregulate an innate immune response and activate the expression of genes and multiple pathways, the production of cytokines, and modulators associated with the progression of mucositis.
   D. Ulceration phase—Mucositis becomes clinically apparent with loss of mucosal integrity, painful lesions, submucosal breach with a risk of bacterial colonization, secondary infection, and sepsis.
   E. Healing occurs 2–4 weeks after CT or RT (may take longer to heal) stopped; submucosa and mesenchyme signal the mucosa to reepithelialize. The mucosa appears normal.
IV. Consequences of mucositis include pain, poor nutrition, reduced QOL, dysphagia, and therapy disruptions.
V. Targeted therapies can cause stomatitis: not well documented, different pathogenesis, etiology unclear.
VI. Stomatitis—oral tissue inflammatory condition unrelated to CT or RT; targeted therapy—associated oral sensitivity or pain (without lesions), xerostomia, taste change
   A. Usually occurs in the first cycle. Superficial aphthous ulcers (herpes simplex–like)—single or multiple small (≤0.5 cm) superficial, discrete, well-demarcated ulcers with erythematous borders and covered with grayish-white pseudomembrane.
   B. Ulcers develop within 5 days on inner aspect of lips, the ventral and lateral tongue surfaces, and soft palate; usually resolve in 1 week.
   C. Drug classes
      1. mTOR inhibitors (e.g., everolimus, temsirolimus, and ridaforolimus)—small shallow and painful ulcers, start 5 days after cycle one begins, improve/resolve spontaneously, severity based on disease being treated
      2. Some epidermal growth factor receptor (EGFR) inhibitors (e.g., bevacizumab and erlotinib)—aphthous-like lesions, begin with cycle 1, may resolve on their own
      3. Tyrosine kinase inhibitors (TKIs; e.g., sorafenib, gefitinib, lapatinib, and sunitinib)—worse with multikinase inhibitors, worse with combination CT
      4. Ado-trastuzumab emtansine—mucosal telangiectasia
      5. Cyclin-dependent kinase 4/6 inhibitors
      6. Antiangiogenesis agents—mucosal hypersensitivity, redness, inflammation, and pain
      7. CAR-T-cell therapy

VII. Clinical manifestations of OM
- A. Cycled or conditioning CT regimens: mild erythema starts 3–4 days after CT; ulcers thereafter; peak intensity days 7 and 14; usually resolves in next week.
- B. RT for HNC (fractionated: 2 grays [Gy]/day, total 10 Gy/week)
  1. Oral mucosal erythema and soreness start around the end of week.
  2. Cumulative dose 20–30 Gy: frank ulcers, pain worsens, and oral intake decreases.
  3. Continued RT (to a total of 60–70 Gy): increased cumulative damage; difficult-to-control pain.
  4. OM typically persists for 2–4 weeks after RT completion, may take up to 6 weeks after the last dose of RT to resolve.

VIII. Progressive ulcerative OM: more diffuse, ulcers may coalesce and be accompanied by
- A. Thick secretions that induce coughing, aspiration, and disturb sleep
- B. Pain that necessitates opioid analgesics
- C. Impaired speaking, eating, drinking, swallowing, taste changes, and weight loss
- D. High risk—gram-negative bacterial, viral or yeast infections, and septic complications

IX. Causes and risk factors
- A. CT—drugs with the highest risk for OM: alkylating agents such as cyclophosphamide, anthracyclines such as doxorubicin, etoposide, ifosfamide, methotrexate, docetaxel, paclitaxel, cisplatin, carboplatin, oxaliplatin, irinotecan, and antimetabolites such as 5-fluorouracil (5-FU)
- B. May also be drug dose and dosing frequency related
- C. High-dose CT, as with conditioning regimens for hematopoietic stem cell transplant (HSCT)
- D. Methotrexate to prevent acute graft-versus-host disease (GVHD) increases the risk
- E. RT for HNC—combined CT/RT increases risk with 90% of patients being affected. Baseline nutritional status below average—body mass index <18.5.
- F. Unintentional pretherapy weight loss (>5% over 1 month or >10% last 6 months), malnutrition
- G. Poor oral hygiene, periodontal disease
- H. Smoking or alcohol use
- I. Xerostomia
- J. Impaired renal function (high serum creatinine) may increase the risk.
- K. Genetic susceptibility
- L. Younger age
- M. Prolonged neutrophil recovery time

Assessment

(Brown & Gupta, 2020; King, Carulli, & Estfan, 2022; NCI, 2017; Zecha et al., 2019)

I. History—ask patient about
- A. Current cancer therapy regimen, particularly CT or RT for HNC; previous OM
- B. Usual oral hygiene, dentures, and dental visits
- C. Any changes in eating, swallowing, coughing, or choking
- D. Weight loss/nutritional/oral intake assessment
  1. Weight loss: >2% in 1 week, 5% in 1 month, or 7.5% in 3 months
  2. Obvious noticeable muscle wasting
  3. Loss of subcutaneous fat
  4. Nutritional intake <50% of recommended for ≥2 weeks
  5. Significantly reduced functional capacity or bedridden
- E. Use OM grading scale on consistent basis to document progression/resolution.
  1. NCI-CTCAE (NCI, 2017)
  2. World Health Organization Mucositis Grading
  3. Radiation Therapy Oncology Group
- F. Oral pain/discomfort: severity/intensity, adequacy of current analgesic
- G. Mouth dryness

II. Physical examination
- A. Recommended: regularly assess OM—at least once a week (instruct patient to report worsening OM symptoms between examinations).
- B. Use a penlight to examine mouth for redness, swelling, discrete or confluent ulceration, white patches; note saliva—thick and sticky. Remove dentures to assess. Look for altered mucosal integrity on the cheeks, lips, tongue, floor of mouth and soft palate. Severity may range from redness to ulceration. Look for periodontal disease and infected teeth.
- C. Auscultate lungs because of potential for aspiration.

III. Psychosocial assessment—ask patient
- A. Does sore mouth interfere with eating, drinking, talking; make them feel depressed
- B. If they no longer enjoy the social interaction of eating with others
- C. If they eat alone because it takes much longer to finish a meal than others because of difficulty chewing, swallowing, coughing, or pain while eating

IV. Imaging and laboratory tests:
- A. Complete blood count (CBC); CMP

Management

(Brown et al., 2020; Correa et al., 2020; Daugėlaitė et al., 2019; Hong et al., 2019; Huang et al., 2018; Lalla et al., 2019; ONS, 2019a; Pulito et al., 2020; Rugo et al., 2017; Saigal et al., 2018; Yu et al., 2020; Yüce et al., 2019)

I. Pharmacologic management
- A. Palifermin (keratinocyte growth factor)—FDA–approved for patients with hematologic malignancy receiving high-dose CT/total body irradiation (TBI), followed by autologous HCST; 60 µg/kg per day 3 days before and after conditioning regimen (very costly) to reduce incidence and severity of OM

B. Supportive care drugs—analgesics (opioids and adjuvants) to relieve severe pain
   1. Analgesics (opioids and adjuvants to reduce pain)—over 97% of patients with ulcerative OM require opioid analgesics (usually morphine equivalent) by week 4. Opioid doses increase to week 7. Usually needed for 6 weeks after treatment completion. Oral, parenteral, or mouth rinses/washed with morphine. Topical morphine 0.2% mouthwash. Swish and spit, not to be swallowed.
   2. Adding adjuvant medications may be opioid sparing.
   3. Doxepin 0.5% mouthwash
   4. Benzydamine (NSAID mouthwash 15 mL, swish 30 seconds, and spit) provides temporary pain relief for H/N RT doses up to 50 Gy.
C. Low-level laser therapy recommended for high-dose CT for HSCT. Suggested for H/N RT but more research needed. Reduces OM prevalence, severity, duration, and associated pain.
D. Cryotherapy; significantly reduces OM severity
   1. Instruct patient to hold ice chips in mouth for 5 minutes before CT or RT, during CT/RT, and up to 30 minutes total.
   2. Bolus 5-FU and high-dose melphalan
   3. Contraindicated with oxaliplatin because of risk for laryngopharyngeal dysesthesia
II. Nonpharmacologic management
A. Preventive oral care regimen—pretreatment with professional dental examination and oral hygiene. Provide patient education and instruction (oral and written) for oral hygiene regimen. Includes brushing and flossing with a soft toothbrush twice a day.
B. Dietary tips for painful OM: avoid coarse, rough, hot and spicy food, hot or acidic foods and/or drinks, and to eat soft or moistened foods. Add liquid nutritional supplements. Consult dietician.
C. Topical protective/coating agent—benzocaine (Orabase, Oratect Gel, Hurricane)±analgesic (e.g., viscous lidocaine) may give some temporary relief. Topical analgesics that numb the mouth increase the risk of oral injury due to reduced sensation in the oral structures. Use with caution and provide patient education. Magic mouthwashes are not evidence based and are not recommended, although they may be prescribed. Provide patient education related to the risk of oral structure injury and aspiration.
D. Use of normal saline, salt, and baking soda (0.5 teaspoon each in 1 cup of warm water), or plain water rinses. Educate patient to use four times a day. Saline rinses and education provided to H/N RT patients improved QOL.
E. Patient education on an oral care regimen improved QOL for patients receiving CT.
   1. Education should include oral care (brushing, flossing unless it causes pain and bleeding), diet modifications, and use of salt/baking soda oral rinses.

NAUSEA AND VOMITING

Overview

(Clemmons et al., 2021; Gan et al., 2020; Gupta, Walton, & Kataria, 2021; Khunger & Estfan, 2022; National Comprehensive Cancer Network® [NCCN], 2022; Navari, 2020; ONS, 2019b; Wickham, 2020a; 2020b)

I. Definitions
A. Nausea—uniquely unpleasant sensory and emotional experience; feeling epigastric or upper abdominal queasiness or need to vomit.
B. Retching—spasmodic inspiratory movements with glottis closed and abdominal muscle contractions, no expulsion of stomach contents.
C. Vomiting—autonomic and motor reflex, coordinated contraction of abdominal muscles and diaphragm with forceful expulsion of gastric contents from mouth.
   1. Acute vomiting—occurs within the first 24 hours after CT.
   2. Delayed vomiting—occurs after the first 24 hours after CT.
   3. Breakthrough vomiting—occurs in spite of appropriate antiemetic therapy.
   4. Refractory vomiting—unresponsible to antiemetic therapy.
   5. Anticipatory vomiting—conditioned response.
D. Nausea usually precedes vomiting, but either can occur alone.
II. Physiology of nausea and vomiting (N&V)
A. N&V reflexes protect against accidental ingestion of toxic substances, cause oral expulsion and GI dysrhythmia with slowed passage of stomach contents to the intestine, hepatic circulation, and bloodstream.
B. The "vomiting center" (VC), a group of neurons in the medulla in the brainstem, is the final common pathway for vomiting from any cause.
C. Neurotransmitters and neuroreceptors in peripheral and central pathways carry signals to the VC.
   1. The GI tract—primarily via the vagus nerve (and stretch receptors in obstruction).
   2. The CT trigger zone (CTZ) is near the VC and receives chemical signals from the bloodstream and cerebrospinal fluid.
   3. The cerebral cortex and limbic region add subjective and emotional responses.
   4. The vestibular apparatus (middle ear) plays the major role in motion sickness.
   5. The endocannabinoid system, activated by peripheral or central emetic stimuli, modulates N&V via cannabinoid-1 receptors in the brain.
   6. Multiple GI tract, brain neurotransmitters, and receptors have roles in N&V and thus antiemetic selection .
   7. Understanding of nausea is poor. A unique nausea "threshold" may rapidly respond to intrinsic

cognitive, GI, CNS and autonomic influences, and emotional centers.

D. Chemotherapy induced nausea and vomiting (CINV), which is best understood, involves two major pathways:

1. Emetogenic CT damages GI mucosal cells and releases serotonin (5-HT) from enterochromaffin cells. 5-HT binds to and activates 5-HT3 receptors on vagus nerve, initiating emetic signal and acute CINV during the first 24 hours after CT.

2. Substance P (SP) and neurokinin-1 (NK1) receptors are abundant in the brain. Emetic stimuli cause SP binding at NK1 receptors in the CTZ, amplifying the emetic message—particularly during delayed CINV that may persist for a few to many days.

3. If antiemetics inadequate for CINV, patients may experience breakthrough CINV.

4. Anticipatory nausea (AN)—conditioned response to poorly controlled CINV; 8%–14% of patients have AN before subsequent CT; can become more intense over successive CT cycles.

5. AN and CINV can lead to refractory CINV not responsive to standard antiemetics.

III. Risk factors

A. Iatrogenic

B. CT emetogenicity: highly emetogenic (HEC: >90%, e.g., cisplatin, anthracycline–cyclophosphamide combination); moderately emetogenic (MEC: 30%–90%, e.g., carboplatin, oxaliplatin); low emetogenic (10%–30%, e.g., cetuximab, docetaxel, and paclitaxel); and minimal emetogenic (<10%, e.g., fludarabine, rituximab, and vincristine). Dose dependent—cyclophosphamide, cytarabine, and doxorubicin.

C. RT: total body RT (TBI >90%), upper abdominal (30%–90%), cranium, thorax, pelvis (10%–30%), breast, and extremities (<10%).

D. Concurrent CT-RT. Combination CT regimens. Drug route and frequency.

E. Inhalational anesthesia Postoperative nausea and vomiting (PONV); type of surgical intervention

F. Opioids and other narcotics

G. Patient related

1. Female gender: greater incidence, lower response rates to antiemetics than men

2. Younger individuals (age 5–60) at greater risk

3. CINV with prior CT (strong predictor for CINV and PONV)

4. AN and vomiting; prechemotherapy anxiety or expectations

5. No history of significant alcohol consumption

6. History of hyperemesis with pregnancy; history of motion sickness

7. Pharmacogenomic differences, particularly in 5-HT3 receptor antagonist (RA) metabolism

8. Anxiety

H. Disease-related (often multifactorial)—may affect over 60% of patient with advanced malignancy.

1. Partial, intermittent, or complete bowel obstruction; constipation, obstipation

2. Metabolic imbalance: hypercalcemia, hyponatremia, hyperglycemia, and uremia

3. Gastric outlet obstruction or delayed emptying

4. Increased intracranial pressure, brain primary tumors or metastases, meningeal disease, and vestibular dysfunction

5. Anxiety, depression

6. Ascites

7. Pancreatitis

Assessment

(NCI, 2017; Navari, 2020; Wickham, 2020a)

I. Assessment goals may vary, depending on the start of CT or RT (identify and incorporate risk factors into management plan) or from another problem (reversible cause vs. palliation)

II. History

A. Ask about N&V separately

1. Onset, pattern over time, frequency (intermittent or constant)

2. Severity (e.g., 0–10 scale or verbal descriptor scale [none, mild, moderate, severe], NCI-CTCAE)

3. Any associated symptoms (e.g., appetite changes, anorexia, constipation, bloating, early satiety, and sense of stomach fullness) or activities (such as food or medications) that affect nausea or vomiting

4. Review risk factors (see earlier) with patient, especially past or current CT or RT, antiemetics used and effectiveness, any remedies, medications, or OTC medications successfully used.

III. Physical examination

A. Nausea may induce parasympathetic manifestations: pallor, perspiration, tachycardia, and feeling dizzy and weak.

B. Assess for signs of dehydration, orthostasis.

C. Abdominal assessment (e.g., for ascites, large stool in colon, and enlarged organs); bowel sounds, weight change, and abdominal tenderness or distention

IV. Psychosocial assessment

A. Ask patient if nausea (or vomiting) affects work, roles and responsibilities, and mood.

B. Ask if inadequate control of N&V has had negative effects on their partner or other family members.

V. Imaging and laboratory tests

A. Imaging only to identify underlying treatable cause

B. Laboratory—chemistries: electrolytes and ions, hepatic and renal function tests, intake and output

Management

(Clemmons et al., 2021; Gan et al., 2020; Hesketh et al., 2020; Khunger & Estfan, 2022; Navari, 2020; NCCN, 2022; ONS, 2019b; Razvi et al., 2019)

I. Pharmacologic management

A. Principles of antiemetic management—use a nationally recognized antiemetic guideline. (See Table 38.2 for a list of antiemetics and their actions.)

TABLE 38.2 List of Antiemetics and Their Actions

Neurotransmitter	Binds to	Site of Action CNS	Site of Action GI	Action of medication	Medication	Examples of Uses
Serotonin (5-HT)	5-HT3	X	X	Antagonist	Ondansetron Granisetron Palonosetron Olanzapine	CINV PONV[a]
Dopamine-2	5-HT4	X	X	Antagonist	Metoclopramide Chlorpromazine	Delayed CINV Gastroparesis
SP	NK1	X	X	Antagonist	Aprepitant/fosaprepitant Netupitant (combined with palonosetron—NEPA) Rolapitant (half-life 180 h)	CINV PONV[a]
Dopamine-2 (D)	D2	X	X	Antagonist	Droperidol, haloperidol Prochlorperazine, metoclopramide Olanzapine, mirtazapine	CINV CINV: rescue PONV Palliative
Unknown	NA	X	X	Unclear, works with 5-HT3 antagonists	Dexamethasone	CINV PONV Palliative
CB-1 and -2	CB-1	X		Poorly understood	Dronabinol (Marinol, Syndros)	Rescue CINV
Ach	M		✓	Antagonist	Hyoscine (Scopolamine) Glycopyrrolate	Bowel obstruction PONV
Dopamine	H1			Antagonist	Cyclizine Prochlorperazine Olanzapine	Bowel obstruction
Dopamine	GABA, CTZ	X		Anxiolytic	Lorazepam	Anxiolytic

Ach, Acetyl-choline; *CB*, cannabinoid; *CTZ*, chemotherapy trigger zone; *GABA*, gamma-Aminobutyric acid; *NEPA*, netupitant-palonosetron; *NK1*, neurokinin-1; *SP*, substance P.
[a]Smaller doses used for PONV than CINV.
Data from *National Cancer Institute (NCI)*. (2022). *Nausea and vomiting related to cancer treatment (PDQ®)–health professional version*. https://www.cancer.gov/about-cancer/treatment/side-effects/nausea/nausea-hp-pdq#_699_toc; Athavale, A., Athavale, T., & Roberts, D. M. (2020). Antiemetic drugs: What to prescribe and when. *Australian Prescriber, 43*(2), 49–56. https://doi.org/10.18773/austprescr.2020.011.

B. Goal: prevention for the entire expected period of N&V.

C. CINV or RINV: select antiemetics based on emetogenicity of regimen. Use combination antiemetic therapy.

D. Consider additional risk factors (see earlier) that may increase likelihood of N&V.

E. N&V from other causes: antiemetic selected on suspected etiology.

F. If N&V persist, add another antiemetic.

G. Use PO antiemetics when possible (nauseated patients may not be able to take).

H. Use adjunct agents (e.g., H2 blocker to prevent dyspepsia/nausea, or lorazepam to decrease anxiety) as needed.

I. CINV standard-of-care (SOC) antiemetics. Use combination therapy when indicated.
1. 5-HT3 RAs: ondansetron (oral—PO, intravenous—IV), granisetron (PO, IV, transdermal, and depot injection), palonosetron (IV), and dolasetron (PO), SOC for RINV
2. NK1 RAs: aprepitant/fosaprepitant (PO/IV), netupitant (fixed PO dose with palonosetron), and rolapitant (IV/PO)

3. Corticosteroid: dexamethasone (antiemetic mechanism unknown); may be used with 5-HT3 RAs for RINV

4. Olanzapine—binds to multiple receptors involved in N&V (5-HT3, dopamine, histamine, and muscarinic); clinically significant decreases in nausea

5. Other antiemetics (e.g., adjunct, rescue, palliative, opioid)
a. CB agonists: dronabinol (Marinol, Syndros), nabilone (Cesamet)—rescue
b. Dopamine (D2) RAs: metoclopramide (prokinetic—avoid in patients with GI obstruction), haloperidol, and prochlorperazine—for palliative care, rescue antiemetics; amisulpride (PONV)
c. Antisecretory drugs (e.g., hyoscine or octreotide)—not antiemetics but useful for GI obstruction
d. Scopolamine—excessive secretions, position changes, or movement-induced nausea/vomiting
e. Benzodiazepines (e.g., lorazepam, alprazolam [Xanax]); not antiemetics—decrease anxiety, help with AN/vomiting

II. Nonpharmacologic management—adjuncts to antiemetics
   A. Ask patient about any nondrug measures that have been helpful for past nausea or N&V.
   B. Ginger—reverses cisplatin-induced delayed gastric emptying, may alleviate or relieve GI dysmotility, muscarinic and histaminergic antagonistic properties.
   C. Dietary strategies (e.g., smaller, more frequent meals; bland diet, avoid fatty, fried, spicy or very sweet foods, eat cold or room-temperature foods, eat foods with little to no odor, avoid strong odors).
   D. Dietary consultation
   E. Relaxation techniques
   F. Patient education
      1. Educate both patient and family using both oral and written instructions on the management of N&V.
      2. Educate patient/family to notify health care provider of nausea/vomiting not controlled by prescribed medications or any drug-related side effects, reduced urine output, or inability to consume fluids/foods.

ASCITES

Overview

(Bleicher & Lambert, 2021; Eitan et al., 2018; Hodge & Badgwell, 2019; Kietpeerakool, Rattanakanokchai, Jampathong, Srisomboon, & Lumbiganon, 2019; Knight et al., 2018; Matsusaki et al., 2022; Robson et al., 2019; Stukan, 2017)

I. Definition: Ascites—abnormal accumulation of fluid in the peritoneal cavity, occurs with some cancers (80% of cases occur with end-stage cirrhosis). Considered refractory when diuretics and sodium restriction are not effective.
   A. Normally, 5–20 mL of peritoneal fluid lubricate organ and bowel surfaces; 50–100 mL/h diffuses from serum to peritoneum, back to circulation (via lymphatics)
II. Malignant ascites (MA) incidence
   A. Ovarian cancer ≈38% of women have MA at diagnosis
   B. Pancreatobiliary (21%), unknown primary (20%), and gastric cancer (18%)
   C. Can occur in tumors that metastasize to the liver or peritoneum (e.g., gastric, colon, pancreas, lung, adrenal, bladder, and breast); pseudomyxoma
III. Pathogenesis of MA is multifactorial.
   A. Changes in vascular permeability caused by primary tumor production of vascular endothelial growth factor causing increased vascular permeability and ascites fluid production
   B. Blocked lymphatic drainage
   C. Hepatic metastases
      1. Due to peripheral arterial vasodilation
      2. Sinusoidal portal hypertension
      3. Vasodilators produced along with nitrous oxide
      4. Reduced arterial blood flow
      5. Sodium retention
      6. Increased capillary permeability
      7. Ascites forms

IV. Any or a combination of these events overwhelms the capacity to drain peritoneal fluid and leads to refractory MA (persists or recurs after drainage).
V. Symptoms of ascites are often more distressing than the underlying cancer, reducing QOL.
   A. Abdominal distension and pain
   B. Nausea, anorexia, vomiting, constipation, early satiety, and weight change
   C. Fatigue
   D. Dyspnea, shortness of breath (SOB)
   E. Urinary frequency
   F. Impaired mobility
VI. Patients with refractory MA have symptoms that reflect advanced cancer as well as MA. Prognoses for those with nonovarian cancer are 1–6 months, and for those with ovarian cancer are 10–24 months (27% are alive at 5 years). Considered a poor prognostic indicator.

Assessment

(Eitan et al., 2018; Knight et al., 2018; NCI, 2017; Rudralingam, Footitt, & Layton, 2017; Stukan, 2017)

I. History
   A. Does the patient have suspected cancer or a confirmed diagnosis?
   B. Ask patient about the presence of MA symptoms (e.g., abdominal fullness or feeling bloated, increased waist size, discomfort or pain, changed appetite or nausea, feeling short of breath, or change in activity).
   C. Ascites Symptom Mini-Scale—assesses ovarian cancer–related MA symptoms; useful to monitor worsening symptoms and relief after MA drainage. A 5-item 1–5 scale tool asking patient to rate: SOB, distended abdomen, reduced mobility, fatigue, and loss of appetite.
   D. Grading scale CTCAE (NCI, 2017)
II. Physical examination
   A. Physical examination cannot identify small MA (≤100 mL) in asymptomatic patients.
   B. Ascites of ≥1500 mL is clinically evident.
   C. Larger ascites: abdomen may appear distended; could be obscured in an obese person.
   D. Palpate/percuss abdomen for fluid wave, shifting dullness, bulging flanks, everted umbilicus, and stretched skin
III. Psychosocial assessment
   A. Ask patient if they feel depressed or anxious, or have difficulty thinking or concentrating (do not usually improve with drainage of ascites).
   B. If they report SOB, ask if they feel anxious or fearful.
   C. Embarrassed because they "look pregnant," have problem finding clothes that fit
   D. Ask if MA has altered their mobility, independence, family, and social activities.
IV. Imaging and laboratory tests
   A. Ultrasound of the abdomen—screen for MA; can detect ≥100 cm³ of fluid.

B. CT or magnetic resonance imaging of abdomen to identify primary malignancy; position emission tomography occult metastases.

C. Ascites cytology analysis—diagnostic gold standard to identify/rule out tumor; protein concentration, ascites character—exudative (from malignancy) versus transudative, bacteria.

D. Tumors that do not shed into peritoneum require biopsy to confirm diagnosis.

E. Coagulation screen may be done before paracentesis.

F. Chemistry panel, CBC: hypoalbuminemia, liver/renal dysfunction, anemia, and infection.

Management

(Bleicher & Lambert, 2021; Eitan et al., 2018; Hodge & Badgwell, 2019; Kietpeerakool et al., 2019; Knight et al., 2018; Matsusaki et al., 2022; Robson et al., 2019; Stukan, 2017)

I. Pharmacologic management aims: relieve symptoms, improve QOL, and treat primary cause, if feasible. Must be individualized to patient's performance status and expected overall prognosis.

II. Pharmacologic management

A. Diuretics (spironolactone and furosemide, titrated as needed and used with caution) may be used for MA secondary to liver metastases and portal hypertension; possible adverse effects are systemic volume depletion, electrolyte abnormalities, renal dysfunction, and N&V.

B. Adjunct or palliative CT or targeted therapy (systemic or intraperitoneal) indicated for some patients with ovarian or gastric cancer.

C. Paracentesis—first-line interventional management for refractory ascites; fine tube inserted into peritoneum under ultrasound guidance; connected to collection bag, ascites freely drained, and catheter removed.

1. Safe, well tolerated; 90% symptom relief (e.g., decreased abdominal distension and discomfort, dyspnea, nausea, anorexia, fatigue, and mobility).

2. Low risk of complications (pain, hypotension, peritonitis, loculation of ascites, bowel perforation, loss of protein and electrolytes, bleeding, and development of adhesions).

3. May be repeated as needed.

D. Volume that can safely be removed depends on the type of ascites.

1. Exudative MA (peritoneal carcinomatosis)—up to 9 L.

2. Transudative (liver metastases with portal hypertension)—rapid, large-volume drainage may cause hemodynamic instability (IV fluids may prevent hypotension).

E. MA may reaccumulate rapidly; average symptom relief 10 days (range 4–45 days).

F. Permanent subcutaneously tunneled abdominal catheter alternative to intermittent paracentesis for some patients. Improves QOL and provides symptom relief.

1. Tenckhoff (peritoneal dialysis) double-cuffed, PleurX single-cuffed, or Aspira double-cuffed vacuum system catheters.

2. Low risk for manageable complications: exit-site infection, cellulitis, ascites leakage at catheter exit, catheter occlusion, fibrin sleeve formation at catheter tip that impedes drainage, catheter dislodgment, hypotension or peritonitis.

3. Patient can drain catheter at home—not to dryness, but to symptom relief when needed. Vendors provide dressing and drainage supplies.

4. Vacuum system catheters—maximum drainage (1000 mL) in ≥15 minutes; usual drainage every other day, 1–2 L.

5. Certain permanent catheters can be used for intraperitoneal CT.

6. Nontunneled catheters should be avoided due to a higher complication rate (cellulitis, blockage, leakage, and infection) but may be used in patients with very limited life expectancy.

7. Implanted intraperitoneal ports

8. Peritoneovenous shunts—not as effective, more complications

G. Surgery with hyperthermic intraperitoneal CT—only for very selected patients with longer expected survival.

H. Clinical trial

I. Palliative care

CONSTIPATION

Overview

(Khunger & Estfan, 2022; Davis et al., 2020; Larkin et al., 2018; LeFebvre, Rogers, & Wolles, 2020; Rogers et al., 2020)

I. Constipation is slow fecal movement.

II. Chronic constipation includes any two of the following for a minimum of 12 weeks:

A. Straining

B. Lumpy, hard stool

C. Less than three stools (BM) per week

D. Disimpaction

E. Feeling of incomplete bowel movement of feeling of blockage

III. Constipation is one of the most frequent symptoms in patients receiving therapy.

IV. Disease progression may be accompanied by worsening bowel symptoms, along with increased fatigue and impaired ability to communicate.

V. Constipation can progress to impaction, stool packing in distal colon and rectum, with overflow diarrhea.

VI. Physiology—extended bowel transit time allows greater absorption of water from feces through the bowel wall, results in hard and dry stools that are difficult to pass along with impaired sphincter function

VII. Potential etiologic factors (often multicausal)

A. Organic

B. Cancer related (e.g., GI tumor, abdominal/pelvic tumor mass, spinal cord involvement, GI obstruction, autonomic dysfunction, brain tumor, and radiation fibrosis)

C. Metabolic causes (dehydration, hypercalcemia, hypokalemia, hyponatremia, hypothyroidism, uremia, and diabetes)

D. Other diseases (diabetes, Parkinson disease, chronic obstructive pulmonary disease, and heart disease)

E. Other GI: small-bowel bacteria overgrowth, diverticulitis, anorectal fissures, and irritable bowel syndrome

F. Female gender

G. Pain

H. Functional
   1. Environmental/cultural (lack of privacy, comfort, or assistance with toileting; cultural sensitivities regarding BMs)
   2. Dietary: insufficient fluid intake, low-fiber diet
   3. Pain with defecation (anorectal pain, bone pain, and other cancer pain)
   4. Other (advanced age, inactivity, decreased mobility, confined to bed, depression, sedation, and progressive cachexia)
   5. Weakness/fatigue (proximal or central myopathy), inactivity
   6. Lower performance status is related to a higher likelihood of constipation
   7. Drug related (polypharmacy is more significant than single drugs)
      a. Opioids—constipation must be managed proactively
      b. Anticholinergics (antihistamines, belladonna, antiparkinsonian drugs, antipsychotics, antispasmodics, monoamine oxidase inhibitors, and tricyclic antidepressants)
      c. Antineoplastic agents (alkylating agents, such as cisplatin, carboplatin; vinca alkaloids; thalidomide and its analogs)
      d. 5-HT3 RA antiemetics
      e. NSAIDs, anticonvulsants (carbamazepine), antihypertensives (beta-blockers, calcium channel blockers, central-acting antiarrhythmics, and diuretics)
      f. Metal ion–containing agents (aluminum, antacids, bismuth, calcium, iron supplements, lithium, and sucralfate)

Assessment

(ALMouaalamy, 2021; Bharucha & Lacy 2020; Larkin et al., 2018; LeFebvre et al., 2020; Mesía et al., 2019; Rogers et al., 2020; NCI, 2017)

I. History—ask patient about their bowel habits:
   A. What they consider "normal" BMs and "constipation" (agree on definitions)
   B. What is their usual BM pattern—frequency, straining
   C. Use a constipation assessment tool
      1. NCI-CTCAE
   2. What are their BMs like (e.g., small or large; rocks or marbles; soft, hard, or liquid; color, odor, blood, or mucus)
      a. Do they have any bowel diseases, hemorrhoids, or other rectal problems, such as a fissure?
      b. Do they have abdominal fullness or bloating, nausea, diarrhea, or a constant feeling of having to move their bowels with an empty colon (tenesmus)?
      c. Do they take laxatives or use suppositories or enemas? Which, how much, and how often? How much do laxatives help?
      d. Medication list including OTC medications.
      e. Activity level: altered mobility, fatigue, or weakness—may interfere with usual BMs.
      f. Current diet and appetite, fiber intake (can patient consume fiber 30 g per day with sufficient fluids to maximize bulk effects and avoid exacerbating constipation).
      g. Medical conditions affecting laxative selection (e.g., vocal cord paralysis precludes mineral oil, or impaired renal function contraindicates magnesium salts).

II. Physical examination
   A. Abdomen
   B. Inspect abdomen for symmetry, distention, bulges, and visible peristalsis
   C. Auscultate all quadrants for normal, hyperactive, or absent bowel sounds
   D. Palpate for masses to distinguish stool (indents) from tumors (do not)
   E. Percuss for gas or fluid with ascites; tympany and distention
   F. Rectal examination (avoid in neutropenic or thrombocytopenic patient); ensure privacy and consider cultural norms. Include perineal area in assessment.
      1. Poor anal sphincter tone—may indicate spinal cord problem
      2. Hard, dry stool in the rectum (fecal impaction)—patient may need disimpaction before starting oral laxative therapy
      3. Hemorrhoids or fissures—stool softener may be indicated

III. Psychosocial assessment
   A. Ask patient if constipation affects their comfort, activities of daily living, and mood
   B. Does the patient avoid taking opioid analgesics because some pain is better than feeling constipated?
   C. Does constipation add to anxiety or depression?

IV. Imaging and laboratory tests
   A. Tests to identify contributing factors (e.g., hypercalcemia or diabetes) or risks from interventions (e.g., blood urea nitrogen, creatinine to assess renal function, white blood cells [WBCs], and platelets to identify risks with manual disimpaction).
   B. Flat plate of abdomen radiograph may distinguish severe constipation, fecal impaction, and obstruction.

Management

(ALMouaalamy, 2021; Bharucha & Lacy, 2020; Khunger & Estfan, 2022; Davies et al., 2020; Larkin et al., 2018; Mesía et al., 2019; Rogers et al., 2020)

I. Pharmacologic management
  A. Oral (PO) laxatives
    1. Stimulant—senna or bisacodyl
    2. Osmotic—lactulose (prescription agent), polyethylene glycol (superior to lactulose), sorbitol—indigestible and nonabsorbable sugars.
    3. Directly stimulate bowel wall neurons that induce forceful peristalsis and release water and electrolytes into the intestine.
    4. First-line laxatives, particularly for opioid-induced constipation (OIC). Administer proactively and titrate doses to effect; however, these agents may not be effective.
  B. PO stool softeners—docusate (Colace, Surfak), mineral oil
    1. Lower surface tension, soften and lubricate stools
    2. Ineffective for established constipation and OIC; less effective than psyllium
    3. Must increase fluid intake to soften stools; contraindicated in advanced cancer
  C. PO bulking agents: soluble—psyllium (e.g., Metamucil), insoluble—methylcellulose (e.g., Citrucel)
    1. Worsen slow-transit opioid– or anticholinergic-related constipation and not recommended.
    2. Avoid in patients with advanced disease; insufficient PO fluids may lead to fecal impaction or GI obstruction.
    3. Do not use for OIC.
  D. Peripherally acting mu-opioid RA (methylnaltrexone oral or subcutaneous or oral naloxegol); safe and effective for OIC. May be started with opioid therapy or used when patients do not respond to maximized laxative doses.
    1. Other medications approved for OIC include—lubiprostone (intestinal secretagogue) and naldemedine (intestinal lubricant).
  E. Rectally administered agents—avoid use in patients with neutropenia or thrombocytopenia or a bowel obstruction
    1. Suppository: bisacodyl, glycerin (hyperosmotic, lubricant)
    2. Enemas: phosphate (Fleet), microenema, mineral oil
    3. Preferred for rapid and predictable evacuation of stool from rectum and distal colon, such as patients with fecal impaction
  F. Nonpharmacologic management
    1. Meager evidence that most nondrug measures (e.g., recommending trying to have BM same time each morning) are helpful for cancer patients. However, it is important to provide privacy and have the patient use correct positioning for defecation.
    2. Dietary fiber, increasing oral fluids, and exercise depend on performance status and prognosis; may or may not be useful (or possible).
      a. Fiber may increase the number of BMs but not change stool consistency, laxative use, or painful BMs.
      b. Dietary fiber might be effective for mild or moderate but not severe constipation in relatively healthy patients.
      c. Fiber can worsen early satiety, increase constipation in patients with limited fluid intake.
    3. Cachectic patients may be unable to consume sufficient food and liquids for effective gut transit and feces consistency.
    4. Increasing activity is often not possible with advanced disease.
    5. Patient education
      a. Report constipation to health care team (HCT).
      b. Report any signs and symptoms of nausea, vomiting, bleeding, pain, cramping, and associated symptoms to HCT.
      c. Provide information on constipation and its management when opioid therapy is initiated.
      d. Increase motility and fluid consumption.
      e. Increase dietary fiber if possible.
      f. Avoid caffeine.

DIARRHEA

Overview

(Abu-Sbeih, Johnson, & Wang, 2019; Abu-Sbeih, Ali, & Wang, 2020; Brahmer et al., 2018; Cherny & Werman, 2019; Khunger & Estfan, 2022; Puzanov et al., 2017; Secombe et al., 2020)

I. Diarrhea is the passage of more than three unformed stools in 24 hours.
II. Objective definition: passing stools of >200 g or >200 mL per 24 hours.
III. Diarrhea key manifestation of GI tract mucositis (GIM) after CT or RT to abdomen/pelvis.
IV. Severity of GIM depends on drug/regimen, dose, and administration schedule and can be classified as follows:
  A. Nonpersistent (existing for <4 weeks) or persistent (lasting >4 weeks); may persist for years posttreatment
  B. Early onset (<24 hours after administration) or late onset (>24 hours after administration)
  C. Uncomplicated (grades 1 and 2, usually manageable at home) or complicated (grades 3 and 4, generally require hospitalization)
V. CT drugs commonly causing GIM: fluoropyrimidines such as capecitabine, 5-FU; irinotecan, gemcitabine, methotrexate, cyclophosphamide, cisplatin, oxaliplatin, carboplatin, doxorubicin, paclitaxel, docetaxel, and cabazitaxel.
  A. Bolus 5-FU causes more diarrhea than continuous infusion 5-FU.
  B. Irinotecan causes early-onset diarrhea and late-onset diarrhea and is worse with 5-FU.

VI. RT-induced GIM can occur after RT to the anus, rectum, cervix, uterus, prostate, urinary bladder, or testes; TBI conditioning for HSCT increases GIM throughout the GI tract.
  A. Small-bowel complications related to the volume of small intestine in the RT field.
  B. RT-related GIM is usually grade 1 or 2.
VII. List of targeted therapies causing diarrhea growing; includes TKIs, EGFR-TKIs, monoclonal antibodies, mammalian target of rapamycin (mTOR) inhibitors, and mitogen-activated protein kinases signaling cascade inhibitors.
  A. Usually mild, but grade 3 diarrhea sometimes occurs. Drug-dependent severity and frequency.
  B. Mechanisms may differ by class, not identified.
  C. GIM is more frequent with combination therapies.
VIII. Immune checkpoint inhibitors (ICIs) including cytotoxic T-lymphocyte antigen-4 (CTLA-4) agents, programmed cell death 1 (PD-1) or PD-1 ligand (PD-L1) agents.
  A. Incidence higher with CTLA-4 therapy and is dose dependent.
  B. Severity ranges from mile to severe and may progress to life-threatening colitis if untreated.
  C. First infusion may produce transient diarrhea. Usual onset is after dose three.
  D. Patients are at risk for immune-related diarrhea/colitis after treatment is completed.
  E. Colitis is accompanied by abdominal pain, rectal bleeding, mucous in stool and fever.
IX. Other causes of diarrhea.
  A. Fecal impaction with overflow diarrhea
  B. Paraneoplastic, secondary to a neuroendocrine tumor
  C. GVHD
  D. *Clostridium difficile* diarrhea, secondary to antibiotics, prolonged NGT, GI surgery, repeated enemas, or CT
  E. Enteral tube feedings
  F. Unrelated to cancer
    1. Lactose intolerance, food poisoning
    2. Viral gastroenteritis
    3. Inflammatory bowel disease or irritable bowel syndrome
    4. Excessive dosing (laxatives, magnesium-based antacids, nutritional supplements, antibiotics, proton pump inhibitors, selective serotonin reuptake inhibitors, and NSAIDs)
X. Neutropenic enterocolitis
XI. Dihydropyrimidine dehydrogenase deficiency—causes unexpected and serious adverse events from 5-FU.
XII. The hallmarks of diarrhea from any cause are GI tract water and electrolyte imbalance.
  A. Damaged villi less able to absorb fluid and nutrients from small bowel into circulation.
  B. Nonabsorbable nutrients exert osmotic pressure to pull water into the intestine.
  C. Greater numbers of immature secretory cells increase GI secretion.
  D. These factors exceed colon's capacity to absorb water from feces, diarrhea results.
XIII. Pathogenesis of CT- and RT-induced GIM
  A. CT and RT diarrhea/GIM occur by the same mechanisms as oral mucositis.
  B. CT induced diarrhea five-phase model
    1. Injury to rapidly dividing GI epithelium and submucosa initiates GIM cascade. The small intestine (single-cell-layer mucosa) is particularly vulnerable.
    2. Transcription factors generate messengers to activate immune response and upregulate proinflammatory cytokines.
    3. Signal amplification activates other pathways, with inflammation and apoptosis of GI epithelial stem cells.
    4. Ulceration phase: superficial and submucosal GI damage causes shift in bacteria when WBCs decreasing; increased risk for secondary infection. Bacterial translocation from thin mucosal layer. Loss of fluid absorption.
    5. Healing occurs after CT or RT complete.
      a. Targeted therapy—multifactorial including inflammation, multikinase inhibitors has a higher incidence of diarrhea. EGFR-TKI diarrhea is common. Associated with an increase in chloride section producing secretory diarrhea.
      b. ICI—due to loss of self-tolerance.
XIV. Diarrhea can range from bothersome to life threatening. Severe GIM can lead to the following:
  A. Treatment interruptions, dose reductions, or early discontinuation.
  B. Hospitalization and readmission, and significant economic burden.
  C. Profound dehydration, electrolyte imbalance, and hypovolemia; severe CT-induced GIM may lead to 4–6 L of diarrhea stools/day.
  D. Other possible complications—hemorrhoids, perianal skin breakdown, malnutrition, cachexia and weight loss, fatigue, declining immune function, renal failure, and systemic infection.
  E. Reduced QOL

Assessment

(Abu-Sbeih et al., 2019; Abu-Sbeih et al., 2020; Brahmer et al., 2018; Cherny & Werman, 2019; Diaz et al., 2021; Khunger & Estfan, 2022; ANCI, 2017)
  I. History
    A. Thoroughly documented bowel history is crucial for timely follow-up interventions.
    B. Is the patient at risk for or experiencing CT- or RT-related diarrhea now?
    C. What "normal" bowel habit was before cancer diagnosis?
    D. If bowel habit changed since diagnosis.

E. What BMs are like now: frequency, color, watery, bloody, mucus-filled, amount, odor, stool consistency. Abdominal and rectal (or stoma) pain.

F. Sense of diarrhea: does patient wake at night because they have to move their bowels, do they have any steatorrhea (stools with excessive fat—are often pale, foamy, foul-smelling, float in toilet bowl, and flush poorly), do they have urgency to move bowels or any BM incontinence (urgent GI consult indicated)?

G. Associated abdominal symptoms: cramping, abdominal pain, bloating, and passing gas.

H. Current cancer treatment, if any; which and last treatment.

I. Review medications (Rx and OTC)—any of these started in the last 10–14 days?

J. Associated symptoms of dehydration.
   1. Any change in urinating (less frequently or smaller amounts, urine color, odor)?
   2. More thirsty than usual?
   3. Sudden, rapid weight loss (1-L weighs 1 kg).
   4. Any dizziness, falling down, or fainting (orthostasis)?
   5. Any change in their thinking (mental status)?

K. Dietary factors.
   1. Recent changes (e.g., more fiber or roughage, fried or fatty foods)
   2. Fluids: fruit juices, coffee, and alcohol

L. Particularly worrying symptom constellation:
   1. Abdominal cramps not relieved by loperamide
   2. Unable to eat
   3. Worsening fatigue or weakness
   4. Chest pain
   5. N&V not controlled by antiemetics
   6. Dehydration with decreased urine output, fever (temperature >100.5°F)
   7. GI bleeding
   8. Previous admission for diarrhea

M. Grading scale.
   1. NCI-CTCAE severity of diarrhea

II. Physical examination—assess the degree of patient's dehydration
   A. General appearance (ill, listless)
   B. Mucous membranes (dry, normal), skin turgor
   C. Circulatory: any delayed capillary refill time, tachycardia, and orthostasis (blood pressure decreases <40 mm Hg systolic and/or 20 mm Hg diastolic in <15 seconds after standing)
   D. Any acute abdominal processes, such as hyperactive bowel sounds
   E. Rectal examination: assess for perineal skin irritation, rectal tenderness, blood, and stool consistency (any hard, dry stool in rectum [fecal impaction]); loose stool may flow around stool (overflow) and reported as diarrhea

III. Psychosocial assessment
   A. Ask patient if diarrhea interferes with social activities, such as going out to dinner with friends, because of concerns of uncontrollable diarrhea.
   B. Ask patient if they feel depressed, anxious, or embarrassed because of diarrhea.
   C. Ask if diarrhea has caused change/limited usual home or work activities.

IV. Imaging and laboratory tests
   A. Flat plate of abdomen, abdominal ultrasound, abdominal CT if indicated and to evaluate bowel obstruction
   B. Fecal occult blood testing
   C. Stool for *C. difficile* toxins (patients who develop unexplained diarrhea after 3 days of hospitalization; positive in 15%–20%)
   D. CBC, serum chemistries, and electrolytes and ions
   E. Immune-related diarrhea
      1. Stool specimens for culture, CMV and other viruses, *C. difficile*, ova and parasites, fecal calprotectin, and lactoferrin
      2. CT scan abdomen/pelvis if patient has fever, abdominal pain/distention, or blood/mucous in stool
      3. Colonoscopy with biopsy
      4. Additional lab studies—CRP, ESR, and TSH

Management

(Abu-Sbeih et al., 2019; Abu-Sbeih et al., 2020; Cherny & Werman, 2019; Gandhi, Gupta, & Ernstoff, 2022; Khunger & Estfan, 2022; Puzanov et al., 2017)

I. Pharmacologic management
   A. Opioid antidiarrheals
      1. Loperamide—first line for CT GIM (minimal systemic absorption, does not cross the blood–brain barrier into the CNS). Patients must call oncology provider if eight 2-mg tablets in 24 hours have no effect on diarrhea. Irinotecan-induced diarrhea requires a more aggressive regimen. Deodorized tincture of opium—second-line opioid antidiarrheal agent; inhibits peristalsis, increases GI transit time, promotes fluid reabsorption.
   B. Octreotide—synthetic somatostatin analog, inhibits gut hormones, increases gut transit time. Second line if unresponsive to loperamide after 48 hours.
   C. Steroids (prednisone 1 mg/kg/day) for ICI colitis Grade 2. Dose increased to 2 mg if lower dose not effective in 48 hours. After 48 hours, infliximab infusion administered for ongoing colitis. Steroids tapered over 4–6 weeks. For Grades 3 and 4, IV steroids administered. Vedolizumab may be used if infliximab not effective or for Grade 3 and 4 diarrhea.
   D. Atropine SC for acute onset (cholinergic) diarrhea from irinotecan. Can also be used prophylactically.
   E. Hydration and electrolyte/ion replacement.
   F. Diphenoxylate/atropine may be used as a second-line agent for targeted therapy–induced diarrhea.

II. Nonpharmacologic management
   A. Rehydration—first priority to manage acute GIM/diarrhea (grades 1 and 2 at home).
   B. Approximate fluid deficit (excludes electrolyte imbalance): patient's usual weight minus present weight (e.g., 70−68 kg=2 kg=2-L deficit).

C. Continue maintenance fluids and replace ongoing losses with PO commercial (Pedialyte or similar) or homemade oral rehydration solution: mix 0.5 teaspoon of salt, 6 teaspoons of sugar, and 1 L of water.

D. Hospitalization, IV rehydration necessary if PO rehydration not feasible or sufficient, grade 3–4 diarrhea.

E. Patient/family teaching critical; patients hesitant to take medicines and "bother" clinicians. Patients and caregivers need verbal, written information; verbalize understanding.

1. Before CT started, emphasize diarrhea/GIM/colitis can potentially become life threatening, and optimal management is critically important.

2. Provide regimen-based information sheet: treatment schedule, possible adverse effects, including need for IV fluids and other treatment measures for diarrhea.

3. Use large font, simple language. Confirm patient, caregiver comprehension.

4. Send patient home with antidiarrheal tablets; instruct them to keep pills with them in case diarrhea starts when they go out.

5. Encourage patient to self-medicate and keep a record of use.

6. Reiterate/reinforce information at every clinical visit throughout treatment.

7. ICI patient education specific—patient to call provider immediately for change in bowel habits, onset of diarrhea, abdominal pain or distention, nausea, constipation, obstipation, cramping, fever, blood/mucous in stool.

8. Dietary modifications may help decrease diarrhea symptoms—bland diet.

9. Avoid foods: spicy, fatty, greasy, or fried; vegetables (especially cruciferous, gas-forming); high fiber, high sugar, and stone fruits (e.g., apricots, cherries, and peaches).

   a. Avoid beverages that may worsen diarrhea: caffeine, alcohol, fruit juices, high-osmolar dietary supplements, lactose-containing dairy products, hot liquids.

   b. Avoid foods, beverages sweetened with sorbitol or xylitol, and tobacco.

   c. Do eat low-fat, high-potassium diet; 6–8 small meals and snacks per day; drink room-temperature clear liquids.

   d. BRAT diet (bananas, rice, apples, and toast) may reduce the frequency of stools.

REFERENCES

Abu-Sbeih, H., Ali, F. S., & Wang, Y. (2020). Immune-checkpoint inhibitors induced diarrhea and colitis: A review of incidence, pathogenesis and management. *Current Opinion in Gastroenterology, 36*(1), 25–32. https://doi.org/10.1097/MOG.0000000000000593.

Abu-Sbeih, H., Johnson, D. H., & Wang, Y. (2019). Immune-related gastrointestinal toxicities. In M. S. Ernstoff, I. Puzanov, C. Robert, A. Diab, & P. Hersey (Eds.), *SITC's guide to managing immunotherapy toxicity* (pp. 93–99). New York: Demos Medical Publishing.

ALMouaalamy, N. (2021). Opioid-induced constipation in advanced cancer patients. *Cureus, 13*(4), e14386. https://doi.org/10.7759/cureus.14386.

Beck, A. M., Kjaersgaard, A., Hansen, T., & Poulsen, I. (2018). Systematic review and evidence based recommendations on texture modified foods and thickened liquids for adults (above 17 years) with oropharyngeal dysphagia – An updated clinical guideline. *Clinical Nutrition, 37*(6), 1980–1991. https://doi.org/10.1016/j.clnu.2017.09.002.

Bharucha, A. E., & Lacy, B. E. (2020). Mechanisms, evaluation, and management of chronic constipation. *Gastroenterology, 158*(5), 1232–1249.E3. https://doi.org/10.1053/j.gastro.2019.12.034.

Bleicher, J., & Lambert, L. A. (2021). A palliative approach to management of peritoneal carcinomatosis and malignant ascites. *Surgical Oncology Clinics of North America, 30*(3), 475–490. https://doi.org/10.1016/j.soc.2021.02.004.

Brahmer, J. R., Lacchetti, C., Schneider, B. J., Atkins, M. B., Brassil, K. J., Caterino, J. M., et al. (2018). Management of immune-related adverse events in patients treated with immune checkpoint inhibitor therapy. *Journal of Clinical Oncology, 36*(17), 1714–1768. https://doi.org/10.1200/JCO.2017.77.6385.

Bressan, V., Bagnasco, A., Aleo, G., Catania, G., Zanini, M. P., Timmins, F., et al. (2017). The life experience of nutrition impact symptoms during treatment for head and neck cancer patients: A systematic review and meta-synthesis. *Supportive Care in Cancer, 25*, 1699–1712. https://doi.org/10.1007/s00520-017-3618-7.

Brown, T. J., & Gupta, A. (2020). Management of cancer therapy-associated oral mucositis. *Journal of Clinical Oncology Practice, 16*(3), 103–109. https://doi.org/10.1200/JOP.19.00652.

Carvalho, C. G., Medeiros-Filho, J., & Ferreira, M. C. (2018). Guide for health professionals addressing oral care for individuals in oncological treatment based on scientific evidence. *Supportive Care in Cancer, 26*, 2651–2661. https://doi.org/10.1007/s00520-018-4111-7.

Cherny, N. I., & Werman, B. (2019). Diarrhea and constipation. In V. T. DeVita, T. S. Lawrence, & S. A. Rosenberg (Eds.), *Cancer principles and practice of oncology* (11th ed.), pp. 2085–2094. Alphen aan den Rijn: Wolters Kluwer.

Chilukuri, P., Odufalu, F., & Hachem, C. (2018). Dysphagia. *Missouri Medicine, 115*(3), 206–210.

Clark, S., & Ebersole, B. (2018). Understanding the role of speech language pathologists in managing dysphagia. *Nursing 2018, 48*(12), 42–46. https://doi.org/10.1097/01.NURSE.0000547723.69610.20.

Clemmons, A., Gandhi, A., Clarke, A., Jimenez, S., Le, T., & Ajebo, G. (2021). Premedications for cancer therapies: A primer for the hematology/oncology provider. *Journal of the Advanced Practitioner in Oncology, 12*(8), 810–832. https://doi.org/10.6004/jadpro.2021.12.8.4.

Correa, M. E. P., Cheng, K. K. F., Chiang, K., Kandwal, A., Loprinzi, C. L., Mori, T., et al. (2020). Systematic review of oral cryotherapy for the management of oral mucositis in cancer patients and clinical practice guidelines. *Supportive Care in Cancer, 28*, 2449–2456. https://doi.org/10.1007/s00520-019-05217-x.

Daugėlaitė, G., Užkuraitytė, K., Jagelavičiene, E., & Filipauskas, A. (2019). Prevention and treatment of chemotherapy and radiotherapy induced oral mucositis. *Medicina, 55*(2), 25. https://doi.org/10.3390/medicina55020025.

Davies, A., Leach, C., Caponero, R., Dickman, A., Fuchs, D., Paice, J., et al. (2020). MASCC recommendations on the management of constipation in patients with advanced cancer. *Supportive Care in Cancer, 28*, 23–33. https://doi.org/10.1007/s00520-019-05016-4.

Diaz, R., Kober, K. M., Viele, C., Cooper, B. A., Paul, S. M., Hammer, M., et al. (2021). Distinct diarrhea profiles during outpatient chemotherapy. *Supportive Care in Cancer, 29*, 2363–2373. https://doi.org/10.1007/s00520-020-05753-x.

Eitan, R., Raban, O., Tsoref, D., Jakobson-Setton, A., Sabah, G., Salman, L., et al. (2018). Malignant ascites: Validation of a novel ascites symptom mini-scale for use in patients with ovarian cancer. *International Journal of Gynecological Cancer, 28*(6), 1162–1166. https://doi.org/10.1097/IGC.0000000000001276.

Espitalier, F., Fanous, A., Aviv, J., Bassiouny, S., Desuter, G., Nerurkar, N., et al. (2018). International consensus (ICON) on assessment of oropharyngeal dysphagia. *European Annals of Otorhinolaryngology, Head and Neck Diseases, 135*(1), S17–S21. https://doi.org/10.1016/j.anorl.2017.12.009.

Gan, T. J., Belani, K. G., Bergese, S., Chung, F., Diemunsch, P., Habib, A. S., et al. (2020). Fourth consensus guidelines for the management of postoperative nausea and vomiting. *Anesthesia and Analgesia, 131*(2), 411–448. https://doi.org/10.1213/ANE.0000000000004833.

Gandhi, S., Gupta, A., & Ernstoff, M. S. (2022). Gastrointestinal toxicities of immunotherapy. In V. Velcheti & S. R. Punekar (Eds.), *Handbook of cancer treatment-related symptoms and toxicities* (pp. 201–221). Amsterdam: Elsevier.

Garcia, M. K., Meng, Z., Rosenthal, D. I., Shen, Y., Chambers, M., Yang, P., et al. (2019). Effect of true and sham acupuncture on radiation-induced xerostomia among patients with head and neck cancer: A randomized clinical trial. *JAMA Network Open, 2*(12), e1916910. https://doi.org/10.1001/jamanetworkopen.2019.16910.

Greco, E., Simic, T., Ringash, J., Tomlinson, G., Inamoto, Y., & Martino, R. (2018). Dysphagia treatment for patients with head and neck cancer undergoing radiation therapy: A meta-analysis review. *International Journal of Radiation Oncology • Biology • Physics, 101*(2), 421–444. https://doi.org/10.1016/j.ijrobp.2018.01.097.

Gupta, K., Walton, R., & Kataria, S. P. (2021). Chemotherapy-induced nausea and vomiting: Pathogenesis, recommendations, and new trends. *Cancer Treatment and Research Communications, 26*, 100278. https://doi.org/10.1016/j.ctarc.2020.100278.

Hesketh, P. J., Kris, M. G., Basch, E., Bohlke, K., Barbour, S. Y., Clark-Snow, R. A., et al. (2020). Antiemetics: ASCO Guideline update. *Journal of Clinical Oncology, 38*(24), 2782–2797. https://doi.org/10.1200/JCO.20.01296.

Hodge, C., & Badgwell, B. D. (2019). Palliation of malignant ascites. *Journal of Surgical Oncology, 120*(1), 67–73. https://doi.org/10.1002/jso.25453.

Hong, C. H. L., Gueiros, L. A., Fulton, J. S., Cheng, K. K. F., Kandwal, A., Galiti, D., et al. (2019). Systematic review of basic oral care for the management of oral mucositis in cancer patients and clinical practice guidelines. *Supportive Care in Cancer, 27*(2), 3949–3967. https://doi.org/10.1007/s00520-019-04848-4.

Huang, B.-S., Wu, S.-C., Lin, C.-Y., Fan, K.-H., Chang, J. T.-C., & Chen, S.-C. (2018). The effectiveness of a saline mouth rinse regimen and education programme on radiation-induced oral mucositis and quality of life in oral cavity cancer patients: A randomised controlled trial. *European Journal of Cancer Care, 27*, e12819. https://doi.org/10.1111/ecc.12819.

Jensen, S. B., Vissink, A., Limesand, K. H., & Reyland, M. E. (2019). Salivary gland hypofunction and xerostomia in head and neck radiation patients. *Journal of National Cancer Institute – Monographs, 2019*(53), lgz016. https://doi.org/10.1093/jncimonographs/lgz016.

Kietpeerakool, C., Rattanakanokchai, S., Jampathong, N., Srisomboon, J., & Lumbiganon, P. (2019). Management of drainage for malignant ascites in gynaecological cancer. *Cochrane Database of Systematic Reviews , 12*(12), CD007794. https://doi.org/10.1002/14651858.CD007794.pub3.

Khunger, A., & Estfan, B. (2022). Gastrointestinal complications of chemotherapy. In V. Velcheti & S. R. Punekar (Eds.), *Handbook of cancer treatment-related symptoms and toxicities* (pp. 29–50). Philadelphia, PA: Elsevier.

King, M., Carulli, A., & Estfan, B. (2022). Oral mucositis. In V. Velcheti & S. R. Punekar (Eds.), *Handbook of cancer treatment-related symptoms and toxicities* (pp. 21–27). Philadelphia, PA: Elsevier.

Knight, J. A., Thompson, S. M., Fleming, C. J., Bendel, E. C., Neisen, M. J., Neidert, N. B., et al. (2018). Safety and effectiveness of palliative tunneled peritoneal drainage catheters in the management of refractory malignant and non-malignant ascites. *Cardiovascular and Interventional Radiology, 41*, 753–761. https://doi.org/10.1007/s00270-017-1872-1.

Krisciunas, G. P., Castellano, K., McCulloch, T. M., Lazarus, C. L., Pauloski, B. R., Meyer, T. K., et al. (2017). Impact of compliance on dysphagia rehabilitation in head and neck cancer patients: Results from a multi-center clinical trial. *Dysphagia, 32*, 327–336. https://doi.org/10.1007/s00455-016-9760-4.

Lalla, R. V., Brennan, M. T., Gordon, S. M., Sonis, S. T., Rosenthal, D. I., & Keefe, D. M. (2019). Oral mucositis due to high-dose chemotherapy and/or head and neck radiation therapy. *Journal of the National Cancer Institute – Monographs, 53*. https://doi.org/10.1093/jncimonographs/lgz011.

Larkin, P. J., Cherny, N. I., La Carpia, D., Guglielmo, M., Ostgathe, C., Scotté, F., et al. (2018). Diagnosis, assessment and management of constipation in advance cancer: ESMO Clinical Practice Guidelines. *Annals of Oncology, 29*(Suppl. 4), iv111–iv125. https://doi.org/10.1093/annonc/mdy148.

Lazarescu, A., Chan, W. W., Gyawali, P. C., Lee, Y. Y., Xiao, Y., & Wu, P. (2020). Updates on diagnostic modalities for esophageal dysphagia. *Annals of the New York Academy of Sciences, 1481*(1), 108-116.

LeFebvre, K. B., Rogers, B. B., & Wolles, B. (2020). Cancer constipation: Clinical summary of the ONS Guidelines™ for opioid-induced and non-opioid-related cancer constipation. *Clinical Journal of Oncology Nursing, 24*(6), 685–688. https://doi.org/10.1188/20.CJON.685-688.

Matsusaki, K., Aridome, K., Emoto, S., Kajiyama, H., Takagaki, N., Takahashi, T., et al. (2022). Clinical practice guideline for the treatment of malignant ascites: Section summary in Clinical Practice Guideline for peritoneal dissemination (2021). *International Journal of Clinical Oncology, 27*(1), 1–6. https://doi.org/10.1007/s10147-021-02077-6.

Mercadante, V., Al Hamad, A., Lodi, G., Porter, S., & Fedele, S. (2017). Interventions for the management of radiotherapy-induced xerostomia and hyposalivation: A systematic review and meta-analysis. *Oral Oncology, 66*, 64–74. https://doi.org/10.1016/j.oraloncology.2016.12.031.

Mercadante, V., Jensen, S. B., Smith, D. K., Bohlke, K., Bauman, J., Brennan, M. T., et al. (2021). Salivary gland hypofunction and/or xerostomia induced by nonsurgical cancer therapies: ISOO/MASCC/ASCO guideline. *Journal of Clinical Oncology, 39*(25), 2825–2843. https://doi.org/10.1200/JCO.21.01208.

Mesía, R., Echaburu, J. A. V., Gómez, J., Sauri, T., Serrano, G., & Pujol, E. (2019). Opioid-induced constipation in oncological patients: New strategies of management. *Current Treatment Options in Oncology, 20*(12), 91. https://doi.org/10.1007/s11864-019-0686-6.

Millsop, J. W., Wang, E. A., & Fazel, N. (2017). Etiology, evaluation, and management of xerostomia. *Clinics in Dermatology, 35*(5), 468–476. https://doi.org/10.1016/j.clindermatol.2017.06.010.

National Cancer Institute (NCI). (2017). Common Terminology Criteria for Adverse Events (CTCAE), version 5.0. https://ctep.cancer.gov/protocoldevelopment/electronic_applications/docs/ctcae_v5_quick_reference_5x7.pdf.

National Comprehensive Cancer Network® (NCCN). (2022). Antiemetics. Version 2.2022. https://www.nccn.org/professionals/physician_gls/pdf/antiemesis.pdf.

Navari, R. M. (2020). Nausea and vomiting in advanced cancer. *Current Treatment Options in Oncology, 21*(2), 14. https://doi.org/10.1007/s11864-020-0704-8.

Okuni, I., Otsubo, Y., & Ebihara, S. (2021). Molecular and neural mechanism of dysphagia due to cancer. *International Journal of Molecular Sciences, 22*(13), 7033. https://doi.org/10.3390/ijms22137033.

Oncology Nursing Society (ONS). (2019a). Mucositis. www.ons.org/pep/mucositis.

Oncology Nursing Society (ONS). (2019b). Chemotherapy-induced nausea and vomiting – Adult. https://www.ons.org/pep/chemotherapy-induced-nausea-and-vomiting-adult?display=pepnavigator&sort_by=created&items_per_page=50.

Panebianco, M., Marchese-Ragona, R., Masiero, S., & Restivo, D. A. (2020). Dysphagia in neurological diseases: A literature review. *Neurological Sciences, 41*, 3067–3073. https://doi.org/10.1007/s10072-020-04495-2.

Pezdirec, M., Strojan, P., & Boltezar, I. H. (2019). Swallowing disorders after treatment for head and neck cancer. *Radiology and Oncology, 53*(2), 225–230. https://doi.org/10.2478/raon-2019-0028.

Pulito, C., Cristaudo, A., La Porta, C., Zapperi, S., Blandino, G., Morrone, A., et al. (2020). Oral mucositis: The hidden side of cancer therapy. *Journal of Experimental & Clinical Cancer Research, 39*, 210. https://doi.org/10.1186/s13046-020-01715-7.

Puzanov, I., Diab, A., Abdallah, K., Bingham, C. O., 3rd, Brogdon, C., Dadu, R., et al. (2017). Managing toxicities associated with immune checkpoint inhibitors: Consensus recommendations from the Society for Immunotherapy of Cancer (SITC) Toxicity Management Working Group. *Journal of ImmunoTherapy of Cancer, 5*(1), 95. https://doi.org/10.1186/s40425-017-0300-z.

Razvi, Y., Chan, S., McFarlane, T., McKenzie, E., Zaki, P., DeAngelis, C., et al. (2019). ASCO, NCCN, MASCC/ESMO: A comparison of antiemetic guidelines for the treatment of chemotherapy-induced nausea and vomiting in adult patients. *Supportive Care in Cancer, 27*, 87–95. https://doi.org/10.1007/s00520-018-4464-y.

Robson, P. C., Gonen, M., Ni, A., Brody, L., Brown, K. T., Getrajdman, G., Thom, B., et al. (2019). Quality of life improves after palliative placement of percutaneous tunneled drainage catheter for refractory ascites in prospective study of patients with end-stage cancer. *Palliative & Supportive Care, 17*(6), 677–685. https://doi.org/10.1017/S1478951519000051.

Rogers, B. B., Ginex, P. K., Anbari, A., Hanson, B. J., LeFebvre, K. B., Lopez, R., et al. (2020). ONS Guidelines™ for opioid-induced and non-opioid-related cancer constipation. *Oncology Nursing Forum, 47*(6), 671–691. https://doi.org/10.1188/20.ONF.671-691.

Rudralingam, V., Footitt, C., & Layton, B. (2017). Ascites matters. *Ultrasound, 25*(2), 69–79. https://doi.org/10.1177/1742271X16680653.

Rugo, H. S., Seneviratne, L., Beck, J. T., Glaspy, J. A., Peguero, J. A., Pluard, T. J., et al. (2017). Prevention of everolimus-related stomatitis in women with hormone receptor-positive, HER-2 negative metastatic breast cancer using dexamethasone mouthwash (SWISH): A single-arm, phase 2 trial. *The Lancet, 18*(5), 654–662. https://doi.org/10.1016/S1470-2045(17)30109-2.

Saigal, B., & Guerra, L. (2018). Prevention of stomatitis: Using dexamethasone-based mouthwash to inhibit everolimus-related stomatitis. *Clinical Journal of Oncology Nursing, 22*(2), 211–217. https://doi.org/10.1188/18.CJON.211-217.

Secombe, K. R., Van Sebille, Y. Z. A., Mayo, B. J., Coller, J. K., Gibson, R. J., & Bowen, J. M. (2020). Diarrhea induced by small molecule tyrosine kinase inhibitors compared with chemotherapy: Potential role of the microbiome. *Integrative Cancer Therapies, 19*, 1–12. https://doi.org/10.1177/1534735420928493.

Strojan, P., Hutcheson, K. A., Eisbruch, A., Beitler, J. J., Langendijk, J. A., Lee, A. W. M., et al. (2017). Treatment of late sequelae after radiotherapy for head and neck cancer. *Cancer Treatment Reviews, 59*, 79–92. https://doi.org/10.1016/j.ctrv.2017.07.003.

Stukan, M. (2017). Drainage of malignant ascites: Patient selection and perspectives. *Cancer Management and Research, 9*, 115–130. https://doi.org/10.2147/CMAR.S100210.

Wickham, R. J. (2020a). Nausea and vomiting: A palliative care imperative. *Current Oncology Reports, 22*(1), 1. https://doi.org/10.1007/s11912-020-0871-6.

Wickham, R. J. (2020b). Revisiting the physiology of nausea and vomiting—Challenging the paradigm. *Supportive Care in Cancer, 28*, 13–21. https://doi.org/10.1007/s00520-019-05012-8.

Wolff, A., Joshi, R. K., Ekström, J., Aframian, D., Pedersen, A. M. L., Proctor, G., et al. (2017). A guide to medications inducing salivary gland dysfunction, xerostomia, and subjective sialorrhea: A systematic review sponsored by the World Workshop on Oral Medicine VI. *Drugs in R&D, 17*(1), 1–28. https://doi.org/10.1007/s40268-016-0153-9.

Yu, Y.-T., Deng, J.-L., Jin, X.-R., Zhang, Z.-Z., Zhang, X.-H., & Zhou, X. (2020). Effects of 9 oral care solutions on the prevention of oral mucositis: A network meta-analysis of randomized controlled trials. *Medicine, 99*(16), e19661. https://doi.org/10.1097/MD.0000000000019661.

Yüce, U. O., & Yurtsever, S. (2019). Effect of education about oral mucositis given to the cancer patients having chemotherapy on life quality. *Journal of Cancer Education, 34*, 35–40. https://doi.org/10.1007/s13187-017-1262-z.

Zebralla, V., Wichmann, G., Pirlich, M., Hammermüller, C., Berger, T., Zimmermann, K., et al. (2021). Dysphagia, voice problems, and pain in head and neck cancer patients. *European Archives of Oto-Rhino-Laryngology, 278*, 3985–3994. https://doi.org/10.1007/s00405-020-06584-6.

Zecha, J. A. E. M., Raber-Durlacher, J. E., Laheij, A. M. G. A., Westermann, A. M., Epstein, J. B., de Lange, J., et al. (2019). The impact of the oral cavity in febrile neutropenia and infectious complications in patients treated with myelosuppressive chemotherapy. *Supportive Care in Cancer, 27*, 3667–3679. https://doi.org/10.1007/s00520-019-04925-8.

39

Genitourinary Symptoms

Carla Schaefer

URINARY INCONTINENCE

Overview

I. Physiology (see Chapter 15)
  A. Definition
    1. Urinary incontinence—involuntary loss of urine (Klein, Mollard, & Eisenhauer, 2021; Si, Ding, Huang, Zhang, & Zhang, 2021)
    2. Stress—involuntary loss of urine during tasks or activities such as laughing, coughing, and sneezing, that increase abdominal and bladder pressure to a higher level than the urethra has the capability to stay closed (D'Ancona et al., 2019; Falah-Hassani, Reeves, Shiri, Hickling, & McLean, 2021; Rahnama'i, Marcelissen, Geavlete, Tutolo, & Hüsch, 2021)
    3. Urge—involuntary loss of urine with an abrupt and strong desire to void
    4. Reflex—involuntary loss of urine with no sensation of urge or bladder fullness
    5. Functional—state in which an individual experiences incontinence because of difficulty in reaching or inability to reach the toilet before urination
    6. Total—continuous loss of urine without distention or awareness of bladder fullness
    7. Urinary retention—chronic inability to void followed by involuntary voiding (overflow incontinence) due to overdistention of the bladder (Carr, 2019)
  B. Mechanisms
    1. Storage problems
      a. Involuntary contracting of bladder during filling
      b. Reduced compliance of bladder wall
      c. Sensory urgency
      d. Loss of bladder neck and change in the length of urethra to maintain bladder outlet resistance (Chang, Hung, Hu, & Chiu, 2018; Gresty, Walters, & Rashid, 2019; Rahnama'i et al., 2021)
      e. Intrinsic sphincter dysfunction
    2. Emptying problems
      a. Loss of or impaired contractility
      b. Urethral or prostatic obstruction
II. Risk factors
  A. Disease related
    1. Loss of ability to inhibit bladder or rectal contractions (Samuels, Pezzella, Berenholz, & Alinsod, 2019)

2. Loss of sphincter competency (Samuels et al., 2019)
    a. Impaired or lost sensation of the bladder
    b. Obstruction of the bladder
    c. Immobility commonly associated with chronic degenerative disease
    d. Loss of functional ability
    e. Previous transurethral resection of the prostate, anastomotic stricture, stage of disease, surgical technique, and experience of the surgeon (Gresty et al., 2019; Rahnama'i et al., 2021)
  B. Treatment related (Angulo et al., 2021; Neal et al., 2020)
    1. Surgical intervention that disrupts neural pathways
    2. Inflammatory reaction from radiation therapy (RT) on bladder and bowel
    3. Chemotherapy agents that cause neurotoxic side effects
    4. Fistula formation as a complication of disease, surgery, or RT
    5. Cryosurgery, which may cause urinary incontinence, urethral sloughing, and bladder neck obstruction (National Cancer Institute, 2021)
    6. Medications, including anticholinergics, diuretics, narcotics, sedatives, hypnotics, tranquilizers, and laxatives
    7. Complications associated with indwelling catheter (Newman, 2021)

Assessment

I. History (Denisenko, Clark, D'Amico, & Murphy, 2021; Hu & Pierre, 2019)
  A. Personal history
  B. Cognitive ability
  C. Neurologic disease or symptoms
  D. Motivation to self-care in toileting
  E. Manual dexterity and mobility
  F. Living arrangements
  G. Identification of caregiver and degree of caregiver involvement
  H. Prescription and nonprescription medications
  I. Impact of incontinence on self-esteem and interpersonal relationships
II. Past and present patterns of elimination (Denisenko et al., 2021; Hu & Pierre, 2019)

A. Precipitants of incontinence—caffeine and alcohol consumption, physical activity
   1. Surgery, trauma, and recent illnesses
B. Daily fluid intake
C. Urinary tract symptoms
D. Duration of incontinence
E. Frequency and amount of continence and incontinence
F. Previous treatments and their effects
G. Bladder diary for 3 days
III. Physical findings
A. Presence of abdominal masses
B. Palpation of full bladder
C. Pelvic organ prolapse
D. Fecal impaction to be ruled out
E. Neurologic assessment
F. Presence of incontinence, odor, perineal skin irritation, or breakdown
IV. Diagnostic testing (Denisenko et al., 2021; Hu & Pierre, 2019)
A. Urinalysis and culture and sensitivity
B. Cough stress test
C. Presence and amount of postvoiding residual urine
D. Urodynamic and imaging studies
E. Cystoscopy to identify the site of obstruction

Management

I. Medical management
A. Interventions to promote urinary continence (Denisenko et al., 2021)
   1. Anticholinergics
   2. Tricyclic antidepressants
   3. Potassium channel openers
   4. Electrostimulation
   5. Urology consultation
II. Nursing management
A. Supportive techniques
   1. Assess and minimize barriers to toileting.
   2. Daily assessment of perianal skin
   3. Instruct patient to clean the area after every voiding or bowel movement.
   4. Apply moisture barrier ointment or skin barrier.
   5. Use of absorbent pads or briefs (Gresty et al., 2019; Si et al., 2021; Yates, 2021)
   6. Male slings (Gresty et al., 2019; Rahnama'i et al., 2021)
   7. Use of penile compression devices for males and pessaries for females (Gresty et al., 2019; Rahnama'i et al., 2021)
   8. Use of external condoms and internal catheters (Yates, 2021)
B. Behavioral techniques (Si et al., 2021)
   1. Establish a routine schedule for voiding (habit training).
   2. Ask the patient on a regular basis about voiding (prompt voiding).
   3. Teach the patient to suppress the urge to void (bladder retraining).

4. Teach the patient how to perform Kegel exercises/pelvic floor muscle exercises.
5. Have the patient decrease fluid intake in the evening.
6. Increase foods in diet to help prevent constipation.
7. Have the patient reduce intake of caffeine-containing beverages and other bladder irritants.

OSTOMIES AND URINARY DIVERSIONS

Overview

I. Urinary diversions (Lenis, Lec, & Chamie, 2020)
A. A new surgically created pathway for the urine to leave the body
   1. Performed in situations in which the bladder is removed (radical cystectomy) or radical cystoprostatectomy for cancer of the bladder
   2. Involves removal of the bladder, pelvic lymph nodes, prostate (in men) and uterus, fallopian tubes, ovaries, and anterior vaginal wall, possibly urethra (in women)
   3. Sexual dysfunction common because of neural damage from surgery (Tyler & Profusek, 2018)
B. Types of urinary diversions (Lenis et al., 2020)
   1. Ileal conduit
      a. Created from segment of small bowel; as the proximal end is sutured closed the distal end is brought out through the abdominal wall; a stoma is created, and the ureters are implanted into the small-bowel segment
      b. Urine produced almost continuously
      c. Requires an external collection device
C. Early complications are related to the intestinal anastomosis and resection with paralytic ileus occurring most often. Later complications can be related to stoma stenosis, retraction, infection, prolapse of the stoma, and parastomal hernia (Prcic & Begic, 2017).
D. Continent cutaneous diversion (ileocecal reservoir/Indiana pouch) (Lenis et al., 2020)
   1. Reservoir constructed from ileum or large intestine
   2. Construction of the reservoir via a one-way-flap valve
   3. External collection device not needed
   4. Patient will need to catheterize through the stoma every 4–6 hours
   5. Least-used option
E. Orthoptic neobladder (Lenis et al., 2020; Qu & Lawretschuk, 2019)
   1. A surgically constructed bladder created from the intestine in the original bladder location and attached to urethra
   2. Allows emptying of the bladder (voiding) through the urethra by relaxation of urinary sphincters and simultaneous Valsalva maneuver with training to prevent leakage
   3. Intermittent catheterization may be needed for urinary retention

4. Contraindications to neobladder—cancer extending into urethra, history of inflammatory bowel disease, radiation, or previous bowel resection

II. Risk factors
   A. Pelvic radiation
   B. Chemotherapy
   C. Bladder cancer with muscle invasion (Qu & Lawretschuk, 2019)

III. Effects of treatment to urinary diversions
   A. Pelvic exenteration (radical surgical treatment that removes all organs from a person's pelvic cavity)
   B. Pelvic and abdominal radiation (mucosal damage when the stoma is in the field of radiation) (Srikanth et al., 2022)

Assessment

I. Pertinent personal history (Haywood, Donahue, & Bochner, 2021)
   A. Type of surgery and stoma
   B. Previous pelvic or abdominal radiation or chemotherapy treatments
   C. Changes in patterns of urinary elimination
   D. Recurrent or chronic urinary tract infections
   E. Difficulty in catheterizing a continent diversion
   F. Diet habits and fluid consumption

II. Physical findings (Haywood et al., 2021)
   A. Characteristics of stoma and peristomal skin
   B. Presence of leakage of urine from a continent diversion

Management

I. Nonpharmacologic management (Berti-Hearn & Elliott, 2019)
   A. Interventions regarding the care of urinary diversion
     1. Teach patient how to care for urinary diversion.
       a. Stoma placement
       b. Scars, bony prominences, skin creases, belt line, or hernia to be avoided
     2. Select appliance based on the type of effluent, abdominal contour, manual dexterity, patient preference, and cost.
     3. Change appliance every 5 days and as needed.
     4. Ensure barrier clears stoma by {⅛} inch; protect exposed skin with barrier paste.
     5. Gently remove pouch by pushing down on skin while lifting up on the pouch.
     6. Cleanse peristomal skin with water and pat dry.
     7. Assess stoma and skin around stoma with each appliance change.
     8. Empty pouch when one-third to one-half full and before chemotherapy.
     9. Protect stoma from injury.
     10. Monitor volume, color, and consistency of effluent.
     11. Monitor functioning of new urinary diversion starting 3–5 days after surgery.
     12. Catheterize new continent diversions 3–4 weeks after surgery.
       a. Ureteral stents are irrigated every 6–8 hours several weeks postoperatively.
       b. As urinary output from continent diversion increases, urine output from ureteral stents decreases.
     13. Catheterize through the stoma to drain urine from the reservoir every 4–6 hours.
     14. Recommend referral to the wound, ostomy, and continence nurse if needed.
   B. Interventions to promote body image and self-esteem
     1. Acknowledge normalcy of emotional response to change in urinary function.
     2. Encourage patient to verbalize positive or negative feelings.
     3. Assist patient in incorporating changes into activities of daily living, social life, interpersonal relationships, and occupational activities.
     4. Help patient identify ways to cope that have been useful in the past.
     5. Refer patient and caregivers to support groups and provide resources.

RENAL DYSFUNCTION

Overview

I. Pathophysiology (see Chapter 15)
II. Risk factors
   A. Effects of disease (Klemencic & Perkins, 2019; Thomas, 2019; Wood, 2018)
     1. Compression of ureters by metastatic tumor causing obstruction, resulting in hydronephrosis
     2. Compression of blood vessels by mass or tumor may cause venous occlusion.
       a. Reduction of blood flow may impair kidney function.
     3. Inability of kidneys to concentrate urine occurs in hypercalcemia of malignancy.
       a. Kidneys are attempting to excrete calcium in blood, leading to diuresis and electrolyte disturbances.
       b. Hypercalcemia of malignancy occurs more commonly in breast cancer with metastases, multiple myeloma, squamous cell cancer of the lung and head and neck, renal cell cancer, lymphomas, and leukemia.
       c. Advanced prostate or cervical cancer renal problems are related to post-renal obstructive uropathy.
   B. Treatment related (Klemencic & Perkins, 2019; Thomas, 2019; Wood, 2018)
     1. Radiation to renal structures may lead to permanent fibrosis and atrophy.
     2. Precipitation of uric acid or calcium phosphate crystallization from tumor lysis
     3. Fluid and electrolyte imbalances caused by chemotherapy agents
     4. Nephrotoxic agents cause a direct effect.

Assessment

I. Pertinent personal history to identify risk factors (Chen, Knicely, & Grams, 2019)
   A. Advanced age—60 years and older
   B. Diuretics, NSAIDs, and cardiac and nephrotoxic medications
   C. Type of malignancy
   D. Comorbidities such as hypertension, diabetes insipidus, and diabetes mellitus
   E. Previous pelvic or abdominal radiation or chemotherapy treatments
   F. History of renal stones
   G. Preexisting renal impairment
II. Physical findings (Chen et al., 2019)
   A. Cardiovascular—arrhythmias, rapid thready pulse, and orthostatic hypotension
   B. Neurologic—lethargy, confusion
   C. Poor skin turgor, dry mucous membranes
   D. Gastrointestinal—nausea, vomiting, polydipsia, and splenomegaly
   E. Genitourinary—nocturia, polyuria, oliguria, flank pain, and dysuria
III. Laboratory data
   A. Serum creatinine and blood urea nitrogen levels reflect renal function.
   B. Creatinine clearance study before implementing nephrotoxic treatment
   C. Elevation of serum uric acid and calcium levels and a decrease in potassium and magnesium levels may suggest renal impairment (Klemencic & Perkins, 2019; Wood, 2018).

Management

I. Pharmacologic management
   A. Saline hydration with appropriate diuretic (Duffy, Fitzgerald, Boyle, & Rohatgi, 2018; Klemencic & Perkins, 2019).
   B. Oral or intravenous sodium bicarbonate to maintain alkaline urine (Chen et al., 2019)
   C. Amifostine and sodium thiosulfate for cisplatin nephrotoxicity (Fang et al., 2021)
   D. Replace electrolytes as needed.
   E. Administer diuretics as needed.
II. Nonpharmacologic management
   A. Education for patient and family
      1. Maintain adequate hydration and safe weight-bearing activity.
      2. Signs and symptoms of electrolyte imbalance and fluid volume excess and the appropriate time to seek medical attention
      3. Medications prescribed
   B. Monitor for signs and symptoms of renal toxicity (Chen et al., 2019)
      1. Verify baseline renal function.
      2. Monitor intake and output closely.
         a. Maintain a greater intake than output unless contraindicated.
         b. Monitor for obstructive diuresis after the removal of obstruction.
         c. Strain urine for stones if indicated.
      3. Monitor vital signs and postural blood pressure.
      4. Monitor relevant laboratory data.
      5. Record daily weights.
      6. Maximize mobility.

REFERENCES

Angulo, J., Arance, I., Apesteguy, Y., Felicio, J., Martins, N., & Martins, F. (2021). Urorectal fistula repair using different approaches: Operative results and quality of life issues. *International Brazilian Journal of Urology*, 47(2), 399–412. https://doi.org/10.1590/S1677-5538.IBJU.2020.0476.

Berti-Hearn, L., & Elliott, B. (2019). Urostomy care: A guide for home care clinicians. *Home Healthcare Now*, 37(5), 248–255. https://doi.org/10.1097/NHH.0000000000000792.

Carr, S. (2019). Catheter valves: Retraining the bladder to avoid prolonged catheter use. *Journal of Community Nursing*, 33(3), 46–51.

Chang, L.-W., Hung, S.-C., Hu, J.-C., & Chiu, K.-Y. (2018). Retzius-sparing robotic-assisted prostatectomy associated with less bladder neck descent and better early continence outcome. *Anticancer Research*, 38(1), 345–351. https://doi.org/10.21873/anticanres.12228.

Chen, T. K., Knicely, D. H., & Grams, M. E. (2019). Chronic kidney disease diagnosis and management: A review. *Journal of the American Medical Association*, 322(13), 1294–1304. https://doi.org/10.1001/jama.2019.14745.

D'Ancona, C., Haylen, B., Oelke, M., Abraches-Monteiro, L., Arnold, E., Goldman, H., et al. (2019). The International Continence Society (ICS) report on the terminology for adult male lower urinary tract and pelvic floor symptoms and dysfunction. *Neurourology and Urodynamics*, 38(2), 433–477. https://doi.org/10.1002/nau.23897.

Denisenko, A. A., Clark, C. B., D'Amico, M., & Murphy, A. M. (2021). Evaluation and management of female urinary incontinence. *The Canadian Journal of Urology*, 28(S2), 27–32.

Duffy, E. A., Fitzgerald, W., Boyle, K., & Rohatgi, R. (2018). Nephrotoxicity: Evidence in patients receiving cisplatin therapy. *Clinical Journal of Oncology Nursing*, 22(2), 175–183. https://doi.org/10.1188/18.CJON.175-183.

Falah-Hassani, K., Reeves, J., Shiri, R., Hickling, D., & McLean, L. (2021). The pathophysiology of stress urinary incontinence: A systematic review and meta-analysis. *International Urogynecology Journal*, 32, 501–552. https://doi.org/10.1007/s00192-020-04622-9.

Fang, C.-Y., Lou, D.-Y., Zhou, L.-Q., Wang, J.-C., Yang, B., He, Q.-J., et al. (2021). Natural products: Potential treatments for cisplatin-induced nephrotoxicity. *Acta Pharmacologica Sinica*, 42(12), 1951–1969. https://doi.org/10.1038/s41401-021-00620-9.

Gresty, H., Walters, U., & Rashid, T. (2019). Post-prostatectomy incontinence: Multimodal modern-day management. *British Journal of Community Nursing*, 24(4), 154–159. https://doi.org/10.12968/bjcn.2019.24.4.154.

Haywood, S., Donahue, T., & Bochner, B. (2021). Management of common complications after radical cystectomy, lymph node dissection, and urinary diversion. In A. M. Kamat & P. C. Black (Eds.), *Bladder cancer* (pp. 185–203). Berlin: Springer. https://doi.org/10.1007/978-3-030-70646-3_16.

Hu, J. S., & Pierre, E. F. (2019). Urinary incontinence in women: Evaluation and management. *American Family Physician*, 100(6), 339–348.

Klein, A., Mollard, E., & Eisenhauer, C. (2021). Self-management of urinary incontinence in women: A concept analysis. *Urologic Nursing, 41*(4), 195–207. https://doi.org/10.7257/1053-816X.2021.41.4.195.

Klemencic, S., & Perkins, J. (2019). Diagnosis and management of oncologic emergencies. *Western Journal of Emergency Medicine, 20*(2), 316–322. https://doi.org/10.5811/westjem.2018.12.37335.

Lenis, A., Lec, P., & Chamie, K. (2020). Bladder cancer: A review. *Journal of American Medical Association, 324*(19), 1980–1991. https://doi.org/10.1001/jama.2020.17598.

National Cancer Institute. (2021). Cryosurgery to treat cancer. https://www.cancer.gov/about-cancer/treatment/types/surgery/cryosurgery#side-effects-from-cryosurgery.

Neal, D., Metcalfe, C., Donovan, J., Lane, J., Davis, M., Young, G., et al. (2020). Ten-year mortality, disease progression, and treatment-related side effects in men with localised prostate cancer from the ProtecT randomised controlled trial according to treatment received. *European Urology, 77*(3), 320–330. https://doi.org/10.1016/j.eururo.2019.10.030.

Newman, D. (2021). Methods and types of urinary catheters used for indwelling or intermittent catheterization. *Urologic Nursing, 41*(2), 111–117. https://doi.org/10.7257/1053-816X.2021.41.2.111.

Qu, L., & Lawretschuk, N. (2019). Orthotopic neobladder reconstruction: Patient selection and perspectives. *Research and Reports in Urology, 11*, 333–341. https://doi.org/10.2147/RRU.S181473.

Prcic, A., & Begic, E. (2017). Complications after ileal urinary derivations. *Medical Archives (Sarajevo, Bosnia and Herzegovina), 71*(5), 320–324. https://doi.org/10.5455/medarh.2017.71.320-324.

Rahnama'i, M., Marcelissen, T., Geavlete, B., Tutolo, M., & Hüsch, T. (2021). Current management of post-radical prostatectomy urinary incontinence. *Frontiers in Surgery, 8*(647656), 1–10. https://doi.org/10.3389/fsurg.2021.647656.

Samuels, J., Pezzella, A., Berenholz, J., & Alinsod, R. (2019). Safety and efficacy of a non-invasive high-intensity focused electromagnetic field (HIFEM) device for treatment of urinary incontinence and enhancement of quality of life. *Lasers in Surgery and Medicine, 51*(9), 760–766. https://doi.org/10.1002/lsm.23106.

Si, L., Ding, Y., Huang, Y., Zhang, M., & Zhang, J. (2021). Postprostatectomy incontinence and self-management for urinary incontinence after laparoscopic radical prostatectomy: A cross-sectional study. *Journal of Wound, Ostomy, and Continence Nursing, 48*(5), 440–446. https://doi.org/10.1097/WON.0000000000000793.

Srikanth, P., Kay, H. E., Tijerina, A. N., Srivastava, A. V., Laviana, A. A., Wolf, J. S., Jr., et al. (2022). Review of the current management of radiation-induced ureteral strictures of the pelvis. *AME Medical Journal, 7*(8), 1–17. https://doi.org/10.21037/amj-21-5.

Thomas, N. (2019). *Renal nursing: Care and management of people with kidney disease* (5th ed.). Hoboken, NJ: Wiley.

Tyler, A., & Profusek, P. (2018). Bladder cancer. In C. H. Yarbro, D. Wujcik, & B. H. Gobel (Eds.), *Cancer nursing: Principles and practice* (8th ed., pp. 1228–1242). Burlington, MA: Jones & Bartlett.

Wood, L. S. (2018). Renal cancer. In C. H. Yarbro, D. Wujcik, & B. H. Gobel (Eds.), *Cancer nursing: Principles and practice* (8th ed., pp. 1873–1896). Burlington, MA: Jones & Bartlett.

Yates, A. (2021). Part 4: Management with appropriate devices/products. *Journal of Community Nursing, 35*(6), 20–27.

40

Hematologic and Immune Symptoms

Jennifer Hadjar

OVERVIEW OF HEMATOLOGIC SYMPTOMS

Overview

I. Definition—*myelosuppression*, a significant reduction in bone marrow function that results in a reduced production of red blood cells (RBCs), white blood cells (WBCs), and platelets (Plts) within the bone marrow (Crombez, 2019; Messin & Amrhein, 2019; Wilson, 2019; Yang, Che, Xiao, Zhao, & Liu, 2021)
   A. Manifests as neutropenia, thrombocytopenia, and anemia
   B. Related to the destruction of rapidly dividing cancer cells
II. Physiology (Crombez, 2019; Lordo et al., 2021; Messin & Amrhein, 2019; Wilson, 2019; Yang et al., 2021)
   A. The bone marrow is the primary source for hematopoiesis, the development of blood components, including myeloid and lymphoid progenitor cells
      1. Myeloid cells include granulocytes (neutrophils, eosinophils, basophils, and monocytes), RBCs, and Plts.
      2. Lymphoid cells include B lymphocytes, T lymphocytes, and natural killer cells.
   B. Myelosuppression decreases a patient's quality of life, as well as increasing overall mortality and financial toxicities.
   C. Risk factors for myelotoxicity are broadly categorized into disease-related, patient-related, and treatment-related.
   D. Chemotherapy-induced myelosuppression is a common dose-limiting adverse event in cancer treatment.
      1. Most chemotherapies cause some degree of myelosuppression.
      2. Each chemotherapeutic agent varies with the onset and duration of cytopenias, depending on pharmacokinetic variables: dose, frequency, route of administration, absorption, distribution, metabolism, and excretion.
   E. Treatment-related myeloid cytopenias commonly include neutropenia and thrombocytopenia, and anemia.
      1. Neutropenia—absolute neutrophil count (ANC) below 1500/mm³ places the patient at increased risk of infection and sepsis
      2. Thrombocytopenia—Plt count below the normal range; places the patient at increased risk of bleeding
      3. Anemia—hemoglobin (Hgb) below 11 g/dL places the patient at increased risk of fatigue and tissue hypoxia
   F. The severity of myeloid cytopenias is based on common grading criteria (Table 40.1).
   G. Treatment-related lymphopenia is less common.
      1. Lymphopenia—a reduction in the number of B or T lymphocytes that increases the risk for opportunistic infections

NEUTROPENIA

Overview

I. Definition—a decrease in the number of circulating neutrophils in the blood evidenced by ANC less than the lower limit of normal (LLN)—less than 1000 μL (see Table 40.1; Crombez, 2019; Messin & Amrhein, 2019; Wilson, 2019)
   A. Lifespan of a neutrophil—less than 48 hours on average
   B. How to calculate ANC: total WBC × total neutrophil count (% segmented neutrophil count + % bands) = ANC. Example:
      1. WBC = 3.1 × 1000/μL
      2. Neutrophils (25%) + bands (10%) = 35%
      3. ANC = 3100 × 0.35 = 1085/mm³ = grade 2 neutropenia
II. Physiology (Crombez, 2019; Wilson, 2019)
   A. Chemotherapy-induced neutropenia is one of the most common dose-limiting toxicities associated with systemic treatment for cancer.
   B. Neutrophils divide rapidly and are susceptible to the cytotoxic effects of chemotherapy.
   C. Chemotherapy and radiation therapy may also damage the bone marrow microenvironment.
      1. Cell cycle–specific chemotherapy is typically less damaging.
      2. Radiation to bone marrow–producing regions—pelvis, ribs, sternum, skull, metaphyses of the long bones—may cause prolonged cytopenias.
III. Risk factors (Crombez, 2019; Messin & Amrhein, 2019; Wilson, 2019; Table 40.2)
   A. Patient-related factors
   B. Disease-related factors
   C. Treatment-related factors
      1. Type and dose of chemotherapy
      2. Location of radiation therapy

TABLE 40.1 Overview of Neutropenia

Neutropenia	A decrease in the number of circulating neutrophils in the blood evidenced by an ANC of less than 1000/μL	Grade 1: ANC <LLN—1500/mm³ Grade 2: ANC <500–1000/mm³ Grade 3: ANC <1000–500/mm³ Grade 4: ANC <500/mm³
FN	ANC <1000/mm³ and a single temperature of >38.3°C (101°F) or a sustained temperature of ≥38°C (100.4°F) for more than 1 h	

ANC, Absolute neutrophil count; *FN*, febrile neutropenia; *LLN*, lower limit of normal.
From Wilkes, G., & Barton-Burke, M. (2019). *2020–2021 Oncology nursing drug handbook* (23rd ed.). Burlington, MA: Jones & Bartlett Learning, LLC; Wilson, B. J. (2019). Myelosuppression. In M. M. Olsen, K. B. LeFebvre, & K. J. Brassil (Eds.), *Chemotherapy and immunotherapy guidelines and recommendations for practice* (pp. 273–292). Pittsburgh, PA: Oncology Nursing Society.

TABLE 40.2 Risk Factors Associated With Chemotherapy-Induced Neutropenia

Patient-Related Factors	Disease- and Treatment-Related Factors
Age greater than 65 years	High tumor burden/extensive disease
Female gender	History of chemotherapy or radiation
Body surface area >2 m²	Preexisting cytopenias
ECOG PS ≥2	Bone marrow involvement with tumor (hematologic malignancies)
Malnutrition—serum albumin ≤3.5 g/dL	Type of chemotherapy
Decrease immune function	Dose intensity of chemotherapy
	Elevated LDH level
Comorbidities, especially COPD, diabetes, renal impairment, and liver disease	Neutropenia lasting more than 4 days after an episode of FN
	Concurrent mucositis, colitis, or typhlitis
	DIC
Open wounds or recent surgery	Elevated CRP level greater
	Bleeding severe enough to require transfusion
Active infections or preexisting infections	Arrhythmia or electrocardiographic changes requiring treatment
Drug–drug interactions	Hypoalbuminemia, hyperbilirubinemia
	Increased number of hospitalizations or ICU admissions

COPD, Chronic obstructive–pulmonary disease; *CRP*, cross-reactive protein; *DIC*, disseminated intravascular coagulation; *ECOG*, Eastern Cooperative Oncology Group; *FN*, febrile neutropenia; *ICU*, intensive care unit; *LDH*, lactate dehydrogenase; *PS*, performance scale.
From Crombez, P. (2019). Evidence-based nursing of patients with hematologic malignancies. In F. Charnay-Sonnek, & A. E. Murphy (Eds.), *Principle of nursing in oncology* (pp. 277–308). Berlin: Springer; Messin, C., & Amrhein, C. (2019). Evidence-based nursing in basic anticancer treatment: Management of the most important side effects. In F. Charnay-Sonnek, & A. E. Murphy (Eds.), *Principle of nursing in oncology* (pp. 33–64). Berlin: Springer; Wilson, B. J. (2019). Myelosuppression. In M. M. Olsen, K. B. LeFebvre, & K. J. Brassil (Eds.), *Chemotherapy and immunotherapy guidelines and recommendations for practice* (pp. 273–292). Pittsburgh, PA: Oncology Nursing Society.

Assessment
See Table 40.3.

Management (see Table 40.3)

I. Pharmacologic management (Wilson, 2019)
   A. Intensive care unit admission for patients with febrile neutropenia (FN) at elevated risk for poor prognosis (Table 40.4)
   B. Granulocyte colony–stimulating factor and blood products as indicated
II. Nonpharmacologic management (Crombez, 2019; Wilson, 2019)
   A. Interventions to minimize the occurrence of infection:
      1. Use a strict hand-washing technique.
      2. Encourage daily, taking care to maintain meticulous personal hygiene, including oral and perineal care.
      3. Restrict the presence of vases with fresh flowers or other sources of stagnant water.
      4. Limit visitors to those without communicable illness, especially children.
      5. Change water in pitchers, denture cups, and nebulizers daily.
      6. Encourage good nutrition.
      7. Take precautions to prevent falls and other traumas.
   B. Use aseptic technique for all nursing interventions, including all indwelling catheters (e.g., venous access devices; urinary, biliary, or feeding tubes), wounds, or invasive procedures; specific institutional guidelines to be referred to for management of central catheters.
   C. Monitor for complications (Crombez, 2019; Wilson, 2019; Yang et al., 2021).
      1. Establish a plan for monitoring blood counts based on the patient's individual risk profile (see Table 40.2).
      2. Monitor for nadir (the lowest point of the blood cell levels after cancer treatment).
         a. Nadir becomes apparent as immature cells in the marrow are destroyed and become absent in the bloodstream.
         b. Usually 7–14 days after chemotherapy, with variability for combined modality treatments, nitrosourea agents, and radiation to the pelvis.
         c. Occasional occurrence after biotherapy.
         d. Usually after multimodal treatment; nadir occurring sooner and more severely than from single-modality therapy.
         e. Cancer treatment may be delayed for an ANC less than 1000–1500/mm³.
         f. Monitor for signs and symptoms of infection.
   D. Patient and family education (Wilson, 2019)
      1. Teach about personal hygiene measures to minimize the occurrence of infection.
      2. Educate about infection precautions and how to minimize the risk of infection.
      3. Educate about the administration of hematopoietic growth factors.
      4. Educate about the symptoms for which to call the physician or nurse, such as temperature higher than 100.4°F (38.1°C), productive cough, painful urination, sore throat.

TABLE 40.3 **Assessment and Recommendations for Prevention and Management of Chemotherapy-Induced Neutropenia and Febrile Neutropenia**

Assessment	• See Table 40.2 for risk factors for CIN due to disease-related, host-related, and treatment-related factors • Assess current/previous cancer therapy; chemotherapy, radiation therapy, and multimodal therapy • Assess for previous neutropenia or neutropenic fevers • Assess for hematopoietic growth factor use • Review of bone marrow biopsy report, if available, to determine bone marrow involvement or hypocellularity • Evaluate vital signs; fever most common manifestation of infection, rigors (should be treated immediately), hypotension or tachypnea, evaluate characteristic signs of infection (erythema, induration, drainage, and cough), assess for change in mental status
Laboratory data	• CBC with differential, calculation of ANC, culture and sensitivity of urine, blood, stool, sputum, CSF, wound, catheter sites, drainage tubes, etc.
Radiology	• Chest radiography (PA and lateral)
Prevention	• Patient and caregiver education for infection prevention appropriate to the level of risk
Management of CIN/FN	• Considered a medical emergency • Prompt intervention is critical to avoid morbidity and mortality • Rapid assessment for risk of clinical deterioration • Implement institutional standard of care for CIN/FN, including frequent CBCs with differentials, calculation of ANC, culture and sensitivity of urine, blood, stool, sputum, CSF, wound, catheter sites, drainage tubes, viral swabs if indicated, PA and lateral chest x-ray, and prompt administration of antibiotics (cefepime most common first-line agent) • Advocate for prophylactic antibiotics, antifungals, and antivirals for patients with hematologic malignancies at very high risk for FN • Prophylactic use of G-CSF is recommended in patients with grade 3 and 4 CIN and a high risk of FN (see Table 27.1) • Most common AEs associated with G-CSF agents include bone pain, myalgia, arthralgia, and fever • Bone pain can be effectively managed with naproxen 225 mg and loratadine 10 mg q12h at the onset of bone pain and continue until resolved (generally 48–72 h) • Implement primary prevention as noted earlier • Establish a plan for close monitoring of blood counts in the initial phase of treatment where risk is greatest • Review reportable signs and symptoms with patients and caregivers, including who to contact and how to do so • Subsequent treatment may require dose modification, dose delay, or administration of G-CSF agents as secondary prophylaxis • Low-risk patients with anticipated early recovery can be managed in an outpatient setting • Unstable patients should be transported by emergency medical services equipped with ACLS capabilities • Patients at very high risk for poor-prognosis FN may require ICU admission

ACLS, Advanced cardiac life support; *AE,* adverse event; *ANC,* absolute neutrophil count; *CBC,* complete blood count; *CIN,* chemotherapy-induced neutropenia; *CSF,* cerebrospinal fluid; *CTC-AE,* Common Terminology Criteria for Adverse Events; *FDA,* U.S. Food and Drug Administration; *FN,* febrile neutropenia; *G-CSF,* granulocyte colony–stimulating factor; *Hypotension,* systolic blood pressure <90 mm Hg; *ICU,* intensive care unit; *IV,* intravenous; *PA,* posteroanterior; *Tachypnea,* respiratory rate >24; *VRE,* vancomycin-resistant enterococci.

From Wilkes, G., & Barton-Burke, M. (2019). *2020–2021 Oncology nursing drug handbook* (23rd ed.). Burlington, MA: Jones & Bartlett Learning, LLC; Wilson, B. J. (2019). Myelosuppression. In M. M. Olsen, K. B. LeFebvre, & K. J. Brassil (Eds.), *Chemotherapy and immunotherapy guidelines and recommendations for practice* (pp. 273–292). Pittsburgh, PA: Oncology Nursing Society; Yang, S., Che, H., Xiao, L., Zhao, B., & Liu, S. (2021). Traditional Chinese medicine on treating myelosuppression after chemotherapy: A protocol for systematic review and meta-analysis. *Medicine (Baltimore)*, *100*(4), e24307. https://doi.org/10.1097/MD.0000000000024307.

TABLE 40.4 **General Factors Associated with Poor-Prognosis Febrile Neutropenia (FN)**

Hypotension	SBP less than 90 mm Hg
Tachypnea	RR greater than 24 breaths/min
Serum albumin	Less than 3.3 g/dL
Serum bicarbonate level	Less than 21 mmol/L
High procalcitonin level	Greater than 2.0 ng/mL
CRP level	Greater than 20 mg/L at baseline
Circulating soluble triggering receptor (sTREM-1)	Greater than 100 pg/mL
High PTX3 levels	At the onset of FN

CRP, Cross-reactive protein; *FN,* febrile neutropenia; *PTX3,* pentraxin 3; *RR,* respiratory rate; *SBP,* systolic blood pressure.

ANEMIA

Overview

I. Definition—a disorder characterized by a reduction in the amount of Hgb in 100 mL of blood—Hgb ≤11 g/dL or ≥2 g/dL below the patient's baseline (Bryer, Kallan, Chiu, Scheuba, & Henry, 2020; Crombez, 2019; Wilson, 2019; Tables 40.1 and 40.5)
   A. Lifespan of an RBC—90–120 days
   B. Patients are at increased risk of fatigue, tachycardia, tachypnea, chest pain, dyspnea, and syncope.
   C. Anemia contributes to increased mortality.
   D. Risk of side effects are related to severity of anemia (Table 40.6).

II. Physiology (Wilson, 2019)
   A. Erythrocytes develop from myeloid stem cells in bone marrow and stimulate the stem cells to produce RBCs.
      1. Function of RBCs is to carry oxygen to all cells in the body.
         a. Decrease in oxygen can increase tumor growth by decreasing tumor sensitivity to cancer treatment.
   B. Iron is essential for RBC production.
   C. Anemia is a common adverse event in patients with cancer, with an incidence ranging from 22% to 67%.

III. Risk factors (Crombez, 2019; Messin & Amrhein, 2019; Wilson, 2019; see Table 40.6)
   A. Patient-related factors
   B. Disease-related factors
   C. Treatment-related factors

Assessment

See Table 40.7.

Management
(see Table 40.7)

I. Pharmacologic management (Adelsberg, & Nagelberg, Occiano, 2019; Vemula, 2021; Vega et al., 2021; Wilson, 2019)
   A. RBC transfusions as indicated (see Chapter 30)
   B. Erythropoietin-stimulating proteins (ESAs) as indicated; use with caution in patients with curative goals of treatment (Table 40.7)
      a. ESAs can have a big financial burden for patients.
   C. Prophylactic prevention with folic acid and vitamin B12 for patients receiving pemetrexed
   D. Certain tumor types carry higher risks of anemia.

II. Nonpharmacologic management (Messin & Amrhein, 2019; Wilson, 2019)
   A. Interventions to minimize secondary effects of anemia
      1. Cancer treatment generally held for Hgb less than 7.5 g/dL with the exception of known bone marrow disorders
      2. Management of fatigue and hypoxia
      3. RBC transfusions based on best practices and organizational guidelines
   B. Interventions to monitor for complications (Wilson, 2019)
      1. Establish a plan for monitoring blood counts based on the patient's individual risk profile (Table 40.6).
      2. Monitor lab values closely and look at trends—assessment includes, but not limited to, RBCs, Hgb,

---

TABLE 40.5 Definition of Anemia

Anemia	A disorder characterized by a reduction in the amount of Hgb in 100 mL of blood	Grade 1: Hgb <LLN—10.0 g/dL
	A Hgb value below 10 g/dL places the patient at increased risk of fatigue and tissue hypoxia	Grade 2: Hgb <10.0–8.0 g/dL
	RBC lifespan is 120 days	Grade 3: Hgb <8.0 g/dL, transfusion indicated
	Normal value gender specific:	Grade 4: Life-threatening consequences; urgent intervention indicated
	Female—Hgb: 12–16 g/dL; Hct: 37%–47%	
	Male—Hgb: 13.5–18 g/dL; Hct: 42%–52%	

Hct, Hematocrit; *Hgb*, hemoglobin; *RBC*, red blood cell.
From Bryer, E. J., Kallan, M. J., Chiu, T.-S., Scheuba, K. M., & Henry, D. H. (2020). A retrospective analysis of venous thromboembolism trends in chemotherapy-induced anemia. *Journal of Clinical Oncology, 38*(15_suppl), e15515. https://doi.org/10.1200/JCO.2020.38.15_suppl.e15515; Kizior, R. J., & Hodgson, K. J. (2021). *Saunders nursing drug handbook 2021.* Amsterdam: Elsevier; Wilson, B. J. (2019). Myelosuppression. In M. M. Olsen, K. B. LeFebvre, & K. J. Brassil (Eds.), *Chemotherapy and immunotherapy guidelines and recommendations for practice* (pp. 273–292). Pittsburgh, PA: Oncology Nursing Society; US Department of Health and Human Services. (2017). Common terminology criteria for adverse events. Version 5.0. Retrieved from https://ctep.cancer.gov/protocoldevelopment/electronic_applications/docs/ctcae_v5_quick_reference_5x7.pdf.

TABLE 40.6 Risk Factors Associated With Chemotherapy-Induced Anemia

Patient-Related Factors	Disease- and Treatment-Related Factors
See Table 40.2	Invasion of tumor cells in the bone marrow or cancers involving the bone marrow; multiple myeloma, lymphoma, leukemia, or myelodysplastic syndrome
Advanced age	
Female gender	
Malnutrition—vomiting, anorexia, deficiencies of folic acid, and vitamin B12	
	Erythroid leukemia
Comorbidities, such as chronic renal insufficiency, chronic GI blood loss, alcoholism, cardiopulmonary disease, and genetic disorders that affect RBC production—thalassemia, autoimmune hemolytic anemia	Type of chemotherapy—platinum drugs, immunotherapies, high-dose chemotherapy for HSCT
	Number of chemotherapy doses
	Dose intensity of chemotherapy
	Drug-induced RBC aplasia (rare)
	Radiation therapy

GI, Gastrointestinal; *HSCT*, hematopoietic stem cell transplant; *RBC*, red blood cell.
From Crombez, P. (2019). Evidence-based nursing of patients with hematologic malignancies. In F. Charnay-Sonnek, & A. E. Murphy (Eds.), *Principle of nursing in oncology* (pp. 277–308). Berlin: Springer; Messin, C., & Amrhein, C. (2019). Evidence-based nursing in basic anticancer treatment: Management of the most important side effects. In F. Charnay-Sonnek, & A. E. Murphy (Eds.), *Principle of nursing in oncology* (pp. 33–64). Berlin: Springer; Wilson, B. J. (2019). Myelosuppression. In M. M. Olsen, K. B. LeFebvre, & K. J. Brassil (Eds.), *Chemotherapy and immunotherapy guidelines and recommendations for practice* (pp. 273–292). Pittsburgh, PA: Oncology Nursing Society.

TABLE 40.7 Assessment and Recommendations for Management of Chemotherapy-Induced Anemia

Assessment	• Assess previous cancer treatment history: chemotherapy, radiation therapy, or multimodal therapy • Current medications that could alter RBC function • Assess social history of alcohol and illicit drug use • Assess for bleeding from nose, rectum, ears, and oral cavity; assess blood in stool, urine, and vomit • Assess menstrual bleeding and the number of sanitary napkins or tampons used • Assess for changes that indicate intracranial bleeding: level of consciousness, restlessness, headache, seizures, pupil changes, ataxia
Laboratory data	• CBC with platelets and differential
Prevention	• Evaluation of contributing factors for anemia: iron deficiency, folate deficiency, vitamin B_{12} deficiency, GI blood loss, hemolysis screening, thyroid function, testosterone level, and serum Epo level • Identification of patients at high risk for anemia and the secondary effects • Consideration of individual characteristics of the patient such as underlying comorbidities affected by anemia; cardiovascular and pulmonary diseases
Treatment of CIA	• Patient and caregiver education for conservation of energy, planning of activities, and reportable signs and symptoms • Establish a plan of care for monitoring blood counts and follow-up • Maintain a current type and screen for patients requiring frequent transfusions • Evaluation of symptoms of anemia with consideration of individual patient characteristics, including fatigue, shortness of breath, lightheadedness, headache, tachycardia, pallor, and cyanosis • Treat underlying cause(s)
Transfusion of PRBCs ESAs	• Weigh the risks and benefits of each treatment approach (PRBC transfusion, ESA administration) • Review informed consent if applicable and evaluate patient understanding of associated risks, such as viral transmissions, transfusion reactions, febrile nonhemolytic reactions, iron overload and secondary organ toxicity, and fluid overload • Asymptomatic patients; transfuse to maintain hemodynamic stability • Symptomatic with hemorrhage transfuse to maintain Hgb 8–10 g/dL, or as directed by provider • Symptomatic with Hgb <10 g/dL: transfuse to maintain Hgb >10 g/dL, or as directed by provider • Acute coronary syndromes with anemia: transfuse to maintain Hgb >10 g/dL • Rapid increase in Hgb may improve fatigue in some patients • ESAs require informed consent • Not indicated in patients receiving chemotherapy for curative intent • Goal is to administer the lowest dose necessary to avoid PRBC transfusion not to exceed Hgb of 10 g/dL • If Hgb rises greater than 1 g/dL in any 2-week period, dose reductions are required: see prescribing information • Assists in the avoidance of transfusions • Associated with inferior survival and decreased time to progression, most notably with target Hgb >12 g/dL • Associated with thrombosis: increased risk with the history of coagulopathy, obesity, coronary artery disease, thrombocytosis, hypertension, and hospitalization

CBC, Complete blood count; *CIA*, chemotherapy-induced anemia; *ESA*, erythropoietin-stimulating proteins; *GI*, gastrointestinal; *Hgb*, hemoglobin; *ICU*, intensive care unit; *PRBC*, packed red blood cells; *RBC*, red blood cell.
From Crombez, P. (2019). Evidence-based nursing of patients with hematologic malignancies. In F. Charnay-Sonnek, & A. E. Murphy (Eds.), *Principle of nursing in oncology* (pp. 277–308). Berlin: Springer; Messin, C., & Amrhein, C. (2019). Evidence-based nursing in basic anticancer treatment: Management of the most important side effects. In F. Charnay-Sonnek, & A. E. Murphy (Eds.), *Principle of nursing in oncology* (pp. 33–64). Berlin: Springer; Occiano, P., Nagelberg, M., & Adelsberg, R. (2019). Nutrition and symptom management. In W. Oh, & A. Chari (Eds.), *Mount Sinai expert guides: Oncology* (pp. 528–534). New York: Icahn School of Medicine at Mount Sinai; Vega, A., Zhang, R., Wong, H., Wernecke, M., Alexander, M., Feng, Y., et al. (2021). Trends in erythropoiesis-stimulating agent use and blood transfusions for chemotherapy-induced anemia throughout FDA's risk evaluation and mitigation strategy lifecycle. *Pharmacoepidemiology & Drug Safety*, 30(5), 626–635. https://doi.org/10.1002/pds.5202; Wilson, B. J. (2019). Myelosuppression. In M. M. Olsen, K. B. LeFebvre, & K. J. Brassil (Eds.), *Chemotherapy and immunotherapy guidelines and recommendations for practice* (pp. 273–292). Pittsburgh, PA: Oncology Nursing Society.

hematocrit, ferritin, serum iron, total iron-binding capacity, reticulocyte count, erythropoietin level, serum B12, and serum folate.

C. Interventions to incorporate patient and family in care (Wilson, 2019)

1. Educate about energy conservation and reportable signs and symptoms.
2. Educate about signs of transfusion reactions.
3. Educate about safety measures to decrease the potential for injury caused by syncope or dyspnea during periods of anemia.

THROMBOCYTOPENIA

Overview

I. Definition—decrease in the circulating Plts below the LLN based on institutional laboratory measures—typically of grave concern when levels fall below 50,000 Plts/µL (Table 40.8; Crombez, 2019; Messin & Amrhein, 2019; Wilson, 2019)

A. Lifespan of Plts is approximately 7–8 days.

B. Cancer-related thrombocytopenia occurs 8–14 days after chemotherapy.

TABLE 40.8 Overview of Thrombocytopenia

Thrombocytopenia	A finding based on laboratory test results that indicate a decrease in the number of platelets in a blood specimen that increases the risk of bleeding Lifespan: 7–8 days (as little as 24 h in stressful situations)	Grade 1: Plt <LLN–75,000/mm^3 Grade 2: Plt <75,000–50,000/mm^3 Grade 3: Plt <50,000–25,000/mm^3 Grade 4: Plt <25,000/mm^3

Plt, Platelet.

From Crombez, P. (2019). Evidence-based nursing of patients with hematologic malignancies. In F. Charnay-Sonnek, & A. E. Murphy (Eds.), *Principle of nursing in oncology* (pp. 277–308). Berlin: Springer; Messin, C., & Amrhein, C. (2019). Evidence-based nursing in basic anticancer treatment: Management of the most important side effects. In F. Charnay-Sonnek, & A. E. Murphy (Eds.), *Principle of nursing in oncology* (pp. 33–64). Berlin: Springer; Wilkes, G., & Barton-Burke, M. (2019). *2020–2021 Oncology nursing drug handbook* (23rd ed.). Burlington, MA: Jones & Bartlett Learning, LLC; Wilson, B. J. (2019). Myelosuppression. In M. M. Olsen, K. B. LeFebvre, & K. J. Brassil (Eds.), *Chemotherapy and immunotherapy guidelines and recommendations for practice* (pp. 273–292). Pittsburgh, PA: Oncology Nursing Society.

TABLE 40.9 Risk Factors Associated With Chemotherapy-Induced Thrombocytopenia

Patient-Related Factors	Disease- and Treatment-Related Factors
See Table 40.2 Underlying platelet disorders; idiopathic thrombocytopenic purpura, thrombotic thrombocytopenic purpura Coagulation abnormalities, comorbidities Splenomegaly Hypocoagulation; vitamin K deficiency from malnutrition or from liver disease, which alters the development of prothrombin and several clotting factors	Invasion of tumor cells in the bone marrow or cancers involving the bone marrow; multiple myeloma, lymphoma, leukemia, or myelodysplastic syndrome Megakaryocytic leukemia Hypercoagulation; paraneoplastic syndromes, DIC, and thrombosis Endotoxins released from bacteria during an infection can damage platelets and later platelet aggregation Drug interactions Platelet count usually decreases in 7–14 days after administration of chemotherapy or sooner with multimodal treatment

DIC, Disseminated intravascular coagulation.

From Crombez, P. (2019). Evidence-based nursing of patients with hematologic malignancies. In F. Charnay-Sonnek, & A. E. Murphy (Eds.), *Principle of nursing in oncology* (pp. 277–308). Berlin: Springer; Messin, C., & Amrhein, C. (2019). Evidence-based nursing in basic anticancer treatment: Management of the most important side effects. In F. Charnay-Sonnek, & A. E. Murphy (Eds.), *Principle of nursing in oncology* (pp. 33–64). Berlin: Springer; Wilson, B. J. (2019). Myelosuppression. In M. M. Olsen, K. B. LeFebvre, & K. J. Brassil (Eds.), *Chemotherapy and immunotherapy guidelines and recommendations for practice* (pp. 273–292). Pittsburgh, PA: Oncology Nursing Society.

1. Severity is related to tumor type, stage of disease, and can be a dose-limiting toxicity with certain agents
2. Leading cause of bleeding in patients with hematologic malignancies

II. Physiology (Wilson, 2019)
   A. Megakaryocytes develop and form the myeloid stem cells in bone marrow
   B. Each megakaryocyte produces millions of Plts each day and can be measured in peripheral blood
   C. All Plts are found in the circulating blood—meaning there is no Plt reserve in the bone marrow
   D. The function of Plts is to maintain vascular hemostasis, prevent blood loss through Plt adhesion to block small breaks in blood vessels, and initiate clotting mechanisms

III. Risk factors (Crombez, 2019; Messin & Amrhein, 2019; Wilson, 2019; Table 40.9)
   A. Patient-related factors
   B. Disease-related factors
   C. Treatment-related factors

Assessment

See Table 40.10.

Management

I. Pharmacologic management (Balitsky, Liu, Van der Meer, Heddle, & Arnold, 2021; Crombez, 2019; Wilson, 2019; see Table 40.10)
   A. Prevention of thrombocytopenia
      1. Identification of patients at elevated risk for thrombocytopenia and bleeding for consideration of treatment

   a. World Health Organization (WHO) classification of bleeding severity
      (1) Grade 1—minimal blood loss: petechiae, ecchymosis, occult blood in body secretions, and mild vaginal spotting
      (2) Grade 2—evidence of mild blood loss not requiring RBC transfusion over routine needs: epistaxis, hematuria, and hematemesis
      (3) Grade 3—gross hemorrhage of one or more units of RBCs per day
      (4) Grade 4—debilitating blood loss: life-threatening hemorrhage causing hemodynamic compromise or bleeding into a vital organ (e.g., intracranial, pericardial, or pulmonary hemorrhage)

II. Nonpharmacologic management (Crombez, 2019; Messin & Amrhein, 2019; Wilson, 2019)
   A. Minimize the occurrence of bleeding
      1. Avoid the use or overinflation of a blood pressure (BP) cuff or use of a tourniquet when the Plt count is less than 20,000/mm^3.
      2. Avoid invasive procedures such as enema, taking rectal temperature, administering suppositories,

TABLE 40.10 **Assessment and Recommendations for Management of Chemotherapy-Induced Thrombocytopenia**

Assessment	• Previous cancer treatment history: chemotherapy, radiation therapy, or multimodal therapy. • Current medications that could alter platelet production. • Social history of alcohol and illicit drug use. • Assess for bleeding from nose, rectum, ears, oral cavity; assess blood in stool, urine, and vomit. • Assess menstrual bleeding and the number of sanitary napkins or tampons used. • Assess for changes that indicate intracranial bleeding: level of consciousness, restlessness, headache, seizures, pupil changes, and ataxia. • Assess skin for ecchymosis, purpura, oozing of puncture sites, and petechiae. • Assess for conjunctiva hemorrhage and sclera injection, pallor.
Laboratory data	• Monitor platelet count. • Coagulation values: fibrinogen, prothrombin time, partial thromboplastin time, and platelet antibodies.
Prevention	• Identification of patients at high risk for thrombocytopenia and bleeding. • Consideration of individual characteristics of the patient, including proximity to treatment center, concomitant anticoagulation therapy or antiplatelet drugs, prior response to platelets, concurrent inflammatory process or infection, CNS disease. • Patient and caregiver education for conservation of energy, planning of activities, and reportable signs and symptoms.
Treatment of CIT	• Establish a plan of care for monitoring blood counts and follow-up. • Maintain a current type and screen for patients requiring frequent transfusions. • Progestational agents may decrease menstrual bleeding. • Withholding anticoagulation therapy for platelet count less than 50,000/µL. • Evaluation of symptoms of thrombocytopenia with consideration of individual patient characteristics. • Treat underlying cause(s).
Transfusion of platelets	• Weigh the risks and benefits of each treatment. • Review informed consent if applicable and evaluate patient understanding of associated risks. • WHO bleeding grades; grade 1—petechiae, ecchymosis, occult blood in body secretions, mild vaginal spotting; grade 2—evidence of gross hematuria not requiring RBC transfusion over routine needs: epistaxis, hematuria, hematemesis; grade 3—hemorrhage of one or more units of PRBCs per day; grade 4—life-threatening hemorrhage, defined as massive bleeding causing hemodynamic compromise or bleeding into a vital organ (intracranial, pericardial, or pulmonary hemorrhage). • Platelets less than 10,000/µL—threshold for therapeutic platelet transfusion. Patients with a history of bleeding or active infection may require a higher threshold for transfusion. Surgical or invasive procedure needs to maintain platelets greater than 50,000 µL. Neurosurgical procedures—platelets need to be maintained greater than 10,000 µL. • RDP—common dose is 4–6 random donor units (pooled from multiple units of whole blood). • SDP—larger volume—1 unit = 60 mL; 6 units = 360 mL. Single-donor apheresis platelets = 200 mL, takes 1.5–2 h to process, and costs more than twice the cost of RDP transfusion.
Benefits	• Improvement in bleeding symptoms.
Risks	• RDP exposes results in patient exposure to more donors. • Refractory to platelet transfusions (alloimmunization). • Transfusion reaction or transmitted disease. • Delay in administering treatment on time or dose delays; dose reductions. • Internal bleeding; intracranial, GI, or respiratory tract bleeding.

CIT, Chemotherapy induced thrombocytopenia; *CNS*, central nervous system; *GI*, gastrointestinal; *PRBCs*, packed red blood cells; *RBC*, red blood cell; *RDP*, random donor platelets; *SDP*, single-donor platelets; *WHO*, World Health Organization.
From Balitsky, A. K., Liu, Y., Van der Meer, P. F., Heddle, N. M., & Arnold, D. M. (2021). Exploring the components of bleeding outcomes in transfusion trials for patients with hematologic malignancy. *Transfusion (Philadelphia, PA)*, 61(1), 286–293. https://doi.org/10.1111/trf.16126; Crombez, P. (2019). Evidence-based nursing of patients with hematologic malignancies. In F. Charnay-Sonnek, & A. E. Murphy (Eds.), *Principle of nursing in oncology* (pp. 277–308). Berlin: Springer; Messin, C., & Amrhein, C. (2019). Evidence-based nursing in basic anticancer treatment: Management of the most important side effects. In F. Charnay-Sonnek, & A. E. Murphy (Eds.), *Principle of nursing in oncology* (pp. 33–64). Berlin: Springer; Punekar, S. R. (2021). Cancer treatment infusion reactions. In V. Velcheti, & S. R. Punekar (Eds.), *Handbook of cancer treatment-related symptoms and toxicities* (pp. 17–19). Elsevier; Wilkes, G., & Barton-Burke, M. (2019). *2020–2021 Oncology nursing drug handbook* (23rd ed.). Burlington, MA: Jones & Bartlett Learning, LLC; Wilson, B. J. (2019). Myelosuppression. In M. M. Olsen, K. B. LeFebvre, & K. J. Brassil (Eds.), *Chemotherapy and immunotherapy guidelines and recommendations for practice* (pp. 273–292). Pittsburgh, PA: Oncology Nursing Society.

bladder catheterization, venipuncture, finger stick, use of nasogastric tubes, and administering subcutaneous or intramuscular injection.

3. Preparation of the environment to avoid trauma (e.g., padding side rails, arranging furniture to eliminate sharp corners, and clearing walkways)

4. Apply firm direct pressure to venipuncture site for 5 minutes.

B. Encourage patient to wear shoes during ambulation to maintain skin integrity.

C. Encourage patient to avoid sharp objects such as a straight-edge razor.

D. If bleeding not controlled, apply absorbable gelatin sponges or liquid thrombin.

E. For nosebleeds, place patient in high Fowler position and apply pressure to the nose.

F. Apply ice packs to decrease the bleeding.

G. Implement a bowel elimination regimen to prevent constipation.

H. Use soft toothbrushes to avoid gingival trauma.

I. Instruct patient to avoid physical activity that may lead to trauma.

J. Plt transfusion based on physician orders and WHO guidelines for transfusion

1. Follow guidelines and thresholds prior to administering cancer treatments.

III. Monitor for bleeding complications (Crombez, 2019; Wilson, 2019).

A. Establish a plan for monitoring blood counts based on the patient's individual risk profile (Table 40.9).

1. Monitor lab values closely and look at Plt trends.

B. Cancer treatment(s) typically held with a Plt count less than 50–100,000 Plts/μL.

IV. Patient and caregiver education (Crombez, 2019; Wilson, 2019)

A. Educate about bleeding precautions.

B. Educate about signs of bleeding that should be called to the attention of the physician or nurse.

C. Educate about safety measures to decrease the occurrence of bleeding when performing activities of daily living, including fall prevention.

INFECTION

Overview

I. Definition—invasion by a microorganism (bacteria, virus, and parasites) in the body (Crombez, 2019; Davis, 2021; Table 40.11)

A. Infectious diseases have a crucial factor in morbidity and mortality in cancer patients.

II. Physiology

A. Microorganisms that are not normally present in the body cause body system dysfunction and clinical symptoms.

1. Can remain localized or become systemic by spreading through the circulatory or lymphatic systems

B. Susceptibility to cancer-related infections results from the nature of the malignancy and cancer treatments.

1. Impairment of host defense mechanisms—skin and mucosal barriers (mucositis, dermatologic reactions, invasive procedures), neutropenia, and immunosuppression

2. Increased susceptibility to infections with variable risk throughout the cancer diagnosis

3. Prolonged immunosuppression, which increases the risk of opportunistic infections (viruses, fungi, mycobacteria, and rare bacterial strains) and more severe consequences of common pathogens

C. Most important physical barrier against the invasion of organism—skin, mucosal barriers

D. WBCs, particularly neutrophils, are important defense mechanisms against infection.

TABLE 40.11 Overview of Infection

Infection	When the body or a part of the body is invaded by a microorganism or virus and an infection develops, depending on susceptibility to cancer-related infections, physical barriers against the invasion of an organism, skin and mucosal barriers, and WBCs, specifically, neutrophils, an important defense against infection	WBC important in defense against infection: Impairment of host defense mechanisms—skin and mucosal barriers (mucositis, dermatologic reactions, and invasive procedures), neutropenia, and immunosuppression Increased susceptibility to infections with variable risk throughout the cancer diagnosis Prolonged immunosuppression, which increases the risk of opportunistic infections (viruses, fungi, mycobacteria, and rare bacterial strains) and more severe consequences of common pathogens

WBC, White blood cell.
From Crombez, P. (2019). Evidence-based nursing of patients with hematologic malignancies. In F. Charnay-Sonnek, & A. E. Murphy (Eds.), *Principle of nursing in oncology* (pp. 277–308). Berlin: Springer; Davis, C. P. (2021). *Medical definition of infection.* MedicineNet. Retrieved from https://www.medicinenet.com/infection/definition.htm.

TABLE 40.12 Risk Factors Associated With Chemotherapy-Induced Infection

Patient-Related Factors	Disease- and Treatment-Related Factors
See Table 40.2	Immunodeficiency associated with primary malignancy
Disruption of mucosal barriers	High tumor burden
Splenectomy or functional asplenia	Corticosteroids and other lymphotoxic agents
Comorbid conditions	Cytotoxic chemotherapy
Malnutrition; hypoalbuminemia	T- and B-cell suppressants, steroids, purine analogs, and alemtuzumab
Hypogammaglobulinemia	Radiation therapy
Remission status	Surgical wounds, delayed healing
HIV, or severe immunosuppression	Solid organ transplantation
Barriers breached—VAD, mucositis, surgery	Hematopoietic stem cell transplantation; GVHD

GVHD, Graft-versus-host disease; *VAD,* vascular access device.
From Crombez, P. (2019). Evidence-based nursing of patients with hematologic malignancies. In F. Charnay-Sonnek, & A. E. Murphy (Eds.), *Principle of nursing in oncology* (pp. 277–308). Berlin: Springer; Messin, C., & Amrhein, C. (2019). Evidence-based nursing in basic anticancer treatment: Management of the most important side effects. In F. Charnay-Sonnek, & A. E. Murphy (Eds.), *Principle of nursing in oncology* (pp. 33–64). Berlin: Springer; Wilson, B. J. (2019). Myelosuppression. In M. M. Olsen, K. B. LeFebvre, & K. J. Brassil (Eds.), *Chemotherapy and immunotherapy guidelines and recommendations for practice* (pp. 273–292). Pittsburgh, PA: Oncology Nursing Society.

III. Risk factors (Crombez, 2019; Messin & Amrhein, 2019; Wilson, 2019; Table 40.12)

A. Patient-related factors

B. Disease-related factors

C. Treatment-related factors

TABLE 40.13   Assessment and Recommendations for Management of Chemotherapy-Induced Infection

History	• Previous cancer treatment history: chemotherapy, radiation therapy, or multimodal therapy • Review of infection history • Review of known allergies to medications, especially antibiotics • Review of immunosuppressive therapy
Physical examination	• Complete physical examination to isolate the potential source of infection; skin, mucosa, lungs, sinus, perirectal, abdomen, wounds, and indwelling catheters • Assessment of mental status for orientation, confusion, memory recall, and alertness • Assessment for rapidity of onset of symptoms • Assessment of vital signs every 4–8 h; fever, hypotension, or tachypnea (RR>24) indicative of high risk for clinical deterioration • Assessment of urine or stool for color, consistency or clarity, odor, and presence of blood
Laboratory data	• CBC with differential, culture, and sensitivity testing of urine, blood, stool, sputum, wounds, drainage bags or tubes, rectal swabs for VRE, oral swabs for viruses, stool for *Clostridium difficile*, skin or wound swabs for bacterial, viral, fungal infections, and skin punch biopsy to isolate fungal infections (see "Neutropenia")
Radiology	• Chest radiography (PA and lateral) • Additional radiology testing based on suspected source
Prevention	• Institute preventive antimicrobial treatments for patients at high risk for opportunistic viral, fungal, and bacterial infections
Treatment	• Isolate source if possible • Administer antibiotics according to organism isolated • Administer WBC line growth factors, as appropriate (see "Neutropenia")
Risks	• Delay in treatment or ineligibility for selected treatment because of infection history • Pneumonia and acute respiratory distress • Resistance to antibiotics or superinfection • Septic shock and death are possibilities

CBC, Complete blood count; *PA*, posteroanterior; *RR*, respiratory rate; *VRE*, vancomycin-resistant enterococcus; *WBC*, white blood cell.
From Crombez, P. (2019). Evidence-based nursing of patients with hematologic malignancies. In F. Charnay-Sonnek, & A. E. Murphy (Eds.), *Principle of nursing in oncology* (pp. 277–308). Berlin: Springer; Messin, C., & Amrhein, C. (2019). Evidence-based nursing in basic anticancer treatment: Management of the most important side effects. In F. Charnay-Sonnek, & A. E. Murphy (Eds.), *Principle of nursing in oncology* (pp. 33–64). Berlin: Springer; Wilson, B. J. (2019). Myelosuppression. In M. M. Olsen, K. B. LeFebvre, & K. J. Brassil (Eds.), *Chemotherapy and immunotherapy guidelines and recommendations for practice* (pp. 273–292). Pittsburgh, PA: Oncology Nursing Society.

Assessment

See Table 40.13.

Management

I. Pharmacologic management (Crombez, 2019; Wilson, 2019; see Table 40.13)
   A. Identification of patients at risk
   B. Institute preventive antimicrobial treatments for patients at high risk for viral, fungal, or opportunistic bacterial infections.
   C. Isolation of the source, if possible
   D. Antibiotics according to organism isolated
   E. WBC line growth factors, as appropriate (see "Neutropenia")
   F. Vaccinations as indicated to prevent communicable infections
   G. Obtain appropriate tests as indicated.
      1. Cultures: blood, sputum, stool, urine, and wounds
      2. Chest radiography
II. Nonpharmacologic management (Crombez, 2019; Wilson, 2019)
   A. Minimize infections
      1. Use strict hand washing before and after all contact with patient.
      2. Promote and encourage meticulous personal and oral hygiene, perineal care.
      3. Avoid unnecessary invasive procedures such as giving enemas, taking rectal temperatures, bladder catheterization, and venipuncture.
      4. Use of aseptic technique when performing nursing interventions
      5. Ensure adequate hydration and a high-calorie, high-protein diet.
      6. Report critical changes in patient assessment parameters to physician.
III. Monitor for complications (Crombez, 2019; Wilson, 2019).
      1. Establish a plan for monitoring blood counts and other diagnostic exams based on the patient's individual risk profile (Table 40.12).
      2. Monitor lab values and trends.
IV. Patient and caregiver education (Crombez, 2019; Wilson, 2019)
      1. Educate about signs and symptoms of infection and when to call the physician or nurse.
      2. Educate about FN and related signs and symptoms.

HEMORRHAGE

Overview

I. Definition—the acute loss of blood from damaged blood vessels (Crombez, 2019; Johnson & Burns, 2021; Lemke, 2019; Mistry, 2019; Shelton, 2019)

TABLE 40.14 Risk Factors Associated With Cancer-Related Hemorrhage

Disease-Related Factors	Treatment-Related Factors
Cerebral hemorrhage may occur with severe thrombocytopenia or with brain metastases	Bone marrow or hematopoietic stem cell transplantation may cause a diffuse alveolar hemorrhage characterized by cough, dyspnea, and hypoxemia
Myeloproliferative disorders such as polycythemia vera, myelofibrosis, and thrombocytopenia may cause hemorrhage	DIC may occur as a result of cancer treatment
DIC may result from prostate cancer or acute promyelocytic leukemia	High-dose chemotherapy such as with cyclophosphamide (Cytoxan) and ifosfamide may cause hemorrhagic cystitis or myocardial hemorrhage
Paraneoplastic syndromes may stimulate bleeding	Ibrutinib
Splenomegaly may cause bleeding	All types of surgical procedures pose a risk for hemorrhage, especially if tumor is embedded within arteries or veins

DIC, Disseminated intravascular coagulation.
From Crombez, P. (2019). Evidence-based nursing of patients with hematologic malignancies. In F. Charnay-Sonnek, & A. E. Murphy (Eds.), *Principle of nursing in oncology* (pp. 277–308). Berlin: Springer; Johnson, A. B., & Burns, B. (2021). Hemorrhage. In: *StatPearls [Internet].* Treasure Island, FL: StatPearls Publishing. Retrieved from https://www.ncbi.nlm.nih.gov/books/NBK542273/; Mistry, H. E. (2019). Gastrointestinal and mucosal toxicities. In M. M. Olsen, K. B. LeFebvre, & K. J. Brassil (Eds.), *Chemotherapy and immunotherapy guidelines and recommendations for practice* (pp. 293–352). Pittsburgh, PA: Oncology Nursing Society.

TABLE 40.15 Assessment and Recommendations for Management of Cancer-Related Hemorrhage

History	• Previous cancer treatment history: chemotherapy, radiation therapy, or multimodal therapy • Ascertain recent traumatic events • Review of the cancer • Evidence of metastasis to the brain or bone marrow • Leukemia, especially nonlymphocytic leukemia, may cause hemorrhage as a result of a paraneoplastic process • Review past medical history for the occurrence of peptic or gastric ulcer disease or esophageal varices
Physical examination	• Assess for signs of hemorrhage complications; weak/irregular pulse, pale skin, cold/moist skin • Assess all stool, urine, and sputum for blood • Assess vital signs • Assess for neurologic deficits such as reduced level of alertness or orientation
Laboratory data	• CBC, coagulation factors, occult stool test, bleeding time
Treatment	• Administration of appropriate blood products • Administration of oxygen • Administration of vasopressors—may control severe bleeding • Lavage with iced saline through nasogastric tube—may control bleeding
Risks	• Viral infection from numerous blood transfusions • Transfusion reaction • Septic shock and death are possibilities

CBC, Complete blood count.
From Crombez, P. (2019). Evidence-based nursing of patients with hematologic malignancies. In F. Charnay-Sonnek, & A. E. Murphy (Eds.), *Principle of nursing in oncology* (pp. 277–308). Berlin: Springer; *Mayo Clinic.* (2022). Fever. https://www.mayoclinic.org/diseases-conditions/fever/symptoms-causes/syc-20352759; Lemke, E. A. (2019). Genitourinary toxicities. In M. M. Olsen, K. B. LeFebvre, & K. J. Brassil (Eds.), *Chemotherapy and immunotherapy guidelines and recommendations for practice* (pp. 471–486). Pittsburgh, PA: Oncology Nursing Society; Shelton, B. K. (2019). Pulmonary toxicities. In M. M. Olsen, K. B. LeFebvre, & K. J. Brassil (Eds.), *Chemotherapy and immunotherapy guidelines and recommendations for practice* (pp. 401–444). Pittsburgh, PA: Oncology Nursing Society.

A. Blood loss can be minimal or significant and is graded based on severity (see Thrombocytopenia).

B. Blood loss can be internally or externally.

C. Commonly caused by high-dose alkylating chemotherapy, radiation therapy, or the combination of both

II. Physiology (Crombez, 2019; Johnson & Burns, 2021; Lemke, 2019; Mistry, 2019; Shelton, 2019)

A. Hemostasis is the process of a solid clot forming in the blood from a fluid component.

B. Coagulation is the mechanism of forming a stable fibrin clot.

C. Hemorrhage occurs in cancer patients from alterations in hemostasis or coagulation mechanisms.

D. There are types of hemorrhage, including alveolar hemorrhage, colitis-induced hemorrhage, hemorrhagic cystitis, and disseminated intravascular coagulation.

  1. Hemorrhagic cystitis is inflammation in the bladder that causes the mucosal lining to bleed.

    a. Can be life-threatening

    b. Common complication in bone marrow transplant patients

III. Risk factors (Crombez, 2019; Lemke, 2019; Mistry, 2019; Shelton, 2019; Table 40.14)

A. Disease-related factors

B. Treatment-related factors

Assessment

See Table 40.15.

Management

I. Pharmacologic management (Crombez, 2019; Lemke, 2019; Mistry, 2019; Shelton, 2019; see Table 40.15)

A. Identification of patients at risk and prescribing prophylaxis as appropriate.

II. Nonpharmacologic management

A. Administration of prophylaxis as ordered.

  1. Chemoprotectants (i.e., mesna) for high-risk drug administrations.

B. Minimize bleeding.

  1. Apply occlusive dressings to bleeding wounds after cleansing the area.

2. If applicable, elevate the body part above the heart level and apply firm pressure over the area.
3. Administer blood components as ordered.

III. Monitor for complications (Crombez, 2019; Mistry, 2019).
    A. Establish a plan for monitoring blood counts and other diagnostic exams based on the patient's individual risk profile (Table 40.14).
       a. Serum blood counts and urinalysis
    B. Hemodynamic measurements—BP monitoring
    C. Strict intake and output records to detect negative fluid balance
    D. Report critical changes in the patient's assessment parameters to the physician such as change in mental status, decrease in BP, and increase in bleeding.

IV. Patient and caregiver education (Crombez, 2019; Mistry, 2019; Wilson, 2019)
    1. Educate about signs and symptoms of hemorrhage and when to call the physician or nurse.

FEVER AND CHILLS

Overview

I. Definition—a temporary elevation of body temperature often due to illness above 100.4°F (38°C) to 101.3°F (38.5°C) orally (Crombez, 2019; Mayo Clinic, 2022; Wilson, 2019)

II. Physiology (Crombez, 2019; Mayo Clinic, 2022; Wilson, 2019)
    A. The thermoregulatory center in the hypothalamus controls body temperature.
    B. Various heat loss mechanisms help return temperature to normal levels during fevers.
    C. Chills (shivering) occur as a body's response to heat loss when the body's temperature abruptly increases, as with fever or a drug reaction.
       1. Involuntary contractions of the skeletal muscles occur with shivering.
       2. The internal body temperature is maintained by shivering, which is a thermoregulatory mechanism.
       3. Shivering is a subjective feeling of cold and results in an increase in metabolic activity and oxygen consumption brought about by an increase in muscle tone.
    D. Vasodilation and sweating are physiologic mechanisms used to increase heat loss.
    E. Vasoconstriction and shivering are the body's mechanisms for conserving or producing heat.
       1. Skin temperature drops because of vasoconstriction, which decreases heat loss.
       2. Each degree of temperature Fahrenheit results in a 7% increase in metabolic rate and increases the demands on the heart.

III. Risk factors (Crombez, 2019; Mayo Clinic, 2022; Wilson, 2019; Table 40.16)
    A. Disease-related factors
    B. Treatment-related factors

TABLE 40.16 Risk Factors Associated With Chemotherapy-Induced Fever and Chills

Disease-Related Factors	Treatment-Related Factors
See "Neutropenia" and "Infection"	See "Neutropenia" and "Infection"
Tumor involving the hypothalamus	Chemotherapy side effects causing drug fever or flu-like syndrome (e.g., bleomycin, daunorubicin, thiotepa, methotrexate, dacarbazine, and plicamycin)
Paraneoplastic syndromes	
Pyrogens released by the tumor cells	
Tumors associated with tumor-induced fever; Hodgkin lymphoma, osteogenic sarcoma, lymphoma, and liver metastasis	Blood transfusion reaction
	Immunotherapy side effects (e.g., interferon, monoclonal antibodies, and interleukin)
	Steroid-induced adrenal insufficiency
	Drug-induced fever; vancomycin or amphotericin B
	Invasive procedures

From Crombez, P. (2019). Evidence-based nursing of patients with hematologic malignancies. In F. Charnay-Sonnek, & A. E. Murphy (Eds.), *Principle of nursing in oncology* (pp. 277–308). Berlin: Springer; *Mayo Clinic.* (2022). Fever. https://www.mayoclinic.org/diseases-conditions/fever/symptoms-causes/syc-20352759; Wilson, B. J. (2019). Myelosuppression. In M. M. Olsen, K. B. LeFebvre, & K. J. Brassil (Eds.), *Chemotherapy and immunotherapy guidelines and recommendations for practice* (pp. 273–292). Pittsburgh, PA: Oncology Nursing Society.

Management
(Table 40.17)

I. Pharmacologic management (Crombez, 2019; Mayo Clinic, 2022; Wilson, 2019)
    A. Interventions to locate the source of infection
       1. Obtain cultures from the blood, throat, urine, stool, sputum, and wounds when an infection is suspected, including cultures from all access devices.
    B. Antipyretics as indicated
       1. Acetaminophen—not to exceed 4000 mg in a 24-hour period; to be used with caution in patients with liver disease
       2. Aspirin—to be used with caution in patients with Plt disorders
       3. Ibuprofen—to be used with caution in patients with renal impairment

II. Nonpharmacologic management (Crombez, 2019; Mayo Clinic, 2022; Wilson, 2019)
    A. Promote slow cooling of the skin and mucous membranes.
    B. Tepid sponge baths
    C. Reduce the amount of patient clothing.
    D. Mechanical cooling blankets
    E. Reduction of the environmental temperature
    F. Avoid rapid reduction in body temperature that can cause chilling by providing warm blankets or heating pads at the first sign of chilling.
    G. Change damp clothing immediately to prevent chilling.
    H. Increase fluid intake to prevent dehydration.
    I. Minimize the occurrence of infection in common sites.
       1. Encourage the patient to cough and take deep breaths every 4–8 hours while awake.

TABLE 40.17   Assessment and Recommendations for Management of Cancer-Related Fever and Chills

History	• Previous cancer treatment history: chemotherapy, radiation therapy, or multimodal therapy • Previous exposure to infections • Type of cancer and extent of disease • Previous blood transfusions • Current medications • History of hypersensitivity reactions
Physical examination	• Frequent assessment of vital signs • Complete physical examination to ascertain source of fever
Laboratory data	• Review laboratory data, additional analysis based on suspected cause (e.g., neutropenia-related fevers, drug reaction fevers, drug reactions, and cholangitis)
Treatment	• Administer antipyretics as ordered-acetaminophen alternated with ibuprofen every 2 h to decrease fever and drug toxicity; caution in patients with thrombocytopenia; NSAIDs for tumor-induced fever; caution in patients with thrombocytopenia and renal insufficiency • Treat underlying cause • Assess for the increase in fatigue, muscle weakness, myalgia, dyspnea, cardiopulmonary compromise, and reduced quality of life
Risks	• Septic shock and death are possibilities

NSAIDs, Nonsteroidal antiinflammatory drugs.
From Crombez, P. (2019). Evidence-based nursing of patients with hematologic malignancies. In F. Charnay-Sonnek, & A. E. Murphy (Eds.), *Principle of nursing in oncology* (pp. 277–308). Berlin: Springer; *Mayo Clinic.* (2022). Fever. https://www.mayoclinic.org/diseases-conditions/fever/symptoms-causes/syc-20352759; Wilson, B. J. (2019). Myelosuppression. In M. M. Olsen, K. B. LeFebvre, & K. J. Brassil (Eds.), *Chemotherapy and immunotherapy guidelines and recommendations for practice* (pp. 273–292). Pittsburgh, PA: Oncology Nursing Society.

2. Encourage the patient to perform oral hygiene every 4 hours while awake.
3. Encourage the patient to void frequently.
4. Instruct the patient to avoid the use of douches or tampons.
5. Encourage the patient to eat well-balanced meals and increase fluid intake.

III. Monitor for complications (Crombez, 2019; Mayo Clinic, 2022; Wilson, 2019).
   A. Establish a plan for monitoring for fever based on the patient's individual risk profile (Table 40.16).
   B. Monitor temperature regularly.
   C. Monitor blood counts and diagnostic tests as indicated.
IV. Patient and caregiver education (Crombez, 2019; Wilson, 2019)
   A. Educate about infection, neutropenia, and necessity of prompt management.
   B. Educate patient as to self-care measures for fever or chills, including medication management.

OVERVIEW OF IMMUNE SYMPTOMS

I. Definition—immune-related adverse events (irAEs) are side effects that resemble autoimmune diseases (Fan, Geng, Shen, & Zhang, 2020; Patil & Velcheti, 2021).
   A. irAEs can be delayed and inflammatory and can develop at any time.
   B. Most irAEs are reversible—with the exception of some endocrine side effects (grade 3 or above).
   C. There are two categories—frequently reported and uncommonly reported (Table 40.18).
II. Physiology (Fan et al., 2020; Guerrouahen, Maccalli, Cugno, Rutella, & Akporiaye, 2020; Kramer et al., 2021; Martinez, 2019; Patil & Velcheti, 2021; Sulicka-Grodzicka et al., 2021)
   A. irAEs' physiology is not completely understood; related to an inflammatory process to an immune-mediated intervention.
      1. T-cell mediation and altered humoral responses
   B. Cytokines are proteins that direct the immune response.
      1. Increases systemic inflammation
      2. Severe cases of irAEs can be fatal.
III. Risks
   A. Patient and disease-related risks
      1. irAREs are linked to genetic markers.
      2. Primary tumor sites
         a. Tumors can avoid immune controls—supported by rapid proliferation.
      3. Age-related symptoms influence the incidence of irAEs.
         a. Decrease in T cells, increase in memory B cells, increase in activated memory lymphocytes
      4. Some secondary immune responses can result in autoimmunity.
         a. Thyroid dysfunction, rheumatoid arthritis, cytokine release syndrome (CRS), and dermatosis
   B. Treatment-related risks
      1. Long-term sequelae of chemotherapy and radiation therapies
      2. Activation of the adaptive immune system
      3. Immunotherapy can cause long-term stimulation of the immune system.
         b. Activation of the adaptive immune system
         c. Immune checkpoint inhibitors (ICI) mediate anti-tumor effects and interrupt immune homeostasis.
      1. Disrupts the immunosuppressive process
      2. Impacts all blood lineages
         B. Due to the complexity of irAEs, early identification and intervention is essential.

CYTOKINE STORM AND CYTOKINE RELEASE SYNDROME

Overview

I. Definition—release of cytokines causing systemic inflammation (Fajgenbaum & June, 2020)
   A. Manifests as flu-like syndromes
   B. Related to an increase in immune-cell activation

II. Physiology (Fajgenbaum & June, 2020; Fan et al., 2020; Patel & Velcheti, 2021; St. Jude Children's Research Hospital, 2019)
   A. Not fully understood
   B. Cytokine storm is an umbrella term for several disorders
   C. CRS is a collection of syndromes that activates T cells
   D. Constitutional symptoms
      1. Fever
      2. Fatigue
      3. Headache
      4. Anorexia
      5. Rash
      6. Diarrhea
      7. Arthralgia
      8. Myalgia
      9. Neuropsychiatric findings
   E. Can lead to multiorgan dysfunction
      1. Renal failure
      2. Acute liver injury
      3. Cardiomyopathy
III. Risk factors (Fajgenbaum & June, 2020; Fan et al., 2020; Kramer et al., 2021; Patel & Velcheti, 2021; Visram & Kourelis, 2021; Wallet et al., 2020)
   A. Patient-related risks
      1. Age
      2. Malignancy
      3. Pathogens
      4. Autoimmune conditions
   B. Treatment-related risks
      1. Lymphodepleting chemotherapy
      2. ICI
      3. Chimeric antigen receptor T cells
         a. CRS incidence 42%–100%
      4. Bispecific T-cell engager
      5. Monoclonal antibodies
      6. Immunomodulatory drugs
      7. Oncolytic viruses

Assessment

See Table 40.19.

Management

I. Pharmacologic management (Fajgenbaum & June, 2020; Fan et al., 2020; Kramer et al., 2021; Xiao et al., 2021)
   A. Identification of patients at risk and prescribing prophylaxis as appropriate

TABLE 40.19 Assessment and Recommendations for Management of Cytokine Storm and Cytokine Release Syndrome (CRS)

Assessment	• Previous cancer treatment history: chemotherapy, radiation therapy, or multimodal therapy
	• Assess hemodynamic status with frequent vital signs.
	• Assess for fever, chills, fatigue, nausea, vomiting, diarrhea, headache, myalgia, rash, hypotension, arrythmia, tachycardia, shortness of breath, decreased oxygen saturation
	• Assess for changes that indicate neurological changes: level of consciousness, restlessness, headache, seizures, pupil changes, and ataxia
Laboratory data	• Monitor lab values: blood counts, electrolytes, kidney function, liver enzymes, ferritin, and cytokines
Prevention	• Identification of patients at high risk for cytokine storm/CRS
	• Patient and caregiver education for reportable signs and symptoms
Treatment	• Maintain a current type and screen for patients requiring frequent transfusions
	• Administer prophylaxis supportive care as ordered
	• Treat underlying cause(s)
Benefits	• Weigh the risks and benefits of each treatment
	• Review informed consent if applicable and evaluate patient understanding of associated risks
Risks	• Transfusion reaction or transmitted disease
	• Delay in administering treatment on time or dose delays; dose reductions

From Fajgenbaum, D. C., & June, C. H. (2020). Cytokine storm. *The New England Journal of Medicine, 383*(23), 2255–2273. https://doi.org/10.1056/NEJMra2026131; Fan, Y., Geng, Y., Shen, L., & Zhang, Z. (2021). Advances on immune-related adverse events associated with immune checkpoint inhibitors. *Frontiers of Medicine, 15*(1), 33–42. https://doi.org/10.1007/s11684-019-0735-3; Kramer, R., Zaremba, A., Moreira, A., Ugurel, S., Johnson, D. B., Hassel, J. C., et al. (2021). Hematological immune related adverse events after treatment with immune checkpoint inhibitors. *European Journal of Cancer, 147,* 170–181. https://doi.org/10.1016/j.ejca.2021.01.013; Martinez, A. L. (2019). Immunotherapy. In M. M. Olsen, K. B. LeFebvre, & K. J. Brassil (Eds.), *Chemotherapy and immunotherapy guidelines and recommendations for practice* (pp. 149–189). Pittsburgh, PA: Oncology Nursing Society; Patil, P. D., & Velcheti, V. (2021). Cancer treatment infusion reactions. In V. Velcheti, & S. R. Punekar (Eds.), *Handbook of cancer treatment-related symptoms and toxicities* (pp. 179–185). Amsterdam: Elsevier; Wallet, F., Bachy, E., Vassal, O., Friggeri, A., Bohe, J., Garnier, L., et al. (2020). Extracorporeal cytokine adsorption for treating severe refractory cytokine release syndrome (CRS). *Bone Marrow Transplantation (Basingstoke), 55*(10), 2052–2055. https://doi.org/10.1038/s41409-020-0896-3.

TABLE 40.18 Categories of Immune-Related Adverse Events

Frequently Reported	Uncommonly Reported
Dermatologic: pruritus, rash	Cardiovascular: cardiomyopathy
Gastrointestinal: diarrhea, colitis	Hematologic: B-cell aplasia, cytopenias
Hepatic: hepatitis	
Endocrine: thyroid dysfunction, hypophysitis	Renal: nephritis
Respiratory: pneumonitis	Neurologic: confusion, aphasia, seizures
Rheumatologic	Ophthalmologic
Musculoskeletal	

From Fan, Y., Geng, Y., Shen, L., & Zhang, Z. (2021). Advances on immune-related adverse events associated with immune checkpoint inhibitors. *Frontiers of Medicine, 15*(1), 33–42. https://doi.org/10.1007/s11684-019-0735-3; Martinez, A. L. (2019). Immunotherapy. In M. M. Olsen, K. B. LeFebvre, & K. J. Brassil (Eds.), *Chemotherapy and immunotherapy guidelines and recommendations for practice* (pp. 149–189). Pittsburgh, PA: Oncology Nursing Society; Patil, P. D., & Velcheti, V. (2021). Cancer treatment infusion reactions. In V. Velcheti, & S. R. Punekar (Eds.), *Handbook of cancer treatment-related symptoms and toxicities* (pp. 179–185). Amsterdam: Elsevier.

TABLE 40.20 **American Society of Transplantation and Cellular Therapy Grading for Cytokine Release Syndrome**

	Fever (°C)	Hypotension		Hypoxia
Grade 1	≥38	None	AND/	None
Grade 2	≥38	Responsive to fluids	OR	Low-flow nasal cannula (≤6 L/min)
Grade 3	≥38	Requiring one vasoactive agent		High-flow nasal cannula (≤6 L/min), facemask, nonrebreather, Venturi mask
Grade 4	≥38	Requiring more than one vasoactive agent		Positive pressure ventilation, intubation with mechanical ventilation

From Chou, C. K., & Turtle, C. J. (2020). Assessment and management of cytokine release syndrome and neurotoxicity following CD19 CAR-T cell therapy. *Expert Opinion on Biological Therapy*, *20*(6), 653–664. https://doi.org/10.1080/14712598.2020.1729735; Xiao, X., Huang, S., Chen, S., Wang, Y., Sun, Q., Xu, X., et al. (2021). Mechanisms of cytokine release syndrome and neurotoxicity of CAR T-cell therapy and associated prevention and management strategies. *Journal of Experimental & Clinical Cancer Research*, *40*(1), 367. https://doi.org/10.1186/s13046-021-02148-6.

B. Identification of grades of CRS and managing appropriately (Table 40.20)
C. Anticytokine agents (including, but not limited to)
1. Tocilizumab
2. Siltuximab
3. Anakinra
4. Lenzilumab
5. Ruxolitinib
6. Dasatinib
7. Ibrutinib
D. Vasopressors for severe hypotension
E. Steroids
F. Supportive care is critical
1. Blood products
2. IV hydration
3. Supportive oxygen
4. Electrolyte replacements
5. Hemodialysis if applicable
II. Nonpharmacologic management (Fajgenbaum & June, 2020; Kramer et al., 2021; Martinez, 2019)
A. Administer blood components as ordered.
B. Administer electrolyte replacements and hydration as ordered.
C. Minimize hemodynamic complications.
1. Monitor vital signs frequently.
2. Strict intake and output in records
D. Report critical changes in the patient's assessment parameters to the physician such as change in mental status, decrease in BP, and fever.

III. Monitor for complications (Fajgenbaum & June, 2020; Kramer et al., 2021; Martinez, 2019).
A. Establish a plan for monitoring blood counts based on the patient's individual risk profile and follow trends.
1. Monitor lab values closely and follow trends.
IV. Patient and caregiver education (Martinez, 2019)
A. Educate about systemic inflammation.
B. Educate about infection prevention and how to minimize the risk of infection.
C. Educate about the symptoms for which to call the physician or nurse.

REFERENCES

Balitsky, A. K., Liu, Y., Van der Meer, P. F., Heddle, N. M., & Arnold, D. M. (2021). Exploring the components of bleeding outcomes in transfusion trials for patients with hematologic malignancy. *Transfusion (Philadelphia, PA)*, *61*(1), 286–293. https://doi.org/10.1111/trf.16126.

Bryer, E. J., Kallan, M. J., Chiu, T.-S., Scheuba, K. M., & Henry, D. H. (2020). A retrospective analysis of venous thromboembolism trends in chemotherapy-induced anemia. *Journal of Clinical Oncology*, *38*(15_suppl), e15515. https://doi.org/10.1200/JCO.2020.38.15_suppl.e15515.

Crombez, P. (2019). Evidence-based nursing of patients with hematologic malignancies. In F. Charnay-Sonnek & A. E. Murphy (Eds.), *Principle of nursing in oncology* (pp. 277–308). Berlin: Springer.

Davis, C. P. (2021). Medical definition of infection. *MedicineNet*. Retrieved from https://www.medicinenet.com/infection/definition.htm.

Fajgenbaum, D. C., & June, C. H. (2020). Cytokine storm. *The New England Journal of Medicine*, *383*(23), 2255–2273. https://doi.org/10.1056/NEJMra2026131.

Fan, Y., Geng, Y., Shen, L., & Zhang, Z. (2020). Advances on immune-related adverse events associated with immune checkpoint inhibitors. *Frontiers of Medicine*, *15*(1), 33–42. https://doi.org/10.1007/s11684-019-0735-3.

Guerrouahen, B. S., Maccalli, C., Cugno, C., Rutella, S., & Akporiaye, E. T. (2020). Reverting immune suppression to enhance cancer immunotherapy. *Frontiers in Oncology*, *9*, 1554. https://doi.org/10.3389/fonc.2019.01554.

Johnson, A. B., & Burns, B. (2021). Hemorrhage: *StatPearls [Internet]*. Treasure Island, FL: StatPearls Publishing. Retrieved from https://www.ncbi.nlm.nih.gov/books/NBK542273/.

Kramer, R., Zaremba, A., Moreira, A., Ugurel, S., Johnson, D. B., Hassel, J. C., et al. (2021). Hematological immune related adverse events after treatment with immune checkpoint inhibitors. *European Journal of Cancer*, *147*, 170–181. https://doi.org/10.1016/j.ejca.2021.01.013.

Lemke, E. A. (2019). Genitourinary toxicities. In M. M. Olsen, K. B. LeFebvre, & K. J. Brassil (Eds.), *Chemotherapy and immunotherapy guidelines and recommendations for practice* (pp. 471–486). Pittsburgh, PA: Oncology Nursing Society.

Lordo, M. R., Scoville, S. D., Goel, A., Yu, J., Freud, A. G., Caligiuri, M. A., et al. (2021). Unraveling the role of innate lymphoid cells in acute myeloid leukemia. *Cancers*, *13*(2), 320. https://doi.org/10.3390/cancers13020320.

Martinez, A. L. (2019). Immunotherapy. In M. M. Olsen, K. B. LeFebvre, & K. J. Brassil (Eds.), *Chemotherapy and immunotherapy guidelines and recommendations for practice* (pp. 149–189). Pittsburgh, PA: Oncology Nursing Society.

Mayo Clinic. (2022). Fever. https://www.mayoclinic.org/diseases-conditions/fever/symptoms-causes/syc-20352759.

Messin, C., & Amrhein, C. (2019). Evidence-based nursing in basic anticancer treatment: Management of the most important side effects. In F. Charnay-Sonnek & A. E. Murphy (Eds.), *Principle of nursing in oncology* (pp. 33–64). Berlin: Springer.

Mistry, H. E. (2019). Gastrointestinal and mucosal toxicities. In M. M. Olsen, K. B. LeFebvre, & K. J. Brassil (Eds.), *Chemotherapy and immunotherapy guidelines and recommendations for practice* (pp. 293–352). Pittsburgh, PA: Oncology Nursing Society.

Occiano, P., Nagelberg, M., & Adelsberg, R. (2019). Nutrition and symptom management. In W. Oh & A. Chari (Eds.), *Mount Sinai expert guides: Oncology* (pp. 528–534). New York: Icahn School of Medicine at Mount Sinai.

Patil, P. D., & Velcheti, V. (2021). Mechanisms of immune-related adverse events. In V. Velcheti & S. R. Punekar (Eds.), *Handbook of cancer treatment-related symptoms and toxicities* (pp. 179–185). Amsterdam: Elsevier.

Shelton, B. K. (2019). Pulmonary toxicities. In M. M. Olsen, K. B. LeFebvre, & K. J. Brassil (Eds.), *Chemotherapy and immunotherapy guidelines and recommendations for practice* (pp. 401–444). Pittsburgh, PA: Oncology Nursing Society.

St. Jude Children's Research Hospital. (2019). Cytokine release syndrome (CRS) after immunotherapy. https://together.stjude.org/en-us/diagnosis-treatment/side-effects/cytokine-release-syndrome-crs.html.

Sulicka-Grodzicka, J., Surdacki, A., Seweryn, M., Mikołajczyk, T., Rewiuk, K., Guzik, T., et al. (2021). Low-grade chronic inflammation and immune alterations in childhood and adolescent cancer survivors: A contribution to accelerated aging? *Cancer Medicine (Malden, MA)*, 10(5), 1772–1782. https://doi.org/10.1002/cam4.3788.

Vemula, S. (2021). Cancer treatment related infusion reactions. In V. Velcheti & S. R. Punekar (Eds.), *Handbook of cancer treatment-related symptoms and toxicities* (pp. 107–112). Amsterdam: Elsevier.

Vega, A., Zhang, R., Wong, H., Wernecke, M., Alexander, M., Feng, Y., et al. (2021). Trends in erythropoiesis-stimulating agent use and blood transfusions for chemotherapy-induced anemia throughout FDA's risk evaluation and mitigation strategy lifecycle. *Pharmacoepidemiology & Drug Safety*, 30(5), 626–635. https://doi.org/10.1002/pds.5202.

Visram, A., & Kourelis, T. V. (2021). Aging-associated immune system changes in multiple myeloma: The dark side of the moon. *Cancer Treatment and Research Communications*, 29, 100494. https://doi.org/10.1016/j.ctarc.2021.100494.

Wallet, F., Bachy, E., Vassal, O., Friggeri, A., Bohe, J., Garnier, L., et al. (2020). Extracorporeal cytokine adsorption for treating severe refractory cytokine release syndrome (CRS). *Bone Marrow Transplantation (Basingstoke)*, 55(10), 2052–2055. https://doi.org/10.1038/s41409-020-0896-3.

Wilson, B. J. (2019). Myelosuppression. In M. M. Olsen, K. B. LeFebvre, & K. J. Brassil (Eds.), *Chemotherapy and immunotherapy guidelines and recommendations for practice* (pp. 273–292). Pittsburgh, PA: Oncology Nursing Society.

Xiao, X., Huang, S., Chen, S., Wang, Y., Sun, Q., Xu, X., et al. (2021). Mechanisms of cytokine release syndrome and neurotoxicity of CAR T-cell therapy and associated prevention and management strategies. *Journal of Experimental & Clinical Cancer Research*, 40(1), 367. https://doi.org/10.1186/s13046-021-02148-6.

Yang, S., Che, H., Xiao, L., Zhao, B., & Liu, S. (2021). Traditional Chinese medicine on treating myelosuppression after chemotherapy: A protocol for systematic review and meta-analysis. *Medicine (Baltimore)*, 100(4), e24307. https://doi.org/10.1097/MD.0000000000024307.

41

Integumentary Symptoms

Diane G. Cope

OVERVIEW

I. Physiology (Mohamed & Hargest, 2022)
   A. The skin is composed of three layers—the epidermis, the dermis, and the subcutaneous tissue.
   B. Intact skin protects the body from harmful microbes, temperature changes, physical trauma, and radiation.
   C. Skin is the first line of defense by regulating thermal processes, protecting underlying structures, and excreting waste.
      1. The epidermis is the avascular outer layer, which serves as a barrier to prevent water loss and renews itself continuously through cell division.
      2. The dermis, the inner connective tissue layer, is highly vascular, with afferent sensory nerve receptors, which provides nutritional support to the avascular epidermal layer.
      3. The subcutaneous tissue is composed of adipose tissue, which serves as a cushion to trauma, an insulator to temperature changes, and an energy reservoir.

II. Risk factors (Bennardo et al., 2021; Cesarman et al., 2019; Gruber & Zito, 2021; Kamijo, & Miyagaki, 2021; Kim, Lee, Kwong, & Martires, 2019; Lai, Cranwell, & Sinclair, 2018; Soares & Sokumbi, 2021; Rodrigues, Oliveira-Ribeiro, de Abreu Fiuza Gomes, & Knobler, 2018; Wick & Patterson, 2019)
   A. Disease related (Table 41.1)
      1. Thrombocytopenia
      2. Cutaneous metastases or direct tumor extension (late manifestation in the course of the illness for solid tumors of the breast and lung, squamous cell carcinoma of the head and neck, malignant melanoma, lymphoma, and Kaposi sarcoma)
      3. Primary cutaneous paraneoplastic syndromes—acanthosis nigricans, acquired ichthyosis, Paget disease, telangiectasia, hypertrichosis, lanuginosa acquisita, and erythroderma
      4. Primary malignant skin cancer (melanoma, basal cell carcinoma, squamous cell carcinoma, and Kaposi sarcoma)
      5. Mycosis fungoides (slow, progressive, and cutaneous T-cell lymphoma)
      6. Premalignant lesions (actinic keratosis, leukoplakia, and dysplastic nevus syndrome)
      7. Malnutrition—decreased protein store

      8. Graft-versus-host disease (skin reaction related to bone marrow transplantation)
      9. Malnutrition—decreased protein stores
      10. Other effects—alopecia, immobility, pressure ulcers, (lymph) edema, pruritus, jaundice, incontinence, and infection
         a. Chest tubes, drains, indwelling urinary catheter, and biliary catheters
         b. Feeding tubes—gastrostomy, jejunostomy
   B. Treatment related (Cury-Martins et al., 2020; Kim, Park, Lee, & Cheon, 2020; Silva, Gomes, Lobo, Almeida, & Almeida, 2020)
      1. Desquamative skin reaction (radiation enhancement, radiation recall, and combined modality therapy) as a result of chemotherapy in association with radiation therapy
      2. Fragile skin from steroid therapy
      3. Erythema multiforme (widespread, scattered, and cutaneous vesicles) associated with multiple drugs
      4. Erythema nodosum (tender, subcutaneous, and anterior leg nodules)—hypersensitivity reaction to penicillin or sulfonamides
      5. Graft-versus-host disease (skin reaction related to bone marrow transplantation)
      6. Side effects of targeted therapy, immunotherapy, chemotherapy, and radiation therapy
      7. Extravasation of chemotherapy (anthracyclines, taxanes, and antimetabolites)
      8. Reaction or sensitivity to tape or adhesive dressings (central and peripheral intravenous access)

ASSESSMENT

I. History (Lawton & Turner, 2020; Mitchell, 2022)
   A. Presence of risk factors
   B. Patient's age
   C. General health status
   D. Exposure to infection
   E. Recent treatment and anticipated side effects
   F. Current drug therapy
   G. Past and current skin conditions
   H. Review of personal hygiene practices
   I. Nutritional status
   J. Smoking habits

TABLE 41.1 Etiologic Factors of Skin Reactions (Ng et al., 2018)

Skin Reaction	General Class of Reaction	Drug Class or Mechanism
Skin Reactions Found With Chemotherapy and Radiation Therapy in Combination		
Radiation recall dermatitis	Occurs in previously irradiated skin within 1–2 weeks after chemotherapy; erythema, edema, superficial ulcerations, and superficial skin sloughing	Drugs such as cetuximab, doxorubicin (Doxil, Adriamycin), docetaxel (Taxotere), gemcitabine (Gemzar), paclitaxel (Taxol), capecitabine, and 5-FU
Skin Reactions Found With Chemotherapy alone		
Allergic or Immune Complex Reactions		
Activation of an already existing immune complex reaction in collagen vascular diseases of systemic lupus erythematosus and progressive systemic sclerosis (scleroderma)	Chemotherapy drug activates immune complexes already circulating due to the underlying collagen vascular disease process, causing circular, red, and scaly rash	Taxanes, bleomycin
Contact allergy (activated T cells) and may not develop until 24–36 h after contact with the allergen	Allergic response where drug touches skin (erythema, local swelling, desquamation, blistering, and necrosis possible)	Chemicals found in poison ivy, oak, and sumac Nickel and cobalt in metal jewelry, clothing snaps, zippers, and metal-plated objects Latex in gloves and rubberized clothing Neomycin in antibiotic skin ointments Potassium dichromate, a tanning agent found in leather shoes and clothing
Erythema multiforme (antigen–antibody complexes)	Rash with typical target lesions involving extremities, including palms and soles, can progress to generalized	*Antibiotics*, such as sulfonamides, tetracyclines, amoxicillin, and ampicillin *NSAIDs*, such as ibuprofen Anticonvulsants (used to treat epilepsy), such as phenytoin and barbiturates *Alkylating agents:* treosulfan, alkysufonates, chlorambucil, mustard gas derivatives, nitrogen mustard, temozolomide, hydrazines and triazines, procarbazine, and hydrazines *Plant alkaloids:* paclitaxel, taxanes, and etoposide *Anthracyclines:* doxorubicin *Antimetabolites:* methotrexate, folic acid antagonists, cytarabine, fludarabine, gemcitabine, and capecitabine Cladribine, 6-mercaptopurine, pemetrexed *Antitumor antibiotics:* bleomycin, mithramycin *Miscellaneous:* lenalidomide, thalidomide *EGFR inhibitors:* afatinib, cetuximab, erlotinib, gefitinib, and panitumumab *KIT and BCR-ABL inhibitors:* imatinib, sorafenib, bortezomib, brentuximab, and rituximab *BRAF inhibitors:* vemurafenib *Immunomodulators:* aldesleukin, ipilimumab, nivolumab, pembrolizumab, and denileukin
IgE mediated	Itching, redness, swelling within 1 h after infusion begun; if life threatening, termed *anaphylaxis* and includes decreased blood pressure, decreased level of consciousness, airway, and breathing compromise	Platinum derivatives (cisplatin, carboplatin)
Serum sickness (antigen–antibody complexes)	Flulike symptoms, which may progress to life threatening	Rituximab and other "mab" drugs
Vasculitis (from antigen–antibody complexes)	Generalized vascular inflammation with end-organ damage	Methotrexate
Extravasation injury (drug leaks from IV site into surrounding tissue)	Varying severity depending on specific drug (swelling, redness, irritation, local tissue loss, and necrosis)	Antitumor antibiotics, vinca alkaloids highest risk; many others can cause

Continued

TABLE 41.1 Etiologic Factors of Skin Reactions (Ng et al., 2018)—(cont'd)

Skin Reaction	General Class of Reaction	Drug Class or Mechanism
Skin Reactions Found With Radiation Therapy Alone		
Acute radiation dermatitis	Immediate dermatitis occurring in radiated areas with erythema, pain, dermal swelling, itching, and necrosis	May occur with all radiation therapy Mechanism is free radical damage to tissue
Chronic radiation dermatitis	Long-term effects of radiation therapy in port area with thinning of skin, scarring and contractures, telangiectasias, and long-term skin sensitivity to irritants and environmental agents	May occur with all radiation therapy Mechanism is free radical damage to tissue Severity depends on the port size and total dose
Skin Reactions Found With Chemotherapy and Radiation Therapy in Combination		
Radiation recall dermatitis	Occurs in previously irradiated skin within 1–2 weeks after chemotherapy; erythema, edema, superficial ulcerations, and superficial skin sloughing	Drugs such as cetuximab, doxorubicin (Doxil, Adriamycin), docetaxel (Taxotere), gemcitabine (Gemzar), paclitaxel (Taxol), capecitabine, and 5-FU
Light-Related Reactions		
Photo enhancement	Drug given several days after sunburn causes sunburn to reappear in that area	Antibiotics 5-FU
Photosensitivity	Patient more sensitive to sun in solar-exposed areas and may develop a severe sunburn	Antitumor antibiotics
Phototoxicity	Allergic response on solar-exposed areas may be severe with edema, erythema, blistering; if very severe, may result in permanent hyperpigmentation	Many drugs
Nail Changes		
Beau's lines	Transverse lines in nails, bands corresponding to when drug was given or time when critical illness occurred	Any chemotherapy agent or critical illness
Onycholysis	Nail lifts from base	Paclitaxel, docetaxel, cyclophosphamide, doxorubicin, 5-FU, hydroxyurea, combination of vinblastine + bleomycin
Nail inflammation	Inflammatory changes around nail, including paronychia	EGFR inhibitors (cetuximab, gefitinib), taxanes (docetaxel)
Pigment Changes of Skin, Mucous Membranes, Nails, and Hair		
Drug secreted in sweat may induce pigmentation	Under areas where adhesive tape applied and skin sweats	Docetaxel, thiotepa, and ifosfamide
Flag sign		
Generalized hyperpigmentation of all skin	Pigment loss of hair during time drug is given; all skin involved	Many drugs Busulfan (termed *busulfan tan*), pegylated liposomal doxorubicin, hydroxyurea, methotrexate Cyclophosphamide
Gums	Permanent hyperpigmentation of gums	Cisplatin, hydroxyurea, and bleomycin
Hyperpigmentation in areas of pressure or injury	Injured skin only, although inciting injury may be mild	Tegafur (5-FU derivative)
Hyperpigmentation of palms, soles, and nails	Circular areas of hyperpigmentation in these locations	Daunorubicin

Hyperpigmentation of solar-exposed skin
  Scalp hyperpigmentation
  Variety of pigmentary changes of skin and appendages
  Various types of hyperpigmentation—serpentine, generalized, and others
	Sun-exposed areas only
	  Circular hyperpigmented areas in scalp
	  General types of pigmentary changes especially common with drugs listed
	Generalized hyperpigmentation (all skin), of sun-exposed areas only, serpentine (follows underlying vein where drug infused), mucosa of tongue, nails, and conjunctiva of eyes
		Daunorubicin
		Various cytotoxic drugs (alkylating agents, tumor-directed antibiotics)
		
		5-FU

TABLE 41.1 Etiologic Factors of Skin Reactions (Ng et al., 2018)—(cont'd)

Skin Reaction	General Class of Reaction	Drug Class or Mechanism
Rashes		
Generalized rash of hands and feet	Usually localized but can become more generalized	Tyrosine kinase signal transduction inhibitors (occurs with 50% of patients on higher doses of imatinib)
Acneiform rash	Papules and pustules similar to acne, although this rash contains *no* comedones; commonly involves face and also back, upper chest	EGFR inhibitors (cetuximab, gefitinib, nivolumab, ipilimumab, and pembrolizumab)
Hand–foot syndrome or acral erythema	Erythema of hands and feet, dysesthesias	Various chemotherapy drugs (capecitabine)
Toxicity to rapidly dividing cells	Alopecia, mouth ulcers, GI tract ulcers, GI yeast overgrowth and other infections from decreased mucous production (mucous is protective), bone marrow effects of anemia, decreased platelets, decreased WBCs, decreased production of sperm and ova	Most chemotherapy drugs; probability of occurrence depends on how much the drug affects rapidly dividing cell groups
Xerosis (dry skin)	Common—can progress to chronic xerotic dermatitis and secondary infection	Many drugs

5-FU, 5-Fluorouracil; *EGFR*, epidermal growth factor receptor; *GI*, gastrointestinal; *IgE*, immunoglobulin E; *IV*, intravenous; *NSAIDs*, nonsteroidal antiinflammatory drugs; *WBCs*, white blood cells.

Data from Ng, C. Y., Chen, C., Wu, M., Wu, J., Yang, C., Hui, R., et al. (2018). Anticancer drugs induced severe adverse cutaneous drug reactions: An updated review on the risks associated with anticancer targeted therapy or immunotherapies. *Journal of Immunology Research, 2018.* Article ID 5376476. https://doi.org/10.1155/2018/5376476; DeHaven, C. (2014). Chemotherapy and radiotherapy effects on the skin. *Plastic Surgical Nursing, 34*(4), 192–195. https://doi.org/10.1097/PSN.0000000000000077. Used with permission.

K. Incontinence of bowel or bladder

L. Review of medication history and potential allergies

M. Presence of underlying disease

N. Patterns of pruritus, including circadian occurrence (pruritus typically increases at night), timing, onset, duration, impact on daily activities

O. Aggravating and alleviating factors

P. Patient's self-report

Q. Adjective lists describing pruritus—constant, intermittent, transient, burning, and numbness

II. Physical examination (Lawton & Turner, 2020; Mitchell, 2022)

A. Skin—color, pigmentation, integrity, temperature, texture, turgor, and presence of sloughing

B. Presence of edema

C. Presence of petechiae, petechiae pattern and location, purpura, ecchymosis, and jaundice

D. Presence of erythema, dry desquamation, and moist desquamation and location

E. Presence and grade of rash (Common Toxicity Criteria for Adverse Events)

F. Local inflammation at injection site (erythema, induration, and blisters)

G. Ulcerations of mouth; dry, cracked mucous membranes and lips

H. Presence of alopecia

I. Presence of pruritus, skin excoriation

J. Integrity of tube sites, perirectal tissue, and perineal tissue

K. Presence of pressure ulcers

L. Presence of pain

M. Vaginal discharge and erythema

III. Psychosocial examination

A. New diagnosis of a malignancy—pruritus may be the presenting symptom

B. Presence of stress, anxiety, depression, and confusion/dementia

IV. Laboratory data

A. Complete blood cell count—elevated or decreased white blood cell count, anemia, eosinophilia, polycythemia, and thrombocytopenia or thrombocytosis

B. Blood chemistries—hyperglycemia, hyperuricemia, elevated blood urea nitrogen or creatinine, abnormal liver function tests, bilirubin, and alkaline phosphatase

C. Thyroid function tests—hypoactive or hyperactive thyroid

D. Other—low ferritin level, increased sedimentation rate, C-reactive protein, and human immunodeficiency virus antibody assay (if immunosuppression or lymphoma is a possibility)

E. Urinalysis—glycosuria

F. Pathology—biopsies as indicated

MANAGEMENT

I. Pharmacologic management

A. Prophylactic medications

B. Hold offending agent depending on the grade of rash

C. Medications to manage rash (Table 41.2)

D. Consider dermatology consult for evaluation and management

II. Nonpharmacologic management

A. Interventions to increase or maintain dietary and fluid intake

TABLE 41.2 **Pharmacologic Management of Pruritus (Alam, Buddenkotte, Ahmad, & Steinhoff, 2021; National Comprehensive Cancer Network, 2022; Rupert & Honeycutt, 2022; Tamargo, Funovits, Nguyen, Manudhane, & Montañez-Wiscovich, 2019)**

Pharmacologic Agent	Type of Pruritus	Comments
Diphenhydramine (H1 and H2 antagonists)	Urticaria, allergic drug reactions, and advanced disease	May cause drowsiness
Corticosteroids/steroids	Inflammatory pruritus, local skin reactions, and immune-mediated rash	Can be given orally or topically as a cream rubbed onto the pruritic skin
Naloxone and methylnaltrexone (opioid antagonists), butorphanol (kappa opioid receptor agonist)	Opioid-induced pruritus related to mu-receptor agonists	Pruritus in up to 50% of patients receiving opioids; if pruritus is caused by an opioid and symptom management has failed, consider switching to another opioid. May reverse analgesic effect, so use with caution
Capsaicin Gabapentin Pregabalin	Postherpetic neuralgia, psoriasis	Helpful for treating chronic and localized pruritus
Aprepitant (substance P neurokinin receptors)	Sezary syndrome, cutaneous T-cell lymphoma, metastatic cancer, erlotinib-induced itch	Clinical trials needed to verify the efficacy
Mirtazapine	Cancer-related itch, nocturnal itch	Other antidepressants may help with itch

Adapted from Alam, M., Buddenkotte, J., Ahmad, F., & Steinhoff, M. (2021). Neurokinin 1 receptor antagonists for pruritus. *Drugs, 81*, 621–634. https://doi.org/10.1007/s40265-021-01478-1; *National Comprehensive Cancer Network*. (2022). Management of immunotherapy-related toxicities, version 1.2022. https://www.nccn.org/professionals/physician_gls/pdf/immunotherapy.pdf; Rupert, J., & Honeycutt, J. D. (2022). Pruritus: Diagnosis and management. *American Family Physician, 105*(1), 55–64. https://doi.org/10.1007/s40257-017-0306-9; Tamargo, K., Funovits, A., Nguyen, T. H., Manudhane, A., & Montañez-Wiscovich, M. E. (2019). Evaluation and management of the patient with pruritus. *SN Comprehensive Clinical Medicine, 1*, 797–805. https://doi.org/10.1007/s42399-019-00137-7.

1. Offer small frequent meals with increased protein and calories.
2. Moisten foods with liquids, sauces, and gravy.
3. Have the patient increase fluid intake to 3 L/day if not medically contraindicated (e.g., water and calorie-dense fluids such as protein drinks, milk, and juice).
4. Have the patient rinse the oral cavity with warm salt water gargles or baking soda rinses or a nonalcoholic mouthwash.
5. Good oral hygiene

B. Interventions to decrease inflammation of mucous membranes (see Chapter 28)
C. Interventions to teach self-care techniques and prevent complications
   1. Teach the patient and the caregiver to assess the skin on a daily basis.
   2. Teach patient and caregiver tube and drain management.
   3. Assist with turning and positioning every 2 hours.
   4. Massage uninjured areas gently.
   5. Use of an air mattress, egg-crate mattress, specialty bed, or water mattress for high-risk persons.
   6. Use of dry, clean, and wrinkle-free linens.
   7. Instruct on gentle skin cleansing with a mild pH-balanced skin cleanser.
   8. Rinse soap thoroughly off skin and pat skin dry.
   9. Moisturize and lubricate skin with emollient or vasoline-type creams.
   10. For those at risk of hand/foot syndrome, teach patient to avoid heat extremes, friction, or constricting clothing on palmar/plantar surfaces.

D. Patient education on interventions to protect skin integrity
   1. Teach patient and caregiver risk factors and effects of treatments on skin.
   2. Use of protective film, skin barriers, or collection devices around drains and tubes with copious drainage
   3. Use of sterile technique for invasive procedures such as insertion of tubes
   4. Hand washing
   5. Avoid scratching
   6. Reportable signs and symptoms of infections
E. Keep patient's fingernails smooth and short.
F. Recommend the use of cotton clothing and avoidance of restrictive clothing.
G. Report changes in skin color, integrity, pain, increased pruritus, and drainage (amount, odor, color, and consistency) to health care provider.
H. Interventions for oral, perineal, and general hygiene
   1. Use of soft toothbrush or oral sponges
   2. Apply moisturizers to oral mucosa.
   3. Cleanse the perineal area with mild soap, rinsing thoroughly, patting the area dry, and applying a skin barrier after each bowel movement.
   4. Apply adhesive perineum pad or panty liner without deodorant to the undergarment.
   5. Gently cleanse skin with mild soap and tepid water and pat dry with a soft cloth.
   6. Add emollients to bath water, skin lubricants to skin other than to irradiated sites.
   7. Oatmeal baths

8. Application of cool or warm compresses
9. Avoid scented or alcohol-based skin lotions.
I. Interventions to adapt and cope with hair loss (see Chapter 36)
J. Interventions for radiation-induced acute and chronic skin reactions (see Chapter 28)

REFERENCES

Alam, M., Buddenkotte, J., Ahmad, F., & Steinhoff, M. (2021). Neurokinin 1 receptor antagonists for pruritus. *Drugs, 81*, 621–634. https://doi.org/10.1007/s40265-021-01478-1.

Bennardo, L., Passante, M., Cameli, N., Cristaudo, A., Patruno, C., Nisticò, S. P., et al. (2021). Skin manifestations after ionizing radiation exposure: A systematic review. *Bioengineering, 8*(11), 153. https://doi.org/10.3390/bioengineering8110153.

Cesarman, E., Damania, B., Krown, S. E., Martin, J., Bower, M., & Whitby, D. (2019). Kaposi sarcoma. *Nature Reviews Disease Primers, 5*, 9. https://doi.org/10.1038/s41572-019-0060-9.

Cury-Martins, J., Eris, A., Abdalla, C., de Barros Silva, G., de Moura, V., & Sanches, J. A. (2020). Management of dermatologic adverse events from cancer therapies: Recommendations of an expert panel. *Anais Brasileiros de Dermatologia, 95*(2), 221–237. https://doi.org/10.1016/j.abd.2020.01.001.

Gruber, P., & Zito, P. M. (2021). Skin cancer. In: *StatPearls*. Treasure Island, FL: StatPearls Publishing.

Kamijo, H., & Miyagaki, T. (2021). Mycosis fungoides and Sézary syndrome: Updates and review of current therapy. *Current Treatment Options in Oncology, 22*, 10. https://doi.org/10.1007/s11864-020-00809-w.

Kim, J. T., Park, J. Y., Lee, H. J., & Cheon, Y. J. (2020). Guidelines for the management of extravasation. *Journal of Educational Evaluation for Health Professions, 17*, 21. https://doi.org/10.3352/jeehp.2020.17.21.

Kim, Y. J., Lee, G. H., Kwong, B. Y., & Martires, K. J. (2019). Evidence-based, skin-directed treatments for cutaneous chronic graft-versus-host disease. *Cureus, 11*(12), e6462. https://doi.org/10.7759/cureus.6462.

Lai, V., Cranwell, W., & Sinclair, R. (2018). Epidemiology of skin cancer in the mature patient. *Clinics in Dermatology, 36*(2), 167–176. https://doi.org/10.1016/j.clindermatol.2017.10.008.

Lawton, S., & Turner, V. (2020). Undertaking an assessment of the skin using a holistic approach. *Nursing Times, 116*(10), 44–47.

Mitchell, A. (2022). Skin assessment in adults. *British Journal of Nursing, 31*(5), 274–278. https://doi.org/10.12968/bjon.2022.31.5.274.

Mohamed, S. A., & Hargest, R. (2022). Surgical anatomy of the skin. *Surgery, 40*(1), 1–7. https://doi.org/10.1016/j.mpsur.2021.11.021.

National Comprehensive Cancer Network. (2022). Management of immunotherapy-related toxicities, version 1.2022. https://www.nccn.org/professionals/physician_gls/pdf/immunotherapy.pdf.

Ng, C. Y., Chen, C., Wu, M., Wu, J., Yang, C., Hui, R., et al. (2018). Anticancer drugs induced severe adverse cutaneous drug reactions: An updated review on the risks associated with anticancer targeted therapy or immunotherapies. *Journal of Immunology Research, 2018*. Article ID 5376476. https://doi.org/10.1155/2018/5376476.

Rodrigues, K., Oliveira-Ribeiro, C., de Abreu Fiuza Gomes, S., & Knobler, R. (2018). Cutaneous graft-versus-host disease: Diagnosis and treatment. *American Journal of Clinical Dermatology, 19*(1), 33–50. https://doi.org/10.1007/s40257-017-0306-9.

Rupert, J., & Honeycutt, J. D. (2022). Pruritus: Diagnosis and management. *American Family Physician, 105*(1), 55–64.

Silva, D., Gomes, A., MS, Lobo, J., Almeida, V., & Almeida, I. F. (2020). Management of skin adverse reactions in oncology. *Journal of Oncology Pharmacy Practice, 26*(7), 1703–1714. https://doi.org/10.1177/1078155220936341.

Soares, A., & Sokumbi, O. (2021). Recent updates in the treatment of erythema multiforme. *Medicina* (Kaunas, Lithuania), *57*(9), 921. https://doi.org/10.3390/medicina57090921.

Tamargo, K., Funovits, A., Nguyen, T. H., Manudhane, A., & Montañez-Wiscovich, M. E. (2019). Evaluation and management of the patient with pruritus. *SN Comprehensive Clinical Medicine, 1*, 797–805. https://doi.org/10.1007/s42399-019-00137-7.

Wick, M. R., & Patterson, J. W. (2019). Cutaneous paraneoplastic syndromes. *Seminars in Diagnostic Pathology, 36*(4), 211–228. https://doi.org/10.1053/j.semdp.2019.01.001.

42

Musculoskeletal Symptoms

Deena Damsky Dell

OVERVIEW

I. Definitions
  A. Musculoskeletal alterations—affecting the body's joints, ligaments, muscles, nerves, tendons, and structures that support limbs, neck, and back.
  B. Impaired physical mobility (immobility)—a state in which the patient experiences or is at risk for a limitation in independent, purposeful physical movement of the body or one or more extremities (Howland, 2020)
II. Pathophysiology
  A. Sarcopenia is a muscle-wasting syndrome characterized by loss of skeletal muscle mass, quality, and strength and is commonly observed in patients with malignancy (15%–50% of patients with cancer) (Wiedmer et al., 2021).
  B. Inactivity and limited use or disuse of muscle groups may decrease the muscles' ability to contract and may lead to decreased muscle size, muscle atrophy, and weakness.
  C. Motor impairment (spasticity, muscle weakness, paralysis, hemiparesis, and ataxia) may occur in primary cancer (brain tumors, multiple myeloma) or as a secondary effect in metastatic disease (spinal cord compression), infections, and cancer therapy or in nonmalignant conditions.
III. Risk factors
  A. Skeletal system tumor
  B. Tumors of the brain and spinal cord
  C. Obstruction in lymphatic or systemic circulation
  D. Bone pain, stiffness, fatigue
  E. Spinal cord compression
  F. Sensory–perceptual alterations
  G. Nonmalignant conditions—herniated disks, vertebral fractures secondary to osteoporosis, and ear infections
  H. Ergonomic factors—performing tasks that require force and/or repetition, poor posture
  I. Complications of bed rest
  J. Complications of cardiopulmonary disorders
  K. Dehydration
  L. Side effects of treatment, including corticosteroid therapy, radiation therapy, and chemotherapy/endocrine therapy
  M. Nerve and muscle damage from surgical intervention
  N. Changes in physical activity level
  O. Independent versus dependent personality
  P. Presence or absence of social support
  Q. Depression or high- or low-stress level
  R. Body mass index (BMI) greater than 75th percentile for age and gender (>25 kg/m^2) (Callahan, Leonard, & Powell, 2022)
  S. BMI less than 18.5 kg/m^2 (Callahan et al., 2022)
  T. Insufficient knowledge of the value of physical activity and/or mobility strategies
  U. Alteration in cognition

ASSESSMENT

I. History
  A. Presence of risk factors
  B. Recent treatment and anticipated side effects
  C. Decreased activity level
  D. Functional status using a standardized tool (Tables 42.1 and 42.2; Oken et al., 1982; Schag, Heinrich, & Ganz, 1984)
  E. Presence of pain, muscle weakness, and fatigue
  F. Presence of dyspnea, activity intolerance
  G. Presence of vertigo, ringing in ears, or blurred vision
  H. Evaluation of fall risk
  I. Fracture Risk Assessment Tool (FRAX) for the evaluation of fracture risk
  J. History of alcohol or drug use
  K. Current exercise practice
  L. Current therapy
II. Physical examination
  A. Changes in muscle tone, strength, and muscle mass
  B. Unintentional weight loss
  C. Strength and motor function
  D. Mobility and sensory function
  E. Changes in sexual function
  F. Changes in bowel and bladder function/incontinence and loss of sphincter control
  G. Range of joint motion
  H. Positive Babinski signs and reflexes
  I. Alignment, balance, gait, and joint structure
  J. Difficulty changing position from supine to prone, sitting to standing, or turning
  K. Difficulty writing name or other fine motor skills
III. Psychosocial examination
  A. Depression
  B. Anxiety, including fear of falling

TABLE 42.1 Eastern Cooperative Oncology Group Performance Status

Grade	Performance Status
0	Fully active, able to carry on all predisease performance without restriction
1	Restricted in physically strenuous activity but ambulatory and able to carry out work of a light or sedentary nature (e.g., light housework, office work)
2	Ambulatory and capable of all self-care but unable to carry out any work activities; up and about more than 50% of waking hours
3	Capable of only limited self-care, confined to bed or chair for more than 50% of waking hours
4	Completely disabled; cannot carry on any self-care; totally confined to bed or chair
5	Dead

From Oken, M. M., Creech, R. H., Tormey, D. C., Horton, J., Davis, T. E., McFadden, E. T., et al. (1982). Toxicity and response criteria of the Eastern Cooperative Oncology Group. *American Journal of Clinical Oncology*, 5(6), 649–655.

TABLE 42.2 Karnofsky Performance Scale

Percentage of Normal Performance Status	Definitions
100	Normal; no complaints; no evidence of disease
90	Able to carry on normal activity; minor signs or symptoms of disease
80	Normal activity with effort; some signs or symptoms of disease
70	Cares for self; unable to carry on normal activity or do active work
60	Requires occasional assistance but is able to care for most of the needs
50	Requires considerable assistance and frequent medical care
40	Disabled; requires special care and assistance
30	Severely disabled; hospitalization is indicated, although death is not imminent
10	Moribund; fatal process progressing rapidly
0	Dead

From Karnofsky DA, Burchenal JH: The clinical evaluation of chemotherapeutic agents in cancer, in Macleod CM (ed): Evaluation of Chemotherapeutic Agents. New York, Columbia University Press, 1949 p 199–205.

   C. Lack of motivation
   D. Cultural beliefs about mobility
   E. Presence of caregiver
IV. Laboratory data (Larson & Wilbur, 2020)
   A. Electrolyte abnormalities (hyper or hypo)
     1. Calcium stabilizes blood pressure and controls skeletal muscle contraction. It is also used to build strong bones and teeth.
     2. Chloride is necessary to maintain a proper balance of body fluids.

     3. Magnesium is a critical mineral that regulates many important functions (muscle contraction, heart rhythm, and nerve function).
     4. Phosphate interacts closely with calcium.
     5. Potassium regulates heart function and helps maintain healthy nerves and muscles.
     6. Sodium maintains fluid balance, critical for normal body function, helps regulate nerve function and muscle contraction.
     7. Alkaline phosphatase is an enzyme that catalyzes the breakdown of protein in the body, found mostly in liver and bones.
   B. Lumbar puncture results to evaluate for disease to central nervous system
   C. Creatine kinase to confirm myopathy

MANAGEMENT

I. Pharmacologic management
   A. Manage electrolyte disturbances; replace as needed
   B. Pain management
   C. Bone strengtheners (e.g., bisphosphonates, RANK ligand inhibitors)
II. Nonpharmacologic management (Howland, 2020)
   A. Prehabilitation before planned procedures
   B. Have the patient perform active-range-of-motion (AROM) exercises on unaffected limbs at least three or four times per day and have patient or caregiver perform passive range of motion on affected limbs at least two times a day in hospital or home.
   C. Monitor progress from AROM to functional activities.
   D. Maintain body alignment while the patient is in bed.
   E. Change/have patient change position every 2 hours.
   F. Before activity, access and manage patient's pain.
   G. Observe the patient before, during, and after activity or exercise.
   H. Obtain appropriate assistive devices (e.g., splints, walker, cane, overhead trapeze).
   I. Consult with rehabilitation services for physical and occupational therapy.
   J. Establish a routine for activities of daily living; assist and supervise as needed.
   K. Advocate for specialty bed with turn assist and/or low-airloss pressure mattress if needed (assess if needed in home).
   L. Place the call light within reach when the patient is left alone; a bell can be used for the patient at home.
   M. Protect areas of decreased sensation from extreme heat and cold.
   N. Teach the patient with decreased perception of extremities to check where the limb is placed when changing positions.
   O. Consider patient's self-reported fear of falling.
   P. Discuss risk factors for impaired mobility.
   Q. Place the bed in low position and the two side rails at the head of bed up.
   R. Clear pathways in room and hallways.

S. Consider home care safety assessment.

T. Use night lights or soft lighting at night to enhance vision.

U. Positive reinforcement for behaviors that contribute to positive outcomes

V. Have the patient and family responsible for aspects of care according to capabilities, and use various modalities as needed to teach patient/family to meet patient's home needs regarding rehabilitation and safety.

W. Initiate and follow up with referrals to rehabilitation services.

X. Instruct patient and family about signs and symptoms to report.

REFERENCES

Callahan, A., Leonard, H., & Powell, T. (2022). *Nutrition: Science and everyday application (2nd ed.)*. Pressbooks.

Howland, W. (2020). Impaired physical mobility. In B. Ackley, G. Ladwig, M. B. Makie, M. Martinez-Katz, & M. Zanotti (Eds.), *Nursing diagnosis handbook* (12th ed., pp. 615–624). Amsterdam: Elsevier.

Larson, S., & Wilbur, J. (2020). Muscle weakness in adults: Evaluation and differential diagnosis. *American Family Physician, 101*(2), 95–108.

Oken, M. M., Creech, R. H., Tormey, D. C., Horton, J., Davis, T. E., McFadden, E. T., et al. (1982). Toxicity and response criteria of the Eastern Cooperative Oncology Group. *American Journal of Clinical Oncology, 5*(6), 649–655.

Schag, C., Heinrich, R., & Ganz, P. (1984). Karnofsky performance status revisited: Reliability, validity, and guidelines. *Journal of Clinical Oncology, 2*(3), 187–193. https://doi.org/10.1200/JCO.1984.2.3.187.

Wiedmer, P., Jung, T., Castro, J., Pomatto, L., Sun, P., Davies, K., et al. (2021). Sarcopenia – Molecular mechanisms and open questions. *Aging Research Reviews, 65*. Article 101200. https://doi.org/10.1016/j.arr.2020.101200.

43

Neurological Symptoms

Nijmeh Al-Atiyyat

OVERVIEW

I. Physiology/definitions (Desforges et al., 2022)
   A. Neuropathies—any functional disturbances, pathologic changes, or both in the peripheral nervous system: cranial, sensory, and motor nerves and portions of the autonomic nervous system
   B. Neuropathies of the central nervous system—seizures, encephalopathy, cerebellar dysfunction, ophthalmologic toxicities and ototoxicities, mental status changes, and peripheral neuropathies with sensory and motor dysfunction
   C. Incidence and severity of neuropathies—may vary, depending on the administration of immunosuppressive therapy, surgeries, diagnosis, or other treatments
   D. Toxicities—may be dose related from chemotherapy or other therapies, and reversible on discontinuation of therapy or exposure to poisons

II. Risk factors
   A. Disease related (Briani, Cocito, Campagnolo, Doneddu, & Nobile-Orazio, 2022; Li, Mizrahi, Goldstein, Kiernan, & Park, 2021a; Pisciotta, Saveri, & Pareyson, 2021)
      1. Effects of cancer
      2. Postherpetic neuralgia
      3. Presence of infiltrative emergencies (e.g., spinal cord compression)
      4. Other diseases (e.g., history of hepatic or neurologic dysfunction)
      5. Preexisting neuropathies because of diabetes mellitus, human immunodeficiency virus infection, and preexisting vitamin B complex deficiency may include tingling of fingers and toes, jaw pain, foot drop, and muscular atrophy.
   B. Treatment related (Desforges et al., 2022; Knoerl, 2021; Laforgia et al., 2021; Li, Zhang, & Zhao, 2021b; Omran et al., 2021; Patel & Shah, 2021)
      1. Side effects of chemotherapy and immunotherapy (e.g., cerebellar dysfunction, strokelike reaction, generalized weakness, gait disturbance, numbness of feet, loss of proprioception, and vibratory sensation) (Table 43.1)
      2. Side effects of radiation therapy (e.g., ataxia, dysarthria, nystagmus, and radicular pain) and preexisting peripheral neuropathy related to radiation therapy

   C. Individual (Kanzawa-Lee, 2020; Knoerl, 2021).
      1. Age—older than 60 years
      2. Social issues (malnutrition, alcohol abuse, and repetitive actions)

ASSESSMENT

(Table 43.2)
   I. History (Kanzawa-Lee, 2020; Knoerl, 2021; Loprinzi et al., 2020)
      A. Presence of risk factors or other comorbidities such as diabetes, idiopathic neuropathy before chemotherapy
      B. Psychiatric and current social situation
      C. Acute herpes zoster
      D. Recent chemotherapy treatment and anticipated side effects
      E. Presence of weakness
      F. Presence of burning, numbness, tingling in feet and hands, perioral numbness, and paresthesias—stocking–glove distribution
      G. Presence of paresthesia of hands and feet, constipation, and loss of deep tendon reflex
      H. Presence of cerebellar involvement (e.g., tremors, loss of balance)
      I. Ability to perform activities of daily living (ADLs) and occupational and recreational activities
      J. Current medication therapy
      K. Presence of anxiety, low self-esteem
   II. Physical examination
      A. Vital signs
      B. Baseline sensory, mobility, motor function, autonomic function, cranial nerve assessment, and cerebellar function
      C. Speech or language ability
      D. Sight-related changes (e.g., blurred vision, impaired color perception)
   III. Psychological examination
      A. Anxiety management strategies
      B. Coping style and ability
   IV. Laboratory data
      A. Nerve conduction studies (e.g., electromyography)
      B. Muscle or nerve biopsy

TABLE 43.1	Chemotherapy Agents Associated With Peripheral Neuropathy				
Antineoplastic Agent	**Associated Neuropathy**	**Antineoplastic Agent**	**Associated Neuropathy**	**Antineoplastic Agent**	**Associated Neuropathy**
Bortezomib	Sensory	Etoposide (VP-16)	Sensory Motor	Vinblastine	Sensory Motor Cranial Autonomic
Carboplatin	Sensory Cranial (rare) Autonomic	5-Fluorouracil	Motor (rare)	Vincristine	Sensory Motor Cranial Autonomic
Carmustine (BCNU)	Cranial Automatic	Hexamethylmelamine	Sensory Motor	Vindesine	Sensory Motor Cranial Autonomic
Cisplatin	Sensory Motor Cranial	Methotrexate	Sensory Motor Cranial	Vinorelbine	Sensory Motor Cranial Autonomic (mild)
Cytarabine (Ara-C)	Sensory Motor Cranial	Paclitaxel	Sensory Motor Autonomic (mild)		
Docetaxel	Sensory Motor Autonomic (mild)	Procarbazine	Sensory Motor		
Doxifluridine (5-dFUrd)	Sensory Motor	Teniposide (VM-26)	Sensory Motor		

TABLE 43.2	Assessment of Neuropathy
Function	**Procedure**
Cerebellar and proprioception	• Evaluate rapid alternating movement of hands. • Observe for accurate movement of extremities. • Evaluate balance using Romberg test: have patient stand with feet together, arms at side with eyes closed. A slight sway is normal. • Observe gait for stride and stance.
Sensory function	• Test for response to touch and pain. • Check vibration sense using a tuning fork. • Evaluate position sense: move a finger or great toe up and down while patient's eyes are closed; have patient identify the position of the digit. • Assess for discrimination between sharp and dull sensations. • Evaluate the ability to distinguish the body part being touched. • Evaluate for stereognosis, the ability to distinguish a common object, such as a coin. • Evaluate for graphesthesia, the ability to identify a common letter or number drawn on the hand.
Deep tendon reflexes	• Test deep tendon reflexes (biceps, brachioradial, triceps, patellar, and Achilles). • Check for clonus.

From Waitman, K. (2020). Chemotherapy agents associated with peripheral neuropathy. *Core Curriculum for Oncology Nursing E-Book* (p. 387), Oncology Nursing Society; Knoerl, R. (2021). CE: Chemotherapy-induced peripheral neuropathy. *AJN: The American Journal of Nursing*, 121(4), 26–30.

MANAGEMENT

I. Pharmacologic management (Kanzawa-Lee, 2020; Knoerl, 2021; Loprinzi et al., 2020)
   A. Mild analgesics—acetaminophen (Tylenol) and nonsteroidal antiinflammatory drugs for painful neuropathies
   B. Antidepressants
      a. Duloxetine (Cymbalta) for patients who have peripheral neuropathies from neurotoxic chemotherapy
   C. Anticonvulsants (e.g., gabapentin [Neurontin], pregabalin [Lyrica], and valproic acid [Depakote]) to alleviate painful peripheral neuropathies (should not be offered for the prevention of chemotherapy induced peripheral neuropathy (CIPN) to patients with cancer undergoing treatment with neurotoxic agents)
   D. Lack of data exists to routinely offer patients the following agents for the prevention of CIPN:

a. Acetyl-L-carnitine
b. All-trans-retinoic acid
c. Amifostine
d. Amitriptyline
e. Calcium magnesium
f. Calmangafodipir
g. Cannabinoids
h. Carbamazepine
i. Diethyldithiocarbamate
j. Gabapentin/pregabalin
k. Glutamate
l. Glutathione (GSH) for patients receiving paclitaxel/carboplatin chemotherapy
m. Goshajinkigan
n. Metformin
o. Minocycline
p. *N*-Acetylcysteine
q. Nimodipine
r. Omega-3 fatty acids
s. Org 2766
t. Oxcarbazepine
u. Recombinant human leukemia inhibitory factor
v. Venlafaxine
w. Vitamin B
x. Vitamin E
E. Opioids
F. Lidocaine 5% patch
G. Glutamine
H. Use of creams (e.g., application of capsaicin cream three or four times daily)

II. Nonpharmacologic management
A. Assess the knowledge of early signs and symptoms of neuropathies.
B. Teach about the side effects of chemotherapy.
C. Teach about hand and foot care (use of massage and lotions).
D. Refer to occupational and rehabilitation services.
E. Before chemotherapy, instruct patient about potential neurologic side effects.
F. Instruct patient on how to maintain a safe environment both at home and at work.
G. Give positive feedback and honest reassurance.
H. Empower patient to communicate with physician and nurse about symptoms.
I. Have patient protect hands and feet from cold through the use of gloves and socks.
J. Have patient avoid excess stimulation of skin and avoid tight clothing.
K. Have patient wear gloves for gardening activities.
L. Teach about the inspection of affected areas for burns, cuts, abrasions.
M. Collaborate with physical and occupational rehabilitation services.
N. Develop an exercise and muscle-strengthening program.
O. Use assistive devices to assist with mobilization and fine motor needs.
P. Assist in the performance of ADLs as needed.
Q. Encourage exercise.
R. Consider transcutaneous electrical nerve stimulation.
S. Offer acupuncture and acupressure.
T. Encourage relaxation techniques—yoga, meditation, and guided imagery.
U. Refer for biofeedback.
V. Encourage art and music therapy.

REFERENCES

Briani, C., Cocito, D., Campagnolo, M., Doneddu, P. E., & Nobile-Orazio, E. (2022). Update on therapy of chronic immune-mediated neuropathies. *Neurological Sciences, 43*(Suppl. 2), 605–614. https://doi.org/10.1007/s10072-020-04998-y.

Desforges, A. D., Hebert, C. M., Spence, A. L., Reid, B., Dhaibar, H. A., Cruz-Topete, D., et al. (2022). Treatment and diagnosis of chemotherapy-induced peripheral neuropathy: An update. *Biomedicine & Pharmacotherapy, 147*, 112671. https://doi.org/10.1016/j.biopha.2022.112671.

Kanzawa-Lee, G. (2020). Chemotherapy-induced peripheral neuropathy: Nursing implications. *Journal of Infusion Nursing, 43*(3), 155–166. https://doi.org/10.1097/NAN.0000000000000368.

Knoerl, R. (2021). CE: Chemotherapy-induced peripheral neuropathy. *AJN: The American Journal of Nursing, 121*(4), 26–30. https://doi.org/10.1097/01.NAJ.0000742060.56042.e7.

Laforgia, M., Laface, C., Calabrò, C., Ferraiuolo, S., Ungaro, V., Tricarico, D., et al. (2021). Peripheral neuropathy under oncologic therapies: A literature review on pathogenetic mechanisms. *International Journal of Molecular Sciences, 22*(4), 1980. https://doi.org/10.3390/ijms22041980.

Li, T., Mizrahi, D., Goldstein, D., Kiernan, M. C., & Park, S. B. (2021a). Chemotherapy and peripheral neuropathy. *Neurological Sciences, 42*(10), 4109–4121. https://doi.org/10.1007/s10072-021-05576-6.

Li, Y., Zhang, X., & Zhao, C. (2021b). Guillain-Barré syndrome-like polyneuropathy associated with immune checkpoint inhibitors: A systematic review of 33 cases. *BioMed Research International, 2021*. Article ID 9800488. https://doi.org/10.1155/2021/9800488.

Loprinzi, C. L., Lacchetti, C., Bleeker, J., Cavaletti, G., Chauhan, C., Hertz, D. L., et al. (2020). Prevention and management of chemotherapy-induced peripheral neuropathy in survivors of adult cancers: ASCO guideline update. *Journal of Clinical Oncology, 38*(28), 3325–3348. https://doi.org/10.1200/JCO.20.01399.

Omran, M., Belcher, E. K., Mohile, N. A., Kesler, S. R., Janelsins, M. C., Hohmann, A. G., et al. (2021). Review of the role of the brain in chemotherapy-induced peripheral neuropathy. *Frontiers in Molecular Biosciences, 8*, 693133. https://doi.org/10.3389/fmolb.2021.693133.

Patel, V., & Shah, J. (2021). The current and future aspects of glioblastoma: Immunotherapy a new hope? *European Journal of Neuroscience, 54*(3), 5120–5142. https://doi.org/10.1111/ejn.15343.

Pisciotta, C., Saveri, P., & Pareyson, D. (2021). Challenges in treating Charcot-Marie-Tooth disease and related neuropathies: Current management and future perspectives. *Brain Sciences, 11*(11), 1447. https://doi.org/10.3390/brainsci11111447.

44

Nutritional Issues

Diane G. Cope

WEIGHT CHANGES AND BODY COMPOSITION

Overview

I. Definition (Deluche et al., 2018)
   A. Overnutrition or undernutrition (weight gain, weight loss, and changes in body composition) associated with cancer and cancer treatments, which may negatively affect cancer recurrence, survival, morbidity, and quality of life (QOL).
   B. Body composition is the relative proportions of protein, fat, water, and mineral components in the body.
II. Risk factors for weight gain (Anderson et al., 2021)
   A. Treatment related
      1. Multiagent chemotherapy regimens, regimens containing steroids, or both
      2. Effusions—pleural, pericardial, and abdominal
      3. Edema
      4. Obstruction
      5. Inactivity
      6. Electrolyte imbalances
      7. Hormonal drugs, steroids, and biological medications such as interleukin-2
      8. Metabolic complications
      9. Adjuvant chemotherapy for breast cancer
   B. Risk factors for weight loss (Cunningham, 2018; Gannavarapu et al., 2018; Muscaritoli et al., 2021)
   C. Disease related
      1. Increased risk with non-Hodgkin lymphoma, lung, nasopharyngeal, and gastrointestinal (GI) cancers
      2. Protein-calorie malnutrition caused by the metabolic effects of the tumor
      3. Tumor location—increased weight loss associated with upper respiratory and gastric tumors
      4. Alterations in ability to eat
      5. Disrupted absorption of nutrients
   D. Treatment related
      1. Surgery related
         a. Increased risk with head and neck, esophageal, gastric, pancreatic, or colorectal cancer surgeries
         b. Postprandial dumping syndrome associated with gastric resections
         c. Frequent tests usually needed in surgical oncology patients; may limit intake, require dietary restrictions, or both

         d. Increased calories expended, energy needs increased during perioperative period
      2. Radiation therapy (RT)
         a. Radiation field related with head and neck, lung, and GI cancers
         b. Increased risk for anorexia, diarrhea, nausea, vomiting, mucositis, esophagitis, gastritis, xerostomia, and taste changes
      3. Chemotherapy
         a. Nausea and vomiting with the prevalence of nausea estimated at 40% (Gupta, Walton, & Kataria, 2021)
         b. Indirect effects causing anorexia, fatigue, constipation, taste changes, anxiety, and depression
   E. Multifactorial
      1. Insensible losses (e.g., perspiration, gastric suction, surgical drains, fistulas, and wounds)
      2. Acute or chronic diarrhea caused by drugs (e.g., antibiotics, chemotherapy, and immunotherapy), dietary alterations, infectious processes (e.g., *Clostridium difficile*), intestinal ischemia, fecal impaction, irritable bowel disease, laxative abuse, endocrine disorders, malabsorption, surgery, and radiation colitis
      3. Post–stem cell transplantation acute and chronic graft-versus-host disease
      4. Presence of concurrent symptoms related to cancer treatment, including anorexia, taste alterations, mucositis, pain, anxiety, depression, and fatigue
      5. Medication side effects, including antibiotics, opioids, biological, and targeted therapies

Assessment

(Cunningham, 2018; Reber, Schönenberger, Vasiloglou, & Stanga, 2021)
   I. History
      A. Previous dietary patterns, food preferences, cultural preferences, food allergies, eating habits, and history of weight changes
      B. Patterns of weight changes: type, onset, duration, and severity; early satiety; associated symptoms—nausea, food intolerances, taste abnormalities, mouth/throat pain, dysphagia, vomiting, and diarrhea; other factors—precipitating, aggravating, and alleviating factors

C. Current or recent treatment for cancer and experienced side effects

D. Assessment of patient for associated cultural, socioeconomic, emotional, and motivational factors that may affect weight loss or gain

E. Ability to carry out interventions to maintain weight

F. Use of food, nutritional supplements, and other remedies

II. Physical examination

A. Determine present weight, height, and amount of total weight loss or gain.

B. Assess for dehydration, electrolyte imbalances, serum albumin.

C. Assess mobility, skin tone and turgor, muscle strength.

D. Evaluation and reassessment of nutritional status

1. Assess/screen each patient for changes in nutritional status at each contact (on admission to the hospital and at regular follow-up intervals, during each home visit, or at outpatient clinic visits).

Management

(Compher et al., 2022; Cunningham, 2018)

I. Pharmacologic management

A. Administer pain medications, if needed, 30–60 minutes before meals.

II. Nonpharmacologic management

A. Teach patient and caregiver to do the following:

1. Take oral supplements to increase protein-calorie intake between meals and bedtime.

2. Limit liquids at mealtime because they may cause early satiety and nausea.

3. Discuss taste changes, review liquids and foods that patient may be able to tolerate.

4. Consume nutritionally dense/high-protein foods such as cottage cheese, puddings, and oatmeal.

5. Eat frequent, small portions throughout the day.

6. Maximize food intake during periods of greatest strength and appetite, usually early in the day.

7. Increase kilocalorie (kcal) protein content of foods by adding protein powders, instant nonfat dry milk powder/instant breakfast powders to gravies, puddings, and other foods.

8. Maximize food preferences and access to favorite foods within dietary restrictions.

9. Choose high-protein, high-calorie, and healthy snacks between meals.

10. Try cold, room-temperature, and soft foods to improve intake.

11. Perform oral hygiene before and after meals.

12. Assist patient/caregiver with calculating individualized calorie and protein requirements so realistic goals can be set for weight changes; may need to consult with a nutritionist.

13. Use proper quantities of foods from the food groups that provide a balanced, nutritious diet for weight control.

14. Have the patient engage in regular exercise, if able.

15. Encourage consultation with a dietitian.

TASTE ALTERATIONS

Overview

(Cunningham, 2018; Kaizu et al., 2021)

I. Definition—actual or perceived change in taste sensation or loss of taste

A. Hypogeusesthesia—a decrease in the acuity of the taste sensation

B. Dysgeusia—an unusual taste perception, perceived as unpleasant

C. Ageusia—an absence of the taste sensation, "mouth blindness"

II. Physiology

A. Taste is a chemical sense that is mediated through specialized epithelial cells located in the oral cavity, oropharynx, larynx, and upper third of esophagus.

B. Receptor sites in taste buds on the tongue are innervated by cranial nerves, which send taste information about sweet, sour, salty, and bitter sensations to the medulla and cortex.

C. Taste and smell are integrated functions.

1. Air entering the nostrils ascends to the olfactory cleft, connects with olfactory receptors.

2. During chewing and swallowing, air is pushed from the mouth into the nose, stimulating the olfactory receptor, carrying the signal via cranial nerve I to the cortex and subcortex II.

D. Pathophysiology (Asif, Moore, Yarom, & Popovtzer, 2020; Cunningham, 2018; Hoppe, Kutschan, Dorfler, Buntzel, & Huebner, 2021; Spencer et al., 2021). Cell damage

1. Decrease in the number of normal cell receptors

2. Alteration of cell structure or receptor surface changes

3. Interruption of neural coding

E. Rapidly proliferating cancer cells release a number of cytokines/chemokines, initiating the recruitment of macrophages and neutrophils and an inflammatory state, which may modulate areas of the brain involved in the control of taste and smell perception.

F. Alteration in carbohydrate metabolism and taste perception may be a common mechanism between type 2 diabetes and cancer.

G. Excretion of amino acid–like substances from the tumor cells changes taste-bud sensations (sweet, sour, bitter, and salty).

H. Zinc deficiency caused by oncolytic agents, which bind and chelate zinc, result in loss of taste.

I. Invasion of tumor into the oral cavity or salivary glands

J. Oral infections such as candidiasis

K. Treatment related

1. RT: changes in salivation production and consistency may precede mucositis or xerostomia (Asif et al., 2020). Destruction of the taste buds occurs by

3–4 weeks, commonly affecting all taste modalities, and return to baseline 6–12 months after treatment, or never return to normal.

    2. Saliva may become thick or tenacious early, and membranes may become dry at about days 10–14 during radiation treatment; condition may continue for 2–4 months after completion of RT; beverages or foods that are slightly tart or carbonated may help thin secretions.

  L. Surgical interventions: specific surgical sites—oral cavity, tongue, salivary glands, pathway of the olfactory nerve, and tracheostomy

  M. Chemotherapy (Kaizu et al., 2021)

    1. Certain drugs have a greater effect on taste sensation than others—for example, cisplatin (Platinol), irinotecan (Camptosar), cyclophosphamide (Cytoxan), dacarbazine (DTIC-Dome), dactinomycin (actinomycin D, Cosmegen), mechlorethamine (nitrogen mustard, Mustargen), methotrexate (Mexate), taxanes, vincristine (Oncovin), and fluorouracil (5-fluorouracil)

III. Risk factors

  A. Poor oral hygiene

  B. Nutritional deficiencies—zinc, copper, nickel, niacin, and vitamins A and C

  C. Age-induced degeneration of the taste buds

  D. Learned aversions

    1. Taste changes that develop when a food is associated with unpleasant symptoms such as nausea, vomiting, and pain

    2. Seem to develop most rapidly to new or novel foods

Assessment

I. History

  A. Presence of hypogeusesthesia, ageusia, or dysgeusia

  B. History of risk factors, including degree and duration of taste alterations

  C. Subjective description of changes in taste and impact of taste alterations on nutritional status and usual lifestyle patterns

  D. Constant or intermittent metallic and bitter taste; increased or decreased threshold for the sweetness sensation; increased threshold for salty and sour tastes; decreased threshold for bitter taste; and aversion to meats, coffee, and chocolate

II. Physical examination

  A. Oral assessment

  B. Weight

  C. Presence of other physical problems associated with altered intake

    1. Evaluate the oral cavity and throat for the presence of erythema, desquamation, dryness or excess saliva, and ulceration.

    2. Assess for signs and symptoms of secondary oral infection.

III. Laboratory findings associated with compromised nutritional status

  A. Decreased levels of albumin, transferrin, and total lymphocytes

  B. Decreased levels of zinc, copper, and nickel

  C. Decreased levels of niacin and vitamin A

Management

(Cunningham, 2018; Spencer et al., 2021)

I. Nonpharmacologic management

  A. Institute measures to increase the sensitivity of taste buds, decrease food aversion, increase salivation, and compensate for oral dryness.

    1. Experiment with spices and flavorings to enhance taste.

    2. Use the aroma of foods to stimulate taste.

    3. Increase fluid intake with meals.

    4. Encourage oral hygiene before and after meals.

    5. Add sweeteners to foods and marinate meats in sweet juices.

    6. Substitute other sources of protein for poorly tolerated protein sources such as meats.

    7. Have patient avoid the sight and smell of unpleasant foods.

    8. Have patient consume candies such as lemon drops or chew gum to change taste before meals and before chemotherapy treatment to reduce metallic taste and stimulate saliva.

    9. Increase water or juices at frequent intervals—for example, several times per hour.

    10. Spray water, saline, or artificial saliva on the mucous membranes.

    11. Have patient suck on smooth, flat, and tart candies or lozenges to stimulate saliva.

    12. Have patient avoid alcohol, commercial mouthwashes, and smoking.

    13. Humidify environmental air.

    14. Offer foods that are moist or have gravy or sauces and discourage the intake of dry foods such as toast or crackers.

    15. Weigh patient at regular intervals.

    16. Maintain a daily diet record.

    17. Teach patients the importance of diligent oral care and inspection, and ensure that they are aware of conditions for which they should contact the health care team.

    18. Include caregiver in care.

ANOREXIA

Overview

(Cunningham, 2018; Hariyanto & Kurniawan, 2021; Ravasco, 2019)

I. Definition—loss of appetite accompanied by decreased oral intake; usually accompanied by other symptoms that exacerbate decreased food intake and progressive weight loss, with approximately 80% incidence in patients with cancer from diagnosis to advanced stages

II. Sequelae of anorexia (Berry et al., 2018)
   A. Decreased calorie and protein intake with subsequent loss of fat and muscle mass, weight loss, weakness, and fatigue
      1. May lead to cachexia, which may affect prognosis by making patient less tolerant of therapy, causing dose or schedule changes that may diminish treatment effectiveness
   B. Abnormalities of carbohydrate, protein, and fat metabolism
   C. Visceral and lean body mass depletion—muscle atrophy, visceral organ atrophy, hypoalbuminemia, and anemia
   D. Compromised humoral and cellular immune function—impaired neutrophil function (chemotaxis, fungicidal, and bactericidal) and delayed bone marrow production
      1. Protein-calorie malnutrition interferes with the delivery of oncologic therapy and increases the severity of side effects of treatment

III. Physiology
   A. Food intake is regulated by long- and short-term mediators involved in the transmission of signals between neurotransmitters in the peripheral and central nervous systems
      1. Short-acting mediators in gut are responsible for satiety signals and maintenance of food intake based on energy expenditure and maintenance of body weight.
         a. Increased food intake and reduction of fat utilization stimulated by ghrelin, a gut hormone.
      2. Long-acting mediators consist of insulin and leptin.
         a. Insulin regulates nutrient storage and energy balance.
         b. Leptin regulates adipose energy reserves, with low leptin levels increasing hypothalamic signals that stimulate feeding, decrease appetite-suppressing signals.

IV. Pathophysiology (Hariyanto & Kurniawan, 2021)
   A. Multifactorial
   B. Tumor-related peripheral or central effects
      1. Peripheral
         a. Substances released by the tumor such as proinflammatory cytokines, lactate, and parathormone-related peptide
         b. Tumors causing dysphagia or altering gut function
         c. Tumors altering nutrients such as zinc deficiency
         d. Tumors causing hypoxia
         e. Increased peripheral tryptophan leading to increased central serotonin
         f. Alterations in the release of peripheral hormones that alter feeding such as peptide tyrosine and ghrelin
      2. Central
         a. Tumors causing alterations in neurotransmitters, neuropeptides, and prostaglandins that modulate feeding
      3. Psychological factors
         a. Anxiety, depression, fear, or distress
      4. Social factors
         a. Loss of pleasure previously associated with food
         b. Changes in eating environment
         c. Changes in companionship during eating
      5. Physiologic factors
         a. Presence of concurrent symptoms, including nausea or vomiting, early satiety, diarrhea, constipation, pain, dysphagia, mucositis, ascites, and taste/smell alterations
         b. Metabolic disturbances: hypercalcemia, hypokalemia, uremia, and hyponatremia
         c. Medication side effects associated with opioids, antibiotics, and iron
         d. Treatment-related effects from chemotherapy, RT, surgery, and biotherapy

V. Risk factors (Cunningham, 2018)
   A. Advanced cancer
   B. Pulmonary and cardiac comorbidities
   C. Older age
   D. Multimodal treatment
   E. Solid tumors, especially lung and GI cancers

Assessment

I. History
   A. Previous dietary patterns, food preferences, eating habits, bowel patterns, and history of anorexia with patient and family
   B. Patterns of anorexia—onset, frequency, and severity; associated symptoms—food intolerances, early satiety, nausea, taste abnormalities, mouth or throat pain, and dysphagia; other factors—precipitating, aggravating, and alleviating factors
   C. Previous self-care strategies
   D. Current or recent treatment for cancer and side effects
      1. Ability to implement interventions to relieve anorexia
      2. Use of food and nutritional supplements
      3. Use of alternative or complementary nutritional products

II. Physical examination
   A. Determine present weight and amount of total weight loss
   B. Assess for dehydration, electrolyte imbalances, or both—dry mouth, poor skin turgor, decreased urinary output
   C. Assess for associated ethnic, socioeconomic, emotional, and motivational factors that may affect the loss of weight or decreased oral intake
   D. Assess psychosocial responses to fear, anxiety, stress, depression, and noxious stimuli in the environment

Management

(Cunningham, 2018)

I. Pharmacologic management
   A. Use of medications as ordered by licensed provider—pain medications, vitamin supplements, and medications that may stimulate appetite (e.g., corticosteroids or megestrol acetate [Megace])

II. Nonpharmacologic management
   A. Maintain a daily dietary intake record.
   B. Weigh regularly.
   C. Assess for signs and symptoms of electrolyte imbalances and dehydration.
   D. Assess for overall skin and nail condition for adverse effects of poor nutrition or intake—skin breakdown, dehiscence, or poor wound healing.
   E. Encourage caregiver to provide foods within dietary restrictions; explore the necessity of dietary restrictions when nutritional requirements not being met as a result of restrictions.
   F. Teach caregiver methods to enhance protein-calorie content of foods and methods to enhance food intake.
   G. Teach patient and caregiver about the signs and symptoms of dehydration (dry skin and mucous membranes, poor skin turgor, and decreased urinary output), delayed wound healing, and malnutrition (wasting of skeletal mass, body fat decrease, weight loss, sepsis, and reduced energy), and when to report critical symptoms to the treatment team.
   H. Develop strategies with patient and caregiver to increase protein-calorie intake each day.
      1. Provide a list of high-calorie, high-protein foods.
      2. Offer suggestions for supplementing nutritional value by adding protein or milk powders and supplements.
      3. Plan mealtimes that are relaxed, unhurried, and pleasant.
      4. Encourage a positive eating environment by setting table attractively, listening to music, and avoiding eating from cartons or cans.
      5. Use a variety of foods to avoid taste fatigue.
      6. Avoid fixating on intake to the point that it may become counterproductive.
   I. Provide written/audiovisual materials on nutrition at patient's level of understanding.
   J. Initiate early referral to a dietitian for nutritional assessment or intervention.

CACHEXIA

Overview

I. Definition (Berry et al., 2018; Cunningham, 2018; Ni & Zhang, 2020; Roeland et al., 2020).
   A. Progressive deterioration with muscle wasting that occurs when protein and calorie requirements are not met
   B. Greater than 5% involuntary weight loss over 6 months or a body mass index (BMI) of less than 20 and any degree of weight loss more than 2%, or an appendicular skeletal muscle index with sarcopenia and any degree of weight loss more than 2% (Meza-Valderrama et al., 2021)
   C. Characterized by anorexia, weight loss, skeletal muscle atrophy, and asthenia
   D. Often occurs with anorexia, which constitutes a clinical syndrome known as the cancer anorexia–cachexia syndrome
   E. Associated with poor QOL, impaired functional status, muscle wasting, inflammation, fatigue, and ultimately shortened survival

II. Sequalae of cachexia
   A. Increased morbidity and mortality present in 80% with advanced cancer
   B. Decreased tissue sensitivity to insulin and decreased insulin response to glucose
   C. Impairment of immunocompetence—humoral, cellular, secretory, and mucosal immunity
   D. Poor wound healing and increased infection rates
   E. Protein-calorie malnutrition with resultant weight loss; visceral and somatic protein depletion that compromises enzymatic, structural, and mechanical functions
   F. Constipation caused by lack of food and fluid intake and the effects of cancer treatments

III. Pathophysiology (da Silva, Santos, Costa e Silva, Gil da Costa, & Medeiros, 2020)
   A. Complex process involving anorexia, metabolic alterations, release of cytokines, and other catabolic factors that lead to skeletal muscle wasting
   B. Mediated by proinflammatory cytokines, including tumor necrosis factor, IL-1, IL-6, interferon (IFN)-alpha, and IFN-beta, which may be produced by the tumor itself or by the immune system in response to the tumor
   C. Metabolic alterations—include decreased gluconeogenesis; alterations in glucose metabolism; increased metabolic rate; changed lipid, protein, and carbohydrate metabolism

IV. Risk factors
   A. Disease related—cancer, especially lung and pancreatic cancers and gastric carcinomas, AIDS, infections, sepsis, and inflammatory diseases
   B. Treatment related—chemotherapy; biotherapy; RT; surgery of the head, neck, stomach, pancreas, and bowel
   C. Situation related
      1. Psychological aspects of nutritional intake—cancer cachexia viewed by some to be the hallmark of terminal illness, thus, patients frequently "give up."
      2. Depression, inactivity, absence of an appetite, and functional losses affect the patient's QOL.

Assessment (Miller et al., 2018)

I. History
   A. Previous dietary patterns, food preferences, eating habits, type and quantity of food consumed, and history of anorexia discussed with patient and family
   B. Patterns of anorexia and presence of fatigue and malaise—assessment for onset, frequency, and severity; associated symptoms—food intolerances, taste abnormalities, pain, and dysphagia; other factors—precipitating, aggravating, and alleviating factors

C. Previous self-care strategies—ability to provide for own interventions to relieve anorexia; use of food, nutritional supplements, and other remedies

D. Current or recent treatment for cancer and side effects experienced

E. Associated cultural, socioeconomic, emotional, and motivational factors that may affect the loss of weight

II. Physical examination

A. Determine present weight and amount of total and recent weight loss.

B. Assess for dehydration, electrolyte imbalances, or both.

C. Assess for muscle atrophy, loss of fat deposits, and presence of edema.

D. Anthropometric measurements or consultation with a nutritionist

E. Review of biochemical measurements

1. Triceps skinfolds and midarm muscle circumference

2. Height and weight (weight loss >5% in previous 6 months significant for the diagnosis of protein-calorie malnutrition)

3. Visceral protein stores—serum albumin, prealbumin, total iron-binding capacity, transferrin, electrolytes, nitrogen balance, C-reactive protein, and urine

4. Lean body mass—computed tomography or dual-energy x-ray absorptiometry

5. Degree of anemia

6. Deficiencies in trace metals and vitamins and glucose intolerance

Management

I. Pharmacologic management

A. Treat underlying disease

B. Megestrol acetate (Megace)—has a dose–response effect

C. Medroxyprogesterone—increases appetite

D. Corticosteroids—dexamethasone (Decadron), methylprednisolone (Medrol), and prednisolone (Prednisone) are effective in improving the appetite

E. Metoclopramide (Reglan)—at low doses may stimulate GI motility and decrease early satiety and nausea

F. Metabolic inhibitors—to induce anabolism

G. Other drugs currently being studied with uncertain efficacy—testosterone, nandrolone decanoate, and oxandrolone

H. Enteral feedings—oral or tube feedings will help maintain normal GI flora and prevent atrophy of GI mucosa

I. Total parenteral nutrition to replace nutritional deficiencies during cancer treatment and according to patient goals

II. Nonpharmacologic management

A. Nursing and nutritional support

1. Five or six small meals per day

2. High-protein snacks

3. High-calorie, low-fat snacks

4. Liquids that have calories, such as nutritional shakes, smoothies, or supplements

5. Activities to increase appetite—for example, light exercise

NUTRITION SUPPORT THERAPY

Overview

(Compher et al., 2022; Cotogni, Stragliotto, Ossola, Collo, & Riso, 2021; Cunningham, 2018; Muscaritoli, Arends, & Aapro, 2019; Muscaritoli et al., 2021)

I. Definition: therapy focusing on nutritional supportive approaches that include screening, assessment, and supplemental enteral or parenteral nutritional support

II. Indications

A. Patients who are actively receiving anticancer treatment, are malnourished, and are expected to be unable to ingest and absorb nutrients for a prolonged interval

B. Multifactorial from treatment, tumor, and/or fluid and electrolyte disturbances

1. Treatment

a. Less able to tolerate therapy and receive optimal benefits from treatment

b. More susceptible to infection, debilitation, poor wound healing, skin breakdown, weakness, fatigue, depression, and apathy; poor nutrition affects QOL

c. Metabolic changes may occur as a result of treatment or side effects of treatment such as increased energy demands that result from fever, stress, diarrhea, vomiting, and cell division or destruction.

(1) Inability to feed oneself

(2) Inability to masticate or swallow

(3) Inability to move food through the stomach and bowel

(4) Bowel diversion

(5) Nausea and vomiting

(6) Malabsorption of fat

(7) Gastric hypersecretion of acid

(8) Water and electrolyte loss

(9) Dumping syndrome and changes in gastric motility

(10) Xerostomia

(11) Mucositis

(12) Constipation

(13) Changes in taste and smell

2. Tumor

a. Cancer cells compete with normal cells for nutrients needed for cellular division and growth.

b. Exact demands of the tumor on the host are unknown; the following metabolic changes are proposed:

(1) Cancer cells produce biochemical substances that affect the desire for food, altering taste, causing anorexia (by central mechanisms or neurotransmitters).

(2) Malignant tumors may invade/compress structures and organs vital to the ingestion, digestion, and elimination of food and fluids, or may increase metabolic demands.

(3) Altered carbohydrate metabolism—glucose is mobilized for energy and results in glucose intolerance in selected patients

(4) Altered protein metabolism—muscle tissue mobilized to meet increased metabolic demands and results in muscle wasting, especially in those patients with cachexia, a severe syndrome of malnutrition

3. Fluid and electrolyte disturbances

a. Anaerobic glycolysis—produces two adenosine triphosphate (ATP) molecules where complete oxidation of glucose yields 36 ATP molecules; thus, anaerobic glycolysis used by tumors is less efficient

b. Increased rate of gluconeogenesis—estimated 10% increase in energy expenditure for an individual with cancer

c. Glucose intolerance—evidenced by a delayed clearing of intravenous (IV) or oral glucose, which could be caused by lack of tissue response to insulin or a defect of insulin response to hyperglycemia

d. Prealbumin and serum albumin levels often used to measure protein status

e. Hypoalbuminemia common in patients with cancer—normal albumin level = 4 g/dL; average albumin level in patient with cancer = 2.9 g/dL

f. Increased uptake of amino acids by tumor

g. Hypercalcemia—high calcium levels in blood caused by certain tumors

h. Hyperuricemia—along with hyperphosphatemia and hyperkalemia, result of chemotherapy breakdown of cells in some leukemias and lymphomas leading to tumor lysis syndrome

i. Hyponatremia—common presentation with bronchogenic and small cell carcinoma causing syndrome of inappropriate antidiuretic hormone secretion and causing persistent loss of sodium and excessive retention of water by the kidneys (see Chapter 39)

j. Hypokalemia may be caused by chemotherapy or antifungal therapy.

k. Decreased protein synthesis

l. Increased protein degradation; muscle protein breakdown is accelerated

m. Protein loss by abnormal leakage or exertion, leading to depletion of protein stores and decreased muscle mass

n. Use of protein for energy needs

(1) Protein wasted despite intake of protein

(2) Weight loss that is often difficult to counteract, despite aggressive feeding

(3) Decrease in food intake, with partial starvation caused by conserving lean body mass, host depleting own muscle mass to provide amino acids needed

(4) Loss of appetite, alteration in taste and smell, loss of appealing foods

(5) Weakness, reduction of strength, and decreased functional capacity

C. Nutrition support therapy should not be used routinely in patients undergoing major cancer operations.

1. Perioperative nutrition support therapy may be beneficial in moderately or severely malnourished patients if administered for 7–14 days preoperatively, but the potential benefits of nutrition support must be weighed against the potential risks of the nutrition support therapy itself and of delaying the operation.

2. Immune-enhancing enteral formulas containing mixtures of arginine, nucleic acids, and essential fatty acids may be beneficial in malnourished patients undergoing major cancer operations.

D. Nutrition support therapy should not be used routinely as an adjunct to chemotherapy.

E. Nutrition support therapy should not be used routinely in patients undergoing head and neck, abdominal, or pelvic irradiation.

F. Nutrition support therapy is appropriate in patients receiving active anticancer treatment who are malnourished and who are anticipated to be unable to ingest and/or absorb adequate nutrients for a prolonged period.

G. The palliative use of nutrition support therapy in terminally ill cancer patients is rarely indicated.

H. Omega-3 fatty acid supplementation may help stabilize weight in cancer patients on oral diets experiencing progressive, unintentional weight loss.

I. Patients should not use therapeutic diets to treat cancer.

Assessment

I. Nutritional workup (Compher et al., 2022)

A. Nutritional screening—should be performed before therapy and at intervals during therapy

B. Nutrition history and dietary habits

C. Anthropometric measurements—height, weight, midarm circumference, skinfold thickness, calculation of ideal body weight, and BMI

D. Biochemical measurements of protein status—serum albumin, transferrin, prealbumin; assessing long-term, intermediate-term, and short-term protein status

1. Nutritional assessment—includes an evaluation of the desire and ability of the patient to ingest and process nutritional products

2. Ingestion, digestion, metabolism, and excretion

3. Desire to eat

4. Patterns of dietary intake, ability of patient to prepare food and feed self

5. Food allergies and preferences

6. Dentition

7. Ability of patient to moisten, chew, and swallow nutrients

8. Ability to digest food in stomach and small intestine

9. Ability to move stomach contents through bowel

10. Presence of abnormal carbohydrate, fat, or protein metabolism
11. Presence of vitamin and mineral deficiencies
12. Fecal and urinary elimination patterns, characteristics of urine and stool

II. Nutritional assessment, including evaluation of the effects of dietary intake on the patient
   A. Physical assessment (Compher et al., 2022)
      1. Skin turgor
      2. Weight in comparison with ideal body weight
      3. Muscle mass as measured by the midarm circumference
      4. Fat stores as measured by triceps skinfold thickness
   B. Laboratory data
      1. Serum prealbumin, total protein, and serum transferrin to assess protein stores
      2. Nitrogen balance to assess energy balance
      3. Hemoglobin and hematocrit index
      4. Electrolyte levels

Management

(Compher et al., 2022; Cotogni et al., 2021)

I. Pharmacologic management
   A. Controversies exist in nutritional support therapy for long-term management in patients with cancer.
   B. Nourishing a patient with cancer may enhance tumor growth by improving its nutrient supply.

C. Beneficial effects of nutritional support are temporary.
D. Determination of calorie and protein needs
E. Increase in weight, maintaining weight
F. Improving sense of well-being, prolonging life
G. Function of GI tract
H. Severity of nutritional problem
I. Ability of patient to masticate and swallow
J. Length of proposed oncologic therapy and prognosis
K. Community resources for management at home
L. Cost
M. Enteral therapy—provision of nutritional replacement through the GI tract through an entry other than the mouth—for example, gastrostomy (button), jejunostomy, or nasogastric (temporary) feeding tube or combination gastrostomy and jejunostomy tube (Cotogni et al., 2021; Cunningham, 2018; Muscaritoli et al., 2019)
   1. Maintenance of gut and maintenance of gut ability (including acid balance and luminal microflora) are the first line of defense against invaders into gut.
   2. Enteral or parenteral therapy used only if adequate oral intake cannot be maintained.
   3. Indicated if the need for nutritional support anticipated for more than 1 month, oral intake attempts unsuccessful; at least 30 cm of functioning small bowel required
   4. May require percutaneous endoscopic feeding tube placement
   5. Potential complications of enteral tube placement and feedings included in Table 44.1

TABLE 44.1 Potential Complications of Enteral Tube Placement and Feedings

Complication	Nursing Intervention
Nasogastric	
Malpositioned tube	Verify proper placement via chest radiography.
	Check placement each time before using tube.
	Aspirate gastric contents.
	Observe for air bubbles by placing distal end of tube in water.
	Inject air and listen with stethoscope over stomach.
	Tape tube securely to nose.
Aspiration	Give bolus feeding rather than continuous feeding.
	Administer no more than 350–400 mL over 20 min every 3–4 h while patient is awake.
	Administer initial volume of 240 mL.
	Keep the head of the bed elevated by 30 degrees during and 1 h after infusion.
Contaminated equipment, clogged tube	Change feeding bag and tube daily.
	Flush nasogastric tube with 30 mL of water after each feeding.
	If tube is clogged, flush with hot water or pulsating motions.
Abdominal distention, vomiting, cramping, diarrhea	Regulate infusion accurately over 20 min.
	Give formula at room temperature; you may need to decrease volume of formula given. Diarrhea may be caused by formula, lactose intolerance, bacterial contamination, osmolality, antibiotics, or *Clostridium difficile*.
Nasoduodenal	
Aspiration	Risk of occurrence is less because tube is in the small bowel.
	Give continuous rather than bolus feeding.
	Small bowel is sensitive to osmolarity; therefore, administer at an initial rate of 30–50 mL/h for isotonic formula and increase by 25 mL/h every 12 h until desired volume is reached.
Contaminated equipment	Do not allow the amount of formula in bag to exceed that which can be administered in 4 h.
	Change the entire administration set every 24 h and rinse with hot water every 8 h.

6. Selection of appropriate formula essential; different ones may need to be tried
   a. Choice of formula is based on current nutritional requirements, any abnormalities of GI absorption, motility, or diarrhea loss and other coexisting diseases; also considered are laboratory data, amount of protein needed, nitrogen balance and metabolic rate of patient; lactose tolerance or intolerance.
   b. Polymeric formulas contain nitrogen as a whole protein, carbohydrate is partially hydrolyzed starch, and fat contains long-chain triglycerides; most contain fiber.
   c. Predigested formulas contain nitrogen as short peptides, or, if elemental formula, proteins are free amino acids; carbohydrates provide much of the energy content, and both long-chain and medium-chain triglycerides are present.
   d. Disease-specific formulas are as follows:
      (1) Requires the gut to have some degree of digestive and absorptive capacity
      (2) Indicated in presence of significant malabsorption
      (3) Respiratory failure formulas contain a low carbohydrate-to-fat ratio to minimize carbon dioxide production
      (4) Renal failure formulas contain modified protein, electrolytes, and volume

N. Parenteral therapy provides feeding through an IV route when the GI tract cannot be used for nutritional replacement (Cunningham, 2018; Muscaritoli et al., 2019).
   1. Parenteral therapy requires placement of a central venous line or peripherally inserted central catheter line, although peripheral parenteral nutrition can be given with a lower glucose concentration.
   2. Mixture of amino acids, glucose, fluid, vitamins, minerals, electrolytes, and trace elements. Lipid emulsions can be added to increase calories with smaller volume.
   3. Potential complications of parenteral therapy are presented in Table 44.2.

TABLE 44.2 Potential Complications of Parenteral or Nutritional Therapy

Complications	Nursing Intervention
Technical or Mechanical	
Pneumothorax	May occur during subclavian catheter insertion.
	Observe patient during insertion for chest pain, dyspnea, and cyanosis.
	Perform chest radiography after insertion to verify placement.
	Verify blood return before connecting IV tubing to catheter.
	Pneumothorax may occur during insertion.
Arterial puncture	Observe for bright red blood pulsating from catheter.
	Patient may complain of pain at site.
	Apply pressure to site for 15 min; you may need to apply a sandbag after this.
Malpositioned catheter	Monitor the catheter for migration from the superior vena cava to another vein. Note patient's complaint of neck and shoulder pain and swelling in the surrounding area.
	NOTE: If unable to infuse solution through catheter and unable to obtain blood return, treat catheter occlusion according to institutional policy (see Chapter 30).
Clotted catheter	Infuse 10% dextrose in water solution peripherally or through other lumen of catheter at the same rate as with TPN to prevent hypoglycemia.
Fluid overload	Regulate infusion on a volumetric pump for accuracy.
	Place a time tape on infusion, checking volume infused over each hour.
	Obtain daily weights, monitor input/output.
Air emboli	Secure all IV tubing connections with tape to prevent disconnection.
	If air emboli are suspected, clamp tubing immediately and place patient on left side in the Trendelenburg position.
Metabolic	
Hyperglycemia	Increase the rate of infusion gradually.
	Check urine for sugar, ketones, and acetone every 6 h.
	Monitor serum glucose levels daily.
Hypoglycemia	Administer insulin in TPN as ordered.
	Monitor capillary blood glucose as ordered.
	Observe for signs and symptoms of hypoglycemia.
	Monitor serum glucose levels.
	If sudden cessation of TPN occurs, infuse 10% dextrose in water solution peripherally at same rate as TPN.
	Per physician's order, administer 50 mL of 50% dextrose intravenously.

TABLE 44.2 Potential Complications of Parenteral or Nutritional Therapy — cont'd

Complications	Nursing Intervention
Infections	
Contaminated solution	Do not leave unrefrigerated longer than 4 h.
	Check each bottle or bag before and during infusion for color and clarity of solution.
Contaminated equipment	Change all IV tubing per institutional or agency procedure using aseptic technique.
	Avoid interrupting TPN for other infusions or blood collecting.
Local site infection	Change dressing, using aseptic technique and following institutional procedure.
	Observe site: redness, tenderness, swelling, and exudates.
Fever	Monitor vital signs every 4 h.
	Obtain both peripheral and central line blood cultures to identify the source of infection.

IV, Intravenous; *TPN*, total parenteral nutrition.

O. Administration of nutritional therapy according to institutional protocol

P. Examination of nutritional supplement for abnormalities in color

Q. Check expiration date on nutritional supplement.

R. Confirm feeding tube or catheter placement before administering nutritional supplement.

II. Nonpharmacologic management

A. Infection—fever and redness; swelling, pus, pain along feeding tube, catheter tract, or exit site

B. Respiratory complications—chest pain, dyspnea, cough, and cyanosis

C. Fluid overload—weight gain, edema, shortness of breath, and distended neck veins

D. Hyperglycemia—blood glucose monitoring every 6 hours, pattern of urinary elimination

E. GI—character of stool, bloating, pattern of fecal elimination

F. Electrolyte abnormalities—changes in mental status, weakness, fatigue, and changes in neurologic examination (restlessness, agitation)

G. Interventions to decrease the incidence and severity of complications of nutritional support therapy (see Tables 44.1 and 44.2)

H. Teach patient and caregiver procedures needed to manage the feeding tube or catheter.

I. Teach patient/caregiver about signs and symptoms of nutritional support therapy complications.

J. Encourage patient/caregiver participation in decision-making about nutritional therapy.

REFERENCES

Anderson, A. S., Martin, R. M., Renehan, A. G., Cade, J., Copson, E. R., Cross, A. J., et al. (2021). Cancer survivorship, excess body fatness and weight-loss intervention—Where are we in 2020? *British Journal of Cancer, 124*, 1057–1065. https://doi.org/10.1038/s41416-020-01155-2.

Asif, M., Moore, A., Yarom, N., & Popovtzer, A. (2020). The effect of radiotherapy on taste sensation in head and neck cancer patients – A prospective study. *Radiation Oncology, 15*, 144. https://doi.org/10.1186/s13014-020-01578-4.

Berry, D. L., Blonquist, T., Nayak, M. M., Roper, K., Hilton, N., Lombard, H., et al. (2018). Cancer anorexia and cachexia: Screening in an ambulatory infusion service and nutrition consultation. *Clinical Journal of Oncology Nursing, 22*(1), 63–68. https://doi.org/10.1188/18.CJON.63-68.

Compher, C., Bingham, A. L., McCall, M., Patel, J., Rice, T. W., Braunschweig, C., et al. (2022). Guidelines for the provision of nutrition support therapy in the adult critically ill patient: The American Society for Parenteral and Enteral Nutrition. *Journal of Parenteral and Enteral Nutrition, 46*(1), 12–41. https://doi.org/10.1002/jpen.2267.

Cotogni, P., Stragliotto, S., Ossola, M., Collo, A., & Riso, S. (2021). The role of nutritional support for cancer patients in palliative care. *Nutrients, 13*(2), 306. https://doi.org/10.3390/nu13020306.

Cunningham, R. (2018). Nutritional disturbances. In C. H. Yarbro, D. Wujcik, & B. H. Gobel (Eds.), *Cancer nursing: Principles and practice* (8th ed., pp. 941–969). Sudbury, MA: Jones & Bartlett.

da Silva, S. P., Santos, J. M. O., Costa e Silva, M. P., Gil da Costa, R. M., & Medeiros, R. (2020). Cancer cachexia and its pathophysiology: Links with sarcopenia, anorexia and asthenia. *Journal of Cachexia, Sarcopenia and Muscle, 11*(3), 619–635. https://doi.org/10.1002/jcsm.12528.

Deluche, E., Leobon, S., Desport, J. C., Venat-Bouvet, L., Usseglio, J., & Tubiana-Mathieu, N. (2018). Impact of body composition on outcome in patients with early breast cancer. *Supportive Care in Cancer, 26*(3), 861–868. https://doi.org/10.1007/s00520-017-3902-6.

Gannavarapu, B. S., Lau, S. K. M., Carter, K., Cannon, N. A., Gao, A., Ahn, C., et al. (2018). Prevalence and survival impact of pretreatment cancer-associated weight loss: A tool for guiding early palliative care. *Journal of Oncology Practice, 14*(4), e238–e250. https://doi.org/10.1200/JOP.2017.025221.

Gupta, K., Walton, R., & Kataria, S. P. (2021). Chemotherapy-induced nausea and vomiting: Pathogenesis, recommendations, and new trends. *Cancer Treatment and Research Communications, 26*, 100278. https://doi.org/10.1016/j.ctarc.2020.100278.

Kaizu, M., Komatsu, H., Yamauchi, H., Yamauchi, T., Sumitani, M., & Doorenbos, A. Z. (2021). Characteristics of taste alterations in people receiving taxane-based chemotherapy and their association with appetite, weight, and quality of life. *Supportive Care in, 29*, 5103–5114. https://doi.org/10.1007/s00520-021-06066-3.

Hariyanto, T. I., & Kurniawan, A. (2021). Appetite problem in cancer patients: Pathophysiology, diagnosis, and treatment. *Cancer Treatment and Research Communications, 27*, 100336. https://doi.org/10.1016/j.ctarc.2021.100336.

Hoppe, C., Kutschan, S., Dörfler, J., Buntzel, J., & Huebner, J. (2021). Zinc as a complementary treatment for cancer patients: A systematic review. *Clinical and Experimental Medicine, 21,* 297–313. https://doi.org/10.1007/s10238-020-00677-6.

Meza-Valderrama, D., Marco, E., Dávalos-Yerovi, V., Muns, M. D., Tejero-Sánchez, M., Duarte, E., et al. (2021). Sarcopenia, malnutrition, and cachexia: Adapting definitions and terminology of nutritional disorders in older people with cancer. *Nutrients, 13*(3), 761. https://doi.org/10.3390/nu13030761.

Miller, J., Wells, L., Nwulu, U., Currow, D., Johnson, M. J., & Skipworth, R. J. E. (2018). Validated screening tools for the assessment of cachexia, sarcopenia, and malnutrition: A systematic review. *The American Journal of Clinical Nutrition, 108*(6), 1196–1208. https://doi.org/10.1093/ajcn/nqy244.

Muscaritoli, M., Arends, J., & Aapro, M. (2019). From guidelines to clinical practice: A roadmap for oncologists for nutrition therapy for cancer patients. *Therapeutic advances in medical oncology, 11,* 1758835919880084. https://doi.org/10.1177/1758835919880084.

Muscaritoli, M., Arends, J., Bachmann, P., Baracos, V., Barthelemy, N., Bertz, H., et al. (2021). ESPEN practical guideline: Clinical nutrition in cancer. *Clinical Nutrition, 40*(5), 2898–2913. https://doi.org/10.1016/j.clnu.2021.02.005.

Ni, J., & Zhang, L. (2020). Cancer cachexia: Definition, staging, and emerging treatments. *Cancer Management and Research, 12,* 5597–5605. https://doi.org/10.2147/CMAR.S261585.

Ravasco, P. (2019). Nutrition in cancer patients. *Journal of Clinical Medicine, 8*(8), 1211. https://doi.org/10.3390/jcm8081211.

Reber, E., Schönenberger, K. A., Vasiloglou, M. F., & Stanga, Z. (2021). Nutritional risk screening in cancer patients: The first step toward better clinical outcome. *Frontiers in Nutrition, 8,* 603936. https://www.frontiersin.org/article/10.3389/fnut.2021.603936.

Roeland, E. J., Bohlke, K., Baracos, V. E., Bruera, E., del Fabbro, E., Dixon, S., et al. (2020). Management of cancer cachexia: ASCO guideline. *Journal of Clinical Oncology, 38*(21), 2438–2453. https://doi.org/10.1200/JCO.20.00611.

Spencer, A. S., da Silva Dias, D., Capelas, M. L., Pimentel, F., Santos, T., Neves, P. M., et al. (2021). Managing severe dysgeusia and dysosmia in lung cancer patients: A systematic scoping review. *Frontiers in Oncology, 11,* 774081. https://www.frontiersin.org/article/10.3389/fonc.2021.774081.

45

Pain

Jeannine M. Brant and Annette Brant Isozaki

OVERVIEW

I. Definition
  A. A sensory and emotional experience associated with, or resembling that associated with actual or potential tissue damage—the International Association for the Study of Pain defined pain in 1979 and revised this definition in 2020 (Raja et al., 2020). This definition should accompany the list below.
    1. Pain is a personalized experience; physical, psychological, and social factors play a role in pain and are variable.
    2. Pain and nociception (painful stimuli) are different; pain is not simply the result of activity in sensory neurons.
    3. The concept of pain is learned through life experiences.
    4. Individual report of pain should be respected.
    5. Pain has adverse effects on functioning and well-being.
    6. Pain can be expressed verbally or nonverbally; even those who cannot report pain can experience pain.
II. Characteristics of pain (Brant, 2022)
  A. Acute pain—typically lasts less than 6 months; etiology is often known; pain behaviors are more frequently exhibited.
  B. Chronic pain—typically lasts longer than 3 months; etiology of the pain is often unknown with nonmalignant chronic pain; fatigue and depression are common.
  C. Cancer pain—includes acute and chronic cancer-related pain associated with direct tumor involvement, diagnostic/therapeutic procedures, or cancer treatment; often clusters with fatigue, depression and anxiety, and sleep disturbance.
  D. Breakthrough pain (BTP)—a flare in the pain pattern that occurs in conjunction with well-controlled background pain (Mercadante et al., 2018).
    1. Incident pain—transient pain precipitated by any movement or activity.
    2. Insidious pain—spontaneous pain that occurs without warning
III. Types of pain (Fink & Brant, 2018; Russo & Sundaramurthi, 2019)
  A. Nociceptive pain—from activation of nociceptors (pain fibers) in deep and cutaneous tissues.
    1. Somatic pain—arises from the bone, joint, or connective tissue; described as sharp, throbbing, or pressure; well localized.
    2. Visceral pain—from nociceptor activation related to distention, compression, or infiltration of the thoracic or abdominal tissue (i.e., pancreas, liver, gastrointestinal [GI] tract); characterized by a diffuse, aching, or cramping sensation; poorly localized.
  B. Neuropathic pain—results from compression, inflammation, infiltration, ischemia, or injury to the peripheral, sympathetic, or central nervous system (CNS).
    1. Peripheral neuropathic pain—caused by peripheral nerve injury, often characterized by a numbness and tingling sensation.
    2. Centrally mediated pain—characterized by radiating and shooting sensations with a background of burning and aching.
    3. Sympathetically maintained pain—centrally generated, caused by autonomic dysregulation; complex regional pain syndrome (CRPS).
IV. Physiology (Fig. 45.1; Russo & Sundaramurthi, 2019)
  A. Transduction
    1. Initiated by mechanical, thermal, or chemical noxious stimuli.
    2. Neurotransmitters released at the time of injury include prostaglandins, bradykinin, serotonin (5-HT), substance P, and histamine, which initiate an inflammatory response.
    3. An action potential/depolarization is generated along the neuron; sodium moves into the cell and potassium out; pain message begins its way to the CNS.
  B. Transmission
    1. Action potential continues to the dorsal horn where nociceptors terminate.
    2. Neurotransmitters and excitatory substances are released in the spinal cord that inhibit presynaptic and postsynaptic nociceptive transmission.
    3. Neurons relay the message to the thalamus and other centers in the brain.
    4. The thalamus transmits the message to the cerebral cortex.
  C. Perception—the cerebral cortex processes the experience of pain and responds to the noxious stimuli to reduce pain perception via descending modulating mechanisms

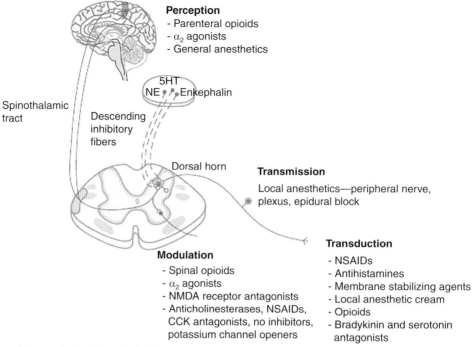

Perception
- Parenteral opioids
- α_2 agonists
- General anesthetics

5HT
NE · Enkephalin

Spinothalamic tract

Descending inhibitory fibers

Dorsal horn

Transmission
Local anesthetics—peripheral nerve, plexus, epidural block

Transduction
- NSAIDs
- Antihistamines
- Membrane stabilizing agents
- Local anesthetic cream
- Opioids
- Bradykinin and serotonin antagonists

Modulation
- Spinal opioids
- α_2 agonists
- NMDA receptor antagonists
- Anticholinesterases, NSAIDs, CCK antagonists, no inhibitors, potassium channel openers

Fig. 45.1 Physiology. From Macres, S. M., Moore, P. G., & Fishman, S. M. (2013). Acute pain management. In P. G. Barash, B. F. Cullen, R. K. Stoelting, et al. (Eds.), *Clinical anesthesia* (7th ed., pp. 1611–1642). Philadelphia, PA: Lippincott Williams & Wilkins.

D. Modulation
1. Neurons in the brainstem (pons and medulla) descend to the dorsal horn and release neuromediators—endogenous opioids, norepinephrine, and serotonin.
2. Neuromediators inhibit the transmission of pain impulses at the dorsal horn.
3. Opioids work at the dorsal horn by binding to receptors and preventing transmission of the pain signal to the higher brain centers.

V. Risk factors (van den Beuken-van Everdingen, Hochstenbach, Joosten, Tjan-Heijnen, & Janssen, 2016)
A. Disease-related factors
1. Types of cancer: prevalence higher in head and neck, lung, and breast cancer
2. Advanced, metastatic, or terminal disease: prevalence 66.4%
B. Treatment-related factors
1. Prevalence
a. 55% of patients have pain during cancer treatment
b. 39.3% of patients have pain after curative treatment
2. Chemotherapy-related side effects causing pain
a. Mucositis—occurs in 40%–70% of patients undergoing chemotherapy, 40%–60% of patients receiving purine analogs or antimetabolites, 80% undergoing hematopoietic stem cell transplantation, 100% of head and neck cancer patients receiving combined chemotherapy and radiation therapy (RT) (Razmara & Khayamzadeh, 2019).
b. Peripheral neuropathies—occur in 20%–85% depending on treatment; characterized by burning, numbness, and tingling of hands/feet (Kanzawa-Lee, Knoerl, Donohoe, Bridges, & Smith, 2019).
3. Postherpetic neuralgia (PHN)—herpes zoster 2–4 times higher among cancer patients and increases the risk of PHN; characterized by burning, aching, and shocklike pain; often occurs due to immunosuppression from the cancer or chemotherapy; topical agents, such as a lidocaine patch/gel and long-acting gabapentin, are indicated for PHN (Svigos, Belum, & Lacouture, 2019).
4. RT-related pain (Brant, 2022)
a. Visceral—chest pain/tightness, dermatitis, cystitis, enteritis, proctitis, and mucositis
b. Somatic—osteoporosis, osteoradionecrosis, and pelvic fractures
c. Neuropathic—myelopathy, peripheral nerve entrapment, and plexopathies
5. Postsurgical pain syndromes (Brant, 2022)
a. Postmastectomy—characterized by tightness in axilla, upper arm, and chest; often exacerbated with movement, extending, reaching, lifting, pulling, and pushing; caused by intercostobrachial nerve damage.
b. Postthoracotomy—characterized by aching, numbness, and/or burning in the incisional area. Believed to be caused by intercostal nerve damage.
c. Postsurgical head and neck cancer pain—characterized by tightness, burning, shocklike pain. Thought to be caused by injury to the accessory and superficial cervical plexus, followed by denervation and atrophy of the trapezius muscle, subsequent

downward and lateral scapula displacement, and thus shoulder dysfunction and pain.

d. Postlimb amputation—phantom or stump pain; may be neuropathic.

e. Lymphedema—characterized as arm/shoulder fullness, heaviness, or tightness. Can result from any cancer surgery that affects the lymphatic system in any body part (e.g., arm, leg). Most common in breast cancer.

C. Genetic risk factors (Yang, Barnes, Lyon, & Dorsey, 2019)

1. Genetic variability exists with the development of different pain syndromes and individual analgesic response.

2. Most common genes associated with response to opioids include opioid receptor mu 1 (OPRM1) and catechol-O-methyl transferase (COMT).

D. Personal, psychosocial, and spiritual factors (Fink, Gates, & Jeffers, 2019)

1. Patient-related fears.

   a. Fear of addiction.

   b. Fear that pain may be a sign of progressive disease; denial prevents patient from taking adequate analgesia.

   c. Desire to be a "good patient"; therefore, pain not reported.

   d. Fear of side effects (e.g., loss of mental clarity).

2. Provider-related—lack of knowledge, fear of addiction, and reluctance to prescribe due to regulations.

3. Culture—influences the perceptions and expression of pain.

4. Suffering—interpretation of the painful event and involves thoughts, beliefs, or judgments about the human experience of pain (Siler, Borneman, & Ferrell, 2019).

ASSESSMENT

I. Special populations (Table 45.1; Fink & Brant, 2018)

A. Older adult population (Cope, 2019)

1. Often have accompanying chronic pain that is unrelated to the cancer or its treatment.

2. High-risk population for falls; increased risk for constipation, delirium, confusion, and other side effects.

3. Obtain a comprehensive medication history—higher risk for polypharmacy and drug interactions in populations over age 70 taking five medications or more.

4. Start with lower doses, titrate slowly, advanced age results in a prolonged half-life and metabolism of the drug.

5. Consider the appropriateness of the pain screening scale; may need to employ the use of a nonverbal pain assessment tool if the patient cannot verbally report pain.

6. Assess for the presence of confusion and poor vision, availability of home supervision, ability to open and safely administer medications, and cost when planning analgesics for older adults.

TABLE 45.1   Pain Assessment Parameters

Domain	Pain Assessment Components
Physical Domain	
WILDA	• **W**ords used to describe the pain
	• **I**ntensity: On a scale of 0–10 what is your pain now, at rest, with movement, worst pain possible in the past 24 h? What is your comfort/function goal?
	• **L**ocation: Where is your pain?
	• **D**uration: Is the pain constant? Does the pain come and go? Do you have both types of pain (one that is constant and one that comes and goes)?
	• **A**ggravating/**A**lleviating factors: What makes the pain worse? What makes the pain better?
PQRST	• **P**rovocation/Palliation: What caused it? What relieves it?
	• **Q**uality: What does it feel like?
	• **R**egion/**R**adiation: Where is the pain located? Does the pain radiate?
	• **S**everity: How severe is the pain on a 0–10 scale?
	• **T**iming: Constant or intermittent?
OLDCART	• **O**nset: When did the pain start?
	• **L**ocation: Where is the pain located? Is there more than one location?
	• **D**uration: How often does the pain occur? Is it constant or intermittent? How long does the pain last?
	• **C**haracteristics: How does the pain feel (intensity)? What words would you use to describe the pain? (Descriptors can aid in diagnosing the pain syndrome.)
	• **A**ggravating factors: What makes your pain worse?
	• **R**elieving factors: What makes your pain better?
	• **T**reatment: What treatments (pharmacologic and/or nonpharmacologic) have you tried to control the pain? How are they working? How do the treatments affect the pain intensity?
Psychological domain	• The meaning of pain to the patient and family.
	• History of anxiety, depression, or other psychological illness.
	• Cognition, including confusion or delirium.
	• Usual coping strategies in response to pain.
	• Psychological responses to pain and illness, such as depression, anxiety, and fear.
	• Past pain experience.
	• Beliefs about opioids, addiction, and other concerns.
	• Willingness to try complementary modalities such as cognitive behavioral therapy.
Social domain	• Functional assessment: interference of pain on daily living, including physical or social withdrawal from activity.
	• Family caregiver communication and response to illness.
	• Support system.
	• Economic impact of the pain and its treatment (e.g., ability to afford analgesics).
Spiritual/ existential domain	• Spiritual beliefs related to pain and illness.
	• Presence of a spiritual community and its role related to pain and illness.
	• Influence of religion or spirituality on coping with pain.
	• Influence of suffering on the pain experience.
	• Use of traditional medicine in healing.

From Fink, R. M., & Brant, J. M. (2018). Complex cancer pain assessment. *Hematology/Oncology Clinics of North America, 32*(3), 353–369. https://doi.org/10.1016/j.hoc.2018.01.001.

B. Pediatric population (Duffy et al., 2019).
   1. Assess pediatric population according to developmental age.
   2. The child's report of pain is the gold standard for pain assessment.
   3. Choose a developmentally appropriate pain scale.
      a. CRIES for neonates—considers oxygenation, vital signs, and behaviors.
      b. Pain faces are usually used in children ages 7 years and younger.
      c. The "0–10" scale may be used for school-aged and older children.
      d. The FLACC scale is used for children who cannot verbalize pain.
      e. Pain Diary can be used in older children and adolescents ages 9–18.
   4. Starting dosage should be calculated according to weight.
C. Patients with substance use disorder (SUD) (Edwards, Foster, & Brant, 2019; Fink & Gallagher, 2019).
   1. Patients should be routinely assessed for the presence of a SUD; establish a good rapport.
   2. Use a standardized assessment tool for SUD.
      a. CAGE for alcohol use disorder—Cut, Annoyed, Guilty, and Eye opener
      b. Current opioid misuse measure, opioid risk tool, or screener and opioid assessment for patients with pain—revised for opioid use disorder
   3. Gather a thorough mental health history, as a dual diagnosis of a mental health disorder is common.
   4. Assessment to include the 5As: analgesic response; activities of daily living; adverse events; aberrant activities that suggest misuse, abuse, or addiction; affect.
II. Clinical pain assessment (Fink & Gallagher, 2019)
   A. Physical domain—onset, location, duration, characteristics, aggravating factors, relieving factors, and treatment.
   B. Psychological domain—meaning of pain to patient/family, how pain affects the patient's affect (e.g., depression, anxiety, and hopelessness); usual coping strategies, beliefs about opioids/addiction, how medications affect cognitive functioning, and willingness to try complementary modalities.
   C. Social domain—how pain/pain medications affect activities of daily living (physical/social withdrawal from activity), support system/family dynamics, and financial impact of pain (i.e., ability to afford analgesics).
   D. Spiritual/existential domain—influence of spiritual/religious beliefs related to pain/illness, presence of spiritual support/community and its role in patient's pain/illness, and use of traditional medicines.
   E. Cultural—assess how culture influences pain expression and management.
III. History and physical examination (Fink & Brant, 2018; Fink et al., 2019)

A. Medical history: current and prior oncologic treatment (e.g., chemo, RT, and surgery), other significant comorbidities, and preexisting chronic pain.
B. Evaluation of imaging studies (computed tomography, magnetic resonance imaging, bone scan, etc.) and laboratory values (tumor markers).
C. Physical and neurologic examination—assess pain behaviors (physical limitations, guarding), changes in muscle tone, and loss of deep tendon reflexes.
D. Assess for alterations in the following systems, which could be related to pain or side effects of analgesics:
   1. Respiratory status—decreased rate and volume, increased CO_2 levels.
   2. CNS changes—sedation/lethargy, euphoria, coordination, and mood.
   3. Cardiovascular system—tachycardia, hypotension.
   4. GI system—constipation, bowel obstruction, inability to evacuate stool, and nausea.
   5. Genitourinary system—urinary retention, difficult urination.
   6. Dermatologic system—diaphoresis, facial flushing, and pruritus.
   7. Endocrine system—decrease in libido and sexual response, hormonal changes.
   8. Musculoskeletal—weakness, muscle rigidity, and potential for falls.
IV. Evaluation and reassessment of pain (National Comprehensive Cancer Network, 2019)
   A. Assess/screen each patient for pain at each contact (on admission to the hospital and at regular follow-up intervals, during each home visit, or at outpatient clinic visits).
   B. Comprehensive pain assessment with each new report of pain.
   C. Pain should be reassessed after appropriate intervals after pain interventions (e.g., evaluate pain approximately 1 hour after oral medication administration).
   D. Evaluate the types of pain experienced including constant, intermittent, insidious, breakthrough, and/or end-of-dose failure at each visit.

MANAGEMENT

I. Medical management (Howard & Brant, 2019)
   A. Tailor pain management according to the patient's individualized pain assessment.
      1. Administer long-acting analgesics around the clock when pain is constant.
      2. Distinguish and manage BTP.
         a. Use BTP analgesics with a rapid onset; consider transmucosal fentanyl.
         b. Oral immediate-release opioids (e.g., morphine, oxycodone): administer 10%–20% of the 24-hour dose; does not apply to transmucosal fentanyl; administer at intervals before anticipated painful activity for incident pain (National Comprehensive Cancer Network, 2019).

3. End-of-dose failure—pain that increases before the next scheduled dose, may be managed by increasing the opioid dose or frequency.

4. Use equianalgesic conversion tables to guide opioid conversion.

5. Begin with least invasive route of administration (oral preferred, transdermal [TD]); change routes or rotate opioids if intolerable side effects or intractable pain occurs despite escalating doses.

6. Implement strategies to minimize side effects of analgesic therapy: bowel regimen that includes stool softener and stimulant, antiemetics, H2 antagonists, and CNS stimulants to counteract sedation.

7. Taper and discontinue opioids when no longer needed.

B. Use the World Health Organization (WHO) analgesic ladder to manage pain (Anekar & Cascellam, 2021; Fig. 45.2).

1. Step 1—nonopioid analgesics
   a. Use for mild pain or as adjuvants with opioid medications.
   b. Examples: acetaminophen, acetylsalicylic acid (ASA) (aspirin), nonsteroidal antiinflammatory drugs (NSAIDs).

2. Step 2—opioid analgesics
   a. Opioids for mild-to-moderate pain.
   b. Examples: hydrocodone and oxycodone in fixed combinations with acetaminophen or aspirin.

3. Step 3—opioid analgesics
   a. Opioids for severe pain.
   b. Step 3 opioids are used most frequently in managing cancer-related pain (e.g., morphine, oxycodone, hydromorphone, and fentanyl).

4. Step 4—this revised step includes the use of invasive and minimally invasive treatments such as epidruals and RT.

5. Analgesic adjuvant: use on each step of the WHO ladder to enhance analgesia, relieve concurrent symptoms that exacerbate pain, and/or relieve side effects.

C. Administer analgesics for safe and effective pain management (Hanna & Senderovich, 2021; Howard & Brant, 2019; Jones et al., 2019; National Comprehensive Cancer Network, 2019).

1. Nonopioids
   a. Acetaminophen should not exceed 3000 mg in 24 hours; use caution in opioid/acetaminophen combinations.
   b. Carefully weigh risk/benefit ratio of NSAIDs; side effects include inhibition of platelet aggregation, renal compromise, and GI toxicity.

2. Opioids
   a. Avoid or use morphine with caution in patients with renal impairment due to potential M3G and M6G metabolite accumulation, which may cause oversedation, respiratory depression, and myoclonus.
   b. Consider delayed onset of TD fentanyl and administer as-needed analgesics until efficacy established.
   c. Administer methadone with caution; its long half-life can lead to accumulation and oversedation.
   d. TD buprenorphine is a partial mu-agonist approved for cancer pain; a ceiling dose exists; may precipitate withdrawal symptoms in patients on pure mu-agonists (e.g., morphine).

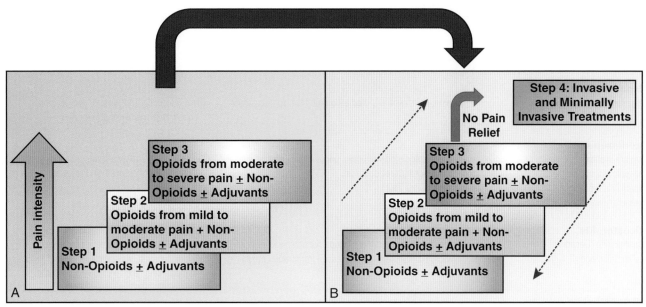

Figure 45.2. Transition from the original WHO three-step analgesic ladder (A) to the revised WHO four-step form (B). The additional step 4 is an "interventional" step and includes invasive and minimally invasive techniques. This updated WHO ladder provides a bidirectional approach. *WHO,* World Health Organization. From Anekar, A. A., Cascella, M. (2022). *WHO analgesic ladder.* In: *StatPearls [Internet].* Treasure Island, FL: StatPearls Publishing. https://www.ncbi.nlm.nih.gov/books/NBK554435/ Updated 15.05.22.

e. Tramadol and tapentadol are weak mu-opioids that block the reuptake of serotonin and norepinephrine; potential for serotonin syndrome; ceiling dose.

3. Adjuvants—use adjuvants specific for individual pain syndromes (e.g., neuropathic pain) (Howard & Brant, 2019; Table 45.2).

4. Bone metastases
   a. Radionuclides (e.g., strontium 89, samarium 153) for pain relief in disseminated metastatic bone cancer (Sierko, Hempel, Zuzda, & Wojtukiewicz, 2019).

b. Bone-modifying agents (e.g., zoledronic acid, denosumab) for pain relief in osteolytic bone metastases (Zajączkowska, Kocot-Kępska, Leppert, & Wordliczek, 2019).

5. Intraspinal analgesia (Sundaramurthi, Gallagher, & Sterling, 2017)
   a. Epidural or intrathecal route—percutaneous catheters, implantable pumps, or Ommaya reservoir.
   b. Indicated for specific pain syndromes; lower doses of opioids used, thus limiting severity and toxicity of side effects.

TABLE 45.2 Adjuvant Analgesics

Drug Classifications	Indications	Side Effects
Acetaminophen (Tylenol)	Mild-to-moderate pain, fever; maximum dose 4000 mg/day	Hepatotoxicity, increased risk with alcohol consumption, liver failure
α_2-Adrenergic agonist: clonidine hydrochloride (Catapres)	Epidural analgesia for neuropathic/postsurgical pain	Hypotension, bradycardia, central nervous system, depression, and dry mouth
CNS Stimulants Caffeine Dextroamphetamine (Dexedrine) Methylphenidate (Ritalin) Modafinil (Provigil) Atomoxetine (Strattera)	Counteract psychomotor retardation, reduce sedation side effects of opioids	Nervousness, sleep disorder, hypertension, palpitations, and anxiety
Anticonvulsants Gabapentin (Neurontin) Pregabalin (Lyrica) (most commonly used)	Neuropathic pain, trigeminal neuralgia, postherpetic neuralgia, and peripheral neuropathy	Sedation, dizziness, ataxia, edema, fatigue, bone marrow depression, nausea, rash, and impaired concentration
Antidepressants TCAs: Amitriptyline (Elavil) Desipramine (Norpramin) Nortriptyline (Pamelor) SNRIs: Venlafaxine (Effexor) Duloxetine (Cymbalta)	Neuropathic pain, postherpetic neuralgia, postsurgical neuropathies, and chemoimmunotherapy-related neuropathies	Dry mouth, sedation, constipation, agitation, delirium, tachycardia, orthostatic hypotension, worsening of cardiac conduction abnormalities, and more side effects with TCAs
Antispasmodics Baclofen (Lioresal)	Spastic pain, centrally mediated pain from spinal lesions	Drowsiness, slurred speech, hypotension, constipation, and urinary retention
Benzodiazepines Alprazolam (Xanax) Clonazepam (Klonopin) Diazepam (Valium) Lorazepam (Ativan)	Anxiety associated with pain, panic attack, muscle spasm, and procedure-related pain	Sedation, dementia, delirium, motor incoordination, hypotension, dizziness, and respiratory depression
Corticosteroids Dexamethasone (Decadron) Methylprednisolone (Solu-Medrol)	Brachial and lumbosacral plexopathies, lymphedema and visceral distention, and increased intracranial pressure	Euphoria/psychosis, increased appetite, hyperglycemia, weight gain, Cushing syndrome, osteoporosis, and GI bleeding, gastritis
Local Anesthetics Lidocaine IV or patch (Lidoderm) Mexilitine (Mexitil) EMLA cream	Lidocaine for postherpetic neuralgia, peripheral neuropathy, postsurgical neuropathies EMLA for dermal anesthesia	Lidocaine patch may cause a mild rash at the application site

TABLE 45.2 Adjuvant Analgesics —cont'd

Drug Classifications	Indications	Side Effects
Muscle Relaxants Cyclobenzaprine (Flexeril) Carisoprodol (Soma) Metaxalone (Skelaxin) Methocarbamol (Robaxin) Tizanidine (Zanaflex)	Should be used short term for musculoskeletal pain, tetanus Tizanidine may be used for longer periods; used for headache or neuropathic pain	Sedation, lightheadedness, blurred vision, hypotension, akathisia (movement disorder characterized by a feeling of inner restlessness and an urgent need to move)
***N*-Methyl-ᴅ-Aspartate Antagonists** Ketamine Amantadine (Symmetrel) Memantine (Namenda)	Neuropathic pain, synergistic with opioids, may be helpful in preventing tolerance to opioids Note: Methadone also has NMDA activity	Psychotomimetic side effects, hallucinations, drowsiness
NSAIDs COX-2 inhibitor: Celecoxib (Celebrex) Nonselective COX inhibitors: Ibuprofen (Advil, Motrin, Nuprin) Indomethacin (Indocin) Ketorolac (Toradol) Naproxen (Naprosyn, Aleve, Anaprox)	Bone metastases, soft tissue infiltration, tumor, fever, inflammation	COX-1 inhibitors may cause inhibition of platelet aggregation, gastric ulceration, renal toxicity, confusion in older adults COX-2 NSAIDs are more selective and cause fewer GI side effects

GI, Gastrointestinal; *TCA*, tricyclic antidepressant; *SNRI*, serotonin and norepinephrine reuptake inhibitors.
Data from Howard, A., & Brant, J. M. (2019). Pharmacologic management of cancer pain. *Seminars in Oncology Nursing, 35*(3), 235–240. https://doi.org/10.1016/j.soncn.2019.04.004; *National Comprehensive Cancer Network.* (2019). Adult cancer pain. v.3. NCCN clinical practice guidelines in oncology. http://www.nccn.org/professionals/physician_gls/PDF/pain.pdf.

II. Management (Farrell, Pereira, Brown, Green, & Aziz, 2021)
  A. RT may alleviate painful bone metastases and reduce large, localized bulky tumors (Sierko et al., 2019).
  B. Nerve blocks and interventional strategies for well-localized pain syndromes (Hofmeister et al., 2020; Piras et al., 2021).
    1. Head and neck—peripheral nerve block.
    2. Upper extremity—brachial plexus neurolysis.
    3. Thoracic wall—epidural, intrathecal, intercostal, and dorsal root ganglion neurolysis.
    4. Abdominal—celiac plexus block, thoracic splanchnicectomy.
    5. Pelvic—superior hypogastric plexus block.
    6. Rectal—intrathecal neurolysis, midline myelotomy, superior hypogastric plexus block, and ganglion impar block.
    7. Unilateral pain—cordotomy.
    8. Neurostimulation for CRPS, neuralgias, and peripheral neuropathy.
  C. Minimally invasive surgical procedures (Mattie et al., 2021).
    1. Percutaneous kyphoplasty/vertebroplasty—for treatment of osteoclastic lesions (spinal metastasis/compressions fractures) to restore spinal stability.
    2. Optimal debulking of tumor to limit pain, or improve or maintain function.
  D. Psychoeducational interventions (Durosier Mertilus, Lengacher, & Rodriguez, 2021; Eaton & Hulett, 2019)
    1. Educate patients and families about strategies to prevent and manage pain.

2. Discuss the importance of good pain management in attaining optimal quality of life and the impact of pain on depression, sleep disturbance, and fatigue.
3. Educate patients and families regarding the use of pain rating scales to communicate pain and the responsiveness to interventions.
4. Encourage the patient to take analgesics early in the pain experience to avoid severe pain; take long-acting analgesics around the clock for constant pain.
5. Educate the patient and family about modalities available to control pain: analgesics, interventional procedures, and complementary techniques.
6. Incorporate patient's social network (family leaders, minister/spiritual leader, healer) as appropriate; manage psychological distress, which can increase pain.
7. Differentiate among tolerance, physical dependence, and addiction.
  a. Analgesic tolerance—physiologic state of adaptation whereby the repeated exposure to a drug results in a diminished effect of the drug over time and a possible need to increase the drug dose to achieve the same level of effect.
  b. Physical dependence—a physiologic state of adaptation manifested by the emergence of a withdrawal syndrome if drug use is abruptly stopped, is rapidly decreased, or an antagonist is administered.
  c. Addiction—a neurobiological disease with genetic, psychosocial, and environmental influences; characterized by psychological dependency, cravings, and compulsive use despite harm.

E. Monitor the patient for safety.
1. Monitor for opioid-related side effects, including respiratory depression.
2. Educate patients who are at high risk for spinal cord compression to notify the health care team if early signs of impending compression occur.
3. Monitor for potential opioid misuse, abuse, and diversion.

REFERENCES

Anekar, A., & Cascellam, M. (2021). WHO analgesic ladder: *StatPearls [Internet]*. Treasure Island, FL: StatPearls Publishing. Retrieved from https://www.ncbi.nlm.nih.gov/books/NBK554435/.

Brant, J. M. (2022). The assessment and management of acute and chronic cancer pain syndromes. *Seminars in Oncology Nursing*, 38(1), 151248. https://doi.org/10.1016/j.soncn.2022.151248.

Cope, D. G. (2019). Cancer pain management considerations in older adults. *Seminars in Oncology Nursing*, 35(3), 274–278. https://doi.org/10.1016/j.soncn.2019.04.008.

Duffy, E. A., Dias, N., Hendricks-Ferguson, V., Hellsten, M., Skeens-Borland, M., Thornton, C., et al. (2019). Perspectives on cancer pain assessment and management in children. *Seminars in Oncology Nursing*, 35(3), 261–273. https://doi.org/10.1016/j.soncn.2019.04.007.

Durosier Mertilus, D. S., Lengacher, C. A., & Rodriguez, C. S. (2022). A review and conceptual analysis of cancer pain self-management. *Pain Management Nursing*, 23(2), 168–173. https://doi.org/10.1016/j.pmn.2021.04.005.

Eaton, L. H., & Hulett, J. M. (2019). Mind-body interventions in the management of chronic cancer pain. *Seminars in Oncology Nursing*, 35(3), 241–252. https://doi.org/10.1016/j.soncn.2019.04.005.

Edwards, T., Foster, T., & Brant, J. M. (2019). Managing cancer pain in patients with opioid and substance use disorders. *Seminars in Oncology Nursing*, 35(3), 279–283. https://doi.org/10.1016/j.soncn.2019.04.009.

Farrell, S. M., Pereira, E. A. C., Brown, M. R. D., Green, A. L., & Aziz, T. Z. (2021). Neuroablative surgical treatments for pain due to cancer. *Neurochirurgie*, 67(2), 176–188. https://doi.org/10.1016/j.neuchi.2020.10.003.

Fink, R. M., & Brant, J. M. (2018). Complex cancer pain assessment. *Hematology/Oncology Clinics of North America*, 32(3), 353–369. https://doi.org/10.1016/j.hoc.2018.01.001.

Fink, R. M., & Gallagher, E. (2019). Cancer pain assessment and measurement. *Seminars in Oncology Nursing*, 35(3), 229–234. https://doi.org/10.1016/j.soncn.2019.04.003.

Fink, R. M., Gates, R. A., & Jeffers, K. D. (2019). Pain assessment in the palliative care setting. In B. R. Ferrell & J. A. Paice (Eds.), *Oxford textbook of palliative nursing* (5th ed.). Oxford: Oxford University Press.

Hanna, V., & Senderovich, H. (2021). Methadone in pain management: A systematic review. *Journal of Pain*, 22(3), 233–245. https://doi.org/10.1016/j.jpain.2020.04.004.

Hofmeister, M., Memedovich, A., Brown, S., Saini, M., Dowsett, L. E., Lorenzetti, D. L., et al. (2020). Effectiveness of neurostimulation technologies for the management of chronic pain: A systematic review. *Neuromodulation*, 23(2), 150–157. https://doi.org/10.1111/ner.13020.

Howard, A., & Brant, J. M. (2019). Pharmacologic management of cancer pain. *Seminars in Oncology Nursing*, 35(3), 235–240. https://doi.org/10.1016/j.soncn.2019.04.004.

Jones, L. K., Lussier, M. E., Brar, J., Byrne, M. C., Durham, M., Kiokemeister, F., et al. (2019). Current interventions to promote safe and appropriate pain management. *American Journal of Health-System Pharmacy*, 76(11), 829–834. https://doi.org/10.1093/ajhp/zxz063.

Kanzawa-Lee, G. A., Knoerl, R., Donohoe, C., Bridges, C. M., & Smith, E. M. L. (2019). Mechanisms, predictors, and challenges in assessing and managing painful chemotherapy-induced peripheral neuropathy. *Seminars in Oncology Nursing*, 35(3), 253–260. https://doi.org/10.1016/j.soncn.2019.04.006.

Mattie, R., Brar, N., Tram, J. T., McCormick, Z. L., Beall, D. P., Fox, A., et al. (2021). Vertebral augmentation of cancer-related spinal compression fractures: A systematic review and meta-analysis. *Spine (Phila PA 1976)*, 46(24), 1729–1737. https://doi.org/10.1097/brs.0000000000004093.

Mercadante, S., Marchetti, P., Cuomo, A., Caraceni, A., Mediati, R. D., Vellucci, R., et al. (2018). Factors influencing the clinical presentation of breakthrough pain in cancer patients. *Cancers (Basel)*, 10(6), 175. https://doi.org/10.3390/cancers10060175.

National Comprehensive Cancer Network. (2019). Adult cancer pain. v.3. NCCN clinical practice guidelines in oncology. http://www.nccn.org/professionals/physician_gls/PDF/pain.pdf.

Piras, A., La Vecchia, M., Boldrini, L., D'Aviero, A., Galanti, D., Guarini, A., et al. (2021). Radiofrequency thermoablation (RFA) and radiotherapy (RT) combined treatment for bone metastases: A systematic review. *European Review for Medical and Pharmacological Sciences*, 25(10), 3647–3654. https://doi.org/10.26355/eurrev_202105_25930.

Raja, S. N., Carr, D. B., Cohen, M., Finnerup, N. B., Flor, H., Gibson, S., et al. (2020). The revised International Association for the Study of Pain definition of pain: Concepts, challenges, and compromises. *Pain*, 161(9), 1976–1982. Retrieved from https://journals.lww.com/pain/Fulltext/2020/09000/The_revised_International_Association_for_the.6.aspx.

Razmara, F., & Khayamzadeh, M. (2019). An investigation into the prevalence and treatment of oral mucositis after cancer treatment. *International Journal of Cancer Management*, 12(11), e88405.

Russo, M. M., & Sundaramurthi, T. (2019). An overview of cancer pain: Epidemiology and pathophysiology. *Seminars in Oncology Nursing*, 35(3), 223–228. https://doi.org/10.1016/j.soncn.2019.04.002.

Sierko, E., Hempel, D., Zuzda, K., & Wojtukiewicz, M. Z. (2019). Personalized radiation therapy in cancer pain management. *Cancers (Basel)*, 11(3), 390. https://doi.org/10.3390/cancers11030390.

Siler, S., Borneman, T., & Ferrell, B. (2019). Pain and suffering. *Seminars in Oncology Nursing*, 35(3), 310–314. https://doi.org/10.1016/j.soncn.2019.04.013.

Sundaramurthi, T., Gallagher, N., & Sterling, B. (2017). Cancer-related acute pain: A systematic review of evidence-based interventions for putting evidence into practice. *Clinical Journal of Oncology Nursing*, 21(3 Suppl), 13–30. https://doi.org/10.1188/17.Cjon.S3.13-30.

Svigos, K., Belum, V. R., & Lacouture, M. E. (2019). Dermatologic cancer pain syndromes. In A. Gulati, V. Puttanniah, B. M. Bruel, W. S. Rosenberg, & J. C. Hung (Eds.), *Essentials of interventional cancer pain management* (pp. 133–138). Cham: Springer International Publishing.

van den Beuken-van Everdingen, M. H., Hochstenbach, L. M., Joosten, E. A., Tjan-Heijnen, V. C., & Janssen, D. J. (2016). Update on prevalence of pain in patients with cancer: Systematic review and meta-analysis. *Journal of Pain and Symptom Management, 51*(6), 1070–1090.E9. https://doi.org/10.1016/j.jpainsymman.2015.12.340.

Yang, G. S., Barnes, N. M., Lyon, D. E., & Dorsey, S. G. (2019). Genetic variants associated with cancer pain and response to opioid analgesics: Implications for precision pain management. *Seminars in Oncology Nursing, 35*(3), 291–299. https://doi.org/10.1016/j.soncn.2019.04.011.

Zajączkowska, R., Kocot-Kępska, M., Leppert, W., & Wordliczek, J. (2019). Bone pain in cancer patients: Mechanisms and current treatment. *International Journal of Molecular Sciences, 20*(23), 6047. https://doi.org/10.3390/ijms20236047.

46

Respiratory Symptoms

Leslie Matthews

ANATOMIC OR SURGICAL ALTERATIONS

Overview

(Hartley, 2018; Lumb & Thomas, 2020)
I. Definition—inadequate ventilation or oxygenation resulting from anatomic or surgical alterations. Alterations in respiratory or cardiovascular systems may cause ventilation/perfusion (V/Q) mismatch causing hypoxemia.
II. Anatomic alterations
   A. Space-occupying lesions within the lung itself or in the pleural space (e.g., from primary or metastatic cancer to the lung)
   B. Airway obstruction of the tracheobronchial tree from direct extension of primary or metastatic tumors or enlarged lymph nodes
   C. Abnormal accumulation of fluid within lung or pleural space
      1. Hemothorax—abnormal accumulation of blood within the pleural space
      2. Hydrothorax (effusion)—abnormal accumulation of fluid within the pleural space
      3. Empyema—abnormal accumulation of infected fluid or pus in the pleural space caused by recent chest surgery, immunocompromise, or lung infection
      4. Compression of tracheobronchial tree from bronchospasm, laryngeal swelling from hypersensitivity reactions related to chemotherapy and/or biotherapy treatments, or superior vena cava syndrome (SVCS) (see Chapter 49)
III. Surgical alterations
   1. Thoracic surgery for the removal of primary or metastatic cancer of the lung
      a. Pneumonectomy—surgical removal of an entire lung
      b. Lobectomy—removal of a lobe of the lung
      c. Segmental resection—removal of one or more segments of a lung lobe
      d. Wedge resection—removal of a small wedge-shaped localized area near the lung surface
   2. Tracheostomy after head and neck surgery, laryngectomy
IV. Risk factors (Lumb & Thomas, 2020)
   A. Primary or metastatic cancer of the lung
   B. Recent surgery (especially thoracic or abdominal), immobility, or situations in which hypoventilation is likely
   C. Cancers associated with SVCS (see Chapter 49)
   D. Thoracic or head and neck surgery
   E. Primary or adjuvant tracheobronchial surgeries
   F. Surgery for palliation, tumor debulking
   G. History of obstructive or restrictive pulmonary disease
   H. History of cardiovascular disease
   I. Smoking history or environmental exposure to irritants such as pollution, pesticides, chemicals, or other irritants

Assessment

(Lumb & Thomas, 2020; Robinson & Scullion, 2021)
I. History
   A. Cough
   B. Sputum production, hemoptysis
   C. Dyspnea—shortness of breath; tachypnea—rapid breathing; orthopnea—difficulty breathing when supine; paroxysmal nocturnal dyspnea—awakening from sleep with shortness of breath
   D. Wheeze, stridor, chest pain, and hoarseness
   E. Ability to carry out activities of daily living (ADLs)
   F. Tobacco use—pack-year history
   G. Chronic obstructive pulmonary disease (COPD)
   H. Exercise or activity tolerance
   I. Number of pillows used for sleep and comfort
   J. Level of consciousness, mental status
   K. Anxiety and apprehension
      1. Acute—less than 2–3 weeks
      2. Chronic—longer than 2 months
   L. Presence of risk factors
II. Diagnostic tests (Sundaralingam, Bedawi, & Rahman, 2020)
   A. Chest radiography, computed tomography (CT), magnetic resonance imaging, and positron emission tomography to delineate anatomic extent of involvement
   B. Pulmonary function tests (PFTs) to quantify air flow limitation
   C. Arterial blood gases (ABGs)
   D. Ventilation–perfusion scans
   E. Bronchoscopy for direct visualization; endobronchial ultrasound
   F. Endobronchial thoracentesis
III. Physical examination (Lumb & Thomas, 2020; Robinson & Scullion, 2021)

A. Abnormal or altered breathing patterns; tachypnea, pursed-lip breathing, or use of accessory muscles of respiration
B. Abnormal breath sounds—wheezes, decreased or absent breath sounds
C. Sputum—amount, color, and presence of blood
D. Cyanosis
E. Vital signs and pulse oximetry; hypoxemia
F. Evaluate airway swelling, oropharyngeal swelling
G. Presence of enlarged lymph nodes or masses in the head and neck area

Management

(Lumb & Thomas, 2020; Robinson & Scullion, 2021; Wong, Galiabovitch, & Bhagwat, 2019)
I. Pharmacologic management
  A. Treat the underlying disease process
    1. Radiation therapy (RT), chemotherapy, biotherapy, and targeted agents for primary or metastatic cancer of the lung or to reduce obstruction of the tracheobronchial tree
    2. Supplemental oxygen administration as indicated for hypoxemia
    3. Incorporate measures to minimize pain, which may contribute to ineffective breathing (see Chapter 45)
    4. Systemic antibiotic treatment for empyema
    5. Thoracentesis to remove abnormally accumulated contents in pleural space
II. Nonpharmacologic management
  A. Use measures to ease and increase the effectiveness of breathing and to promote physical comfort
    1. Proper positioning, use of pillows
  B. Prioritize patient activity and exercise and use energy conservation strategies
  C. Maximize safety
    1. Encourage patient to use supplemental oxygen and assistive devices (e.g., cane, walker, and wheelchair) as needed for ambulation to prevent hypoxia and potential falls
    2. Report critical changes to the oncology provider
  D. Educate patient and caregiver regarding the following:
    1. Prioritize activity and energy conservation strategies
      a. Frequent rest periods
      b. Easy-to-prepare meals
      c. Often-used items within reach
      d. Emergency care, available community resources, and medication management
      e. Signs and symptoms to report to the health care team

PULMONARY TOXICITY RELATED TO CANCER THERAPY

Overview

I. Definition—parenchymal pulmonary disease caused by antineoplastic therapy, radiation, chemotherapy, biological agents, or targeted therapies (Arroyo-Hernandez et al., 2021; Postow, Sidlow, & Hellmann, 2018)

II. Classification
  A. Radiation-induced lung toxicity, pneumonitis (Arroyo-Hernandez et al., 2021; Giuranno, Ient, De Ruysscher, & Vooijs, 2019)
    1. Subacute inflammatory response to radiation exposure to the lung; occurs in 1% to 20% of patients receiving thoracic radiation
    2. Toxic effects are proportionate to the following:
      a. Total radiation dose and volume of lung tissue irradiated
      b. Fractionation schedule; hyperfractionation schedules may cause less RT pneumonitis
      c. Concomitant administration of chemotherapy (Table 46.1)
  B. Chemotherapy-induced pulmonary toxicity (Dhamija et al., 2020; Tilak, Handa, Kumar, Mutreja, & Subramanian, 2021; Table 46.2)
    1. Targets rapidly proliferating cells and may impart direct injury to parenchymal endothelial cell membranes of lung, causing bilateral interstitial infiltrates, or fibrosis, or ground-glass opacities.
    2. Systemic release of cytokines, hypersensitivity reaction, or immune complex–related reaction
    3. Administration of immunotherapy or targeted therapy-induced pulmonary toxicity (Carter, Altan, Shroff, Truong, & Vlahos, 2022; Isono et al., 2021)
      a. May induce overwhelming inflammatory responses and autoimmunity
      b. Inflammation process affects the interstitial lung parenchyma, causing infectious and noninfectious lung injury

TABLE 46.1 Chemotherapy and Biological Agents Predisposing to Radiation Pneumonitis

Chemotherapy Agents	Targeted Therapies
Bleomycin	Alemtuzumab
Busulfan	Bevacizumab
Chlorambucil	Cetuximab
Cyclophosphamide	Rituximab
Doxorubicin	Trastuzumab
Gemcitabine	Idelalisib
Ifosfamide	
Irinotecan	
Methotrexate	
Mitomycin	
Paclitaxel	
Vinblastine	
Vincristine	

From Arroyo-Hernandez, M., Maldonado, F., Lozano-Ruiz, F., Muñoz-Montaño, W., Nunez-Baez, M., & Arrieta, O. (2021). Radiation-induced lung injury: Current evidence. *BMC Pulmonary Medicine, 21*(1),9. https://doi.org/10.1186/S12890-020-01376-4; Giuranno, L., Ient, J., De Ruysscher, D., & Vooijs, M. A. (2019). Radiation-induced lung injury (RILI). *Frontiers in Oncology, 9*, 877. https://doi.org/10.3389/fonc.2019.00877.

TABLE 46.2 Chemotherapy and Targeted Therapy–Related Pulmonary Abnormalities

Pattern of Lung Involvement	Specific Agents	Radiologic Abnormality
Acute pneumonitis	Bortezomib, cetuximab, dasatinib, erlotinib, everolimus, gefitinib, gemcitabine, idelalisib, imatinib, irinotecan, pemetrexed, piritrexim, procarbazine, rituximab, sorafenib, sunitinib, temozolomide, temsirolimus, thalidomide, and trastuzumab	Diffuse, patchy, ground-glass opacities; diffuse reticular pattern
Bronchiolitis	Bortezomib, busulfan, cetuximab, panitumumab, and topotecan	Hyperinflation, air trapping
Hemoptysis	Bevacizumab	Bilateral ground-glass opacities, consolidation
Hypersensitivity reactions	Alpha-interferon, cetuximab, etoposide, gemcitabine, L-asparaginase, obinutuzumab, panitumumab, rituximab, taxanes, and vinca alkaloids	Air flow obstruction, airway hyperreactivity, and hyperinflation
Interstitial pneumonitis	Erlotinib, everolimus, gefitinib, idelalisib, ofatumumab, rituximab, sorafenib, sunitinib, temsirolimus, thalidomide, and trastuzumab	Diffuse, patchy, and ground-glass opacities
Isolated acute chest pain	Bleomycin, doxorubicin, etoposide, and methotrexate	Nonspecific
Isolated cough	Alpha-interferon, IL-2, methotrexate	Nonspecific
Isolated DLCO	BCNU (carmustine), gemcitabine, paclitaxel	Nonspecific
Mediastinal lymphadenopathy	Bleomycin, interferon, and methotrexate	Hilar, mediastinal lymphadenopathy
Pleural effusion	Bleomycin, bortezomib, busulfan, dasatinib, etoposide, fludarabine, gemcitabine, imatinib, IL-2, methotrexate, procarbazine, taxanes, thalidomide, and trametinib	Pleural effusion
Pneumothorax	Carmustine	Pneumothorax
Pulmonary edema	Ara-C, alpha-interferon, azathioprine, decitabine, G-CSF, gemcitabine, imatinib, nitrogen mustard, paclitaxel, vinorelbine	Diffuse alveolar infiltrates, without cardiomegaly or pleural effusion
PE	Axitinib, bevacizumab, dasatinib, imatinib, lenalidomide, thalidomide	Acute PE
Pulmonary hypertension	Dasatinib, Imatinib	Right-sided heart enlargement, acute PE

BCNU, Bischloroethylnitrosourea; DLCO, diminished diffusion capacity of the lungs for carbon monoxide; G-CSF, granulocyte colony-stimulating factor; PE, pulmonary embolus.

From Dhamija, E., Meena, P., Ramalingam, V., Sahoo, R., Rastogi, S., & Thulkar, S. (2020). Chemotherapy-induced pulmonary complications in cancer: Significance of clinicoradiological correlation. *The Indian Journal of Radiology & Imaging*, 30(1), 20–26. https://doi.org/10.4103/ijri.IJRI_178_19; Shannon, V. R. (2019). Cancer treatment-related lung injury. *Oncologic Critical Care*, 531–556. https://doi.org/10.1007/978-3-319-74588-6_52; Tvsvgk, T., Handa, A., Kumar, K, Mutreja, D., & Subramanian, S. (2021). Chemotherapy-associated pulmonary toxicity – Case series from Single Center. *South Asian Journal of Cancer*, 10(4), 255-260. https://doi.org/10.1055/S-0041-1731581.

III. Risk factors
    A. Radiation, chemotherapy, or targeted therapy (Arroyo-Hernandez et al., 2021; Carter et al., 2022)
    B. Occurs in 5%–20% of all patients receiving RT
    C. Concurrent chemotherapy and RT or sequential RT to lungs
    D. Cumulative dose of administered drug
    E. Previous chemo or RT
    F. Biological factors/cytokines, such as transforming growth factor beta-1
    G. Preexisting pulmonary disease, interstitial lung disease (e.g., COPD), renal dysfunction, or cardiovascular disease
    H. Smoking history
    I. Poor performance status
    J. More severe in older adults and females
    K. Age—older than 70 years

Assessment

I. History (Arroyo-Hernandez et al., 2021)
    A. Radiation, chemotherapy, or targeted therapy-induced pulmonary toxicity
       1. Dyspnea is the cardinal symptom; also nonproductive cough, malaise, fatigue, and fever
       2. Generally develops over weeks to months but can also develop quickly (within hours) and may occur years after drug exposure
    B. Early nonspecific symptoms include nonproductive cough, mild dyspnea, low-grade temperature, pleuritic chest pain
       1. May occur 6–12 weeks after completion of RT, although symptoms can range from 1 to 6 months after RT
    C. Exclude other causes of pulmonary infiltrates—infection, recurrent tumors, thromboembolic disease, lymphangitic carcinomatosis
II. Physical examination (Arroyo-Hernandez et al., 2021)
    A. Physical examination—may be unreliable
       1. Respiratory rate, rhythm, and effort
       2. Assess for signs of pulmonary toxicity—dyspnea, dry persistent cough, basilar rales, tachypnea, and pleuritic pain
       3. Moist rales, pleural friction rub
       4. Evidence of pleural fluid heard over the area of irradiation
       5. Low-grade fever, congestion
       6. Tachypnea, cyanosis (late)
       7. Early—diffuse haziness, ground-glass opacification

8. Late—infiltrates or dense consolidation corresponding to the region of radiation exposure
III. Radiographic changes
    A. Results may be normal, early onset, as late as 2 months, or even years after therapy
    B. Diffuse bilateral lung infiltrates
    C. Classic diffuse reticular pattern, ground-glass opacities, usually bilateral
IV. Diagnostic tests and findings (Arroyo-Hernandez et al., 2021)
    A. PFTs—may reveal restrictive defect or obstructive pattern
        1. Decreased lung volume
        2. Decreased restrictive ventilatory pattern, diminished diffusion capacity of the lungs for carbon monoxide (DLCO); DLCO measures the ability of the lungs to transfer gas from inhaled air to the red blood cells in pulmonary capillaries
    B. High-resolution CT
        1. Detection of radiation fibrosis
            a. Early—diffuse haziness, ground-glass opacification
            b. Late—infiltrates or dense consolidation corresponding to the region of radiation exposure
        2. Abnormality is generally nonspecific
    C. ABGs
        1. Hypoxia
        2. Hypocapnia, respiratory alkalosis

Management

I. Pharmacologic management:
    A. Manage treatment-related pulmonary toxicity that is RT induced (Arroyo-Hernandez et al., 2021); chemotherapy induced (Dhamija et al., 2020); targeted therapy induced (Shannon, 2019)
    B. Mild symptoms—cough suppressants, antipyretics, and rest
    C. Severe symptoms and impaired gas exchange—glucocorticoid therapy until symptoms improve, then taper slowly; pneumonitis may flare if taper is too rapid; about 50% respond to glucocorticoid therapy
    D. Monitor baseline PFTs and limit cumulative dose
    E. Discontinue suspected agent or reduce dose for prompt resolution
II. Nonpharmacologic management
    A. Encourage balanced activity training to decrease or prevent adverse effects of therapy
    B. Evaluate cardiorespiratory fitness
    C. Monitor activities to minimize energy expenditure
    D. Monitor for adequate relief of symptoms

DYSPNEA

Overview

I. Definition—a subjective sensation of breathlessness, or air hunger, difficulty breathing, the feeling of inability to get enough air, and the reaction to the sensation (Hui et al., 2021)
II. Risk factors
    A. Disease related
        1. Tumors that impinge on respiratory structures and decrease air flow
        2. Conditions that increase metabolic demands (e.g., fever, infection)
        3. Cerebral metastasis, which affects the respiratory center or stimulates the central and peripheral chemoreceptors
        4. Metastatic effusions in the pleural or cardiac space or abdominal cavity, which compromise lung expansion, gas exchange, or blood flow to the lungs
        5. Coexisting pulmonary, cardiac, or neuromuscular disease, which compromises lung expansion or blood flow to the lungs
        6. Coexisting pulmonary infection or COVID-19 positive
        7. Advanced disease or terminal illness
    B. Treatment related
        1. Incisional pain that may compromise lung expansion
        2. Immediate and long-term effects of RT to the lung fields
            a. May be acute or delayed (up to 10 years after treatment)
            b. May be dose related, reversible, or chronic
        3. Antineoplastic agents that may cause pulmonary toxicity
            a. May be acute or delayed (up to 10 years after treatment)
            b. May be dose related, reversible, or chronic
        4. Anaphylactic reactions to antineoplastic agents, biological response modifiers, or targeted therapy agents
        5. Pneumothorax related to the placement of vascular access catheters, fine-needle aspiration, or thoracentesis
    C. Lifestyle related
        1. Strong emotional responses, particularly anxiety or anger, contribute to the sensation of dyspnea
        2. Tobacco use or exposure to environmental toxic substances—asbestos, chromium, coal products, ionizing radiation, vinyl chloride, and chloromethyl ethers
        3. Obesity

Assessment

(Budhar & Syed, 2020; Hui et al., 2021)
I. History
    A. Presence of risk factors such as smoking, chemical exposure
    B. Subjective reports of shortness of breath, "can't catch breath," "smothering," "air hunger," uncomfortable breathing, anxiety, or panic
    C. Pattern of dyspnea—onset, frequency, severity, associated symptoms, and aggravating or alleviating factors
    D. Impact of dyspnea on ADLs, lifestyle, relationships, role responsibilities, emotional well-being, sexuality, and body image

E. Intake and output

F. Vascular perfusion

II. Physical findings

A. Tachypnea, hypercapnia, and increased respiratory excursion

B. Use of accessory muscles, retraction of intercostal spaces, and nostril flaring

C. Clubbing of digits caused by chronic hypoxemia; cyanosis, pallor, jugular vein distention, upper extremity swelling, and venous congestion in thorax or chest region

III. Diagnostic tests and findings

A. Complete blood cell count—hemoglobin deficiencies

B. Pulse oximetry—severity of hypoxia

C. Chest radiography and CT—structural abnormalities, PFTs

D. Bronchoscopic examination

E. Sputum or bronchial cultures

F. ABGs

G. COVID-19 testing

H. Assessment scales such as a numeric rating scale to measure degree of patient's dyspnea (Campbell, 2018)

IV. Psychological signs and symptoms

A. Concentration difficulties, memory difficulties, or both; confusion

B. Restlessness

Management

(Feliciano et al., 2021; Hui et al., 2021; Oncology Nursing Society [ONS], 2019)

I. Pharmacologic management

A. Supplemental oxygen for patients with hypoxemia who are experiencing dyspnea ($SpO_2 \leq 90\%$ on room air)

B. Treatment of underlying disease with thoracentesis, RT, chemotherapy, and antimicrobial medications

C. Pharmacologic agents

1. Glucocorticoids—decrease local inflammation

2. Opioids and anxiolytics—decrease pain and anxiety

3. Bronchodilators—increase air flow to the lungs

4. Diuretics—decrease fluid overload

D. Manage the discomfort of dyspnea

1. Immediate-release oral and parenteral opioids, which decrease central respiratory drive by reducing ventilatory demand

2. Pharmacologic agents

a. Extended-release morphine

b. Midazolam plus morphine

c. Nebulized opioids

d. Furosemide

e. Lidocaine

E. Benzodiazepines for anxiety

II. Nonpharmacologic management

A. Promote comfort for palliation of dyspnea (Hui et al., 2021; ONS, 2019)

1. Increased ambient air flow directed at the cheek (trigeminal nerve distribution)

2. Cooler temperatures

3. Promotion of relaxation and stress reduction techniques

B. Provide educational, emotional, and psychosocial support to patient and caregiver; referral to other disciplines as appropriate.

C. Further research needed for use of acupuncture and cognitive behavioral approaches.

D. Avoidance of volume overload.

E. Encourage positioning to facilitate breathing—upright position; forward position with elbows on knees, table, or pillows.

F. Instruct patient about diaphragmatic breathing techniques with slow exhalation; may not be effective and may be harmful in patients with pulmonary restrictive disease.

G. Recommend assistive devices such as wheelchair, walker, and portable oxygen as needed.

H. Exercise rehabilitation.

I. Maximize safety.

1. Encourage the use of assistive devices such as cane, walker, or wheelchair as needed for ambulation and ADLs.

2. Use activity limitation, conservation of energy strategies.

a. Frequent rest periods

b. Use of ready-made meals

c. Often-used items within reach

J. Monitor subjective reports of the changes in the pattern of dyspnea or psychological responses to dyspnea such as anxiety or distress.

K. Educate patient and caregiver.

1. Teach about activity limitation, energy conservation strategies.

2. Provide information about accessing emergency care, available community resources.

3. Use of language that is easy to understand (e.g., shortness of breath instead of dyspnea).

L. Decrease the sense of dyspnea and enhance psychosocial well-being.

1. Encourage the use of relaxation techniques, prayer and meditation, and aromatherapy.

2. Use complementary and alternative therapies such as relaxation techniques and stress reduction strategies.

PLEURAL EFFUSIONS

Overview

I. Definition—presence of excess fluid in the pleural space; may be pulmonary or non-pulmonary, and acute or chronic (Kugasia et al., 2019)

II. Classification (Jany & Weite, 2019; Li, Ajmal, Tufail, & Ranchal, 2021)

A. Benign pleural effusion may be caused by the following:

1. Increased hydrostatic pressure (congestive heart failure [CHF])

2. Increased permeability in microvascular circulation (infection, trauma)

3. Increased negative pressure in the pleural space (atelectasis)

4. Decreased oncotic pressure in the microvasculature (nephrotic syndrome, cirrhosis, hypoalbuminemia)
5. Increased permeability caused by inflammation or disruption of the capillary endothelium
6. Altered mucosal lung or mediastinal tissue resulting from RT

B. Malignant pleural effusion, the presence of malignant cells in the pleura that signifies distant spread of disease, may be caused by the following:
1. Direct extension of primary tumor to the pleura or mediastinum or mesothelioma involving the pleura
2. Impaired lymphatic drainage from the pleural space resulting from obstruction caused by tumor

III. Risk factors (Li et al., 2021)
A. Primary tumors of lung, breast, and hematopoietic system
B. Prior pleural effusion
C. Radiation to the chest, thorax, or abdomen
D. Surgical modification of venous or lymphatic vessels

Assessment

(Beaudoin, & Gonzalez, 2018; Jany & Welte, 2019)
I. History
A. Presence of risk factors
B. Symptoms—severity related to the speed of accumulation, not amount; usually caused by pulmonary compression
1. Dyspnea, progressive, and exertional
2. Cough usually dry and nonproductive
3. Chest pain

II. Physical examination
A. Fever, tachypnea
B. Restricted chest wall expansion
C. Dullness to percussion
D. Auscultation—diminished or absent breath sounds, egophony (an increased resonance of voice sounds heard when auscultating the lungs, often caused by lung consolidation and fibrosis), and pleural friction rub
E. General manifestations—compression atelectasis or mediastinal shift if pleural effusion severe

III. Diagnostic tests (Beaudoin, & Gonzalez, 2018; Jany & Welte, 2019).
A. Chest radiography—effusion size, position of mediastinum and diaphragm; blunting of costophrenic angle
B. Chest CT—to identify loculated effusion or alternative diagnosis
C. Ultrasonography—to assess pleural fluid volume; to identify optimal site for ultrasound-guided thoracentesis
D. Gastrointestinal (GI) disease—GI abscess, pancreatic disease, and postabdominal surgery
E. Pleural biopsy—increases diagnostic yield when combined with cytologic studies
F. Thoracentesis—pleural fluid withdrawal for cytology, chemical analysis, and culture (rule out infection); diagnostic and therapeutic

G. Pleural fluid evaluation (lactate dehydrogenase, glucose, protein)—to distinguish transudative or exudative fluid
1. Transudative—systemic factors causing effusion, such as CHF, cirrhosis, nephrotic syndrome, and hypoalbuminemia
2. Exudative—local factors causing effusion
a. Neoplastic—metastatic or primary tumor
b. Infectious—bacterial, fungal, viral, and parasitic
c. Pulmonary embolus

Management

(Dipper et al., 2020; Li et al., 2021)
I. Pharmacologic management
A. Manage pleural effusions (Fig. 46.1)
B. Therapeutic aspiration using intrapleural chemical agent; talc most efficacious, evidence-based
1. Obliterates the pleural space to prevent fluid reaccumulation
2. May improve patient comfort, relieve dyspnea for palliation
3. Reaccumulation of fluid is common
4. Potential for hypoproteinemia, pneumothorax, empyema, and fluid loculation
5. Hydrodissection with irrigation device into the pleural space
6. Talc pleurodesis if large effusion or recurrent
C. Thoracoscopic drainage and talc poudrage
D. Video-assisted thoracoscopic surgery
E. Indwelling pleural catheters—for palliative relief
F. Chemotherapy and mediastinal radiation—may be effective in responsive tumors (lymphoma, small cell lung cancer)

II. Nonpharmacologic management
A. Decrease symptom severity associated with pleural effusion
B. Educate about measures to increase the ease and effectiveness of breathing
C. Incorporate measures to minimize discomfort (e.g., opioid analgesia before chest tube insertion and as needed)
D. Recommend the use of relaxation techniques as indicated for coping with anxiety
E. Maximize safety
1. Encourage the use of assistive devices as needed for ADLs
2. Use the activity limitation and conservation of energy strategies
3. Instruct caregiver in the use of and precautions related to oxygen therapy
4. Instruct caregivers in the appropriate use of medications to manage disease
F. Monitor the consequences of therapy
1. Respiratory rate, rhythm, effort, and adventitious breath sounds
2. Characteristics of pain and relief measures
3. Subjective response to drainage and rate of fluid reaccumulation

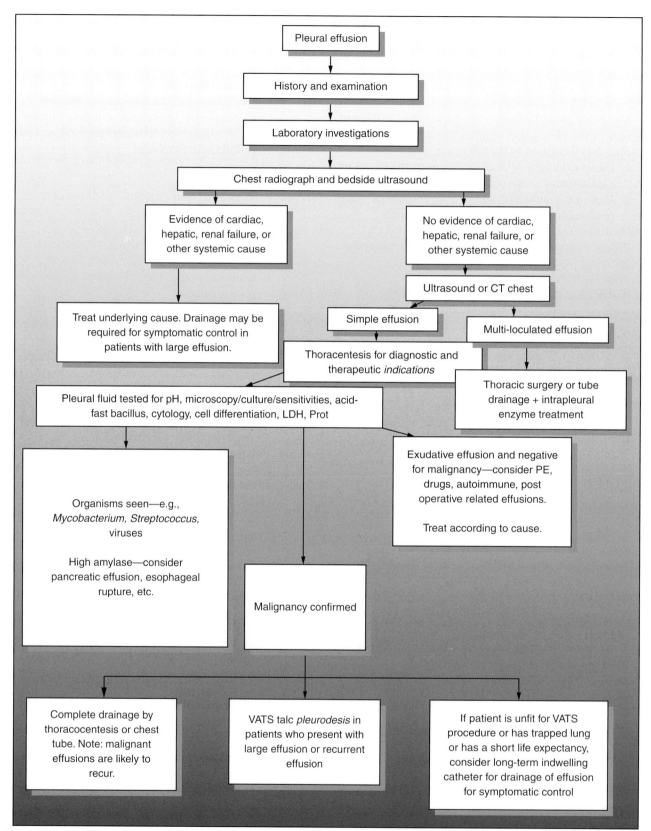

Fig. 46.1 Decision-making and management of pleural effusion. From Quinn, T., Alam, N., Aminazad, A., Marshall, M. B., & Choong, C. K. C. (2013). Decision making and algorithm for the management of pleural effusions. *Thoracic Surgery Clinics, 23*(1), 11–16. https://doi.org/10.1016/j. thorsurg.2012.10.009.

4. Report critical changes to the oncology provider—chest pain, fever, and change in the character of respiration.

G. Educate patient and caregiver regarding the following:
1. Activity limitation, conservation of energy strategies
2. Emergency care, available community resources
3. Signs and symptoms to report to the health care team
4. Procedures that may be required to alleviate pleural effusions

H. Enhance adaptation or rehabilitation
1. Assist the patient to maintain independence within the limitation of symptoms.
2. Encourage the patient and family to express concerns.

REFERENCES

Arroyo-Hernández, M., Maldonado, F., Lozano-Ruiz, F., Munoz-Montano, W., Nuñez-Baez, M., & Arrieta, O. (2021). Radiation-induced lung injury: Current evidence. *BMC Pulmonary Medicine*, 21(1), 9. https://doi.org/10.1186/s12890-020-01376-4.

Beaudoin, S., & Gonzalez, A. V. (2018). Evaluation of the patient with pleural effusion. *Canadian Medical Association Journal*, 190(10), E291–E295. https://doi.org/10.1503/cmaj.170420.

Budhwar, N., & Syed, Z. (2020). Chronic dyspnea: Diagnosis and evaluation. *American Family Physician*, 101(9), 542–548.

Campbell, M. L. (2018). Ensuring breathing comfort at the end of life: The integral role of the critical care nurse. *American Journal of Critical Care*, 27(3), 171. https://doi.org/10.4037/ajcc2018487.

Carter, B. W., Altan, M., Shroff, G. S., Truong, M. T., & Vlahos, I. (2022). Post-chemotherapy and targeted therapy imaging of the chest in lung cancer. *Clinical Radiology*, 77(1), e1–e10. https://doi.org/10.1016/j.crad.2021.08.001.

Dhamija, E., Meena, P., Ramalingam, V., Sahoo, R., Rastogi, S., & Thulkar, S. (2020). Chemotherapy-induced pulmonary complications in cancer: Significance of clinicoradiological correlation. *The Indian Journal of Radiology & Imaging*, 30(1), 20–26. https://doi.org/10.4103/ijri.IJRI_178_19.

Dipper, A., Jones, H. E., Bhatnagar, R., Preston, N. J., Maskell, N., & Clive, A. O. (2020). Interventions for the management of malignant pleural effusions: A network meta-analysis. *Cochrane Database of Systematic Reviews*, 4(4), CD010529. https://doi.org/10.1002/14651858.CD010529.pub3.

Feliciano, J. L., Waldfogel, J. M., Sharma, R., Zhang, A., Gupta, A., Sedhom, R., et al. (2021). Pharmacologic interventions for breathlessness in patients with advanced cancer: A systematic review and meta-analysis. *JAMA Network Open*, 4(2), e2037632. https://doi.org/10.1001/jamanetworkopen.2020.37632.

Giuranno, L., Ient, J., De Ruysscher, D., & Vooijs, M. A. (2019). Radiation-induced lung injury (RILI). *Frontiers in Oncology*, 9, 877. https://doi.org/10.3389/fonc.2019.00877.

Hartley, J. (2018). Respiratory rate 2: Anatomy and physiology of breathing. *Nursing Times*, 104(6), 43–44.

Hui, D. B., Bohlke, K., Bao, T., Campbell, T. C., Coyne, P. J., Currow, D. C., et al. (2021). Management of dyspnea in advanced cancer: ASCO guideline. *Journal of Clinical Oncology*, 39(12), 1389–1411. https://doi.org/10.1200/JCO.20.03465.

Isono, T., Kagiyama, N., Takano, K., Hosoda, C., Nishida, T., Kawate, E., et al. (2021). Outcome and risk factor of immune-related adverse events and pneumonitis in patients with advanced or postoperative recurrent non-small cell lung cancer treated with immune checkpoint inhibitors. *Thoracic Cancer*, 12(2), 153–164. https://doi.org/10.1111/1759-7714.13736.

Jany, B., & Welte, T. (2019). Pleural effusion in adults – Etiology, diagnosis, and treatment. *Deutsches Ärzteblatt International*, 116(21), 377–386. https://doi.org/10.3238/arztebl.2019.0377.

Kugasia, I., Kumar, A., Khatri, A., Saeed, F., Islam, H., & Epelbaum, O. (2019). Primary effusion lymphoma of the pleural space: Report of a rare complication of cardiac transplant with review of the literature. *Transplant Infectious Disease*, 21(1), e13005. https://doi.org/10.1111/tid.13005.

Li, D., Ajmal, S., Tufail, M., & Ranchal, R. K. (2021). Modern day management of a unilateral pleural effusion. *Clinical Medicine, Journal of the Royal College of Physicians of London*, 21(6), e561–e566. https://doi.org/10.7861/clinmed.2021-0617.

Lumb, A. B., & Thomas, C. R. (2020). *Nunn and Lamb's applied respiratory physiology* (9th ed.). Amsterdam: Elsevier.

Oncology Nursing Society (ONS). (2019). Dyspnea. https://www.ons.org/pep/dyspnea?display=pepnavigator&sort_by=created&items_per_page=50.

Postow, M. A., Sidlow, R., & Hellmann, M. D. (2018). Immune-related adverse events associated with immune checkpoint blockade. *New England Journal of Medicine*, 378, 158–168. https://doi.org/10.1056/NEJMra1703481.

Robinson, T., & Scullion, J. (2021). *Oxford handbook of respiratory nursing* (2nd ed.). Oxford: Oxford University Press.

Shannon, V. R. (2019). Cancer treatment-related lung injury. *Oncologic Critical Care*, 531–556. https://doi.org/10.1007/978-3-319-74588-6_52.

Sundaralingam, A., Bedawi, E. O., & Rahman, N. M. (2020). Diagnostics in pleural disease. *Diagnostics*, 10(12), 1046. https://doi.org/10.3390/diagnostics10121046.

Tvsvgk, T., Handa, A., Kumar, K., Mutreja, D., & Subramanian, S. (2021). Chemotherapy-associated pulmonary toxicity – Case series from a single center. *South Asian Journal of Cancer*, 10(4), 255–260. https://doi.org/10.1053/j.seminoncol.2005.11.005.

Wong, A., Galiabovitch, E., & Bhagwat, K. (2019). Management of primary spontaneous pneumothorax: A review. *ANZ Journal of Surgery*, 89(4), 303–308. https://doi.org/10.1111/ans.14713.

47

Sleep Disturbances

Shaunna Kersten and Jeannine M. Brant

OVERVIEW

I. Definition (Matthews, Carter, Page, Dean, & Berger, 2018; National Institute of Neurological Disorders and Stroke, 2019)
   A. Sleep—a dynamic and complex process—biological and behavior aspects to include duration, quality, sense of well-being.
   B. Sleep disturbances—actual or perceived disturbance in the sleep, resulting in daytime impairment and influenced by many factors—environment, sleep–wake regulation, emotions, blood pressure, light exposure, gene mutations, and medical conditions.
   C. Research in sleep and sleep disorders are ongoing.

II. Sleep disturbances—unsatisfactory sleep quantity and sleep quality
   A. Experienced by 30%–75% of cancer patients and is a problem for more than 15 million cancer survivors in the United States (Garland, Mahon, & Irwin, 2019; Matthews et al., 2018).
   B. Disruption of sleep–wake cycle—consequence of not enough sleep at the right time leads to poor sleep—often overlooked by health care professionals (Divani et al., 2022).
      1. Negatively impacts the ability to carry out activities of daily living and significantly diminishes the quality of life (Smith et al., 2018).
   C. Patients may not report symptoms due to thinking it is a normal reaction to the cancer diagnosis or treatment. Health care professionals may perceive sleep disturbances as a low priority (Jeon et al., 2021).
   D. Found to often present in a cluster of symptoms with fatigue, anxiety, and depression (National Comprehensive Cancer Network, 2022; Oh, Kim, Na, Cho, & Chu, 2019).
   E. Commonly referred to as sleep disorders.

III. Common sleep disorders
   A. Insomnia—the most common type of sleep disorder characterized by difficulty getting to sleep, maintaining sleep, frequent awakenings during sleep, and problems returning to sleep or nonrestorative sleep contributing to reduced quality of life. People with cancer report a higher incidence of insomnia (Patel, Steinberg, & Patel, 2018; Roth, 2019).
   B. Circadian rhythm disorder—A disruption in the 24-hour sleep–wake cycle (our "biological clock") that influences the ability to go to sleep, maintain sleep, or waking up too early despite adequate circumstances for sleep (Edinger et al., 2021).
   C. Sleep-related disordered breathing (sleep apnea, snoring)
   D. Hypersomnia—excessive sleepiness (narcolepsy)

IV. Physiology
   A. Sleep–wake cycle (National Cancer Institute 2021)
      1. Consists of two stages
         a. Rapid eye movement (REM)—Fourth stage of sleep where the brain is active—known as dream sleep. Important for concentration, memory, and learning.
         b. Non-REM—quiet or restful sleep—includes three stages from light to deep sleep.
      2. Stages repeat, with each cycle lasting approximately 90 minutes and cycles occurring 4–6 times during a 7- to 8-hour sleep period.
      3. Dictated by an inherent biological clock or circadian rhythm.
   B. Risk factors—several risk factors can increase the prevalence of disturbed sleep (Matthews et al., 2018; National Cancer Institute 2021).
   C. Lifestyle
      1. Sleep hygiene practices: daytime naps, use of caffeine, and/or nicotine close to bedtime, lack of daily exercise, lack of a regular bedtime schedule, and poor nutrition.
   D. Demographic
      1. Older patients may already experience sleep disturbances before diagnosis due to age-related changes in sleep patterns and circadian rhythm (Patel et al., 2018).
      2. Menopause, which may be treatment induced (Otte, Carpenter, Roberts, & Elkins, 2020)
   E. Environment
      1. Disrupted sleep in hospitalized patients—can be due to frequent monitoring.
      2. Temperature of room—cool is preferred between 60- and 67-degrees Fahrenheit.
      3. Room setup—lighting, noise, clutter, television, and sharing space with others.
      4. Electronic devices
   F. Disease related

1. Paraneoplastic syndrome (increased steroid production), tumor invasion symptoms—pain, fever, cough, shortness of breath, fatigue, and pruritus (National Cancer Institute, 2021).
2. Sleep disturbances are common to breast, lung cancer, head and neck, and gynecological cancer (Lin et al., 2019).
3. Psychiatric disorders—depression, anxiety (Roth, 2019).
4. Medications—opioids, caffeine, steroids, dietary supplements, some antidepressants, nicotine, and alcohol.
5. Psychological—pain, loss of function, inability to care for self, cost of treatment, and lost work.
   G. Treatment-related factors
   1. Side effects of systemic chemotherapy (nausea, vomiting, diarrhea, fatigue, depression, and steroids).

ASSESSMENT

I. History and physical information (Matthews et al., 2018; Strik et al., 2021)
   A. Sleep history
   B. Prior or current treatments and side effects—surgical intervention (pain, opioid use), systemic chemotherapy, radiation, hormonal therapy, biologic and targeted therapies, and steroids.
   C. Presence of concurrent psychiatric disorder (depression, anxiety, and delirium).
   D. Current medications—opioids, sedatives/hypnotics, steroids, caffeine/nicotine, alcohol, some antidepressants, decongestants, stimulants, and illegal drugs.
   E. Dietary supplements and alternative therapies—should be addressed.
   F. Environment factors—hospitalization (frequent checks, roommates, lights on/off, and noise) or at home (temperature of room, lights, sounds, and others in room).
   G. Physical stressors—inability to move self, pain, and limited motion.
   H. Psychological stressors—depression, fatigue, cancer fears, fear of loss of income, increased cost of health care, fear of death, and burden on caregiver.
   I. Diet and exercise history—dietary supplement usage, over-the-counter herbal remedies, alternative therapies, regular exercise routine, and nutrition status.
II. Sleep screening
   A. Screening questions (Smith et al., 2018)
   1. Are you having any problems falling asleep or staying asleep?
   2. Are you dissatisfied with your sleep?
   3. Do you feel refreshed in the morning?
   4. Are you experiencing excessive sleepiness?
   5. Have you been told that you snore frequently or stop breathing during sleep?
   6. Do you have an uncomfortable urge to move your legs frequently?
   B. Screen at regular intervals and with any changes in clinical status

C. If yes to screening, conduct a more in-depth assessment—consider using sleep disturbance scales (Epworth Sleepiness Scale, Pittsburgh Sleep Quality Index [PSQI]) (Lin et al., 2019).
III. Characterization of quality sleep (National Sleep Foundation, 2020)
   A. Sleep patterns—usual bedtime, bedtime routine, and how long it takes to fall asleep.
   1. Sleep duration—episodes of being awake, ability to fall back asleep, and feeling restored upon awakening.
   2. Alterations in sleep after cancer diagnosis; sleep changes with treatment as well as hospitalization.
   3. Family/personal history of sleep disturbances.
   4. Others' perceptions of patient sleep quantity and quality.
IV. Objective tools for measuring sleep quality
   A. Polysomnography—diagnostic tool to diagnose sleep disorders such as sleep-related breathing disorders and limb movement disorders (sleep apnea).
   B. Testing can be time-consuming, expensive, and impractical for scheduling.
   C. Actigraphy—noninvasive sensor worn on the wrist over days to weeks to measure sleep–wake patterns and diagnose circadian rhythm disorders—may be helpful to identify sleep disruptions, discrepancies in self-reported data and objective data, and assess response to treatments and guide management (Smith et al., 2018).
   D. Sleep questionnaires and sleep assessment tools—some include Epworth Sleep Scale, PSQI.

MANAGEMENT

I. Pharmacologic management (Fang, Tu, Sheng, & Shao, 2019; Matthews et al., 2018; National Cancer Institute, 2021)
   A. While many agents are Food and Drug Administration approved for sleep, most have not been well tested in patients with cancer; medications are intended for short-term management of sleep disorders, as long term can exacerbate sleep disturbances and depression.
   B. Hypnotics—used for help with getting to sleep. Most widely used to treat insomnia; may be preferred in cancer patients when a hypnotic effect is desired (next-day drowsiness is the major side effect).
   1. Benzodiazepines—commonly used class of hypnotics—associated with a higher risk for tolerance, dependence, withdrawal. May carry a higher risk of loss of motor coordination, falls, increased risk of delirium, and memory impairment in the older adult.
   C. Nonhypnotics
   1. Nonbenzodiazepines (the "Z" drugs)—preferred for their low-risk profile and benefit.
   2. Antihistamines—treats only difficulty falling asleep, limited evidence for insomnia. May be preferred if concerned about cross-dependence; must be used with caution in older adults due to anticholinergic effects. May contribute to brain fog and forgetfulness.

3. Antidepressants—first-line agent when insomnia is associated with depression or anxiety symptoms.
4. Melatonin receptor agonists—endogenous hormone produced by the pineal gland during hours of darkness—may be used for the treatment of difficulties falling asleep and/or circadian sleep disorders. Little to no risk of other impairments/dependence, does not treat difficulties staying asleep.
5. Antipsychotic—sedating effects; generally not preferred and should be considered as last resort due to serious side effect profile.
6. Alpha-adrenergic receptor blocker—may prevent nightmares in PTSD sleep disorders—acts to relax muscles, developed to treat hypertension and benign prostatic hypertrophy.
7. Orexin receptor antagonist—blocks orexin in the brain, to inhibit arousal by decreasing the time it takes to fall asleep and increasing total sleep time. The controlled substance suvorexant is the only agent on the market—long-term data are lacking.
8. Cannabinoids—tetrahydrocannabinol and cannabidiol—efficacy and safety as treatment for sleep disorders remains unclear; further investigation needed.

II. Nonpharmacologic management (National Cancer Institute, 2021)
A. Sleep disturbances can change throughout the cancer continuum—sleep quality should be continually assessed.
B. Determine sleep quality—taking less than 30 minutes to get to sleep, waking up once or less during the night, spending less than 20 minutes awake, and spending 85% of time actually asleep when in bed (National Sleep Foundation 2020).
C. Promote sleep hygiene—interventions which promote quality sleep.
   1. Support patient to establish a routine of only going to bed when sleepy at about the same time each night and waking up at the same time each day. Encourage patient to use the bed and bedroom only for sleep or sex (sleep restriction).
   2. Educate patient on developing a bedtime routine, such as trying to do something relaxing before sleep—meditation, listening to soothing music, taking a warm bath, dim lights, and journaling (relaxation therapy).
   3. Have patient avoid caffeine after noontime, avoid heavy meals in evening, avoid alcohol, and no smoking within 6 hours of bedtime.
   4. Promote a restful environment; comfortable bedding, a bedroom free from distraction; avoid television, phones, texting, tablets, iPad, blue screens, and looking at mail in bed.
D. Provide interventions to maximize patient comfort.
   1. Treat contributing factors; pain, depression, anxiety, delirium, and nausea.
   2. Skin care—protect skin, use of alcohol- and fragrance-free moisturizers and soaps.
   3. Coordinate bedside contacts so as to not interrupt sleep for the hospitalized cancer patient.
E. Cognitive behavior therapy (CBT) (Garland et al., 2019; National Cancer Institute 2021).
   1. CBT—first line of treatment recommended for patients with most sleep disturbances and insomnia sleep disorder.
      a. A technique which helps the individual to recognize negative thoughts and change them into positive thoughts.
      b. Most commonly used for insomnia—involves stress reduction, relaxation, and sleep schedule management; limit role of bed to sleep and sex, restrict time spent in bed, and sleep hygiene (Fang et al., 2019).
      c. CBT combined with relaxation therapies have shown to be as effective as pharmacologic therapies; studies with cancer patients—although limited—demonstrate CBT to improve sleep and have sustained benefit.
   2. Cognitive therapies combined with relaxation therapies have shown to be as effective as pharmacologic therapies—studies with cancer patients are limited, though preliminary research shows improved sleep with sustained benefit.
F. Integrative therapies—alternative methods to promote sleep (Garland et al., 2019).
   1. Meditative therapies—meditation, yoga, qi gong, tai chi, and music therapy.
   2. Body based—massage, acupressure, and acupuncture (shows to deliver sleep benefit in the cancer patient) (Liou et al., 2020).
   3. Light therapy (Wu et al., 2018)
      a. Exposure to natural light for at least 20–30 minutes each day.
      b. Bright light therapy delivered in the morning to reset the sleep–wake cycle.

REFERENCES

Divani, A., Heidari, M. E., Ghavampour, N., Parouhan, A., Ahmadi, S., Charan, O. N., et al. (2022). Effect of cancer treatment on sleep quality in cancer patients: A systematic review and meta-analysis of Pittsburgh Sleep Quality Index. *Supportive Care in Cancer*, *30*(6), 4687–4697. https://pubmed.ncbi.nlm.nih.gov/35079904/.

Edinger, J. D., Arnedt, J. T., Bertisch, S. M., Carney, C. E., Harrington, J. J., Lichstein, K. L., et al. (2021). Behavioral and psychological treatments for chronic insomnia disorder in adults: An American Academy of Sleep Medicine clinical practice guideline. *Journal of Clinical Sleep Medicine*, *17*(2), 255–262. https://doi.org/10.5664/jcsm.8986.

Fang, H., Tu, S., Sheng, J., & Shao, A. (2019). Depression in sleep disturbance: A review on a bidirectional relationship, mechanisms and treatment. *Journal of Cellular and Molecular Medicine*, *23*(4), 2324–2332. https://doi.org/10.1111/jcmm.14170.

Garland, S. N., Mahon, K., & Irwin, M. R. (2019). Integrative approaches for sleep health in cancer survivors. *Cancer Journal* (Sudbury, Mass.), *25*(5), 337–342. https://doi.org/10.1097/PPO.0000000000000398.

Garland, S. N., Xie, S. X., DuHamel, K., Bao, T., Li, Q., Barg, F. K., et al. (2019). Acupuncture versus cognitive behavioral therapy for insomnia in cancer survivors: A randomized clinical trial. *Journal of the National Cancer Institute, 111*(12), 1323–1331. https://doi.org/10.1093/jnci/djz050.

Jeon, M. S., Agar, M. R., Koh, E.-S., Nowak, A. K., Hovey, E. J., & Dhillon, H. M. (2021). Barriers to managing sleep disturbance in people with malignant brain tumours and their caregivers: A qualitative analysis of healthcare professionals' perception. *Supportive Care in Cancer, 29*(7), 3865–3876. https://doi.org/10.1007/s00520-020-05970-4.

Lin, C.-Y., Cheng, A. S. K., Nejati, B., Imani, V., Ulander, M., et al. (2019). A thorough psychometric comparison between Athens Insomnia Scale and Insomnia Severity Index among patients with advanced cancer. *Journal of Sleep Research, 29*(1), e12891. https://doi.org/10.1111/jsr.12891.

Liou, K. T., Root, J. C., Garland, S. N., Green, J., Li, Y., Li, Q. S., et al. (2020). Effects of acupuncture versus cognitive behavioral therapy on cognitive function in cancer survivors with insomnia: A secondary analysis of a randomized clinical trial. *Cancer, 126*(13), 3042–3052. https://doi.org/10.1002/cncr.32847.

Matthews, E., Carter, P., Page, M., Dean, G., & Berger, A. (2018). Sleep-wake disturbance: A systematic review of evidence-based interventions for management in patients with cancer. *Clinical Journal of Oncology Nursing, 22*(1), 37–52. https//doi.org/10.1188/18.CJON.37-52.

National Cancer Institute. (2021). Sleep disorders (PDQ®)—Health professional version. https://www.cancer.gov/about-cancer/treatment/side-effects/sleep-disorders-hp-pdq#_86.

National Comprehensive Cancer Network. (2022). Clinical practice guidelines in oncology. Cancer-related fatigue (version 2.2022). https://www.nccn.org/professionals/physician_gls/pdf/fatigue.pdf.

National Institute of Neurological Disorders and Stroke. (2019). Brain basics: Understanding sleep. https://www.ninds.nih.gov/health-information/public-education/brain-basics/brain-basics-understanding-sleep.

National Sleep Foundation. (2020). What is sleep quality? Sleep and you. https://www.thensf.org/what-is-sleep-quality/#:~:text=Sleep%20quality%20is%20the%20measurement,the%20sleep%20you%20are%20getting.

Oh, C.-M., Kim, H. Y., Na, H. K., Cho, K. H., & Chu, M. K. (2019). The effect of anxiety and depression on sleep quality of individuals with high risk for insomnia: A population-based study. *Frontiers in Neurology, 10*, 849. https://doi.org/10.3389/fneur.2019.00849.

Otte, J. L., Carpenter, J. S., Roberts, L., & Elkins, G. R. (2020). Self-hypnosis for sleep disturbances in menopausal women. *Journal of Women's Health, 29*(3), 461–463. https://doi.org/10.1089/jwh.2020.8327.

Patel, D., Steinberg, J., & Patel, P. (2018). Insomnia in the elderly: A review. *Journal of Clinical Sleep Medicine, 14*(6), 1017–1024. https://doi.org/10.5664/jcsm.7172.

Roth, T. (2007). Insomnia: Definition, prevalence, etiology and consequences. *Journal of Clinical Sleep Medicine, 3*(5 Suppl), S7–S10. https://jcsm.aasm.org/doi/10.5664/jcsm.26929.

Smith, M. T., McCrae, C. S., Cheung, J., Martin, J. L., Harrod, C. G., Heald, J. L., et al. (2018). Use of actigraphy for the evaluation of sleep disorders and circadian rhythm sleep-wake disorders: An American Academy of Sleep Medicine systematic review, meta-analysis, and GRADE assessment. *Journal of Clinical Sleep Medicine, 14*(7), 1209–1230. https://doi.org/10.5664/jcsm.7228.

Strik, H., Cassel, W., Teepker, M., Schulte, T., Riera-Knorrenschild, J., Koehler, U., et al. (2021). Why do our cancer patients sleep so badly? Sleep disorders in cancer patients: A frequent symptom with multiple causes. *Oncology Research and Treatment, 44*(9), 469–475. https://doi.org/10.1159/000518108.

Wu, L. M., Amidi, A., Valdimarsdottir, H., Ancoli-Israel, S., Liu, L., Winkel, G., et al. (2018). The effect of systematic light exposure on sleep in a mixed group of fatigued cancer survivors. *Journal of Clinical Sleep Medicine, 14*(1), 31–39. https://doi.org/10.5664/jcsm.6874.

48

Metabolic Emergencies

Elizabeth Delaney

DISSEMINATED INTRAVASCULAR COAGULATION

Overview

I. Definition—a systemic disorder of coagulation
   A. Disseminated intravascular coagulation (DIC) is usually secondary to an underlying disorder that causes an activation of coagulation which is often overactive (National Institute of Health [NIH], 2019; Smith 2021).
   B. Extensive intravascular thrombi cause end-organ damage.
   C. Hemorrhage due to the consumption of platelets and coagulation factors (Robison, 2017).
   D. According to the NIH (2019), DIC can also be called consumption coagulopathy.
   E. DIC can either be
      1. Acute and start over hours or days. The DIC develops quickly, resulting in widespread blood clots in smaller vessels and dangerous bleeding. Clotting occurs first, followed by bleeding, which is the result of the consumption of clotting factors. Bleeding into organs is a common presenting factor. Blood clots in small vessels may cause dysfunction and organ failure. Examples of affected organs include lungs, kidneys, brain, heart, liver, spleen, adrenals, pancreas, and gastrointestinal (GI) tract.
      2. Chronic and develops slower. The DIC occurs with exposure to smaller amounts of thrombin over a longer period (i.e., weeks). Consumption of platelets and coagulation factors occurs but happens more slowly, which allows the body time to compensate. Patients with chronic DIC may present with more blood-clotting complications or symptoms (Robison, 2017).
      3. Inflammation/sepsis, cancer, and blood transfusion reactions can be common causes (National Institutes of Health, 2019; Robison, 2017; Venes, 2021).

II. Pathophysiology of DIC begins with understanding the normal.
   A. An understanding of the normal physiology of clot formation is essential to understand the pathophysiology of DIC (Smith, 2021; Venes, 2021). Following is a description of normal steps in the coagulation pathway (Table 48.1).
      1. Extrinsic pathway (factor VII) activated with damage to endothelial lining of blood vessels, leading to release of tissue factor
      2. Intrinsic pathway (factor XII) activated with damage to subendothelial tissue
      3. Extrinsic and intrinsic pathways come together; comprise the common pathway
      4. Results in clot formation and activation of coagulation cascade (Fig. 48.1)
      5. With a normal coagulation system, homeostasis is achieved when there is a balance between clot formation and breakdown—a balance between the two (Robison, 2017; Fig. 48.2).
      6. Cofactors can enhance or accelerate this process. Common cofactors in patients with cancer may include cancer procoagulant.

III. Activation of DIC
   A. DIC is usually secondary to an underlying disorder that causes excessive activation of coagulation (NIH, 2019; Smith, 2021).
   B. DIC can be a complication from inflammation/sepsis, cancer, and blood transfusion as stated above; also liver disease, severe tissue injuries such as burns, pregnancy complications, or trauma (Levi, 2020; NIH, 2019).
   C. Cancers associated with DIC include acute and chronic leukemias, especially acute promyelocytic, lymphomas, and solid cancers, such as prostate, lung, breast, stomach, biliary, colon, pancreatic, cholangiocarcinoma, and ovarian. Most are adenocarcinoma (Robison, 2017; Blackburn, Bender, & Brown, 2019).
   D. COVID-induced DIC may be slightly different and mimics other post-viral illness DIC (Frame et al., 2022).

TABLE 48.1 Normal Laboratory Values Related to Coagulation

Laboratory Test	Results
Platelet count	150,000–400,000/mm³
Fibrinogen	1.8–4 g/L
Thrombin time	7–12 s
Protein C level	4 µg/mL
Protein S level	23 µg/mL
Prothrombin time	11–14 s
Activated partial thromboplastin time	30–40 s
International normalized ratio	1–1.2 times normal
Fibrin degradation products	<10 mg/mL
D-Dimer assay	<500 ng/mL
Bilirubin level	0.1–0.2 mg/dL
Blood urea nitrogen	8–21 mg/dL

Adapted from Morton, P. G., Fontaine, D. K., Hudak, C. M., & Gallo, B. M. (Eds.). (2005). *Critical care nursing: A holistic approach* (8th ed.). Philadelphia, PA: Lippincott, Williams and Wilkins.

Assessment

I. Physical examination
  A. Skin symptoms—pallor, petechiae, jaundice, ecchymosis, hematomas, acral cyanosis (irregularly shaped blue or gray discolored areas on extremities), bleeding from any site of invasive procedures (i.e., intravenous [IV], drains or dressing sites), back/flank ecchymoses associated with retroperitoneal hemorrhage. Microvascular symptoms in small vessels become more quickly occluded, for example, digits, earlobes, and genitalia.
    1. Purpura fulminans is a rare and serious condition that is demonstrated by widespread hemorrhagic skin necrosis and tissue thrombosis.
  B. Eyes, ears, mouth, nose, and throat symptoms—visual disturbances, scleral injection, periorbital edema, subconjunctival hemorrhage, eye or ear pain, petechiae on nasal or oral mucosa, epistaxis, tenderness or bleeding from gums.
  C. Cardiac symptoms—tachycardia, hypotension, diminished peripheral pulses, changes in color, and temperature of extremities.
  D. Respiratory symptoms—dyspnea, tachypnea, hypoxia, hemoptysis, cyanosis, shortness of breath.
  E. GI symptoms—tarry stools, hematemesis, abdominal pain, abdominal distention, positive results of guaiac stool test.
  F. Genitourinary (GU) symptoms—hematuria (burning, dysuria, and frequency associated with hematuria), decreased urinary output.
  G. Musculoskeletal symptoms—joint pain and stiffness.
  H. Neurologic symptoms—headache, mental status changes (NIH, 2019; Robison, 2017; Smith, 2021)
II. Diagnostic and laboratory data
  A. Laboratory studies (Table 48.2)

Management

I. Treat the underlying cause; once the underlying cause is managed, DIC will likely correct itself, but this is dependent on the degree of ischemia, necrosis, and organ damage that has occurred (Robison, 2017; NIH, 2019).
  A. Laboratory data, patient condition, and underlying cause should be used to determine effective treatment strategies.
  B. Pharmacologic and hematologic management based on patient assessment.
    1. Avoid medications that affect platelet function.
    2. Transfusion of platelets, fresh frozen plasma (FFP), and cryoprecipitate; should be administered prior to red blood cells or RBCs may bleed out the vasculature (Smith, 2021).
    3. Use of anticoagulants (e.g., heparin, low-molecular-weight heparin)—may be used in DIC when there is continued bleeding and clotting despite ongoing treatment. Anticoagulants should only be considered when the platelet count is at least 50,000/mm³. Contraindications due to increasing risk of hemorrhage include history of acute promyelocytic leukemia, GI bleeding, central nervous system disorders, recent surgery, open wounds, or obstetrical complications that require surgery (Robison, 2017).
    4. Use of fibrinolytic agents (e.g., epsilon–aminocaproic acid, tranexamic acid)—can be used in severe cases in which bleeding does not respond to other therapies (NIH, 2019).
    5. Use of defibrotide with COVID-induced DIC (Frame et al., 2022).
    6. IV fluids, as needed, for volume repletion.
    7. Oxygen therapy, as needed (NIH, 2019).
  C. Nonpharmacologic management
    1. Interventions to manage sites of active bleeding
      a. Application of pressure to bleeding sites via pressure dressing or sandbag, or consider topical hemostatic agents and tissue adhesives.
      b. Manage clotting with warming devices, peripheral limb wrapping, and ensure fluid balance.
      c. Assess the role of spirituality in the patient and the impact of receiving blood products. Discuss blood substitute products for those who do not use blood products.
    2. Interventions for maximizing patient safety
      a. Assistance with activities of daily living to avoid unnecessary skin bumping or scraping, as well as heavy lifting or straining
      b. Use of electric razor instead of straight-edge razor
      c. Educate patient and caregiver
        (1) Possible risks related to injury/falls
        (2) Critical signs and symptoms to report, such as bruising; red rash; headache; black stool; blood in urine or stool; bleeding from gums,

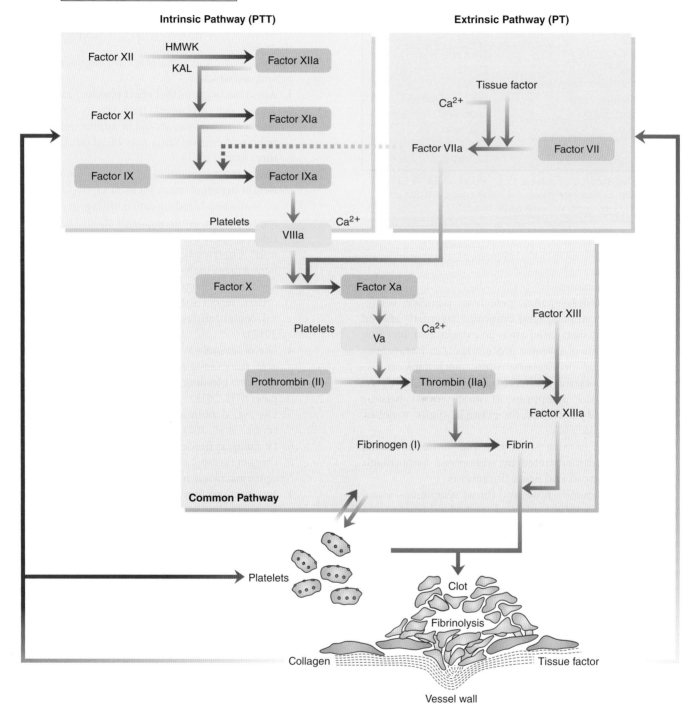

Fig. 48.1 Coagulation cascade. *PT*, Prothrombin time; *PTT*, partial thromboplastin time. From Copstead, L., & Banasik, J. L. (2014). *Pathophysiology* (5th ed.). St. Louis, MO: Elsevier.

nose, eyes, vagina, rectum, wound(s), or central venous access device

(3) Avoidance of over-the-counter medications that may interfere with normal platelet function such as aspirin and nonsteroidal antiinflammatory drugs (NSAIDs)

d. Provide close supervision for mobilization with appropriate device and footwear needed for ambulation.

e. If hospitalized, place bed in low locked position, two side rails up, call bell within reach, with clear pathways for ambulation.

A primary condition such as septicemia, obstetric complication, severe burns, or trauma causes

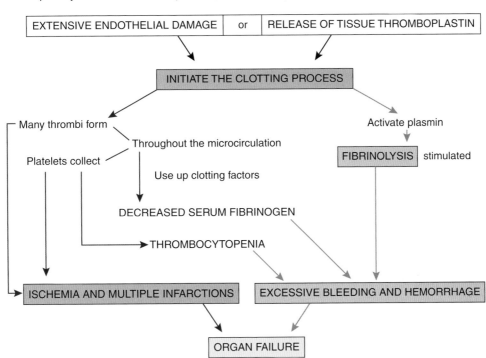

Fig. 48.2 DIC cascade. *DIC,* Disseminated intravascular coagulation. From VanMeter, K. C., & Hubert, R. J. (2018). *Gould's pathophysiology for the health professions* (6th ed.). St. Louis, MO: Elsevier.

TABLE 48.2 Laboratory Results With Disseminated Intravascular Coagulation

Increased Values	Decreased Values	Other
Thrombin time	Platelet count	Schistocytes present on peripheral smear
Prothrombin time	Fibrinogen level	
Activated partial thromboplastin time	Protein C level	
International normalized ratio	Protein S level	
Fibrin degradation products	Antithrombin III level	
D-Dimer assay	Hemoglobin if anemia present	
Bilirubin level		
Blood urea nitrogen		

From Boral, B. M., Williams, D. J., & Boral, L. I. (2016). Disseminated intravascular coagulation. *American Journal of Clinical Pathology, 146*(6), 670–680. https://doi.org/10.1093/ajcp/aqw195.

    f. If appropriate, schedule a home assessment with home nursing care and physical therapy (Robison, 2017).

  3. Interventions to assist in coping

    a. Assess available resources for patient and caregivers.

    b. Provide emotional support for patient and caregivers.

THROMBOTIC THROMBOCYTOPENIC PURPURA

Overview

I. Definition—thrombotic thrombocytopenic purpura (TTP) is a thrombotic microangiopathy, a disorder of blood clotting related to endothelial injury in which platelet-rich thrombi are created in the microvasculature leading to microangiopathic hemolytic anemia, severe thrombocytopenia, and ischemic end–organ damage (Chiasakul & Cuker, 2018).

II. Pathogenesis of TTP

  A. von Willebrand factor (VWF) is a central component of hemostasis, serving both as a carrier for factor VIII and as an adhesive link between platelets and the injured blood vessel wall (Johnson & Ginsburg, 2021).

  B. The ADAMTS13 enzyme is responsible for cleaving and breaking down the ultra-large VWF into small components (Hoffman, 2020).

    a. An anti-ADAMTS13 antibody inactivates the enzyme for an unknown reason.

  C. There is a lack of ADAMTS13, either hereditary or acquired, leading to ultra-large amounts of VWF not being broken down and instead continuing to stick to the endothelium, collecting platelets that pass by, which results in the formation of thrombi in small vessels (Hoffman, 2020).

  D. These increased clumps cause RBCs passing over them to be damaged, resulting in fragmented RBCs or schistocytes (Hoffman, 2020).

III. TTP occurs secondary to hereditary or acquired causes.
   A. Hereditary (Shatzel & Taylor, 2017)
      1. Hereditary TTP is an autosomal-recessive disorder and very rare.
      2. Hereditary TTP is caused by a deficiency of ADAMTS13, a regulator of VWF secreted by endothelial cells, and manifests in childhood or young adulthood, typically after an event (e.g., surgery or infectious process).
      3. ADAMTS13 multiple mutations have been linked to TTP.
   B. Acquired (Shatzel & Taylor, 2017)
      1. Acquired TTP is consistent with severe VWF cleaving protease deficiency and can be caused by
         a. Cancer
         b. Infection, HIV
         c. Autoimmune diseases such as systemic lupus erythematosus
         d. Drug induced (such as quinine, ticlopidine, and clopidogrel)
         e. Chemotherapeutic agents (such as mitomycin-C, cisplatin, gemcitabine, bleomycin, and pentostatin)
         f. Anticancer agents (such as bevacizumab)
         g. Pregnancy

Assessment

I. Physical examination (Scully, 2021)
   A. General—fever and overall weakness
   B. Skin symptoms—jaundice, pallor, mucosal bleeding, petechiae, and ecchymosis
   C. Cardiac symptoms—arrhythmia, chest pain, and tachycardia
   D. Respiratory symptoms—shortness of breath due to anemia
   E. Head, eyes, ears, nose, throat (HEENT) symptoms—visual disturbance, aphasia, epistaxis, and retinal hemorrhage
   F. GI symptoms—nausea, vomiting, diarrhea, and abdominal pain
   G. Neurologic symptoms—highest incidence of adverse effects including headache, confusion, cerebral vascular events, dizziness, seizures, paresthesia, fever, and altered level of consciousness
   H. Musculoskeletal symptoms—weakness
   I. Renal symptoms—oliguria, renal compromise
II. Diagnostic and laboratory data
   A. ADAMTS13 assays important in diagnosis; however, multiple versions of the assay exist, and testing takes time (Hoffman, 2020).
   B. Laboratory studies
      1. Improved reliability and timeliness of ADAMTS13 testing
      2. Complete blood cell count (CBC) (Scully, 2021)
         a. Decreased hemoglobin or hematocrit
         b. Decreased platelet count (<50,000 or 50% decrease from the previous count)
         c. Elevated reticulocyte count or lactate dehydrogenase (LDH)
      3. Coombs test can help rule out hemolytic anemia.
      4. Coagulation studies
         a. INR less than 1.5 (Hoffman, 2020)
      5. Peripheral blood smear
         a. Schistocytes likely on peripheral smear (Chiasakul & Cuker, 2018)
      6. Metabolic panel
         a. Indications of hemolysis on the metabolic panel
            (1) Elevated LDH
            (2) Elevated bilirubin
            (3) Elevated blood urea nitrogen and creatinine (Hoffman, 2020)
      7. Urinalysis
         a. Presence of RBCs and proteinuria in urinalysis may occur

Management

I. Medical management (Scully, 2021; Chiasakul & Cuker, 2018; Hoffman, 2020)
   A. Plasma exchange (plasmapheresis) was the first method to use in management of TTP, continues to be an option
   B. FFP used to replace the plasma removed in plasma exchange
   C. Other blood products as needed
   D. High-dose steroids shown to be effective in treatment; need to proceed with caution with an ill cancer patient due to toxicities
   E. Platelet transfusions should only be used in life-threatening emergencies in which the patient has severe bleeding or hemorrhage.
   F. Rituximab—used in patients with autoimmune TTP; other promising agents in development
   G. Cyclosporine is a potential prophylactic treatment; can be used in conjunction with plasma exchange.
   H. Discontinue drugs that may prompt TTP.
   I. IV fluids as needed for volume repletion
   J. Oxygen therapy as needed
II. Nursing management
   A. Monitor ongoing for bleeding and clotting complications.
      1. Monitor laboratory values, specifically platelet count.
      2. Inspect skin, wounds, and insertion sites for bleeding.
      3. Apply pressure to sites of bleeding via pressure dressing or sandbag.
      4. Monitor for neurologic symptoms and renal failure.
   B. Assist with coping.
      1. Assess the available resources for patient and caregiver support.
      2. Provide education specific to TTP and its signs and symptoms.
      3. Assess and employ the strategies for fatigue if anemia is present.
      4. Provide positive feedback to patients and caregivers through coaching and listening.
      5. Suggest resources such as psychological counseling and pastoral care services for emotional and spiritual support (Saha, McDaniel, & Zheng, 2017).

SYNDROME OF INAPPROPRIATE ANTIDIURETIC HORMONE

Overview

I. Definition—syndrome or secretion of inappropriate antidiuretic hormone (SIADH) is a condition in which antidiuretic hormone (ADH), in activated form called *arginine vasopressin* (*AVP*), is inappropriately excreted resulting in water retention and excess excretion of electrolytes, ultimately leading to hypotonic hyponatremia. This can be a result of cancers (Harrois & Anstey, 2019).

II. Pathophysiology of SIADH (Mount, 2022; Maloney, 2017)
   A. ADH is converted to AVP as its active form throughout the body.
   B. AVP or Vasopressin is an antidiuretic hormone synthesized by the posterior pituitary gland to maintain a proper water balance between 280 and 295 mOsm/kg. ADH is released in its activated form (AVP) when stimulated, causing renal tubules to absorb more sodium and water.
   C. In SIADH, ADH is secreted even though the osmolality is normal, causing a dilutional hyponatremia. In addition, aldosterone secretion is decreased, and atrial natriuretic peptide is secreted, which combine to worsen hyponatremia. Potassium loss also occurs. In addition, SIADH stimulates the thirst mechanism, which adds to the imbalance of intake and output, contributing to hyponatremia.
   D. Cancer cells can cause an abnormal release of AVP released in response to
      1. Changes in plasma osmolality
      2. Changes in plasma volume
         a. Results in an increase in free water in extracellular fluid
         b. Causes plasma hypo-osmolality and serum hyponatremia
         c. Sodium excreted from the kidneys
         d. Intracellular edema—as fluid shifts from extracellular to intracellular spaces, cerebral edema occurs

III. Causes of SIADH (Harrois & Anstey, 2019)
   A. Nervous system disorders—infections (abscess, meningitis, and encephalitis), bleeding (subdural hematoma, subarachnoid hemorrhage, and traumatic brain injury), brain tumors, multiple sclerosis, or thrombosis.
   B. Lung disease—infections (bacterial, viral, abscess, tuberculosis, and aspergillosis), cystic fibrosis, or positive pressure ventilation
   C. Drug induced (those that stimulate AVP release, enhance action of AVP, or have unknown mechanism of action). Numerous medications may be responsible.
      1. Antidepressant agents (selective serotonin reuptake inhibitors, tricyclic antidepressants)
      2. Neuroleptics (clofibrate, carbamazepine, sodium valproate, and chlorpropamide)
      3. Chemotherapeutic agents, including vincristine, ifosfamide, and cyclophosphamide
      4. NSAIDs
      5. Nicotine
      6. Amiodarone
      7. Proton pump inhibitors
      8. Vasopressin analogs (desmopressin, oxytocin, terlipressin, and vasopressin)
   D. Cancer (Yeung et al., 2022)
      1. Etiology of SIADH in cancer patients—cancer causes the release of a similar protein to ADH, called atrial natriuretic factor. This mimics the ADH, causing the renal excretion of sodium leading to water retention in the system.
         a. Cancers most likely to cause SIADH (Harrois & Anstey, 2019; Yeung et al., 2022)
            (1) Small-cell lung cancer
            (2) Non–small-cell lung cancer
            (3) Oropharyngeal
            (4) GI and pancreatic
            (5) GU
            (6) Head and neck cancer
            (7) Mesothelioma
            (8) Lymphoma
            (9) Sarcoma

Assessment

I. Physical examination (Mentrasti et al., 2020)
   A. Presentation—based on the severity of hyponatremia and how rapid the onset
      1. Acute—onset less than 48 hours
         a. Leads to more symptoms and an increased risk of cerebral edema and herniation.
      2. Chronic—onset happens over 48 hours
         a. More insidious onset leading to symptoms.
   B. Signs and symptoms of SIADH—primarily neurologic and GI systems
      1. Neurologic—symptoms include personality changes, headache, decreased mentation, lethargy, fatigue, weight gain, disorientation, and confusion related to osmotic shift and increased intracranial pressure. Severe neurologic symptoms: seizures and coma. Cerebral edema can result from acute hyponatremia manifested by irritability, confusion, coma, seizures, and respiratory arrest.
      2. Decreased urine output secondary to hyponatremia, fluid retention, weight gain, and anasarca.
      3. GI—abdominal cramps, nausea, vomiting, diarrhea, and anorexia.

II. Diagnostic and laboratory data (Mentrasti et al., 2020)
   A. Basic metabolic panel
      1. Sodium, decreased, remaining electrolytes normal, indicating the sample is not diluted.
   B. Serum sodium (<135 mEq/L)
      1. Mild: 130–134 mmol/L
      2. Moderate: 125–129 mmol/L
   C. Serum Osmolality (<275 mOsm/kg)
   D. Urine osmolality greater than serum osmolality; urine electrolytes

E. Urine sodium: >30 mEq/L

F. Blood glucose

G. Thyroid-stimulating hormone, severe hypothyroidism can cause hyponatremia

  1. Plasma AVP—decreased with hypotonic state

Management

I. Medical management (Mentrasti et al., 2020; Harrois & Anstey, 2019)

  A. Asymptomatic patients with mild hyponatremia should be treated with a fluid restriction (500–800 cm³ a day).

  B. Pharmacologic management indicated severe symptoms (seizures, obtundation); most likely to occur in patients with serum sodium <120 mEq/L in less than 48 hours leading to potentially lethal cerebral edema.

  1. 3% hypertonic saline infusion

    a. Considered in acute situations in which neurological symptoms are present.

    b. Infused 100–150 mL bolus over 10 minutes, which can be repeated 2–3 times to increase by 5 mmol.

      (1) Giving this way helps to prevent an increase of serum sodium too rapidly and to prevent pulmonary edema, and osmotic demyelination leading to severe damage to the CNS.

      (2) Use a central line to administer 3% saline; 2% saline can be given peripherally.

      (3) Correct serum sodium slowly, not more than 0.5 mEq/h.

  2. Demeclocycline may be used for long-term management.

  3. Enteral urea

  4. Vaptans or vasopressin V2 receptor antagonists

  5. Employ medications to treat the underlying cause.

II. Nursing management

  A. Primarily for mild symptoms

    1. Fluid restriction to 500–800 mL/day; water intake should not exceed the urine output.

    2. Increase salt intake.

  B. Place patient on seizure precautions when SIADH is severe.

  C. Aspiration precautions with impaired mental status.

  D. Monitor the sodium levels.

  E. Weigh daily.

  F. Maintain accurate intake and output records.

HYPERSENSITIVITY AND ANAPHYLAXIS

Overview

I. Definitions

  A. Hypersensitivity—hypersensitivity reactions in cancer care are most often associated with chemotherapy or other drugs. Drug hypersensitivity is an immune-mediated reaction. Symptoms range from mild to severe. Drug hypersensitivities may occur with anticancer treatments, especially with immune and targeted therapies. The terms *drug reaction*, *drug allergy*, and *drug hypersensitivity* may be used interchangeably (Fernandez, 2018b; O'Leary, 2017).

  B. Anaphylaxis—an acute, potentially fatal, multiorgan system reaction caused by the release of chemical mediators from mast cells and basophils. Involves prior sensitization to an allergen with later re-exposure, producing symptoms via an immunologic mechanism.

II. Pathophysiology

  A. Hypersensitivity reactions are divided into four categories (Gell and Coombs classification—UpToDate, 2022):

    1. Type I—immediate (usually within 1 hour) immunoglobulin E (IgE) mediated

      a. Most common type associated with antineoplastic agents

      b. Results from exposure to an antigen with the formation of IgE antibodies, attached to receptors on mast cells and basophils

      c. Further exposure to the same antigen—creates an escalated reaction due to memory cell release of histamines, leukotrienes, prostaglandins, and other inflammatory mediators

    2. Type II—IgG or IgM antibody mediated

    3. Type III—immune complex mediated

    4. Type IV—cell-mediated or delayed

    5. Some emerging cancer treatments are not falling under the traditional classification system; therefore, different classification systems are emerging (O'Leary, 2017).

  B. Anaphylaxis

    1. IgE antibody is developed after the first exposure to an antigen.

    2. At next exposure, the IgE antibody binds to mast cells and basophils.

    3. This triggers the release of inflammatory mediators, including histamine, tryptase, leukotrienes, prostaglandins, and platelet-activating factor (Kemp, 2021).

    4. The release of substances causes systemic vasodilation, increased capillary permeability, bronchoconstriction, and coronary vasoconstriction.

    5. The term "anaphylaxis" typically describes anaphylactic reactions mediated by IgE. Historically, anaphylactoid reaction was a term used for non–IgE-mediated reactions. The World Allergy Organization has recommended replacing this terminology with immunologic (IgE-mediated and non–IgE-mediated [e.g., IgG and immune complex complement mediated]) and nonimmunologic anaphylaxis. Grading systems for systemic allergic reactions continue to evolve (Cox, Sanchez-Borges, & Lockey, 2017).

  C. In general, hypersensitivity reactions are mediated by IgE. However, B and T cells play a significant role in the development of involved antibodies. These components initiate a cytokine cascade response. The cytokine cascade begins at the exposure of the allergen and then concludes with an immune reaction (Chan, Rundell, & Aring, 2018; Table 48.3).

TABLE 48.3 Classification of Drug Hypersensitivity Reactions

Type	Mechanism	Clinical Features	Timing of Reactions	Examples
Type I (IgE mediated)	Drug–IgE complex binds to mast cells	Urticaria, angioedema, bronchospasm, pruritus, GI symptoms, and anaphylaxis	Immediate (minutes to hours after drug exposure, depending on the route of administration)	β-Lactam antibiotic
Type II (cytotoxic)	Specific IgG or IgM antibodies directed at drug–hapten-coated cells	Hemolytic anemia, neutropenia, and thrombocytopenia	Variable	Penicillin (hemolytic anemia), heparin (thrombocytopenia)
Type III (immune complex)	Antigen–antibody complexes	Serum sickness, vasculitis, and drug fever	1–3 weeks after drug exposure	Penicillin (serum sickness), sulfonamides (vasculitis), and azathioprine (drug fever)
Type IV (delayed, cell mediated)	Activation and expansion of drug-specific T cell	Prominent skin findings: contact dermatitis, morbilliform eruptions	2–7 days after exposure	Topical antihistamine, penicillin, and sulfonamides

GI, Gastrointestinal; *Ig*, immunoglobulin.
From Chan, M., Rundell, K., & Aring, A. M. (2018). Drug hypersensitivity reactions. In R. D. Kellerman, & E. T. Bope (Eds.), *Conn's current therapy 2018*. Philadelphia, PA: Elsevier.

III. Risk factors
  A. Chemotherapeutic agents have the potential to induce a hypersensitivity reaction (O'Leary, 2017).
    1. Platinums (e.g., cisplatin, carboplatin, and oxaliplatin)
      a. Consistent with type I reactions because most typically occur after multiple cycles of therapy.
      b. Most reactions to oxaliplatin occur within the first minutes of infusion.
      c. Desensitization protocols for platinum agents can be successful to decrease the risk.
    2. Taxanes (e.g., paclitaxel, docetaxel)
      a. Paclitaxel treatment—should include premedication to prevent reactions, as well as a longer infusion time
      b. Unclear if reaction is to drug or diluent
      c. Desensitization protocols used for paclitaxel administration
      d. Most severe reactions—occur with the first or second dose within the first minutes of infusion
    3. L-Asparaginase
      a. Higher risk when given intermittently rather than daily; IV administration poses a higher risk than intramuscular or subcutaneous route
      b. Intradermal skin testing performed before administration
    4. Procarbazine
      a. Corticosteroid recommended before infusion
    5. Epipodophyllotoxins (e.g., etoposide, teniposide)
      a. Reactions within the first few minutes or hours after infusion; more commonly occur after multiple doses
    6. Pegylated liposomal doxorubicin—"acute infusion-related reactions consisting of, but not limited to, flushing, shortness of breath, facial swelling, headache, chills, back pain, tightness in the chest or throat, and/or hypotension occurred in 11% of patients with solid tumors treated with doxorubicin (liposomal). Serious, life-threatening, and fatal infusion reactions have been reported" (National Library of Medicine, 2023c).
    7. Cytarabine—allergic reaction and anaphylaxis are reported (National Library of Medicine, 2023a).
    8. Monoclonal antibodies (MoABs, e.g., rituximab, cetuximab, trastuzumab, bevacizumab, obinutuzumab, and ofatumumab) and checkpoint inhibitors (e.g., pembrolizumab, nivolumab, atezolizumab, avelumab, durvalumab, and ipilimumab)
      a. Type of biotherapy—murine (mouse protein), chimeric (7%–9% mouse protein), humanized or fully humanized; makeup of the MoABs may lead to hypersensitivity reaction; higher content of murine protein correlates with a higher risk of reaction.
      b. Most infusion reactions occur with the first dose and are related to cytokine release rather than murine exposure.
    9. Ixabepilone—hypersensitivity reaction (National Library of Medicine, 2023b)
  B. Other factors that indicate a greater risk
    1. History of other drug allergies, regardless of drug class
    2. History of hypersensitivity and history of reaction in the same drug class
    3. IV administration
    4. After several cycles of certain agents (e.g., oxaliplatin)
  C. Additional risk factors for anaphylaxis
    1. Antibiotics (most common are beta-lactams [e.g., penicillins, cephalosporins])
    2. Anesthetics or anesthetic adjuncts
    3. Antineoplastic agents (e.g., chemotherapy, biotherapy)
  D. Examples include carboplatin, paclitaxel (Horita et al., 2021)
    1. Blood products
    2. Contrast media used for radiographic testing

3. Foods (e.g., eggs, fish, food additives, peanuts, shell-fish, and milk)
4. Insect venom
5. Latex

Assessment

I. Physical examination
   A. Hypersensitivity reactions are often patient and drug dependent. Signs and symptoms of hypersensitivity may be very similar to, yet not as severe as, those of anaphylaxis.
   B. Symptoms of hypersensitivity and anaphylaxis reactions (allergic reaction) (O'Leary, 2017; Lockey, 2019; Kelso, 2021)
      1. Dermatologic symptoms—flushing, itching, urticaria, morbilliform rash, and angioedema
      2. Oral symptoms—itching and edema of tongue and lips
      3. Ophthalmologic symptoms—periorbital edema, infected conjunctiva, and tears
      4. Respiratory symptoms—bronchospasm, chest tightness, tachypnea, throat or nasal itching, congestion, sneezing, dysphonia, hoarseness, dry cough, stridor, cyanosis, rhinitis, and respiratory arrest
      5. Cardiovascular symptoms—chest pain, tachycardia, diaphoresis, faintness, hypotension, cyanosis, dysrhythmias, palpitations, and shock
      6. GI symptoms—nausea, vomiting, diarrhea, abdominal pain, and hyperperistalsis with fecal/urinary urgency
      7. Neurologic symptoms—headache, dizziness, uneasiness, lightheadedness, confusion, tunnel vision, and loss of consciousness
      8. Other symptoms—metallic taste, feeling of impending doom (Kelso, 2021)
      9. Reaction severity
         a. Mild—hives, rash, itching, scratchy throat, watery or scratchy eyes
         b. Moderate—swelling of lips, face, and eyes
         c. Severe—angioedema, bronchospasm, chest tightness, tachypnea, stridor, cyanosis, respiratory arrest, chest pain, tachycardia, cyanosis, dysrhythmias, palpitations, shock, loss of consciousness, and feeling of impending doom (Kelso, 2021)
   C. There is an association of symptom onset with drug administration (Fernandez, 2018b).
II. Diagnostic and laboratory data
   A. Test dose via skin testing (e.g., carboplatin, oxaliplatin, and bleomycin).
      1. Determine if skin test is positive or negative, which could predict potential for reaction.
   B. A drug provocation test—controlled administration of a drug to diagnose immune- or nonimmune-mediated drug hypersensitivity. This should be the last step for accurate recognition of drug hypersensitivity reactions; only perform when previous diagnostic evaluations are negative or unavailable.
   C. Possibly direct and indirect antiglobulin assays (Fernandez, 2018b). 24-hour urinary levels of n-methylhistamine or serum levels of tryptase may be performed (Fernandez, 2018a).

Management

I. Medical management
   A. Administer pharmacologic management used for pre-therapy delivery to assist in the prevention of a reaction when appropriate, 30 minutes to 24 hours in advance. Longer intervals for premeds should occur if the patient has experienced previous reactions (Fernandez, 2018b; O'Leary, 2017).
      1. Corticosteroids
      2. Histamine 1 (H_1) antagonists (e.g., diphenhydramine)
      3. H_2 antagonists (e.g., ranitidine, famotidine)
      4. Antipyretics (e.g., acetaminophen)
   B. Possible pharmacologic interventions in the event of a hypersensitivity reaction.
      1. Epinephrine (Vemula, 2021)
         a. Works through α- and β-adrenergic properties; increases peripheral vasoconstriction and bronchodilation, reduction of mast cells
         b. Begins working within seconds to minutes of administration
         c. Can be administered intravenously by health care provider trained in the management of vasopressors; also given intramuscularly in the anterolateral aspect of the thigh
         d. Injection may be repeated
      2. H_1 antagonists—to improve cutaneous erythema and decrease itching
      3. H_2 antagonists
      4. Corticosteroids—for example, dexamethasone or hydrocortisone—to prevent biphasic reactions
      5. Albuterol (for inhalation)
      6. Opioids (for rigors)
      7. Oxygen
      8. IV fluids and sometimes vasopressors for persistent hypotension
      9. Inhaled β-agonists for bronchoconstriction
II. Nursing management (Fernandez, 2018b; O'Leary, 2017; Lockey, 2019)
   A. Identify risk for allergy response
   B. Lockey suggests a helpful memory cue regarding anaphylaxis:
      1. Quickly assess and treat
         a. A=Airway
         b. B=Breathing
         c. Circulation
      2. Possible pharmacologic treatments could be remembered similarly.
         a. A=Adrenalin
         b. B=Benadryl-diphenhydramine
         c. C=Corticosteroids
   C. Know the patient's past medical history information regarding hypersensitivity reactions.
      1. Baseline knowledge of hypersensitivity risk associated with medications to be administered

2. Awareness of the patient's current allergies

3. Provide avoidance education for patient/significant other should hypersensitivity or anaphylaxis occur; inform patient to wear Medic-Alert bracelet if indicated.

4. Obtain baseline vital signs and additional vital signs per infusion protocol for specific medication.

D. Use premedication when appropriate.

E. Cease current infusion and be prepared for initiation of IV fluids if signs and symptoms of reaction occur.

F. Have emergency equipment easily accessible to the patient in addition to emergency drugs, oxygen, tracheostomy supplies, and automated external defibrillator/defibrillator.

G. Maintain patent airway

H. Notify oncology care provider about signs and symptoms observed.

I. Administer supportive medications when ordered (e.g., antihistamine, epinephrine, corticosteroids, and NSAID).

J. Continue monitoring the airway for potential compromise.

K. Restart infusion, potentially at a slower rate, based on orders.

L. Rechallenge or desensitize when appropriate for subsequent administrations.

M. Manage potential anxiety or fear of patient/significant other.

N. Assist patient in identifying appropriate coping strategies.

1. Encourage patient/significant other to verbalize potential signs and symptoms of hypersensitivity.

2. Provide relaxation methods as appropriate.

3. Acknowledge the patient's feelings as they are expressed.

4. Suggest resources such as psychological counseling and pastoral care services for emotional and spiritual support (Saha et al., 2017).

SEPSIS AND SEPTIC SHOCK

Overview

I. Definitions

A. Early sepsis—patients with infection and bacteremia are at risk for developing sepsis. No formal definition for early sepsis exists; however, early identification of those at risk is critical for prevention and to decrease mortality (Neviere, 2022).

B. Sepsis—sepsis is a syndrome that is caused by a dysregulated host or a body's extreme response to infection and can be life threatening (CDC, 2021; Tavakoli & Carannante, 2021).

C. Septic shock—subset of those with sepsis causing serious metabolic, cellular, and circulatory compromise. Fluid resuscitation attempted without success (Tavakoli & Carannante, 2021; Evans et al., 2021).

II. Pathophysiology (Gyawali, Ramakrishna, & Dhamoon, 2019)

A. A circulating pathogen (e.g., bacterial, viral, or fungal products) releases toxins and cell components into the bloodstream where there is activation of immune cells such as macrophages, monocytes, neutrophils, and natural killer cells. Chemotherapy and radiation can cause impaired production of white blood cells (WBCs), especially neutrophils, which can make one more vulnerable (Gyawali et al., 2019).

B. Then there is a progression to dysregulation of hemostasis. See "Septic Shock"—Science Direct (Fig. 48.3).

C. Pathogens

1. Gram-positive organisms most common in the United States (increase in prevalence because of increased use of access devices), for example, *Staphylococcus aureus* and *Streptococcus pneumoniae* (Boucher & Carpenter, 2020).

2. Gram-negative organisms remain a substantial contributor. The most common include *Escherichia coli*, *Klebsiella pneumoniae*, and *S. pneumoniae*. Over 50% of cases are culture negative (Boucher & Carpenter, 2020).

3. Viral infections, for example, COVID-19 or influenza (CDC, 2021).

4. Fungal infections

5. Mycobacterium

III. Risk factors for sepsis or septic shock (CDC, 2021; Tavakoli & Carannante, 2021)

A. Compromised immune system—possibly those with a cancer diagnosis (e.g., acute leukemia) or undergoing treatments for cancer

B. Medical devices—central venous catheter, urinary catheter, and drains

C. Bacteremia, community-acquired pneumonia

D. Advanced age, older than 65

E. Intensive care unit admission, previous hospitalization, or sepsis

F. History of diabetes, COPD, cancer, obesity, kidney disease, autoimmune disease, or other chronic medical conditions

G. Skin and mucosal barrier breeches—mucositis, open wounds

H. Genetic factors or social determinants of health challenges

I. Four types of infections most often associated with sepsis: lung, urinary tract infection, skin, and gut

IV. Physical manifestations (Evans et al., 2021)

A. Signs and symptoms of sepsis

1. Fever >100.4°F or >100 sustained for at least two hours; oncology patients are at increased risk of neutropenic fever due to chemotherapy and/or radiation.

2. Constitutional symptoms—fatigue, malaise, arthralgias, and myalgias.

3. Infection-specific symptoms (e.g., cough or dyspnea suggesting pneumonia; purulent drainage from a wound).

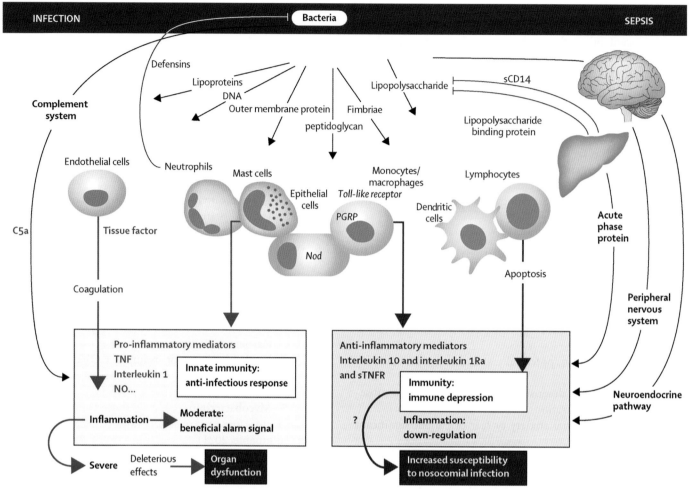

Fig. 48.3 Septic shock cascade. From Annane, D., Bellissant, E., & Cavaillon, J.-M. (2005). Septic shock. *The Lancet, 365*(9453), 63–78. https://doi.org/10.1016/s0140-6736 (04)17667-8.

4. Vital signs: hypotension ≤90 mm Hg; mean arterial pressure (MAP) <70 mm Hg; temperature >101°F or <96.8°F; heart rate >90 bpm; respiratory rate >20 respirations/min or respiratory distress.

5. GI: abdominal pain, distention, firmness, and guarding.

6. GU: lesions or abscess, decreased urine output.

7. Skin: lesions, erythema, tenderness, and breaks in skin integrity.

8. Oral mucosa: erythema, ulceration, and tenderness.

9. Catheter sites: erythema, purulent drainage, inflammation, and tenderness.

10. In early sepsis, skin may be warm/flushed. Progressive sepsis may result in cool skin allowing blood to be diverted to vital organs.

11. Neurologic: confusion or disorientation, and somnolence.

12. Extremities: edema

13. Extreme pain or discomfort

B. Signs and symptoms of septic shock
1. Patient requires vasopressors to maintain MAP ≥65 mm Hg despite adequate fluid status.
2. Elevated lactate level

C. Organ dysfunction in sepsis/septic shock may manifest as:
1. Central nervous system—confusion, agitation, obtundation, and coma
2. Cardiovascular—tachycardia, dysrhythmias, and hypotension
3. Respiratory—tachypnea, hypoxia, shortness of breath, decreased breath sounds, crackles or wheezes, pulmonary edema, and acute respiratory distress syndrome
4. Renal—azotemia, oliguria, or anuria. Urine output <0.5 mL/kg per hour for at least 2 hours without hypovolemia.
5. Skin—dry, warm, flushed; may progress to cold, pale, decreased perfusion, and mottling
6. Hepatic—elevated liver enzymes, jaundice
7. GI—nausea, vomiting, ileus, and GI blood loss
8. Hematologic—neutropenia or neutrophilia, thrombocytopenia, DIC (Rhodes et al., 2017)

D. Abnormal laboratory (Rhodes et al., 2017; Tavakoli & Carannante, 2021)
1. Indicative of sepsis in addition to suspected or documented infection

a. Leukocytosis or leukopenia (neutropenia); WBC can be normal with left shift
b. Prolonged prothrombin time (PT) or activated partial thromboplastin time
c. Arterial hypoxemia
d. Decreased platelets
e. Decreased fibrinogen
f. Hyperglycemia
g. Increased lactic acid
h. Positive blood cultures
i. Elevated creatinine
2. Indicative of septic shock (in addition)
a. Elevated liver function
b. Elevated lactate
c. Urine output <0.5 mL/kg per hour for at least 2 hours without hypovolemia
d. Increased creatinine >2.0 mg/dL
e. Anemia, thrombocytopenia <100,000 cells/μL
f. Hypoglycemia

Assessment

I. Physical exam
A. Evaluation of mental status
B. Capillary refill
C. Skin changes
1. Discoloration
2. Mottling
3. Bruising
4. Lymphadenopathy
5. Necrotizing fasciitis
D. Respiratory: cough, hypoxia, dyspnea, hyperventilation, rales, rhonchi, and decreased breath sounds (bilateral or unilateral)
E. Cardiac: tachycardia, decreased capillary refill, cool extremities, and diminished peripheral pulses
F. GI: abdominal rigidity, pain, distention, decreased bowel sounds, and jaundice
G. GU: costovertebral angle tenderness, pelvic pain, dysuria, hematuria, and vaginal discharge
II. Laboratory and radiologic analysis
A. CBC, comprehensive metabolic panel, coagulation studies including D-dimer, serum lactate, arterial blood gas, blood cultures, wound cultures, bodily fluid cultures (sputum, urine) to look for the source of infection, fungal assays, for example, beta D-glucan, galactomannan
B. Chest x-ray, chest/abdomen computed tomography, abdominal ultrasound, and MRI

Management

I. Medical management
A. Control possible infectious sources—remove infected lines, drain abscesses
B. Fluid resuscitation
C. Employ empiric antibiotic therapy with one or more antibiotics administered within the first hour of presentation; additional antibiotics given if fever nonresponsive.
D. Provide vasopressor therapy as ordered to maintain an MAP of 65 mm Hg and monitor for urine output of >0.5 mL/kg per hour.

E. Administer glucocorticoids.
F. Blood transfusions as indicated
II. Nursing management
A. Manage sepsis urgently.
B. Establish/maintain airway for supplemental oxygen and to address hypoxia.
C. Secure venous access and begin rapid fluid replacement.
D. Obtain cultures before giving antibiotics.
E. Monitor respiratory status. Begin oxygen therapy to maintain SpO_2 at >90% (e.g., nasal cannula, nonrebreather mask, or mechanical ventilation if needed).
F. Monitor clinical response.
1. Vital signs
2. MAP
3. Urine output
4. Skin color
5. Pulse oximetry
6. Mental status

TUMOR LYSIS SYNDROME

Overview

I. Definition—an oncologic emergency which is caused by the rapid lysis of cells, usually as a result of cytotoxic therapy. This results in the release of potentially toxic intracellular contents leading to hyperuricemia, hyperkalemia, hyperphosphatemia, hypocalcemia, and acidosis. Usually associated with high count leukemias and high tissue burden lymphomas; however, can occur with any regimen using more potent chemoradiation (Lichtman, 2021).
II. Pathophysiology (Williams & Killeen, 2019)
A. Tumor lysis generally occurs 12–72 hours (has been reported for up to 5–7 days) following the initiation of cytotoxic therapy; causes brisk lysis and massive destruction of tumor cells. This leads to leakage of intracellular contents including nucleic acids, electrolytes, and cytokines into systemic circulation. This influx can lead to multiorgan failure, most notable in the cardiac and renal systems.
1. Hyperuricemia: Release of nucleic acids are catabolized to uric acid: causing crystallization in the kidneys, leading to obstruction and compromised renal function.
2. Hyperkalemia: Potassium is a primary intracellular electrolyte; when cell lysis occurs, potassium is released into circulation. Manifesting in muscle weakness and cardiac dysrhythmia.
3. Hyperphosphatemia: Released when cell lysis occurs, and renal excretion cannot manage increased serum contents. May cause GI symptoms such as nausea, vomiting, and diarrhea.
4. Hypocalcemia: Results from binding of phosphate to calcium cations. Symptoms include cramps, hypotension, tetany, and arrhythmias. Bound phosphate–calcium also accumulates in renal tissue.
B. Patients at highest risk (Gucalp & Dutcher, 2018)
1. Cancers: Burkitt lymphoma, acute lymphoblastic leukemia, acute myeloid leukemia, diffuse large

B-cell lymphoma, testicular, small-cell lung cancer, and other high-grade lymphomas
   2. Tumor lysis syndrome (TLS) can occur in other cancers with a rapid proliferation rate.
   3. Tumors with a high sensitivity to chemotherapy or radiotherapy
   4. Large volume of disease as evidenced by
      a. Elevated LDH
      b. WBC >50,000/mm^3
      c. Significant liver metastasis
      d. Involvement of the bone marrow
      e. Cancer stage, proliferative rate
   C. Patient comorbidities contribute to the development of TLS (Webster & Kaplow, 2021).
      1. Preexisting renal dysfunction
      2. Increased uric acid levels (gout)
      3. Dehydration or insufficient fluid resuscitation
      4. Extensive lymphadenopathy
   D. Treatment with high risk for the development of TLS (Webster & Kaplow, 2021)
      1. High-risk chemotherapy
         a. Cisplatin
         b. Fludarabine
         c. Etoposide
         d. Paclitaxel
         e. Doxorubicin, daunorubicin
         f. Bendamustine
         g. Mitoxantrone
      2. Radiation therapy
         a. Total body irradiation or targeted radiation in high tumor burden of a radiosensitive tumor
      3. MoABs
      4. Tyrosine kinase inhibitors
      5. Chimeric antigen receptor T cells (CAR-T cells)
      6. Corticosteroids

Assessment

(Webster & Kaplow, 2021)
   I. Hyperkalemia
      A. Cardiac dysrhythmias
      B. Muscle weakness
      C. Ileus and abdominal distention or diarrhea
   II. Hypocalcemia
      A. Paresthesia and tetany
      B. Anxiety
      C. Bronchospasm
      D. Seizures
      E. Cardiac arrest
   III. Calcium deposited in tissue may cause
      A. Itching
      B. Iritis
      C. Arthritis
   IV. Uremia
      A. Fatigue
      B. Weakness
      C. Nausea and vomiting
      D. Anorexia
      E. Difficulty concentrating or confusion

   F. Fluid overload
   V. Hyperphosphatemia
      A. Likely asymptomatic
   VI. Acidosis
      A. Secondary to the hyperinflammatory state caused by TLS and renal failure results in
         1. Fatigue
   VII. Diagnosis based on laboratory studies
      A. Basic metabolic panel
      B. Liver function tests
      C. Phosphorous
      D. Urinalysis
      E. LDH

Management

   I. Medical management
      A. Reduce the risk of TLS (Webster & Kaplow, 2021)
         1. Administer IV hydration 24–48 hours before treatment initiation if possible to facilitate renal perfusion and increase urine output, minimizing the risk of uric acid and calcium–phosphate deposition in the renal tubules.
         2. Employ uric acid-lowering agents (i.e., allopurinol, febuxostat)
            a. Used to decrease the uric acid in the blood to decrease the risk of hyperuricemia from TLS.
      B. Promptly manage confirmed TLS—withhold treatment until resolution of TLS
      C. Manage hyperkalemia (Williams & Killeen, 2019).
         1. Mild
            a. Hydration
            b. Calcium (allows stabilization of cardiac tissue)
            c. Sodium polystyrene sulfonate (oral or rectal administration)
         2. Severe—same as mild plus the following:
            a. Hypertonic glucose, insulin—shift potassium from intracellular to extracellular space
            b. Sodium bicarbonate—shifts potassium intracellularly
      D. Manage hyperphosphatemia (Webster & Kaplow, 2021).
         1. Administer aggressive fluid resuscitation.
         2. Treat with phosphate binder.
      E. Hypocalcemia (Webster & Kaplow, 2021).
         1. Self-limiting once phosphorus is corrected
         2. Calcium replacement with calcium gluconate if needed
      F. Manage hyperuricemia (Williams & Killeen, 2019).
         1. Allopurinol, for levels of uric acid <8 mg/dL—reduces the production of new uric acid.
         2. Febuxostat—decreases the production of uric acid.
         3. Rasburicase—administered intravenously. Converts uric acid to an inactive and soluble metabolite of uric acid to allow excretion.
   II. Nonpharmacologic management
      A. High-acuity patients require continuous monitoring of cardiac status, intensive monitoring of electrolytes, renal status, and uric acid every 4–6 hours.

B. Monitor cardiac status with hyperkalemia, and review medications that contribute to elevated potassium levels.

C. Monitor electrocardiography changes.

D. Monitor intake and output, daily weights.

E. Monitor indications for dialysis, and prepare patient and family for this potential (Webster & Kaplow, 2021).

1. Severe oliguria or anuria
2. Persistent fluid overload
3. Intractable hyperkalemia
4. Symptomatic hypocalcemia due to hyperphosphatemia
5. Calcium–phosphate precipitate value ≥ 70 mg^2/dL

HYPERCALCEMIA

Overview

I. Definition—abnormally high level of calcium (>10.5 mg/dL) when corrected with serum albumin; the most common oncologic emergency occurring in 20%–30% of all cancer patients; reduced incidence due to prophylactic use of bisphosphonates in patients with bone metastases.

A. Mild: Serum calcium levels between 12 and 14 mg/dL or ionized Ca 5.6–8 mg/dL

B. Severe: Serum calcium levels elevated above 14 mg/dL or ionized Ca 8–10 mg/dL

II. Physiology and pathophysiology

A. Calcium and bone metabolism regulated by parathyroid hormone (PTH), 1,25-dihydroxyvitamin D (calcitriol), and calcitonin (Khosla et al., 2018). These hormones influence bone, kidney, and small intestine to maintain calcium homeostasis.

B. PTH stimulates calcium reabsorption from bones and kidneys.

C. When the body detects low calcium levels, 1,25-dihydroxyvitamin D works on the gut and stimulates the absorption of dietary calcium intake for body needs.

D. Calcitonin works to decrease serum calcium levels by suppressing bone and renal reabsorption of calcium.

III. Causes of hypercalcemia (Potts & Jüpper, 2018)

A. Cancers posing a risk for hypercalcemia

1. Solid tumors—Secondary to increased PTH or those that commonly metastasize to the bone
   a. Breast
   b. Lung
   c. Prostate
   d. Renal carcinoma
   e. Squamous cell cancers
2. Hematologic malignancies
   a. Multiple myeloma
   b. Lymphoma

B. Hyperparathyroidism

C. Vitamin D intoxication

D. Chronic granulomatous disorders (e.g., sarcoidosis, tuberculosis)

E. Medications (e.g., thiazide diuretics, lithium), contrast media, bisphosphonates, antibiotics, and antiepileptics

Assessment

I. Physical examination (Khosla et al., 2018)

A. Signs and symptoms of hypercalcemia

1. Mild hypercalcemia (<12 mg/dL) may be asymptomatic or have vague symptoms of constipation, fatigue, and depression.
2. Severe hypercalcemia (12–14 mg/dL)
   a. Patients with chronic elevation may not exhibit significant symptoms.
   b. Acute elevation may cause patient to have marked symptoms.
      (1) GI symptoms—anorexia, abdominal cramping, and loss of appetite. Severe: nausea, vomiting, pancreatitis, and peptic ulcer.
      (2) Neurologic symptoms—restlessness, difficulty concentrating, lethargy, and confusion. Severe: seizures, coma.
      (3) Muscular symptoms—fatigue and generalized weakness. Severe: ataxia and pathologic fractures.
      (4) Renal symptoms—frequent urination, nocturia, and polydipsia. Severe: renal failure.
      (5) Cardiovascular symptoms—bradycardia, orthostatic hypotension, shortened QT interval, and heart block. Severe: ventricular arrhythmia, ST segment elevation.

II. Diagnosis

A. Initial testing (Khosla et al., 2018).

1. Chemistry panel, including a serum calcium or ionized calcium.
2. Serum albumin and prealbumin. Important to adjust serum calcium for low serum albumin, as is experienced by many patients with cancer.
3. PTH level

B. Additional testing may include

1. Phosphorus, 1,25 (OH)$_2$D
2. PTH-related protein
3. Alkaline phosphatase
4. Serum and urine electrophoresis

Management

In addition to acute management of the hypercalcemia, treating the underlying malignancy is crucial to the resolution of the hypercalcemia. Patients with a serum calcium below 12 mg/dL and asymptomatic do not require immediate therapy (Arora & Jefferson, 2022).

I. Medical management (Arora & Jefferson, 2022)

A. Reduce serum calcium with IV hydration—0.9% normal saline, 200–300 cm^3/h, to increase renal clearance of circulating calcium, until the patient is euvolemic.

B. Maintain calcium in the bone/inhibit mobilization of calcium from bone.

1. Bisphosphonates: zoledronic acid

a. Work by inhibiting bone resorption and suppressing the activity of osteoclasts.

b. May cause tubular and glomerular damage. Dose should be reduced for patients with renal compromise, or avoided in severe renal disease.

c. Zoledronic acid proven to be more effective than pamidronate.

2. Denosumab

a. MoAB against RANKL, inhibits osteoclasts, inhibiting bone resorption.

b. Utilized in patients unable to receive or refractory to bisphosphonates.

c. Not excreted through kidneys; therefore, may be used in patients with renal insufficiency. Also used in patients who are refractory to bisphosphonate therapy.

d. Potential to cause severe hypocalcemia.

3. Calcitonin

a. Enhances renal excretion of calcium.

b. Interferes with osteoclast function.

c. Limited efficacy as only effective in lowering calcium for 48 hours.

d. Traditionally given in combination with bisphosphonates to acutely lower calcium.

4. Glucocorticoids

a. Reduce absorption of calcium through intestines.

b. Inhibit 1,25-dihydroxyvitamin D production.

5. Loop diuretics—may be used carefully in patients with renal dysfunction or heart failure for volume overload

C. Dialysis can be considered in refractory and severe cases.

II. Nursing management

A. Monitor intake and output closely, mental status, and symptoms related to hypercalcemia.

B. Weigh daily.

C. Administer IV fluids for hydration as ordered.

D. Monitor heart and rhythm when hypercalcemia severe.

E. Provide psychosocial support when changes in the level of consciousness occur.

REFERENCES

Arora, N., & Jefferson, J. (2022). Hypercalcemia. In M. A. Papadakis, S. J. McPhee, M. W. Rabow, & K. R. McQuaid (Eds.), *Current medical diagnosis & treatment 2022*. New York: McGraw Hill. https://accessmedicine.mhmedical.com/content.aspx?bookid=3081&sectionid=258968969.

Blackburn, L. M., Bender, S., & Brown, S. (2019). Acute leukemia: Diagnosis and treatment. *Seminars in Oncology Nursing, 35*(6), 150950. https://doi.org/10.1016/j.soncn.2019.150950.

Boucher, J. E., & Carpenter, D. (2020). Sepsis: Symptoms, assessment, diagnosis, and the Hour-1 bundle in patients with cancer. *Clinical Journal of Oncology Nursing, 24*(1), 99–102.

Centers for Disease Control. (2021). What is sepsis? https://www.cdc.gov/sepsis/what-is-sepsis.html. Retrieved 04.04.22.

Chan, M., Rundell, K., & Aring, A. M. (2018). Drug hypersensitivity reactions. In R. D. Kellerman & E. T. Bope (Eds.), *Conn's current therapy 2018*. Philadelphia, PA: Elsevier.

Chiasakul, T., & Cuker, A. (2018). Clinical and laboratory diagnosis of TTP: An integrated approach. *Hematology. American Society of Hematology. Education Program, 2018*(1), 530–538. https://doi.org/10.1182/asheducation-2018.1.530.

Cox, L. S., Sanchez-Borges, M., & Lockey, R. F. (2017). World Allergy Organization systemic allergic reaction grading system: Is a modification needed? *Journal of Allergy and Clinical Immunology In Practice, 5*(1), 58–62.e5. https://doi.org/10.1016/j.jaip.2016.11.009.

Evans, L., Rhodes, A., Alhazzani, W., Antonelli, M., Coopersmith, C. M., French, C., et al. (2021). Surviving sepsis campaign: International guidelines for management of sepsis and septic shock 2021. *Intensive Care Medicine, 47*(11), 1181–1247. https://doi.org/10.1007/s00134-021-06506-y.

Fernandez, J. (2018a). *Anaphylaxis Merck Manuals*. Rahaway, NJ: Merck & Co., Inc. Retrieved from https://www.merckmanuals.com/professional/immunology-allergic-disorders/allergic,-autoimmune,-and-other-hypersensitivity-disorders/anaphylaxis.

Fernandez, J. (2018b). *Drug hypersensitivity Merck Manuals*. Rahaway, NJ: Merck & Co., Inc. Retrieved from https://www.merckmanuals.com/professional/immunology-allergic-disorders/allergic,-autoimmune,-and-other-hypersensitivity-disorders/drug-hypersensitivity.

Frame, D., Scappaticci, G. B., Braun, T. M., Maliarik, M., Sisson, T. H., Pipe, S. W., et al. (2022). Defibrotide therapy for SARS-CoV-2 ARDS. *Chest Journal, 162*(2), 346–355. https://doi.org/10.1016/j.chest.2022.03.046. Epub ahead of print.

Gucalp, R., & Dutcher, J. P. (2018). Oncologic emergencies. In J. L. Jameson, A. S. Fauci, D. L. Kasper, S. L. Hauser, D. L. Longo, & J. Loscalzo (Eds.), *Harrison's principles of internal medicine* (20e). New York: McGraw Hill. https://accessmedicine.mhmedical.com/content.aspx?bookid=2129&sectionid=192015258.

Gyawali, B., Ramakrishna, K., & Dhamoon, A. S. (2019). Sepsis: The evolution in definition, pathophysiology, and management. *SAGE Open Medicine, 7*, 2050312119835043. https://doi.org/10.1177/2050312119835043.

Harrois, A., & Anstey, J. R. (2019). Diabetes insipidus and syndrome of inappropriate antidiuretic hormone in critically ill patients. *Critical care clinics, 35*(2), 187–200. https://doi.org/10.1016/j.ccc.2018.11.001.

Hoffman, P. (2020). Thrombotic thrombocytopenic purpura (TTP). In S. D. C. Stern, A. S. Cifu, & D. Altkorn (Eds.), *Symptom to diagnosis: An evidence-based guide* (4e). New York: McGraw Hill. https://accessmedicine.mhmedical.com/content.aspx?bookid=2715&sectionid=249058804.

Horita, N., Miyagi, E., Mizushima, T., Hagihara, M., Hata, C., Hattori, Y., et al. (2021). Severe anaphylaxis caused by intravenous anti-cancer drugs. *Cancer Medicine, 10*(20), 7174–7183.

Johnsen, J. M., & Ginsburg, D. (2021). von willebrand disease. In K. Kaushansky, J. T. Prchal, L. J. Burns, M. A. Lichtman, M. Levi, & D. C. Linch (Eds.), *Williams Hematology* (10e). McGraw Hill. https://accessmedicine.mhmedical.com/content.aspx?bookid=2962&sectionid=252538379.

Kelso, J. M. (2021). *Patient education: Anaphylaxis symptoms and diagnosis (Beyond the basics)*. Waltham, MA: UpToDate. https://www.uptodate.com/contents/anaphylaxis-symptoms-and-diagnosis-beyond-the-basics/print. Retrieved 04.04.22.

Kemp, S. F. (2021). *Pathophysiology of anaphylaxis*. Waltham, MA: UpToDate.

Khosla, S. (2018). Hypercalcemia and hypocalcemia. In J. L. Jameson, A. S. Fauci, D. L. Kasper, S. L. Hauser, D. L. Longo, & J. Loscalzo (Eds.), *Harrison's principles of internal medicine* (20e). New York: McGraw Hill. https://accessmedicine.mhmedical.com/content.aspx?bookid=2129&sectionid=192013331.

Levi, M. M. (2020). Disseminated intravascular coagulation (DIC). *Medscape*. https://emedicine.medscape.com/article/199627-overview#a7 Retrieved 12.03.22.

Lichtman, M. A. (2021). Classification and clinical manifestations of the clonal myeloid disorders. In K. Kaushansky, J. T. Prchal, L. J. Burns, M. A. Lichtman, M. Levi, & D. C. Linch (Eds.), *Williams hematology* (10e). New York: McGraw Hill. https://accessmedicine.mhmedical.com/content.aspx?bookid=2962&sectionid=252541292.

Lockey, R.F. (2019). *Anaphylaxis: Synopsis*. World Allergy Organization. https://www.worldallergy.org/education-and-programs/education/allergic-disease-resource-center/professionals/anaphylaxis-synopsis. Retrieved 04.04.22.

Maloney, K. W. (2017). Metabolic emergencies. In S. Newton, M. Hickey, & J. M. Brant (Eds.), *Mosby's oncology nursing advisor* (pp. 367–376). St. Louis, MO: Elsevier.

Mentrasti, G., Scortichini, L., Torniai, M., Giampieri, R., Morgese, F., Rinaldi, S., et al. (2020). Syndrome of inappropriate antidiuretic hormone secretion (SIADH): Optimal management. *Therapeutics and Clinical Risk Management*, 16, 663–672. https://doi.org/10.2147/TCRM.S206066.

Mount, D. B. (2022). Fluid and electrolyte disturbances. In J. Loscalzo, A. Fauci, D. Kasper, S. Hauser, D. Longo, & J. L. Jameson (Eds.), *Harrison's principles of internal medicine* (21e). New York: McGraw Hill. https://accessmedicine.mhmedical.com/content.aspx?bookid=3095&sectionid=265471636.

Neviere, R. (2022). Sepsis syndromes in adults: Epidemiology, definitions, clinical presentation, diagnosis and prognosis. Waltham, MA: *UpToDate*. https://www.uptodate.com/contents/sepsis-syndromes-in-adults-epidemiology-definitions-clinical-presentation-diagnosis-and-prognosis. Retrieved 04.04.22.

National Institute of Health (NIH). (2019). What are blood clotting disorders? https://www.nhlbi.nih.gov/health-topics/disseminated-intravascular-coagulation#:~:text=Signs%20and%20symptoms%20of%20DIC,has%20no%20signs%20or%20symptoms. Retrieved 07.03.22.

National Library of Medicine (2023a). *Cytarabine*. https://medlineplus.gov/druginfo/meds/a682222.html. Accessed Accessed 27.03.23.

National Library of Medicine (2023b). *Ixabepilone*. https://medlineplus.gov/druginfo/meds/a608042.html. Accessed 27.03.23.

National Library of Medicine (2023c). *Doxorubicin Lipid Complex Injection*. https://medlineplus.gov/druginfo/meds/a612001.html. Accessed 27.03.23.

O'Leary, C. (2017). Hypersensitivity reactions. In S. Newton, M. Hickey, & J. M. Brant (Eds.), *Mosby's oncology nursing advisor* (pp. 315–317). St. Louis, MO: Elsevier.

Potts, J. T., Jr., & Jüppner, H. (2018). Disorders of the parathyroid gland and calcium homeostasis. In J. L. Jameson, A. S. Fauci, D. L. Kasper, S. L. Hauser, D. L. Longo, & J. Loscalzo (Eds.), *Harrison's principles of internal medicine* (20e.). New York: McGraw Hill. https://accessmedicine.mhmedical.com/content.aspx?bookid=2129&sectionid=192530415.

Rhodes, A., Evans, L. E., Alhazzani, W., Levy, M. M., Antonelli, M., Ferrer, R., et al. (2017). Surviving sepsis campaign: International guidelines for management of sepsis and septic shock: 2016. *Intensive Care Medicine*, 43(3), 304–377. https://doi.org/10.1007/s00134-017-4683-6.

Robison, J. (2017). Hematologic emergencies. In S. Newton, M. Hickey, & J. M. Brant (Eds.), *Mosby's oncology nursing advisor* (pp. 377–398). St. Louis, MO: Elsevier.

Saha, M., McDaniel, J. K., & Zheng, X. L. (2017). Thrombotic thrombocytopenic purpura: Pathogenesis, diagnosis and potential novel therapeutics. *Journal of Thrombosis and Haemostasis*, 15(10), 1889–1900. https://doi.org/10.1111/jth.13764.

Scully, M. (2021). Thrombotic microangiopathies. In K. Kaushansky, J. T. Prchal, L. J. Burns, M. A. Lichtman, M. Levi, & D. C. Linch (Eds.), *Williams hematology* (10e). McGraw Hill. https://accessmedicine.mhmedical.com/content.aspx?bookid=2962&sectionid=252538768.

Shatzel, J. J., & Taylor, J. A. (2017). Syndromes of thrombotic microangiopathy. *Medical Clinics of North America*, 101(2), 395–415. https://doi.org/10.1016/j.mcna.2016.09.010. Epub 2016 Dec 27. PMID: 28189178.

Smith, L. (2021). Disseminated intravascular coagulation. *Seminars in Oncology Nursing*, 37(2),151135. https://doi.org/10.1016/j.soncn.2021.151135.

Tavakoli, A., & Carannante, A. (2021). Nursing care of oncology patients with sepsis. *Seminars in Oncology Nursing*, 37(2), 151130. https://doi-org.cedarville.ohionet.org/10.1016/j.soncn.2021.151130.

UpToDate. (2022). Gell and Coombs classification of immunologic drug reactions. https://www.uptodate.com/contents/image?imageKey=PULM%2F80466. Retrieved 28.03.22.

Vemula, S. (2021). Cancer treatment infusion reactions: *Handbook of cancer treatment-related symptoms and toxicities e-book* (pp. 107–112). Amsterdam: Elsevier.

Venes, D. (Ed.), (2021). *Taber's cyclopedic medical dictionary* (24th ed.). Philadelphia, PA: F.A. Davis Company.

Webster, J. S., & Kaplow, R. (2021). Tumor lysis syndrome: Implications for oncology nursing practice. *Seminars in Oncology Nursing*, 37(2), 151136. https://doi.org/10.1016/j.soncn.2021.151136.

Williams, S. M., & Killeen, A. A. (2019). Tumor lysis syndrome. *Archives of Pathology & Laboratory Medicine*, 143(3), 386–393. https://doi.org/10.5858/arpa.2017-0278-RS.

Yeung, S., Manzullo, E. F., & Chaftari, P. (2022). Oncologic emergencies. In H. M. Kantarjian, R. A. Wolff, & A. G. Rieber (Eds.), *The MD Anderson manual of medical oncology* (4e). New York: McGraw Hill. https://accessmedicine.mhmedical.com/content.aspx?bookid=3151&sectionid=264031134.

49

Structural Emergencies

Nimian Bauder

INCREASED INTRACRANIAL PRESSURE

Overview

I. Definition—a potentially life-threatening neurologic event that occurs with an increase in brain tissue, blood, cerebrospinal fluid (CSF), or all of these in the intracranial cavity, resulting in nerve cell damage, permanent neurologic deficits, and death (Saría, & Kesari, 2021).

II. Pathophysiology

  A. The intracranial cavity is a nonexpandable chamber that contains brain tissue, blood, and CSF. An increase in intracranial pressure (ICP) (with or without displacement of intracranial structures) occurs with an increase in the volume of any of the three components or due to mass effect (Allen, 2018). An increase of pressure >20 mm Hg in adults is considered pathologic (Smith & Amin-Hanjani, 2019).

  B. Causes of ICP in the oncology setting include primary or metastatic tumors within the intracranial cavity, leptomeningeal metastases, intracranial hemorrhage, encephalopathy syndromes, radiation necrosis, opportunistic infections, or a metabolic disorder (Shelton, Skinner, & Baynes, 2018; Smith & Amin-Hanjani, 2019).

  C. Brain injury results from brainstem compression and/or reduction in cerebral blood flow; leads to tissue necrosis (Smith & Amin-Hanjani, 2019).

    1. Displacement or edema of brain tissue
    2. Obstruction of CSF outflow
    3. Increased vascularity associated with tumor growth

Assessment

I. Identification of patients at risk

  A. Patients with cancers of the lung, breast, and kidney, as well as melanoma, who have an increased risk for metastases to the brain.

  B. Patients with primary tumors of the brain or spinal cord.

  C. Patients with a diagnosis of leukemia, lymphoma, or neuroblastoma.

  D. Oncology patients with thrombocytopenia, platelet dysfunction, or disseminated intravascular coagulation may have bleeding that may cause increased ICP.

  E. Patients with infections such as encephalitis, meningitis, or systemic candidiasis, especially immunocompromised patients.

  F. Patients with syndrome of inappropriate antidiuretic hormone secretion (see Chapter 52).

  G. Patients with the history of radiation therapy (RT) to the brain.

  H. Patients with occluded Ommaya reservoir.

  I. Patients treated with high-dose cytosine arabinoside (Nurgat et al., 2017).

  J. Patients treated with drugs for risk of posterior reversible encephalopathy syndrome (PRES) (e.g., immunosuppressants, immune checkpoint inhibitors, tyrosine kinase inhibitors, certain chemotherapeutic agents) (Brydges & Brydges, 2021; Saría & Kesari, 2021).

II. Signs and symptoms depend on volume, location, and rate of ICP

  A. Early signs and symptoms: may be subtle and include headaches (worse in the mornings, bending over, or during Valsalva maneuvers), nausea, vomiting, and weakness. Altered mental status with new onset of confusion or increased somnolence (Allen, 2018; Shelton et al., 2018).

  B. Later signs and symptoms (Allen, 2018; Shelton et al., 2018; Smith & Amin-Hanjani, 2019)

    1. Neurologic: headaches, cranial nerve abnormalities, and papilledema

      a. Headache pain may be initiated or aggravated by Valsalva maneuver, coughing, vomiting, exercise, or bending over

      b. Headache pain may be described as dull, sharp, or throbbing, and may increase in severity, frequency, and duration over time

      c. Blurred vision (diplopia), photophobia, contralateral pupillary dilation, and decreased visual fields

      d. Extremity drifts and ipsilateral weakness

      e. Lethargy, apathy, confusion, and restlessness

      f. Speech alterations such as slowed or delayed responses, word confusion

      g. Level of consciousness—sensitive index of the patient's neurologic status: decreased ability to concentrate, personality changes, hemiplegia, hemiparesis, seizures, and pupillary changes

      h. Papilledema (considered a cardinal sign of increased ICP), which is a swelling of the optic nerve where it meets the eye (the optic disk) and usually noted bilaterally

i. Glasgow Coma Scale score less than 8 (Table 49.1); the Full Outline of Unresponsiveness scale is another reliable neurological assessment tool (Sacco & Davis, 2019).
j. Abnormal posturing
k. Temperature elevations

2. Gastrointestinal (GI)
   a. Nausea/vomiting: often worse in the early morning; moderate to severe in intensity; global or localized; may be projectile, sudden, unexpected, not related to food intake
   b. Loss of appetite
3. Cardiovascular—bradycardia, widening pulse pressure; as ICP increases, blood pressure rises, and ST-segment elevation noted across all leads
4. Respiratory—slow, shallow respirations; tachypnea; Cheyne–Stokes respirations
5. Cushing triad (bradycardia, respiratory depression, and hypertension)—late and poor prognostic sign

III. Diagnostic testing
   A. May include contrast-enhanced magnetic resonance imaging (MRI) (often preferred), computed tomography (CT), cerebral angiography, or positron emission tomography (PET) with CT. Gadolinium-enhanced MRI has surpassed CT as the method of choice to evaluate tumors and increased ICP. A negative finding does not rule out increased ICP (Smith & Amin-Hanjani, 2019; Shelton et al., 2018).

TABLE 49.1 Glasgow Coma Scale

	Score
Eye Opening	
Spontaneous	4
Response to verbal command	3
Response to pain	2
No eye opening	1
Best Verbal Response	
Oriented	5
Confused	4
Inappropriate words	3
Incomprehensible sounds	2
No verbal response	1
Best Motor Response	
Obeys commands	6
Localizing response to pain	5
Withdrawal response to pain	4
Flexion to pain	3
Extension to pain	2
No motor response	1

Glasgow Coma Scale score—lowest score is 3 (worst) and highest is 15 (best). Record by the three parameters: eye opening (E), verbal response (V), and motor response (M). (Example: E4V4M4 is a score of 12.) A score of 13 or higher correlates with mild brain injury, scores of 9–12 correlate with moderate brain injury, and a score of 8 or less correlates with severe brain injury.

B. ICP monitoring—per intraventricular, intraparenchymal, subarachnoid, or epidural site (Smith & Amin-Hanjani, 2019); most reliable method to diagnose ICP; goal is to keep ICP at less than 20 mm Hg and cerebral perfusion pressure between 60 and 70 mm Hg; risks of ICP monitoring include central nervous system (CNS) infection and intracranial hemorrhage (Sacco & Davis, 2019).
C. CT- or MRI-guided stereotactic biopsy for tissue diagnosis if malignancy is suspected cause (Shelton et al., 2018).
D. CSF examination if leptomeningeal metastasis or meningitis is suspected (Shelton et al., 2018).

Management

I. Medical management
   A. Surgery
      1. Remove offending cause (such as tumor or hematoma)
      2. Shunt placement: provides an alternative pathway for CSF
      3. Ommaya reservoir placement for intrathecal chemotherapy administration
   B. RT—if radiosensitive tumor is cause; however, RT should be used with caution if the elevation of ICP is uncontrolled, as this may cause acute herniation and death (Lin & Avila, 2017). Radiation techniques such as stereotactic radiosurgery, including CyberKnife or brachytherapy, could be utilized.
   C. Hyperventilation: the most rapid method to decrease ICP by causing vasoconstriction; decreases cerebral blood volume and ICP; requires patient to be sedated, intubated, and ventilated to a partial pressure of carbon dioxide (PCO_2) between 26 and 30 mm Hg; contraindicated in traumatic brain injury and acute stroke (Smith & Amin-Hanjani, 2019). Affects short-lived, and prolonged hyperventilation could lead to increased ICP due to compensating metabolic alkalosis (Allen, 2018).
   D. Pharmacologic measures.
      1. Discontinue offending agent as in cases of PRES
      2. Treatment of tumor with chemotherapy or targeted agents
         a. Regional drug delivery such as through the intrathecal or intraventricular (via CSF) routes, circumvents the blood–brain barrier
      3. Corticosteroids may be indicated in the setting of brain tumor or CNS infection but could be contraindicated in head injuries, cerebral infarction, or intracranial hemorrhage (Allen, 2018; Smith & Amin-Hanjani, 2019).
      4. Osmotherapy—to maintain euvolemia and normo-osmolality to hyperosmolality (Brydges & Brydges, 2021; Han, Yang, Guo, & Zhang, 2022)
         a. Isotonic fluids such as normal saline. Hypertonic saline expands the intravascular volume, increases blood pressure, and increases cerebral blood flow. Continuous infusion or bolus may

be utilized. Observe for renal failure, electrolyte disturbances, acute red blood cell lysis, or phlebitis (Smith & Amin-Hanjani, 2019).

     b. Mannitol bolus—decreases reabsorption of water and sodium across renal tubules, creating a diuretic effect. Monitor the blood pressure carefully, observe for signs of cardiac overload, and caution in patients with renal dysfunction.

5. Anticonvulsant therapy if indicated
6. Antipyretic therapy to reduce fever
7. Sedative agents
8. Loop diuretics (e.g., furosemide) may be given with mannitol to potentiate effect; however, this may exacerbate dehydration and hypokalemia.
9. Stool softeners/stimulants as ordered to prevent constipation and straining
10. Antiemetics if indicated

II. Nursing management
  A. Position to reduce ICP by maximizing venous outflow from head
    1. Head elevation—usually about 30 degrees
    2. Avoid excessive flexion or rotation of neck and restrictive neck taping.
    3. Use of log-roll technique when turning patients, keeping patient passive
    4. Avoid prone position or activities that exert pressure on the abdomen.
    5. Avoid Valsalva maneuver.
  B. Provide mechanical cooling.
  C. Minimize endotracheal suctioning.
  D. Avoid rectal temperatures.
  E. Maintain a calm environment:
    1. Minimizing external stimulation—light, noise, touch, and temperature extremes
    2. Encouraging calm interactions between the patient and others
    3. Teaching stress reduction strategies to patient and family
    4. Developing a daily schedule of activities with appropriate rest periods
  F. Maintain bed rest with increasing ICP and progressive symptoms.
  G. Prevent injury.
    1. Keep bed in lowest position with side rails elevated.
    2. Use assistive devices as needed.
    3. Use bed alarms to monitor patient activity.
  H. Facilitate physical mobility and prevent injury.
    1. Assess skin integrity regularly; inspect pressure points and immobile extremities.
    2. Use pressure-distributing devices or padding as needed.
    3. Change position every 2 hours.
    4. Instruct patient about the proper use of assistive devices.
    5. Assist patient and family to set realistic goals to maintain optimal activity and self-care levels within limitations imposed by the disease.

I. Address knowledge deficit.
  1. Instruct patient on signs and symptoms that might indicate progressive disease.
  2. Include family or significant other in educational process.
  3. Assess readiness to learn and preferred learning method
  4. Instruct patient about self-care, community resources, and emergency contacts.
  5. Provide information about disease process, interventions, and expected outcomes.

J. Monitoring
  1. Monitor for mental status changes.
  2. Monitor for changes of decreasing cardiac output (changes in vital signs, decreased urinary output, and changes in mentation).
  3. Monitor for sensory or motor changes—changes in visual acuity, pupil reactions, and verbal expression; decrease in muscle strength, coordination, and movement.
  4. Monitor for associated symptoms such as nausea, vomiting, and headache.
  5. Monitor for seizure activity.
  6. Any negative changes of neurologic function require immediate action (Allen, 2018; Sacco & Davis, 2019; Schizodimos, Soulountsi, Iasonidou, & Kapravelos, 2020).

SPINAL CORD COMPRESSION

Overview

I. Definition—a neurologic emergency that occurs when the spinal cord or cauda equina is compromised by direct pressure, vertebral collapse, or both caused by metastatic spread or direct extension of a malignancy; compression results in compromised neurologic function if not treated promptly (Rucker, 2018).

II. Pathophysiology (Rucker, 2018)
  A. The spinal cord is a cylindric body of nervous tissue that occupies the upper two-thirds of the vertebral canal. The spinal cord is surrounded by protective bones (vertebral bodies, lamina and pedicles, and spinous processes) (Laufer, Schiff, Kelly, & Bilsky, 2021).
  B. The spinal cord has motor, sensory, and autonomic functions.
  C. Compression of the spinal cord may occur because of tumor invasion of the vertebrae and results from subsequent collapse of the spinal cord that causes increased pressure, or because of primary tumors of the spinal cord.
  D. Compression of the spinal cord may result in minor changes in motor, sensory, and autonomic function or complete paralysis. Spinal cord compression (SCC) is the second most frequent neurologic complication of metastatic cancer.
  E. Ambulatory status and extent of neurologic compromise at diagnosis are directly related to prognosis and quality of life.
  F. SCC is a poor prognostic sign, and most patients die within a year of diagnosis (Rucker, 2018).

Assessment

I. Identification of patients at risk (Kaplan, 2018a; Lawton et al., 2019; Macdonald, Lynch, Garbett, & Nazeer, 2019; Rucker, 2018; Laufer et al., 2021):
  A. Cancers that have a natural history for metastasizing to the bone—breast, lung, prostate, renal, melanoma, non-Hodgkin lymphoma, and myeloma
  B. Cancers that metastasize to the brain and spinal cord—lymphoma, seminoma
  C. Primary cancers of the spinal cord—ependymoma, astrocytoma, and glioma
  D. History of vertebral compression fractures
  E. Metastatic disease at presentation
II. History
  A. Histology of primary tumor, date of diagnosis, stage at diagnosis, treatment history, history of metastatic disease; responses to treatment and survival following treatment vary among types of cancer
  B. Time since the onset of symptoms; level and degree of compression
  C. Comprehensive pain assessment, including onset, duration, location, intensity, description, and exacerbating and relieving factors
  D. Preexisting medical problems and current medications
III. Physical examination—presenting signs and symptoms vary, depending on the location and severity of the compression (Kaplan, 2018a; Lawton et al., 2019; Rucker, 2018)
  A. Early signs and symptoms:
    1. Localized pain is the most common initial symptom (96% of patients), often described as dull or achy. Pain may precede other symptoms by up to 2 months (Rucker, 2018).
    2. Neck or back pain—always requires prompt evaluation in cancer patients
  B. Late signs and symptoms (Kaplan, 2018a; Rucker, 2018)—ominous; treatment must be instituted on an emergent basis.
    1. As SCC compression progresses, pain may become radiating or radicular, and may increase when supine, coughing, sneezing, or with Valsalva maneuvers.
    2. Gentle percussion and palpation of the vertebral column, neck flexion, and straight-leg raises—may indicate the level of cord compression.
    3. Motor weakness or dysfunction is the second most common symptom and may present as heaviness, stiffness, or weakness of extremities and lead to loss of coordination and ataxia. Once patient has progressed to paraplegia, very few will regain mobility. Muscle atrophy can occur (Table 49.2).
    4. Sensory loss—regarding light touch, pain, or temperature (occurs less often than motor deficits) (see Table 49.2).
      a. Loss of sensation for deep pressure, vibrations, position
      b. Changes begin distally and move proximally
    5. Autonomic dysfunction

TABLE 49.2	Assessment of Motor and Sensory Function
Function	**Assessment Techniques**
Muscle strength	Upper extremities—ask patient to grip your finger as firmly as possible.
	Lower extremities—ask patient to resist plantar flexion of his or her feet.
Coordination of hands and feet	Ask patient to touch each finger to his or her thumb in rapid sequence.
	Ask patient to turn hand over and back as quickly as possible.
	Ask patient to tap your hand as quickly as possible with the ball of each foot.
Sensory perception	Touch patient along the length of extremities and trunk with the blunt and sharp ends of a safety pin, and ask patient to identify as either sharp or dull.
	Ask patient to report the sensation of touch when touched with a wisp of cotton.
	Move one of the patient's fingers and ask if the finger is being moved up or down.
	Touch skin of patient with test tube of hot water and then cold water; ask the patient to describe the temperature.

    a. Incontinence or retention of urine or stool
    b. Sexual impotence
    c. Loss of sweating below lesion
  C. Grade peripheral sensory neuropathy and motor neuropathy and document according to Common Toxicity Criteria for Adverse Events (CTCAE) criteria.
IV. Diagnostic testing
  A. Laboratory testing: no diagnostic laboratory tests exist; however, calcium and serum albumin tests should be examined in patients with bone metastases due to potential hypercalcemia (Kaplan, 2018a; see Chapter 52).
  B. Diagnostic studies (Kaplan, 2018a; Laufer et al., 2021; Lawton et al., 2019; Rucker, 2018)
    1. MRI—diagnostic procedure of choice for evaluating SCC; entire spine should be assessed, as multiple sites of metastasis may exist
    2. CT—alternative when MRI unavailable or contraindicated; less sensitive
    3. Myelography—used with or without CT when MRI and other imaging modalities are nondiagnostic
    4. Spinal radiography—shows bone abnormalities or soft tissue masses; should not be used to diagnose or rule out spinal metastasis
    5. PET—both sensitive and specific but less available than MRI; should not be used alone for diagnosis or treatment guidance

Management

I. Medical management (Kaplan, 2018a; Lawton et al., 2019; Rucker, 2018; Schiff, Brown, Bilsky, & Laufer, 2021)
  A. Radiation

1. For radiosensitive tumors such as lymphoma, myeloma, breast, prostate cancers, and small-cell lung cancers (SCLCs)
2. Treatment of choice for most epidural metastases and cord compressions
3. Used alone when no evidence of spinal instability
4. Most common dose is 30 Gy given in 10 fractions
5. Helpful in managing pain even in patients with poor prognosis
6. Stereotactic body RT standard of care for areas of previous radiation
7. If performed after decompressing surgery, radiation is delayed at least a week

B. Surgery
   1. Laminectomy used to decompress a vertebral body in patients with spinal instability and for tumors not responsive to RT
   2. Urgency of surgery dependent on neurologic compromise
   3. May be used if recurrent tumor is in an area that has received a maximal safe radiation dose

C. Pharmacologic interventions
   1. Corticosteroids
      a. Immediate high initial dose given intravenously (IV); patients may experience a sudden, intense burning or tingling perineal discomfort; slow IV administration may lessen or eliminate this sensation. Taper corticosteroids when discontinued.
      b. Monitor blood glucose and assess for other adverse events such as mania and insomnia.
      c. GI prophylaxis with proton pump inhibitors
   2. Analgesics
      a. More than 95% of patients with SCC have pain; opioids commonly employed
      b. Coanalgesics for neuropathic pain
         (1) Anticonvulsants
         (2) Antidepressants
      c. Observe for adverse events such as constipation, nausea, somnolence, and pruritus
   3. Chemotherapeutic agents
      a. For chemosensitive tumors (such as lymphomas, neuroblastoma, germ cell neoplasms, and breast cancers)
      b. Also manages malignancy in other parts of the body
   4. Anticoagulation
      a. Patients with SCC have an increased risk of thrombus
      b. Low-molecular-weight heparin prophylaxis
   5. Bowel regimen
      a. Needs vary depending upon the extent of SCC
   6. Bone-remodeling agents to reduce the incidence of skeletal-related events

II. Nursing management
   A. Treat emergently within 24 hours of signs of neurologic compromise.
   B. Promote physical mobility.

1. Mobilize the patient based on findings of stable or unstable spine.
2. Maintain neutral spine alignment by using the log-roll technique until neurologically stable.
3. Assist patient to maintain a safe level of independence within the limitations imposed by the cord compression.
4. Encourage patient and family to express concerns about the effect of residual limitations on activities of daily living (ADLs) and lifestyle.

C. Improve or maintain neurologic function (Kaplan, 2018a).
   1. Monitor for progression of motor or sensory deficits every 8 hours.
   2. Monitor bowel and urinary elimination patterns and effectiveness.
      a. Palpation for bladder distention if interval between voiding increases.
      b. Record frequency and characteristics of stool with each bowel movement.
      c. Conduct gentle digital rectal examination to check for impaction if no bowel movement within 3 days, unless neutropenic or thrombocytopenic.
      d. Record intake and output every 8 hours.
   3. Monitor for
      a. Decrease in muscle strength and coordination
      b. Decrease in the perception of temperature, touch, and position
      c. Change in the level of consciousness
   4. Improve or maintain skin integrity.
      a. Regularly assess skin integrity and evaluate intervention.
      b. Institute a skin care regimen.
      c. Provide instructions to the patient and family about assessing the pressure and temperature of objects, contact with areas of compromised feeling or sensation.
   5. Increase the knowledge of disease process and therapeutic interventions.
      a. Provide education about reporting any changes in bowel and urinary elimination patterns; pain, sensory and motor function; skin integrity; or sexual dysfunction.
      b. Provide education about treatment modalities, potential adverse events, and self-care.

SUPERIOR VENA CAVA SYNDROME

Overview

I. Definition: results from compromised venous drainage of the head, neck, upper extremities, and thorax through the superior vena cava (SVC) because of compression or obstruction of the vessel such as by tumor, lymph nodes, or thrombus

II. Pathophysiology (Drews and Rabkin, 2022; McNally, 2018; Shelton, 2018; Zimmerman & Davis, 2018)
   A. The SVC is a thin-walled major vessel that carries venous drainage from the head, neck, upper extremities, and upper thorax to the heart.

B. The SVC is located in the mediastinum; surrounded by structures of the sternum, trachea, vertebrae, aorta, right bronchus, lymph nodes, and pulmonary artery.

C. The SVC is a low-pressure vessel easily compressed; compression (acute or gradual) can occur from multiple causes. Right-sided lung cancers are responsible for most cases of SVC syndrome (SVCS).

D. When obstruction of the SVC occurs, venous return to the heart from the head, neck, thorax, and upper extremities is impaired.

 1. Venous pressure and congestion in head, neck, upper extremities, and upper thorax increase but eventually decrease over time as blood flow diverts to multiple smaller collaterals to the azygos vein or the inferior vena cava.

 2. Rapid tumor growth often does not allow time to develop collateral flow.

 3. Decreased cardiac filling and output may ensue.

 4. Hemodynamic compromise occurs from mass effect on the heart.

 5. Concomitant thrombosis often occurs.

Assessment

I. Identification of patients at risk (Drews & Rabkin, 2022)

 A. Presence of chest malignancy, most often non–SCLC (NSCLC) and SCLC, followed by lymphoma. Other malignancies can cause SVC syndrome.

 B. Presence of central venous catheters and pacemakers.

 C. Previous RT to the mediastinum secondary to vascular fibrosis.

 D. Associated conditions (e.g., fungal infection, benign tumors, and aortic aneurysm).

 E. Cardiovascular disease.

II. History (McNally, 2018; Shelton, 2018; Zimmerman & Davis, 2018)

 A. Assess for risk factors.

 B. Assess the rapidity of symptom onset.

 C. Symptoms more pronounced in the morning or when bending over and improve after being upright for several hours.

 D. Assess for symptoms such as dyspnea (most common symptom), sensation of head fullness, headache, blurred vision, nasal stuffiness, hoarseness, dysphagia, nonproductive cough, need to sleep in an upright position, and chest pain.

 E. Mild symptoms may disappear after patient has been upright for a few hours.

III. Physical examination (McNally, 2018; Shelton, 2018; Zimmerman & Davis, 2018)

 A. Redness and edema in conjunctivae and around the eyes and face

 B. Swelling of the neck, arms, and hands; men may have problems buttoning shirt collars (Stokes sign)

 C. Neck and thoracic vein distention—with visible collateral veins

 D. Hoarseness

 E. Women may experience swelling of their breasts.

F. Dysphagia, hoarseness, and hemoptysis

G. Horner syndrome—the combination of drooping of the eyelid (ptosis) and constriction of the pupil (miosis), sometimes accompanied by decreased sweating (anhidrosis) of the face on the same side

H. Later signs:

 1. Cyanosis of upper torso

 2. Symptoms of increased ICP—severe headache, visual disturbances, blurred vision, dizziness, syncope, irritability, and changes in mental status

 3. Stridor, signs of congestive heart failure

 4. Tachycardia, tachypnea, and orthopnea

 5. Hypotension, absence of peripheral pulses

I. Grade toxicities according to CTCAE criteria

IV. Diagnostic testing (Drews & Rabkin, 2022; McNally, 2018; Zimmerman & Davis, 2018)

 A. CT of the thorax (contrast or helical)—the preferred diagnostic test; often identifies the cause of SVCS and presence of collateral vessels

 B. MRI—sensitive for SVCS, beneficial in those who cannot tolerate contrast; may be complicated by inability to tolerate supine position, longer scanning time, and higher cost

 C. PET useful when planning the radiation field and to determine if the cause is malignant or benign

 D. Contrast venography is more invasive but useful to determine the extent of thrombus formation and if stent placement or surgery is planned.

 E. Chest radiography results are usually abnormal, showing mediastinal widening and pleural effusion.

 F. Additional tests to determine the histologic diagnosis of the primary condition include bronchoscopy, bone marrow biopsy, mediastinoscopy, thoracentesis, sputum analysis, and needle biopsy of palpable lymph nodes.

 G. Evaluation of laboratory data—comparison of available laboratory data against previous and normal values.

 1. Arterial blood gases

 2. Electrolytes, kidney function

 3. Complete blood cell (CBC) count

 4. Coagulation studies

Management

I. Medical management (Drews & Rabkin, 2022; McNally, 2018; Shelton, 2018)

 A. Goals of treatment include relief of the obstruction and treatment of the underlying cause and presenting symptoms (Drews & Rabkin, 2022; Richardson, Rupasov, & Sharma, 2018; Shelton, 2018).

 1. Treatment and prognosis determined by the rapidity of onset and cause of obstruction.

 2. Histologic diagnosis necessary for the treatment of the causes of the primary tumor, but treatment of airway obstruction or laryngeal edema should not be delayed.

 B. Thrombolytic therapy or tissue plasminogen activators may be used to treat a thrombosis that is catheter induced.

1. Systemic anticoagulation may also be indicated, especially after stent placement.
2. Observe for complications related to stent placement, such as infection, pulmonary embolus, stent migration, hematoma at insertion site, and bleeding or perforation of the SVC.

C. Corticosteroids—may reduce edema or inflammation (e.g., to prevent postradiation edema); useful in steroid-responsive malignancies. Blood glucose should be monitored closely.

D. Diuretics—may reduce edema and intravascular volume.

E. Antineoplastic therapy alone or in conjunction with radiation in patients who have chemosensitive diseases such as SCLC, non-Hodgkin lymphoma, or germ cell cancer.
   1. Antineoplastic therapy may follow initial emergent treatment.
   2. Alternative sites of administration (such as femoral vein port-a-cath or dorsal foot vein) may be utilized. If vesicant agents are prescribed, great care must be taken to avoid extravasation.

F. RT
   1. The primary treatment for SVCS if the patient has NSCLC but often used in other types of malignancies.
   2. RT also used as initial treatment if a histologic diagnosis cannot be made or the clinical status of the patient is deteriorating.

G. Percutaneous intravascular stent placement.
   1. Most effective treatment modality when urgent intervention needed; restores blood flow, and symptoms rapidly resolve.
   2. Percutaneous balloon angioplasty may be necessary to enlarge the vascular lumen prior to stent placement.
   3. Stent placement will require at least short-term anticoagulation (Calsina Juscafresa, Bazo, Grochowicz, Paramo Alfaro, & Lopez-Picazo Gonzalez, 2017; Khan, Shanholtz, & McCurdy, 2017; Niu, Xu, Cheng, & Cao, 2017).
   4. Observe for procedure complications such as acute pulmonary edema and bleeding (Morin et al., 2017).

H. Remove the central venous catheter to avoid embolization.

I. Surgical reconstruction of SVC is rarely required because of the effectiveness of stent placement. Surgical resection of the tumor is rare because of the poor prognosis in many patients with SVCS.

II. Nursing management (Drews & Rabkin, 2022; McNally, 2018; Shelton, 2018)

A. Maintain adequate gas exchange (Drews & Rabkin, 2022; Shelton, 2018).
   1. Maintain airway.
   2. Position in Fowler or semi-Fowler position to decrease edema, dyspnea, and hydrostatic pressure.
   3. Instruct patient to avoid Valsalva maneuver or other straining activities.
   4. Assist with ADLs to conserve breathing and energy.
   5. Assess for progressive respiratory distress.
   6. Administer oxygen as ordered.

B. Maintain adequate cardiac output (Shelton, 2018).
   1. Monitor for changes in tissue perfusion (decreased peripheral pulses, decrease in blood pressure, and cyanosis).
   2. Monitor for changes of decreasing cardiac output (changes in vital signs, decreased urinary output, and changes in mentation).
   3. Monitor intake, output, and weight.

C. Increase the knowledge of disease process and therapeutic interventions (Shelton, 2018).
   1. Provide information about critical signs and symptoms that might indicate progressive disease.
   2. Include family or significant other in educational process.
   3. Assess the readiness to learn and preferred learning method.
   4. Instruct patient in self-care measures, community resources, and emergent contacts.
   5. Educate about disease process, interventions, and expectations of outcome.

D. Prevent injury (Drews & Rabkin, 2022; Shelton, 2018).
   1. Avoid venipunctures, IV fluid administration, intramuscular injections, or measurement of blood pressure in the upper extremities.
   2. Remove jewelry (e.g., rings) and restrictive clothing.
   3. Assess for changes in neurologic or mental status.
   4. Monitor for signs and symptoms of adverse effects of anticoagulant therapy—petechiae; ecchymosis; bleeding—gums, nose, urinary tract, and GI system.
   5. Monitor for signs and symptoms of adverse effects of steroid therapy—muscle weakness, mood swings, steroid-induced glycosuria, dyspepsia, and insomnia.

CARDIAC TAMPONADE

Overview

I. Definition—a life-threatening situation of excessive accumulation of fluid in the pericardial sac exerting extrinsic pressure on the cardiac chambers, resulting in impaired intracardiac filling, decreased cardiac output, and compromised cardiac function

II. Pathophysiology (Appleton, Gillam, & Koulogiannis, 2017; Hoit, 2017; Kearns & Walley, 2017; Khan et al., 2017)

A. The pericardium is a two-layered sac (parietal and visceral layers) surrounding the heart.

B. As intrapericardial pressure increases, the following occur:
   1. The space between the two layers is the pericardial cavity.
   2. The cavity normally is filled with 10–50 mL of fluid produced by the mesothelial cells of the visceral pericardium. This fluid between opposing layers of the heart allows the heart to move without friction.

3. Recesses and sinuses may accommodate a limited increase of pericardial fluid.
4. Fluid accumulation in the pericardial sac occurs secondary to the following:
   a. Direct or metastatic tumor invasion to the pericardial sac
   b. Fibrosis of the pericardial sac related to RT
   c. Infections causing pericardial effusions
   d. Obstruction of mediastinal lymph nodes
   e. Increased capillary permeability from chemotherapy or biotherapy
   f. Direct trauma to the chest
   g. Improper insertion of central line or pacemaker
5. Cardiac chambers are compressed, and left ventricular filling decreases.
6. The ability of the heart to pump decreases.
7. Cardiac output decreases, and blood pressure falls.
8. Impaired systemic perfusion occurs, and cardiogenic shock may follow.

III. Rate of pericardial fluid increase is more important than the volume accrued because the slow accumulation allows time for the pericardium to expand. Acute increases may cause severe symptoms, even with a small amount of fluid (Khan et al., 2017).

IV. Malignant pericardial involvement has a poor prognosis.

Assessment

I. Identification of patients at risk (Kaplan, 2018b; Kearns & Walley, 2017)
   A. Patients with primary tumors of the heart, including mesothelioma and sarcomas (including Kaposi sarcoma)
   B. Patients with metastatic tumors to the pericardium—lung, breast, GI tract, leukemia, Hodgkin or non-Hodgkin lymphoma, sarcoma, and melanoma
   C. Patients who have received more than 4000 cGy of radiation to a field in which the heart is included
   D. Patients receiving chemotherapy or biotherapy associated with increased capillary permeability (e.g., anthracyclines, interferon, interleukin, and granulocyte-macrophage colony-stimulating factor)
   E. Those with comorbidities such as heart disease, connective tissue disorders, myxedema (dry, waxy, non-pitting edema with abnormal deposits of mucin in the skin often associated with hypothyroidism), tuberculosis, aneurysms, renal failure, and history of cardiac surgery (e.g., valve surgery)

II. History
   A. Early signs and symptoms (Appleton et al., 2017; Kaplan 2018b; Kearns & Walley, 2017; Khan et al., 2017)
      1. May be nonspecific
      2. Exertional dyspnea
      3. Tachycardia, chest pain
      4. Restlessness
      5. Fatigue, malaise
   B. Late signs and symptoms (Appleton et al., 2017; Kaplan, 2018b; Kearns & Walley, 2017)
      1. Retrosternal chest pain relieved by leaning forward and intensified when lying supine or by inspiration; may radiate to neck and jaw; chest pain may be difficult to differentiate from a myocardial infarction.
      2. Oliguria
      3. Peripheral edema
      4. Diaphoresis
      5. Anxiety and agitation, mental status changes
      6. Hiccups
      7. Hoarseness, dysphagia
      8. Chest pain—may disappear
      9. Vague, right upper quadrant pain resulting from hepatic venous congestion

III. Physical examination (Appleton et al., 2017; Kaplan, 2018b; Kearns & Walley, 2017; Khan et al., 2017)
   A. Beck triad: muffled heart sounds, hypotension, and increased jugular venous pressure may be seen in about one-third of patients, less common in chronic effusions.
   B. Pulsus paradoxus (decrease in blood pressure of more than 10 mm Hg with inspiration) is found in over 75% of patients with tamponade (Appleton et al., 2017). An ominous finding.
   C. Decreased systolic pressure and rising diastolic pressure (narrow pulse pressure)
   D. Pericardial friction rub is common but may be absent in large pericardial effusions.
   E. Jugular venous distention.
   F. Tachycardia—more than 100 beats/min; a protective mechanism
   G. Weak or absent apical and peripheral pulses, heart palpitations
   H. Tachypnea, orthopnea
   I. Increased central venous pressure
   J. Altered levels of consciousness
   K. Cyanosis, central and peripheral; mottled, cool skin
   L. Delayed capillary refill

IV. Diagnostic testing (Appleton et al., 2017; Kaplan, 2018b; Kearns & Walley, 2017; Khan et al., 2017)
   A. Chest radiography shows enlarged transverse pericardial diameter (water bottle heart) after more than 200 mL of fluid has accumulated; however, it is not a definitive diagnostic tool.
   B. CT is very useful because it can also reveal pleural effusion, masses, or pericardial thickening; however, it may overestimate the volume of effusion. It can reveal whether effusion is hemorrhagic and estimate pericardial thickness.
   C. Echocardiography is the initial and most precise diagnostic test and should be repeated frequently to monitor for progression. Effusion, collapse of right or left atrium, respiratory variation in flow velocities, and dilation of inferior vena cava may be seen.
   D. Electrocardiography results vary, depending on the extent of the tamponade; signs similar to pericarditis (elevation of ST segments with reciprocal ST depression

in aVR T-wave inversions may be seen with large pericardial effusions) may be seen. Typically, sinus tachycardia, low QRS voltage, and electrical alternans are present.

E. Cardiac catheterization may demonstrate right-sided pressures and equalizations of the right atrial, right ventricular, and pulmonary capillary wedge pressures.

F. MRI is very sensitive in the detection of effusions as small as 30 mL; however, it requires more time and involves increased cost.

G. Evaluation of laboratory data
　1. Arterial blood gas values if patient has respiratory distress
　2. Electrolyte values

Management

I. Medical management (Kaplan, 2018b; Kearns & Walley, 2017; Khan et al., 2017; McCanny & Colreavy, 2017)

A. Emergent pericardiocentesis is the treatment for acute pericardial tamponade.
　1. Pericardiocentesis is the temporary removal of excess pericardial fluid.
　2. Usually performed under ultrasound.
　3. Cytology testing of fluid may be performed.
　　a. Bloody fluid is associated with a positive cytology test result.
　　b. Cytology testing has a significant false-negative rate.
　4. About half of malignant pericardial effusions will reaccumulate; continue to monitor for tamponade.
　5. Observe for complications such as bleeding, change in vital signs, cardiac arrhythmias, infection, and abdominal or shoulder pain.

B. Pericardial window is a surgical opening of the pericardium to allow fluid drainage. Alternatively, an indwelling catheter may be placed.

C. Total pericardiectomy is the removal of the pericardial sac for patients with constrictive or chronic pericarditis.

D. Percutaneous balloon pericardiotomy (an alternative to surgical pericardial window) involves a balloon being used to create a pericardial window by stretching the pericardium.

E. For surgical interventions, it is important to be aware of a possible delay in scheduling the procedure and to ensure patient stability. Local anesthesia is preferred because anesthesia with endotracheal intubation may cause life-threatening hypotension and cardiac arrest. Surgical procedures may be contraindicated in thrombocytopenia and with anticoagulation therapy.

F. RT may be performed to treat radiosensitive tumors of the pericardium. RT is contraindicated in radiation pericarditis and when area involved has previously received radiation.

G. Volume resuscitation is done to correct hypovolemia. Monitor for negative changes in hemodynamic stability due to fluid overload.

H. Pericardial sclerosis (to prevent recurrence of pericardial effusion) is an instillation through a pericardial catheter of an agent (e.g., doxycycline [Doxy 100], thiotepa [Thioplex], bleomycin [Blenoxane], mitomycin C [Mitomycin], and sterile talc) that causes inflammation and subsequent fibrosis.

I. Pharmacologic interventions (Kaplan, 2018b; Kearns & Walley, 2017; Khan et al., 2017; McCanny & Colreavy, 2017)
　1. Systemic antineoplastic therapy may be used for treating chemotherapy-sensitive malignancies such as lymphoma, breast cancer, or SCLC.
　2. Corticosteroids may be used after drainage of the effusion but are not used in urgent treatment.
　3. Analgesics as indicated.
　4. Any intervention that lowers the heart rate (e.g., beta-blocker or anesthesia) could cause a dangerous decrease in cardiac output.

II. Nursing management
A. Conduct frequent, regular assessment of cardiovascular status, evaluating for instability (e.g., sinus tachycardia, drop in blood pressure).
B. Assess character and amount of drainage from pericardial catheter if present.
C. Assess catheter site for signs and symptoms of infection.
D. Conduct frequent, regular assessment of respiratory status, and evaluating for changes.
E. Administer oxygen therapy as ordered.
F. Position with the head of bed (HOB) elevated.

BOWEL OBSTRUCTION

Overview

I. Definition: cessation of forward movement of bowel contents

II. Pathophysiology (Rami Reddy & Cappell, 2017; Yeh & Bordeianou, 2021)
A. Mechanical obstruction—most common in end-stage cancer, may be partial or complete and may be caused by extrinsic or intrinsic factors.
B. Functional obstructions—caused by changes to peristalsis such as by infiltration of bowel muscle by tumor; includes fecal impaction.
C. Small-intestine obstructions are more common.
D. Large-bowel obstructions (about 25% of bowel obstructions) most often at or distal to the transverse colon.
E. Bowel dilation occurs proximal to the obstruction due to intestinal stasis that increases gas from bacterial proliferation and fermentation of ingested food. Mural edema occurs, and the bowel loses its absorptive ability, leading to the accumulation of fluids. This leads to bowel distention because of the stationary solids, intestinal fluids, and gas. Tension increases in the intestinal wall, and an increased risk for bowel perforation exists (see the "Bowel Perforation" section). Transudative fluid leakage from the intestinal lumen

to the peritoneal cavity may occur. Loss of fluids in addition to emesis secondary to the obstruction may lead to hypovolemia and electrolyte disturbance. If obstruction is not relieved, bowel ischemia and necrosis may result.

F. Colorectal obstruction may lead to perforation, colonic necrosis, and septic shock.

G. Causes of obstructions:
1. Cancer, most often colorectal cancer and may be the presenting symptom
   a. Malignant obstruction occurs in 8%–29% of colorectal cancers and 10%–50% of ovarian cancers.
   b. Cholangiocarcinoma, pancreatic, and gallbladder carcinoma are the most common tumors causing duodenal obstruction.
   c. Intraluminal tumors that may occlude the lumen or act as a point of intussusception.
   d. Intramural tumors that may extend to the mucosa and obstruct the lumen or impair peristalsis.
   e. Mesenteric and omental masses or malignant adhesions that may kink or angulate the bowel, creating an extramural obstruction.
   f. Tumors that infiltrate into the mesentery bowel muscle or the enteric or celiac plexus and cause dysmotility.
2. Postoperative intra-abdominal adhesions—entrap a loop of intestine and contract, causing an obstruction and possibly strangulation; may develop a few days after surgery or many years later
3. Nonsurgical adhesions after an infection such as peritonitis or after RT; may occur at any time after the infection or completion of RT
4. Hernias with colonic incarceration
5. Miscellaneous conditions such as inflammatory bowel disease
6. Volvulus: twisting of the intestine that may cut off blood flow; most common benign cause of bowel obstruction
7. Diverticulitis—repetitive bouts causing strictures
8. Pseudo-obstruction from paraneoplastic destruction of enteric neurons in rare cases
9. Severe ileus caused by:
   a. Pharmacologic agents: anticholinergic drugs, opioids, certain antineoplastic agents and antihypertensive agents, and antidiarrheals/antispasmodics
   b. Medical conditions: pancreatitis, gastroenteritis, spinal cord injury, hypokalemia, diabetic ketoacidosis, myocardial infarction, stroke, and other comorbid conditions
10. Objects blocking the intestinal lumen—for example, foreign bodies and fecal or barium impaction

III. Poor prognostic factor in colorectal cancer

Assessment

I. Identification of patients at risk (Yeh & Bordeianou, 2021)
A. Disease related: cancers such as colorectal, ovarian, and pancreatic most common
B. Treatment related
1. Prior abdominal surgery due to adhesive bowel disease (more common in small-bowel obstructions)
2. Stricture formation from prior colorectal resection
3. Surgical trauma to neurogenic pathways to intestines, rectum, or both
4. RT to abdominal area
C. Previous intestinal obstruction
D. Frequent intestinal inflammation from diseases such as diverticulitis, colitis, and inflammatory bowel disease
E. Abdominal wall hernia
F. Chronic constipation, fecal impaction
G. Peritoneal carcinomatosis (Lambert & Wiseman, 2018)

II. History (Yeh & Bordeianou, 2021)
A. Abdominal pain and intestinal colic from intestinal stretching and pressure of peristalsis as the bowel tries to push its contents past the obstruction.
1. Assess characteristics of pain (description, timing, duration, location, intensity, and associated symptoms).
2. May describe as cramping and spasmodic in mechanical obstructions (every 20–30 minutes) or as diffuse, constant, and less intense pain (may be described as pressure or fullness) in functional obstructions.
3. In partial obstructions, pain may be described as cramping pain after eating.
4. In complete obstructions, pain intensifies and comes in waves or spasms as the bowel tries to push intestinal contents past the obstruction.
5. With strangulation pain is constant and severe pain intensified with movement.
6. A sudden relief of pain followed by more severe pain may indicate bowel perforation (see the "Bowel Perforation" section).
B. Nausea and vomiting
1. Small-bowel obstructions—more severe nausea and vomiting
2. Gastric outlet obstruction—sour emesis that is not bile-colored and often contains undigested food
3. Proximal small-intestine obstruction—rapid-onset, bitter, and bile-stained emesis that may be projectile
4. Distal small-intestine obstruction or colonic obstruction with an incompetent ileocecal valve—orange-brown, malodorous, and feculent emesis
C. Anorexia, appetite changes
D. Change in bowel habits—constipation to obstipation
1. May experience lack of bowel movements and flatus or may have paradoxical diarrhea (if partial blockage exists)
2. Bowel may evacuate below an obstruction
E. Bloating, abdominal distention

F. Assess current medications

G. Note endocrine and immunologic history

H. Dietary history

III. Physical examination (Lambert & Wiseman, 2018; Rami Reddy & Cappell, 2017; Yeh & Bordeianou, 2021)

A. Immediate assessment for signs of dehydration, shock, or abdominal compartment syndrome

B. Presentation will vary according to severity, location, duration, and etiology of the bowel obstruction

C. Abdominal

1. Distention: baseline measurement of abdominal girth should be obtained and section of measurement marked. Serial exams are needed.

2. Abnormal bowel sounds:

a. Mechanical obstruction: intermittent borborygmi (loud prolonged gurgles of hyperperistalsis)

b. Nonmechanical:

(1) Proximal to obstruction—high-pitched, tinkling, or hyperactive bowel sounds that may be heard in clusters or rushes

(2) Distal to the obstruction—bowel sounds hypoactive or absent

(3) Hypoactive, low-pitched gurgles or weak tinkles

(4) Absent bowel sounds indicating a paralytic ileus

3. Abdominal palpation:

a. Boardlike abdomen may indicate peritonitis

b. Abdominal tympany noted over air-filled bowel

c. Abdominal dullness noted over fluid-filled bowel

d. Abdominal tenderness often present but does not correlate well with the location of obstruction

e. Note surgical scars

f. Assess for abdominal hernia, abdominal mass, hepatomegaly, and lymphadenopathy

g. Rebound tenderness, guarding may indicate ischemia or bowel perforation

4. Rectal examination may note fecal impaction or rectal mass

D. Vital signs:

1. Pyrexia may indicate mucosal ischemia and sepsis

2. Tachycardia, hypotension, and orthostasis could indicate dehydration

E. Dry mucous membranes and poor skin turgor may indicate dehydration

F. May appear restless and acutely ill

IV. Diagnostic testing (Ramanathan, Ojili, Vassa, & Nagar, 2017; Rami Reddy & Cappell, 2017; Yeh & Bordeianou, 2021)

A. Abdominal radiography: less sensitive than CT

B. CT of the abdomen: highly sensitive and specific

1. Can identify multifocal disease, metastatic disease, ascites, or carcinomatosis

2. Can identify ischemia, necrosis, or perforation

C. Lower endoscopy may assist in patients with chronic symptoms or with nondiagnostic CT

D. MRI:

1. More time consuming and expensive

2. Useful in persons with Crohn disease and when radiation is a concern, such as pregnant patients

E. Abdominal ultrasound

1. Useful in pregnancy and in children

2. Poor diagnostic ability in early obstruction

F. Laboratory studies: CBC with differential, electrolyte panel; carcinoembryonic antigen if imaging shows mass consistent with colorectal malignancy

Management

I. Medical management (Lambert & Wiseman, 2018; Obita, Boland, Currow, Johnson, & Boland, 2016; Shimura & Joh, 2016; Yeh & Bordeianou, 2021)

A. Initial management is supportive care, and subsequent management depends on etiology, location, comorbidities, prognosis, and goals of treatment (Obita et al., 2016; Rami Reddy & Cappell, 2017; Shimura & Joh, 2016; Yeh & Bordeianou, 2021).

B. Chemotherapy/targeted therapy

1. If surgery cannot be performed, or before surgery as neoadjuvant treatment, or after surgery as adjuvant treatment

2. After a stent placement

C. IV fluid therapy for dehydration and correction of electrolyte abnormalities

D. Pharmacologic management

1. Low-dose steroids to decreased bowel wall edema and to decrease nausea

2. Antiemetic agents

3. Octreotide to decrease intestinal secretions and stretching of bowel wall, thus decreasing pain

4. Hyoscine butylbromide or scopolamine butylbromide

5. Metoclopramide

E. Flexible sigmoidoscopy to initially decompress colon allowing time for planning surgical intervention

F. GI stenting allows time to plan surgical intervention or for palliation in advanced disease

G. Surgical management:

1. Ostomy alone for fecal diversion

2. Colectomy with primary anastomosis with or without ostomy

3. Hartmann procedure: resection of the rectosigmoid colon with closure of the rectal stump and formation of an end colostomy

4. Emergent surgery has worse outcomes than elective surgery with more complications (such as sepsis and organ failure) and higher rates of local recurrence, as well as metastatic disease and lower 5-year survival rates.

II. Nursing management

A. Obtain dietary consultation for possible total parenteral nutrition.

B. Provide patient comfort measures.

1. Ensure a relaxing environment.

2. Position patient on side and support with pillows.
3. Provide frequent oral care; use of moistened sponge sticks; avoidance of lemon or glycerin swabs.

C. Provide nasogastric tube care:
1. Assess pressure around nostrils every shift.
2. Apply a water-soluble lubricant to nasal mucosa.
3. Irrigate the tube with normal saline.
4. Elevate HOB to 45 degrees to improve ventilation and prevent aspiration.

D. Monitor for complications related to bowel obstruction.
1. Assess for signs and symptoms of dehydration—dry mouth and lips, poor skin turgor, decreased urinary output.
2. Assess for interference with deep breathing related to abdominal distention.
3. Assess for signs and symptoms of peritonitis—boardlike abdomen, increased pain on movement, shallow respirations, and tachycardia.
4. Measure abdominal girth during every shift.
5. Monitor intake and output ratio, including gastric output.

BOWEL PERFORATION

Overview

I. Definition: a full-thickness injury of the bowel wall allowing bowel contents to leak out
II. Pathophysiology (Odom, 2021; Lee-Kong & Lisle, 2015; Li et al., 2016; Rogalski, Daniluk, Baniukiewicz, Wroblewski, & Dabrowski, 2015)
   A. Perforation of the bowel may happen acutely or indolently. Perforation may be due to direct trauma or spontaneously.
   B. When the bowel perforates, leakage of fluids into the abdominal cavity may cause peritonitis, or the fluid may be contained, as with an abscess or fistula formation. This depends on the location of the perforation and the patient's immune response. Inflammation after perforation could lead to abdominal compartment syndrome.
   C. Clinical presentation depends on the organ affected, what is released from the bowel, and the immune response.
   D. Causes:
      1. Tumor—most commonly colorectal cancers; poorer outcomes are noted in patients with colorectal cancer who present with perforation
      2. Instrumentation—includes endoscopies, stent placement, endoscopic sclerotherapy, nasogastric intubation, and esophageal dilation
      3. Procedures not directly related to the bowel such as chest tube insertion, peritoneal dialysis catheter insertion, paracentesis, peritoneal lavage, percutaneous drainage of fluid collections/abscesses
      4. Surgery
      5. Blunt, penetrating injury
      6. Bowel obstruction (see the earlier section)
         a. Perforation usually occurs proximal to the obstruction.
         b. Pressure increases, exceeding intestinal perfusion pressure. This leads to ischemia and then necrosis, breaking down the bowel wall.
         c. Diastatic rupture occurs when pressure increases, causing the bowel wall to split with no necrosis present.
      7. Inflammation
      8. Peptic ulcer disease
      9. Corrosive medications/agents
         a. Acetylsalicylic acid and nonsteroidal antiinflammatory drugs
         b. Glucocorticoids
         c. Antibiotics
         d. Potassium supplements
         e. Immunosuppression therapy
         f. Chemotherapy
         g. Bevacizumab
         h. Iron supplementation
      10. Violent retching
      11. Hernia
      12. Inflammatory bowel disease such as Crohn disease
   E. Immunosuppression increases the risk for perforation.
   F. Serious complications of GI tract perforations are abdominal compartment syndrome, tension pneumothorax, tension pneumoperitoneum, subcutaneous emphysema, and peritonitis.

Assessment

I. Identification of patients at risk (Odom, 2021; Teixeira et al., 2015)
   A. Colorectal cancers or other abdominal cancers or metastatic disease
   B. Bowel obstruction
   C. Recent GI procedures such as endoscopy, stent placement
   D. History of diverticula
   E. Comorbid diseases such as immunosuppression, diabetes, cirrhosis, HIV, and inflammatory bowel disease
   F. Recent abdominal surgery, particularly emergent surgery
   G. Certain medication use (see the "Causes" section earlier)
   H. Severe nausea and vomiting with violent retching
   I. Hernia
II. History (Odom, 20216; Schmidt, Fuchs, Caca, Kullmer, & Meining, 2016)
   A. Carefully assess patients complaining of neck, chest, or abdominal pain.
      1. Assess characteristics of pain (description, timing, duration, location, intensity, and associated symptoms).
      2. Patients may be able to pinpoint the precise time of perforation, noting a sudden relief of pain, followed by more severe pain, which may indicate bowel perforation.
      3. Pain may be present in the shoulder or psoas muscles.

B. Assess for dysphagia.

C. Medication review

D. Assess for risk factors as noted earlier.

E. Assess for the history of surgery (recent or remote), procedures, and prior malignancies.

F. Assess postoperative wounds for drainage.

III. Physical examination (Odom, 2021)

A. Abdomen

1. Mass may be palpated.

2. Abdomen may be tender and/or distended (distention more common in small-bowel perforation).

B. Rectal—mass or abscess may be palpable on digital rectal exam.

C. Signs of sepsis

1. Hemodynamic instability, may or may not be febrile

2. Mental status changes

3. Organ dysfunction

4. Ill appearing

5. Initially vital signs may be normal or mildly tachycardic or hypothermic

D. Neck and chest

1. Assess for facial swelling

2. Palpate/percuss/auscultate for any signs of effusion.

IV. Diagnostic testing (Odom, 2021)

A. Laboratory studies: CBC, electrolytes, blood urea nitrogen, creatinine, liver function tests, amylase, lipase, and C-reactive protein

B. Radiograph of the chest and abdomen—however, cannot rule out a perforation or determine the location of perforation.

C. CT is the most sensitive and specific modality.

D. Endoscopy may be useful in certain situations.

E. Barium should not be used as an oral contrast agent.

F. Abdominal surgical exploration

Management

I. Medical management (Odom, 2021; Rogalski et al., 2015)

A. Initial management will likely occur in intensive care unit.

B. Antibiotics—broad spectrum until the known suspected site of perforation

C. Proton pump inhibitors for patients with upper GI tract perforations

D. Analgesics

E. Stent placement

F. Endoscopic procedure—closure of perforation (Li et al., 2016; Schmidt et al., 2016)

G. Surgery—immediate consult if perforation is suspected

II. Nursing management (Odom, 2021; Rogalski et al., 2015; Schmidt et al., 2016)

A. Monitor the drainage of effusion or abscess.

B. Provide nutritional support.

C. Stent placement

D. Position the patient to reduce the risk of intraluminal content leakage.

PNEUMONITIS

Overview

I. Definition: inflammation of the interstitial lung parenchyma with interstitial and alveolar infiltrates caused by a noninfectious source such as a chemical or radiation treatment

II. Pathophysiology (King, 2021a, 2021b; Maldonado, Limper, & Cass, 2021a, 2021b; Postow, 2022)

A. Pharmacologic treatment–induced pneumonitis pathogenesis is not well understood. It is postulated that lung injury results from direct cytotoxicity.

1. Injury to pneumocytes and alveolar epithelial cells causes the release of cytokines resulting in endothelial dysfunction, capillary leak syndrome, and pulmonary edema.

2. Inflammatory cells recruited to the site of injury, causing further cellular damage.

3. Oxidative injury from free oxygen radicals and proteases may occur.

4. Certain agents that target epidermal growth factor receptor (EGFR) may impair alveolar repair mechanisms.

5. Fibroblasts proliferate, leading to the production of collagen, widening of alveolar septae, and subsequent alveolar exudate. Resolution occurs here with some patients, although others will continue to have fibrotic progression.

6. Alveolar hemorrhage may occur.

B. Pathophysiology of radiation pneumonitis (Bledsoe, Nath, & Decker, 2017; Kroschinsky et al., 2017)

1. Direct cytotoxic damage to type II pneumocytes and vascular endothelial cells occurs and subsequently:

a. Immediate phase—an inflammatory response that causes leukocyte infiltration, resulting in intra-alveolar edema and vascular congestion.

b. Latent phase—thick secretions are produced due to an increase in goblet cells and ciliary malfunction.

c. Acute exudate phase—hyaline membrane formation, proliferation of type II pneumocytes, sloughing of epithelial and endothelium. Patient begins having symptoms of radiation pneumonitis usually within 4–12 weeks of completion of radiation.

d. Intermediate phase—repair of the lung begins; dissolution of hyaline membranes, migration of fibroblasts, and capillary regeneration occur.

e. Fibrotic phase—fibrosis is progressive as fibroblasts deposit collagen resulting in diminished lung volume.

2. Radiation recall pneumonitis may occur when a subsequent injury occurs, such as with cytotoxic chemotherapy (such as carmustine, doxorubicin, etoposide, gefitinib, gemcitabine, paclitaxel, and trastuzumab).

C. Several subtypes of pneumonitis have been identified.

1. Cryptogenic
2. Ground-glass opacities
3. Interstitial—most acute onset and rapidly progresses (King, 2021c)
4. Hypersensitivity
5. Not otherwise specified
D. Causes
   1. Radiation to chest (Bledsoe et al., 2017; Peikert & Owen, 2021)
      a. Risk varies by type of radiation given, dose, dose–time factor, use of induction or concomitant chemotherapy, and volume of lung irradiated.
   2. Pharmacologic agents:
      a. ALK inhibitors (Maldonado et al., 2021a)
      b. Bcr-Abl tyrosine kinase inhibitors (Maldonado et al., 2021a)
      c. Checkpoint inhibitor immunotherapy (Postow, 2022)
      d. EGFR inhibitors (Maldonado et al., 2021a)
      e. Immunotherapeutics such as rituximab (Kroschinsky et al., 2017)
      f. MEK inhibitors (Maldonado et al., 2021a)
      g. mTOR inhibitors (Willemsen et al., 2015)
      h. PD-1/PD-L1 immune checkpoint inhibitors (Cuellar, 2017)
      i. PI3K inhibitors such as idelalisib (Kroschinsky et al., 2017)
      j. Taxanes (King, 2021b)
      k. Tyrosine kinase inhibitors (Kroschinsky et al., 2017)
      l. Vascular endothelial growth factor inhibitors (Maldonado et al., 2021a)

Assessment

I. Identification of patients at risk (King, 2021a, 2021c; Postow, 2022)
   A. Immunosuppression
   B. Preexisting autoimmune disorder
   C. Prior immune-related toxicity
   D. Preexisting lung disease
   E. Occupational and environmental exposures such as silicates, carbon, metals, and organic or inorganic dusts
   F. Those undergoing concomitant therapy or combination therapy
II. History (King, 2021a; Peikert & Owen, 2021)
   A. Review medication list.
   B. Assess for risk factors noted earlier.
   C. Inquire about current/past oncologic treatments.
   D. Document any comorbidities.
   E. Ask about dyspnea, cough, and other pulmonary symptoms—inquire whether this is an acute onset or exacerbation of a chronic problem. Patients may describe being unable to take a deep breath.
   F. Assess for low-grade fever and hypoxia.
   G. Assess for weight loss, anorexia, fatigue, and malaise.
   H. Assess timing of symptoms—early in course of therapy or later; assess the time of treatments, including past treatments.

1. Radiation pneumonitis usually develops about 4–12 weeks after radiation completion (Peikert & Owen, 2021).
I. Patients may complain of pleuritic or substernal chest pain.
III. Physical examination (Maldonado et al., 2021a; Peikert & Owen, 2021)
   A. Evaluate hemodynamic status stability.
   B. Vital signs: low-grade fever may be present.
   C. Pulse oximetry—hypoxia may be present; oxygen saturation below 90% or more than a 4% decrease from baseline with worsening clinical status should be reported immediately. Tachypnea and cyanosis may be present in more severe cases.
   D. Pulmonary: may be normal, but bibasilar crackles or a pleural rub are often heard. Wheezing is rare.
   E. Assess for rash, which could indicate a hypersensitivity reaction.
   F. Grade and document pneumonitis according to CTCAE criteria.
IV. Diagnostic testing (King, 2021a, 2021c; Maldonado et al., 2021a; Peikert & Owen, 2021; Postow, 2022)
   A. Laboratory testing: CBC, chemistry panel, liver and kidney function, arterial blood gases; consider antinuclear antibody and rheumatoid factor.
   B. Chest radiography—compare with previous to assess the rate of change; chest radiography can be normal in 10% of patients with interstitial lung disease.
   C. High-resolution CT: more accurate than chest radiography, generally preferred.
   D. PET scanning is not as useful as CT scanning.
   E. Pulmonary function testing, possible bronchoscopy and bronchoalveolar lavage (to rule out other causes).
   F. Cardiac evaluation is useful in some patients.
   G. Lung biopsy in certain situations, such as progressive or severe disease and when etiology of pneumonitis is uncertain.
   H. No specific test will establish the diagnosis of anticancer drug–induced pneumonitis, as this is primarily a diagnosis of exclusion; consider rechallenging with suspected agent after patient recovers; decision is made on a case-by-case basis.
   I. It is important to rule out infectious causes of the pneumonitis.

Management

I. Medical management (King, 2021a, 2021b; Maldonado et al., 2021a)
   A. Management principles.
      1. Stop offending agent/therapy for any grade 3 or 4 pneumonitis.
      2. Prevent complications such as thromboembolism, GI bleeding, and nosocomial pneumonia.
   B. Glucocorticoid therapy may be considered, depending on the severity of symptoms and progressiveness of the pneumonitis. Monitor blood glucose in diabetics, and ensure infectious cause has been excluded. Tapering of glucocorticoid will likely occur over 1 to 2 months.

C. Proton pump inhibitors may be indicated for patients on steroids.

D. Inhaled bronchodilators.

E. For severe, immunotherapy-related pneumonitis, immunosuppression with infliximab with/without cyclophosphamide may be considered (Postow, 2022).

F. For those patients who will be receiving steroids long term, prophylaxis for Pneumocystis pneumonia should be considered.

G. Antibiotics for any subsequent opportunistic infection.

H. Mechanical ventilation may be indicated in severe compromise.

II. Nursing management (King, 2021b; Maldonado et al., 2021a, 2021b)

A. Provide oxygen therapy.

B. Provide supportive care for dyspnea, discomfort.

REFERENCES

Allen, D. (2018). Increased intracranial pressure. In C. Yarbro, D. Wujcik, & B. Gobel (Eds.), *Cancer nursing: Principles and practice* (8th ed., pp. 1169–1185). Burlington, MA: Jones & Bartlett Learning.

Appleton, C., Gillam, L., & Koulogiannis, K. (2017). Cardiac tamponade. *Cardiol Clin, 35*(4), 525–537. https://doi.org/10.1016/j.ccl.2017.07.006.

Bledsoe, T., Nath, S., & Decker, R. (2017). Radiation pneumonitis. *Clinics in Chest Medicine, 38*(2), 201–208. https://doi.org/10.1016/j.ccm.2016.12.004.

Brydges, N., & Brydges, G. J. (2021). Oncologic emergencies. *AACN Advanced Critical Care, 32*(3), 306–314. https://doi.org/10.4037/aacnacc2021832.

Calsina Juscafresa, L., Bazo, I. G., Grochowicz, L., Páramo Alfaro, M., López-Picazo González, J., et al. (2017). Endovascular treatment of malignant superior vena cava syndrome secondary to lung cancer. *Hospital Practice, 45*(3), 70–75. https://doi.org/10.1080/21548331.2017.1342507.

Cuellar, S. (2017). Unleashing the immune system with checkpoint inhibitors in non–small cell lung cancer: Clinical review of adverse events. *Journal of the Advanced Practitioner in Oncology, 8*, 65–75. https://doi.org/10.6004/jadpro.2017.8.5.18.

Drews, R. & Rabkin, D. (2022). In E. Bruera, J. Eidt, J. Mills, & N. Muller (Eds.), *Malignancy-related superior vena cava syndrome.* Waltham, MA: UpToDate. https://www.uptodate.com/contents/malignancy-related-superior-vena-cava-syndrome?search=malignancy%20related%20superior%20vena%20cava%20syndrome&source=search_result&selectedTitle=1~150&usage_type=default&display_rank=1. Accessed 19.03.22.

Han, C., Yang, F., Guo, S., & Zhang, J. (2022). Hypertonic saline compared to mannitol for the management of elevated intracranial pressure in traumatic brain injury: A meta-analysis. *Frontiers in Surgery*, 8. https://doi.org/10.3389/fsurg.2021.765784.

Hoit, B. (2017). Pathophysiology of the pericardium. *Progress in Cardiovascular Diseases, 59*(4), 341–348. https://doi.org/10.1016/j.pcad.2016.11.001.

Kaplan, M. (2018a). Spinal cord compression. In M. Kaplan (Ed.), *Understanding and managing oncologic emergences* (3rd ed., pp. 509–557). Oncology Nursing Society.

Kaplan, M. (2018b). Cardiac tamponade. In M. Kaplan (Ed.), *Understanding and managing oncologic emergencies* (3rd ed., pp. 45–101). Pittsburgh, PA: Oncology Nursing Society.

Kearns, M., & Walley, K. (2018). Tamponade: Hemodynamic and echocardiographic diagnosis. *Chest Journal, 153*(5), 1266–1275. https://doi.org/10.1016/j.chest.2017.11.003.

Khan, U., Shanholtz, C., & McCurdy, M. (2017). Oncologic mechanical emergencies. *Hematology/Oncology Clinics of North American, 31*(6), 927–940. https://doi.org/10.1016/j.hoc.2017.08.001.

King, T. (2021a). In K. Flaherty (Ed.), *Acute interstitial pneumonia (Hamman-Rich syndrome).* Waltham, MA: UpToDate. https://www.uptodate.com/contents/acute-interstitial-pneumonia-hamman-rich-syndrome?search=acute%20interstitial%20pneumonia&source=search_result&selectedTitle=1~62&usage_type=default&display_rank=1. Accessed 26.03.22.

King, T. (2021b). In K. Flaherty, & R. Drews (Eds.), *Taxane-induced pulmonary toxicity.* Waltham, MA: UpToDate. https://www.uptodate.com/contents/taxane-induced-pulmonary-toxicity?search=Taxane-induced%20pulmonary%20toxicity&source=search_result&selectedTitle=1~150&usage_type=default&display_rank=1. Accessed 26.03.22.

King, T. (2021c). In K. Flaherty (Ed.), *Approach to the adult with interstitial lung disease: Diagnostic testing.* Waltham, MA: UpToDate. https://www.uptodate.com/contents/approach-to-the-adult-with-interstitial-lung-disease-diagnostic-testing?search=approach%20to%20the%20adult%20with%20interstitial%20lung%20disease&source=search_result&selectedTitle=2~150&usage_type=default&display_rank=2. Accessed 26.03.22.

Kroschinsky, F., Stölzel, F., von Bonin, S., Beutel, G., Kochanek, M., Kiehl, M., et al. (2017). New drugs, new toxicities: Severe side effects of modern targeted and immunotherapy of cancer and their management. *Critical Care, 21*, 89. https://doi.org/10.1186/s13054-017-1678-1.

Lambert, L., & Wiseman, J. (2018). Palliative management of peritoneal metastases. *Annals of Surgical Oncology, 25*, 2165–2171. https://doi.org/10.1245/s10434-018-6335-7.

Laufer, I., Schiff, D., Kelly, H., & Bilsky, M. (2021). In R. Drews, & P. Wen (Eds.), *Clinical features and diagnosis of neoplastic epidural spinal cord compression.* Waltham, MA: UpToDate. https://www.uptodate.com/contents/clinical-features-and-diagnosis-of-neoplastic-epidural-spinal-cord-compression. Accessed 22.3.23.

Lawton, A. J., Lee, K. A., Cheville, A. L., Ferrone, M. L., Rades, D., Balboni, T. A., et al. (2019). Assessment and management of patients with metastatic spinal cord compression: A multidisciplinary review. *Journal of Clinical Oncology, 37*(1), 61–71. https://doi.org/10.1200/jco.2018.78.1211.

Lee-Kong, S., & Lisle, D. (2015). Surgical management of complicated colon cancer. *Clinics in Colon and Rectal Surgery, 28*(4), 228–233. https://doi.org/10.1055/s-0035-1564621.

Li, Y., Wu, J., Meng, Y., Zhang, Q., Gong, W., & Liu, S. (2016). New devices and techniques for endoscopic closure of gastrointestinal perforations. *World Journal of Gastroenterology, 22*(33), 7453–7462. https://doi.org/10.3748/wjg.v22.i33.7453.

Lin, A. L., & Avila, E. K. (2016). Neurologic emergencies in the patients with cancer: Diagnosis and management. *Journal of Intensive Care Medicine, 32*(2), 99–115. https://doi.org/10.1177/0885066615619582.

Macdonald, A. G., Lynch, D., Garbett, I., & Nazeer, N. (2019). Malignant spinal cord compression. *Journal of the Royal College of Physicians of Edinburgh, 49*(2), 151–156. https://doi.org/10.4997/jrcpe.2019.217.

Maldonado, F., Limper, A., & Cass, A. (2021a). In K. Flaherty (Ed.), *Pulmonary toxicity associated with antineoplastic therapy: Molecularly targeted agents.* Waltham, MA: UpToDate. https://www.uptodate.com/contents/pulmonary-toxicity-associated-with-antineoplastic-therapy-molecularly-targeted-agents?search=Pulmonary%20toxicity%20associated%20with%20 antineoplastic%20therapy:%20Molecularly%20targeted%20 agents&source=search_result&selectedTitle=1~150&usage_ type=default&display_rank=1. Accessed 26.03.22.

Maldonado, F., Limper, A., & Cass, A. (2021b). In K. Flaherty (Ed.), *Pulmonary toxicity associated with systemic antineoplastic therapy: Clinical presentation, diagnosis, and treatment.* Waltham, MA: UpToDate. https://www.uptodate.com/contents/pulmonary-toxicity-associated-with-systemic-antineoplastic-therapy-clinical-presentation-diagnosis-and-treatment?search=Pulmonary%20 toxicity%20associated%20with%20antineoplastic%20therapy:%20 clinical%20presentation&source=search_result&selectedTitle=1~1 50&usage_type=default&display_rank=1. Accessed 26.03.22.

McCanny, P., & Colreavy, F. (2017). Echocardiographic approach to cardiac tamponade in critically ill patients. *Journal of Critical Care, 39,* 271–277. https://doi.org/10.1016/j.jcrc.2016.12.008.

McNally, G. (2018). Superior vena cava syndrome. In C. Yarbro, D. Wujcik, & B. Gobel (Eds.), *Cancer nursing: Principles and practice* (8th ed., pp. 1187–1196). Burlington, MA: Jones & Bartlett Learning.

Morin, S., Grateau, A., Reuter, D., de Kerviler, E., de Margerie-Mellon, C., de Bazelaire, C., et al. (2018). Management of superior vena cava syndrome in critically ill cancer patients. *Supportive Care in Cancer, 26,* 521–528. https://doi.org/10.1007/s00520-017-3860-z.

Niu, S., Xu, Y., Cheng, L., & Cao, C. (2017). Stent insertion for malignant superior vena cava syndrome: Effectiveness and long-term outcome. *La Radiologia Medica, 122*(8), 633–638. https://doi.org/10.1007/s11547-017-0767-1.

Nurgat, Z., Alzahrani, H., Lawrence, M., Mannan, A., Rasheed, W., & Aliurf, M. (2017). Intracranial hypertension secondary to high dose cytosine arabinoside – A case study. *Journal of Infection and Chemotherapy, 23*(5), 319–322. https://doi.org/10.1016/j.jiac.2016.11.005.

Obita, G., Boland, E., Currow, D., Johnson, M., & Boland, J. (2016). Somatostatin analogues compared with placebo and other pharmacologic agents in the management of symptoms of inoperable malignant bowel obstruction: A systematic review. *Journal of Pain and Symptom Management, 52*(6), 901–919.

Odom, S. (2021). In M. Weiser, & K. Raghavendran (Eds.), *Overview of gastrointestinal tract perforation.* Waltham, MA: UpToDate. https://www.uptodate.com/contents/overview-of-gastrointestinal-tract-perforation?search=Overview%20of%20gastrointestinal%20 tract%20perforation.&source=search_result&selectedTitle=1~150 &usage_type=default&display_rank=1. Accessed 27.03.22.

Peikert, T. & Owen, D. (2021). In J. Jett, & S. Schild (Eds.), *Radiation-induced lung injury.* Waltham, MA: UpToDate. https://www.uptodate.com/contents/radiation-induced-lung-injury?search=Radiation-induced%20lung%20 injury.&source=search_result&selectedTitle=1~27&usage_ type=default&display_rank=1. Accessed 26.03.22.

Postow, M. (2022). In M. Atkins, & H. West (Eds.), *Toxicities associated with immune checkpoint inhibitors.* Waltham, MA: UpToDate. https://www.uptodate.com/contents/toxicities-associated-with-immune-checkpoint-inhibitors?search=Toxicities%20associated%20with%20 checkpoint%20inhibitor%20immuno%20therapy.&source=search_re sult&selectedTitle=1~150&usage_type=default&display_rank=1. Accessed 26.03.22.

Ramanathan, S., Ojili, V., Vassa, R., & Nagar, A. (2017). Large bowel obstruction in the emergency department: Imaging spectrum of common and uncommon causes. *Journal of Clinical Imaging Science, 7,* 15.

Rami Reddy, S., & Cappell, M. (2017). A systematic review of the clinical presentation, diagnosis, and treatment of small bowel obstruction. *Current Gastroenterology Reports, 19*(28). https://doi.org/10.1007/s11894-017-0566-9.

Richardson, B., Rupasov, A., & Sharma, A. (2018). Superior vena cava syndrome. *Journal of Radiology Nursing, 37*(1), 36–40. https://doi.org/10.1016/j.jradnu.2017.11.002.

Rogalski, P., Daniluk, J., Baniukiewicz, A., Wroblewski, E., & Dabrowski, A. (2015). Endoscopic management of gastrointestinal perforations, leaks and fistulas. *World Journal of Gastroenterology, 21*(37), 10542–10552. https://doi.org/10.3748/wjg.v21.i37.10542.

Rucker, Y. (2018). Spinal cord compression. In C. Yarbro, D. Wujcik, & B. Gobel (Eds.), *Cancer nursing: Principles and practice* (8th ed., pp. 1153–1167). Burlington, MA: Jones & Bartlett Learning.

Sacco, T. L., & Davis, J. G. (2019). Management of intracranial pressure part II: Nonpharmacologic interventions. *Dimensions of Critical Care Nursing, 38*(2), 61–69. https://doi.org/10.1097/dcc.0000000000000341.

Saría, M. G., & Kesari, S. (2021). Increased intracranial pressure: The use of an individualized ladder approach. *Seminars in Oncology Nursing, 37*(2), 151133. https://doi.org/10.1016/j.soncn.2021.151133.

Schiff, D., Brown, P., Bilsky, M., & Laufer, I. (2021). In P. Wen (Ed.), *Treatment and prognosis of neoplastic epidural spinal cord compression.* Waltham, MA: UpToDate. https://www.uptodate.com/contents/treatment-and-prognosis-of-neoplastic-epidural-spinal-cord-compression Accessed 22.3.23.

Schizodimos, T., Soulountsi, V., Iasonidou, C., & Kapravelos, N. (2020). An overview of management of intracranial hypertension in the intensive care unit. *Journal of Anesthesia, 34*(5), 741–757. https://doi.org/10.1007/s00540-020-02795-7.

Schmidt, A., Fuchs, K. H., Caca, K., Küllmer, A., & Meining, A. (2016). The endoscopic treatment of iatrogenic gastrointestinal perforation. *Deutsches Arzteblatt International, 113*(8), 121–128. https://doi.org/10.3238/arztebl.2016.0121.

Shelton, B. (2018). Superior vena cava syndrome. In M. Kaplan (Ed.), *Understanding and managing oncologic emergencies* (3rd ed., pp. 561–584). Oncology Nursing Society.

Shelton, B., Skinner, J., & Baynes, M. (2018). Increased intracranial pressure. In M. Kaplan (Ed.), *Understanding and managing oncologic emergencies* (3rd ed., pp. 277–323). Oncology Nursing Society.

Shimura, T., & Joh, T. (2016). Evidence-based clinical management of acute malignant colorectal obstruction. *Journal of Clinical Gastroenterology, 50*(4), 273–285.

Smith, E. & Amin-Hanjani, S. (2019). In M. Aminoff, & J. Wilterdink (Eds.), *Evaluation and management of elevated intracranial pressure in adults.* Waltham, MA: UpToDate. https://www.uptodate.com/contents/evaluation-and-management-of-elevated-intracranial-pressure-in-adults?search=Evaluation%20and%20 management%20of%20elevated%20intracranial%20pressure%20 in%20adults&source=search_result&selectedTitle=1~150&usa ge_type=default&display_rank=1. Accessed 19.03.22.

Teixeira, F., Akaishi, E., Ushinohama, A., Dutra, T., Netto, S., Utiyama, E., et al. (2015). Can we respect the principles of oncologic resection in an emergency surgery to treat colon cancer? *World Journal of Emergency Surgery, 10,* 5. https://doi.org/10.1186/1749-7922-10-5.

Willemsen, A., Grutters, J., Gerritsen, W., van Erp, N., van Herpen, C., & Tol, J. (2015). *International Journal of Cancer, 138*(10), 2312–2321. https://doi.org/10.1002/ijc.29887.

Yeh, D. & Bordeianou, L. (2021). In M. Weiser (Ed.), *Large bowel obstruction.* Waltham, MA: UpToDate. https://www.uptodate.com/contents/large-bowel-obstruction?search=Large%20bowel%20 obstruction&source=search_result&selectedTitle=1~110&usag e_type=default&display_rank=1. Accessed 27.03.22.

Zimmerman, S., & Davis, M. (2018). Rapid fire: Superior vena cava syndrome. *Emergency Medicine Clinics of North America, 36*(3), 577–584. https://doi.org/10.1016/j.emc.2018.04.011.

50

Body Image Considerations

Elizabeth Freitas

OVERVIEW

I. Body image disturbance (Rhoten, 2017)
   A. Self-perception related to an actual or perceived change in appearance.
   B. Change in function that may be visible in cancer status or physiological mechanisms (Boland, Brady, & Drury, 2020):
      1. Alopecia: most is transitory; incidence depends on the type of treatment delivered—14% of childhood cancer treatments and 30% of breast cancer treatments result in persistent or permanent alopecia (Ding et al., 2020; Freites-Martinez et al., 2019).
         a. Chemotherapy (incidence 10%–100%, average 65%): total hair loss (e.g., eyelashes, nose hair, and pubic hair); typically starts 1–3 weeks after chemotherapy, may occur over a day to weeks, and occurs later with low dose chemotherapy. Hair regrowth usually starts 3–6 months after the completion of treatment. Hair may come back slowly, thinner, or take up to a year.
         b. Radiation therapy will cause temporary or may cause permanent hair loss, in the field of treatment, starting 1–3 weeks after the first treatment and regrowth 2–6 months after completion.
         c. Mild diffuse alopecia with epidermal growth factor receptor inhibitors.
         d. Stem cell transplantation results in 100% alopecia with chemotherapy induction and may result in continued hair changes due to graft-versus-host. Total body irradiation can also impact hair loss.
      2. Changes in body composition and appearance due to:
         a. Cachexia due to inadequate nutritional intake.
         b. Weight gain due to steroids or loss of estrogen.
         c. Moon face due to high-dose corticosteroids.
      3. Sensory change such as neuropathic pain or numbness associated with neurotoxic chemotherapeutic agents.
      4. Amputation/mastectomy, surgical scar, or lymphedema.
   C. Body changes can result in psychological distress and/or changes in social interactions due to changes in appearance and/or function.

ASSESSMENT

I. Risk factors of altered body image—reactions are individual and may be related to the following:
   A. Age: Young individuals may be at increased risk for altered body image.
   B. Sex: Body image issues are a concern for both males and females (Reynolds & Harris, 2021).
   C. Treatment type: Body image issues are more significant for individuals who experience multiple treatment modalities and more radical surgeries.
   D. Time since diagnosis: Body image satisfaction is not dependent on time since diagnosis (Brederecke, Heise, & Zimmermann, 2021).
II. Physical examination
   A. Hair loss: WHO classifications of alopecia: grade 0—no alopecia; grade 1—minimal hair loss; grade 2—moderate, patchy hair loss; grade 3—complete alopecia but reversible; grade 4—irreversible alopecia (Freites-Martinez et al., 2019).
   B. Function: Assess for functional limitations that may impact body image such as lymphedema, a colostomy, or presence of neuropathy.
   C. Surgical site: wound healing, scaring, or amputation.
   D. Weight: cachexia or weight gain.
III. Psychosocial assessment: Many assessment tools are available to measure altered body image with significant variation in assessment methods, and several are cancer site specific (Muzzattii & Annuziata, 2017). Assessment tools need to be valid for the culture of the population being assessed. Body image disturbance can result in psychological distress manifesting in changes in:
   A. Coping often occurs by avoidance (Cohee et al., 2021).
   B. Increased distress can result from the reaction of others (Reynolds & Harris, 2021).

C. Role changes and changes in sexuality can result from body image changes: wife/mother, husband/father (Hovén et al., 2021; Stanca, Căpîlna, Trâmbițaș, & Căpîlna, 2022).

D. Body image changes may lead to decreased self-confidence and depressive thoughts (Boland et al., 2020).

MANAGEMENT

I. Pharmacologic management
  A. Topical minoxidil used to minimize or shorten the period of alopecia due to cytotoxic agents (Williams et al., 2020).
  B. Antianxiety or antidepressants may be recommended in combination with psychotherapy if body image distress is impactful to well-being, prolonged, and unresponsive to nonpharmacologic management.

II. Nonpharmacologic management
  A. Nurses should ask about individuals' body image throughout the pretreatment, treatment, and survivorship continuum.
  B. Interventions to enhance psychological adaptation and rehabilitation throughout the cancer continuum:
    1. Educate patient, partner, and family about potential body implications. For example: presurgery counseling regarding prothesis—breast and testicular implants, or nipple-sparing surgery for eligible patients (Parks, 2021).
    2. Concealment: wigs, hats, and clothing.
    3. Cognitive therapy: adjustment to physical changes (Graboyes et al., 2020) and sexual counseling (Farnam, Khakbazan, Nedjat, Razavi Dizaji, & Barjasteh, 2021).
    4. Hypnotic relaxation, progressive muscle relaxation, and exercise interventions may improve body image (Barton et al., 2019; Langelier et al., 2019).
    5. Interventions to incorporate individual, partner (encourage communication between partners), and social (Vani, Sabiston, Trinh, & Santa Mina, 2022) and spiritual support (Olasehinde et al., 2019).
  C. Lymphedema (Hasenöhrl, Palma, Huber, Zdravkovic, & Crevenna, 2021).
    1. Physical therapy and lymphedema experts can help to prevent and/or manage lymphedema.
    2. Exercise may decrease arm symptoms; wearing a lymphedema sleeve and long sleeves may help conceal the swollen arm.
  D. Scalp cooling for alopecia prevention (Williams et al., 2020).
    1. Types: automatic (start 30–45 minutes before and 20–150 minutes after) and manual (start 30 minutes before).
    2. Effectiveness based on the type of chemotherapy treatment, contact with scalp, hair type, and liver function.
    3. Side effect: headache can be mitigated with acetaminophen.
    4. No evidence that scalp cooling increases scalp metastases.

REFERENCES

Barton, D. L., Brooks, T. M., Cieslak, A., Elkins, G. R., Clark, P. M., Baydoun, M., et al. (2019). Phase II randomized controlled trial of hypnosis versus progressive muscle relaxation for body image after breast or gynecologic cancer. *Breast Cancer Research and Treatment, 178*(2), 357–365. https://doi.org/10.1007/s10549-019-05395-6.

Boland, V., Brady, A.-M., & Drury, A. (2020). The physical, psychological and social experiences of alopecia among women receiving chemotherapy: An integrative literature review. *European Journal of Oncology Nursing, 49*, 101840. https://doi.org/10.1016/j.ejon.2020.101840.

Brederecke, J., Heise, A., & Zimmermann, T. (2021). Body image in patients with different types of cancer. *PLoS ONE, 16*(11), e0260602. https://doi.org/10.1371/journal.pone.0260602.

Cohee, A., Johns, S. A., Alwine, J. S., Talib, T., Monahan, P. O., Stump, T. E., et al. (2021). The mediating role of avoidant coping in the relationships between physical, psychological, and social wellbeing and distress in breast cancer survivors. *Psycho-Oncology, 30*(7), 1129–1136. https://doi.org/10.1002/pon.5663.

Ding, J., Farah, M. H., Nayfeh, T., Malandris, K., Manolopoulos, A., Ginex, P. K., et al. (2020). Targeted therapy- and chemotherapy-associated skin toxicities: Systematic review and meta-analysis. *Oncology Nursing Forum, 47*(5), E149–E160. https://doi.org/10.1188/20.ONF.E149-E160.

Farnam, F., Khakbazan, Z., Nedjat, S., Razavi Dizaji, S., & Barjasteh, S. (2021). The effect of Good Enough Sex (GES) model-based sexual counseling intervention on the body image in women surviving breast cancer: A randomized clinical trial. *Asian Pacific Journal of Cancer Prevention, 22*(7), 2303–2310. https://doi.org/10.31557/APJCP.2021.22.7.2303.

Freites-Martinez, A., Shapiro, J., Goldfarb, S., Nangia, J., Jimenez, J. J., Paus, R., et al. (2019). Hair disorders in patients with cancer. *Journal of the American Academy of Dermatology, 80*(5), 1179–1196. https://doi.org/10.1016/j.jaad.2018.03.055.

Graboyes, E. M., Maurer, S., Park, Y., Marsh, C. H., McElligott, J. T., Day, T. A., et al. (2020). Evaluation of a novel telemedicine-based intervention to manage body image disturbance in head and neck cancer survivors. *Psycho-Oncology, 29*(12), 1988–1994. https://doi.org/10.1002/pon.5399.

Hasenöhrl, T., Palma, S., Huber, D. F., Zdravkovic, A., & Crevenna, R. (2021). Effects of a structured exercise program on physical performance and function, quality of life and work ability of physically active breast cancer survivors: A retrospective data analysis. *Wiener klinische Wochenschrift, 133*(1–2), 1–5. https://doi.org/10.1007/s00508-020-01739-1.

Hovén, E., Fagerkvist, K., Jahnukainen, K., Ljungman, L., Lähteenmäki, P. M., Axelsson, O., et al. (2021). Sexual dysfunction in young adult survivors of childhood cancer – A population-based study. *European Journal of Cancer (Oxford, England: 1990), 154*, 147–156.

Langelier, D. M., D'Silva, A., Shank, J., Grant, C., Bridel, W., & Culos-Reed, S. N. (2019). Exercise interventions and their effect on masculinity, body image, and personal identity in prostate cancer – A systematic qualitative review. *Psycho-Oncology, 28*(6), 1184–1196. https://doi.org/10.1002/pon.5060.

Muzzatti, B., & Annunziata, M. A. (2017). Body image assessment in oncology: An update review. *Supportive Care in Cancer, 25*(3), 1019–1029. https://doi.org/10.1007/s00520-016-3538-y.

Olasehinde, O., Arije, O., Wuraola, F. O., Samson, M., Olajide, O., Alabi, T., et al. (2019). Life without a breast: Exploring the experiences of young Nigerian women after mastectomy for breast cancer. *Journal of Global Oncology, 5,* 1–6. https://doi.org/10.1200/JGO.18.00248.

Parks, L. (2021). Nipple-sparing mastectomy in breast cancer: Impact on surgical resection, oncologic safety, and psychological well-being. *Journal of the Advanced Practitioner in Oncology, 12*(5), 499–506. https://doi.org/10.6004/jadpro.2021.12.5.5.

Reynolds, L. M., & Harris, L. (2021). Stigma in the face of cancer disfigurement: A systematic review and research agenda. *European Journal of Cancer Care, 30*(1), e13327. https://doi.org/10.1111/ecc.13327.

Rhoten, B. A. (2017). Conceptual issues surrounding body image for oncology nurses. *Oncology Nursing Forum, 44*(5), 534–536. https://doi.org/10.1188/17.ONF.534-536.

Stanca, M., Căpîlna, D. M., Trâmbiţaş, C., & Căpîlna, M. E. (2022). The overall quality of life and oncological outcomes following radical hysterectomy in cervical cancer survivors results from a large long-term single-institution study. *Cancers, 14*(2), 317. https://doi.org/10.3390/cancers14020317.

Vani, M. F., Sabiston, C. M., Trinh, L., & Santa Mina, D. S. (2022). Testing the associations between body image, social support, and physical activity among adolescents and young adults diagnosed with cancer. *Frontiers in Psychology, 12,* 800314. https://doi.org/10.3389/fpsyg.2021.800314.

Williams, L. A., Ginex, P. K., Ebanks, G. L., Jr., Ganstwig, K., Ciccolini, K., Kwong, B. K., et al. (2020). ONS Guidelines™ for cancer treatment-related skin toxicity. *Oncology Nursing Forum, 47*(5), 539–556. https://doi.org/10.1188/20.ONF.539-556.

51

Caregiver Burden

Geline J. Tamayo

OVERVIEW

I. Definition
  A. Caregiver: a trained or untrained spouse, family member, or friend who assumes a typically uncompensated, allied role in domestically supporting the health management and well-being of another person, involving significant amounts of time and energy for months or years, and performing tasks requiring physical, emotional, social, or financial demands (Watabashi et al., 2020).
    1. Primary caregiver: mainly provides and/or assists the care recipient with day-to-day care, activities of daily living (ADLs), facilitates health care delivery, and participates in decisions regarding care (Thompson, Wilson-Genderson, & Siminoff, 2022).
    2. Secondary caregiver: assists the primary caregiver with caregiving or provides support to patients (Thompson et al., 2022).
  B. Caregiving: a complex and dynamic process of assisting with the continuum of health care activities for someone unable to independently care for themselves or who needs help/assistance to manage their care (Al-Daken & Ahmad, 2018).
    1. An aging and growing population has made caregiving a major public health concern (National Alliance for Caregiving & AARP, 2020).
      a. Imposes time-sensitive, life-changing commitment/experience
      b. Includes shifting and evolving existing, often long-standing, and relationships
    2. Caregiving is associated with significant physical, psychosocial, relationship, and economic burden (Bardley, 2019; Trevino, Prigerson, & Maciejewski, 2018; Watabashi et al., 2020).
    3. Caregivers often cite positive aspects of the experience, including:
      a. The caregiver feels good about themselves, as if they are needed
      b. Gives meaning to their lives
      c. Enables them to learn new skills
      d. Strengthens their relationships with others
    4. Dependency creates an environmental stressor; caregiver and recipient at high risk for depression (Trevino et al., 2018).
      a. Change in the dynamic of close relationships
      b. Impact of the disease increases dependency, further limiting caregiver control over the caregiving situation

II. Epidemiology of family caregiving and caregiver burden (Statistics regarding family caregivers ar available at https://www.aarp.org/content/dam/aarp/ppi/2020/05/infographic-caregiving-in-the-united-states.doi.10.26419-2Fppi.00103.002.pdf)
  A. Caregiver demographic
    1. Most are women
    2. Number of caregivers is growing
    3. Caregivers are commonly providing care for more than one person
  B. Challenges (Table 51.1)
    1. Difficulty coordinating care
    2. Caregiver burden: emotional, physical, social, financial, and spiritual impact perceived by a caregiver (Johansen, Cvancarova, & Ruland, 2018; Watabashi et al., 2020); caregiver burden is influenced by patient comorbidities, depression, and symptoms (Johansen et al., 2018)
    3. Caregiver fatigue, depression, sleep disturbance, low self-efficacy, and low social support affect caregiver burden (Al-Daken & Ahmad, 2018; Johansen et al., 2018)

III. Factors that may influence the impact of caregiving (Alam, Hannon, & Zimmermann, 2020; Sun, Qin, & Hengudomsub, 2020)
  A. Caregiver resilience
  B. Relationship with the patient
  C. Presence of difficult-to-manage symptoms
  D. Degree of challenge (e.g., physical assistance required or the presence of dementia)
  E. Financial impact of patient and caregiver income, costs of medical care
  F. Lack of information and professional support. This may include the following:
    1. Quality of interface between health care team, patient, and caregiver
    2. Implementation and integration of relevant caregiver legislation
    3. Access to patient advocacy/support/respite care groups

TABLE 51.1.	**Risk Factors of Caregiving**
Domain/Feature	**Risk Factor and/or Outcome Status of Caregiving**
Demographic	
Female sex	Women experience a higher burden of care than men (Ketcher et al., 2020).
	Older female caregivers have a higher risk of experiencing burden and worst physical health (Spatuzzi et al., 2021).
Low education	Associated with the highest levels of caregiver burden in various conditions (Xu et al., 2021).
Cohabitation with care recipient	Associated with caregiver burden (La et al., 2021).
Younger caregiver	Added responsibilities of younger caregiver, increased risk of disrupted schedule and financial problems (La et al., 2021).
Physiological	
Cardiometabolic risk	Caregivers with poor health have a higher cardiometabolic risk (Steel et al., 2019).
Pro-inflammatory cytokines	Inflammatory cytokine levels were negatively correlated with caregiving distress (Kim et al., 2022).
Clinical and Physical Outcomes of Caregiver Burden	
Mortality	Identified as a predictor of mortality; 63% increased risk of death in caregiver spouses. Recent population-based studies examining actual mortality appear to suggest the opposite (Steel et al., 2019).
Self-care needs	Caregivers are more interested in conversations about self-care needs.
	Caregivers who live alone (34%); African American (32%); caregivers who live with care recipient (26%); and LGBTQ (34%) (American Association of Retired Persons, 2023).
Sleep deprivation	Moderate-to-severe sleep disturbance reported. Reduction in total sleep time appears to be the biggest issue (Steel et al., 2019).
Fatigue, loss of physical strength and pain	Decrease motivation, ability to concentrate, relationship affected, and inability to perform usual actvities (Yiin, Chen, & Lee, 2021).
Psychosocial	
Depression and depressive symptoms	Identified as a risk factor for and outcome of caregiver burden (Jansen et al., 2021).
Coping strategies	Absence of an alternate caregiver, family support (La et al., 2021).
Perceived patient distress	Patient's emotional distress increases caregiver-perceived burden (Yang, Pan, Allen, & Hendrix, 2019).
Social isolation and decreased social activity	Lack of social support and greater disruption in schedules (Xu et al., 2021).
Anxiety	An outcome of caregiving (Garcia-Torres et al., 2020).
Suicide	An outcome of caregiver burden (Adelman et al., 2014).
Caregiving Context	
Caregiving time and effort	Caregivers have less time to spend on self-care (La et al., 2021).
Financial stress	A risk factor for caregiver burden and an outcome of caregiver burden (La et al., 2021)
Lack of choice	Lack of choice (53%) in becoming a caregiver associated with caregiver burden (American Association of Retired Persons, 2023).
Inability to continue regular employment	Work conflicts for spousal caregivers was significant due to caregiving (Jeong, Shin, Park, & Park, 2020).
	Caregiver productivity loss associated with intensive cancer treatment, travel for treatment, costs associated with treatment, and change of work hours during treatment (Kamal et al., 2017).
Travel	Cost to travel, inaccessible transportation for both the caregiver and recipient (Xu et al., 2021).
Personal/family obligations	Disruption of social life and family obligations.
	Changes in family and other relationships due to caregiving demands and limited time (Xu et al., 2021).

G. Degree to which caregivers think that they are carrying out patients' wishes

H. Social support available to the caregiver

I. Five key themes that increased demands on caregivers during COVID-19 (Carer Well-Being Index)
1. Rising demands
2. Changed responsibilities
3. The toll on caregivers
4. Inequities in caregiving
5. Path to solutions

IV. Family caregiving legislation
A. Recognize, Assist, Include, Support, and Engage Family Caregivers Act of 2017, or the RAISE Family Caregivers Act, provides for the establishment and maintenance of a family caregiving strategy (American Association of Retired Persons, 2023)

B. CARE (Caregiver Advise, Record, and Enable) Act (National Alliance for Caregiving, 2023)
1. Enables family caregivers to provide safe and effective home care to older adults
2. Requires hospitals to record family caregiver name with hospital admission
3. The hospital is required to notify the caregiver when the patient is discharged
4. Provides instructions of medical tasks for transitions of care

C. The Credit for Caring Act (American Association of Retired Persons, 2023)
1. Supports family caregivers who work
2. Helps address the financial challenges of family caregiving and assists family caregivers to stay in the workforce and be more financially secure
3. Gives eligible family caregivers the opportunity to receive a tax credit for 30% of the qualified expenses above $2000 paid to help a loved one, up to a maximum credit amount of $3000

D. The Family and Medical Leave Act
1. Federal law that allows employees to take up to 12 weeks of unpaid leave per year to care for themselves, or for a seriously ill family member, or for a new child without losing their jobs or health care insurance.

E. Kupuna Caregivers Act, Hawaii:
1. Provides financial assistance to support employed carers to remain in the workforce

ASSESSMENT

I. Family caregivers should be assessed for their needs, especially when care plans are dependent upon them (Alam et al., 2020).
   A. Identify designated caregiver with patient; document in the electronic health record
   B. Identify the problems, needs, strengths, and resources of the caregiver, and the ability of the caregiver to contribute to the needs of the care recipient (Alam et al., 2020; Table 51.2).

II. Caregiver clinical measurement tools (Table 51.3)
   A. Generalized findings are based on a wide variety of measures available to assess caregiving tasks, burden, and health outcomes (Halpern et al., 2017).

TABLE 51.3 Caregiver Clinical Measurement Tools

Name of Tool	Number of Items	Domain
Zarit Burden Interview	22	Burden (health, psychological well-being, finances, social life, and relationship with impaired person)
Caregiver Reaction Assessment	24	Burden (self-esteem, lack of family support, and impact on finances, schedule, and health)
CG QOL Scale-Cancer (CQOL-C)	35	QOL (burden, disruptiveness, positive adaptation, and financial concerns)
Preparedness for Caregiving Scale	8	Needs assessment
Caregiver Strain Index	13	Burden (employment, financial, physical, social, and time aspects)
Caregiver Burden Scale	15	Burden (patient needs, caregiver tasks, and caregiver burden)

From Eaton, L. H., Tipton, J. M., & Irwin, M. (Eds.). (2011). *Putting evidence into practice: Improving oncology patient outcomes* (Vol. 2). Pittsburgh, PA: Oncology Nursing Society.

TABLE 51.2 The CARES Framework for Family Caregivers

Domain	Description
Consider caregivers as part of the unit of care	Consider caregivers as part of the unit as well as part of the care team
	Acknowledge the importance of the caregiving role
	Respect the patient's wishes regarding the nature and degree of caregiver participation in decision-making
Assess the caregiver's situation, perceptions, and needs	Document the caregiver's relationship to the patient, their living situation, employment, and whether care is being provided by other dependents (e.g., children)
	Assess the caregiver's capacity and willingness to provide care
	Inquire about the caregiver's physical and mental health
	Assess the impact of caregiving, including social isolation and financial strain
	Inquiry about the caregiver's perception of the patient's status and the ability for self-care
Refer to appropriate services and resources	Refer the caregiver to locally available resources:
	Palliative care teams, hospice
	Home care services, respite care
	Social work, psychology, and spiritual care
	Community resources, support groups, and online resources
Educate about practical aspects of caregiving	Ensure the caregiver and patient have a joint understanding of the patient's cancer, its treatment, its typical causes, and signs of advancing disease
	Check understanding of pain control (e.g., dosing, adverse effects, and addiction potential)
	Ensure education for practical skills (e.g., dressing changes, injections, and lifting/transferring)
	Highlight the importance of personal health and self-care and the availability of benefits and services for caregivers
Support caregivers through bereavement	Clarify when it is important to call and who should be called
	Be available by phone or in person to discuss caregiver concerns
	Offer referral to local bereavement support services
	Call or send a card to the caregiver after bereavement

From Alam, S., Hannon, B., & Zimmerman, C. (2020). Palliative car for family caregivers. *Journal of Clinical Oncology, 38*(9), 926–936.

B. Selected caregiver assessment measures (https://www.caregiver.org/selected-caregiver-assessment-measures-resource-inventory-practitioners-2012).

MANAGEMENT

(Oncology Nursing Society, 2017)

I. Medical management
   A. Prescribe assistive devices that make caregiving less strenuous
   B. Refer to physical or occupational therapy to teach caregiver safe transfer techniques and to encourage as much self-care by the patient within the limits of the disease

II. Nursing management (https://www.caregiver.org/caregiver-resources/all-resources/; Table 51.4)
   A. Incorporate needs and preferences of patients and caregiver in care planning
   B. Improve caregivers' understanding of their role; teach skills necessary
   C. Facilitate caregiver coping
      1. Provide written instructions for reinforcement
      2. Reinforce teaching with each interaction
      3. Ensure that caregiver knows who to call with questions
   4. Provide clear instruction on when and how to use medications and nonpharmacologic interventions for symptom control
   5. Ensure caregiver knows who to call if the plan of care for symptom control is not working or a new symptom develops, whatever the time of day
   6. Provide information to clarify any misperceptions or misunderstandings
   D. Provide continuous therapeutic communication with caregivers
      1. Clarify patient and family goals, including advance care planning, to ensure the plan of care is congruent with patient and family goals
      2. Communicate changes in patient condition, especially signs and symptoms of imminent death, so that caregivers feel as prepared as possible
   E. Provide psychosocial support and refer to appropriate resources as needed
      1. Actively listen to fears, concerns, and expressions of grief
      2. Encourage caregiver interventions, including respite options:
         a. Caregiver support services: in-person and online support groups

TABLE 51.4	Caregiver Assessment for Needs and Preferences
Category	**Question**
Context of Care	
Caregiver relationship	What is the caregiver's relationship with the patient?
	How long has the caregiver been in this role?
Caregiver profile	What is the educational background of the caregiver?
	Is the caregiver employed?
	Does the caregiver have dependents who require care as well?
Additional caregivers	Are other family members or friends involved in providing care?
	Are paid caregivers (e.g., home health aides) involved?
Living arrangements	Does the caregiver live in the same household?
	If the caregiver lives elsewhere, how far away are they and do they have access to dependable transportation?
Physical environment	Does the care recipient's home have grab bars and other adaptive devices and necessary equipment to assist with care?
	Is the care recipient homebound?
	Other concerns (i.e., laundry, grocery shopping, meal prep, medication pick-ups from the pharmacy)?
	Is there a readily accessible bathroom on the same floor that the care recipient spends most of the day? Stairs?
	Is the care recipient a pet owner? Can they handle pet care?
Caregiver's Perception of Care Recipient's Overall Health	
Cognitive status	Is the patient cognitively impaired?
	How does this affect care provision?
Health perceptions	What medical problems does the care recipient have?
	What is the caregiver's perception of the care recipient's medical problems and prognosis and goals of care?
Caregiving needs	Is the care recipient totally dependent 24/7 or only partially?
	Is there evidence that the caregiver is providing adequate care?
Assessment of Caregiver Values	
Willingness	Is the caregiver willing to undertake the caregiver role?
	Is the care recipient willing to accept care provision?
Cultural norms	What care arrangements are considered culturally acceptable for family (i.e., ethnicity, personal beliefs, religion, language barriers, values, communication, and decision-making)

TABLE 51.4 Caregiver Assessment for Needs and Preferences —Cont'd

Category	Question
Assessment of Caregiver Health	
Caregiver health	How does the caregiver assess his or her own health?
	Does the caregiver have limitations that affect the ability to give care?
	Does the caregiver feel she or he is under a lot of stress?
	Is there evidence of anxiety, depression, and suicidal ideation?
	How does the caregiver rate his or her quality of life?
Impact of caregiving	Is the caregiver socially isolated?
	Does the caregiver feel health has suffered because of caregiving?
Assessment of Caregiver Knowledge and Skills	
Caregiving confidence	How knowledgeable does the caregiver feel about care recipient's condition?
Caregiver competence	Does the caregiver have appropriate knowledge of medical tasks required to provide care (e.g., wound care, transferring patient, and health literacy for administrating complex medication regimen)?
Assessment of Caregiver Resources	
Social support	Do friends and family assist with care so that the caregiver has time off?
	Are there additional support systems given (e.g., dates, times, and expectations for stepping in to assist)?
Coping	What does the caregiver do to relieve stress and tension?
Financial resources	Does the caregiver feel financial strain associated with caregiving?
	Does the caregiver have access to insurance coverage information?
Community resources and services	Have providers (nurses and social workers) given the caregiver information about available community resources and services (caregiver support programs, religious organizations, volunteer agencies, and respite services)?

From https://www.caregiver.org/caregiver-resources/all-resources/.

b. Counseling

c. Family meetings

F. Facilitate physical support

1. Demonstrate physical caregiving (e.g., changing sheets on occupied bed, catheter care, and dressing change); have the caregiver do a return demonstration with home health aide available for coaching and support

2. Encourage caregivers to accept assistance so that they have time for self-care, including sleeping, eating, and other restorative activities

G. Mobilize resources

1. Augment caregiving with home health aides, personal care assistants, and home services

2. Make referrals to social workers, chaplains, counselors, and community resources

a. Aging Life Care Association: https://www.aginglifecare.org//

b. American Cancer Society: https://www.cancer.org; (800) 227-2345

c. Association of Jewish Family and Children's Agencies (AJFCA): http://www.ajfca.org; ajfca@ajfca.org

d. CancerCare: http://www.cancercare.org; (800) 813-4673

e. **Cancer Support Community:** http://www.cancersupportcommunity.org/; **(888) 793-WELL (888) 793-9355 (202) 659-9709**

f. **Caregiver Action Network:** https://caregiveraction.org/; **(202) 454-3970**

g. **Caring.com:** http://www.caring.com/; **(866) 824-8174**

h. **Catholic Charities:** http://www.catholiccharitiesusa.org/

i. Eldercare Locator: eldercarelocator@n4a.org; https://eldercare.acl.gov; 800-677-1116

j. Family Caregiver Alliance (FCA): http://www.caregiver.org; (800) 44 8106

k. National Brain Tumor Foundation: http://www.braintumor.org; (800) 93 2873

l. National Brain Tumor Society: http://www.braintumor.org/; (800) 770-TBTS (800-770-8287)

m. **National Respite Locator Service:** www.archrespite.org/respitelocator

n. Well Spouse Association: (toll-free) info@wellspouse.org; www.wellspouse.org; 800-838-0879

H. Referral to financial counseling and navigation partners:

1. Access to Health Insurance/Resources for Care: http://www.ahirc.org/; (800) 798-8447 Ext. 265

a. Benefits Checkup: http://www.benefitscheckup.org

b. Benefits.gov: http://www.benefits.gov/

c. Consumer Education and Training Services (CENTS): www.centsprogram.org

d. Medi-Care Waiver Programs or Statewide Equivalents: https://www.payingforseniorcare.com/longtermcare/resources/cash-and-counseling-program.html

e. National Adult Day Services Association (NADSA): http://www.nadsa.org; (877) 745-1440

f. Patient Advocate Foundation (PAF): www.patientadvocate.org

2. Encourage the caregiver to call on extended family members, friends, and faith community networks for assistance with direct caregiving or household tasks

3. Increase the level of care if symptoms are not responding to usual treatment (e.g., palliative care or hospice referral, transfer to an inpatient facility, and initiation of continuous hospice care at home)

4. Provide resources on anticipatory grief as losses occur throughout the disease trajectory; for example, loss of roles, loss of function, and death

5. Family caregivers should have access to relevant information through technology
    a. Able Project.org: http://www.ableproject.org; (408) 263-8000
    b. ABLEDATA: https://abledata.acl.gov/; (800) 227-0216
    c. AssistiveTech.net: http://www.assistivetech.net; (800) 726-9119
    d. Comfort Zone: http://www.alz.org/comfortzone/index.asp; 1-877-259-4850

REFERENCES

American Association of Retired Persons (2023). Family Caregiving. https://www.aarp.org/caregiving/ Accessed at 15.01.23.

Al-Daken, L. I., & Ahmad, M. M. (2018). Predictors of burden and quality of sleep among family caregivers of patients with cancer. *Supportive Care in Cancer, 26*, 3967–3973.

Alam, S., Hannon, B., & Zimmerman, C. (2020). Palliative car for family caregivers. *Journal of Clinical Oncology, 38*(9), 926–936.

Bradley, C. J. (2019). Economic burden associated with cancer caregiving. *Seminars in Oncology Nursing, 35*, 333–336.

Garcia-Torres, F., Jablonski, M. J., Gomez Solis, A., Jaen-Moreno, M. J., Galvez-Lara, M., Moriana, J. A., et al. (2020). Caregiver burden domains and their relationship with anxiety and depression in the first six months of cancer diagnosis. *International Journal of Environmental Research an Public Health, 17*(11), 4101.

Halpern, M. T., Fiero, M. H., & Bell, M. L. (2017). Impact of caregiver activities and social supports on multidimensional caregiver burden: Analyses from nationally-representative surveys of cancer patients and their caregivers. *Quality of Life Research, 26*(6), 1587–1595. https://doi.org/10.1007/s11136-017-1505-9. https://www.caregiver.org/caregiver-resources/all-resources/ Retrieved 14.03.22.

Jansen, L., Dauphin, S., De Burghgraeve, T., Schoenmakers, B., Buntinx, F., & van den Akker, M. (2021). Caregiver burden: An increasing problem related to an aging population. *Journal of Health Psychology, 26*(11), 1833–1849.

Jeong, A., Shin, D., Park, H. J., & Parl, K. (2020). Attributes of caregivers' quality of life: A perspective comparison between spousal and non-spousal caregivers of older patients with cancer. *Journal of Geriatric Oncology, 11*, 82–87.

Johansen, S., Cvancarova, M., & Ruland, C. (2018). The effect of cancer patients' and their family caregivers' physical and emotional symptoms on caregiver burden. *Cancer Nursing, 41*(2), 91–99. https://doi.org/10.1097/NCC.0000000000000493.

Kamal, K. M., Covvey, J. R., Dashputre, A., Ghosh, S., Shah, S., Bhosle, M., et al. (2017). A systematic review of the effect of cancer treatment on work productivity of patients and caregivers. *Journal of Managed Care & Specialty Pharmacy, 23*(2), 136–162. https://doi.org/10.18553/jmcp.2017.23.2.136.

Ketcher, D., Trettevik, R., Vadaparampil, S. T., et al. (2020). Caring for a spouse with advanced cancer: Similarities and differences for male and female caregivers. *Journal of Behavioral Medicine, 43*(5), 817–828.

Kim, Y., Kim, H., Suh, S. -Y., Park, H., & Lee, H. (2022). Association between inflammatory cytokines and caregiving distress in family caregivers of cancer patients. *Supportive Care in Cancer, 30*, 1715–1722.

La, I. S., Johantgen, M., Storr, C. L., Zhu, S., Cagle, J. G., & Ross, A. (2021). Caregiver burden and related factors during active cancer treatment: A latent growth curve analysis. *European Journal of Oncology Nursing, 52*, 101962. https://doi.org/10.1016/j.ejon.2021.101962.

National Alliance for Caregiving (2023). Share Care Act. https://www.caregiving.org/advocacy/care-act/ Accessed 15.02.23.

National Alliance for Caregiving & AARP. (2020). *Caregiving in the U.S.* https://www.caregiving.org/wp-content/uploads/2020/08/AARP1316_ExecSum_CaregivingintheUS_508.pdf Accessed 08.02.22.

Oncology Nursing Society. (2017). *Putting evidence into practice: Caregiver strain and burden*. https://www.ons.org/practice-resources/pep/caregiver-strain-and-burden.

Spatuzzi, R., Giulietti, M. V., Romito, F., Reggiardo, G., Genovese, C., Passarella, M., et al. (2021). Becoming an older caregiver: A study of gender differences in family caregiving at the end of life. *Palliative and Supportive Care, 1–7.* https://doi.org/10.1017/S1478951521000274.

Steel, J. L., Cheng, H., Pathak, R., Wang, Y., Miceli, J., Hecht, C. L., et al. (2019). Psychosocial and behavioral pathways of metabolic syndrome in cancer caregivers. *Psycho-Oncology, 28*(8), 1735–1742.

Sun, H., Qin, Y., & Henguddomsub, P. (2020). Factors associated with resilience in spousal caregivers of patients with cancer: An integrative review. *Nursing Open, 8*, 2131–2141.

Thompson, M.D., Wilson-Genderson, M., & Siminoff, L.A. (2022). The presence of a secondary caregiver differentiates primary cancer caregiver well-being. *Supportive Care in Cancer, 30*, 1597–1605.

Trevino, K. M., Prigerson, H. G., & Maciejewski, P. K. (2018). Advanced cancer caregiving as a risk for major depressive episodes and generalized anxiety disorder. *Psychooncology, 27*(1), 243–249.

Watabashi, K., Steelquist, J., Overstreet, K. A., Leahy, A., Bradshaw, E., Gallagher, K. D., et al. (2020). A pilot study of a comprehensive financial navigation program in patients with cancer and caregivers. *Journal of the National Comprehensive Cancer Network, 18*(10), 1366–1373.

Xu, H., Kadambi, S., Mohile, S.G., Yang, S., Kehoe, L.A., Wells, M., et al. (2021). Caregiving burden of informal caregivers of older adults with advanced cancer: The effects of rurality and education. *Journal of Geriatric Oncology, 12*, 1015–1021.

Yang, Y., Pan, W., Allen, D., & Hendrix, C. C. (2019). Caregiver burden as a mediator between emotional distress and concentration problems in patients with cancer. *Oncology Nursing Forum, 46*(6), E180–E184.

Yiin, J. -J., Chen, Y. -Y., & Lee, K. -C. (2021). Fatigue and vigilance-related factors in family caregivers of patients with advanced cancer: A cross-sectional study. *Cancer Nursing, 45*(2), E621–E627.

52

Social Determinants of Health and Financial Toxicity

Rachel Hirschey

OVERVIEW

I. Social determinants of health (SDOH) are the circumstance in which people are born, live, work, play, learn, worship and age and comprise five domains: (1) economic stability, (2) neighborhood and built environment, (3) education access and quality, (4) health care access and quality, and (5) social and community context (see Fig. 52.1) (U.S. Department of Health and Human Services).

1. SDOH, such as access to programs, discrimination, and provider bias, are significant contributors to inequities in the early detection and treatment of cancer (Cousin, Roper, & Nolan, 2021).

2. SDOH decrease African American patient participation in cancer clinical trials (Hernandez et al., 2022).

II. SDOH and structural racism are inextricably connected in the United States, leading to significant cancer health disparities between patients of different races (Cousin et al., 2021; Hamilton, 2021).

A. Structural racism refers to practices that disproportionality distribute and sustain access to power and resources between groups assigned to different racial categories (Jones, 2000). These practices are normative, often legal practices that are engrained into society. Structural racism is also sometimes called systemic or institutionalized racism.

III. An understanding of the social, environmental, and economic factors that impact patient outcomes is foundational for delivering quality and equitable oncology nursing care (Gehlert, Hudson, & Sacks, 2021).

A. Socioeconomic factors, environmental conditions, and health behaviors determine about 80% of a person's health (Robert Wood Johnson Foundation, 2019).

B. A focus on social risks is needed in health care because these hazards are associated with decreased treatment compliance, poor health outcomes, and increased care costs (Gusoff, Fichtenberg, & Gottlieb, 2018).

C. Nurses should develop an understanding of how the SDOH are impacting a patient, when advising them to engage in healthy behaviors (e.g., physical activity, healthy diet, and cancer screening) (Gehlert et al., 2021; Hirschey, Tan, Petermann, & Leak Bryant, 2021).

D. Psychological distress treatment can be ineffective for underserved populations when health care providers do address SDOH, especially those related to the social and community context (Hamilton, 2021).

E. Cancer screening interventions that are focused on the SDOH are effective for underserved and vulnerable populations (Mohan & Chattopadhyay, 2020).

IV. SDOH domains

A. Economic stability

1. Economic stability (i.e., access to resources necessary for a healthy life) is an especially important SDOH in oncology due to the high costs of cancer treatment causing financial toxicity (i.e., "the harmful personal financial burden faced by patients receiving cancer treatment") (Zafar et al., 2015).

2. It is critical that oncology nurses discuss and help manage patients' financial concerns (Carrera, Kantarjian, & Blinder, 2018).

3. Proactive and early assessment is needed because patients may be embarrassed or ashamed to share their financial concerns with nurses (Edward et al., 2021).

4. Frequent address changes may be a signal of housing insecurity that should prompt an in-depth nursing assessment.

a. Up to 48% of cancer survivors report financial toxicity due to out-of-pocket expenses (Gordon, Merollini, Lowe, & Chan, 2017).

b. Financial toxicity leads to poor cancer treatment completion rates and increased medical problems (Chan & Gordon, 2021).

c. Survivors of cancer who are experiencing financial toxicity are at significantly greater risk for depression and anxiety (Chan et al., 2019).

d. Patients may need to prioritize paying for basic needs of food and shelter over seeking medical care.

e. See Chapter 53 for further discussion on poverty and cancer.

B. Neighborhood and built environment

1. The neighborhood and built environment refer to the location and physical aspects that one interacts with where they live. Current-day residential segregation stemming from Jim Crow laws and redlining puts patients of color at higher risk of living in an unsafe and underserved neighborhood with less access to health care, transportation, healthy food,

Social Determinants of Health

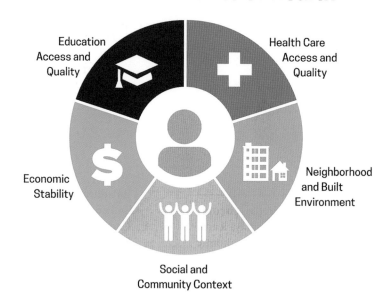

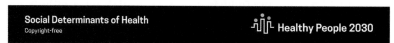

Fig. 52.1 Healthy People 2030 social determinants of health. From *U.S. Department of Health and Human Services. (2023). Healthy people 2030.* https://health.gov/healthypeople/objectives-and-data/social-determinants-health.

safe spaces for physical activity, and quality education (Hamilton, 2021).

2. Safe housing considerations include the assessment of one's neighborhood characteristics.
   a. Presence of crime and exposure to violence.
   b. Access to healthy food/distance to grocery store.
   c. Safe spaces to be physically active—sidewalks, parks, streetlights, and cross walks.
   d. Transportation—distance and availability of bus lines and routes to grocery stores and public and medical services.
   e. Presence of polluted air and water.

C. Education access and quality
   1. Racist policies have led to present-day educational achievement gaps that place patients of color at higher risk for low access and quality education (Hamilton, 2021).
   2. Several measures may inform nursing assessment of education access and quality:
      a. Literacy and language spoken.
      b. Quality of schools attended.
      c. Early childhood education.
      d. High school completion.
      e. Higher education.

D. Health care access and quality
   1. Patients of color are at risk for lower access and utilization of health care due to residential segregation and medical systems being untrustworthy for certain racial and ethnic populations.

   a. Cancer centers and medical systems that generally deliver high-quality care can be untrustworthy to patients of color. This can lead to patients of color not wanting to receive care in these settings. Additionally, patients of color may have negative and harmful experiences when being treated in these systems. These negative experiences may stem from clinician's lack of structural awareness, cultural humility, and bias management (Cahn, 2020; Tucker-Seeley, 2021).

2. Patients may need to travel significant distances to receive medical care.

3. About 20% of people in the United States do not have broadband internet (Zahnd, Bell, & Larson, 2021).
   a. People without broadband are not able to use telehealth and policies that require a camera to be used for telehealth may further limit access for those with poor Internet connectivity.

4. Health literacy (i.e., the extent to which individuals can understand information to inform their health-related decisions) impacts patient's decision-making and outcomes.
   a. Patients with high literacy levels may have low health literacy.
   b. Health literacy does not refer to only the written word. Health literacy encompasses all forms of information transfer.

5. It is recommended that patient education materials be at a sixth-grade reading level.

6. Most patients facing cancer-related educational materials are above the eighth-grade reading level (Rooney et al., 2021).
7. Nurses should review educational materials with patients.
E. Social and community context
1. Several social factors can negatively or positively influence health
a. Social support
b. Experiences of discrimination
c. Racism
d. Social isolation
e. Culture (see Chapter 53)

ASSESSMENT

I. Several barriers to nursing assessment of SDOH have been identified (Kostelanetz et al., 2021; Persaud, 2018; Phillips et al., 2020).
A. Lack of resources to address identified needs
B. Lack of time
C. Personal discomfort
D. Anticipated patient discomfort
II. Nurses are more comfortable and more often discuss social and structural concerns related to access to care and are less comfortable and less often discuss concerns related to the other SDOH domains (i.e., economic stability, neighborhood and built environment, education access and quality, and social and community context) (Phillips et al., 2020).
III. Nurse leaders should provide structures and systems to integrate SDOH assessment into nursing workflow and integration with the electronic medical record (Tiase, Crookston, Schoenbaum, & Valu, 2022).
A. Many SDOH screening measures are available for nurses to consider implementing in practice (Table 52.1).

B. Nurse leaders can guide the implementation of SDOH screening using these published examples (LaForge et al., 2018).
IV. Nurses may also integrate questions related to SDOH into all interactions with patients (see Table 52.2).

MANAGEMENT

I. Addressing patient needs related to SDOH begins with nurses' personal education about structural awareness (Metzl & Hansen, 2014; Ruth, SturtzSreetharan, Brewis, & Wutich, 2020).
A. Structural awareness refers to one's understanding of how policies and environments impact health outcomes.
B. Nurses with structural awareness are prepared to provide better patient care through an understanding of how policies, residential patterns, and environmental inputs are impacting patients' engagement with the health system, health behaviors, and health outcomes.
C. Nurses can increase their structural awareness through antiracism education provided by organizations such as the Racial Equity Institute (The Racial Equity Institute, 2023).
II. Nurses must practice cultural humility when addressing SDOH (Nolan, Alston, Choto, & Moss, 2021).
A. To be equipped to practice cultural humility, nurses can begin with their bias using the Harvard IAT test (Project Implicit, 2011).
B. The Oncology Navigation Standards of Professional Practice requires that all navigators practice cultural humility; these standards can be applied to all oncology nurses (Franklin, Burke, Dean, & Johnson, 2022).
C. See Chapter 53 for improving care with spiritual, religious, and cultural considerations.

TABLE 52.1	**Social Determinants of Health Screening Tools**
Tool	**Brief Description**
PREPARE: Protocol for Responding to and Assessing Patient's Assets, Risks, and Experiences (American Academy of Family Physicians, 2019)	Contains 15 questions that identify needs related to housing, food, transportation, utilities, childcare, employment, education, finances, and personal safety. An 11-item short form is also available (American Academy of Family Physicians, 2017).
WellRx Questionnaire (Page-Reeves et al., 2016)	Contains 11 questions that identify needs related to food insecurity, housing, utilities, income, employment, transportation, education, substance abuse, childcare, safety, and abuse. Available in English or Spanish. Designed with literacy specialist to develop questions for people with low literacy.
YCLS shorter form (Your Current Life Situation) (Kaiser Permanente, 2016)	Contains nine questions designed to identify needs recommended by the Institute of Medicine. Also includes an additional item bank for a more detailed assessment. Kaiser Permanente seeks feedback for ongoing developing and sharing of best implementation practices as the tool is used by others.
AHC HRSN (Accountable Health Communities Health-Related Social Needs) (Billioux, Verlander, Anthony, & Alley, 2017)	Contains 10 questions to help identify patient needs around housing instability, food insecurity, transportation problems, utility help needs, and interpersonal safety. Also includes eight supplemental questions to assess financial strain, employment, family and community support, education, physical activity, substance abuse, and mental health and disabilities (Centers for Medicare & Medicaid Service, 2016).
OCHIN (Gold et al., 2017)	Designed for SDOH assessment integrated through the electronic health record. Includes items from the PREPARE tool, IOM recommendations and pulls data already contained in the EHR (e.g., race).

TABLE 52.2   Example Questions Nurses Can Integrate Into Common Patient Conversations to Identify Need for Detailed Social Determinant of Health (SDOH) Assessment or Referral

SDOH Domain	Examples Questions
Neighborhood and built environment	• What is it like where you are living? • How do you travel to your medical appointments? • What safety concerns do you have where you live? • Where do you get most of your food?/How do you get there? • Are you able to safely do physically near where you live?
Health care access and quality	• What questions do you have about your treatments? • What is your understanding of the cancer? • Do you have a doctor who you see for regular check-ups?/When do you usually see them?/How do you get there? • How far away is this hospital/clinic from where you live?/How do you get here?
Social and community context	• What is an average day like for you? • What do you do on a regular day? • Who do you take care of in your family and community? • How do others in your family/community support you? • In what ways may it be helpful for you to have more support? • What are some of the foods you enjoy most or eat regularly? • Do you have spiritual or religious beliefs that are important for me to understand? • What language do you speak at home? • Will you tell me about your family? • I'm interested to understand what your community is like, will you tell me about it?
Education	• Will you tell me about your work or the work you used to do? • What was your education like when you were younger? • Do you read? • Do you read English or do you prefer to read another language? • Did you go to high school?/What was it like?
Economic stability	• Have you been able to meet with someone to talk about financial concerns yet? • Have you been able to buy food recently?/What types of food have you been able to buy? • How long have you been where you are living?/Where were you before that?/How long will you be able to stay there? • What concerns may you have about your job given the cancer?

III. It is important for nurses to establish professional relationships with social workers and nurse navigators (Phillips et al., 2020).

   A. Oncology nurses should assess SDOH for all patients and provide referrals to social workers or case managers for a more detailed assessment and identification of resources (Kostelanetz et al., 2021).

   B. Collaboration with social workers, navigators, and case managers can increase nursing knowledge about resources to share with patients.

      1. Nurse navigators focus on eliminating financial, psychological, logistical, and communication-related barriers to improve outcomes for patients (Oncology Nursing Society, 2018).

      2. Oncology nurse navigators can comprehensively assess patient needs using the ONN Patient Assessment (Flucke & Sullivan-Moore, 2021).

         a. All navigators must work from an understanding of how systems of inequitable power distribution impact patient's ability to access services and their health outcomes.

         b. Be prepared to provide sensitive and appropriate care for all races, ethnicities, gender identities, sexual orientations, religions, abilities, ages, and more.

         c. All navigators must engage in continuous personal education about providing culturally appropriate and affirming care.

         d. Understand how different cultural beliefs and practices may impact patient recovery and outcomes.

IV. Organizational support can help establish community partnerships and provide regularly updated patient resources and education (Edward et al., 2021).

V. Nurses can look up resources for a patient near their home by using the neighborhood navigator tool from the EveryONE project which identifies resources by zip code (The EveryONE Project, 2023).

   A. Resources and education should be provided in a variety of formats including, but not limited to, written and spoken word, demonstration, videos, and voice memos.

VI. Implementation of SDH screening and responsive systems must be done through equity lens to integrate social needs into cancer care (Tucker-Seeley, 2021).

REFERENCES

American Academy of Family Physicians. (2017). *Social needs screening tool patient form (short version)*. The EveryONE Project. https://www.aafp.org/dam/AAFP/documents/patient_care/everyone_project/hops19-physician-form-sdoh.pdf

American Academy of Family Physicians. (2019). *Social needs screening tool*. The EveryONE Project. https://www.aafp.org/dam/AAFP/documents/patient_care/everyone_project/hops19-physician-form-sdoh.pdf.

Billioux, A., Verlander, K., Anthony, S., & Alley, D. (2017). Standardized screening for health-related social needs in clinical settings: The accountable health communities screening tool. In: *NAM perspectives. Discussion paper, issue*. National Academy of Medicine. https://doi.org/10.31478/201705b.

Cahn, P. S. (2020). How interprofessional collaborative practice can help dismantle systemic racism. *Journal of Interprofessional Care, 34*(4), 431–443. https://doi.org/10.1080/13561820.2020.1790224.

Carrera, P. M., Kantarjian, H. M., & Blinder, V. S. (2018). The financial burden and distress of patients with cancer: Understanding and stepping-up action on the financial toxicity of cancer treatment. *CA: A Cancer Journal for Clinicians, 68*(2), 153–165. https://doi.org/10.3322/caac.21443.

Centers for Medicare & Medicaid Service. (2016). *The accountable health communities health-related social needs screening tool*. https://innovation.cms.gov/files/worksheets/ahcm-screeningtool.pdf.

Chan, R. J., & Gordon, L. G. (2021). Screening for financial toxicity in clinical care with finance-related outcome measures. *Cancer Nursing, 44*(2), 87–88. https://doi.org/10.1097/NCC.0000000000000926.

Chan, R. J., Gordon, L. G., Tan, C. J., Chan, A., Bradford, N. K., Yates, P., et al. (2019). Relationships between financial toxicity and symptom burden in cancer survivors: A systematic review. *Journal of Pain and Symptom Management, 57*(3), 646–660.e1. https://doi.org/10.1016/j.jpainsymman.2018.12.003.

Cousin, L., Roper, N., & Nolan, T. S. (2021). Cardio-oncology health disparities: Social determinants of health and care for black breast cancer survivors. *Clinical Journal of Oncology Nursing, 25*(5), 36–41. https://doi.org/10.1188/21.CJON.S1.36-41.

Edward, J., Petermann, V. M., Eberth, J. M., Zahnd, W. E., Vanderpool, R. C., Askelson, N., et al. (2021). Interventions to address cancer-related financial toxicity: Recommendations from the field. *The Journal of Rural Health, 38*(4), 817–826. https://doi.org/10.1111/jrh.12637.

Flucke, N., & Sullivan-Moore, C. (2021). Patient assessment: Using the oncology nurse navigator patient assessment for rural and other resource-poor settings. *Clinical Journal of Oncology Nursing, 25*(6), 729–734. https://doi.org/10.1188/21.Cjon.729-734.

Franklin, E., Burke, S., Dean, M., & Johnson, D. (2022). Oncology navigation standards of professional practice. *Clinical Journal of Oncology Nursing, 26*

Gehlert, S., Hudson, D., & Sacks, T. (2021). A critical theoretical approach to cancer disparities: Breast cancer and the social determinants of health. *Frontiers in Public Health, 9*, 674736. https://doi.org/10.3389/fpubh.2021.674736.

Gold, R., Cottrell, E., Bunce, A., Middendorf, M., Hollombe, C., Cowburn, S., et al. (2017). Developing electronic health record (EHR) strategies related to health center patients' social determinants of health. *Journal of the American Board of Family Medicine, 30*(4), 428–447. https://doi.org/10.3122/jabfm.2017.04.170046.

Gordon, L. G., Merollini, K. M. D., Lowe, A., & Chan, R. J. (2017). A systematic review of financial toxicity among cancer survivors: We can't pay the co-pay. *Patient, 10*(3), 295–309. https://doi.org/10.1007/s40271-016-0204-x.

Gusoff, G., Fichtenberg, C., & Gottlieb, L. M. (2018). Professional medical association policy statements on social health assessments and interventions. *The Permanente Journal, 22*, 18–092. https://doi.org/10.7812/TPP/18-092.

Hamilton, J. B. (2021). Social determinants of health-using a holistic approach to cancer care. *Journal of Cancer Education, 36*(6), 1131–1133. https://doi.org/10.1007/s13187-021-02104-0.

Hernandez, N. D., Durant, R., Lisovicz, N., Nweke, C., Belizaire, C., Cooper, D., et al. (2022). African American Cancer Survivors' perspectives on cancer clinical trial participation in a safety-net hospital: Considering the role of the social determinants of health. *Journal of Cancer Education, 37*(6), 1589–1597. https://doi.org/10.1007/s13187-021-01994-4.

Hirschey, R., Tan, K., Petermann, V. M., & Leak Bryant, A. (2021). Healthy lifestyle behaviors: Nursing considerations for social determinants of health. *Clinical Journal of Oncology Nursing, 25*(5), 42–48. https://doi.org/10.1188/21.CJON.S1.42-48.

Jones, C. P. (2000). Levels of racism: A theoretic framework and a gardener's tale. *American Journal of Public Health, 90*, 1212–1215.

Kaiser Permanente. (2016). *Your current life situation (shorter form)*. https://sirenetwork.ucsf.edu/sites/default/files/Your%20Current%20Life%20Situation%20Questionnaire%20v2-0%20%28Core%20and%20supplemental%29%20no%20highlights.pdf.

Kostelanetz, S., Pettapiece-Phillips, M., Weems, J., Spalding, T., Roumie, C., Wilkins, C. H., et al. (2021). Health care professionals' perspectives on universal screening of social determinants of health: A mixed-methods study. *Population Health Management, 25*(3), 367–374. https://doi.org/10.1089/pop.2021.0176.

LaForge, K., Gold, R., Cottrell, E., Bunce, A. E., Proser, M., Hollombe, C., et al. (2018). How 6 organizations developed tools and processes for social determinants of health screening in primary care: An overview. *The Journal of Ambulatory Care Management, 41*(1), 2–14. https://doi.org/10.1097/JAC.0000000000000221.

Metzl, J. M., & Hansen, H. (2014). Structural competency: Theorizing a new medical engagement with stigma and inequality. *Social Science & Medicine, 103*, 126–133. https://doi.org/10.1016/j.socscimed.2013.06.032.

Mohan, G., & Chattopadhyay, S. (2020). Cost-effectiveness of leveraging social determinants of health to improve breast, cervical, and colorectal cancer screening: A systematic review. *JAMA Oncology, 6*(9), 1434–1444. https://doi.org/10.1001/jamaoncol.2020.1460.

Nolan, T. S., Alston, A., Choto, R., & Moss, K. O. (2021). Cultural humility: Retraining and retooling nurses to provide equitable cancer care. *Clinical Journal of Oncology Nursing, 25*(5), 3–9. https://doi.org/10.1188/21.Cjon.S1.3-9.

Oncology Nursing Society. (2018). Role of the oncology nurse navigator throughout the cancer trajectory. *Oncology Nursing Forum, 45*(3), 283. https://doi.org/10.1188/18.ONF.283.

Page-Reeves, J., Kaufman, W., Bleecker, M., Norris, J., McCalmont, K., Ianakieva, V., et al. (2016). Addressing social determinants of health in a clinic setting: The WellRx Pilot in Albuquerque, New Mexico. *Journal of the American Board of Family Medicine, 29*(3), 414–418. https://doi.org/10.3122/jabfm.2016.03.150272.

Persaud, S. (2018). Addressing social determinants of health through advocacy. *Nursing Administration Quarterly, 42*(2), 123–128. https://doi.org/10.1097/naq.0000000000000277.

Phillips, J., Richard, A., Mayer, K. M., Shilkaitis, M., Fogg, L. F., & Vondracek, H. (2020). Integrating the social determinants of health into nursing practice: Nurses' perspectives. *Journal of*

Nursing Scholarship, 52(5), 497–505. https://doi.org/10.1111/jnu.12584.

Project Implicit. (2011). *Implicit Association Test.* https://implicit.harvard.edu/implicit/takeatest.html.

Robert Wood Johnson Foundation. (2019). *Medicaid's role in addressing social determinants of health.* https://www.rwjf.org/en/library/research/2019/02/medicaid-s-role-in-addressing-social-determinants-of-health.html.

Rooney, M. K., Santiago, G., Perni, S., Horowitz, D. P., McCall, A. R., Einstein, A. J., et al. (2021). Readability of patient education materials from high-impact medical journals: A 20-year analysis. *Journal of Patient Experience, 8,* 2374373521998847. https://doi.org/10.1177/2374373521998847.

Ruth, A., SturtzSreetharan, C., Brewis, A., & Wutich, A. (2020). Structural competency of pre-health students: Can a single course lead to meaningful change? *Medical Science Educator, 30*(1), 331–337. https://doi.org/10.1007/s40670-019-00909-9.

The EveryONE Project. (2023). *Project neighborhood navigator.* American Academy of Family Physicians Foundation. https://www.aafp.org/family-physician/patient-care/the-everyone-project/neighborhood-navigator.html.

The Racial Equity Institute. (2023). Services *and workshops.* https://www.racialequityinstitute.com/ourservices.

Tiase, V., Crookston, C. D., Schoenbaum, A., & Valu, M. (2022). Nurses' role in addressing social determinants of health. *Nursing, 52*(4), 32–37. https://doi.org/10.1097/01.NURSE.0000823284.16666.96.

Tucker-Seeley, R. D. (2021). Social determinants of health and disparities in cancer care for black people in the United States. *JCO Oncology Practice, 17*(5), 261–263. https://doi.org/10.1200/OP.21.00229.

Zafar, S. Y., Chino, F., Ubel, P. A., Rushing, C., Samsa, G., Altomare, I., et al. (2015). The utility of cost discussions between patients with cancer and oncologists. *The American Journal of Managed Care, 21*(9), 607–615.

Zahnd, W. E., Bell, N., & Larson, A. E. (2021). Geographic, racial/ethnic, and socioeconomic inequities in broadband access. *The Journal of Rural Health, 38*(3), 519–526. https://doi.org/10.1111/jrh.12635.

53

Cultural and Spiritual Care

Emily A. Haozous

OVERVIEW

I. Human beings are unique individuals. Each of us interacts with our world according to values, beliefs, and social norms that are influenced by our spiritual, religious, and cultural perspectives.

II. Oncology nurses should recognize the importance of spiritual, religious, and cultural diversity and apply the nursing process to meet the unique needs of patients and caregivers with sensitivity and an understanding of interventions that support optimal outcomes.

III. Definitions—understanding diversity in health care begins with establishing a common language to ensure clear communication among different people. Cross-cultural health care delivery requires an appreciation for the dynamic nature of communication, particularly language. Operationalization of terms allows for clarity, which then translates to meaningful and focused information for oncology nurses providing patient- and family-centered care.

A. Diversity.
1. Condition of being composed of differing elements, especially the inclusion of people of different races or cultures in a group (Merriam-Webster, 2022).

B. Culture.
1. A shared set of beliefs, values, customs, behaviors, and perspectives on the world specific to a racial, religious, or social group in a place or time (Centers for Disease Control and Prevention, 2021; Saint Arnault & Sinko, 2021).
2. Learned and passed from one generation to the next and, as such, responds to larger societal and environmental influences.
3. Encompasses the religious and economic views, language use, social structure, and use of technology within a shared group: for example, youth culture is often cited as strikingly different from previous generations in their use of technology, language, spending habits, and preferred manner of interpersonal communication.
4. Although frequently considered in the context of race or ethnicity, cultural traits are observed across diverse groups; for example, nursing culture varies from one practice area to another.

C. Race and ethnicity: according to the US Census Bureau, ethnicity and race are defined by the federal government via the Office of Management and Budget as two distinct concepts, shaping how American society and demographers conceptualize what are in practice social definitions without any biological foundations (United States Census Bureau, 2022).
1. Race: a social construct in which groups of people are clustered according to shared physical traits, and having no basis in one's biological, anthropological, or genetic composition (Flanagin, Frey, Christiansen, & Bauchner, 2021).
2. Ethnicity: cultural heritage; historical, cultural, contextual, and geographic experiences of a specific community or population (Flanagin et al., 2021).
   a. Ethnic groups may comprise more than one racial group. For example, people who identify as Hispanic or Latino/a have wide racial diversity but share characteristics based on geographic, historic, contextual, and cultural groups of origin. Race and ethnicity can provide some health-related information about a person, such as a predisposition for sickle cell disease in populations who originated in sub-Saharan Africa, India, Saudi Arabia, and Mediterranean countries, yet caution must be taken to avoid generalizations based on external appearance alone (Flanagin et al., 2021).

D. Sexuality: sexual diversity includes sexual preference (heterosexual, homosexual, lesbian, gay, bisexual, asexual, pansexual, and queer), sexual identity, and gender identity (transgender, nonbinary, cisgender, and intersex), gender expression, and those who feel their sexual identity does not or should not fit into a label (Ventriglio, Kelly, & Bhugra, 2021).

E. Spirituality.
1. A lifelong process of discovery that brings meaning, purpose, and connection between a person and the greater world around them; inclusive of a personal search for understanding and insight into one's essential questions on their reason for being (Badanta, Rivilla-García, Lucchetti, & de Diego-Cordero, 2021; Miller et al., 2021).

2. Spiritual distress is defined as an impairment in one's ability to create or find meaning in life "through connection with self, others, the world, or a higher being" (Smiechowski et al., 2021).

F. Religion—personal set or institutionalized system of religious attitudes, beliefs, and practices, often linked to a defined system of worship or faith-based organization and believed to have a sacred purpose or component that brings meaning (Merriam-Webster, 2022; Nissen & Andersen, 2022).

  1. Sacred—dedicated and distinguished as being made in service to a deity; entitled to special recognition and respect. Although similar in ends to religion, what is sacred exists (Merriam-Webster, 2022) outside established religion; for example, in Native American traditions, knowledge about traditional medicine is considered sacred and protected knowledge but is not associated with a specific organized religious practice, nor is it typically published in any religiously oriented text.

G. Socioeconomic status—a person's position in the social hierarchy, this term typically encompasses social class, occupation, level of educational achievement, and annual income (American Psychological Association, 2023).

H. Poverty

  1. In the United States, the federal poverty guidelines refer to a single person earning $13,590 or less per year (all amounts are as of January 12, 2022). Federal poverty guidelines vary based on household size and are adjusted to accommodate higher costs of living in Alaska and Hawaii (Department of Health and Human Services, 2022).

  2. The culture of poverty crosses racial and ethnic groups and has a major impact on health status (National Academies of Sciences, Engineering, and Medicine [NASEM], 2021).

IV. Cultural diversity.

A. Health care consumers in the United States include increasingly diverse populations.

  1. The US Census Bureau defines the Hispanic or Latino population as "a person of Cuban, Mexican, Puerto Rican, South or Central American, or other Spanish culture or origin regardless of race" (United States Census Bureau, 2021a, 2021b).

  2. Hispanics account for 18.7% of the US population (United States Census Bureau, 2021b).

  3. Asians account for 6% of the total population.

  4. Native Hawaiian and other Pacific Islanders represent 0.2% of the total population.

  5. 10.2% of the US population identifies itself as being of two or more races.

  6. Although projections are complicated by trends in births, deaths, immigration, and overall population growth, it is projected that there will be an overall demographic shift in the United States. By the year 2045, the majority of the US population will identify with a race or ethnicity other than non-Hispanic White (Vespa, Medina, & Armstrong, 2020).

B. Cultural norms influence relationships between health care practitioners and patients or caregivers.

  1. Culture is intersectoral, influenced by race, ethnicity, gender, sexual orientation, age, geography, and income (NASEM, 2021).

  2. Although traditions and trends can emerge in various groups, generalizing across populations is inappropriate.

  3. Culture affects time orientation to past, present, or future. In some cultures, time is fluid and flexible, and the process takes priority over the task at hand.

C. Cultural norms vary widely (Blaszko Helming et al., 2022). Examples include the following:

  1. Cultures hold wide-ranging beliefs about personal space and eye contact.

    a. Closeness of personal space, eye contact, touching, and even shaking hands is either respectful and comforting or intrusive and violating.

    b. Facial expressions have a wide range of meanings; smiling may be inviting and indicate an emotional connection or happiness, or it may be a nervous or socially accepted response to unpleasant news.

    c. Winking means different things in different cultures.

     (1) As a sexual invitation

     (2) To convey a shared joke

     (3) A rude or patronizing gesture

  2. Hand gestures hold meanings unique to a culture.

    a. The hand signal that people in the United States use to mean "OK" is the symbol for money in some cultures, and in other cultures it is used as an offensive gesture to indicate a bodily orifice.

    b. The "thumbs up" gesture widely recognized in the United States as a congratulatory gesture has vulgar connotations in other cultures.

    c. Many cultures view pointing with a single finger as rude and prefer using the entire hand or a gesture with the face, lips, or chin to point to something or indicate direction.

  3. Posture and physical position have varying significance in different cultures.

    a. Showing the bottom of the feet to others is rude in some cultures.

    b. In some cultures, it is important to be facing the person to whom you are speaking, whereas others see this as overly assertive or aggressive.

    c. In some cultures, placing hands on the hips while speaking to someone is indicative of anger or confrontation.

  4. Some cultures are more modest than others.

    a. Nudity may be acceptable and even embraced in some cultures.

b. In some cultures, it is taboo for people from the opposite gender to see or touch their body, even when coming from a health care provider.

D. Human sexuality contributes to health and well-being (Gianotten, Alley, & Diamond, 2021).

1. Recognition of sexual diversity includes rejecting heteronormative assumptions that all people are heterosexual and/or happily conforming to the gender conventions of the dominant culture.

2. If unsure, best practice is to ask a patient's preferred pronouns (she/her/hers, he/him/his, and they/theirs).

V. Poverty and cancer (see Chapter 52).

A. Access to health care is a major determinant of health.

1. Cancer prevention through early screening is harder to access for people without access to primary care (Moss, Pinto, Srinivasan, Cronin, & Croyle, 2022).

a. Poor people may lack access to quality health care.

b. Pursuit of food and shelter takes priority over seeking care for cancer diagnosis or treatment unless symptoms prohibit basic activities of daily living.

c. Poor people have a higher risk for illness, including cancer, due to higher exposure to poor nutrition, workplace carcinogens, and modifiable risk factors such as habitual tobacco use.

d. People living in poverty and/or without health insurance are more often diagnosed with cancer in advanced stages (Lin, Soni, Sabik, & Drake, 2021).

2. Cancer prevention, defined as health-seeking behaviors, genetic testing, awareness of environmental exposures, and access to regular screening, is a determinant of prevention and early diagnosis (National Cancer Institute, 2022).

VI. Racial/ethnic diversity in cancer (see Chapter 1)

VII. Responses to the cancer experience

A. The meaning of a life-threatening illness (e.g., cancer) is influenced by culture.

B. Cultural norms and behaviors have a major impact on all aspects of the cancer experience, including screening, seeking diagnosis, treatment options, symptom management, response to advanced cancer, hospice use, and end-of-life care (Silbermann, Berger, & Berger, 2022).

C. Cancer prevention behaviors.

1. Cultures that do not trust the conventional medicine system in the United States may not participate consistently in cancer prevention, screening, or treatment.

2. Some cultures rely heavily on traditional healers and may choose not to pursue allopathic/conventional models of health and wellness.

3. Individuals or groups who are recent immigrants to the United States may lack knowledge about cancer screening.

4. Some populations may expect that cancer is inevitably fatal. This expectation is based on the poor cancer outcomes in their communities and limited exposure to cancer survivors. This belief may keep people from those communities from participating in screening.

D. Response to the diagnosis of cancer.

1. Diagnosis of cancer is often considered devastating news.

a. Depending on an individual's culture, the response may range from one of stoic acceptance to one that is highly demonstrative.

b. Regardless of demonstrative emotional response, it is incumbent on nurses to assist all patients with positive coping strategies.

E. Participation in clinical trials.

1. Cultural influences determine the response to clinical trials as a health care option; cultural factors, such as lack of trust, present barriers to patient participation in clinical trials.

2. Patients may resist clinical trials based on the historical precedent of unethical research conducted with people from their ethnic/racial group (Vince & Spratt, 2021).

F. Coping with advanced cancer and end of life.

1. Cultural and religious beliefs and norms influence responses to advanced cancer and end of life.

2. These responses range on a continuum from fearing and fighting cancer as an enemy to acceptance and integrative therapies to assist with symptom management, including psychosocial symptoms (Larson et al., 2021; Lu, Liu, & Yuan, 2021).

VIII. Spiritual and religious diversity.

A. *Spirituality* is the relationship or connection to the sacred, giving a broader meaning and purpose that is experienced through personal or communal devotions or through meditation, art, nature, or ceremony (Badanta et al., 2021; Miller et al., 2021).

B. *Religion* describes organized systems of faith and worship that follow regulated practices intended to enhance spirituality.

1. For this reason, religiosity is rarely discussed without spirituality being at the core of the discussion.

2. A person may consider himself or herself a spiritual being without belonging to an organized religion.

3. As defined in this chapter, spirituality applies to all persons, whether they consider themselves spiritual or not.

C. Spiritual care is an important component of comprehensive, patient-centered nursing care in the following ways (Badanta et al., 2021; Miller et al., 2021; Smiechowski et al., 2021):

1. Strongly influences health-related decision-making.

2. May influence a person's health-seeking behaviors (e.g., cancer prevention).

3. Delays in seeking medical care may stem from religious/spiritual (R/S) beliefs associated with fatalism or disease attribution.

4. May have a positive impact on the patient's response to cancer and treatment.

5. Patients may experience R/S distress associated with a cancer diagnosis, with feelings of abandonment, meaning-making, identity, and existential distress.

D. The patient with cancer may experience a heightened sense of spirituality associated with a cancer diagnosis. Patients may:
   1. Discover an intensified sense of spirituality or faith, which may include closer relationships with friends, family, and community, and a greater connection to the simple pleasures of life.
   2. Experience a sense of betrayal linked to their R/S beliefs.

E. R/S and cultural beliefs may influence how people respond to cancer across the spectrum of care; for some R/S inspires active participation, yet others may feel it more appropriate to respond with a passive or fatalistic perspective on cancer treatment, seeing cancer death as "the will of God" (Cohen, 2022).

F. R/S also influences how caregivers perceive the cancer experience.
   1. As with patients, R/S may be a source of strength for caregivers; they may also feel betrayed, punished, or abandoned in their time of need.
   2. Healthy caregivers may experience guilt when their loved one is suffering.

G. R/S may have a beneficial or harmful impact on the patient's and caregiver's adjustment to cancer and their participation in treatment (Cohen, 2022).
   1. Relying on faith as a coping mechanism may help patients overcome the initial shock and distress related to a new diagnosis of cancer.
   2. Acceptance of the cancer diagnosis related to a belief in a higher power in control of life and death has been shown to correlate with better adjustment to illness.
   3. Patients may transfer their faith in a higher power to faith in their physician to be able to cure their disease.
   4. Feeling punished, abandoned, or both has been shown to contribute to higher levels of distress for patients; may be a barrier to active participation in treatment.

H. R/S may have a beneficial or harmful influence on responses to end-of-life issues.
   1. Patients who believe in existence after death may find joy in prospect of afterlife.
   2. Patients whose belief system does not include an afterlife may or may not feel despondent about the finality of death.

ASSESSMENT

I. Assessment includes socioeconomic needs, sexuality concerns, cultural components of care, and pertinent spiritual and religious beliefs of their patients and caregivers; and incorporates assessment findings into their nursing diagnoses, nursing plan of care, and interdisciplinary care planning, where appropriate (Deshields et al., 2021),
   A. The oncology nurse should first recognize his or her own culture, sexual orientation, spirituality, and religiosity and how this may affect his or her perception of others.
   B. The oncology nurse recognizes culture, sexual orientation, spirituality, and religiosity as part of the whole person, which are assessed in the context of the human experience (Christensen, 2019).
   C. Assessment of the patient and caregivers includes, but is not limited to, the patient's support system and chosen community, cultural beliefs and practices, philosophical or religious belief system, sense of belonging, and love for self and others (Deshields et al., 2021).
   D. The oncology nurse's spiritual assessment is performed without judgment and includes the following in both patient and caregiver(s) (Badanta et al., 2021):
      1. Identification of R/S background, preferences, beliefs, rituals, and preferred practices.
      2. Identification of possible symptoms of R/S distress, such as emotional pain, guilt, resentment, despair, despondency, and hopelessness.
      3. Ways that the oncology nurse may support the patient's and caregivers' spiritual needs include deep listening, holding a presence, bearing witness, and practicing compassion (Badanta et al., 2021).

MANAGEMENT

I. Provide interventions to enhance cultural comfort, R/S, and hopefulness.
   A. Identify patient's cultural identity and any needs that may affect cancer care.
      1. Plan treatment around cultural holidays or events when possible.
      2. Ask before assuming stereotypes.
      3. Make space for extended family, appreciating cultural norms regarding modesty, physical space, gestures, and contact.
   B. Respect patient's R/S beliefs and plan care that honors these beliefs.
      1. Create time, space, and privacy, as needed, for spiritual or religious rituals.
      2. When appropriate (per patient request), pray with patient, caregivers, or both as a sincere, genuine gesture.
      3. Encourage patient and caregivers to speak with their R/S leader.
   C. Avoid proselytizing—the nurse does not impose his or her own spiritual or religious beliefs on patients and caregivers.
   D. Support the patient's use of spiritual coping.
      1. Refer the patient and caregiver to a hospital chaplain or group that can support coping with spiritual issues as needed.

E. Assist the patient in exploring modalities to enhance spiritual well-being.
   1. Meditation (e.g., mindfulness meditation), yoga, and prayer
   2. Expressive therapies
      a. Art therapy
      b. Music therapy
      c. Journaling: gratitude or expressive journaling

REFERENCES

American Psychological Association. (2023). *Socioeconomic status.* https://www.apa.org/topics/socioeconomic-status/.

Badanta, B., Rivilla-García, E., Lucchetti, G., & de Diego-Cordero, R. (2021). The influence of spirituality and religion on critical care nursing: An integrative review. *Nursing in Critical Care, 27*(3), 348–366. https://doi.org/10.1111/nicc.12645.

Blaszko Helming, M. A., Shields, D. A., Avino, K. M., & Rosa, W. E. (2022). *Dossey & Keegan's Holistic Nursing: A Handbook for Practice,* (8th ed.). Boston: Jones & Bartlett.

Centers for Disease Control and Prevention. (2021). *Culture and language.* https://www.cdc.gov/healthliteracy/culture.html.

Christensen, D. (2019). Cultivate cultural humility in yourself and your practice: *ONS Voice* https://voice.ons.org/news-and-views/cultivate-cultural-humility-in-yourself-and-your-practice.

Cohen, M. (2022). Cancer fatalism: Attitudes toward screening and care. In J. L. Steel & B. I. Carr (Eds.), *Psychological aspects of cancer* (pp. 301–318). Cham: Springer.

Department of Health and Human Services. (2022). *Annual update of the HHS poverty guidelines, § 42 U.S.C. 9902(2).* https://www.govinfo.gov/content/pkg/FR-2022-01-21/pdf/2022-01166.pdf.

Deshields, T. L., Wells-Di Gregorio, S., Flowers, S. R., Irwin, K. E., Nipp, R., Padgett, L., et al. (2021). Addressing distress management challenges: Recommendations from the consensus panel of the American Psychosocial Oncology Society and the Association of Oncology Social Work. *CA: A Cancer Journal for Clinicians, 71*(5), 407–436. https://doi.org/10.3322/caac.21672.

Flanagin, A., Frey, T., Christiansen, S. L., & Bauchner, H. (2021). The reporting of race and ethnicity in medical and science journals: Comments invited. *Journal of the American Medical Association, 325*(11), 1049–1052. https://doi.org/10.1001/jama.2021.2104.

Gianotten, W. L., Alley, J. C., & Diamond, L. M. (2021). The health benefits of sexual expression. *International Journal of Sexual Health, 33*(4), 478–493. https://doi.org/10.1080/19317611.2021.1966564.

Larson, K. L., Mathews, H. F., Moye, J. P., Congema, M. R., Hoffman, S. J., Murrieta, K. M., et al. (2021). Four kinds of hard: An understanding of cancer and death among Latino community leaders. *Global Qualitative Nursing Research, 8,* 233339362110035. https://doi.org/10.1177/23333936211003557.

Lin, L., Soni, A., Sabik, L. M., & Drake, C. (2021). Early- and late-stage cancer diagnosis under 3 years of Medicaid expansion. *American Journal of Preventive Medicine, 60*(1), 104–109. https://doi.org/10.1016/j.amepre.2020.06.020.

Lu, L., Liu, J., & Yuan, Y. C. (2021). Cultural differences in cancer information acquisition: Cancer risk perceptions, fatalistic beliefs, and worry as predictors of cancer information seeking and avoidance in the U.S. and China. *Health Communication, 37,* 1–10. https://doi.org/10.1080/10410236.2021.1901422.

Merriam-Webster. (2022). Merriam-Webster, Inc. https://www.merriam-webster.com/

Miller, M., Xu, D., Lehto, R., Moser, J., Wu, H.-S., & Wyatt, G. (2021). Pain and spirituality outcomes among women with advanced breast cancer participating in a foot reflexology trial. *Oncology Nursing Forum, 48*(1), 31–43. https://doi.org/10.1188/21.onf.31-43.

Moss, J. L., Pinto, C. N., Srinivasan, S., Cronin, K. A., & Croyle, R. T. (2022). Enduring cancer disparities by persistent poverty, rurality, and race: 1990-1992 to 2014-2018. *Journal of the National Cancer Institute, 114*(6), 829–836. http://10.1093/jnci/djac038.

National Academies of Sciences, Engineering, and Medicine (NASEM). (2021). *The future of nursing 2020-2030: Charting a path to achieve health equity.* The National Academies Press. https://doi.org/10.17226/25982.

National Cancer Institute. (2022). *Prevention: Cancer trends progress report.* https://progressreport.cancer.gov/prevention.

Nissen, R. D., & Andersen, A. H. (2022). Addressing religion in secular healthcare: Existential communication and the post-secular negotiation. *Religions, 13*(1), 34. https://www.mdpi.com/2077-1444/13/1/34.

Saint Arnault, D., & Sinko, L. (2021). Comparative ethnographic narrative analysis method: Comparing culture in narratives. *Global Qualitative Nursing Research, 8,* 23333936211020722.

Silbermann, M., Berger, A. M., & Berger, C. P. P. C. A. (2022). *Global perspectives in cancer care: Religion, spirituality, and cultural diversity in health and healing.* Oxford: Oxford University Press. https://books.google.com/books?id=ot5eEAAAQBAJ.

Smiechowski, J., Stelfox, H., Sinclair, S., Sinuff, T., Grindrod-Millar, K., Roze des Ordons, A., et al. (2021). Vicarious spiritual distress in intensive care unit healthcare providers: A qualitative study. *Intensive and Critical Care Nursing, 63,* 102982. https://doi.org/10.1016/j.iccn.2020.102982.

United States Census Bureau. (2021a). *About the Hispanic population and its origin.* https://www.census.gov/topics/population/hispanic-origin/about.html.

United States Census Bureau. (2021b). *Race and ethnicity in the United States: 2010 census and 2020 census.* https://www.census.gov/library/visualizations/interactive/race-and-ethnicity-in-the-united-state-2010-and-2020-census.html.

United States Census Bureau. (2022). *About the topic of race.* https://www.census.gov/topics/population/race/about.html.

Ventriglio, A., Kelly, M., & Bhugra, D. (2021). *Sexual diversity and transcultural context: Psychiatry and sexual medicine.* Berlin: Springer.

Vespa, J., Medina, L., & Armstrong, D. M. (2020). Demographic Turning Points for the United States: Population Projections for 2020 to 2060. Current Population Reports, P25-1144. Washington, DC: U.S. Census Bureau.

Vince, R., & Spratt, D. E. (2021). Drivers of racial disparities in prostate cancer trial enrollment. *Prostate Cancer and Prostatic Diseases, 24*(4), 946–947. https://doi.org/10.1038/s41391-021-00427-z.

54

Psychosocial Disturbances and Coping

Kathleen Murphy-Ende

EMOTIONAL DISTRESS

Overview

I. Distress
  A. Psychosocial distress and existential concerns are common in patients with cancer
  B. A psychological (cognitive, behavioral, and emotional), social, and spiritual nature may interfere with the ability to cope effectively with cancer, its physical symptoms, and its treatment. Distress extends along a continuum, ranging from common normal feelings of vulnerability, sadness, and fears to problems that may become disabilities, such as depression, anxiety, panic, social isolation, and existential and spiritual crises (National Comprehensive Cancer Network [NCCN], 2018)
  C. Psychological, social, spiritual, physical, and financial stressors that strain the individual's and family's coping abilities
  D. Used to describe the unpleasant emotional experience associated with the stressors that patients face when living with cancer
  E. Reflects a normative response different from psychological or psychiatric diagnoses such as clinical depression, adjustment disorder, posttraumatic stress disorder (PTSD), delirium, and anxiety disorder
  F. Depression and anxiety are associated with a significantly increased risk of cancer incidence, cancer-specific mortality, and all-cause mortality in cancer patients (Wang et al., 2020)

II. Risk factors
  A. All patients experience some form or level of distress related to their diagnosis or treatment, and so are faced with coping challenges (Cohen & White, 2018; NCCN, 2018).
    1. Disease and stage (Cohen & White, 2018)
      a. Highest level of distress reported in patients with lung cancer
      b. Higher level of distress in patients in the advanced stage of disease
      c. Impact of physical symptoms such as poor pain control
    2. Situational
      a. Personal meaning of the diagnosis
      b. Resources—emotional and practical support, spiritual guidance, and financial security
      c. Changes in roles—occupation, within family, between friends, altered physical capacity, and cognitive functioning
    3. Developmental
      a. Developmental life tasks disrupted by diagnosis and treatment
      b. Personality and coping style

III. General treatment approaches
  A. Psychotherapeutic interventions that have been effective in the cancer population—individual supportive psychotherapy, cognitive behavioral therapy, group therapy (Antoni, Moreno, & Penedo, 2023; https://www.ons.org/practice-resources/pep/anxiety), and bibliotherapy (Malibiran, Tairman, & Amer, 2018)
  B. Family psychotherapy
  C. Psychoeducational approaches
  D. Spiritual counseling
  E. Support groups
  F. Relaxation exercises, including meditation and guided imagery (Antoni et al., 2023; https://www.ons.org/intervention/cognitive-behavioral-interventionsapproach-2)

IV. Potential sequelae of emotional distress
  A. Ineffective coping—may occur in crisis and may lead to suicidal ideation (Cohen & White, 2018)
  B. Chronic emotional distress
  C. Development of major psychiatric disorders—anxiety, depression, adjustment disorder, and suicidal ideation or suicide
  D. Acute stress disorder or PTSD. Traumatic event or experience prompting responses. PTSD may occur in cancer survivors with similar experiences to those in military combat or natural disasters. Diagnostic criteria for PTSD and acute stress disorder are different. Symptoms are similar and in general include the following:
    1. Cognitive (e.g., forgetful, distracted, and cannot concentrate)
    2. Behavioral (e.g., fight-or-flight response, avoidance, and isolation)
    3. Emotional (e.g., numbing feeling, irritable, and angry outbursts)
    4. Physiologic (e.g., insomnia, nightmares, and agitated) (American Psychiatric Association [APA], 2013)

E. Somatic symptoms such as sleep disturbance, fatigue, loss of appetite, and gastrointestinal (GI) disturbances

F. Declined performance at home, school, or work

G. Nonadherence or misunderstanding of health information

Assessment

I. Screening

A. National Comprehensive Cancer Network Guideline (NCCN, 2018)

1. Screen patients routinely to identify the level and source of their distress so that further evaluation can be completed.

2. Identifying and treating psychological issues is a complex process; appropriate referrals should be made to mental health specialists such as licensed clinical psychologists or psychiatrists.

3. Psychological needs vary, depending on the individual, developmental stage, phase of disease trajectory, past coping skills, and available emotional and practical resources.

B. Screening tools for distress

1. Information obtained from screening checklists useful for identifying specific concerns and needs, rather than identifying a clinical diagnosis

2. Distress Thermometer (DT), developed in the late 1990s, is still used today (Roth et al., 1998)—a unidimensional screening tool in which the patient is asked to indicate the severity of distress in the domains of emotional, spiritual, physical, practical, and family matters

a. Designed for rapid assessment of patient distress; well validated in patients with cancer

b. Can be used as a one-item scale assessing the level of distress

c. Contains a problem list; the source of distress can be identified

d. Sensitive to changes over time; takes a few minutes to complete

e. Not useful for identifying specific psychiatric disorders

f. Clinical pathways for the DT available to guide the follow-up assessment and management of distress (National Cancer Institute [NCI], 2017); can be downloaded as part of the Distress Guidelines through the website for the NCCN (NCCN, 2018)

C. Screening for suicide

1. Strategies nurses use include assessing the situation, offering end-of-life or palliative care, treating symptoms, and referring for further assessment.

2. Barriers to assessing suicidality include lack of training, stigma, lack of time, or access to mental health professionals (Granek, Nakash, Ariad, Shapira, & Ben-David, 2019).

3. Screening instruments, which are easy to administer and are reliable and cost-effective, include the Columbia Suicide Severity Rating Scale, the Ask Suicide-Screening Questions from the National Institute of Mental Health, the Suicide Behavior Questionnaire-Revised, and the Patient Health Questionnaire-0 (PHQ-9) Depression Scale.

II. History

A. Age, diagnosis, stage of disease, and treatment regimen

B. Presence of risk factors

C. Distressing thoughts, feelings, and behaviors such as nervousness, worry, jitteriness, tearfulness, hopelessness, difficulty concentrating, irritability, social withdrawal, ruminating, thoughts of death, suicidal ideation, self-harm, or harm to others

III. Pattern of emotional distress

A. Distress occurs across the disease continuum, accompanied by vulnerability, sadness, fear of disability, worry of becoming a burden to others, depression, anxiety, panic, social isolation, and existential and spiritual crises.

B. For each specific distressing symptom, assess the frequency and intensity of specific distress, associated symptoms, and precipitating and alleviating factors.

C. Duration of symptoms to determine if symptoms are episodic or prolonged.

1. Episodic symptoms often occur during disease transitions such as diagnosis or relapse.

2. Persistent symptoms may represent a psychiatric disorder, and the patient should be referred to a psychologist or psychiatrist.

IV. Impact on functional status—physical, interpersonal, occupational, academic performance, and spiritual practices

Management

I. Nonpharmacologic

A. Address hopelessness

1. Identify which dimension (affective, cognitive, behavioral, affiliative, temporal, or contextual) applies to the patient; support and facilitate the individual's hope; professionals may increase cancer patients' sense of hope by being present, giving accurate information, and showing care

2. Assist patient to explore his or her value system, purpose, and life meaning

3. Promote goal setting

4. Offer psychological support programs grounded on the construct of hope and have successfully helped cancer patients to gain hope

B. Address PTSD

1. Assist the patient in identifying perceived threats and providing accurate information on actual risks

2. Provide an opportunity for patients to give a narrative of their experience with support in the form of family and friends, nursing staff, support groups, and individual psychotherapy

3. Offer supportive and expressive group therapy

C. Address ineffective role performance

1. Assist the patient in identifying realistic goals based on what he or she wants to accomplish in the current role

2. Ask the patient to list the priorities within his or her personal, professional, and social roles

3. Refer the patient to his or her employer's human resource department to assist with job schedule and duty changes
4. Refer to occupational rehabilitation psychologist, if indicated

ANXIETY

Overview

I. Definition—anxiety is a "mood state characterized by apprehension and somatic symptoms of tension in which an individual anticipates impending danger, catastrophe, or misfortune. The future threat may be real or imagined, internal or external. It may be an identifiable situation or a vaguer fear of the unknown" (APA, 2022a).
   A. Commonly associated with cancer.
   B. Characterized by a high negative effect in which the patient may experience feeling distressed, fearful, hostile, jittery, nervous, and scornful.
   C. Anxiety frequently occurs with depression.
II. Risk factors
   A. Disease related
      1. Disease trajectory points—new diagnosis, treatment initiation, completion of treatment, recurrent disease, advanced phase, and end of life
      2. Physical symptoms—pain, insomnia, dyspnea, urinary retention, and pruritus
      3. Abnormal metabolic states—hyperthyroidism, hormone-secreting tumors, paraneoplastic syndromes, electrolyte imbalance, hypoxia, sepsis, delirium, and hypoglycemia
      4. Scans, tumor marker tests, and disease surveillance studies often precipitate anxiety
      5. Psychiatric disorders such as depression, delirium, paranoia, and persecution delusions, which may predispose the patient to anxiety
      6. Preexisting anxiety disorders, genetics, age, and gender influence the expression and manifestation of anxiety (Murphy-Ende, 2019)
      7. Immunocompromised may be afraid of infection or exposure to coronavirus disease (COVID)
   B. Treatment related
      1. Starting treatment (preoperative time, initial chemotherapy/biotherapy, and initial radiation treatment)
      2. Prolonged treatment and hospitalization, blood and marrow transplantation, major surgery, or prolonged phase of recovery
      3. Medications—corticosteroids, neuroleptics causing akathisia, thyroxine, bronchodilators, antihistamines, decongestants, beta-adrenergic stimulants, and opioids that induce hallucinations
      4. Opioid, alcohol, or benzodiazepine withdrawal
      5. Body image changes from mastectomy, orchiectomy, colostomy, alopecia, skin changes, amputation, and weight loss or gain
      6. Failure of therapy, progression of disease, or relapse
   C. Intrapersonal related

1. Concern about future health, relationships, finances, and social or occupational roles and responsibilities
2. Loss of independence and perceived loss of sense of control
3. Limited coping skills
4. Cumulative losses that contribute to social isolation
5. Limited social resources

III. General treatment approaches
   A. Treatment should be aimed at the exact cause whenever possible.
   B. Physical symptoms such as pain, insomnia, pruritus, urinary retention, dyspnea, and infection should be treated.
   C. Psychoeducational interventions, including a focus on providing information about the medical system and treatment process and anticipatory guidance, are likely to reduce anxiety (Murphy-Ende, 2019).
      1. Orientation to the health care setting and oncology team
      2. Providing information about support groups may reduce anxiety
   D. Written or Internet-based education materials about specific types of cancer, treatment, and side effects should be provided.
   E. Self-care and relaxation techniques need to be taught to the patient.
   F. The patient and family should be instructed about managing and treating the side effects of chemotherapy and radiation therapy.
   G. Refer to a licensed psychologist for individual cognitive behavioral therapy, cognitive existential group psychotherapy, or family psychotherapy and counseling.
   H. Refer to cancer support groups to provide anxiety management techniques and coping skills.
   I. Pharmacologic management is accomplished with anxiolytics, azapirones, antihistamines, antidepressants, or atypical neuroleptics.
   J. Complementary therapies such as exercise, art therapy, massage, music therapy, meditation, and progressive muscle relaxation.
IV. Potential sequelae of anxiety (APA, 2013)
   A. Somatic symptoms—nausea, vomiting, headaches, and change in bowel habits
   B. Behavioral issues—substance use, altered eating habits, self-harm, suicide, and social dysfunction
   C. Cognitive effects—difficulty concentrating and making decisions, poor attention span, and impaired memory
   D. Anxiety disorders—may occur as a maladaptive response; include adjustment disorder with anxious mood, generalized anxiety disorder, panic attacks, phobias, obsessive–compulsive disorder, PTSD, and depression
   E. Interference with performance at home, school, or work

Assessment

I. Presence of risk factors
II. Subjective symptoms

A. Persistently tense, unable to relax, worried, easily excitable, having poor concentration or poor attention, indecisive, easily overwhelmed, and irritable; experiencing panic attacks, loss of control, insomnia, eating disturbances, palpitations, feelings of suffocation, dizziness, fatigue or exhaustion, difficulty swallowing, and a sense of impending doom; crying easily

III. Objective symptoms and measurement
   A. Facial tension or flushing, pallor, tremors, twitches, pacing, restlessness, nail biting, wringing of hands, voice quivering, rapid heart rate, increased respirations, increased blood pressure, constricted pupils, and cold hands.
   B. Screening tool: General Anxiety Disorder-7 scale measures the severity of anxiety over the past 2 weeks.

Management

I. Pharmacologic
   A. Antidepressants: serotonin reuptake inhibitors, serotonin and norepinephrine reuptake inhibitors, and tricyclic antidepressants and atypical antidepressants (Table 54.1)
   B. Anticonvulsants
   C. Benzodiazepines (low dose and short term for situational anxiety)
   D. Antipsychotics
   E. Administer medications, monitor for side effects, and evaluate effectiveness
      1. Explain the rationale for medications provided, including psychopharmacology
      2. Provide information to patient and family
II. Nonpharmacologic
   A. Interventions to address anxiety

TABLE 54.1	Most Commonly Used Antidepressants
Tricyclic antidepressants	• Amitriptyline (Elavil)
	• Clomipramine (Anafranil)
	• Desipramine (Norpramin)
	• Doxepin (Sinequan)
	• Imipramine (Tofranil)
	• Nortriptyline (Pamelor)
Selective serotonin reuptake inhibitors	• Citalopram (Celexa)
	• Fluoxetine (Prozac)
	• Fluvoxamine (Luvox)
	• Paroxetine (Paxil)
	• Sertraline (Zoloft)
Serotonin and norepinephrine reuptake inhibitors	• Venlafaxine (Effexor)
	• Duloxetine (Cymbalta)
Monoamine oxidase inhibitors	• Tranylcypromine (Parnate)
	• Phenelzine (Nardil)
Atypical antidepressants	• Bupropion (Wellbutrin)
	• Trazodone (Desyrel)
	• Nefazodone (Serzone)
	• Mirtazapine (Remeron)
	• Maprotiline (Ludiomil)

   1. Provide a safe environment
      a. Assess the potential for self-harm
      b. Provide a subdued space with reduced stimuli
   B. Use active and empathic listening skills
      1. Use positive interpersonal skills
      2. Use a calm demeanor, speaking slowly with an even voice, listening, encouraging the identification of the cause of anxiety, normalizing or affirming fears, and assisting the patient to identify past effective coping skills
      3. Assist patient to identify overwhelming feelings such as vulnerability, hopelessness, helplessness, fear, loss of control, and fear of the unknown
   C. Provide information about psychological resources
   D. Provide information as appropriate for relaxation resources to minimize anxiety: massage, distraction, Reiki, music, and prayer
   E. Address iatrogenic causes of anxiety (medications, physical symptoms)
   F. Address spiritual needs
   G. Provide interventions to address death anxiety
      1. Consider the developmental differences in conceptualizing death
      2. Establish a nurturing and supportive relationship
         a. Provide continuity of care by assigning the same staff and encouraging consistent care
      3. Assist the patient to contain the anxiety associated with impending death by listening to the concerns and being present
         a. Allow patient to have discussions about fears concerning dying
         b. Facilitate open communication with family
      4. Encourage family and friends to visit if the patient okay with visitors
         a. Facilitate open communication
         b. Provide privacy
      5. Assist the patient to identify and address practical concerns of death
      6. Assist the patient in finding pleasure in short-term goals
         a. Provide information about predictable physical symptoms
         b. Reassure patient that pain/symptoms will be assessed and addressed
      7. Explain common emotional phases that patients may face
         a. Acknowledge defense mechanisms as denial, which is a possible adaptive response to impending death
      8. Encourage the patient to identify his or her spiritual belief system that helps face the transition of death
         a. Offer to arrange for clergy services, as needed
         b. Ask how faith-based interventions can be incorporated into care
      9. Refer to palliative care or a psychologist to provide short-term psychological interventions

DEPRESSION

Overview

I. Depression
   A. A mood state of feeling sad, discouraged, hopeless, and worthless
      1. May vary from mild and transient emotional distress to a major psychiatric illness
      2. Several types of depressive disorders may affect one's physical, affective, cognitive, and social well-being
      3. Reactive depression—a normal response to a precipitating event or situation and can be a response to the cancer diagnosis, prognosis, treatment, fear of the unknown, cumulative losses, or fear of death
      4. Depression characterized by low positive affect, with symptoms of anhedonia and cognitive and motor slowing
   B. Patient evaluation by a qualified mental health practitioner such as a psychologist or psychiatrist critical for accurate diagnosis and treatment
      1. Clinicians and patients may believe depression is normal in cancer, which may be one barrier to accurate evaluation and effective treatment.
      2. Nurses may underestimate the level of depressive symptoms in patients with moderate or severe depression; nurses are key to identify patients who are at risk and make referrals for further evaluation.
      3. The *Diagnostic and Statistical Manual of Mental Disorders* (DSM-V) criteria for a diagnosis of a major depressive disorder are as follows:
         a. Depressed mood or loss of interest in pleasure in nearly all activities for at least 2 weeks.
         b. Have five or more of the following symptoms— change in appetite or weight change (5% or more in a month), insomnia or hypersomnia nearly every day, psychomotor agitation or retardation nearly every day (observable by others), decreased energy, feelings of worthlessness or guilt, difficulty concentrating or making decisions, recurrent thoughts of death or suicidal ideation, or plans or attempts (APA, 2013).
      4. The symptoms listed here do not meet the diagnostic criteria if they are caused by the direct physiologic effects of a substance or a general medical condition, or if the symptoms are accounted for by bereavement.
      5. It is often difficult to determine if physical symptoms are caused by cancer and its treatment or by a mood disorder such as major depression.
         a. Many patients with cancer have physical symptoms and anxiety; psychologists should use clinical judgment and other diagnostic criteria besides the DSM-V.
      6. Depression indicators that require more focused interventions (Box 54.1).
      7. Possible medical causes of cancer-related depression (Table 54.2).

II. Mood disorder
   A. Caused by a medical condition with depressive features
   B. Defined as depression that has a cause in a medical illness or is caused by a direct biological condition and the full criteria for a major depressive episode are not met (APA, 2013)

III. Adjustment disorder with depressed mood
   A. Considered acute if lasts less than 6 months
   B. Considered chronic when symptoms last for 6 months or longer (APA, 2013)

IV. Demoralization
   A. Described as subjective incompetence along with distress in an environment of social isolation (deFigueiredo, 2013). This is a different construct from depression and should be considered a separate syndrome.
   B. Characterized by the loss of meaning, purpose, hope, low morale, and limited sense of coping.
   C. There is a strong positive correlation between depression and demoralization with a small cohort of those with low depression and high demoralization (deFigueiredo, 2013).

BOX 54.1　Depression Indicators

Indicators of Depression Requiring More Focused or Involved Interventions

- History of depression
- Weak social support system (e.g., not married, few friends, and solitary work environment)
- Evidence of persistent irrational beliefs, negativistic thinking about the diagnosis
- More serious prognosis
- Greater dysfunction related to cancer
- Depressed mood for most of the day on most days

General Symptoms for More Than 2 Weeks

- Diminished pleasure or interest in most activities
- Significant change in appetite and sleep patterns
- Psychomotor agitation or slowing
- Fatigue
- Feelings of worthlessness or excessive, inappropriate guilt
- Poor concentration
- Recurrent thoughts of death or suicide

Because suicide risk is elevated in patients with cancer, those whose screens suggest suicide risk should be asked about suicidal ideation as part of their clinical evaluation.

Adapted from Cohen, M., & Bankston, S. (2011). Cancer-related distress. In C. H. Yarbro, D. Wujick, & B. H. Gobel (Eds.), *Cancer nursing: principles and practice* (7th ed., pp. 667–684). Sudbury, MA: Jones and Bartlett.

TABLE 54.2	**Possible Medical Causes of Cancer-Related Depression**
Mood-affecting treatments	• Corticosteroids • Methyldopa • Reserpine • Barbiturates • Propranolol • Antibiotics (e.g., amphotericin B)
Chemotherapy and immunotherapy	• Procarbazine • L-Asparaginase • Interferon-alpha • Aldesleukin (IL-2)
Metabolic changes	• Hypercalcemia • Sodium or potassium imbalance • Anemia • Vitamin B_{12} or folate deficiency • Fever
Endocrine abnormalities	• Hyperthyroidism or hypothyroidism • Adrenal insufficiency

IL-2, Interleukin-2.
Adapted from *National Cancer Institute*. (2011). *Depression (PDQ)*. www.cancer.gov/cancertopics/pdq/supportivecare/depression/Patient; Lee, H. Y., & Jin, S. W. (2013). Older Korean cancer survivors' depression and coping: directions toward culturally competent interventions. *Journal of Psychosocial Oncology, 31*(4), 357–376. https://doi.org/10.1080/07347332.2013.798756; Boyajian, R. (2010). Depression's impact on survival in patients with cancer. *Clinical Journal of Oncology Nursing, 14*(5), 649–652. https://doi.org/10.1188/10.CJON.649-652.

D. For those who have low depression and high demoralization, meaning centered psychotherapy is more likely to be helpful rather than antidepressants. Those who have both depression and demoralization will likely benefit from antidepressants and meaning centered psychotherapy (Ignatius & De La Garza, 2019).

V. Risk factors for depression
  A. History and situational
    1. Personal history of major depression
    2. Previous suicide attempt
    3. Family history of depression
    4. Comorbid conditions (e.g., chronic illness, substance use disorder)
    5. Sleep deprivation
    6. Social isolation
    7. Other unexpected life events (e.g., changes in role, relationships, occupation, or living arrangement)
    8. Spouse with an illness
    9. Cumulative losses of friends and family members
  B. Disease and treatment related
    1. Severe active disease—may lead to feelings of uncertainty about the future
    2. Depression can occur with any cancer; pancreatic, lung, central nervous system tumors, and head and neck cancer may be at higher risk
    3. Body image issues
    4. Poorly controlled pain, nausea, or dyspnea
    5. Physical limitations or restrictions
    6. Prolonged treatment or treatment failure
    7. Medications—use of biological agents, chemotherapy, hormone therapy (antiestrogens), corticosteroids, benzodiazepines, and opioids
  C. General treatment approaches
    1. Refer patients who express thoughts of suicide or desire to hasten death for immediate psychological evaluation
    2. Treat underlying medical conditions and physical symptoms
    3. Provide patient and family with education about depression, treatment, and reason for referral for further evaluation and treatment
    4. Coordinate psychological or psychiatric care
    5. Provide education about prescribed medications and expected effects, time for response, importance of regular dosing, and side effects
      a. Explain the rationale for not stopping the medication without first discussing this with the prescriber
    6. Monitor the patient for side effects and assess for positive response to medication, such as improved mood, appetite, and sleep
    7. Facilitate individual cognitive behavioral or psychotherapy or family therapy by a highly trained mental health specialist
    8. Provide pharmacologic management of depression with selective serotonin reuptake inhibitors, tricyclic antidepressants, serotonin–norepinephrine reuptake inhibitors, atypical antipsychotics, and central nervous system stimulants
  D. Potential sequelae of depression
    1. Suicide or self-harm
    2. Altered sleep patterns
    3. Inability to maintain current role—functional disability
    4. Poor quality of life (QOL) and social withdrawal
    5. Adherence issue

Assessment

(Choi, 2018)
I. History
  A. Presence of risk factors for depression
  B. Presence of either a depressed mood or loss of interest or pleasure, and at least five of the defining symptoms of depression for a period of 2 consecutive weeks or more (see the "Overview" section earlier)
  C. Variation in cultural groups in their interpretations about the meaning of depressive symptoms and use of different terms to describe symptoms
  D. Suicidal ideation, suicide attempt, and suicide plan with means such as firearms or medication. Protective factors: Spiritual beliefs, social and emotional support, satisfaction with life, children in home, pets, and meaning and purpose
  E. Past use of effective or noneffective treatment for depression including medications and therapy

F. Concept and meaning of depression

G. Impact of depressive symptoms on individual role and interpersonal communications or relationships

II. Symptoms and signs (APA, 2013)

A. Subjective symptoms—report of depressed mood or anhedonia, insomnia, social withdrawal, fatigue, sense of worthlessness or guilt, difficulty concentrating, thoughts of death, suicide ideation, irritability, and somatic complaints without cause

B. Objective symptoms—depressed or flat affect, crying, weight loss or gain, slow speech, and psychomotor excitation or retardation

III. Laboratory or measurement findings

A. Medical laboratory testing—cortisol level, thyroid-stimulating hormone, complete blood cell count, or chemistry panel

B. Mental status examination—changes may indicate depression, early delirium

C. Depression screening instruments—Geriatric Depression Scale, Zung Self-Rating Depression Scale, Beck Depression Inventory, Hospital Anxiety and Depression Scale (HADS), and the PHQ-9

D. Functional rating scales—Eastern Cooperative Oncology Group (ECOG Scale), Karnofsky Rating Scale, and Palliative Performance Scale

Management

I. Pharmacologic

A. Antidepressant therapy—serotonin reuptake inhibitors, serotonin-norepinephrine reuptake inhibitors, tricyclics, norepinephrine-dopamine reuptake inhibitors, mixed serotonin receptor agonist/antagonists, and alpha-adrenergic receptor antagonists (see Table 54.1)

II. Nonpharmacologic

A. Address the risk of suicide

B. Stay with the patient and keep him or her safe from self-harm

C. Obtain an immediate psychological or psychiatric referral

D. Provide the patient and family with information on suicide prevention and a contact number for a clinician who is available 24 hours a day

E. Identify and modify patient's psychological pain by assisting to alter the stressful environment and obtain aid from significant other, family, or friends

F. Build a trusting relationship and offer realistic support by recognizing or validating the patient's concerns and struggles

1. Recommend support groups

2. If patient dies, survivor guilt of other support group members may occur

G. Coordinate care with mental health providers

III. Interventions to address situational low self-esteem

A. Facilitate expression of feelings by acknowledging the patient's pain and despair, and engaging in active listening

B. Reinforce depression may be self-limiting and that effective treatment exists

C. Assist the patient to identify his or her strengths and accomplishments

D. Collaborate with patient to identify factors that cause low self-esteem (e.g., interpersonal deficits, role transitions, role disputes, marital conflict, and grief)

E. Assist patient to identify personal growth goals and problem-solving strategies

LOSS OF PERSONAL CONTROL

Overview

I. Loss of personal control

A. People facing cancer often feel a loss of control over their situation, a loss of ability to cope with current and future events, or both.

1. Loss of personal control is the perception that one's own actions will not significantly affect an event or an outcome.

2. Having a perceived lack of control may influence one's level of optimism, motivation level, and goals.

3. The concept of internal–external locus of control, which is a personality trait conceptualized by Rotter (1966), considers how much an individual believes that outcomes depend on his or her own actions or on circumstances outside the individual's control.

4. Self-efficacy is the perceived ability to cope with specific situations.

5. Concept of powerlessness is often situationally determined.

B. People tend to be strongly motivated to gain control over their circumstances.

C. Perception of lack of control has negative effects on well-being.

D. Belief that an event or one's reaction can be controlled may facilitate adjustment.

E. Personal control is correlated with better emotional well-being and health outcomes, enhanced ability to cope with stress, and improved motor and intellectual tasks in those living with a serious illness.

F. Some patients may have a perceived sense of control to inappropriately blame themselves for negative outcomes, which may result in guilt, remorse, and emotional distress.

G. The response to the situation and level of perceived control is influenced by the meaning of the event, comparison of similar events, patterns of coping, personality, support system, and available resources.

II. Risk factors

A. Disease related

1. Unexpected diagnosis; lack of understanding of disease and treatment

2. Uncertainty of the prognosis

3. Inability to perform usual activities or a change in routine

4. Physical disability or cognitive impairment

5. Frequent hospitalizations or placement in an intensive care unit
6. Terminal phase of illness

B. Treatment related
1. Insufficient understanding about treatment, side effects, and outcomes
2. Lengthy treatment course, travel to treatment site, and need for assistance with occupation and domestic responsibilities during treatment phase
3. Unexpected or poorly controlled side effects of treatment
4. Treatment failure
5. Body image issues such as weight loss or gain, alopecia, and loss of limb

C. Situation related
1. Dependency on others and loss of independence
2. Loss of decision-making capacity
3. Lack of privacy

D. Developmental, personality, and culture related
1. Age-specific considerations
   a. Young children tend to be externally controlled.
   b. Adolescents tend to depend on peers for approval and test their independence.
   c. Young adults concerned about launching often conceptualize illness as a disruption of roles.
   d. Adults may be responsible for family members (children and aging parents) and conceptualize illness as a disruption of productivity in family and work.
   e. Older adults often facing retirement and comorbid illnesses; conceptualize illness and possible death as separation from family and friends.
2. Personality—degree of internal–external locus of control and other traits such as neuroticism, extraversion, openness, agreeableness, and conscientiousness
3. Cultural differences from health care providers or health care system may affect communication and choices—dominant language, gender roles, high-risk behaviors, spiritual concerns, basic value, and belief system

III. General treatment approaches
A. Patient and family education
1. Encouraging questions and providing time for it
2. Explaining that education is an ongoing process

B. Assist patient/family in decision-making—explain options, risks, and benefits

C. Offer to arrange for individual counseling with a mental health specialist

D. For the pediatric population, provide opportunities to make choices and express concerns through play and expressive arts (e.g., art therapy)

E. Encourage verbalization of feelings, providing emotional support and assisting in basic problem-solving

IV. Potential sequelae of prolonged loss of personal control
A. Lowered self-esteem
B. Helplessness and hopelessness

C. Nonadherence or delay in treatment
D. Depression, anxiety, or both
E. Cancer fatalism with avoidance of health-promoting behaviors and cancer-screening practices

Assessment

I. History and presence of risk factors
II. Symptoms and signs
A. Subjective characteristics of loss of personal control
1. Overt or covert statements that suggest a loss of control
2. Expressed frustration or dissatisfaction with care
3. Anger or criticism toward staff

B. Presence of objective characteristics of loss of personal control
1. Refusal or reluctance to participate in decision-making
2. Refusal or reluctance to participate in activities of daily living (ADLs)
3. Reluctance to express emotions
4. Behavioral responses may include apathy, resignation, withdrawal, uneasiness, anxiety, and aggression
5. Responses to limitations on personal control may include attempts to circumvent limits, increased attempts to exercise control, and ignoring limits
6. Nonadherence with the medical treatment regimen

III. Patient's problem-solving abilities
A. Ability to identify the sense of powerlessness, insight into contributing factors
B. Past coping behaviors during other uncontrollable events
C. Ability to identify aspects of care that the individual can make choices about
D. Identification of other people or events that reduce feelings of powerlessness

Management

I. Nonpharmacologic interventions
A. Provide patient and family with orientation to the health care system and health education on the diagnosis, treatment, and expected outcomes
B. Provide updated information on the current plan of care
C. Provide opportunities for the patient to control decisions
D. Assist patient to identify the factors that can be controlled
E. Reassure patient or power of attorney for health care that he or she has the right to make decisions regarding medical care and will be assisted in the decision-making process

II. Interventions to address impaired individual resilience
A. Assist the patient in identifying past successful coping techniques
B. Ask the patient to list his or her coping strengths
C. Provide positive reinforcement when patient demonstrates resilient behavior

LOSS AND GRIEF

Overview

I. Loss, grief, bereavement, and anticipatory grief
   A. Loss involves any perceived or experienced change in function, role, relationship, or lifestyle and implies separation from the people and things that are meaningful (Kubler-Ross, 1969).
      1. Although loss is a part of normal growth and development as attachments are given up, the sudden or cumulative losses associated with cancer are often distressing.
   B. Grief is the active, adaptive process of recognizing, coping with, and reconciling loss (Kubler-Ross, 1969).
      1. The individual's reaction to the loss is often based on his or her perception of the loss.
      2. Grief response may be affected by personality, coping skills, and available supportive resources.
   C. Bereavement is deprivation of something or someone, such as a relation or friend, especially by death (APA, 2022b)
      1. A bereft person is deprived of nonmaterial assets and may feel robbed of someone or something important, and future plans.
   D. Anticipatory grief begins in response to the awareness of the impending loss of a loved one and acknowledgment of future losses.

II. Risk factors
   A. Disease and treatment related
      1. Unexpected diagnosis, high-risk of recurrence, advanced disease, and poor prognosis
      2. Changes in body structure, function, or image (e.g., amputation, mastectomy, colostomy, alopecia, cachexia, or cognition)
      3. Poor pain control or chronic pain
      4. History of psychiatric illness
   B. Situational and social
      1. Loss of a person through death, divorce, or separation
      2. Loss of something considered valuable, such as pet, home, and possessions
      3. Nature of the relationship with lost person
      4. Cumulative losses
      5. Limited social support
      6. Occupational or employment restrictions
   C. Developmental (Loney & Murphy-Ende, 2009; Table 54.3)
   D. Risk for complicated grief
      1. Perception of death as preventable
      2. Ambivalent relationship to the deceased
      3. Coexisting medical conditions
      4. Coexisting financial or legal problems
   E. General treatment approaches
      1. Provide basic information (verbal and written) on the grief process
      2. Explore spiritual beliefs that may offer a sense of comfort and referral to spiritual care
      3. Refer to grief counselor or psychologist for individual or family counseling

TABLE 54.3	**Developmental Grief and Loss Responses**
Age	**Concept of Loss**
Younger than 2 years	Self-centered and sees loss as deprivation of needs or separation
2–5 years	Concept is temporary and concrete; may express little distress of not being loved
5–9 years	Concept is concrete and logical; may see loss as fear of punishment or bodily harm
9–12 years	Concept is realistic; may perceive loss as separation
12–18 years	Concept is abstract and realistic; may perceive loss as a threat to independence
18–25 years	Impact of loss is complex, with disruption in lifestyle
25–45 years	Impact of loss may represent a threat to future
45–65 years	Loss or death represents disruption of productivity in family or work
65 to death	Concept of loss may be philosophical, with death perceived as separation

      4. Refer to support groups in the community
      5. Offer music or art therapy
      6. Provide pharmacologic management of severe symptoms
   F. Potential sequelae of loss and grief
      1. Complicated grief
      2. Depression or anxiety
      3. Denial
      4. Self-neglect or inability to take care of others
      5. Social isolation
      6. Physical symptoms
      7. Cognitive symptoms
      8. Substance abuse
      9. Suicidal ideation or attempt

Assessment

I. History
   A. Presence of risk factors, including previous losses
   B. Nature and meaning of the loss
   C. Personality and past coping responses
   D. Family characteristics and communication style
   E. Symptoms and signs of grief
      1. Cognitive—lack of concentration, distractibility, preoccupation with loss, searching for meaning, intrusive thoughts, or psychiatric symptoms
      2. Physical—fatigue, headache, shortness of breath, GI complaints, sleep disturbance, cardiac symptoms, fatigue, or exhaustion
      3. Psychological—shock, denial, guilt, anger, hostility, ambivalence, sadness, shame, depression, preoccupation, ruminating, anxiety, or dulled senses
      4. Social—dependency on or avoidance of others and occupational lapses
      5. Spiritual distress—searching for meaning or change in views or beliefs

II. Stage of grief
   A. Alarm—a physiologic response

B. Searching—psychological pain with obtrusive wish for the lost person
C. Mitigation—feeling comfort in sensing the presence of the deceased
D. Anger and guilt—may be angry at others or self
E. Gaining a new identity—recovery of lost functions, adaptation to new roles

III. Patient and family level of understanding of their grief
IV. Meaning of the loss
V. Impact of losses and grief on routine, roles, relationships, occupation, and school

Management

I. Nonpharmacologic
A. Interventions to address grieving
1. Establish a trusting relationship and encourage the patient and family to share their grief without imposing own values or judgment
2. Validate the grief and encourage ways to express it
3. Be prepared for negative affect such as anger, increased demands, irritability, sarcasm, and blaming
4. Remain calm during patient's behavioral outbursts and set limits on inappropriate or dangerous behavior
5. Convey acceptance and empathetic concern
6. Assist patient and family in exploring coping methods
7. Provide anticipatory guidance before loss—discuss impending loss, review significance of past losses and responses to those losses, provide information on mourning process, and assist in formulating coping strategies
B. Interventions to address interrupted family processes
1. Provide privacy for the expression of feelings
2. Encourage family members to share their perceptions with each other and remind them that everyone grieves in unique ways
3. Validate each member's grief
4. Consider cultural, religious, and social customs of mourning
5. Refer family to professional family or individual bereavement counseling

COPING

Overview

I. Definitions
A. Coping—use of cognitive and behavioral strategies to manage demands of a situation when demands are appraised as taxing or exceeding one's resources; to reduce the negative emotions and conflict caused by stress (APA, 2022a).
B. Coping mechanism—conscious or unconscious adjustment or adaptation that decreases tensions/anxiety in a stressful experience or situation (APA, 2022c).
C. Coping behavior—characteristic and often automatic action(s) in dealing with stressful/threatening situations (APA, 2022c); adaptive or maladaptive.

II. Types of coping identified by Folkman (2013)
A. Problem focused—directed toward reducing or eliminating a stressor
B. Emotion focused—directed toward changing one's own emotional reaction
C. Meaning focused—deriving meaning from the stressful experience
D. Primary appraisal—coping-based beliefs, values, and goals (Folkman, 2013; Seib et al., 2018)
E. Secondary appraisal—coping based on one's belief and conception of being able to reduce or minimize the threat (Folkman, 2013)
F. Problem focused—directed toward reducing or eliminating the stressor
G. Situational coping—directed at the specific situational factors that are causing stress (Krok, & Telka, 2019)
H. Posttraumatic growth—positive psychological change from a traumatic life event (Cormio, Muzzatti, Romito, Mattioli, & Annunziata, 2017)
I. Commonsense model of self-regulation and health and illness (CMS-9)—psychological model of the process underlying health and coping in those with chronic illness. Individual representation of health threats (Diefenbach & Leventhal, 1996)

III. Adaptation
A. Ability to minimize disruptions to social roles, regulate experience of emotional distress, and maintain active engagement in meaningful life activities (Cohen & White, 2018)
B. According to Jean Piaget's theory of cognitive development, adaptation is the process of adjusting one's cognitive structures to meet environmental demands, involving the complementary process of assimilation and accommodation

IV. Factors influencing coping in oncology patients and their family members (Cohen & White, 2018; NCI, 2017)
A. Cancer diagnosis related (Oberoi et al., 2017)—prevailing perception that diagnosis of cancer is a death sentence
B. Lack of knowledge of the disease process
C. Effects of the treatments
1. Fear of the effects of treatment
a. Chemotherapy
b. Biotherapy
c. Immunotherapy
d. Radiation therapy
e. Surgery
f. Clinical trials
2. Posttreatment (survivorship)
3. Psychological
4. Comorbidities—psychiatric history such as neurodevelopmental, psychotic, depressive, anxiety, obsessive–compulsive, personality, somatic symptom, eating, sleep–wake and substance use, illness anxiety disorders, sexual dysfunction, PTSD, and other minor/major mental illness
5. Adjustment disorders—criteria or symptoms based on American Psychiatric Association's DSM-5 (APA, 2013)

D. Social factors
1. Roles—maintaining or changing
2. Routine health tasks, family issues, financial management, and living conditions that affect the individual's ability to cope
3. Family influences
4. Cultural factors, beliefs, values, and health practices
5. Community resources issues
6. Factors influenced by gender

V. Ineffective coping
A. The conscious or unconscious attempt to deny the knowledge or meaning of an event to reduce anxiety or fear but leading to the detriment of health
1. Delays seeking health care attention
2. Displaced fears of the impact of the disease
3. Limited perception of relevance of symptoms
B. Risk assessment and interventions
C. Suicidal ideation screen for risk factors: Risk factors for suicide outcomes among cancer patients were male sex and older age, a cancer diagnosis within the prior year, and some specific cancer sites (Calati et al., 2021)
D. Denial
1. Conscious or unconscious attempt to deny the knowledge or meaning of an event to reduce anxiety or fear but leading to the detriment of health
   a. Delays seeking health care attention
   b. Displaces fears of the impact of the disease
   c. Does not perceive personal relevance of symptoms
   d. Uses self-treatment
2. Denial not necessarily considered dysfunctional coping
3. Assessment of coping distress and coping status

Assessment

I. Assessment tools—interview, questionnaire, checklists, psychological tests, observation, and metrics (biofeedback, psychoneuroimmunology)
II. Commonly used assessment tools
A. NCCN DT (NCCN, 2018)
1. 0 (no distress) to 10 (severe distress) measurement, with accompanying simple questions identifying the source of distress
2. Recommendation that score of 4 or more triggers further physician or nurse evaluation, referral to psychosocial services, or both
B. HADS (Annunziata et al., 2020)
1. 14-item scale (7 questions: anxiety; 7 questions: depression)
2. Score from 0 to 21 (0–3 per question) to evaluate anxiety or depression levels
III. Components of assessment
A. Assess psychosocial distress
B. Identify psychosocial needs that affect QOL, ADLs
C. Identify patterns of coping
D. Observe for contributing factors to ineffective coping (see the "Ineffective Coping" section earlier)
1. Anxiety, depression, and insomnia
2. Previous stressors and the coping mechanisms used

3. Diagnosis of mental disorders
E. Provide opportunities for patient to discuss the meaning of the situation
1. Self-described definitions of well-being and QOL
F. Identifying contributors to distress
1. Social factors contributing to distress
2. Presence of family and community support
3. Management
4. Nonpharmacologic

Management

I. Provide effective communication and emotional support.
A. Use verbal and nonverbal therapeutic communication approaches, including empathy, active listening, and confrontation, to encourage patient and family to express emotions and solve problems
1. Encourage the patient to express feelings and thoughts.
2. Explore the meaning of the person's illness experience on their physical, psychological, social, and spiritual functioning and needs.
3. Provide honest perception about symptoms and response to symptoms.
4. Encourage the patient to explore and try adaptive behaviors to optimize functioning and accomplish ADLs.
B. Encourage the patient to identify stressors
1. Ability to relate the facts of the contributing stress factors
2. Ability to recognize the source of the stressors
3. Assisting the patient to expand personal skills and knowledge
C. Assist patient to identify strengths and positive/alternative coping behaviors
1. Identify past methods used to self-manage distress
2. Assist patient to set realistic expectations of emotional response to stress
3. List strengths and identify how these can be used to cope with situation
4. Participate in planning care and scheduled activities
   a. Support decisions regarding patient's method of integrating therapeutic regimens
   b. Validate difficulty of the situation
   c. Find a new sense of normal and routine
   d. Provide positive reinforcement on behaviors that minimize distress and maximize independence
5. Encourage opportunities for social support
   a. Support groups
   b. Brief visits with friends or phone/social media connection
6. Support spiritual needs
   a. Hospital chaplain services
   b. Spiritual readings or music
7. Initiate and coordinate referrals to clinical psychologist or counselor
II. Patient and family education
A. Provide verbal and written information to the patient and family about the disease, process, therapy, expected

effects of therapy, side effects, and management. Offer instructions regarding common and simple brief coping strategies
B. Provide and explain the types of available resources
C. Provide the patient and family with a list of appropriate community-based resources (e.g., housing, home health care, hospice care, and community meals)
III. Referrals or counseling
A. Coordinate referral appointments
B. Provide documentation/assessment to support counseling or therapy referral
IV. Support groups
A. Psychosocial support groups and resources are available to patients across the continuum of cancer care. Consider patient's preference for the following: disease specific (type of cancer), spiritual beliefs, cultural concerns, age specific, caregivers, and ongoing open group or time-limited group.
B. General support groups provide patients and caregivers a place to share experiences and obtain knowledge from those with similar situations.
C. Support groups may have a positive effect on an individual's coping.
D. Support groups may offer inspiration through witnessing the motivation to survive, experiencing the courage of others, and exposure to role modeling of others with similar problems.
E. Participation in online support groups may provide easy access to patients.
V. Self-care
A. Self-care skill building
1. Multifocused education programs may build coping skills (preparatory education, cognitive restructuring, building current coping skills, and guided imagery) (Chen et al., 2018)
2. Identifying strengths and recognizing and managing the source of stressors
B. Offer complementary and alternative medicine and treatment
1. Various strategies effective; individual preference
2. Types include massage, yoga, aromatherapy, exercise groups, mindfulness meditation, guided imagery, nutrition, animal-facilitated therapy, art therapy, and music therapy
3. Psychoeducational and complementary interventions—review the literature and make recommendations accordingly

PUBLIC AND COMMUNITY HEALTH'S IMPACT ON MENTAL HEALTH

Overview

I. Pandemic: COVID
A. COVID was declared a pandemic by the World Health Organization in March 2020
II. Cancer-specific concerns

A. Cancer and the burden of COVID in this population is more pronounced in cancer patients from racial and ethnic minorities and underserved populations (American Association for Cancer Research, 2022)
B. Cancer survivors reported mental health symptoms during the pandemic including anxiety, depression, hopelessness, and loneliness compared to adults without cancer (Islam, Vidot, & Camacho-Riveria, 2021)
C. Cancer patients undergoing treatment experience fear with concerns regarding delayed diagnosis, cancellations, missed treatments, and weakened immunity (Moraliyage et al., 2021)

Assessment

I. Evaluate patients' mental health symptoms at each visit and determine the patients' most distressing symptom or concern.
II. Ask patient what has been helpful in managing their mental well-being.
III. Assess for loneliness and isolation.

Management

I. Offer access to care by telehealth or phone.
II. Discuss the benefits of COVID vaccination and concerns if unvaccinated.
III. Work with health care leaders to develop COVID education, wellness, and support for staff.

REFERENCES

American Association for Cancer Research. (2022). *AACR.org #AACROVIDReports*. Washington, DC: American Psychiatric Association. https://cancerprogressreport.aacr.org/covid/c19c-contents/c19c-cancer-in-the-midst-of-covid-19-and-beyond/.

American Psychiatric Association (APA). (2013). *Diagnostic and statistical manual of mental disorders (DSM-5)* (5th ed.). Washington, DC: American Psychiatric Association.

American Psychological Association (APA). (2022a). *APA dictionary of psychology* (p. 17). Washington, DC: American Psychological Association. https://dictionary.apa.org/anxiety.

American Psychological Association (APA). (2022b). *APA dictionary of psychology* (p. 17). Washington, DC: American Psychological Association. https://dictionary.apa.org/bereavement.

American Psychological Association (APA). (2022c). *APA dictionary of psychology* (p. 17). Washington, DC: American Psychological Association. https://dictionary.apa.org/coping.

Annunziata, M. A., Muzzatti, B., Bidoli, E., Flaiban, C., Bomben, F., Piccinin, M., et al. (2020). Hospital Anxiety and Depression Scale (HADS) accuracy in cancer patients. *Supportive Care in Cancer, 28*(8), 3921–3926.

Antoni, M. H., Moreno, P. I., & Penedo, F. J. (2023). Stress management interventions to facilitate psychological and physiological adaptation and optimal health outcomes in cancer patients and survivors. *Annual review of psychology, 74*, 423–455. https://doi.org/10.1146/annurev-psych-030122-124119.

Calati, R., Filliponi, C., Mansi, W., Casu, D., Peviani, G., Gentile, G., et al. (2021). Cancer diagnosis and suicide outcomes: Umbrella review and methodological considerations. *Journal of*

Affective Disorders, 295, 1201–1214. https://doi.org/10.1016/j.jad.2021.08.13.

Chen, X., Gong, X., Shi, C., Sun, L., Tang, Z., Yuan, Z., et al. (2018). Multi-focused psychosocial residential rehabilitation interventions improve quality of life among cancer survivors: A community-based controlled trial. *Journal of Translational Medicine, 16*(1), 250. https://doi.org/10.1186/s12967-018-1618-0.

Choi, S., & Ryu, E. (2018). Effects of symptom clusters and depression on the quality of life in patients with advanced lung cancer. *European Journal of Cancer Care (England), 27*(1). https://doi.org/10.1111/ecc.12508. Epub 2016 Apr 26. PMID: 27112232.

Cohen, M. Z., & White, L. (2018). Cancer-related distress. In C. H. Yarbro, D. Wujcik, & B. H. Gobel (Eds.), *Cancer nursing: Principles and practice* (8th ed., pp. 759–779). Sudbury, MA: Jones and Bartlett.

Cormio, C., Muzzatti, B., Romito, F., Mattioli, V., & Annunziata, M. A. (2017). Posttraumatic growth and cancer: A study 5 years after treatment end. *Supportive Care in Cancer: Official Journal of the Multinational Association of Supportive Care in Cancer, 25*(4), 1087–1096. https://doi.org/10.1007/s00520-016-3496-4.

De Figueiredo, J. M. (2013). Distress, demoralization and psychopathology: Diagnostic boundaries. *The European Journal of Psychiatry, 27*(1), 61–73.

Diefenbach, M. A., & Leventhal, H. (1996). The common-sense model of illness representation: Theoretical and practical considerations. *Journal of Social Distress and Homelessness, 5*(1), 11–38. https://doi.org/10.1007/BF02090456.

Folkman, S. (2013). Psychological aspects of cancer: A guide to emotional and psychological consequences of cancer, their causes and management. In B. I. Carr & J. Steel (Eds.), *Stress, coping, and hope* (pp. 119–127). New York: Springer.

Granek, L., Nakash, O., Ariad, S., Shapira, S., & Ben-David, M. (2019). Strategies and barriers in addressing mental health and suicidality in patients with cancer. *Oncology Nursing Forum, 46*(5), 561–571. https://doi.org/10.1188/19.ONF.561-571.

Ignatius, J., & De La Garza, R. (2019). Frequency of demoralization and depression in cancer patients. *General Hospital Psychiatry, 60,* 137–140. https://doi.org/10.1016/j.genhosppsych.2019.04.013. Epub 2019 Apr 26. PMID: 31103216.

Islam, J., Vidot, D., & Camacho-Riveria, M. (2021). Evaluating mental health-related symptoms among cancer survivors during the COVID-19 pandemic: An analysis of the COVID impact survey. *JCO Oncology Practice, 17*(9). https://doi.org/10.1200/OP.20.0075.

Krok, D., & Telka, E. (2019). The role of meaning in gastric cancer patients: Relationships among meaning structures, coping, and psychological well-being. *Anxiety, Stress, & Coping, 32*(5), 522–533.

Kubler-Ross, E. (1969). *On death and dying.* New York: Macmillan. https://www.liebertpub.com/toc/jayao/4/4. https://doi.org/10.1089/jayao.2015.0005.

Loney, M., & Murphy-Ende, K. (2009). Death, dying, and grief in the face of cancer. In C. Burke (Ed.), *Psychosocial dimensions of oncology nursing care* (pp. 159–185). Pittsburgh, PA: Oncology Nursing Society.

Malibiran, R., Tairman, J., & Amer, K. (2018). Bibliotherapy: Appraisal of evidence for patients diagnosed with cancer. *Clinical Journal of Oncology Nursing, 22*(4), 377–380. https://doi.org/10.1188/18.CJON.377-380.

Moraliyage, H., De Silva, D., Ranasinghe, W., Adikari, A., Alahakoon, D., Prasad, R., et al. (2021). *The Oncologist, 26*(2), e342–e344. https://doi.org/10.1002/onco.13604.

Murphy-Ende, K. (2019). Mental health issues in cancer. In J. Payne & K. Murphy-Ende (Eds.), *Current trends in oncology nursing* (pp. 215–242). Pittsburgh, PA: Oncology Nursing Society.

National Cancer Institute (NCI). (2017). *Adjustment to cancer: Anxiety and distress (PDQ).* www.cancer.gov/cancertopics/pdq/supportivecare/adjustment/HealthProfessional.

National Comprehensive Cancer Network (NCCN). (2018). *Distress management. Ver 2.2018.* https://www.nccn.org/professionals/physician_gls/pdf/distress.pdf.

Oberoi, D. V., White, V. M., Seymour, J. F., Prince, H. M., Harrison, S., Jefford, M., et al. (2017). Distress and unmet needs during treatment and quality of life in early cancer survivorship: A longitudinal study of haematological cancer patients. *European Journal of Haematology, 99*(5), 423–430. https://doi.org/10.1111/ejh.12941.

Roth, A. J., Kornblith, A. B., Batel-Copel, L., Peabody, E., Scher, H., & Holland, J. (1998). Rapid screening for psychological distress in men with prostate carcinoma: A pilot study. *Cancer, 82*(10), 1904–1908. https://doi.org/10.1002/(SICI)1097-0142(19980515)82:10<1904::AID-CNCR13>3.0.CO;2-X.

Rotter, J. (1966). Generalized expectations for internal versus external control of reinforcement. *Psychological Monographs, 80*(1), 1–28. https://doi.org/10.1037/h0092976.

Seib, C., Porter-Steele, J., Ng, S. K., Turner, J., McGuire, A., McDonald, N., et al. (2018). Life stress and symptoms of anxiety and depression in women after cancer: The mediating effect of stress appraisal and coping. *Psychooncology, 27*(7), 1787–1794. https://doi.org/10.1002/pon.4728.

Wang, Y. H., Li, J. Q., Shi, J. F., Que, J. Y., Liu, J. J., Lappin, J. M., et al. (2020). Depression and anxiety in relation to cancer incidence and mortality: A systematic review and meta-analysis of cohort studies. *Mol Psychiatry, 25*(7), 1487–1499. https://doi.org/10.1038/s41380-019-0595-x. Epub 2019 Nov 19. PMID: 31745237.

55

Sexuality and Sexual Dysfunction

Sari Williams

OVERVIEW

I. Sexuality

A. Prevalence rates of sexual dysfunction associated with cancer and respective treatments vary depending on the cancer diagnosis, treatment modality, assessment methods, and type of sexual dysfunction, estimates are reported to range from 40% to 100%. Patients with low socioeconomic statuses in general have a higher prevalence of sexual problems, and evidence points to the notion that cancer survivors in underserved areas have high rates of sexual dysfunction (Carter et al., 2018). Surgery, radiation, chemotherapy, and endocrine therapies, while shown to improve clinical outcomes, all impact sexual function (Melisko & Narus, 2016; Miaja, Platas, & Martinez-Cannon, 2017).

B. Sexuality is a component of survivorship that can significantly affect the quality of life (QOL) (Rhoten, 2017). Sexual health and body image are integral to QOL, and cancer survivors who experience sexual morbidity are at an increased risk of distress and poor QOL (Carter et al., 2018; Miaja et al., 2017).

C. Discussions about sexuality related to cancer/cancer treatment normalize it as a part of routine care, increase support and guidance (Carter et al., 2018), provide comfort, relieve suffering, and facilitate connections (Nelson, 2017). Intimate relationships as part of a patient's social support may reduce cancer-related stress, and good quality relationships can lower the risk of sexual dysfunction in female cancer patients (Jonsdottir, Vilhjalmsson, & Svavarsdottir, 2021).

D. Discussions of potential threats to fertility and family planning should be initiated prior to starting cancer-directed treatment so as to allow for the most options for fertility preservation (Oktay et al., 2018).

E. The Oncology Nursing Society's (ONS) Sexuality Standard of Care reinforces nursing responsibility of addressing sexuality changes (Lubejko & Wilson, 2019). The American Society of Clinical Oncology (ASCO) recommends that a member of the healthcare team initiates discussion with the patient regarding sexual health and dysfunction that may occur as a result of cancer or cancer-directed treatment at the time of diagnosis and obtain periodic reassessments to address any changes. Discussions should be at the patient's literacy level and be sensitive to patient's cultural/religious beliefs and sexual orientation (Carter et al., 2018).

1. Despite the ONS Standard, patients frequently initiate the conversation rather than the nurse, and female cancer survivors were less likely to have sexual side effects discussed than their male survivor counterparts (Taylor et al., 2020).

2. See Boxes 55.1 and 55.2 for patient/provider hesitation (Carter et al., 2018).

3. Risks of not addressing sexual concerns include blaming dysfunction on the partner, use of unsafe "home remedies," decreased QOL (Rhoten, 2017), relationship discord, isolation, emotional morbidity (Vermeer, Bakker, Kenter, Stiggelbout, & ter Kuile, 2016), perception of an unsupportive provider (Leonardi-Warren et al., 2016), and decreased sexual function (Hoyt, McCann, Savone, Saigal, & Stanton, 2015).

4. Adolescents, the elderly, and the terminally ill are those at greatest risk if not given the opportunity to discuss their concerns about sexuality.

   a. For any age group, intimacy or self-perception as a sexual being does not end when given a terminal prognosis (Wang et al., 2017).

   b. Intimacy is identified as "very important" in those with recurrent or advanced diseases (Reese & Haythornthwaite, 2016).

F. Nurses tend to focus on the medical–technical aspects when discussing sexuality or providing psychosexual support (Vermeer et al., 2015).

1. Sexuality is not limited to only intercourse or orgasm but also includes sexual response, sexual self-concept, and sexual/intimate relationships related to intimacy and communication. Relationship quality seems to be proportional to how close the couple is, how they get along and how content they are in their relationship (Jonsdottir et al., 2021).

2. Psychosexual support includes intimacy, partner concerns, and relationship satisfaction by emphasizing a sex-positive message (Vermeer et al., 2016).

G. Basic knowledge of potential treatment-related changes is critical (Table 55.1).

1. Chemotherapy and radiation therapy can cause long-term sexual changes in 30%–100% of survivors

BOX 55.1 Reasons Survivors/Patients Hesitate to Ask Questions About Sexual Functioning

- Embarrassment, anxiety
- Unaware treatment is possible
- Concern questions will be considered secondary to treatment or that their sexual health concerns are an expected and untreatable sequelae of their disease and treatment (Williams & Addis, 2021)
- Belief that it is the clinician's responsibility to bring up the topic
- Belief that they are the only one who has this concern
- Cultural/religious beliefs
- Patient age (if a minor, concern physician will tell parents that questions were asked)
- Sexual orientation
- Unpartnered at the time of treatment (Miaja et al., 2017)
- Time, cost, and transportation for a separate consultation (Dizon et al., 2018)

BOX 55.2 Reasons Nurses/Physicians May Hesitate to Ask About Sexuality

- Lack of knowledge and poor confidence levels (Williams & Addis, 2021)
- Cultural/religious beliefs (Williams & Addis, 2021)
- Biased beliefs about age, interest, culture, partner availability, gender, sexual identity, or prognosis, or not seeing a patient as a sexual person (Williams & Addis, 2021)
- Lack of time or privacy for counseling, discomfort using psychosocial counseling interventions (Melisko & Narus, 2016).
- Feeling it is not their responsibility; for example, nurses believed it was the medical team's responsibility and the medical team felt it was psychology's role (Rhoten, 2017; Williams & Addis, 2021)
- Concerns about making patients feel uncomfortable or embarrassed (Williams & Addis, 2021)
- Lack of training or insufficient skill in sexual medicine issues (Melisko & Narus, 2016).

TABLE 55.1 Potential Physiological Changes Due to Cancer Treatments That Affect Sexual Function

Treatment	Possible Changes Due to Cancer Treatments
Endocrine therapy for men	Gynecomastia, feminization, ED, decreased fertility, penile or testicular atrophy, decrease/loss of libido.
Endocrine therapy for women	Estrogen deprivation can lead to sleep disturbances, decreased vaginal lubrication, vaginal atrophy, urinary frequency, incontinence or UTIs, decreased libido, masculinization, amenorrhea, temporary or permanent menopause, mood changes, hair and skin changes, weight gain, inability to orgasm, hot flashes, and myalgias/arthralgias (Melisko & Narus, 2016).
Immunotherapy for men or women	Fatigue, fever, and flulike symptoms can affect libido. Chest pain, shortness of breath, diarrhea, and mouth sores can affect sexual behavior.
Pelvic radiation therapy for men	Vascular or nerve damage causing temporary or permanent ED, absent or weak orgasm, painful ejaculation, decreased ejaculate volume. Brachytherapy for prostate cancer causes ED in 6%–61% of patients.
Radiation therapy to penile bulb	Destruction of nitric oxide–producing cells.
Radiation to brain, body, or pelvis	Can cause hypogonadism.
Pelvic radiation therapy for women	Decreased vaginal lubrication, hardened clitoris, dyspareunia, vaginal sensation changes, vaginal atrophy/vault shortening, decreased vaginal elasticity/stenosis. It can create concern of partner "safety" after therapy (Garcia et al., 2018). Sclerosis of vascular structures in uterus, leading to defective placentation and placental abruption, and preeclampsia, along with increased risk for IUGR and mid-trimester abortion (American Society for Reproductive Medicine, 2019). Irradiation of 2 Gy will destroy half of the follicular pool (Condorelli et al., 2019).
Chemotherapy for men	Decreased/loss of libido, delayed or inhibited ejaculation, ED (Catamero et al., 2017), and hair loss.
Chemotherapy for women	Premature menopause, decreased libido, body image changes, decreased vaginal lubrication, dyspareunia, vaginal stomatitis (Catamero et al., 2017), and hair loss.
Chemotherapy for men or women	Oral stomatitis, dry mouth, taste bud changes, nausea/vomiting, fluid retention, fatigue, pain, skin changes, and alopecia to include pubic hair, infertility, and diarrhea/constipation (Melisko & Narus, 2016). Taxane- and platinum-based chemotherapy regimens cause peripheral neurologic symptoms that affect sexual functioning (Westin et al., 2016).
Steroids	Hyperglycemia can result in reduced sexual function, mood dysregulation, ED, decreased desire, hypoactive arousal, dyspareunia, thinning of vaginal wall, and orgasm dysfunction (Catamero et al., 2017). Can cause weight gain which in turn can affect body image (Miaja et al., 2017).
Surgery	When surgery disrupts the vascular, sympathetic nervous, or parasympathetic nervous systems, it can affect the sexual response cycle. Surgery in breast cancer patients can result in loss of breast(s), surgical scars, lymphedema, all potentially affecting body image and quality of life (Miaja et al., 2017).
Prostatectomy	Retrograde ejaculation, ED if damage to autonomic nerve plexus (ED rates anywhere from 12% to 96% [Melisko & Narus, 2016]), diminished orgasm intensity, and urinary incontinence (Barocas et al., 2017). Risk for Peyronie's curvature following radical prostatectomy due to nerve damage of reduced blood flow (Melisko & Narus, 2016).
Orchiectomy	Changes in orgasm, infertility, decreased sexual confidence, decreased self-image, and decreased sexual satisfaction (Hoyt et al., 2015). Unilateral may not result in infertility or sexual dysfunction if contralateral testis is normal; bilateral may decrease libido, cause penile atrophy.
Oophorectomy	Results in acute estrogen and testosterone deprivation.
Hysterectomy	May result in changes in vaginal length/size, dyspareunia, lack of sexual interest, and decreased lubrication (Melisko & Narus, 2016).
Rectal Surgery	Decreased body image and self-esteem. Libido was the most commonly reported sexual dysfunction experienced in both women (41%) and men (47%) (Melisko & Narus, 2016).
Pharmacotherapies related to cancer and cancer-directed treatment side effects	Opioids prescribed to mitigate cancer and treatment-related pain can reduce libido, cause ED. Antidepressants prescribed to address mood concerns may also cause decreased libido.

ED, Erectile dysfunction; *UTI*, urinary tract infection.

BOX 55.3 Potential Risky Sexual Practices When Receiving Treatment

- Increased risk of infection with shared sex toys, anal/rectal stimulation, multiple partners
- Stoma coitus
- Laryngectomy and water play
- Nipple or penile rings when thrombocytopenic
- Vaginal stimulation without lubrication when neutropenic
- Penile ring/rubber band around penis base if experiencing neurotoxicity
- Home remedies—may interact with medication
- Potential risk to partner of shared body fluids when within 3 days of chemotherapy

From Kelvin, J. F., Steed, R., & Jarrrett, J. (2014). Discussing safe sexual practices during cancer treatment. *Clinical Journal of Oncology Nursing, 18*(4), 449–453.

BOX 55.4 Discussion Models to Enhance Sexual Health Communication

Plissit
- Give **permission** to discuss the topic.
- Provide **limited information**.
- Provide **specific suggestions**.
- Refer for **intensive therapy**.

5As
- *Ask:* Bring the topic up.
- *Advise:* Normalize symptoms and acknowledge the problems.
- *Assess:* Ask about sexual functioning and use standardized assessments if needed.
- *Assist:* Provide information and resources, and refer as needed.
- *Arrange:* Provide follow-up to check how the patient is doing.

Better
- *Bring* up the topic.
- *Explain* that sexuality is part of the quality of life and that patients can talk about any concerns they have.
- *Tell* the patients about resources.
- *Time* the discussion to the patients' preferences.
- *Educate* patients about side effects that may affect sexuality.
- *Record* assessments and interventions in the medical record.

From Kelvin, J. F., Steed, R., & Jarrett, J. (2014). Discussing safe sexual practices during cancer treatment. *Clinical Journal of Oncology Nursing, 18*(4), 449–453.

(Leonardi-Warren et al., 2016) and can occur years after treatment (Dizon, Katz, Ganz, & Vora, 2018). Surgery can negatively affect erectile functioning and orgasm intensity (Barocas et al., 2017) and causes issues with urinary incontinence (Wilson, McGuire, Rodgers, Elswick, & Temkin, 2021). Systemic chemo and/or radiation directed at the gonads, hypothalamus, or pituitary gland can lead to infertility in men 30%–75% of the time (Grabowski, Spitzer, Stutzman, & Olson, 2017).

2. Physiological changes can negatively alter self-perceptions as a sexual being. Sexual dysfunction and negative affect are often intertwined (Benedict et al., 2015).
3. Relationship problems that existed before treatment are often exacerbated during treatment (Olsson, Sandin-Bojo, Bjuresater, & Larsson, 2016).
4. Alterations in nonsexual organ function can affect sexual functioning, for example, taste bud changes or fingertip tenderness due to peripheral neuropathy.
5. For women, menopausal symptoms such as changes to the atrophic urogenital and vaginal areas, sleep, mood, body image, sense of femininity, and weight can affect sexuality (Melisko & Narus, 2016). Men can experience retrograde ejaculation, infertility, diminished self-image, and orgasm changes (Barocas et al., 2017) that could negatively affect sexuality.
6. Nurses need to balance safety without unnecessary constraints (Box 55.3).

ASSESSMENT

I. Multiple models are used to begin the conversation with patients about changes in sexual functioning due to a cancer diagnosis or treatment (Box 55.4). The ONS standards of nursing practice include systematic assessment and data collection about the health status of each patient, which includes their sexuality.
II. A study done in 2017–2019 by Jonsdottir et al. (2021) showed that implementation of a Couple-Strengths-Oriented

Therapeutic conversation intervention was effective in supporting sexual adjustment, improving confidence in how illness beliefs affect sexuality and intimacy, and increasing the quality of intimate relationships. Miaja et al. (2017) discussed the importance of structure, safety, and support within relationships as key in preserving sexual functioning and health.
III. While fertility preservation interventions may not be appropriate or available for all patients, every patient is a candidate for the conversation and counseling (Holman, 2019).
IV. The specific model used depends on the clinician's comfort with the topic. Studies on the use of psychoeducational interventions have consistently shown positive results in patient outcomes and reveal the need for their use in practice (Gondim de Almeida et al., 2020).

MANAGEMENT

I. Medical management (Box 55.5).
   A. Pharmacologic and medical management strategies are available; however, sexuality is most effectively addressed using a biopsychosocial model of care.
   B. When issues are not proactively addressed, patients may try unsafe practices (Box 55.6).
II. Nursing management—implications for nursing.
   A. Oncology nurses should ensure fertility risk disclosure and consent regarding options related to treatment plans for patients newly diagnosed with cancer in their childbearing years. There are five domains that define

BOX 55.5   Pharmacologic/Medical Interventions

- Penile prostheses for erectile dysfunction or testicular prosthesis for men who are s/p orchiectomy (Carter et al., 2018) are third-line therapy options (Melisko & Narus, 2016).
- Hormone replacement for vasomotor symptoms in patients with non-hormone-sensitive cancers (Vermeulen et al., 2017).
- Phosphodiesterase type 5 inhibitors (oral agents are the first-line therapy [Melisko & Narus, 2016]).
- Intracavernosal injection therapy or intraurethral suppository are second-line therapy options (Melisko & Narus, 2016).
- External devices: Penile prosthesis vacuum or constriction device at base of penis.
- Penile implants: Semirigid rod, fully inflatable, or self-contained inflatable unit.
- Vaginal moisturizers and lubricants, vaginal dilators, and low-dose vaginal estrogen (Carter et al., 2018). Eros therapy—improves clitoral and genital blood flow, improves sensation, lubrication, ability to achieve orgasm, and an overall increase in sexual satisfaction. FDA approved in 2000 to improve sexual response in women.
- Ospemifene/Osphena (daily oral tablet), intravaginal dehydroepiandrosterone (Prasterone), or lidocaine for painful sexual intercourse in women (Carter et al., 2018). Testosterone vaginal cream studies showed improvements in sexual functioning, vaginal dryness (Melisko & Narus, 2016).
- Testosterone repletion if total AM testosterone is <300 ng/dL (Melisko & Narus, 2016).
- Microablative CO_2 laser for vaginal dryness (Melisko & Narus, 2016).
- Hot flashes treatment includes low-dose antidepressants, clonidine, gabapentinoids, vitamin E, soy supplementation, and black cohosh (Melisko & Narus, 2016).

BOX 55.6   Pharmacologic Interventions That Can Be Unsafe

- Intracavernous and transurethral injections for erectile dysfunction—contraindicated for men with multiple myeloma due to the risk of priapism (Leonardi-Warren et al., 2016).
- Herbs—may interact with medication.
- Hormone-containing agents if patient has hormone-positive malignancy (Leonardi-Warren et al., 2016).
- Medication for female sexual interest/arousal disorder—can be unsafe if taken with alcohol.
- Testosterone repletion can increase the risk for heart attack or stroke and should be avoided altogether in men with prostate cancer on active surveillance or those undergoing androgen deprivation therapies (Melisko & Narus, 2016).
- Lubricants—oil based can damage latex condoms, disrupt the normal vaginal bacteria, and increase risk of bacterial vaginosis; glycerin based can increase risk of yeast infection; silicone based can irritate, as can perfumed/flavored lubricants.

BOX 55.7   Nonpharmacologic Measures

- Lifestyle modifications such as regular exercise, stress reduction, therapy with a sexual health specialist, and couples counseling to improve emotional intimacy (Melisko & Narus, 2016).
- Pelvic floor physiotherapy with occupational therapy and Kegel exercises (Vermeer et al., 2016).
- Nonhormone-based lubricants: coconut, olive, mineral oil, and topical Vitamin D or E (Melisko & Narus, 2016).
- Cognitive behavioral stress management intervention for anxiety reduction (Carter et al., 2018) and other integrative therapies such as yoga or meditation (Melisko & Narus, 2016).
- Sensate focus with exercises focused on sexual touch.
- Positioning.
- Hypnosis for hot flashes in women (Carter et al., 2018).

TABLE 55.2   Sexuality Resources for Cancer Survivors

American Cancer Society	Women: www.cancer.org/treatment/treatments-and-side-effects/physical-side-effects/fertility-and-sexual-side-effects/sexuality-for-women-with-cancer.html
	Men: www.cancer.org/treatment/treatments-and-side-effects/physical-side-effects/fertility-and-sexual-side-effects/sexuality-for-men-with-cancer.html
Will2Love	https://www.will2love.com/
Planned Parenthood	https://www.plannedparenthood.org/learn/stds-hiv-safer-sex/safer-sex
Oncolink	www.oncolink.org/oncolife
Mautner Project	www.mautnerproject.org (same-sex partners for women)
Sloan-Kettering Sexual Health Program	www.mskcc.org/mskcc/html/13814.cfm

the scope of barriers oncology nurses must overcome to improve compliance with fertility preservation recommendations, and these include confidence, self-awareness, and treatment barriers (external, time, and perceived) (Grabowski et al., 2017; Box 55.7).

   B. Nurses are expected to recognize the importance of early fertility preservation counseling, provide patient specific education about the gonadotoxic effects of cancer-directed care, and place referrals to reproductive endocrinologists for evaluation (Holman, 2019) as part of a holistic care approach.

   C. Sexual functioning can be improved through interventions targeting communication and couple dynamics (Reese & Haythornthwaite, 2016); Table 55.2 provides several resources.

III. Fertility preservation is a key survivorship issue, and the psychological impact of losing fertility may be as remarkable as the initial cancer diagnosis.

   A. Women who receive pre–cancer-treatment fertility preservation counseling report higher posttreatment QOL (Holman, 2019).

   B. When a person loses the ability to "choose" conception, it can affect personhood (Croson & Keim-Malpass, 2016) and cause existential questioning. For many patients, the ability to bear one's own genetic offspring is a central aspect of survivorship and the distress of losing childbearing abilities may affect patient's

BOX 55.8 Benefits of Fertility Preservation Counseling

- Decreased decisional regret (Grabowski et al., 2017; Holman, 2019).
- Decreased stress (de Carvalho, Kliemchen, & Woodruff, 2017; Pereira & Schattman, 2017)
- Decreased depressive symptomatology, decrease in incidence of distrust in and resentment towards medical staff (Grabowski et al., 2017)
- Reduction in distress and improved posttreatment QOL (Holman, 2019; Oktay et al., 2018)

BOX 55.9 Factors to Discuss With Patient Surrounding Fertility Preservation

- Cancer diagnosis and prognosis.
- Treatment options and risk to fertility with each option.
- Will fertility preservation delay treatment start date, and will that time affect outcome/prognosis?
- Is preservation experimental or standard procedure?
- Cost of preservation, storage, and implantation fee.
- Insurance reimbursement, available moneys, or discount programs (e.g., Livestrong Foundation).
- Applicable laws and regulations of length of storage and custody of biological materials if donor dies.
- Success rate.
- Planning/timing for the safe initiation of pregnancy following cancer treatment.

BOX 55.10 Ethical/Legal Issues of Fertility Preservation

- Privacy/confidentiality of patient, family, and progeny of stored tissue
- Assent of minors
- Safeguards to prevent conflation of research and therapy
- Terminally ill at time of diagnosis (Meyer & Farrell, 2015)
- Addressing experimental status of oncofertility strategies with unknown efficacy, low viability, or possible safety risks to survivors or progeny
- Potential conflicts of interest between patients, parents, clinicians, researchers, and institutions
- Stored tissue issues: number of children that may be conceived from stored tissue; unused tissue disposition (e.g., research or termination); desired length of viable storage (de Carvalho et al., 2017)
- "Noncontingent biographies" (where couple may break up in the future) (Gracia & Crockin, 2016) or "biographical acceleration" (new relationship) (Fournier, 2016)
- Single women may refuse sperm donation for embryo cryopreservation (Massarotti et al., 2017)

BOX 55.11 Fertility Resources for Patients

- Alliance for Fertility Preservation—www.allianceforfertilitypreservation.org
- American Society for Reproductive Medicine—www.reproductivefacts.org
- LIVESTRONG Foundation—www.livestrong.org
- RESOLVE: The National Infertility Association—www.resolve.org
- Save My Fertility—www.savemyfertility.org

BOX 55.12 Why Is Fertility Preservation Not Done? Complex and Intricate Decision-Making

- Higher patient out-of-pocket costs are a barrier to treatment, and these costs depend on insurance coverage (Oktay et al., 2018).
- Lack of information—patient/provider (Woodruff, 2017).
- Provider concerns of age—prepubertal or over 50 years, socioeconomic status, partnership status, existing children, sexual orientation (Russell, Galvin, Harper, & Clayman, 2016), religion (Linkeviciute, Boniolo, Chiavari, & Perccatori, 2014).
- Gender disparity (males counseled more frequently than females) (Holman, 2019; Taylor et al., 2020).
- Too ill to discuss option or too ill to qualify for fertility preservation (Holman, 2019).
- Sense of urgency on part of patient or provider that delay would affect prognosis (Holman, 2019).
- Risk for reimplanting occult cancer cells during ovarian tissue cryopreservation, especially in ovarian and leukemic patients (Holman, 2019). Parental values can affect the decision of adolescents (Klosky, Flynn et al., 2017; Klosky, Wang et al., 2017).

decision-making in that they would opt for less invasive therapies (Holman, 2019). Box 55.8 provides the benefits of fertility counseling.

1. Nurses should recognize and acknowledge grief issues of infertility.
2. Grieving can be interrupted when there is too much focus on medical treatment (Croson & Keim-Malpass, 2016).

C. Risks to fertility are based on type and stage of cancer, drug class/cumulative dose, radiation field/cumulative dose, extent of surgery, age, gender, and genetic factors (Cardonick, 2017). Box 55.9 lists fertility resources.

D. The importance of fertility counseling is recognized by the ASCO, the American Society for Reproductive Medicine, and the American Academy of Pediatrics (Bann et al., 2015). Boxes 55.10 and 55.11 list factors to discuss.

E. Oncofertility discussion is the standard of care even if emergency treatment is needed (Massarotti et al., 2017; Box 55.12).

1. Ideally, patients meet with an oncofertility specialist to increase the use of fertility preservation interventions (Klosky, Flynn et al., 2017; Klosky, Wang et al., 2017). Boxes 55.13 and 55.14 provide fertility options.

F. Due to complexities of fertility preservation, it is recommended that donors and partners meet with legal representatives for written documentation of disposition rights (Fournier, 2016) and that fertility clinics update their consent forms (Gracia & Crockin, 2016).

IV. Birth control measures while on treatment are a vital component of counseling (Box 55.15).

A. If pregnant, patient needs to be informed of risks to the fetus from treatment or diagnostic tests.

BOX 55.13 Fertility Preservation Options for Males

- Sperm cryopreservation (if unable to masturbate, use testicular sperm extraction [TESE], micro-TESE, or electroejaculation) (Saraf & Nahata, 2017)
- Single intracytoplasmic sperm injection, which allows future use of a limited quantity of sperm (Oktay et al., 2018)
- Gonadal shielding during external radiation therapy
- Spermatogonial diploid stem cells—question if could reseed malignancy (Linkeviciute et al., 2014)
- Testicular cryopreservation is the only option for prepubertal pediatric patients, although it still remains investigational (Oktay et al., 2018)

BOX 55.14 Fertility Preservation Options for Females

- Embryo cryopreservation—may require a delay, although less so with newer protocols in place and partner availability.
- Ovarian transposition (oophoropexy) for radiation therapy to the pelvis. Not effective for whole-body external radiation therapy (approximately 90% effective in preserving ovarian function). Due to radiation scatter, ovaries are not always protected, and because of the risk of ovarian remigration, this procedure should be done as close to irradiation as possible (Oktay et al., 2018).
- Oocyte cryopreservation—allows flexibility to fertilize with future partner/donor and sensitivity for patients who have moral/ethical objections to embryo freezing (Oktay et al., 2018).
- Of note, breast cancer patients with BRCA mutation have less oocytes retrieved and less embryos obtained during controlled ovarian hyperstimulation treatments (Condorelli et al., 2019).
- Conservative fertility-sparing surgery with early-stage gynecologic malignancies such as radical trachelectomy (surgical removal of the cervix) or ovarian cystectomy (Oktay et al., 2018).
- Fertoprotective neoadjuvant therapies (Woodruff, 2017).
- Ovarian tissue cryopreservation for future use does not require ovarian stimulation nor does it require sexual maturity, and may therefore be the only method available in female pediatric patients. Currently, it is still experimental in the United States (Oktay et al., 2018).
- Suboptimal option when hormonal stimulation undesirable (transgender) (Saraf & Nahata, 2017).
- Ovarian suppression via gonadotropin-releasing hormone agonist—controversial with questionable safety for lymphoma and estrogen receptor–positive breast cancer patients (Bortoletto, Confinio, Smitch, Woodruss, & Pavone, 2017; Oktay et al., 2018). When oocyte, embryo, or ovarian tissue cryopreservation is not an option, and in younger breast cancer patients, GnRHA may be offered to mitigate the chemotherapy-induced ovarian insufficiency, but it should not be used instead of proven fertility preservation interventions (Oktay et al., 2018).
- Ovarian stimulation/phase start techniques—wide variation in practice (Bortoletto et al., 2017).

BOX 55.15 Risks of Birth Control Methods

- Hormonal birth control (implant/pill/shot/patch) contraindicated for:
  - Hormone-sensitive malignancies are a contraindication to using systemic hormone therapy (Carter et al., 2018)
  - History of venous thromboembolism, migraines with aura, or cardiovascular or cerebrovascular disease
  - Impaired liver function
  - Women >35 years and a smoker
- Increased risk of infection at time of intrauterine device insertion and for a 20-day period after insertion
- Condoms: use latex unless latex allergy (although polyurethane condoms more likely to break)

BOX 55.16 Factors When Considering Pregnancy After Cancer Treatment

- Optimal time depends on diagnosis, treatment, and individual patient factors.
- Length of time for repair of damaged gametes: 6–12 months usually recommended.
- When aggressive cancer or at the highest risk of recurrence, consider waiting 2–3 years.
- In the setting of preexisting infertility issues, patients should strongly consider earlier fertility evaluation, work up and management with a Reproductive Endocrinologist (Holman, 2019). All women with a history of cancer and cancer-directed care that are considering pregnancy should first be cleared by their oncologist and preferentially referred to a Maternal Fetal Medicine specialist for preconception evaluation and risk counseling (Holman, 2019).

---

1. The challenge is that many pregnancy symptoms can mimic symptoms of malignancy, such as bloating, weight changes, fatigue, and menstrual changes.
2. In general, most diagnostic radiology tests expose the embryo to less than 5.0 mSv (500 mrem) with little to no risk to the fetus. Using a lead shield decreases that risk.

V. Deciding when to have children after treatment.
   A. A safe interval of time from completion of systemic chemotherapy to pregnancy has not been determined, but there does not appear to be a risk of congenital malformations in children that are spontaneously conceived in survivorship versus the general population (Holman, 2019; Box 55.16).
   B. "Window of fertility" (i.e., premature ovarian failure that is shortened due to the damage to primordial follicle pool) (Roness, Kalich-Philosoph, & Meirow, 2014) may affect decision to conceive.
   C. Women on long-term hormonal therapy will weigh the risk of stopping treatment to conceive against the risk of stopping treatment (Roness et al., 2014). Part of a survivorship plan is to decide whether to stop hormonal treatment for pregnancy and then restart after giving birth (Waimey et al., 2015).
      1. There may not be physical restrictions for pregnancy if the cancer is surgically resected, less aggressive, and there is a low risk of recurrence, but

B. Surgery that affects the bladder, large intestine, or rectum can increase the risk of miscarriage (Waimey, Smith, Confino, Jeruss, & Pavone, 2015).
C. Mutagenic changes in gametes and/or teratogenic effects can occur if the fetus is exposed to chemotherapy or external radiation therapy.
D. Safety and how to decrease exposure to the fetus from diagnostic tests.

it is still important to discuss waiting 6–12 months to psychologically recover from the cancer diagnosis. General guidelines recommend waiting at least 1 year after cancer treatment before attempting to conceive (Hartnett et al., 2018). The most reliable strategy to assess ovarian reserve/predict the onset of menopause is the serum anti-Mullerian hormone (AMH) and antral follicle count (AFC) levels, both of which decline with age, mirroring the decline in fertility (Cardonick, 2017; Holman, 2019). AFC and AMH results can help provide guidance for triaging the urgency of fertility preservation situations in each female patient (Holman, 2019). Serum AMH may not be helpful in adolescent and young adult childhood survivors, as ovarian reserve is most robust in women's 2nd decade of life (Holman, 2019).

2. Menses can continue for 10–15 years after the onset of infertility (Pereira & Schattman, 2017).

REFERENCES

American Society for Reproductive Medicine. (2019). Fertility preservation in patients undergoing gonadotoxic therapy or gonadectomy: A committee opinion. *Fertility and Sterility, 112*(6), 1022–1033.

Bann, C. M., Treiman, K., Squiers, L., Tzeng, J., Nutt, S., Arvey, S., et al. (2015). Cancer survivors' use of fertility preservation. *Journal of Women's Health, 24*(12), 1030–1037.

Barocas, D. A., Alverez, J., Resnick, M. J., Koyama, T., Hoffman, K. E., Tyson, M. D., et al. (2017). Association between radiation therapy, surgery, or observation for localized prostate cancer and patient-reported outcomes after 3 years. *Journal of the American Medical Association, 317*(11), 1126–1140.

Benedict, C., Philip, E. J., Baser, R. E., Carter, J., Schuler, T. A., Jandorf, L., et al. (2015). Body image and sexual function in women after treatment for anal and rectal cancer. *Psycho-Oncology, 25*(3), 316–323.

Bortoletto, P., Confinio, R., Smitch, B. M., Woodruss, T. K., & Pavone, M. E. (2017). Practices and attitudes regarding women undergoing fertility preservation: A survey of the national physician's cooperative. *Journal of Adolescent and Young Adult Oncology, 6*(3), 444–449.

Cardonick, E.H. (2017). *Overview of infertility and pregnancy outcome in cancer survivors.* Waltham, MA: UpToDate. Retrieved from https://www.uptodate.com/contents/overview-of-infertility-and-pregnancy-outcome-in-cancer-survivors.

Carter, J., Lacchetti, C., Andersen, B. L., Barton, D. L., Bolte, S., Damast, S., et al. (2018). Interventions to address sexual problems in people with cancer: American Society of Clinical Oncology clinical practice guideline adaptation of cancer care Ontario guideline. *Journal of Clinical Oncology, 36*(5), 492–511.

Catamero, D., Noonan, K., Richards, T., Faiman, B., Manchulenko, C., Devine, H., et al. (2017). Distress, fatigue, and sexuality: Understanding and treating concerns and symptoms in patients with multiple myeloma. *Clinical Journal of Oncology Nursing, 21*(5), 7–18.

Condorelli, M., Lambertini, M., Del Mastro, L., Boccardo, F., Demeestere, I., & Bober, S. L. (2019). Fertility, sexuality and cancer in young adult women. *Current Opinion in Oncology, 31*(4), 259–267.

Croson, E., & Keim-Malpass, J. (2016). Grief and gracefulness regarding cancer experiences among young women. *Oncology Nursing Forum, 43*(6), 747–753.

de Carvalho, B. R., Kliemchen, J., & Woodruff, T. K. (2017). Ethical, moral and other aspects related to fertility preservation in cancer patients. *Jornal Brasileiro de Reproducao Assistida, 21*(1), 45–48.

Dizon, D.S., Katz, A., Ganz, P.A., & Vora, S.R. (2018). *Overview of sexual dysfunction in male cancer survivors.* Waltham, MA: UpToDate. www.uptodate.com.

Fournier, E. (2016). Oncofertility and the rights to future fertility. *JAMA Oncology, 2*(2), 249–252.

Garcia, R. M., Hanlon, A., Small, W., Jr., et al., Strauss, J. B., Lin, L., Wells, J., et al. (2018). The relationship between body mass index and sexual function in endometrial cancer. *Oncology Nursing Forum, 45*(1), 25–32.

Gondim de Almeida, N., Knobf, T. M., Renato de Oliveira, M., De Goes Salvetti, M., Oliveira Batista Oria, M., & Virginia de Melo Fialho, A. (2020). A pilot intervention study to improve sexuality outcomes in breast cancer survivors. *Asia-Pacific Journal of Oncology Nursing, 7*(2), 161–166. https://doi.org/10.4103/apjon.apjon_56_19.

Grabowski, M. C., Spitzer, D. A., Stutzman, S. E., & Olson, D. M. (2017). Development of an instrument to examine nursing attitudes toward fertility preservation in oncology. *Oncology Nursing Forum, 44*(4), 497–502.

Gracia, C. R., & Crockin, S. L. (2016). Legal battles over embryos after in vitro fertilization: Is there a way to avoid them? *Journal of the American Medical Association, 2*(2), 182–184.

Hartnett, K. P., Mertens, A. C., Kramer, M. R., Lash, T. L., Spencer, J. B., Ward, K., et al. (2018). Pregnancy after cancer: Does timing of conception affect infant health? *Cancer, 124*(22), 4401–4407.

Holman, D. A. (2019). Fertility preservation in gynecologic cancer. *Seminars in Oncology Nursing, 35*(2), 202–210.

Hoyt, M. A., McCann, C., Savone, M., Saigal, C. S., & Stanton, A. L. (2015). Interpersonal sensitivity and sexual functioning in young men with testicular cancer: The moderating role of coping. *International Journal of Behavioral Medicine, 22*(6), 709–716.

Jonsdottir, J. I., Vilhjalmsson, R., & Svavarsdottir, E. K. (2021). Effectiveness of a couple-based intervention on sexuality and intimacy among women in active cancer treatment: A quasi-experimental study. *European Journal of Oncology Nursing, 52*, 101975.

Klosky, J. L., Flynn, J. S., Lehmann, V., Russell, K. M., Wang, F., Hardin, R. N., et al. (2017). Parental influences on sperm banking attempts among adolescent males newly diagnosed with cancer. *Fertility and Sterility, 108*(6), 1043–1049.

Klosky, J. L., Wang, F., Russell, K. M., Zhang, H., Flynn, J. S., Huang, L., et al. (2017). Prevalence and predictors of sperm banking in adolescents newly diagnosed with cancer: Examination of adolescent, parent, and provider factors influencing fertility preservation outcomes. *Journal of Clinical Oncology, 35*(34), 3830–3836.

Leonardi-Warren, K., Neff, I., Mancuso, M., Wenger, B., Galbraith, M., & Fink, R. (2016). Sexual health: Exploring patient needs and healthcare provider comfort and knowledge. *Clinical Journal of Oncology Nursing, 20*(6), E162–E167.

Linkeviciute, A., Boniolo, G., Chiavari, L., & Perccatori, F. A. (2014). Fertility preservation in cancer patients: The global framework. *Cancer Treatment Reviews, 40*(8), 1019–1027.

Lubejko, B. G., & Wilson, B. J. (2019). *Oncology nursing: Scope and standards of practice.* Pittsburgh, PA: Oncology Nursing Society.

Massarotti, C., Scaruffi, P., Lambertini, M., Remorgida, V., DelMastro, L., & Anserini, P. (2017). State of the art on oocyte cryopreservation in female cancer patients: A critical review of the literature. *Cancer Treatment Reviews, 57*, 50–57.

Melisko, M. E., & Narus, J. B. (2016). Sexual function in cancer survivors: Updates to the NCCN guidelines for survivorship. *Journal of the National Comprehensive Cancer Network, 14*(5.5), 685–689.

Meyer, F., & Farrell, E. (2015). Ethical dilemmas in palliative care: A case study of fertility preservation in the context of metastatic cancer. *Journal of Palliative Medicine, 18*(8), 661.

Miaja, M., Platas, A., & Martinez-Cannon, B. A. (2017). Psychological impact of alterations in sexuality, fertility, and body image in young breast cancer patients and their partners. *Revista de Investigacion Clinica, 69*(4), 204–209.

Nelson, R. (2017). *Time to have the talk! Sex and the cancer patient.* Medscape. Retrieved from https://www.medscape.com/viewarticle/888119.

Oktay, K., Harvey, B. E., Partridge, A. H., Quinn, G. P., Reinecke, J., Taylor, H. S., et al. (2018). Fertility preservation in patients with cancer: ASCO clinical practice guideline update. *Journal of Clinical Oncology, 36*(19), 1994–2001.

Olsson, C., Sandin-Bojo, A. K., Bjuresater, K., & Larsson, M. (2016). Changes in sexuality, body image and health related quality of life in patients treated for hematologic malignancies: A longitudinal study. *Sexuality and Disability, 34*(4), 367–388.

Pereira, N., & Schattman, G. L. (2017). Fertility preservation and sexual health after cancer therapy. *Journal of Oncology Practice, 13*(10), 643–651.

Reese, J. B., & Haythornthwaite, J. A. (2016). Importance of sexuality in colorectal cancer: Predictors, changes, and response to an intimacy enhancement intervention. *Supportive Care in Cancer, 24*(10), 4309–4317.

Rhoten, B. A. (2017). Conceptual issues surrounding body image for oncology nurses. *Oncology Nursing Forum, 44*(5), 534–536.

Roness, H., Kalich-Philosoph, L., & Meirow, D. (2014). Prevention of chemotherapy-induced ovarian damage: Possible roles for hormonal and non-hormonal attenuating agents. *Human Reproduction Update, 20*(5), 759–774.

Russell, A. M., Galvin, K. M., Harper, M. M., & Clayman, M. L. (2016). A comparison of heterosexual and LGBTQ cancer survivors' outlooks on relationships, family building, possible infertility, and patient-doctor fertility risk communication. *Journal of Cancer Survivorship, 10*(5), 935–942.

Saraf, A. J., & Nahata, L. (2017). Fertility counseling and preservation: Considerations for the pediatric endocrinologist. *Translational Pediatrics, 6*(4), 313–322.

Taylor, J., Ruggiero, M., Maity, A., Ko, K., Greenberger, B.A., Donofree, D., et al. (2020). Sexual health toxicity in cancer survivors: Is there a gender disparity in physician evaluation and intervention? ASTRO Annual Meeting. Abstract 1042.

Vermeer, W. M., Bakker, R. M., Kenter, G. G., Stiggelbout, A. M., Creutzberg, C. L., Kenter, G. G., et al. (2015). Psychosexual support for gynecological cancer survivors: Professionals' current practices and need for assistance. *Supportive Care in Cancer, 23*(3), 831–839.

Vermeer, W. M., Bakker, R. M., Kenter, G. G., Stiggelbout, A. M., & ter Kuile, M. M. (2016). Cervical cancer survivors' and partners' experiences with sexual dysfunction and psychosexual support. *Supportive Care in Cancer, 24*, 1679–1687.

Vermeulen, R. F., Beurden, M. V., Kieffer, J. M., Bleiker, E. M., Valdimarsdottir, H. B., Massuger, L. F., et al. (2017). Hormone replacement therapy after risk-reducing salpingo-oophorectomy minimizes endocrine and sexual problems: A prospective study. *European Journal of Cancer.* https://doi.org/10.1016/j.ejca.2017.07.018.

Waimey, K. E., Smith, B. M., Confino, R., Jeruss, J. S., & Pavone, M. E. (2015). Understanding fertility in young female cancer patients. *Journal of Women's Health, 24*(10), 812–818.

Wang, K., Ariello, K., Choi, M., Turner, A., Wan, B. A., Yee, C., et al. (2017). Sexual healthcare for cancer patients receiving palliative care: A narrative review. *Annals of Palliative Medicine.* https://doi.org/10.21037/apm.2017.10.05.

Westin, S. N., Sun, C. C., Tung, C. S., Lacour, R. A., Meyer, L. A., Urbauer, D. L., et al. (2016). Survivors of gynecologic malignancies: Impact of treatment on health and well-being. *Journal of Cancer Survivorship, 10*(2), 261–270.

Williams, M., & Addis, G. (2021). Addressing patient sexuality in cancer and palliative care. *British Journal of Nursing, 30*(10), s24–s28.

Wilson, C., McGuire, D. B., Rodgers, B. L., Elswick, R. K., & Temkin, S. M. (2021). Body image, sexuality, and sexual functioning in women with gynecologic cancer. *Cancer Nursing, 44*(5), E252–E286. https://doi.org/10.1097/NCC.0000000000000818.

Woodruff, T. K. (2017). A win-win for women's reproductive health: A nonsteroidal contraceptive and fertoprotective neoadjuvant. *Proceedings of the National Academy of Sciences of the United States of America, 114*(9), 2101–2102.

56

Standards of Practice and Professional Performance

Barbara Wilson

I. Definition of standards
  A. Nursing and other health care organizations develop standards and guidelines for practice. Standards and guidelines are not the same and are differentiated by expectations of compliance. Standards for professional nursing practice are defined as "authoritative statements of the duties that all registered nurses [RNs], regardless of role, population, or specialty, are expected to competently perform" (American Nurses Association [ANA], 2021).
  B. Clinical practice guidelines differ from guidelines. Guidelines are related to broader systems whereas clinical practice guidelines are used by health care providers or those with clinic management responsibilities to address clinical conditions.
    1. Best-practice guidelines cover screening, diagnosis, management, or monitoring best practices (Kredo et al., 2016).

II. Need for published standards
  A. Nursing standards of practice and professional performance (NSPPP) set expectations for competent nursing practice.
  B. NSPPP apply to all nursing roles in all settings where nurses care for patients. When implementing the standards, consider the characteristics of the practice setting as well as current health care and nursing trends (ANA, 2021).
  C. NSPPP guide evidence-based, quality nursing care and provide direction to nurses and their employers' expectations about skills and competence.
  D. NSPPP provide the public with information about what they can expect from nursing care related to professional competence.

III. Who defines nursing standards in the United States?
  A. Professional nursing organizations establish standards and how standards are applied to:
    1. Specialty practice
    2. Professional accountability
  B. American Nurses Association (ANA, 2021): The ANA develops:
    1. Nursing: Scope and Standards of Practice
    2. Code of Ethics for Nurses with Interpretive Statements
  C. Oncology Nursing Society (ONS): Defines standards for oncology nursing practice across settings, patient populations, and subspecialties.
    1. Standards for oncology nursing focus on helping people at risk for or with a cancer diagnosis achieve the best quality of life and outcomes.
    2. ONS publishes a variety of standards based on the best available evidence to guide oncology nursing practice.

IV. Oncology Nursing Scope and Standards of Practice
  A. Description
    1. ONS first released NSPPP in 1979, and it has been periodically updated. The latest version was released in 2019 (Lubjeko & Wilson, 2019).
  B. Scope of oncology nursing practice
    1. Addresses "the 'who,' 'what,' 'where,' 'when,' 'why,' and 'how' of nursing practice" (ANA, 2021).
    2. Defines the practice of nursing as it is performed within the specialty area of oncology.
    3. Addresses all levels of oncology nursing from the generalist RN to graduate-level prepared and advanced practice RNs.
    4. Concepts addressed within an oncology scope of practice include (Lubjeko & Wilson, 2019):
      a. History of cancer care and oncology nursing
      b. Populations and practice settings that are the focus of oncology nursing qualifications for oncology nurses include educational background, professional development, and certification
      c. Code of ethics as applied to oncology nursing
      d. Oncology and nursing practice trends that affect oncology nursing practice
  C. Oncology Nursing Standards of Practice
    1. Performance
      a. Describe the expectations for oncology nursing practice across care settings.
      b. Include standards of practice and standards of professional performance (Table 56.1).

TABLE 56.1	**Standards of Oncology Nursing Practice and Professional Performance**
Standards of Practice	**Description**
Assessment	The oncology nurse systematically and continually collects data regarding the physical, psychological, social, spiritual, and cultural health status of the patient, including in-depth data specific to the disease and treatment experience of the patient with cancer.
Diagnosis	The oncology nurse analyzes assessment data to determine nursing diagnoses, problems, and issues related to health concerns of people with cancer.
Outcomes identification	The oncology nurse identifies expected outcomes individualized to the patient, caregiver, or both with a focus on symptom management, survivorship, or a comfortable death.
Planning	The oncology nurse develops an individualized and holistic plan of care that prescribes interventions to attain expected outcomes.
Implementation	The oncology nurse implements the plan of care to achieve the identified expected outcomes for the patient.
Coordination of care	The oncology nurse ensures that care is coordinated throughout the cancer care continuum.
Health teaching and health promotion	The oncology nurse uses evidence-based strategies to engage patients in learning to promote health and safety.
Evaluation	The oncology nurse systematically and regularly evaluates the patient's response to interventions to determine progress toward achievement of expected outcomes.
Standards of Professional Performance	**Description**
Ethics	The oncology nurse uses ethical principles as a basis for decision-making and patient advocacy.
Culturally Congruent Care	The oncology nurse considers cultural diversity and inclusion principles with planning and providing care.
Communication	The oncology nurse uses evidence-based strategies to foster mutual respect and shared decision-making that enhance clinical outcomes and patient satisfaction in all practice settings.
Collaboration	The oncology nurse partners with the patient and family, the interprofessional team, and community resources to optimize cancer care.
Leadership	The oncology nurse demonstrates leadership in the practice setting and in the nursing profession by acknowledging the dynamic nature of cancer care and the necessity to prepare for advances in technologies, modalities of treatment, and supportive care.
Education	The oncology nurse seeks and expands personal knowledge and competence that reflect the current evidence-based state of cancer care and oncology nursing, and contributes to the professional development of peers, assistive personnel, and interprofessional colleagues.
Evidence-based practice and research	The oncology nurse integrates relevant research into clinical practice and identifies clinical dilemmas and problems appropriate for study while supporting research efforts.
Quality of practice	The oncology nurse systematically evaluates the quality, safety, and effectiveness of oncology nursing practice within all practice settings and across the continuum of cancer care.
Professional practice evaluation	The oncology nurse consistently evaluates his or her own nursing practice and that of their peers and other health care providers.
Resource utilization	The oncology nurse considers factors related to safety, efficiency, effectiveness, and cost in planning and delivering care to patients.
Environmental health	The oncology nurse practices in an environmentally safe and healthy manner.

Adapted from Lubjeko, B. G., & Wilson, B. J. (2019). *Oncology nursing scope & standards of practice*. Pittsburgh, PA: Oncology Nursing Society; American Nurses Association (ANA). (2021). *Nursing: Scope and standards of practice* (4th ed.) Silver Spring, MD: American Nurses Association.

c. For each standard at the RN level, criteria to demonstrate competence apply to all nurses who provide care to patients with cancer or practice in an oncology setting.
   (1) Additional standards apply to graduate-level prepared nurses and advanced practice RNs.
2. Application in practice: the Oncology Nursing Scope and Standards of Practice can be used to define oncology nursing roles, develop individual competence, and highlight the contribution oncology nurses make to quality cancer care, such as:
   a. Development of job descriptions, performance appraisals, evaluation instruments, and peer reviews.
   b. Self-assessment to identify professional development needs.
   c. Basis for organizational policies, procedures, and protocols.
   d. Inform patients, public, legislators, and regulatory bodies about the impact of oncology nursing on safe, high-quality cancer care.
   e. Inform quality assessment and quality improvement projects and initiatives.
   f. Reveal organizational, regional, or national evidence gaps that provide appropriate questions for nursing research.
   g. Identify quality outcomes that can be used to demonstrate the impact of oncology nursing on patient outcomes.

h. Promote ways oncology nursing can contribute to evolving health care delivery and reimbursement models.

i. Develop a curriculum to prepare nursing students and practicing nurses for oncology nursing–specific role responsibilities (ANA, 2021; Lubjeko & Wilson, 2019).

3. Education: generalist/advanced practice

a. Provide guidance to educators in schools of nursing and clinical settings about preparing students and practicing nurses to meet the care needs of cancer survivors across care settings.

b. Address educational structure, process, and outcomes at the generalist and advanced practice levels, including faculty qualifications, clinical and educational resources, relevant curriculum, and teaching–learning process and expectations.

c. Practice application, used by individuals and organizations when:

(1) Plan, update, and evaluate education offered in prelicensure and graduate-level nursing programs.

(2) Plan and evaluate cancer-related continuing education for nurses at all levels of practice (Jacobs & Mayer, 2015).

4. Education: patient, significant other, and public

a. Defines expectations for the oncology nurse, resources, curriculum, the teaching–learning process, and different types of learners.

b. Standards set expectations for patient and caregiver quality education.

(1) Education covers all phases of cancer care

(2) Engages public to promote health behaviors (Blecher, Ireland, & Watson, 2016).

c. Application in practice: can be used by individuals and organizations to:

(1) Develop education for nurses new to oncology practice about needs and evidence-based interventions recommended for teaching patients, caregivers, and the public about cancer-related topics.

(2) Develop, implement, and evaluate education plans for individual patients or populations.

(3) Provide direction to develop, implement, and evaluate educational programs for patients, caregivers, and the public.

(4) Perform a self-evaluation of the educational content, techniques, and outcomes provided to patients, caregivers, and the public.

(5) Identify education that supports personal–professional development related to educating patients, caregivers, and the public about cancer-related topics.

D. ONS nursing documentation—treatment (Wiley, Galioto, Matey, & Wyant, 2016)

1. Nursing documentation requirements for people with cancer undergoing treatment and requiring supportive care.

2. Goal is to use standardized health care terminology.

a. Includes minimal description and explanation about people receiving treatment for cancer

b. Documentation builds over time

c. Documentation includes individual, updated patient assessment

d. Documentation supports patient's plan of care

3. Sections of these standards address the following:

a. Chemotherapy and biotherapy administration (Olsen, LeFebvre, & Brassil, 2019)

b. Radiation therapy (McQuestion, Drapek, & Witt, 2021)

c. Blood and marrow transplantation

d. Surgery

e. Treatment with a central venous access device (Camp-Sorrell & Matey, 2017)

f. Blood product transfusion

g. Extravasation management (Olsen et al., 2019; Wiley et al., 2016)

4. Application in practice:

a. Develop and evaluate current policies and procedures and develop new organizational policies and procedures related to documentation requirements for oncology nursing care.

b. Develop orientation and professional development programs related to documentation in oncology settings.

c. Compare standards to current documentation processes and platforms to identify gaps.

d. Evaluate the adequacy of one's own documentation in relation to the criteria addressed in the standards.

e. Provide structure for documentation audits to identify areas for improvement.

E. Application in practice—documentation: access device standards of practice for oncology nursing

1. Provide guidance on best practices in the care of people with cancer who have access devices.

2. Practices are categorized according to the strength of the evidence.

a. Practice standard: strong evidence to accept practice.

b. Practice recommendation: evidence less strong, but use suggested based on expert opinion, common practice, and nursing judgment.

c. No definitive recommendations: adequate evidence is lacking.

3. Includes standards and recommendations for venous and specialty access devices.

4. Application in practice: used by individuals and organizations to:

a. Develop and evaluate current and develop new organizational policies and procedures related to the use and management of access devices in people with cancer.

b. Develop didactic and clinical educational programs for nurses who care for people with access devices.

c. Evaluate the initial and ongoing competence of nurses caring for people with access devices.

d. Evaluate own knowledge and skills related to access devices and identify needs for professional development.

e. Guide quality assessment and improvement projects to identify, address, and reevaluate gaps in practice (Camp-Sorrell & Matey, 2017).

F. ASCO/ONS Chemotherapy Administration Safety Standards

1. Interprofessional standards outline best practices to reduce the risk of error during chemotherapy delivery.

2. Detailed standards address
   a. Appropriate staff and policies
   b. Planning, consent, and education for patients and caregivers
   c. Order, prepare, administer and, document chemotherapy via parenteral and oral routes
   d. Monitor adherence, side effects, and complications (Neuss et al., 2016)

3. Application in practice: can be used by organizations and individuals to:
   a. Develop and evaluate new organizational policies and procedures associated with chemotherapy administration.
   b. Develop didactic and clinical educational programs for health care professionals involved in the administration of chemotherapy.
   c. Evaluate the initial and ongoing competence of health care professionals involved in the administration of chemotherapy.
   d. Self-evaluation of knowledge and skills associated with chemotherapy administration; identify professional development plan related to chemotherapy administration.
   e. Guide quality assessment and improvement projects to identify, address, and reevaluate gaps in practice.
   f. To measure and identify quality outcomes to improve practice and support quality research, collect data. Provide evidence required for reporting quality outcomes metrics and identify topics for quality outcomes research.

G. Oncology Navigation Standards of Professional Practice (Professional Oncology Navigation Task Force, 2022)

1. Oncology Navigation Standards address:
   a. Enhance the quality of professional navigation services provided to people impacted by cancer
   b. Advocate with and on behalf of people at risk for cancer, cancer patients, survivors, families, and caregivers to protect and promote the needs and interests of people impacted by cancer

c. Encourage navigator participation in the creation, implementation, and evaluation of best practices and quality improvement in oncology care

d. Promote navigator participation in the development, analysis, and refinement of public policy at all levels to best support the interests of people impacted by cancer and to protect and promote the profession of navigation

e. Educate all stakeholders about the essential role of navigators in oncology systems

REFERENCES

American Nurses Association (ANA). (2021). *Nursing: Scope and standards of practice* (4th ed.). Silver Spring, MD: American Nurses Association.

Blecher, C. S., Ireland, A. M., & Watson, J. L. (2016). *Standards of oncology education: Patient/significant other and public* (4th ed.). Pittsburgh, PA: Oncology Nursing Society.

Camp-Sorrell, D., & Matey, L. (2017). *Access device standards of practice for oncology nursing*. Pittsburgh, PA: Oncology Nursing Society.

Jacobs, L. A., & Mayer, D. K. (2015). *Standards of oncology nursing education: Generalist and advanced practice levels*. Pittsburgh, PA: Oncology Nursing Society.

Kredo, T., Bernhardsson, S., Machingaidze, S., Young, T., Louw, Q., Ochodo, E., et al. (2016). Guide to clinical practice guidelines: The current state of play. *International Journal for Quality in Health Care, 28*(1), 122–128. https://doi.org/10.1093/intqhc/mzv115.

Lubejko, B. G., & Wilson, B. J. (2019). *Oncology nursing scope & standards of practice*. Pittsburgh, PA: Oncology Nursing Society.

McQuestion, M., Drapek, L., & Witt, M. E. (2021). *Manual for radiation oncology nursing practice and education* (5th ed.). Pittsburgh, PA: Oncology Nursing Society.

Neuss, M., Gilmore, T. R., Belderson, K. M., Billett, A. L., Conti-Kalchik, T., Harvey, B. E., et al. (2016). 2016 Updated American Society of Clinical Oncology/Oncology Nursing Society Chemotherapy Administration Safety Standards, including standards for pediatric oncology. *Oncology Nursing Forum, 44*, 31–43. https://doi.org/10.1188/17.ONF.31-43.

Olsen, M. M., LeFebvre, K. B., & Brassil, K. J. (2019). *Chemotherapy and immunotherapy guidelines and recommendations for practice*. Pittsburgh, PA: Oncology Nursing Society.

Professional Oncology Navigation Task Force. (2022). Oncology navigation standards of professional practice. *Journal of Oncology Navigation & Survivorship, 13*(3). Retrieved from https://www.jons-online.com/issues/2022/march-2022-vol-13-no-3/4399-oncology-navigation-standards-of-professional-practice.

Wiley, K., Galioto, M., Matey, L., & Wyant, T. (2016). *Oncology nursing society documentation standards for cancer treatment*. Pittsburgh, PA: Oncology Nursing Society.

57

Evidence-Based Practice

Jennifer Hadjar

I. Overview: evidence-based practice (EBP)
   A. Key to delivering high-quality health care, empowering clinicians, improved patient outcomes, and decreased health care costs (Melnyk & Fineout-Overholt, 2019).
   B. First developed as a method for clinical learning in evidence-based medicine in the 1980s at McMaster University in Hamilton, Ontario, Canada.
   C. Goal is to guide oncology nursing interventions and practices that are evidence based and improve the quality and outcomes of cancer care (Arthur et al., 2019).
      1. Quality and Safety Education for Nurses established EBP as a quality and safety competency necessary to prepare nurses to deliver safe and high-quality care (Cengiz & Yoder, 2020; Young, Ball, Flott, Goodman, & Hercinger, 2021).
      2. The oncology nursing profession, and regulatory agencies, mandates the inclusion of EBP in curricula and professional standards—a component of each of the six Standards of Care and five of the Standards of Professional Practice (Arthur et al., 2019; Saunders, Gallagher-Ford, Kvist, & Vehviläinen-Julkunen, 2019).
   D. A professional obligation exists for oncology nurses to value research-guided practices (Arthur et al., 2019). Definitions and components of EBP include the following:
      1. Intentional use of current evidence in decision-making in patient care (Melnyk & Fineout-Overholt, 2019).
      2. Utilizing research as a form of evidence in proposed practice changes (Jolley, 2020).
      3. A paradigm and lifelong problem-solving approach to clinical practice that integrates individual clinical expertise, patient preference and actions, clinical circumstance, and the best available external evidence to improve outcomes. (Melnyk & Fineout-Overholt, 2019).
      4. A systematic approach to practice that emphasizes using the best evidence in combination with clinical experience and patient preferences and values to make decisions about care and treatment (Esteban-Sepulveda et al., 2021; Melnyk & Fineout-Overholt, 2019).
      5. Essential components—a systematic review and synthesis of research that results in a systematic process

for change, including rigorous assessment, implementation, and evaluation of outcomes (Melnyk & Fineout-Overholt, 2019).

II. Need for EBP based on the following:
   A. Cancer care is a continuous mode of change and nursing practices should adapt and be evidence based (Arthur et al., 2019).
   B. EBP is the cornerstone of effective clinical care and optimal patient outcomes (O'Rourke et al., 2019).
   C. The Institute of Medicine has mandated that 90% of all health care decisions in the United States will be evidence based by 2020 (Cengiz & Yoder, 2020).
   D. Evidence continues to evolve on a continual basis and can take decades to transition into practice without the use of EBP (Melnyk & Fineout-Overholt, 2019).
   E. EBP-enriched culture can increase nurse satisfaction and retention, as well as decrease turnover and burnout (Melnyk & Fineout-Overholt, 2019).
   F. Pay-for-performance programs, nonpayment for complications when evidence-based guidelines are not followed, and patients and family members seeking the latest evidence online are increasing (Melnyk & Fineout-Overholt, 2019).
   G. EBP is not consistently implemented at health care institutions throughout the United States and globally (Melnyk & Fineout-Overholt, 2019).

III. EBP competencies for registered nurse and advanced practicing nurses (Melnyk & Raderstorf, 2019)
   A. To promote an EBP culture and provide high-quality health care, the registered nurse is expected to maintain the following knowledge, skills, and attitude:
      1. Question clinical practice for improving health care quality
      2. Utilize internal evidence to describe clinical problems (assessment data, quality indicators)
      3. Apply the PICOT format to ask clinical questions (see Section IV)
      4. Search external evidence to answer clinical questions
      5. Critically appraise evidence using practice guidelines and literature synthesis
      6. Critically appraise research studies; determine the strength of evidence and applicability to clinical practice

7. Evaluate evidence and consider applicability to clinical practice
8. Collect data for decision-making in the care of individuals, groups, or populations
9. Use internal and external evidence to plan EBP changes
10. Implement practice change based on evidence, clinical expertise, and patient preference to improve the quality of care and patient outcomes
11. Evaluate outcomes of EBP to determine best practice
12. Disseminate best practices to improve the quality of care and patient outcomes
13. Sustain and promote an EBP culture

B. Using evidence to support clinical practice change is a multistep process (Melnyk & Fineout-Overholt, 2019).
1. Cultivate a sense of inquiry and create an EBP culture
2. Question current practice—gap analysis, observational research
3. Journal clubs, ongoing EBP education, access to key databases
4. National Nursing Standards & Recommendations for Best Practice including, but not limited to, National Cancer Institute, National Comprehensive Cancer Network, Oncology Nursing Society, Agency for Healthcare Research & Quality, and American Nurses Association (ANA)
5. Organizational and/or unit-based shared governance
6. Collaborate with other health care professionals and members of the interdisciplinary team who have in-depth knowledge of EBP
7. Administrative and leadership support and mentorship
8. Regular recognition of EBP values and implementation

C. Identify a problem or trigger
1. Problem-focused: existing data that show an opportunity for improvement (financial data, quality data, benchmark data, and clinical problems [e.g., patient falls])
2. Knowledge-focused: new research or practice guidelines that warrant practice change
3. Problems with higher volume or cost association will have higher organizational priority

D. Identification of information and stakeholders needed to solve the problem

E. Stakeholders develop, implement, and evaluate change with other disciplines

F. Search and critique of the literature for relevant studies (Jolley, 2020; Melnyk & Fineout-Overholt, 2019)
1. Use a clinical question to develop a list of keywords
   a. Using the PICOT format for clinical questions will yield the most relevant evidence:
      (1) P—Patient population or disease of interest
      (2) I—Intervention or issue of interest
      (3) C—Comparison intervention or control group
      (4) O—Outcomes
      (5) T—Time frame to achieve outcomes
2. Data sources for EBP include but are not limited to the following:
   a. Electronic health records
   b. Benchmark data/national standards
   c. Textbooks
   d. Nursing theories and frameworks
   e. Peer-reviewed journals
      (1) Systematic reviews
      (2) Research articles (randomized control trials [RCTs])
      (3) Expert opinion/editorials
      (4) Case studies, case reports
      (5) Clinical practice guidelines
   f. Databases
      (1) MEDLINE, CINAHL, PsychINFO, Cochrane Database, EBSCO, UpToDate, ClinicalKey for Nursing, PubMed, Embase, Ovid, National Guideline Clearinghouse, and Google Scholar

G. Critically appraise the evidence (Jolley, 2020; Melnyk & Fineout-Overholt, 2019)
1. Quantitative evidence (numerical data with statistical analysis)
   a. Why was this study done?
   b. Does the evidence answer or support the clinical question?
   c. What was the sample size?
   d. Are the measures/tools valid and reliable?
   e. How was the data analyzed?
   f. Did any unpredictable events occur during the study?
   g. Are the results valid and reliable?
   h. What do the results mean for current clinical practice?
   i. Determine the strength of the evidence (Melnyk & Fineout-Overholt, 2019)
      (1) Level 1: systematic review or metaanalysis of RCTs—highest level of evidence on which to base practice change
      (2) Level 2: single-site RCT studies
      (3) Level 3: quasi-experimental studies
      (4) Level 4: case or cohort studies
      (5) Level 5: systematic review of descriptive or qualitative studies
      (6) Level 6: single descriptive or qualitative study
      (7) Level 7: expert opinion—lowest level on which to base practice change
2. Qualitative evidence (nonnumeric data)
   a. Are the results of the study valid/credible?
   b. Are the implications of the research noted?
   c. What are the results/outcomes?
   d. How does the researcher identify the approach of the study?

e. Is the significance of the study clear?

f. Is the strategy for sampling guided by the desired outcome?

g. Are procedures for data collection clear?

h. How are the findings presented?

i. How will the results help address the clinical problem?

3. Develop an evidence table to organize data, compare results, and identify themes

4. Critical appraisal of the evidence should occur before piloting a practice change

5. Evidence should be integrated with clinical expertise and patient preferences/values

H. Pilot a practice change in the clinical setting

1. Practice changes should first be implemented in one or two practice areas to ensure feasibility, sustainability, and outcomes

2. If the implementation is successful, it can be implemented across the organization

I. Evaluate practice change and outcomes

1. Evaluation of practice changes is an important step to determine if the impact on health care quality, cost, or patient outcomes was achieved in the clinical setting due to EBP

2. Consider using existing data sources for demonstrating improvement in outcomes

a. Quality indicators (nurse-sensitive indicators, incident reports, sentinel events, and patient satisfaction)

b. Financial/cost–benefit analysis

c. Electronic health records, dashboards, and/or scorecards

d. Survey of staff, patients and family, and/or environment

3. Evaluation tools should be validated and reliable to ensure the accuracy of results

4. Determine if practice change should be implemented across the organization based on reported outcomes or results

5. Monitor for any deviations in practice or changes in outcomes

J. Disseminate outcomes and results

1. EBP is most valuable when clinical practice changes and impact on patient outcomes are communicated effectively and adopted into the current literature

2. Information gained from EBP should be shared with colleagues through, but not limited to, the following methods:

a. Oral and poster presentations at national, regional, or local conferences

b. Panel presentations

c. Roundtable discussions

d. EBP grand rounds

e. Nursing journal publications

f. Institutional or national health care policies

g. News conferences

K. An EBP model can assist nurses with designing, implementing, and sustaining an EBP change

1. Stetler Model of Evidence-Based Practice (Anderson & Jenson, 2019)

2. The Iowa Model of Evidence-Based Practice (Hanrahan, Fowler, & McCarthy, 2019)

3. Model for Evidence-Based Practice Change (Loma Linda University, 2021)

4. The Evidence-Based Advancing Research & Clinical Practice Through Close Collaboration (ACRR) Model (Southern New Hampshire University, 2021)

5. iPARIHS framework (Promoting Action on Research Implementation in Health Services) (Roberts et al., 2020)

6. Clinical Scholar Model (Saunders & Vehviläinen-Julkunen, 2017)

7. The Johns Hopkins Evidence-Based Practice Model (Dang, Dearholt, Bissett, Ascenzi, & Whalen, 2022)

8. ACE Star Model of Knowledge Transformation (Song, Park, Lee, & Stevens, 2021)

IV. Potential roles of the oncology nurse generalist that can facilitate EBP:

A. Identify practice problems by observing patient populations and quality improvement activities. Examples of practice problems include the following:

1. Develop and evaluate a nurse-led intervention to enhance medication knowledge of and adherence to oral chemotherapy (Coyne et al., 2019)

2. Develop, implement, and evaluate an infection–prevention process to reduce hospital-acquired *Clostridium difficile* in oncology patients (Nielsen, Sanchez-Vargas, & Perez, 2019)

B. Participate in the evaluation of existing research or clinical evidence.

1. Use identified measurement criteria to outline staff nurse roles and responsibilities in oncology nursing research (Melnyk & Raderstorf, 2019).

a. ANA Scope and Standards of Practice and Code of Ethics (American Nurses Association, 2021)

b. Nursing practice act of state in which staff nurse is practicing

c. 2016 Oncology Nursing Society Oncology Clinical Trials Nurse Competencies

d. EBP Competencies for Registered Nurses & Advanced Practice Nurses (Melnyk & Raderstorf, 2019)

2. Assist in studies related to high-incidence problem areas or oncology nursing priorities (Von Ah et al., 2019)

a. Consider which nursing interventions promote excellence in oncology nursing and quality cancer care

b. Assist in studies in high-priority research areas and cross-cutting themes in oncology nursing research (Von Ah et al., 2019):

(1) Symptom science

(2) Disparities

(3) Palliative and psychosocial care

(4) Cross-cutting themes

(5) Aging

(6) Survivorship

(7) Health care delivery

(8) Research methodologies

c. Use of standards to identify possible oncology nursing–related research questions (Von Ah et al., 2019):

(1) Standardize assessments and strengthen commonalities among symptom science

(2) Develop and pilot interventions to include vulnerable populations in cancer care and research

(3) Determine interventions that are most effective to improve patient health-related quality of life

C. Collaborate with other health care providers or nurse researchers to identify and implement a potential solution to a specific clinical problem

D. Participate in research activities or research training programs under the guidance of competent nursing researchers that may lead to practice changes and add to EBP (Melnyk & Raderstorf, 2019).

1. Conceptualization and design of a research study

a. Establish that the problem is clinically significant and that a gap exists in the current literature and practice

b. Assess the feasibility of the methods and procedures for the proposed study

2. Implementation of a nursing research study

a. Identify and enroll patients

b. Implement protocol-specific orders

c. Collect study data

d. Educate patients, caregivers, and other health care team members about the study

E. Role of oncology nurses in clinical trials (see Chapter 11)

V. Critiquing research reports for applicability to EBP (Melnyk & Fineout-Overholt, 2019)

A. Guidelines and exact questions for completing a critique vary, depending on the study methodology, and include evaluation of the following:

1. Research problem or purpose

a. What clinical question does the study address? Are the purpose, study variables, and population to be studied explicitly stated?

b. Does the problem have significance for nursing?

2. Are there formally stated hypotheses or research questions that directly relate to the research problem?

3. Theoretic framework (most common in nursing research)

a. Is a theoretic framework identified?

b. Does the framework support the hypothesis, research statement, or question?

4. Design or method

a. What is the study design, and is it well suited to the research problem?

(1) Qualitative research to describe or explore phenomena, gain understanding.

(a) Characteristics—process focused, subjective, and not generalizable

(b) Types—descriptive, survey, phenomenology, and content analysis

(2) Quantitative research to describe relationships between variables, examine cause and effect, and identify facts.

(a) Characteristics—outcome focused, objective, may be generalizable

(b) Types—quasi-experimental, experimental, and correlational

b. Is the method adequate to answer the research question or phenomenon studied?

5. Sampling

a. Are criteria for participant selection clearly identified? For a qualitative study, was purposive sampling done?

b. Is participant selection appropriate for the research purpose and method?

c. Is the sample representative of a larger population?

6. Data collection

a. Are data collection criteria and procedures clearly identified?

b. Do data collection tools seem appropriate for the research question and methodology?

c. Are the tools valid and reliable, and is information about this clear?

d. Is protection of human subjects (e.g., informed consent, protected health information) clearly addressed?

e. For qualitative research, is data saturation described?

7. Data analysis—differs depending on the qualitative or quantitative methodology used

a. Qualitative

(1) Is the data analysis strategy compatible with the study purpose?

(2) Are the findings presented in a manner that allows the reader to verify the researcher's theoretic conclusions?

(3) Do conclusions, implications, and recommendations reflect the findings of the study?

(4) Would a quantitative approach be more appropriate?

b. Quantitative

(1) Does the report include the appropriate statistics?

(2) Were the results of any statistical tests significant, and was this information adequately reported?

(3) Could the study have been strengthened by including qualitative data?

8. Findings, implications, and recommendations
   a. Are important results presented; is their interpretation consistent with the results?
   b. Are specific limitations of the study presented?
   c. Are identified implications appropriate as related to specified study limitations?
   d. Are implications for nursing practice discussed?
   e. Are specific recommendations for future research discussed?
VI. Questions to ask before implementing research findings into nursing practice (Melnyk & Fineout-Overholt, 2019)
   A. Are the results clinically significant and can they be generalized?
   B. Are implementation strategies discussed by the researcher desirable/feasible in practice?
   C. Are institutional support and resources adequate to implement the study findings?
   D. Can the outcome of implementing study findings be measured?

REFERENCES

Anderson, K. K., & Jenson, C. E. (2019). Violence risk–assessment screening tools for acute care mental health settings: Literature review. *Archives of Psychiatric Nursing, 33*(1), 112–119. https://doi.org/10.1016/j.apnu.2018.08.012.

American Nurses Association. (2021). *American Nurses Association recognition of a nursing specialty, approval of a specialty nursing scope of practice statement, acknowledgement of specialty nursing standards of practice, and affirmation of focused practice competencies.* https://www.nursingworld.org/~49d755/globalassets/practiceandpolicy/scope-of-practice/3sc-booklet-2021-june.pdf.

Arthur, E. K., Brown, C. G., Martz, L., Weatherby, L., Purcell, T., Dove, J., et al. (2019). Oncology nurses' attitudes and engagement in nursing research. *Oncology Nursing Forum, 46*(6), 727–737. https://doi.org/10.1188/19.ONF.727-737.

Cengiz, A., & Yoder, L. H. (2020). Assessing nursing students' perceptions of the QSEN competencies: A systematic review of the literature with implications for academic programs. *Worldviews on Evidence-Based Nursing, 17*(4), 275–282. https://doi.org/10.1111/wvn.12458.

Coyne, K. D., Trimble, K. A., Lloyd, A., Petrando, L., Pentz, J., Van Namen, K., et al. (2019). Interventions to promote oral medication adherence in the pediatric chronic illness population: A systematic review from the Children's Oncology Group. *Journal of Pediatric Oncology Nursing, 36*(3), 219–235. https://doi.org/10.1177/1043454219835451.

Dang, D., Dearholt, S., Bissett, K., Ascenzi, J., & Whalen, M. (2022). *Johns Hopkins evidence-based practice for nurses and healthcare professionals: Model and guidelines* (4th ed.). Indianapolis, IN: Sigma Theta Tau International.

Esteban-Sepúlveda, S., Sesé-Abad, A., Lacueva-Pérez, L., Domingo-Pozo, M., Alonso-Fernandez, S., Aquilue-Ballarin, M., et al. (2021). Impact of the implementation of best practice guidelines on nurse's evidence-based practice and on nurses' work environment: Research protocol. *Journal of Advanced Nursing, 77*(1), 448–460. https://doi.org/10.1111/jan.14598.

Hanrahan, K., Fowler, C., & McCarthy, A. M. (2019). Iowa Model revised: Research and evidence-based practice application. *Journal of Pediatric Nursing, 48*, 121–122. https://doi.org/10.1016/j.pedn.2019.04.023.

Jolley, J. (2020). *Introducing research and evidence-based practice for nursing and healthcare professionals* (3rd ed.). London: Taylor & Francis. https://doi.org/10.4324/9780429329456.

Loma Linda University. (2021). *Nurses' guide to evidence-based practice.* https://libguides.llu.edu/evidence/modelsframeworks.

Melnyk, B. M., & Fineout-Overholt, E. (2019). Evidence-based practice in nursing &: *healthcare: A guide to best practice* (4th ed.). Philadelphia, PA: Wolters Kluwer.

Melnyk, B. M., & Raderstorf, T. (2019). *Evidence-based leadership, innovation and entrepreneurship in nursing and healthcare: A practical guide to success.* New York: Springer Publishing Company.

Nielsen, C. S. R., Sanchez-Vargas, R., & Perez, A. (2019). *Clostridium difficile*: Reducing infections using an evidence-based practice initiative. *Clinical Journal of Oncology Nursing, 23*(5), 482–487. https://doi.org/10.1188/19.CJON.482-487.

O'Rourke, N., Lehane, E., Agreli, H., O'Connor, S., Hegarty, J., Leahy-Warren, P., et al. (2019). 16 Adding capacity: Getting EBP into the curriculum for all health professionals in Ireland. *BMJ Evidence-Based Medicine, 24*(Suppl. 1), A12. https://doi.org/10.1136/bmjebm-2019-EBMLive.24.

Roberts, N. A., Janda, M., Stover, A. M., Alexander, K. E., Wyld, D., & Mudge, A. (2020). The utility of the implementation science framework "Integrated Promoting Action on Research Implementation in Health Services" (i-PARIHS) and the facilitator role for introducing patient-reported outcome measures (PROMs) in a medical oncology outpatient department. *Quality of Life Research, 30*(11), 3063–3071. https://doi.org/10.1007/s11136-020-02669-1.

Saunders, H., Gallagher-Ford, L., Kvist, T., & Vehviläinen-Julkunen, K. (2019). Practicing healthcare professionals' evidence-based practice competencies: An overview of systematic reviews. *Worldviews on Evidence-Based Nursing, 16*(3), 176–185. https://doi.org/10.1111/wvn.12363.

Saunders, H., & Vehviläinen-Julkunen, K. (2017). Nurses' evidence-based practice beliefs and the role of evidence-based practice mentors at university hospitals in Finland. *Worldviews on Evidence-Based Nursing, 14*(1), 35–45. https://doi.org/10.1111/wvn.12189.

Song, C. E., Park, H., Lee, M., & Stevens, K. R. (2021). Integrating EBP into an undergraduate research methodology course using the Star Model of Knowledge Transformation: A mixed-method study. *Nurse Education Today, 105*, 105021. https://doi.org/10.1016/j.nedt.2021.105021.

Southern New Hampshire University. (2021). *Evidence based nursing: Models for implementation.* https://libguides.snhu.edu/c.php?g=92409&p=5033539.

Von Ah, D., Brown, C. G., Brown, S. J., Bryant, A. L., Davies, M., Dodd, M., et al. (2019). Research agenda of the Oncology Nursing Society: 2019-2022. *Oncology Nursing Forum, 46*(6), 654–669. https://doi.org/10.1188/19.ONF.654-669.

Young, C., Ball, S., Flott, E., Goodman, J., & Hercinger, M. (2021). Threading QSEN competencies across a baccalaureate nursing program: The development of dedicated QSEN labs. *The Journal of Nursing Education, 60*(9), 526–528. https://doi.org/10.3928/01484834-20210719-02.

58

Principles of Education and Learning

Diane G. Cope

I. Education and learning principles
  A. Educational theory provides the foundation for any formal and informal educational interventions, whether aimed at an individual patient, staff, nurse, or community.
  B. Learning theories can be useful for formulating teaching strategies in clinical practice (Table 58.1; Miller & Stoeckel, 2019).
  C. Definitions.
    1. Education—the process of receiving or giving systematic instruction
    2. Learning—knowledge acquired through experience, study, or being taught
    3. Teaching—encouraging someone to accept something as a fact or principle
II. Patient education principles
  A. Needs assessment (Kitchie, 2023; Miller & Stoeckel, 2019)
    1. What does the patient know and from what source? The patient needs to be asked what he or she understands about the diagnosis, tests, treatment, needed self-care, and follow-up.
    2. What does the patient want to know? This may be different from what the nurse thinks the patient wants to know.
    3. Will any cultural, ethnic, social inequalities, or religious/spiritual beliefs affect the teaching or learning process (Miller & Stoeckel, 2019)? For example, alternative supplements may be a traditional and important part of the patient's belief system, but these supplements may interfere with chemotherapy drugs.
    4. What is the preferred language for providers to relay education content? If the nurse does not speak the same language, what is the alternative teaching plan (Miller & Stoeckel, 2019)? The availability of translators on site should be explored.
    5. Does the patient have a physical (e.g., hearing, vision, mobility, and dexterity) or cognitive (e.g., stroke, confusion, and somnolence) impairment that might impede learning?
    6. Does the patient have a preferred learning style (e.g., visual, aural, or kinesthetic—seeing, hearing, doing; global or analytic—big picture, component parts)?
    7. Assess educational background and level of literacy and health literacy.
  B. Assessment considerations
    1. Individual assessment involves specific questions such as the following: What is the most important thing you want to learn now? Do you have concerns about continuing your normal activities during chemotherapy treatments?
    2. Caregiver assessment. Are you able to assist the patient? What information do you want to learn to assist in your care?
    3. Community assessment before the development of targeted patient education programs or materials (Miller & Stoeckel, 2019)
      a. Survey or checklist
      b. Interested party analysis
      c. Interview and key informant
      d. Focus group
  C. Education goals and objectives; also called *outcome criteria* or *outcome objectives* (Bastable & Capacci, 2023; Miller & Stoeckel, 2019)
    1. Objectives: specific assessment criteria; for example, ability to state four foods with high iron content after reading information regarding foods with high iron content
    2. SMART: acronym for intended outcomes—for example, ability for self-care after discharge
      a. S—specific
      b. M—measurable
      c. A—attainable
      d. R—realistic
      e. T—timely
    3. ABCD: acronym that represents factors affecting education plan
      a. A—audience (who the learner is)
      b. B—behavior (what the learner is to do)
      c. C—condition (under what circumstances)
      d. D—degree (how much; to what extent the learner is to perform)
  D. Teaching plan: decisions about the content (Miller & Stoeckel, 2019)
    1. Who will teach (e.g., staff nurse, patient educator, and patient-to-patient volunteer)?
    2. Methods to teach content based on patient's preference, health literacy, and availability of alternative methods (e.g., one-on-one, group, demonstration

TABLE 58.1	Learning Theories
Learning Theory	**Description**
Behavioral learning theory (operant conditioning, classical conditioning) (Miller & Stoeckel, 2019; Schunk, 2019)	Learning based on observable behaviors that are reinforced to improve the strength of the behavior. Examples of behavioral intervention include relaxation techniques, biofeedback, and visual imagery. Often applied to help pediatric patients with cancer cope with painful procedures; adult patients with cancer can apply them to reduce stress, pain, and anxiety, and to increase coping ability.
Cognitive learning theory (Miller & Stoeckel, 2019; Schunk, 2019)	For knowledge acquisition, internal processes require attention thought, and reasoning for information to be retrieved and applied. An example of cognitive learning is establishing a mnemonic for symptoms to trigger a phone call to the physician or other health care provider. A patient's ability to differentiate systemic from local treatment demonstrates cognitive learning.
Social learning theory (Bandura, 1977; Schunk, 2019)	For learning to lead to knowledge acquisition, an individual may observe and imitate others. Core concepts of social learning theory include attention, retention, reproduction, and motivation.
Motivational learning theory (Schunk, 2019)	Concerned with the processes that describe why and how human behavior is activated and directed. Motivation can result from internal cues or drive (e.g., "I want to be here for my children, so I've got to stop smoking") or environmental (external) cues (e.g., "I have to stop smoking because my workplace has a nonsmoking policy and I hate sneaking out for a cigarette") that activate behavior.
Humanistic learning theory (Braungart & Braungart, 2023)	Everyone is unique, and all individuals have the desire to learn and grow in a positive manner. A learner-directed approach is based on spontaneity, the importance of emotions and feelings, the right of individuals to make their own choices, and human creativity.
Adult learning theory (andragogy) (Knowles et al., 2020)	The adult learner is self-directed, independent, and problem centered. Learning that leads to knowledge acquisition is based on past experience. An example of an adult learning experience would be an independent Internet search for information related to a new cancer diagnosis.

and return demonstration, self-instruction activities, video, computer, print, and combination)?

3. Prepare to teach by reviewing evidence-based teaching practices in the literature (professional journal articles or recent textbooks), standards of care, and hospital procedure manuals and consulting experts (e.g., advanced practice nurses, physicians).

4. Organize and practice all teaching sessions before the actual teaching.

5. Plan teaching to coincide with a teachable moment when the learner might be most likely to be receptive to the message (e.g., smoking cessation in caregivers when a patient is diagnosed with lung cancer; self-care skills before discharge; cancer screening to coincide with a public awareness campaign).

6. Measure learning (e.g., learner explains in own words, return demonstration, quiz, and behavior change).

7. Document learning outcomes (e.g., patient can state the side effects of the medication; patient can demonstrate correct catheter care technique) on care plan, documentation form, or nursing notes.

8. Reassess and reinforce teaching and learning at next available opportunity.

E. Evaluate education (Kitchie, 2023; Miller & Stoeckel, 2019; Worral, 2023)
   1. Assessing knowledge can be done through testing in a variety of ways such as multiple choice, essay, or short answer.
   2. Skills can be assessed through case studies, case presentations, discussions, and written questions.
   3. Knowledge application can be assessed through simulation and observation in a variety of settings.

III. Caregiver education principles
   A. Caregivers may have the same or different learning needs; addressing these learning needs is especially important if the caregiver has a role in caring for the patient at home (Miller & Stoeckel, 2019)
   B. Assess caregiver needs
      1. Assess caregiver needs with or independent of the patient
      2. Identify overlapping separate needs
      3. Confirm patient's permission to include the caregiver in teaching (Health Insurance Portability and Accountability Act)
   C. Scheduling teaching sessions when caregiver can be available
      1. Assess learning; reinforce as necessary
      2. Document caregiver learning needs, as indicated by needs and relationship with patient

IV. Staff education principles (Bastable & Rosario-Gonzalez, 2023)
   A. Assessment: identify staff learning needs, learning styles, and readiness to learn
      1. Target needs assessment to learning objectives, such as those related to critical events, new or revised policies or procedures, and new treatment or orientation of new staff nurses
      2. Institution
         a. New staff nurses must understand hospital and organizational policies and sign off on learning
         b. Staff nurses must be informed when nursing policies or procedures change

3. Self-assessment
   a. Nurses evaluate their own learning needs based on the type of patient for whom they will provide care
   b. Nurses identify learning needs based on interest
B. Establish education objectives (e.g., nurse will demonstrate venipuncture technique; nurse will identify components of a patient's admission assessment)
C. Develop teaching plan
   1. Apply principles of adult learning (Knowles, Holton, Swanson, & Robinson, 2020).
   2. When teaching adults, adults understand rationale for learning content, are self-directed to want to learn content.
   3. Consider prior education and experiences of the learner.
   4. Develop specific content.
   5. Determine teaching method (e.g., class, one-on-one, print or computer, self-directed or teacher-directed, games and simulations, grand rounds, panels and seminars, case studies, and webinars).
   6. Provide staff opportunities in a learning environment.
   7. Establish evaluation criteria (e.g., test, observation, dialog, learner satisfaction, performance improvement, and patient satisfaction).
D. Evaluation
   1. Establish criteria (e.g., test, observation, dialog, learner satisfaction, performance improvement, and patient satisfaction).
   2. Performance analysis (e.g., information is obtained from quality improvement and incident reports; infection control data are analyzed)
   3. Diagnostic methods (e.g., nurses are tested for competence in specific areas; nurses are observed in practice)
V. Community education principles
A. Healthy People 2030—national priorities established by the US Department of Health and Human Services (United States Department of Health and Human, 2020) to improve health and reduce health disparity
B. Community assessment (Williams, 2020)
   1. Analyze data such as descriptive data (e.g., demographics, history, ethnicity, values and beliefs, physical environment, and health and social services) and illness prevalence data; community can be defined geographically (e.g., New York City, state of Missouri), by ethnic or religious group (e.g., African Americans, evangelical Christians), and by interest or characteristics (e.g., sexual orientation, occupation), among many others.
   2. Assess health learning needs (e.g., human immunodeficiency virus and acquired immunodeficiency syndrome prevention, smoking prevention in teens)
   3. Identify common health problems (e.g., high incidence of heart disease, tuberculosis)
   4. Develop a community health diagnosis; for example, senior citizens at risk for social isolation due to lack of public transportation—generally aimed at primary, secondary, and tertiary prevention
C. Community intervention
   1. Work with community (e.g., key informants, leaders, health care community, schools) to prioritize and develop interventions to meet health needs identified in assessment
   2. Implement plan using community resources, advocates, and agencies
   3. Modify intervention for ongoing health needs.
      a. Is it cost-effective?
      b. Were objectives met?
      c. What are the long-term implications of continuing or not continuing the intervention?
D. Community evaluation
   1. Define the role of nurse as educator in the community. Many definitions include the word "populations" as the target of nursing interventions. Definitions include:
      a. American Nurses Association (http://www.ana.org).
      b. American Public Health Association (http://www.apha.org).
      c. State and local departments of health.
   2. Evaluate intervention for impact on identified health need.
      a. Intervention may be modified for ongoing health needs.
      b. Is it cost-effective?
      c. Were objectives met?
   3. What are the long-term implications of continuing or not continuing the intervention? Intervention is evaluated for impact on identified health need.

REFERENCES

Bandura, A. (1977). *Social learning theory*. Hoboken, NJ: Prentice Hall.

Bastable, S. B., & Capacci, N. M. (2023). Behavioral objectives and teaching plans. In S. B. Bastable (Ed.), *Nurse as educator: Principles of teaching and learning* (6th ed., pp. 441–478). Burlington, MA: Jones and Bartlett.

Bastable, S. B., & Rosario-Gonzalez, K. M. (2023). Overview of education in health care. In S. B. Bastable (Ed.), *Nurse as educator: Principles of teaching and learning* (6th ed., pp. 3–38). Burlington, MA: Jones and Bartlett.

Braungart, M. M., & Braungart, R. G. (2023). Applying learning theories to healthcare practice. In S. B. Bastable (Ed.), *Nurse as educator: Principles of teaching and learning for nursing practice* (pp. 75–124). Burlington, MA: Jones and Bartlett.

Kitchie, S. (2023). Determinants of learning. In S. B. Bastable (Ed.), *Nurse as educator: Principles of teaching and learning* (6th ed., pp. 127–180). Burlington, MA: Jones and Bartlett.

Knowles, M. S., Holton, E. F., Swanson, R. A., & Robinson, P. A. (2020). *The adult learner: The definitive classic in adult education and human resource development.* Oxfordshire: Routledge.

Miller, M. A., & Stoeckel, P. R. (2019). *Client education: theory and practice* (3rd ed.). Burlington, MA: Jones and Bartlett.

Schunk, D. H. (2019). *Learning theories: An educational perspective* (8th ed.). London: Pearson Education.

United States Department of Health and Human Services. (2020). *Healthy people 2030.* https://health.gov/healthypeople.

Williams, C. A. (2020). Public health foundations and population health. In M. Stanford & J. Lancaster (Eds.), *Public health nursing: Population-centered health care in the community* (10th ed.). Amsterdam: Elsevier.

Worral, P. S. (2023). Evaluation in healthcare education. In S. B. Bastable (Ed.), *Nurse as educator: Principles of teaching and learning* (6th ed., pp. 629–664). Burlington, MA: Jones and Bartlett.

59

Legal Issues

Nezar Ahmed Salim

I. Overview
  A. Legal liability terms and definitions (https://dictionary.law.com/)
    1. Negligence—deviation from the acceptable standard of care that a reasonable person would use in a specific situation
    2. Malpractice—deviation from a professional standard of care
    3. Duty—care relationship between patient and provider
    4. Breach of duty—failure to meet an acceptable standard of care
    5. Defamation—the act of harming the reputation of another by making false statements to a third person
    6. False imprisonment—a restraint of a person in a bounded area without justification or consent
    7. Slander—a defamatory statement expressed in a transitory form, especially speech
    8. Proximate cause—the cause that directly produces an event and without which the event would not have occurred
    9. Civil—of or pertaining to private rights and remedies that are sought by action or suit but distinct from criminal proceedings
    10. Assault—the threat of, or use of, force on another that causes that person to have a reasonable apprehension of imminent harmful or offensive contact
  B. Nurse practice (Russell, 2017)
    1. Interact with individuals who may be most vulnerable
    2. Nurses are among the most trusted professionals
    3. Legal, regulatory, and practice standards are the foundation of practice
      a. Standards ensure that nurses are well-prepared, competent nurses
      b. Adhering to legal principles and standards can help mitigate risks and unintended negative outcomes
      c. Nurses are individually licensed and are consequently responsible for their nursing actions
  C. Common causes of litigation against nurses
    1. In the United States a patient may allege medical malpractice against nurses, which is typically defined by the failure to provide the degree of care which could result in injury to the patient (Bono, Wermuth, & Hipskind, 2021; Cheluvappa & Selvendran, 2020)
    2. Examples of litigation:
      a. Lack of informed consent
      b. Negligence or breach of duty
      c. Improper medical device use
      d. Not following standards of care
      e. Failure to communicate effectively/appropriately
      f. Inadequate or inappropriate patient assessment, monitoring, or teaching
      g. Lack of patient advocacy
      h. Failure to communicate/report changes in patient condition
      i. Inadequate or inappropriate treatment or care
      j. Medication errors
      k. Inappropriate delegation or supervision—lack of consideration for delegating the right task, to the right person, at the right time, under the right circumstances, and providing the right supervision
      l. Inadequate documentation
      m. Working while impaired (substance use, fatigue)

II. Regulation of nursing practice: State Board of Nursing (BON) Jurisdiction
  (Stoelting-Gettelfinger, 2018)
  A. State BONs—provide oversight of nursing practice by enforcing the state nurse practice act to protect the health, welfare, and safety of the public
    1. State BONs typically have employed staff (e.g., executive officer, attorney, and administrative staff) and appointed or elected representatives of various nursing groups (e.g., registered nurses, licensed practical or vocational nurses, and advanced practice registered nurses).
    2. Board membership, selection, and length of term of appointed or elected members are determined by the state and vary by state.
    3. Nurse can influence health care policy and nursing practice via the state BON.
      a. Appointed or elected BON member
      b. Attend BON public meetings
      c. Advocate for issues before the BON—issues important to cancer care and cancer nursing

B. National Council of State Boards of Nursing
   1. Develops the National Council Licensure for Registered Nurses examination
   2. Encourages consistency among state BONs (e.g., provides model language for nurse practice acts) (National Council of State Boards of Nursing [NCSBN], 2022a)
C. Nursing Licensure Compact
   1. Allows nurses to practice (physically, electronically, and telephonically) in multiple states without obtaining multiple nursing licenses (NCSBN, 2022b)
   2. Approximately 39 states currently have this legislation, with additional states pursuing compact membership
   3. Affects traveling nurses, nurses who live near state lines, nurses who move, large health care organizations with sites in multiple states, and distance and online nursing education students/programs
D. Nurse practice acts
   1. Define nursing roles, titles, and scopes of practice
   2. Define educational program standards, requirements for licensure, and grounds for disciplinary action

III. Laws govern nursing practice (Cassiani, Lecorps, Rojas Cañaveral, da Silva, & Fitzgerald, 2020)
   A. Primary law
      1. Constitutions, legislation, rules, and cases are the primary sources of law. Lawmaking powers are divided among three branches of government: executive; legislative; and judicial. These three departments of government, whether federal or state, create fundamental sources of legislation.
   B. Administrative law
      1. Definitions of regulatory terms.
         a. Nursing regulation ensures that safe nursing care is provided to the public.
         b. Regulation mechanism:
            (1) The initial review of credentials during registration
            (2) The periodic professional registration renewal, competency exams
            (3) Continuing education serve as mechanisms to safeguard the public
      2. Rules, regulation, executive order, and directive.
         a. The President of the United States issues executive orders.
         b. Government administrative agencies (such as the Environmental Protection Agency) create rules and regulations.
      3. Statement issued by a government-sanctioned agency (e.g., BON) with the intent to clarify a law (e.g., the nursing practice act) or explain the agency's structure or processes.
      4. For specific legislation, there is a public comment process.
      5. Once adopted, these regulations and rules have the power and effect of law.

6. When there is an alleged breach of the states' nursing practice legislation, the BON is involved (NCSBN, 2022c; Nguyen, 2019).
C. Branches that affect nursing practice
   1. Legislative
   2. Judicial
      a. Issues decisions (opinions, cases), published in case reports
      b. Common law shaped by judges
         (1) From judges interpreting specific cases, common law evolves as doctrine rather than based on abstract principles
         (2) Changes over time
   3. Important element: stare decisis, which means that courts are bound to follow earlier decisions ("precedents") (University of California Hasting Law, 2022)
      a. Secondary sources of judicial actions
      b. Plain-language publications; main sources of basic law, used as a basis for legal studies
      c. Not enforceable in any court; not laws
      d. Accessible and intelligible, they arrange and explain; provide direction to key legislation
      e. Can cite in briefs, memoranda
      f. Examples: treatises, practice guides, legal encyclopedias, and law journal articles
      g. Legal journals may have an impact on legislation. (University of California Hasting Law, 2022)

IV. Disciplining nursing practice: State BON Jurisdiction (NCSBN, 2022c):
   A. Practice related
      1. Failure to uphold standard of care (e.g., failure to assess patients or document care, practicing outside the scope of practice or without a license).
      2. Substance abuse (e.g., impairment related to controlled substances or alcohol).
      3. Diversion of controlled substances—misuse of controlled substances intended for patients (e.g., stealing pain medications from work for own personal use, to give to others, or for financial gain).
         a. Professional boundary violations—extending therapeutic relationship for personal benefit (e.g., flirting, showing favoritism, and keeping secrets with patients)
         b. Sexual misconduct—inappropriate sexual contact between nurse and patient (e.g., behaviors considered seductive, sexually demeaning, and harassing)
         c. Abuse—physical, mental, or emotional maltreatment of patients/clients
         d. Fraud—misrepresenting the truth (e.g., overstating own credentials or experience, falsely documenting care, and submitting/authorizing inaccurate records for billing)
         e. Positive criminal background checks—rules vary according to the extent of past criminal activity and potential future risk to patients (e.g., the

more severe the past criminal activity, the more extensive potential consequences on licensure).

    f. Improper social media use—unethical, unprofessional, insensitive use of social media (e.g., posting disparaging comments about patients even without using the patient name, posting photos of work settings, breaching patient privacy or confidentiality, and texting information about patients to coworkers).

B. Potential disciplinary action by BONs (NCSBN, 2022c).
1. Fine or civil penalty
2. Referral to alternative-to-discipline program
3. Public reprimand or censure
4. Requirements for monitoring, remediation, and education
5. Limitation or restriction of practice
6. Separation from practice (e.g., suspension, loss of license)
7. Remediation (various educational content or exercises)

V. Health Care: Patient's Bill of Rights in Health Care
A. A variety of documents from national organizations and health care institutions outline what consumers can expect from the health care environment.
B. The Affordable Care Act legislated patient's rights in the health care environment (U.S. Department of Health & Human Services, 2022).
1. Provides coverage to Americans with preexisting conditions
2. Mandates insurers to offer dependent coverage for children to age 26
3. Prohibits annual and lifetime limits on coverage
4. Prohibits preexisting condition exclusions for children
5. Prohibits arbitrary withdrawals of insurance coverage
6. Mandates essential health services (e.g., screening, vaccination)
7. Provides four tiers of benefit coverage (e.g., low to high monthly premiums and out-of-pocket costs).
8. Established individual mandate for insurance coverage (later repealed)
C. Rights for hospitalized individuals (Olejarczyk, 2021).
1. To be treated justly.
2. To receive information about care.
3. To refuse treatment.
4. To have confidential medical care.
5. To have continuity of care.
6. To have pain treated to a level of toleration.
7. To be free from physical restraints (unless the patient is thought to be likely to hurt himself or others).
8. To view medical records.
9. To have explanations about bills.
10. To provide advanced directives.
VI. Standards of Practice in Context of Legal Issues
A. Intent of Standards of Practice (Russell, 2017)

1. National scope
2. Practice expectations for organizations and individuals
3. Guide nurses, employers, and educators
4. Foundational reference for legal situations to determine whether an individual or organization met established standard of care
B. Nursing Professional Practice Standards
1. Nursing—scope and standards of practice (American Nurses Association [ANA], 2021a)
2. Code of ethics for nurses—with interpretative statements (ANA, 2015a)
3. Nursing's social policy statement—the essence of the profession (ANA, 2015b)
C. Health Care Institutions: accreditation and certification agencies or programs
1. Outline nationally determined practice expectations for individuals or organizations
2. Provide guidance for nurses, employers, and educators and are often used in legal situations to determine whether an individual or organization met what is regarded as the standard of care
D. Oncology nursing practice standards (Table 59.1; Blecher, Ireland, & Watson, 2016; Camp-Sorrell & Matey, 2017; Jacobs & Mayer, 2015; Lubejko & Wilson, 2019; Neuss et al., 2017; Oncology Nursing Society [ONS], n.d.a., n.d.b; Wiley, Galioto, Matey, & Wyant, 2017)
1. Practice standards can be used by individual nurses, health care organizations, and educational programs to promote and support high-quality cancer care
E. Oncology-specific accreditation and certification agencies and programs (Table 59.1)
1. Oncology Nursing Certification Corporation (ONCC) (https://www.oncc.org/)
2. American College of Surgeons—Commission on Cancer (https://www.facs.org/quality-programs/cancer/coc)
3. Quality Oncology Practice Initiative (QOPI) (https://practice.asco.org/quality-improvement/quality-programs/quality-oncology-practice-initiative)
F. Health Care Institutions: Accreditation and certification agencies or programs
1. The Joint Commission (https://www.jointcommission.org)
2. National Patient Safety Goals (https://www.jointcommission.org/standards_information/npsgs.aspx)
3. Magnet Recognition Program (https://www.nursingworld.org/organizational-programs/magnet)
4. Occupational Safety and Health Administration (OSHA) (https://www.osha.gov)
5. Centers for Disease Control and Prevention (https://www.cdc.gov/)
6. Department of Health and Human Services (www.hhs.gov)

TABLE 59.1 Oncology Nursing Society Standards for Practice

Standard Title	Standard Description	Link
Access Device Standards of Practice for Oncology Nursing (Camp-Sorrell & Matey, 2017)	Provides an overview of literature and standards of practice related to device selection, care, optimal use, and legal implications in oncology care.	Access device standards of practice for oncology nursing—Memorial Sloan Kettering Cancer Center (exlibrisgroup.com)
ONS Nursing Documentation Standards for Cancer Treatment (Wiley et al., 2017)	Provides a comprehensive overview of documentation standards for multiple cancer treatments, use of vascular access devices, blood product transfusion, and chemotherapy extravasation.	Oncology Nursing Society | e-Books https://www.ons.org/sites/default/files/publication_pdfs/ONS%20Nursing%20Documentation%20Standards%20-%20DRAFT.pdf
ONS Standard for Educating Nurses Who Administer Chemotherapy and Biotherapy (ONS, n.d.a)	Describes pathways for chemotherapy/biotherapy course and/or certificate completion based on administration volume or number of chemotherapy and/or biotherapy agents.	https://www.ons.org/sites/default/files/ONS_Standard_Educating_Nurses_Chemo_Pathway_Web_111016.pdf
Statement on the Scope and Standards of Oncology Nursing Practice Generalist and Advanced Practice (Lubejko & Wilson, 2019)	Describes the scope of oncology nursing practice, standards of care for RNs and advanced practice RNs, and professional performance issues.	https://www.ons.org/standards-and-reports/scope-and-standards-oncology-nursing-practice
Standards of Oncology Education: Patient/Significant Other and Public (4th ed.) (Blecher et al., 2016)	Describes formal and informal education standards that oncology nurses can use for planning and evaluating education for patients and significant others.	https://www.ons.org/sites/default/files/StandardsPatientEducation_PublicComment.pdf
Standards of Oncology Nursing Education: Generalist and Advanced Practice Levels (4th ed.) (Jacobs & Mayer, 2015)	Addresses standards of oncology nursing academic and clinical education for faculty and/or clinical educators.	https://www.ons.org/sites/default/files/Public%20Comment%20Standards%20Nursing%20Education%204th%20Edition.pdf
Survivorship Care Standards for Accreditation (ONS, n.d.b)	Describes the CoC and NAPBC survivorship care plans requirements, including documentation, implementation, and key elements of the care plan.	https://www.cancer.northwestern.edu/docs/news-docs/JCSO_May_192_Garcia.pdf Creating and Sustaining Survivorship Care Plans in Practice | ONS Voice (https://voice.ons.org/news-and-views/survivorship-care-plans-in-practice)
2016 Updated American Society of Clinical Oncology/Oncology Nursing Society chemotherapy administration safety standards, including standards for pediatric oncology (Neuss et al., 2017)	This paper describes the recommended components of safe administration of enteral and parenteral chemotherapy, including policies and procedures outlining staff training and continuing education, chemotherapy preparation, chemotherapy administration, and patient education and management guidelines.	https://www.ons.org/sites/default/files/2016%20ASCO_ONS%20Chemo%20Standards.pdf

CoC, Commission on Cancer; *NAPBC*, National Accreditation Program for Breast Centers; *RNs*, Registered Nurses.

7. National Institutes of Health (https://www.nih.gov)
8. Centers for Medicare and Medicaid (https://www.cms.gov/)
9. National Institute for Occupational Safety and Health (https://www.cdc.gov/niosh/index.htm)

VII. Legal issues: individuals for cancer (Ponto, 2018; Schulmeister, 2018; Zablow, 2022)
   A. Advance care planning (e.g., advance directives, orders for life-sustaining treatment)
   B. Bankruptcy—3% of cancer survivors file for bankruptcy (Cavallo, 2022; Yabroff, Bradley, & Shih, 2020)
   C. Competence for decision-making
   D. Disability insurance
   E. Employment discrimination
   F. Genetic testing and discrimination
   G. Health insurance
   H. Hospital-acquired conditions (HACs) (CMS, 2021).
   I. Informed consent for chemotherapy (oral and parenteral)
   J. Lesbian, gay, bisexual, and transgender discrimination (Cahill, 2018; CancerCare, 2021)
   K. Medical errors
   L. Organ and tissue donation
   M. Privacy and confidentiality
   N. Survivorship care planning
   O. Time off from work (Family & Medical Leave Act)
   P. Withdrawing treatment—right to receive or discontinue treatment

VIII. Oncology Nursing Practice: legal implications (Ponto, 2018; Salim et al., 2018; Schulmeister, 2018)
   A. Patient-related issues
      1. Adverse drug events
      2. Iatrogenic/HACs (e.g., falls, infection)
      3. Inadequate patient/family education
      4. Proper use of telephone triage
      5. Treatment-related errors (e.g., chemotherapy administration errors)

6. Vesicant administration
7. Withholding and withdrawing life support

B. Professional practice/nursing issues
1. Drug or substance diversion
2. Documentation errors/omissions (e.g., inadequate/nonexistent informed consent, patient/family education, or telephone triage documentation)
3. Exposure to occupational and environmental hazards
4. Improper risk evaluation and mitigation strategies reporting
5. Lack of competency/lack of competency documentation (e.g., chemotherapy administration, patient safety, and preventing iatrogenic conditions)
6. Malpractice
7. Mandatory reporting (state regulations requiring nurses and other health care providers to report certain conditions or events, e.g., suspected child, sexual, domestic, or elder abuse; communicable diseases; death)
8. Misuse of social media (NCSBN, 2018)
9. Off-label drug or device use (Oregon State Board of Nursing, 2018)
10. Practicing outside of authorized scope of practice
11. Workplace behavior and performance issues—lateral violence, bullying, and verbal intimidation (Verschuren, Tims, & de Lange, 2021)
    a. Can range in severity from disruptive behaviors to assault
    b. Negative work behavior (NWB) defined as an "exposure to ongoing negative and unwanted behavior by superiors or colleagues" (Glambek, Skogstad, & Einarsen, 2020)
       (1) NWB is harmful to employees and the organization (Van Steijn et al., 2019)
       (2) NWB includes: bullying, unwanted sexual attention, mobbing, physical and verbal assaults, sexual violence, verbal discrimination, verbal and sexual harassment, stalking, and assaults by internal and external actor types (Magnavita et al., 2019)
       (3) Currently no national workplace laws governing workplace bullying, but some state laws have established penalties

C. OSHA—requires employers to provide a workplace free from hazards and recommends policies and procedures that reflect "zero-tolerance for all forms of violence from all sources" (Occupational Safety and Health Administration, 2019)

D. Support staff education to understand their role in situations involving lateral violence, bullying, and intimidation

IX. Legislative policy issues: oncology care (ONS, n.d.c)
A. Quality cancer care
B. Patient/staff safety
C. Workforce/education
D. Value of oncology nurses
E. Scope of practice (ASCO, 2022)
F. Access to care
G. Clinical trials
H. Drug shortage
I. Federal funding for cancer research

X. Minimizing the risk of malpractice or disciplinary action (Bono et al., 2021)
A. Develop skills in interpersonal communication—positive relationships with patients and families reduce the likelihood of a patient or family complaint
   1. Communicate clearly when educating patients and families
   2. Listen carefully to family members' questions and concerns

B. Maintain knowledge and skills
   1. Attend relevant continuing education programs
   2. Obtain specialty certification
   3. Obtain an advanced or graduate degree
   4. Join relevant professional associations (e.g., Oncology Nursing Society)
   5. Become involved in advocacy initiatives with nursing professional organizations
   6. Verify that job description fits within state-defined scope of practice
   7. Maintain individual professional liability insurance—can protect a nurse beyond what employer policies may cover
   8. Maintain a "job well done" file—keeping letters of commendation, thank-you notes or cards from patients and family members, colleagues, and supervisors
   9. Keep a list of community service activities which demonstrate civic-mindedness (e.g., participation in cancer screening activities; teaching community basic life support classes; leading cancer support groups)
   10. Maintain positive relationship with supervisor—demonstrating willingness to contribute to the professional environment (e.g., serving on unit or institutional committees; leading journal club)
   11. Keep abreast of current regulatory and practice issues through state BON
   12. Maintain professional boundaries with patients
   13. Respect physical limitations (e.g., fatigue related to rotating shifts, overtime)
   14. Respond quickly to a medical emergency
   15. Always think about the worst-case scenario
   16. Never skip monitoring vital signs during procedures
   17. Talk directly to the doctor
   18. Document nursing on time

XI. Documentation and legal risk
A. Reflects the quality of care
B. Can be used in legal disputes to determine whether a standard of care was met

1. Nurses may be deposed and questioned about own or others' documentation
2. In court of law, patient's health record is the legal record of treatment delivered to that patient
3. Accrediting bodies and risk managers assess the quality of treatment provided to patients
4. To verify patient care provided, insurance firms employ documentation systems. Nurses may be deposed and questioned about own or others' documentation

C. Nursing documentation
   1. Accurate, complete documentation demonstrates the scope and quality of the nursing care provided; includes:
      a. Results of patient care
      b. Patient treatment
      c. Patient and family education
      d. Additional documentation: patient's vital signs, assessment results, care plan, and interventions and response to interventions
   2. Documentation is an important tool to effectively communicate with the health care team.
   3. Accurate documentation.
   4. Evidence that nurse has applied professional nursing standards, using nursing knowledge, skills, and judgment (Craven, Hirnle, & Henshaw, 2021).
   5. Reduces the risk of misunderstandings and errors.
   6. Patient documentation time stamp:
      a. Clearly indicates the date/time of events
         (1) Electronic medical records (EMR) post date and time of note (Accreditation Association for Hospitals and Health Systems, 2020).
         (2) Time is posted according to facility requirements, 24-hour military time or "a.m." or "p.m."
   7. Actions and interventions.
      a. Use approved abbreviations (Joint Commission, 2020)
   8. Ensure personal security when documenting:
      a. Privacy when documenting nurse note
      b. Log off when EMR documentation complete
      c. Never give password to others (Joint Commission, 2021)
   9. Follow facility's error-correction procedures (i.e., recording note in incorrect chart)
      a. Rather than leave a field blank, enter "N/A" (not applicable) if information does not apply to the patient.
      b. Do not tamper with paperwork or the clinical record.

XII. Resources
   A. American Association of Legal Nurse Consultants—www.aalnc.org
   B. American Hospital Association—www.aha.org
   C. American Nurses Association—nursingworld.org
   D. Cancer Legal Resource Center—thedrlc.org
   E. National Cancer Legal Services Network—askjan.org
   F. National Council of State Board of Nursing—www.ncsbn.org
   G. Oncology Nursing Society—ons.org
   H. ONCC—oncc.org
   I. QOPI—https://practice.asco.org/quality-improvement/quality-programs/quality-oncology-practice-initiative
   J. National Cancer Institute—cancer.gov/research

REFERENCES

Accreditation Association for Hospitals and Health Systems. (2020). *Standard 10.00.03. Healthcare Facilities Accreditation Program: Accreditation requirements for acute care hospitals.* Chicago, IL: Accreditation Association for Hospitals and Health Systems. (Level VII).

American Nurses Association (ANA). (2015a). *Code of ethics for nurses with interpretive statements.* Silver Spring, MD: American Nurses Association.

American Nurses Association (ANA). (2015b). *Nursing's social policy statement: The essence of the profession.* Silver Spring, MD: American Nurses Association.

American Nurses Association (ANA). (2021a). *Nursing: Scope and standards of practice* (4th ed.). Silver Spring, MD: American Nurses Association.

American Society of Clinical Oncology (ASCO). (2022). *Public policy advocacy.* https://www.cancer.net/research-and-advocacy/public-policy-advocacy.

Blecher, C. S., Ireland, A. M., & Watson, J. L. (Eds.), (2016). *Standards of oncology education: Patient/significant other and public* (4th ed.). Pittsburgh, PA: Oncology Nursing Society.

Bono, M.J., Wermuth, H.R., & Hipskind, J.E. (2021). Medical malpractice. In: *StatPearls.* Treasure Island, FL: StatPearls Publishing. Retrieved from https://www.ncbi.nlm.nih.gov/books/NBK470573/.

Cahill, S. R. (2018). Legal and policy issues for LGBT patients with cancer or at elevated risk of cancer. *Seminars in Oncology Nursing, 34*(1), 90–98. https://doi.org/10.1016/j.soncn.2017.12.006.

Camp-Sorrell, D., & Matey, L. (2017). *Access device standards of practice for oncology nursing.* Pittsburgh, PA: Oncology Nursing Society.

Cancer Care. (2021). *Coping with cancer as an LGBTQ+ person.* https://www.cancercare.org/publications/209-coping_with_cancer_as_an_lgbtq_person.

Cassiani, S., Lecorps, K., Rojas Cañaveral, L. K., da Silva, F., & Fitzgerald, J. (2020). Regulation of nursing practice in the Region of the Americas. *Pan American Journal of Public Health, 44*, e93. https://doi.org/10.26633/RPSP.2020.93.

Cavallo, J. (2022). Cancer survivors face substantial medical financial hardship. *The ASCO Post.* https://ascopost.com/news/january-2020/cancer-survivors-face-substantial-medical-financial-hardship/.

Cheluvappa, R., & Selvendran, S. (2020). Medical negligence—Key cases and application of legislation. *Annals of Medicine and Surgery, 57*, 205–211. https://doi.org/10.1016/j.amsu.2020.07.017.

CMS. (2021). *Hospital acquired conditions.* https://www.cms.gov/Medicare/Quality-Initiatives-Patient-Assessment-Instruments/Value-Based-Programs/HAC/Hospital-Acquired-Conditions.

Craven, R. F., Hirnle, C. J., & Henshaw, C. M. (2021). *Fundamentals of nursing: Human health and function* (9th ed.). Alphen aan den Rijn: Wolters Kluwer.

Glambek, M., Skogstad, A., & Einarsen, S. V. (2020). Does the number of perpetrators matter? An extension and re-analysis of workplace bullying as a risk factor for exclusion from working life. *Journal of Community and Applied Social Psychology, 1*, 1–8. https://doi.org/10.1002/casp.2456.

Jacobs, L. A., & Mayer, D. K. (2015). *Standards of oncology nursing education: Generalist and advanced practice levels* (4th ed.). Pittsburgh, PA: Oncology Nursing Society.

Lubejko, B. G., & Wilson, B. J. (2019). *Oncology nursing scope & standards of practice* . Pittsburgh, PA: Oncology Nursing Society.

Magnavita, N., Di Stasio, E., Capitanelli, I., Lops, E. A., Chirico, F., & Garbarino, S. (2019). Sleep problems and workplace violence: A systematic review and meta-analysis. *Frontiers in Neuroscience, 13*, 997. https://doi.org/10.3389/fnins.2019.00997.

National Council of State Boards of Nursing (NCSBN). (2022a). *NCLEX and other exams.* https://www.ncsbn.org/index.htm.

National Council of State Boards of Nursing (NCSBN). (2022b). *Nurse licensure compact (NLC).* https://www.ncsbn.org/nurse-licensure-compact.htm.

National Council of State Boards of Nursing (NCSBN). (2022c). *Initial review of complaint.* https://www.ncsbn.org/1616.htm#6038.

National Council of State Boards of Nursing (NCSBN). (2018). *A nurse's guide to the use of social media.* https://www.ncsbn.org/NCSBN_SocialMedia.pdf.

Neuss, M. N., Gilmore, T. R., Belderson, K. M., Billett, A. L., Conti-Kalchik, T., Harvey, B. E., et al. (2017). 2016 Updated American Society of Clinical Oncology/Oncology Nursing Society Chemotherapy Administration Safety Standards, Including Standards for Pediatric Oncology. *Oncology Nursing Forum, 44*(1), A1–A13. https://doi.org/10.1200/JOP.2016.017905.

Nguyen, J. (2019). *Legal and ethical issues for health professions* (4th ed.). Amsterdam: Elsevier.

Occupational Safety and Health Administration. (2019). *Workers' rights booklet.* https://www.osha.gov/publications/publication-products?publication_title=Workers%27+Rights+Booklet.

Olejarczyk, J.P., & Young, M. (2021). Patient rights and ethics. In: *StatPearls.* Treasure Island, FL: StatPearls Publishing. Retrieved from https://www.ncbi.nlm.nih.gov/books/NBK538279/.

Oncology Nursing Society (ONS). (n.d.a). *ONS standard for educating nurses who administer chemotherapy and biotherapy.* Pittsburgh, PA: Oncology Nursing Society.

Oncology Nursing Society (ONS). (n.d.b). *Survivorship care standards for accreditation.* Pittsburgh, PA: Oncology Nursing Society.

Oncology Nursing Society (ONS). (n.d.c). *Legislative and regulatory health policy agenda 115th congress, 1st session.* Retrieved from https://www.ons.org/sites/default/files/ONS_HP_Agenda_115th_1st_Session_012317.pdf.

Oregon State Board of Nursing. (2018). *Prescriptive and dispensing authority in Oregon: For advanced practice registered nurses.* https://www.oregon.gov/osbn/Documents/Booklet_prescriptive_authority.pdf.

Ponto, J. (2018). Legal issues in cancer care. In M. M. Gullatte (Ed.), *Clinical guide to antineoplastic therapy: A chemotherapy handbook* (4th ed.). Pittsburgh, PA: Oncology Nursing Society.

Russell, K. A. (2017). Nurse practice acts guide and govern: Update 2017. *Journal of Nursing Regulation, 8*(3), 18–25. https://doi.org/10.1016/S2155-8256(17)30156-4.

Salim, A., Nematollahi, R., Tuffaha, M., Chehab, F. H., Nigim, H. A., Al, A. A., et al. (2018). Legal and ethical issues among oncology nurses toward end of life care. *Advanced Practices in Nursing, 3*(1), 149. https://doi.org/10.4172/2573-0347.1000149.

Schulmeister, L. C. (2018). Legal and safety issues. In C. H. Yarbro, D. Wujcik, & B. H. Gobel (Eds.), *Cancer nursing: Principles and practice* (8th ed.). Burlington, MA: Jones and Bartlett.

Stoelting-Gettelfinger, W. (2018). Nursing licensure and certification. In G. Roux & J.A. Halstead (Eds.), *Issues and trends in nursing: Practice, policy, and leadership* (pp. 63–83). Burlington, MA: Jones & Bartlett.

The Joint Commission. (2020). *Do not use list: The Joint Commission fact sheet.* https://www.jointcommission.org/resources/news-and-multimedia/fact-sheets/facts-about-do-not-use-list/.

The Joint Commission. (2021). *Standard RC.01.03.01. Comprehensive accreditation manual for hospitals.* Oakbrook Terrace, IL: The Joint Commission. (Level VII).

U.S. Department of Health & Human Services. (2022). *Affordable care act.* https://www.hhs.gov/healthcare/about-the-aca/index.html.

University of California Hasting Law. (2022). *Academic success resources for students: Sources of law: Cases, statutes, secondary sources and more.* https://libguides.uchastings.edu/academic-success/sourcesoflaw.

Van Steijn, M. E., Scheepstra, K. W. F., Yasar, G., Olff, M., de Vries, M. C., & van Pampus, M. G. (2019). Occupational well-being in pediatricians: A survey about work-related posttraumatic stress, depression, and anxiety. *European Journal of Pediatrics, 178*, 681–693. https://doi.org/10.1007/s00431-019-03334-7.

Verschuren, C. M., Tims, M., & de Lange, A. H. (2021). A systematic review of negative work behavior: Toward an integrated definition. *Frontiers in Psychology, 12*, 726973. https://doi.org/10.3389/fpsyg.2021.726973.

Wiley, K., Galioto, M., Matey, L., & Wyant, T. (2017). *Oncology Nursing Society Documentation standards for cancer treatment.* Pittsburgh, PA: Oncology Nursing Society.

Yabroff, K. R., Bradley, C., & Shih, Y. T. (2020). Understanding financial hardship among cancer survivors in the United States: Strategies for prevention and mitigation. *Journal of Clinical Oncology, 38*(4), 292–301. https://doi.org/10.1200/JCO.19.01564.

Zablow, S. (2022). Legal assistance and cancer. New York: CancerCare. Retrieved from https://www.cancercare.org/publications/331legal_assistance_finding_resources_and_support.

60

Ethical Issues

Jeanne Marie Erickson and Joshua Hardin

I. Ethics overview
  A. Concepts and definitions
    1. Ethics is the study about what is morally good, whether actions are judged to be right or wrong, and how people and institutions choose ethical actions and implement those actions. Ethics influence all nursing interactions—ethical dilemmas are not isolated or sporadic (Hoskins, Grady, & Ulrich, 2018).
  B. Ethics and oncology nurses
    1. Oncology nurses can frequently experience ethical issues, since they care for cancer patients who are diagnosed with life-threatening diseases and undergo complex treatments (Neumann, Counts, & Jernigan, 2019).
    2. Oncology nurses may experience ethical dilemmas in practice at a prevalence rate of 27.8% or 1 in 90 patient encounters (Tuca et al., 2021).
    3. Ethics constantly evolves due to changes in professional roles, codes, and legislation, as well as changes in society and culture (Rainer, Schneider, & Lorenz, 2018).
  C. Relevant ethical concepts and definitions
    1. *Ethical conflict* describes the tension created when moral notions of what is right are compromised or ethical choices incompatible with personal, disciplinary, or organizational values occur leading to intractable moral–ethical dilemmas (Liu et al., 2021).
      a. Common causes of ethical conflict involve the type and quantity of information provided, disagreements about therapy, treatment declination, clinical trial expectations, assisted suicide, and withdrawal of care (Tuca et al., 2021).
    2. When ethical conflicts are not adequately resolved, nurses may experience *moral distress*, a "painful" experience that "occurs when a nurse cannot follow through with moral actions" and feels their professional integrity has been compromised (McAndrew, Leske, & Schroeter, 2018, p. 522).
      a. Nurses experience moral distress when they witness patient suffering. Distress can be prompted by:
        (1) Lack of communication among clinicians

        (a) Aggressive and prolonged care that is not in the best interest of patients, and a lack of organizational support (McAndrew & Hardin, 2020).
      b. Moral distress is associated with work avoidance behaviors and burnout (Fumis, Junqueira Amarante, de Fatima Nascimento, & Vieira Junior, 2017; Marturano, Hermann, Giordano, & Trotta, 2020).
      c. When caring for patients, the nurse's ability or inability to act as a free moral agent directly impacts the health and well-being of patients and families (Ulrich, 2018).
    3. *Moral residue* is the lasting negative emotional and physical effects of moral distress that accumulate and remain with nurses over time, leading to negative effects on patient care and job resignations (Henrich et al., 2017).
    4. *Moral injury* is psychological distress caused by a traumatic violation of one's ethical code or values.
      a. Although not a mental health diagnosis, moral injury can lead to depression, suicidal thoughts, and posttraumatic stress disorder (Greenberg, Docherty, Gnanapragasam, & Wessely, 2020).
      b. During the COVID-19 pandemic, clinicians may have experienced sustained and demanding stress when providing direct patient care; this may have resulted in moral injury (see Box 60.1).
  D. Individuals perceive ethical issues differently, based on their individual values, knowledge, reflective thinking, and reasoning.
II. American Nurses Association (ANA) Code of Ethics
  A. Overview
    1. The *Code of Ethics for Nurses with Interpretive Statements* (American Nurses Association [ANA], 2015), referred to here as *the code*, may be accessed free online via the ANA's website (www.nursing world.org) or purchased through most book distributors.
    2. The code (ANA, 2015) articulates nursing's core values to the public and the discipline. The ANA's, (2015) ethical code outlines general provisions followed by interpretive statements to help nurses

---

BOX 60.1   Moral Injury and the COVID-19 Pandemic

- The unprecedented and sometimes devastating ethical choices required during the COVID-19 pandemic will have lasting and unforeseen consequences for the well-being of oncology clinicians (Nickitas, 2021).
- The experiences shared by front-line clinicians during the pandemic that include mass death, absence of family at the bedside, shifting treatment protocols, powerlessness and fear, and care rationing constitute a traumatic experience (Hossain & Clatty, 2021).
- The consequences of the COVID-19 crisis will likely affect nursing as a discipline. In a letter to the Department of Health and Human Services, the American Nurses Association (ANA) expressed concern that the nursing staff shortage has been exacerbated by the COVID-19 pandemic. The ANA suggests that the current staffing crisis "will have long-term repercussions for the profession, the entire health care delivery system, and ultimately, on the health of the nation" (Grant, 2021, p. 10).
- The ANA launched the "Well Being Initiative" during the COVID-19 crisis to provide self-care resources tailored to the needs of nursing professionals (ANA Enterprise, COVID-19 Resource Center. n.d.).

---

better understand the deeper meaning underlying each provision and how each nurse might best embody the code.

B. Code provisions
  1. The Code's first four provisions are based on core values, duties, and accountabilities (Winland-Brown, Lachman, & Swanson, 2015). They are:
      a. *The nurse practices with compassion and respect for the inherent dignity, worth, and unique attributes of every person.*
      b. *The nurse's primary commitment is to the patient whether an individual, family, group, community, or population.*
      c. *The nurse promotes, advocates for, and protects the rights, health, and safety of the patient.*
      d. *The nurse has authority, accountability, and responsibility for nursing practice; makes decisions; and takes action consistent with the obligation to promote health and to provide optimal care.*
  2. Provisions 5–9 of the code establish boundaries of duty and loyalty, and delineate nursing's responsibilities toward social justice, health policy, and advancement of nursing as a science and profession, and include (Lachman, Swanson, & Winland-Brown, 2015):
      a. *The nurse owes the same duties to self as to others, including the responsibility to promote health and safety, preserve wholeness of character and integrity, maintain competence, and continue personal and professional growth.*
      b. *The nurse, through individual and collective effort, establishes, maintains, and improves the ethical environment of the work setting and conditions*

of employment that are conducive to safe, quality health care.
      c. *The nurse, in all roles and settings, advances the profession through research and scholarly inquiry, professional standards development, and the generation of both nursing and health policy.*
      d. *The nurse collaborates with other health professionals and the public to protect human rights, promote health diplomacy, and reduce health disparities.*
      e. *The profession of nursing, collectively through its professional organizations, must articulate nursing values, maintain integrity of the profession, and integrate principles of social justice into nursing and health policy.*

III. Ethical theories and approaches
  A. Philosophical underpinnings
    1. Ethical theories provide a common frame of reference that facilitates ethical discourse. Examples of ethical theories are:
        a. Utilitarianism. This theory identifies what is good as what will result in the most good for the most people. Proponents of utilitarianism choose actions based on what will generate the most good or, as is often the case, the least harm (Stone, 2018).
        b. Deontology. This theory argues that an action's goodness is derived from intention. From this perspective, certain actions are *intrinsically* right or wrong. Deontology is traditionally associated with notions of duty (Holland, 2019).
  B. Approaches to health care ethics
    1. Currently, the dominant approach to health care ethics is the bioethical model (Naidoo, Turner, & McNeill, 2020).
        a. The bioethical model is strongly associated with medicine as a discipline and principlist approaches to ethics.
        b. A principlist ethical approach entails determining the salient ethical principles related to an ethical dilemma and balancing those principles to achieve a justifiable resolution that maximizes good.
    2. Beauchamp and Childress (2019) propose that the ethical principles of nonmaleficence, beneficence, autonomy, and justice are universally applicable to health care. These principles are summarized in Box 60.2.
    3. Virtue- and care-based ethics provide alternative approaches to health care ethics.
        a. Virtue-based approaches propose that dynamic character traits motivate actions. If nurses acquire qualities like courage, fidelity, and veracity, they will make ethically sound decisions (Holland, 2019).
        b. Care-based ethical approaches centralize the relationship between nurse and patient/family as the locus of moral decision-making.

BOX 60.2 Ethical Principles

Beneficence—The duty to do good or do what is of benefit. However, the duty is more complex than the simple definition implies. What is good for one patient may not be for another patient, and the options available for doing good may be scarce. Compassion is a defining quality of beneficence.

Nonmaleficence—The duty to not harm others. Sometimes, this means ensuring that the benefits of a treatment outweigh the harm. Exemplified by the Hippocratic admonition, "First, do no harm."

Autonomy—The respect for another person's right to choose, or self-determination. Autonomy stems from the core value of dignity (ANA, 2015).

Justice—In relation to health care ethics, justice refers to the fair allocation of resources. This concept is referred to as distributive justice (Beauchamp & Childress, 2019).

This approach suggests that nurses form connections with patients that allow them to interpret what decisions create the most good (Maykut & Wild, 2019).

4. For the good of the community, public health ethics are the basis for ethical decisions from a community-based perspective.
   a. Autonomy may be weighted differently against beneficence or justice, relative virtues are applied differently, and care is group-based rather than administered toward individuals.
   b. In public health ethics, limiting individual liberties may be necessary to safeguard the health and safety of the public, but such limitations must be publicly justified and adjusted according to established benchmarks (Holland, 2019).

IV. Ethical issues in nursing
   A. Communication with patients and families
      1. For effective nurse–patient communication, nurses develop a trusting relationship that relays compassion and respect.
      2. To support patient autonomy, nurses are the source of truth and accurate information.
      3. Truth-telling and ensuring the patient has adequate information are critical to support patient autonomy.
      4. Ineffective communication leads to increased distress and poorer outcomes in patients and increased stress and burnout in oncology nurses. Oncology nurses report that communication challenges that may raise ethical concerns (Wittenberg, Goldsmith, Buller, Ragan, & Ferrell, 2019).
         a. Nurses may be aware of bad news before that news is relayed to the patient
            (1) Perhaps the patient did not fully understand the content and consequences of bad news
            (2) In some cases, providers did not honestly relay the news
      5. Nurses may feel they lack skills to communicate with empathy—not knowing the best thing to provide comfort.

      a. Nurses can be troubled by some patients and families who are angry or disrespectful.
      b. Patient and families may not welcome the nurse relaying empathy.
      6. Communication between nurses and patients is challenging in difficult situations. Communication is affected by
         a. Differences in age
         b. Cultural differences
         c. Different personalities
      7. Nurses may feel constrained to communicate effectively due to a lack of time, being left out of team discussions, and feeling uncertain about goals of care.
   B. Confidentiality and privacy
      1. Privacy and confidentiality are issues of autonomy; respecting confidentiality and privacy is part of respecting human dignity.
         a. Privacy is an expectation and a right codified by law, while confidentiality is a professional and personal duty to keep certain types of information private.
         b. In the United States, confidentiality and privacy as they relate to protected health information (PHI) is protected. It is defined by the Health Insurance Portability and Accountability Act (Health Insurance Portability and Accountability Act [HIPAA], 1996).
         c. For health care providers, HIPAA requires that only the minimum amount of PHI required to care for patients be accessed or shared; the law requires that (PHI) be kept private and held in confidence by health care providers (HIPAA, 1996).
         d. In the interest of public safety as mandated by the law, PHI disclosures without authorization may be waived (Oyeleye, 2021)
            (1) Public health crises such as the COVID-19 pandemic allowed PHI disclosures
      2. Genomics, personalized medicine, and genetically developed pharmacotherapeutics are rapidly evolving fields, creating new ethical challenges involving autonomy, beneficence, veracity, and justice.
         a. Nurses will need to develop the competency of providing patient education about the risks and benefits of genetic tests, and genomic data collection.
         b. Confidentiality of genetic information is protected by law, but risks include discrimination and unequal treatment associated with sharing of genetic test results (Hammer, 2019).
         c. Consumers and health care professionals have access to social media and social networking sites.
            (1) Patients use social media to research their conditions, interact with other people in similar situations, and become better-informed health care consumers.

(2) Using social media platforms, health care professionals can also learn and engage with each other and conduct research.

d. The use of social media platforms can have negative consequences.

(1) Information provided can be incorrect or inaccurate

(2) Nurses as professionals can breach patients' privacy and confidentiality, since it is difficult to completely deidentify data online (Watson, 2018).

(a) Posting deidentified information about a patient encounter may erode patients' trust in nursing as a discipline, places patients at risk of identification (Watson, 2018).

e. Social media can blur professional boundaries; ethically questionable to connect with patients on social media outside nurse–patient relationship (Watson, 2018).

C. Ethics in the practice environment

1. For nurses, a poor ethical climate environment reflects lack of support from peers and managers, lack of respect between colleagues, lack of involvement in decision-making, and poor nurse–physician collaboration (Lamiani, Borghi, & Argentero, 2017).

a. Intimidating behavior ranges from incivility and disruptive conduct to bullying and to physical and emotional assault (Crawford et al., 2019).

b. Horizontal/lateral violence is rude or derogatory remarks or condescending behavior toward (or about) a coworker.

(1) If the coworker is at a comparable level within the organization, the violence is lateral.

(2) If the behavior is directed at someone above or below the aggressor's organizational level, the conduct is vertical.

2. Nurses may perceive inadequate resources and support in their setting that prevents them from practicing according to their values and fulfilling their professional duties.

a. Nurses who report stressors in their work environment, such as increasing acuity, concerns about quality, and unsafe staffing levels, may have higher moral distress (Sheppard et al., 2022).

D. Ethics: patient care

1. End-of-life care

a. End-of-life situations commonly raise ethical issues for nurses and cause moral distress (Gallagher, Neel, & Sotomayor, 2018).

b. Due to increased technology and life-support measures, patients may receive aggressive care for a longer period of time. Care can be considered:

(1) Overtreatment.

(2) Inappropriate treatment.

(3) The reason patient experiences a prolonged dying process (Wolf, White, Epstein, & Enfield, 2019).

c. Advance directives may improve the likelihood that patients receive their preferred end-of-life care, but end-of-life decisions are emotionally charged and dynamic. Nurses may also lack the knowledge and time to help patients with advanced directives. These difficult situations threaten patient autonomy (ANA, 2015; Croson, Malpass, Bohnenkamp, & LeBaron, 2018; Fry, 2018).

d. Despite advances in palliative care, nurses report challenges when caring for "difficult patients."

(1) Patients may decline to follow recommended treatments.

(2) For nurses, these patients may remind them of themselves or their own life situation.

(3) Patient symptoms may be difficult to manage (Dobrina, Chialchia, & Palese, 2020).

2. Medical aid in dying

a. Nurses may encounter patients at the end of life who express a desire to die and who make requests related to assisted dying, assisted suicide, and euthanasia.

b. Nurses should assess for any mental disorder, such as depression, or for psychological or physical suffering in patients who express a desire to die (Granek, Nakash, Ariad, Shapira, & Ben-David, 2019).

c. Although controversial, assisted dying is legal in several countries and in several US states. Nurses need to be prepared to discuss options and resources with patients who desire death (Wright et al., 2017).

d. Oncology nurses may be most likely to experience moral distress when care requires continued life-support efforts or the initiation of life-sustaining treatment.

(1) Nurses may feel such actions are not in the patient's best interest (Marturano et al., 2020).

(2) End-of-life care is more difficult when patients are from different cultures, when language barriers require translation, and when providers lack cultural training.

(a) Cultural awareness is the foundation for managing end-of-life situations (Herbstsomer & Stahl, 2021).

3. Decision-making

a. Shared decision-making is the contemporary model where patients and health care professionals make decisions together based on the best medical evidence as well as the patients' values and preferences.

(1) This model of care can be applied when there are a variety of options and/or difficult decisions (Steffensen et al., 2018).

b. Informed consent process

(1) Ensures the patient has an adequate understanding of risks, benefits, alternatives, and consequences of treatment.

(2) Supports autonomy and human dignity.

(3) Relies on beneficence, justice, and veracity (Regan, 2018).

c. Rational autonomy

(1) Rational autonomy: When seriously ill patients make decisions considering the values and preference of their family members in addition to or instead of their own values (Gómez-Vírseda, De Maeseneer, & Gastmans, 2019).

(2) When indicated, any concerns about the patient's decision-making ability should be evaluated using a formal assessment of capacity (Anandaiah & Rock, 2019).

(3) In the best situations, the decision-maker is the patient, but this may not be possible due to the patient's illness, physical or psychological status.

(4) Patients may voluntarily give the power of decision-making to others. This designation is power of attorney (POA).

(a) If no POA is available, the patient's next of kin is the decision-maker.

(b) Courts may select a guardian or proxy to make decisions on the patient's behalf.

d. Pediatric patients younger than 18 years of age cannot legally consent to treatments or procedures. Therefore their parents or guardians make decisions on the child's behalf.

(1) For patients as young as 7 years, the nurse confirms assent for procedures.

(2) Assent is the approval or agreement for planned intervention.

(3) On behalf of children, evidence-based methods to enhance the assent process include

(a) Planning an individual and tailored assent session

(b) At the assent session, using multimedia (i.e., videos) and relaying stories (Weisleder, 2020).

4. Health disparities

a. Health disparities persist in cancer care and affect groups of people based on age, race, ethnicity, culture, gender identity, socioeconomic status, and other characteristics.

b. To address health inequities, nurses can approach issues using a foundation of social justice.

(1) Provides "culturally sensitive empowering care" to individuals at risk for being marginalized

(2) Considers social determinants of health to develop group interventions for vulnerable populations

(3) As leaders, advocates, and policymakers, nurses can address inequities in societal structures (Truant, 2017)

V. Addressing ethical issues

A. Ethical issues: a priority

1. Moral distress in nurses is associated with burnout, lower job satisfaction, and intention to leave a position (Sandberg, Beuer, Reich, & Mason, 2021)

2. When providers are focused on their own moral struggles or interprofessional conflicts, they may miss the needs of patients and families (Sandberg et al., 2021).

B. Everyday professional comportment

1. Nurses can take responsibility and ownership for their professional behaviors, words, and practice. This type of conduct is exemplified by the concept of *everyday professional comportment* and includes attributes of mutual respect, harmony in beliefs and actions, commitment to colleagues and patients, and collaboration (Goodolf & Godfrey, 2021).

2. The concept of everyday ethical comportment refers to practice-based knowledge, skills, and reasoning that nurses can learn through lived clinical experiences of caring for patients and developing an ethical sense of what is right and good (Hardin, 2018).

C. Create an ethical community

1. Moral communities include respectful team relationships, open and honest communication, ethics-minded leadership, and readily available ethics resources that are used by providers (Epstein et al., 2020).

2. As a management style, leaders focus on people and relationships rather than policies may reduce moral distress in staff (Gillet et al., 2018).

D. Framework for ethical decision-making

1. Doherty and Purtilo (2015) outline one process to address ethical concerns and facilitate a decision or resolution to the problem

a. Clinical and advanced practice nurses can provide resources in clinical settings, and serve as ethics consultants in their facilities (Box 60.3).

E. Education

1. Nurses establish an ethical foundation

BOX 60.3 Identifying and Addressing Ethical Concerns

Step 1. Gather information from key participants and obtain facts to understand the multiple, complex perspectives of the ethical problem.

Step 2. Identify the type of ethical problem that exists. Define what makes this an ethical problem.

Step 3. Analyze the problem using ethical theories or approaches. Discuss what principles, codes, laws, or perspectives are relevant.

Step 4. Explore practical alternatives. Discuss possible courses of action, with the goal of an action that is ethically reasonable and most likely to achieve the desired outcome with the least harm.

Step 5. Take action. Implement the chosen course of action involving team members and key stakeholders.

Step 6. Evaluate the process and outcome. Debriefing sessions with those involved are critical for exploring whether the problem was adequately resolved, to addressing emotions and distress, and to discuss implications for future similar situations.

a. Builds over a career

b. Develops from the intersection of philosophical and applied ethical theory

c. Evolves from discipline-specific norms and experience

d. Is based on reflection, mentoring, and communication

2. Continuing education in ethics

a. Participate in ethics committees, conferences, and educational programs (Neumann et al., 2019).

b. Review professional journals

(1) Journals can include content about ethical issues in nursing

(2) Journal issues can focus on ethical issues

(3) Example of journals: *Nursing Ethics*

F. Ethics consultation/committees

1. All hospitals should have access to ethics consultation services.

2. Functions of hospital ethics committees are education, policy development, and case consultation (Neumann et al., 2019). Additional functions include difficult situation debriefing, organization and operational ethics leadership, and risk management related to ethics.

3. Review of ethics cases

a. Ethics session: review and reflect about specific issue or dilemma

b. May provide helpful moral insight, especially if the session is held at the right time for ethical deliberation

c. Allows space for interprofessional reflections

d. Includes the patient's perspectives (Bartholdson, Molewijk, Lutzen, Blomgren, & Pergert, 2018)

G. Mental health and self-care support

1. Nurses need to identify and practice self-care strategies to mitigate the effects of the multiple stressors they experience while working on the front lines of health care.

2. Self-care practices are a joint responsibility of individual nurses and health care organizations.

a. Evidence-based resources can be readily available to nurses in their workplace

b. Self-care is a priority to promote mental health, build resilience, and decrease burnout (Blackburn, Thompson, Frankenfield, Harding, & Lindsey, 2020).

REFERENCES

American Nurses Association (ANA). (2015). *Code of ethics for nurses with interpretive statements*. Silver Spring, MD: American Nurses Association.

ANA Enterprise, COVID-19 Resource Center. (n.d.) What you need to know. https://www.nursingworld.org/practice-policy/work-environment/health-safety/disaster-preparedness/coronavirus/what-you-need-to-know/the-well-being-initiative/

Anandaiah, A., & Rock, L. (2019). Twelve tips for teaching the informed consent conversation. *Medical Teacher, 41*(4), 465–470. https://doi.org/10.1080/0142159X.2018.1426844.

Bartholdson, C., Molewijk, B., Lutzen, K., Blomgren, K., & Pergert, P. (2018). Ethics case reflection sessions: Enablers and barriers. *Nursing Ethics, 25*(2), 199–211. https://doi.org/10.1177/0969733017693471.

Beauchamp, T. L., & Childress, J. F. (2019). *Principles of biomedical ethics* (8th ed.). New York: Oxford University Press.

Blackburn, L. M., Thompson, K., Frankenfield, R., Harding, A., & Lindsey, A. (2020). The THRIVE(c) program: Building oncology nurse resilience through self-care strategies. *Oncology Nursing Forum, 47*(1), E25–E34. https://doi.org/10.1188/20.ONF.E25-E34.

Croson, E., Malpass, J. K., Bohnenkamp, S., & LeBaron, V. (2018). The medical-surgical nurse's guide to understanding palliative care and hospice. *Medsurg Nursing, 27*(4), 215–222. https://search-ebscohost-com.ezproxy.lib.uwm.edu/login.aspx?direct=true&AuthType=ip,uid&db=epref&AN=MN.BG.BAE.CROSON.MNGUPC&site=ehost-live&scope=site.

Crawford, C. L., Chu, F., Judson, L. H., Cuenca, E., Jadalla, A. A., Tze-Polo, L., et al. (2019). An integrative review of nurse-to-nurse incivility, hostility, and workplace violence: A GPS for nurse leaders. *Nursing Administration Quarterly, 43*(2), 138–156. https://doi.org/10.1097/NAQ.0000000000000338.

Dobrina, R., Chialchia, S., & Palese, A. (2020). "Difficult patients" in the advanced stages of cancer as experienced by nursing staff. *European Journal of Oncology Nursing, 46*, 101766. https://doi.org/10.1016/j.ejon.2020.101766.

Doherty, R. F., & Purtilo, R. B. (2015). *Ethical dimensions in the health professions—E-book. Elsevier health sciences*. St. Louis, MO: Elsevier.

Epstein, E. G., Haizlip, J., Liaschenko, J., Zhao, D., Bennett, R., & Marshall, M. F. (2020). Moral distress, mattering, and secondary traumatic stress in provider burnout: A call for moral community. *AACN Advanced Critical Care, 31*(2), 146–157. https://doi.org/10.4037/aacnacc2020285.

Fry, A. (2018). Advance directives: An oncology nurse's personal experience with end-of-life decision making and its complexities. *Clinical Journal of Oncology Nursing, 22*(4), 375–376. https://doi.org/10.1188/18.CJON.375-376.

Fumis, R. R. L., Junqueira Amarante, G. A., de Fatima Nascimento, A., & Vieira Junior, J. M. (2017). Moral distress and its contribution to the development of burnout syndrome among critical care providers. *Annals of Intensive Care, 7*(1), 71. https://doi.org/10.1186/s13613-017-0293-2.

Gallagher, C. M., Neel, M. B., & Sotomayor, C. R. (2018). A retrospective review of clinical ethics consultations requested by nurses for oncology patients. *Journal of Nursing, 7*(1), 1–7. https://doi.org/10.18686/jn.v7i1.137.

Gillet, N., Fouquereau, E., Coillot, H., Bonnetain, F., Dupont, S., Moret, L., et al. (2018). Ethical leadership, professional caregivers' well-being, and patients' perceptions of quality of care in oncology. *European Journal of Oncology Nursing, 33*, 1–7. https://doi.org/10.1016/j.ejon.2018.01.002.

Gómez-Vírseda, C., De Maeseneer, Y., & Gastmans, C. (2019). Relational autonomy: What does it mean and how is it used in end-of-life care? A systematic review of argument-based ethics literature. *BMC Medical Ethics, 20*(1), 1–15. https://doi.org/10.1186/s12910-019-0417-3.

Goodolf, D. M., & Godfrey, N. (2021). A think tank in action: Building new knowledge about professional identity in nursing. *Journal of Professional Nursing, 37*(2), 493–499. https://doi.org/10.1016/j.profnurs.2020.10.007.

Granek, L., Nakash, O., Ariad, S., Shapira, S., & Ben-David, M. (2019). Strategies and barriers in addressing mental health and suicidality in patients with cancer. *Oncology Nursing Forum, 46*(5), 561–571. https://doi.org/10.1188/19.ONF.561-571.

Grant, E. (2021). ANA letter to HHS. *Alabama Nurse, 48*(4), 15. https://search-ebscohost-com.ezproxy.lib.uwm.edu/login.aspx?direct=true&AuthType=ip,uid&db=rzh&AN=153915666&site=ehost-live&scope=site.

Greenberg, N., Docherty, M., Gnanapragasam, S., & Wessely, S. (2020). Managing mental health challenges faced by healthcare workers during covid-19 pandemic. *British Medical Journal, 368*, m1211. https://doi.org/10.1136/bmj.m1211.

Hammer, M. J. (2019). Beyond the helix: Ethical, legal, and social implications in genomics. *Seminars in Oncology Nursing, 35*(1), 93–106. https://doi.org/10.1016/j.soncn.2018.12.007.

Hardin, J. (2018). Everyday ethical comportment: An evolutionary concept analysis. *Journal of Nursing Education, 57*(8), 460–468. https://doi.org/10.3928/01484834-20180720-03.

Henrich, N. J., Dodek, P. M., Gladstone, E., Alden, L., Keenan, S. P., Reynolds, S., et al. (2017). Consequences of moral distress in the intensive care unit: A qualitative study. *American Journal of Critical Care, 26*(4), e48–e57. https://doi.org/10.4037/ajcc2017786.

Herbstsomer, R. A., & Stahl, S. T. (2021). Cross-cultural experiences of hospice and palliative care services: A thematic analysis. *Omega (Westport), 84*(2), 551–566. https://doi.org/10.1177/0030222820904205.

Health Insurance Portability and Accountability Act (HIPAA). (1996). *Public law no. 104-191.* https://www.gpo.gov/fdsys/pkg/PLAW-104publ191/content-detail.html.

Holland, S. (2019). *Public health ethics.* Boston: Polity.

Hoskins, K., Grady, C., & Ulrich, C. M. (2018). Ethics education in nursing: Instructions for future generations of nurses. *The Online Journal of Issues in Nursing, 23*(1), 1–4. https://doi.org/10.3912/OJIN.Vol23No01Man03.

Hossain, F., & Clatty, A. (2021). Self-care strategies in response to nurses' moral injury during COVID-19 pandemic. *Nursing Ethics, 28*(1), 23–32. https://doi.org/10.1177/0969733020961825.

Lachman, V. D., Swanson, E. O., & Winland-Brown, J. (2015). The new 'code of ethics for nurses with interpretative statements' (2015): Practical clinical application, part II. *Medsurg Nursing, 24*(5), 363.

Lamiani, G., Borghi, L., & Argentero, P. (2017). When healthcare professionals cannot do the right thing: A systematic review of moral distress and its correlates. *Journal of Health Psychology, 22*(1), 51–67. https://doi.org/10.1177/1359105315595120.

Liu, Y., Cui, N., Zhang, Y., Wang, X., Zhang, H., Chen, D., et al. (2021). Psychometric properties of the ethical conflict in nursing questionnaire critical care version among Chinese nurses: A cross-sectional study. *BMC Nursing, 20*(1), 133. https://doi.org/10.1186/s12912-021-00651-x.

Marturano, E. T., Hermann, R. M., Giordano, N. A., & Trotta, R. L. (2020). Moral distress: Identification among inpatient oncology nurses in an academic health system. *Clinical Journal of Oncology Nursing, 24*(5), 500–508. https://doi.org/10.1188/20.CJON.500-508.

Maykut, C., & Wild, C. (2019). Relational comportment: Embodying caring as a contemplative journey. *International Journal for Human Caring, 23*(4), 295–301. https://doi.org/10.20467/1091-5710.23.4.295.

McAndrew, N. S., & Hardin, J. B. (2020). Giving nurses a voice during ethical conflict in the ICU. *Nursing Ethics*, 969733020934148. https://doi.org/10.1177/0969733020934148.

McAndrew, N. S., Leske, J., & Schroeter, K. (2018). Moral distress in critical care nursing: The state of the science. *Nursing Ethics, 25*(5), 552–570. https://doi.org/10.1177/0969733016664975.

Naidoo, S., Turner, K. M., & McNeill, D. B. (2020). Ethics and interprofessional education: An exploration across health professions education programs. *Journal of Interprofessional Care, 34*(6), 829–831. https://doi.org/10.1080/13561820.2019.1696288.

Neumann, J., Counts, V., & Jernigan, C. (2019). The role of oncology nurses as ethicists: Training, opportunities, and implications for practice. *Clinical Journal of Oncology Nursing, 23*(1), 103–107. https://doi.org/10.1188/19.CJON.103-107.

Nickitas, D. M. (2021). Confronting the truth and trauma of the COVID-19 pandemic. *Nursing Economic$, 39*(2), 57–58. https://search-ebscohost-com.ezproxy.lib.uwm.edu/login.aspx?direct=true&AuthType=ip,uid&db=rzh&AN=149855700&site=ehost-live&scope=site.

Oyeleye, O. A. (2021). The HIPAA privacy rule, COVID-19, and nurses' privacy rights. *Nursing2021, 51*(2), 11–14. https://doi.org/10.1097/01.NURS.0000731892.59941.a9.

Rainer, J., Schneider, J. K., & Lorenz, R. A. (2018). Ethical dilemmas in nursing: An integrative review. *Journal of Clinical Nursing, 27*(19–20), 3446–3461. https://doi.org/10.1111/jocn.14542.

Regan, E. M. (2018). Clinical trials informed consent: An educational intervention to improve nurses' knowledge and communications skills. *Clinical Journal of Oncology Nursing, 22*(6), E152–E158. https://doi.org/10.1188/18.CJON.E152-E158.

Sandberg, A. D., Beuer, G., Reich, R. R., & Mason, T. M. (2021). Moral distress among interdisciplinary critical care team members at a comprehensive cancer center. *Dimensions of Critical Care Nursing, 40*(5), 301–307. https://doi.org/10.1097/DCC.0000000000000490.

Sheppard, K. N., Runk, B. G., Maduro, R. S., Fancher, M., Mayo, A. N., Wilmoth, D. D., et al. (2022). Nursing moral distress and intent to leave employment during the COVID-19 pandemic. *Journal of Nursing Care Quality, 37*(1), 28–34. https://doi.org/10.1097/NCQ.0000000000000596.

Steffensen, K. D., Vinter, M., Crüger, D., Dankl, K., Coulter, A., Stuart, B., et al. (2018). Lessons in integrating shared decision-making into cancer care. *Journal of Oncology Practice, 14*(4), 229–235. https://doi.org/10.1200/JOP.18.00019.

Stone, E. G. (2018). Evidence-based medicine and bioethics: Implications for health care organizations, clinicians, and patients. *The Permanente Journal, 22*, 18–30. https://doi.org/10.7812/TPP/18-030.

Truant, T. (2017). Equity in cancer care: Strategies for oncology nurses. *Nursing Clinics of North America, 52*(1), 211–225. https://doi.org/10.1016/j.cnur.2016.11.003.

Tuca, A., Viladot, M., Barrera, C., Chicote, M., Casablancas, I., Cruz, C., et al. (2021). Prevalence of ethical dilemmas in advanced cancer patients (secondary analysis of the PALCOM study). *Supportive Care in Cancer, 29*(7), 3667–3675. https://doi.org/10.1007/s00520-020-05885-0.

Ulrich, B. (2018). Nurse fatigue: Dangerous for nurses and patients. *Nephrology Nursing Journal, 45*(3), 239. Retrieved from https://www.ncbi.nlm.nih.gov/pubmed/30304615.

Watson, J. (2018). Social media use in cancer care. *Seminars in Oncology Nursing, 34*(2), 126–131. https://doi.org/10.1016/j.soncn.2018.03.003.

Weisleder, P. (2020). Helping them decide: A scoping review of interventions used to help minors understand the concept and process of assent. *Frontiers in Pediatrics, 8*, 25. https://doi.org/10.3389/fped.2020.00025.

Winland-Brown, J., Lachman, V. D., & Swanson, E. O. (2015). The new 'code of ethics for nurses with interpretive statements' (2015): Practical clinical application, part I. *Medsurg Nursing, 24*(4), 268.

Wittenberg, E., Goldsmith, J., Buller, H., Ragan, S. L., & Ferrell, B. (2019). Communication training: Needs among oncology nurses across the cancer continuum. *Clinical Journal of Oncology Nursing*, *23*(1), 82–91. https://doi.org/10.1188/19.CJON.82-91.

Wolf, A. T., White, K. R., Epstein, E. G., & Enfield, K. B. (2019). Palliative care and moral distress: An institutional survey of critical care nurses. *Critical Care Nurse*, *39*(5), 38–49. https://doi.org/10.4037/ccn2019645.

Wright, D. K., Chirchikova, M., Daniel, V., Bitzas, V., Elmore, J., & Fortin, M. L. (2017). Engaging with patients who desire death: Interpretation, presence, and constraint. *Canadian Oncology Nursing Journal*, *27*(1), 56–64. https://doi.org/10.5737/236880762715664.

61

Professional Issues

Kerri Stuart

Quality Improvement

I. Impact of medical errors
   A. Approximately 160,000 people die in hospitals each year because of preventable medical errors (Austin & Derk, 2019).
   B. The United States spends more than $3.5 trillion per year on health care and has a lower life expectancy than many other developed countries with similar wealth (Emmanuel et al., 2021).
   C. A total of 1.3 million patients visit emergency departments each year due to adverse drug events resulting in longer hospital stays, increased medical costs, permanent disability, and death for approximately 350,000 of these patients each year (Centers for Disease Control and Prevention, 2017).
   D. Nonfinancial costs of medical errors include loss of trust in the health care system, low hospital employee morale, and lower levels of health in the general population.

II. Types of errors
   A. Diagnostic—error or delay in diagnosis
   B. Treatment—error in administering or an avoidable delay in treatment
   C. Preventive—inadequate risk assessment (falls, suicide, infection, etc.)
   D. Other—communication or equipment failure

III. Several strategies for improvement provided by the Institute of Medicine (IOM) report, *To Err Is Human: Building a Safer Health System* (Institute of Medicine [IOM], 1999)
   A. National focus to increase the knowledge about safety—creation of Center for Patient Safety tasked with setting national safety goals and tracking their progress
   B. Improved identification of errors—both mandated and confidential voluntary reporting systems to improve participation
      1. In 2017, registered nurse (RN) RaDonda Vaught admitted to making a medication error that resulted in the death of her 75-year-old patient. In 2022, the case went to trial and Ms. Vaught was convicted for her error, despite calls by her colleagues and clinicians nationwide to consider a just culture.

IV. The American Nurses Association (2022) released a joint statement after the verdict with the following key takeaways:

A. Health care delivery is highly complex; mistakes will happen and systems will fail.
B. The criminalization of medical errors sets into motion a dangerous precedent, where nurses and physicians will stop reporting errors for fear of punishment.
C. More effective and just mechanisms to examine errors and establish system improvements need to be implemented.
D. Nonintentional acts of individual nurses should not be criminalized to ensure patient safety.

V. Implementing safety systems and developing a "culture of safety" where safety is an explicit organizational goal. Key to a culture of safety/just culture is the establishment of processes amenable to building trust and accountability throughout all levels of professional collaboration in health care settings (Wyant, 2017). This should include:
   A. Policies and procedures supporting safe care
   B. Confidential, nonpunitive investigatory processes involving peers
   C. Training in event prevention strategies
   D. Effective and efficient response to identified issues

VI. Strategies to prevent errors in oncology settings (Mahoney-Newton, 2022):
   A. Establish a culture that values the safety
   B. General safety measures
   C. Standard operating procedures
   D. Technology
   E. Practice interventions including evaluating every error and near miss

VII. Patient's role in safety (Mahoney-Newton, 2022):
   A. Inform patient about the plan of care
   B. Patient education
   C. Include patient in dual RN verification prior to administration of chemotherapy: five rights of medication administration: correct patient, correct medication, correct dose, correct route, and correct time
   D. Encourage patient to pay attention and question unexpected changes

VIII. *Delivering High-Quality Cancer Care: Charting a New Course for a System in Crisis* (IOM, 2011)
   A. Conceptual framework for high-quality cancer care delivery system with six key elements of the model (IOM, 2013)

1. Engaged patients
2. Optimally trained and coordinated workforce for team-based cancer care
3. Evidence-based cancer care
4. A health care information technology system for cancer care that meets "meaningful use" criteria
5. Translation of evidence into clinical practice, quality measurement, and performance improvement
6. Accessible, affordable cancer care to reduce disparities and reform traditional fee-for-service payment reimbursements to new payment models
   a. The Affordable Care Act (or "Obamacare") 2010 made significant advancements in this area with an estimated 30% of traditional Medicare payments flowing through alternative payment models like bundled payments and accountable care organizations (O'Mahen & Petersen, 2021)
   b. The individual mandate, stating that individuals must sign up for health insurance or face a tax penalty, was repealed in late 2017
      (1) Without a higher number of healthy members to stabilize risk pools, premiums will go up as the balance shifts toward less healthy, higher-cost beneficiaries
B. The American Rescue Plan Act of 2021 lowers health care premiums for millions of Americans, eliminating premiums for some who participate in the health insurance marketplace established in 2016 (White House, 2021).
C. Implementing and sustaining improvements in health care can be accomplished with a systematic approach (Mate & Rakover, 2019) in four proposed steps:
   1. Choose a pilot unit within the organization
   2. Start with the immediate supervisor and front-line staff at the point of care delivery
   3. Use early wins to build momentum
   4. Motivate front-line clinical managers by tracking current challenges and opportunities for improvement
D. Patient family advisors (PFAs)—recognized by The Joint Commission as essential in supporting organizational performance improvement, engaging PFAs in decisions around health care delivery where possible leads to measurably improved outcomes in quality and safety (Agency for Healthcare Research and Quality, 2022). Their participation provides:
   1. Insight regarding an organization's strengths and where opportunities for improvement reside
   2. Input on policy, procedure, and practices that patients and their caregivers find helpful in staying engaged their plan of care
   3. More robust input in real-time context and dialog with health care professionals than a patient engagement survey provides
IX. Model for quality improvement
A. Plan–Do–Study–Act model (Connelly, 2021) developed by Associates in Process Improvement:
B. Three fundamental questions:

1. What is our goal?
2. What changes can we make that will result in improvement?
3. Set measurable goals.

Interdisciplinary Collaboration

I. Oncology Nursing Society (ONS) *Statement on the Scope and Standards of Oncology Nursing Practice: Generalist and Advanced Practice* (Lubjeko & Wilson, 2019). Collaboration involves a partnership between the oncology nurse and the patients, families, interdisciplinary team, and community resources to provide optimal care for complex cancer patients.
II. Barriers to the development of collaborative relationships (Zajac, Woods, Tannenbaum, Salas, & Holladay, 2021):
   A. Lack of clearly defined, distinct domain of influence
   B. Lack of understanding regarding the scope of practice
   C. Overlapping and changing domains of practice that produces competition
   D. Lack of recognition for knowledge and expertise
   E. Legal responsibility
III. Opportunities for collaboration.
   A. Potential for collaboration among health care providers and agencies exists whenever and with whomever the patient and family have contact.
   B. Although emphasis is often placed on physician–nurse collaboration, nurses have the opportunity for collaborative relationships with any member of the multidisciplinary health care team.
IV. During interdisciplinary tumor boards, some information (e.g., biomedical factors) dominates other information, such as patient comorbidities and psychosocial factors.
   A. A recent study showed that input from surgeons, radiologists, pathologists, and oncologists positively affected the team's ability to make a decision; patient comorbidity information and nursing inputs were negative predictors of decision-making ability (Soukup et al., 2016).
V. There are many opportunities for nurse-to-nurse collaboration within different domains of responsibility, practice settings including telehealth and subspecialities.
   A. Collaboration among nurses in different subspecialty and practice settings to include inpatient and ambulatory care may lead to the development of comprehensive educational cancer care materials
VI. The future of oncology nursing depends on critical collaborative partnerships being formed within the clinical practice arenas and with other organizations.

Patient Advocacy

I. For 20 consecutive years, Americans rated nurses the highest on honesty and ethical standards in the Gallup survey (Gaines, 2022); thus nurses are in an excellent position to advocate for patients
II. Definition
   A. In the broadest terms, advocacy is support for a particular cause.
   B. Nurses are natural advocates as they are on the front lines of patient care.

C. Advocacy involves the use of ethical principles.

D. Advocacy is a core value of many professional organizations.

   1. ONS promotes advocating for patients.

      a. Maximizing quality of life and patient safety.

      b. Optimizing patient access to excellent care.

      c. Advocating for public policy, especially with respect to health equity and the contributing factors to poor health (Pittman, 2019).

   2. ONS promotes advocating for nurses.

      a. Supporting and respecting oncology nurses.

      b. Promoting access to continuing education.

      c. Emphasizing a safe work environment and fair compensation.

E. Oncology nursing and the promotion of patient self-advocacy (Alsbrook, Donovan, Wesmiller, & Hagan Thomas, 2022).

   1. Assist patient with clarifying their goals of care, priorities, and needs.

   2. Assess patient's ability to be a self-advocate, including communicating needs to care team, assessing ability to learn and make informed decisions about their care.

   3. Build upon patient's strengths in self-advocacy using past examples as shared by patient, use these examples to demonstrate how patient might frame future dialog with care team around patient needs, priorities, and goals of care.

   4. Support patients who struggle with self-advocacy: assess barriers to advocacy, reassure patient that knowing their goals of care is important to the care team.

   5. Encourage continued self-advocacy: prepare patient for crucial conversations during pivotal points in care, including treatment options and progression of disease.

F. Barriers to advocacy (Nsiah, Siakwa, & Ninnoni, 2019).

   1. Nurses may lack autonomy to take moral actions.

   2. Conflicting demands of different patients, family, or other care team members/providers may create ethical conflicts.

   3. Independent action may be restricted by conflicting accountability to public, employer, and patients.

   4. Supporting ideas or well-being of another person may lead to personal difficulty and sacrifice.

   5. Oncology nurses often must deal with very difficult and controversial issues such as pain management, end-of-life care, and ethical decision-making.

G. Avenues to be advocates.

   1. Within one's own work setting

      a. By listening and speaking out for the needs expressed by patients and their families, thereby empowering patients and their families

      b. By keeping current on clinical trials, newly available evidence-based treatments, health legislation that affects practice and health care delivery, hospice, and other resources that can benefit patients and families under their care

   2. Within one's own community

      a. By volunteering or practicing in minority, underserved, medically disadvantaged, or vulnerable populations to decrease health disparities in cancer and other areas that affect health and well-being

      b. By becoming active politically to ensure that legislation protects the health of his or her community, state, and nation

   3. Within professional organizations

      a. By becoming actively involved in organizational legislative committees advocating for nurses, cancer care, and patients

      b. By using avenues available to ONS, American Nurses Association (ANA), and other professional organizations to provide testimony or letters to state legislators, congressional representatives, or both groups to support health care and health care initiatives and reform

Educational and Professional Development

I. Synopsis

A. Nursing training evolves to keep pace with our health care system, patient needs and expectations, technological advances, and increasing specialization.

B. Key recommendations of the IOM report, *The Future of Nursing: Leading Change, Advancing Health* (IOM, 2011), are as follows:

   1. Nurses practice to the full potential of their education and training.

   2. Nurses achieve higher levels of education and training through improved education systems.

   3. Nurses engage as full partners with physicians and health care professionals in redesigning health care.

   4. Nurses develop effective workforce planning and policymaking through better data collection and information infrastructure.

C. Over the next 10 years (2020–2030) nursing will need to evolve to become a much more diversified workforce, prepared to deliver care in a variety of settings, promote health and well-being for patients, communities, and nursing as a whole, and advocate to change disproportionate health inequities through collaboration within the public health domain, health care, and public health policy (National Academies of Sciences, Engineering, and Medicine [NASEM], 2021)

D. Key recommendations of *The Future of Nursing 2020-2030: Charting a Path to Achieve Health Equity* (NASEM, 2021):

   1. Nurses are prepared to act individually, through teams, and across sectors to meet challenges associated with an aging population, access to primary care, mental and behavioral health problems, structural racism, high maternal mortality and morbidity, and elimination of the disproportionate disease burden carried by specific segments of the US population.

2. Nurses are fully engaged in addressing the underlying causes of poor health. Individually and in partnership with other disciplines and sectors, nurses act on a wide range of factors that influence how well and long people live, helping to create individual- and community-targeted solutions, including a health in all policies orientation.

3. Nurses reflect the people and communities served throughout the nation, helping to ensure that individuals receive culturally competent, equitable health care services.

4. Health care systems enable and support nurses to tailor care to meet the specific medical and social needs of diverse patients to optimize their health.

5. Nurses' overarching contributions are quantified, extended, and strengthened, including the removal of institutional and regulatory barriers that have prevented nurses from working to the full extent of their education and training. Practice settings that were historically undercompensated, such as public health and school nursing, are reimbursed for nursing services in a manner comparable to that of other settings.

6. Nurses and other leaders in health care and public health create organizational structures and processes that facilitate the profession's expedited acquisition of relevant content expertise to serve flexibly in areas of greatest need in times of public health emergencies and disasters.

7. Nurses consistently incorporate a health equity lens learned through academic and continuing education.

8. Nurses collaborate across their affiliated organizations to develop and deploy a shared agenda to contribute to substantial, measurable improvement in health equity. National nursing organizations reflect an orientation of diversity, equity, and inclusion within and across their organizations.

9. Nurses focus on preventive person-centered care, focus on innovation in care delivery, always seeking new opportunities for growth and development. Nurses expand their roles, work in new settings and in new ways, and markedly expand their partnerships connecting health and health care with all individuals and communities.

10. Nurses attend to their own self-care and help to ensure that nurse well-being is addressed in educational and employment settings through the implementation of evidence-based strategies.

E. Barriers to practice
   1. Variability in educational pathways leading to entry-level RN licensure
   2. State variability in licensure requirements of RNs and advanced practice RNs
   3. Variability in advanced certification requirements across specialties
   4. Limited capacity in nursing schools for new nurses (LPN/LVN, Associate Degree (AD) RN, and BSN)
   5. Individual institutional limits to nursing practice as described per institutional policy and procedure

II. Educational development
   A. Nationally the 2011 IOM target of having 80% of graduating RNs graduating with a BSN by the year 2020 has not been met. Thus a revised target of 80% of newly graduated RNs doing so with a BSN by 2030 may be met through some of the following strategies (Spetz, 2018):
      1. Increased offering of baccalaureate programs through community colleges.
      2. Expanding part-time BSN program offerings in remote locations.
   B. In 2020, the American Association of Colleges of Nursing (American Association of Colleges of Nursing, 2021) shifted to competency-based essentials for nursing education for BSN, Master of Science in Nursing (MSN), DNP, and PhD preparedness:
      1. Knowledge for nursing practice
      2. Quality and safety
      3. Person-centered care
      4. Population health
      5. Scholarship for nursing discipline
      6. Interprofessional partnerships
      7. System-based practice
      8. Informatics and health care technologies
      9. Professionalism
      10. Personal, professional, and leadership development
   C. Strategies include the following:
      1. RN to BSN or MSN degree programs—some nursing schools offer these programs to provide an efficient bridge for nurses with an AD to obtain their BSN or MSN degree.
      2. BSN at community colleges—some community colleges offer AD students a streamlined, automatic transition to universities to obtain BSN degrees.
      3. Participation in organizational, local, and national educational and professional seminars, webinars, workshops, and conferences to expand the knowledge base in oncology and to obtain continuing education credits for relicensure.
      4. Graduate education.
         a. Formalized university or college education to increase the depth of professional knowledge and skills
         b. Formalized university/college education to redirect career path or fulfill career development plan
   D. Implementation of oncology nurse practitioner fellowships at academic centers is a potential solution for those seeking training in managing patients with cancer (Alencar, Butler, MacIntyre, & Wempe, 2018)

III. Professional development
   A. Obtaining certification in oncology nursing (Oncology Nursing Certification Corporation [ONCC], 2021a)

1. Certification—assures public that the certified nurse has the knowledge and qualifications needed to practice in his or her clinical area of nursing
2. Six certifications available in oncology nursing (ONCC, 2021b)—Oncology Certified Nurse, Advanced Oncology Certified Nurse Practitioner, Advanced Oncology Certified Clinical Nurse Specialist, Certified Pediatric Hematology Oncology Nurse, Certified Breast Care Nurse, and the Blood and Marrow Transplant Certified Nurse
3. Initial certifications in Certified Pediatric Oncology Nurse and Advanced Oncology Certified Nurse no longer available, but renewals are available for nurses who currently hold these credentials

B. Membership and participation in local, state, national, and international professional organizations such as the ONS, ANA, American Society of Clinical Oncology, and American Society of Hematology

REFERENCES

Agency for Healthcare Research and Quality. (2022). 2021 National healthcare quality and disparities report. https://www.ahrq.gov/research/findings/nhqrdr/nhqdr21/index.html.

Alencar, M. C., Butler, E., MacIntyre, J., & Wempe, E. P. (2018). Nurse practitioner fellowship: Developing a program to address gaps in practice. *Clinical Journal of Oncology Nursing, 22*(2), 142–145. https://doi.org/10.1188/18.CJON.142-145.

Alsbrook, K., Donovan, H., Wesmiller, S., & Hagan Thomas, T. (2022). Oncology nurses' role in promoting patient self advocacy. *Clinical Journal of Oncology Nursing, 26*(3), 239–244. https://doi.org/10.1188/22.CJON.239-243.

American Association of Colleges of Nursing. (2021). *The essentials: Core competencies for professional nursing education.* https://www.aacnnursing.org/Portals/42/AcademicNursing/pdf/Essentials-2021.pdf.

American Nurses Association. (2022). *Statement in response to the conviction of nurse RaDonda Vaught.* https://www.nursingworld.org/news/news-releases/2022-news-releases/statement-in-response-to-the-conviction-of-nurse-radonda-vaught/.

Austin, M., & Derk, J. (2019). *Lives lost, lives saved: An updated comparative analysis of avoidable deaths at hospitals graded by the leapfrog group.* Armstrong Institute for Patient Safety and Quality, Johns Hopkins Medicine. hopkinsmedicine.org/armstrong_institute/.

Centers for Disease Control. (2017). *Adverse drug events in adults.* https://www.cdc.gov/medicationsafety/adult_adversedrugevents.html.

Connelly, L. M. (2021). Using the PDSA model correctly. *Medsurg Nursing, 30*(1), 61–64.

Emanuel, E., Gudbranson, E., Van Parys, J., Gortz, M., Helgeland, J., & Skinner, J. (2021). Comparing health outcomes of privileged U.S. citizens with those of average residents of other developed countries. *JAMA Internal Medicine, 181*(3), 339–344. https://doi.org/10.1001/jamainternmed.2020.7484.

Gaines, K. (2021). *Nursing ranked as the most trusted profession for 20th year in a row.* https://nurse.org/articles/nursing-ranked-most-honest-profession/.

Institute of Medicine. (1999). *To err is human: Building a safer health system.* Washington, DC: National Academies Press.

Institute of Medicine. (2011). *The future of nursing: Leading change, advancing health.* Washington, DC: National Academies Press.

Institute of Medicine. (2013). *Delivering high-quality cancer care: Charting a new course for a system in crisis.* Washington, DC: National Academies Press.

Lubejko, B. G., & Wilson, B. J. (2019). *Oncology nursing: Scope and standards of practice.* Pittsburgh: Oncology Nursing Society.

Maloney-Newton, S. (2022). Creating a culture of safety. In: *47th Annual ONS congress,* Anaheim, CA. https://ons.confex.com/ons/2022/meetingapp.cgi/Session/4293.

Mate, K.S., & Rakover, J. (2019). *The answer to culture change: Everyday management tactics.* NEJM Catalyst. https://catalyst.nejm.org/doi/full/10.1056/CAT.19.0004.

National Academies of Sciences, Engineering, and Medicine (NASEM). (2021). *The future of nursing 2020-2030: Charting a path to achieve health equity.* The National Academies Press. https://doi.org/10.17226/25982.

Nsiah, C., Siakwa, M., & Ninnoni, J. (2019). Barriers to practicing patient advocacy in healthcare setting. *Nursing Open, 20*(7), 650–659. https://doi.org/10.1002/nop2.436.

O'Mahen, P., & Petersen, L. (2021). Will the American Rescue Plan overcome opposition to Medicaid expansion. *Journal of General Internal Medicine, 36*(11), 3550–3552. https://doi.org/10.1007/s11606-021-07084-x.

Oncology Nursing Certification Corporation (ONCC). (2021a). *General information.* www.oncc.org/TakeTest.

Oncology Nursing Certification Corporation (ONCC). (2021b). *Eligibility.* www.oncc.org/Eligibility.

Pittman, P. (2019). Rising to the challenge: Re-embracing the Wald model of nursing. *American Journal of Nursing, 119*(7), 46–52.

Soukup, T., Lamb, B. W., Sarkar, S., Arora, S., Shah, S., Darzi, A., et al. (2016). Predictors of treatment decisions in multidisciplinary oncology meetings: A quantitative observational study. *Annals of Surgical Oncology, 23*(13), 4410–4417. https://doi.org/10.1245/s10434-016-5347-44410-4417.

Spetz, J. (2018). Projections of progress toward the 80% bachelor of science in nursing recommendation and strategies to accelerate change. *Nursing Outlook, 66*(4), 394–400. https://doi.org/10.1016/j.outlook.2018.04.012.

The White House. (2021). *American Rescue Plan.* https://www.whitehouse.gov/american-rescue-plan/.

Wyant, T. (2017). Safety culture: Establishing processes to support trust and accountability for risk reduction. *Clinical Journal of Oncology Nursing, 21*(4), 499–501. https://doi.org/10.1188/17.CJON.499-501.

Zajac, S., Woods, A., Tannenbaum, S., Salas, E., & Holladay, C. L. (2021). Overcoming challenges to teamwork in healthcare: A team effectiveness framework and evidence-based guidance. *Frontiers in Communication, 6.* https://doi.org/10.3389/fcomm.2021.606445.

62

Compassion Fatigue

Susie Maloney-Newton

OVERVIEW

(Arimon-Pagès, Torres-Puig-Gros, Fernández-Ortega, & Canela-Soler, 2019)

I. People who are attracted to professions that involve caring for others, such as nursing, are prone to compassion fatigue by the nature of their tendency to put others' needs ahead of their own.

II. Oncology nurses are even more likely to experience compassion fatigue because they care for patients who may be facing a terminal disease.

III. Compassion fatigue is often correlated with burnout, but there are differences between the two phenomena.

IV. Job stress and burnout occur in approximately 40% of nurses. Although rates vary by study, oncology nurses are at particularly high risk for compassion fatigue (Xie et al., 2021).

V. It is beneficial to invest in strategies to reduce compassion fatigue and burnout in nurses, as it has been shown to reduce turnover, increase job satisfaction, increase the ability to provide quality care, and decrease overall health care expenditures.

VI. Personal resilience has been shown to protect against compassion fatigue (Sullivan et al., 2019). Adaptability may serve as a protective mechanism.

VII. The COVID-19 epidemic has nurses and other health care providers working non-stop to care for COVID-19 patients, while concurrently determining how to meet the needs of their other patients (Ross, 2020).

VIII. Definitions.

A. Compassion fatigue is defined as fatigue, emotional distress, or apathy resulting from the constant demands of caring for others. It explains the exhaustion that results from prolonged exposure to compassion stress among those who work in a caring profession. Compassion fatigue is also described as the diminished ability to feel compassion or empathize when providing care (Baqeas, Davis, & Copnell, 2021). Compassion fatigue is often referred to as *secondary traumatic stress*.

B. Burnout develops gradually as physical, emotional, behavioral, professional, and interpersonal symptoms progressively worsen (Cross, 2019). Burnout is a syndrome involving exhaustion, cynicism, and inefficacy that arises in response to chronic stressors on the job and evolves slowly over a prolonged period of stress.

Compassion fatigue is related to both burnout and secondary traumatic stress.

1. Exhaustion: including physical, emotional, and cognitive fatigue. Tends to occur over an extended period as opposed to after one long day.

2. Cynicism: feelings of detachment, depersonalization, and a lack of engagement. Distancing from work or from personal interactions.

3. Inefficacy: feelings of incompetence, feeling overwhelmed, and a lack of achievement and productivity.

C. Compassion satisfaction is the positive feelings derived from helping others, and the alleviation of patient suffering (Baqeas et al., 2021). This concept explains the pleasure derived from work.

ASSESSMENT

I. Assessment tools

A. Professional Quality of Life Scale V (Baqeas et al., 2021; Stamm, 2010; Sullivan et al., 2019). The most common tool used for assessing and measuring compassion fatigue and is easy to use and score. Includes three subscales:

1. Secondary traumatic stress
2. Burnout
3. Compassion satisfaction

B. Self-care assessment

II. Risk factors for compassion fatigue (Sullivan et al., 2019)

A. Younger age (under 40).

B. Single.

C. Less than 5 years in the nursing profession.

D. High job expectations: corporate or self-imposed.

E. Blurred professional boundaries.

F. Ineffective coping strategies.

G. Work setting issues such as an inpatient setting, a heavy caseload, high stress levels, and prolonged periods of working with high-acuity patients.

H. Numerous studies have shown that the COVID-19 pandemic is having a significant impact on health care worker's mental well-being, and the data demonstrate that nurses are suffering in record numbers (Gee, Weston, Harshman, & Kelly, 2022).

I. Predictors of compassion fatigue and burnout (Sullivan et al., 2019).

1. Personal distress or traumatic life events
2. Psychological inflexibility
3. High level of being self-judgmental
4. Empathy-based guilt feelings
5. Environmental factors: feeling overworked, poor communication between nurses and physicians, staffing issues, high patient acuity, rapidly changing technology, and lack of administrative support

J. Symptoms of compassion fatigue: physical, behavioral or emotional, and work related (Cross, 2019).
   1. Physical: frequent headaches, digestive problems such as constipation or diarrhea, muscle tension, sleep disturbances, fatigue, cardiac issues such as chest pain, tachycardia or palpitations, and experiencing frequent illness.
   2. Behavioral/emotional: mood swings/irritability; anxiety; abuse of alcohol, food, illicit drugs, or nicotine; lack of joyfulness; memory issues; poor judgment; overextension issues; poor concentration; and anger or resentment.
   3. Work related: dread of going to work, frequent use of sick days, decreased ability to empathize with patients or families, and avoiding working with certain patients (Sullivan et al., 2019).

MANAGEMENT

I. Nonpharmacologic management
   A. Components of prevention and management include personal, professional, and organizational support (Baqeas et al., 2021; Sullivan et al., 2019)
   B. Personal
      1. Emphasize self-care
      2. Good sleep habits
      3. Exercise (recommend three to four times weekly for 20–30 minutes)
      4. Nutrition/eating well
      5. Massage
      6. Enjoying a hobby, listening to music, humor, and enjoying nature
      7. Schedule preventive and medical care appointments
      8. Set aside time each day to do something for self
      9. Self-reflection exercises
      10. Make time for prayer and meditation
      11. Keep a self-care journal
      12. Work–life balance
      13. Grief support and counseling (Zajac, Moran, & Groh, 2017)
      14. Verbalization with others such as family members, friends, and other nurses (Ko & Kiser-Larson, 2016). Many nursing units involve the use of social workers or chaplains to assist in this area
      15. Mindfulness-based interventions (Baqeas et al., 2021; Duarte & Pinto-Gouveia, 2017)
         a. Activities that focus a person's attention on the present experience, becoming more aware of one's physical, mental, and emotional condition,

in a way that is nonjudgmental. Mindfulness has been shown to be effective at reducing stress. The interventions can be offered individually or in a group setting (Green & Kinchen, 2021).
   C. Professional
      1. Verbalization with others such as family members, friends, and others
      2. Nurses. Many nursing units involve the use of social workers or chaplains to assist in this area
      3. Boundary setting
      4. Peer consultation
      5. Awareness of workloads
      6. Team building
      7. Positive work environment (Ross, 2020)
   D. Organizational: Healthy and supportive work environments that promote teamwork and cohesiveness and engaged leadership styles
      1. Increased staffing
      2. Providing and encouraging frequent breaks (Ross, 2020)
      3. Grief meeting or huddle after the loss of a patient
      4. Fun gatherings outside of work
      5. Mentoring novice nurses
      6. Encouraging verbalization of feelings and grief support
      7. Send cards to the family, reminisce about time spent with patients, and sometimes attend the funeral of patients with whom there has been a close bond
      8. Individualized staff bereavement programs (Cross, 2019)
      9. Respite rooms (Sullivan et al., 2019)

REFERENCES

Arimon-Pagès, E., Torres-Puig-Gros, J., Fernández-Ortega, P., & Canela-Soler, J. (2019). Emotional impact and compassion fatigue in oncology nurses: Results of a multicenter study. *European Journal of Oncology Nursing, 43*, 101666. https://doi.org/10.1016/j.ejon.2019.09.007.

Baqeas, M. H., Davis, J., & Copnell, B. (2021). Compassion fatigue and compassion satisfaction among palliative care health providers: A scoping review. *BMC Palliative Care, 20*(1), 88. https://doi.org/10.1186/s12904-021-00784-5.

Cross, L. A. (2019). Compassion fatigue in palliative care nursing: A concept analysis. *Journal of Hospice and Palliative Nursing, 21*(1), 21–28. https://doi.org/10.1097/NJH.0000000000000477.

Duarte, J., & Pinto-Gouveia, J. (2017). Mindfulness, self-compassion and psychological inflexibility mediate the effects of a mindfulness-based intervention in a sample of oncology nurses. *Journal of Contextual Behavioral Science, 6*, 125–133.

Gee, P. M., Weston, M. J., Harshman, T., & Kelly, L. A. (2022). Beyond burnout and resilience: The disillusionment phase of COVID-19. *AACN Advances in Critical Care, 33*(2), 134–142. https://doi.org/10.4037/aacnacc2022248.

Green, A. A., & Kinchen, E. V. (2021). The effects of mindfulness meditation on stress and burnout in nurses. *Journal of Holistic Nursing, 39*(4), 356–368. https://doi.org/10.1177/08980101211015818.

Ko, W., & Kiser-Larson, N. (2016). Stress levels of nurses in oncology outpatient units. *Clinical Journal of Oncology Nursing, 20*(2), 158–164. https://doi.org/10.1188/16.CJON.158-164.

Stamm, B. H. (2010). *The concise ProQOL manual* (2nd ed.). Pocatello, ID: ProQOL.org.

Ross, J. (2020). The exacerbation of burnout during COVID-19: A major concern for nurse safety. *Journal of PeriAnesthesia Nursing, 35*(4), 439–440. https://doi.org/10.1016/j.jopan.2020. 04.001.

Sullivan, C. E., King, A. R., Holdiness, J., Durrell, J., Roberts, K. K., Spencer, C., et al. (2019). Reducing compassion fatigue in inpatient pediatric oncology nurses. *Oncology Nursing Forum, 46*(3), 338–347. https://doi.org/10.1188/19.ONF.338-347.

Xie, W., Wang, J., Zhang, Y., Zuo, M., Kang, H., Tang, P., et al. (2021). The levels, prevalence and related factors of compassion fatigue among oncology nurses: A systematic review and meta-analysis. *Journal of Clinical Nursing, 30*(5–6), 615–632. https://doi. org/10.1111/jocn.15565.

Zajac, L.M., Moran, K.J., & Groh, C.J. (2017) Confronting compassion fatigue: Assessment and intervention in inpatient oncology. Clinical Journal of Oncology Nursing, 21(4), 446-453. https://doi. org/10.1188/17.CJON.446-453.

Note: Page numbers followed by f indicate figures, t indicate tables, and b indicate boxes.